ASCO-SEP™

MEDICAL ONCOLOGY SELF-EVALUATION PROGRAM

Editor

Anne Moore, MD

Associate Editors

Fredrick R. Appelbaum, MD, Charles L. Loprinizi, MD, and Joseph T. Ruggiero, MD

David Aboulafia, MD

Jan C. Buckner, MD

Lisa A. Carey, MD

Bruce D. Cheson, MD

Bruce E. Clurman, MD, PhD

Arlene A. Forastiere, MD

Matthew P. Goetz, MD

Axel Grothey, MD

Robert G. Maki, MD, PhD

Maurie Markman, MD

Matthew I. Milowsky, MD

Joanne Mortimer, MD

David M. Nanus, MD

Alfred I. Neugut, MD, PhD

Joan H. Schiller, MD

Lynn M. Schuchter, MD

Pierre L. Triozzi, MD

Requests for permission to reprint abstracts should be directed to Intellectual Property Rights Manager, American Society of Clinical Oncology, 330 John Carlyle St., Suite 300, Alexandria, VA 22314. Tel: 703-299-0150; fax 703-518-8157; e-mail permissions@asco.org. Editorial correspondence and production questions should be addressed to Publications Department—*ASCO-SEP*™, American Society of Clinical Oncology, 330 John Carlyle St., Suite 300, Alexandria, VA 22314. Tel: 703-299-0150; fax: 703-518-8157.

LETTER FROM THE ASCO-SEP EDITOR

Dear Participant:

On behalf of ASCO, I am pleased to present the first edition of *ASCO-SEP™: Medical Oncology Self-evaluation Program.* This is a self-assessment resource designed to help physicians assess their level of knowledge in various areas of oncology as preparation for the certification exam and to assist physicians moving through the maintenance of certification process.

Available in print and online formats, *ASCO-SEP™* is a comprehensive learning tool that includes more than 180 multiple-choice questions that can be used for self study.

The success of this publication has relied on the time and talents of many. I would like to thank my colleagues who graciously shared their expertise as they wrote and reviewed these chapters. I would also like to thank past contributors to the previous edition, especially the Editor, Bruce D. Cheson, MD. ASCO staff have contributed an enormous amount of time, effort, and expertise to the publication, and I would especially like to thank Michal Tibbits and Heather Drummond for their work on our behalf. Lastly, I am tremendously grateful for the dedication and commitment of the three Associate Editors on this project: Frederick R. Appelbaum, MD, Charles L. Loprinzi, MD, and Joseph T. Ruggiero, MD.

Thank you for participating in this worthwhile continuing medical education program. If you have comments or suggestions regarding *ASCO-SEP™*, please send an e-mail to cme@asco.org.

Sincerely,

Anne Moore, MD
Editor, *ASCO-SEP™*

CONTRIBUTORS

EDITOR

Anne Moore, MD
Weill Cornell Medical College
New York-
Presbyterian Hospital
New York, NY

ASSOCIATE EDITORS

Frederick R. Appelbaum, MD
Fred Hutchinson Cancer Research Center
Seattle, WA

Charles L. Loprinzi, MD
Mayo Clinic
Rochester, MN

Joseph T. Ruggiero, MD
Weill Cornell Medical College
New York-
Presbyterian Hospital
New York, NY

AUTHORS

David Aboulafia, MD
Virginia Mason Medical Center
Seattle, WA

Frederick R. Appelbaum, MD
Fred Hutchinson Cancer Research Center
Seattle, WA

Jan C. Buckner, MD
Mayo Clinic
Rochester, MN

Lisa A. Carey, MD
University of North Carolina
Chapel Hill, NC

Bruce D. Cheson, MD
Georgetown University Hospital
Washington, DC

Bruce E. Clurman, MD, PhD
Fred Hutchinson Cancer Research Center
Seattle, WA

Arlene A. Forastiere, MD
Johns Hopkins University
Baltimore, MD

Matthew P. Goetz, MD
Mayo Clinic
Rochester, MN

Axel Grothey, MD
Mayo Clinic
Rochester, MN

Charles L. Loprinzi, MD
Mayo Clinic
Rochester, MN

Robert G. Maki, MD, PhD
Memorial Sloan-Kettering Cancer Center
New York, NY

Maurie Markman, MD
M. D. Anderson Cancer Center
Houston, TX

Matthew I. Milowsky, MD
Memorial Sloan-Kettering Cancer Center
New York, NY

Joanne Mortimer, MD
City of Hope
Duarte, CA

David M. Nanus, MD
Weill Cornell Medical College
New York-
Presbyterian Hospital
New York, NY

Alfred I. Neugut, MD, PhD
Columbia University Medical Center
New York, NY

Joan H. Schiller, MD
University of Texas Southwestern Medical School
Dallas, TX

Lynn M. Schuchter, MD
University of Pennsylvania Cancer Center
Philadelphia, PA

Pierre L. Triozzi, MD
Cleveland Clinic Foundation
Cleveland, OH

PEER REVIEWERS

Shantanu Banerji, MD, FRCPC
Cancer Care Manitoba
Winnipeg, Manitoba

Thomas Beck, MD
St. Luke's Mountain States Tumor Institute
Boise, ID

Kathleen Beekman, MD
Providence Cancer Institute
Novi, MI

Al Benson III, MD
Northwestern University
Chicago, IL

Don M. Benson, Jr., MD, PhD
Ohio State University
Columbus, OH

José Bines, MD
Instituto Nacional de Cancer
Rio de Janeiro, Brazil

Stephanie V. Blank, MD
New York University
New York, NY

Sean P. Bohen, MD, PhD
Genentech, Inc.
South San Francisco, CA

Jonathan C. Britell, MD
Southlake Clinic
Renton, WA

Robert W. Carlson, MD
Stanford University
Stanford, CA

Priya Chakravarthi, MD
Palo Alto Medical Foundation
Palo Alto, CA

Kelly Cooke, DO
Scott and White Memorial Hospital
Temple, TX

Mary B. Daly, MD, PhD
Fox Chase Cancer Center
Philadelphia, PA

Lisa M. DeAngelis, MD
Memorial Sloan-Kettering Cancer Center
New York, NY

George Demetri, MD
Dana-Farber Cancer Institure
Boston, MA

Patrick J. Donovan, MD, FACP
Scottsdale Medical Specialists
Scottsdale, AZ

Eric R. Fearon, MD, PhD
University of Michigan School of Medicine
Ann Arbor, MI

Stuart P. Feldman, MD
Westchester Medical Group PC
White Plains, NY

Richard Fisher, MD
University of Rochester
Rochester, NY

Dean Gesme, MD
Minnesota Hematology Oncology
Minnetonka, MN

Stacey M. Gore, MD
Harvard Vanguard Medical Association
Boston, MA

Sharad Goyal, MD
UMDNJ/Robert Wood Johnson
New Brunswick, NJ

Peter R. Graze, MD
Annapolis Oncology Center
Annapolis, MD

Robert Haddad, MD
Dana-Farber Cancer Institute
Boston, MA

Nora Lynn Henry, MD, PhD
University of Michigan Medical Center
Ann Arbor, MI

Martee Leigh Hensley, MD, MSc
Memorial Sloan-Kettering Cancer Center
New York, NY
Weill Cornell Medical College
New York-
Presbyterian Hospital
New York, NY

Jade Homsi, MD
H. Lee Moffitt Cancer Center & Research Institute
Tampa, FL

Aminah Jatoi, MD
Mayo Clinic
Rochester, MN

Brandon Johnson, MD
Mayo Clinic
Jacksonville, FL

Anthony Joshua, MBBS
Princess Margaret Hospital
Toronto, ON

Mark Klein, MD
University of Minnesota
Minneapolis, MN

Mark G. Kris, MD
Memorial Sloan-Kettering Cancer Center
New York, NY

Richard A. Larson, MD
University of Chicago
Chicago, IL

Hillard M. Lazarus, MD
Case Western Reserve University
Cleveland, OH

Alexandra M. Levine, MD
City of Hope National Medical Center
Duarte, CA

Steven K. Libutti, MD
National Cancer Institute
National Institutes of Health
Bethesda, MD

Gilberto Lopes, MD
Johns Hopkins Singapore International Medical Center
Singapore
Thomas A. Marsland, MD
Orange Park Cancer Center
Orange Park, FL

Robert S. Miller, MD
Sacramento Center for Hematology and Medical Oncology
Sacramento, CA

Timothy J. Moynihan, MD
Mayo Clinic
Rochester, MN

Joseph O'Connell, MD
Connecticut Oncology & Hematology
Milford, CT

Thomas P. O'Connor Jr., MD
Commonwealth Hematology Oncology
Weymouth, MA

Bimal Patel, MD
East Bay Medical Oncology & Hematology Associates
Lafayette, CA

Daniel P. Petrylak, MD
Columbia University
New York, NY

Lawrence D. Piro, MD
The Angeles Clinic and Research Institute
Los Angeles, CA

W. Thomas Purcell, MD, MBA
Billings Clinic Cancer Center
Billings, MT

W. Kimryn Rathmell, MD, PhD
University of North Carolina at Chapel Hill
Chapel Hill, NC

Gregory J. Riely, MD, PhD
Memorial Sloan-Kettering Cancer Center
New York, NY

Peter J. Rosen, MD
Tower Center Cancer Research Foundation
Beverly Hills, CA

Vered Stearns, MD
Johns Hopkins University
Baltimore, MD

Shelby Terstriep, MD
Mayo Clinic
Rochester, MN

Stephan Thome, MD, FACP
Oncology Hematology West PC
Papillion, NE

Steven Tucker, MD, FACP
The West Clinic International
Singapore

James A. Wallace, MD
University of Chicago
Chicago, IL

Ronald S. Walters, MD, MBA, MS
M. D. Anderson Cancer Center
Houston, TX

Jedd Wolchok, MD, PhD
Memorial Sloan-Kettering Cancer Center
New York, NY

Ruth T. Young, MD, MA
Vanderbilt Ingram Cancer Center
Franklin, TN

Dan Zuckerman, MD
Dana-Farber Cancer Institute
Boston, MA

ASCO STAFF

Content Development and Continuing Medical Education

Michal Tibbits — *Senior Program Coordinator*
Heather Drummond — *Program Assistant*

Editorial and Publishing Services

Joy Curzio — *Assistant Director, Meeting Publications*
Doug Byrnes — *Assistant Director, Production*
Andrea Smiley — *Editorial Coordinator*
Allie Moore — *Editorial Assistant*

DISCLOSURES

Editorial Board Disclosure Index

Financial relationships reported by members of the *ASCO-SEP*™ Editorial Board. During all phases of planning for the *ASCO-SEP*™, areas of conflict were managed through a peer-review process and/or through individual recusal when appropriate.

Editor

ANNE MOORE, MD
No significant financial relationship to disclose

Associate Editors

CHARLES L. LOPRINZI, MD
Consultant, Par Pharmaceuticals, Quality Oncology
Research funding, Aventis, Amgen, Roche, Centocor, Ortho Biotech, Novartis, MOVC

JOSEPH T. RUGGIERO, MD
No significant financial relationship to disclose

FREDERICK R. APPELBAUM, MD
Advisory board, Kanisa Pharmaceuticals, Cellerent Therapeutics, Zymogenetics, Merck & Co., Genzyme
Honoraria, Swedish Providence Medical Center, Acute Leukemia Forum

Author Disclosure Index

The *ASCO-SEP*™ Editorial Board has reviewed all author disclosure reports, identified potential conflicts of interest and implemented strategies to manage those areas of conflict, where they exist.

DAVID ABOULAFIA, MD
Research funding, SWOG, AIDS Mahoney Consortium

FREDERICK R. APPELBAUM, MD
Advisory board, Kanisa Pharmaceuticals, Cellerent Therapeutics, Zymogenetics, Merck & Co., Genzyme
Honoraria, Swedish Providence Medical Center, Acute Leukemia Forum

JAN C. BUCKNER, MD
Consultant, Amgen, NeoPharm, AntiSense Pharma, Genentech

LISA CAREY, MD
Consultant, Genentech, BMS, GSK

BRUCE D. CHESON, MD
No significant financial relationship to disclose

BRUCE E. CLURMAN, MD, PHD
No significant financial relationship to disclose

ARLENE A. FORASTIERE, MD
Advisory board, Imclone, BMS
Research funding, Pfizer

MATTHEW P. GOETZ, MD
Research funding, Aviara Dx

AXEL GROTHEY, MD
Consultant, sanofi-aventis, Genentech, BMS, Roche
Honoraria, sanofi-aventis, Genentech, Roche
Research funding, Sanofi-aventis

CHARLES L. LOPRINZI, MD
Consultant, Par Pharmaceuticals, Quality Oncology
Research funding, Aventis, Amgen, Roche, Centocor, Ortho Biotech, Novartis, MOVC

ROBERT G. MAKI, MD, PHD
Advisory board, Novartis
Honoraria, Novartis, Pfizer
Research funding, Pfizer, Novartis, Lilly

MAURIE MARKMAN, MD
Advisory board, Eli Lilly, Cell Therapeutics, Telik, Bibuteci, GSK, Genentech

MATTHEW I. MILOWSKY, MD
Consultant, sanofi-aventis
Honoraria, sanofi-aventis

JOANNE MORTIMER, MD
Research funding, Novartis

DAVID M. NANUS, MD
Stock ownership, Amgen

ALFRED I. NEUGUT, MD, PHD
Consultant, Executive Health Exams in NYC,
Expert testimony, Expert testimony in malpractice cases related to cancer screening

JOAN H. SCHILLER, MD
Advisory board, Genentech, AstraZeneca, Taiho, sanofi-aventis, Lilly, GSK, Pfizer, Novartis
Honoraria, Genentech, AstraZeneca, Taiho, sanofi-aventis, Lilly, GSK, Pfizer, Novartis
Research funding, Pfizer, Amgen, Taiho, AstraZeneca

LYNN M. SCHUCHTER, MD
No significant financial relationship to disclose

PIERRE L. TRIOZZI, MD
No significant financial relationship to disclose

JOSEPH T. RUGGIERO, MD
No significant financial relationship to disclose

ANNE MOORE, MD
No significant financial relationship to disclose

Peer Reviewer Disclosure Index

The *ASCO-SEP*™ Editorial Board has reviewed all peer reviewer disclosure reports, identified potential conflicts of interest and implemented strategies to manage those areas of conflict, where they exist.

DAVID ABOULAFIA, MD
Research funding, AIDS Mahoney Consortium, SWOG

FREDERICK R. APPELBAUM, MD
Advisory board, Kanisa Pharmaceuticals, Cellerent Therapeutics, Zymogenetics, Merck & Co., Genzyme
Honoraria, Swedish Providence Medical Center, Acute Leukemia Forum

SHANTANU BANERJI, MD, FRCPC
No significant financial relationship to disclose

THOMAS BECK, MD
No significant financial relationship to disclose

KATHLEEN BEEKMAN, MD
No significant financial relationship to disclose

AL BENSON, III, MD
Advisory board, Amgen, Bristol-Myers Squibb, Genentech, ImClone, Novartis, Pfizer, Roche, sanofi-aventis
Honoraria, sanofi-aventis
Research funding, Amgen, Bristol-Myers Squibb, Genentech, ImClone, Novartis, Pfizer, Roche, sanofi-aventis

DON M. BENSON, JR., MD, PHD
No significant financial relationship to disclose

JOSÉ BINES, MD
Honoraria, AstraZeneca

STEPHANIE V. BLANK, MD
No significant financial relationship to disclose

SEAN P. BOHEN, MD, PHD
Leader, Genentech, Inc.
Stock ownership, Genentech, Inc., Johnson & Johnson, Inc., Pharmacyclics, Inc.

JONATHAN C. BRITELL, MD
Honoraria, Celgene
Research funding, Novartis, Gist Registry

JAN C. BUCKNER, MD
Consultant, Amgen, NeoPharm, AntiSense Pharma, Genentech

LISA A. CAREY, MD
Consultant, Genentech, Bristol-Myers Squibb, GlaxoSmithKline

ROBERT W. CARLSON, MD
Consultant, Pfizer, AstraZeneca, Novartis, Genentech, Genomic Health, Bristol-Myers Squibb
Honoraria, Pfizer, AstraZeneca, Novartis, Genentech, Genomic Health, Bristol-Myers Squibb
Research funding, AstraZeneca, Aventis, Taiho

PRIYA CHAKRAVARTHI, MD
No significant financial relationship to disclose

BRUCE D. CHESON, MD
No significant financial relationship to disclose

BRUCE E. CLURMAN, MD, PHD
No significant financial relationship to disclose

KELLY COOKE, DO
No significant financial relationship to disclose

MARY D. DALY, MD, PHD
No significant financial relationship to disclose

LISA M. DEANGELIS, MD
Consultant, Schering-Plough, MGI Pharma

GEORGE DEMETRI, MD
Advisory board, Novartis, Pfizer, Johnson & Johnson, Pharmamar, Abbott, Ariad, Infinity, Phenomix, Idera, Genentech
Honoraria, Novartis, Pfizer
Research funding, Bristol-Myers Squibb, Johnson & Johnson, Pharmamar, Ariad, Abbott, Infinity
Expert testimony, Novartis, Pfizer, Johnson & Johnson

PATRICK J. DONOVAN, MD, FACP
No significant financial relationship to disclose

ERIC R. FEARON, MD, PHD
No significant financial relationship to disclose

STUART P. FELDMAN, MD
No significant financial relationship to disclose

RICHARD FISHER, MD
Advisory board, GlaxoSmithKline, Millennium, Genentech
Honoraria, GlaxoSmithKline, Millennium, Genentech

ARLENE A. FORASTIERE, MD
Advisory board, ImClone, Bristol-Myers Squibb
Research funding, Pfizer

DEAN GESME, MD
No significant financial relationship to disclose

MATTHEW P. GOETZ, MD
Consultant, Amgen, Bayer

STACEY M. GORE, MD
No significant financial relationship to disclose

SHARAD GOYAL, MD
No significant financial relationship to disclose

PETER R. GRAZE, MD
No significant financial relationship to disclose

AXEL GROTHEY, MD
Advisory board, Genentech, Roche, Bristol-Myers Squibb, Amgen, sanofi-aventis
Honoraria, Amgen, Roche, Genentech

ROBERT HADDAD, MD
Honoraria, Bristol-Myers Squibb, Amgen, sanofi-aventis
Research funding, Medimmune Oncology

NORAH LYNN HENRY, MD, PHD
No significant financial relationship to disclose

MARTEE LEIGH HENSLEY, MD, MSc
Employment, Bristol-Myers Squibb (Significant other)

JADE HOMSI, MD
No significant financial relationship to disclose

AMINAH JATOI, MD
Consultant, Amgen

BRANDON JOHNSON, MD
No significant financial relationship to disclose

ANTHONY JOSHUA, MBBS
No significant financial relationship to disclose

MARK KLEIN, MD
No significant financial relationship to disclose

MARK G. KRIS, MD
Consultant, Bristol-Myers Squibb
Expert testimony, AstraZeneca – FDA Hearing Appearance (no compensation)

RICHARD A. LARSON, MD
Consultant, Amgen, Genta, LymphoSign, Enzon, Celgene, Wyeth, GlaxoSmithKline, BioCryst, MGI Pharma, Hana Bioscience
Stock ownership, Amgen, Bristol-Myers Squibb, GlaxoSmithKline, Merck, MedCo Health, Pfizer
Research funding, Amgen, Bristol-Myers Squibb, Celgene, Kanisa, Novartis, Telik, Wyeth
Expert testimony, GlaxoSmith Kline, Novartis
Other remuneration, UpToDate, Inc.

HILLARD M. LAZARUS, MD
Honoraria, Enzon, Celgene, Genentech, IDEC

ALEXANDRA M. LEVINE, MD
No significant financial relationship to disclose

STEVEN K. LIBUTTI, MD
No significant financial relationship to disclose

GILBERTO LOPES, MD
Advisory board, Pfizer
Research funding, Abraxis, Bristol-Myers Squibb, Amgen

CHARLES L. LOPRINZI, MD
Consultant, Par Pharmaceuticals, Quality Oncology
Research funding, Aventis, Amgen, Roche, Centocor, Ortho Biotech, Novartis, MOVC

ROBERT G. MAKI, MD, PHD
Honoraria, Pfizer, Novartis
Research funding, Pfizer, Lilly

MAURIE MARKMAN, MD
Consultant, Eli Lilly, Genentech, Celgene, CTI, GlaxoSmithKline, Tibutec, Wyeth, Merck

THOMAS A. MARSLAND, MD
Consultant, Genentech, Lilly
Stock ownership, Amgen, Genentech

ROBERT S. MILLER, MD
No significant financial relationship to disclose

MATTHEW I. MILOWSKY, MD
No significant financial relationship to disclose

ANNE MOORE, MD
No significant financial relationship to disclose

TIMOTHY J. MOYNIHAN, MD
No significant financial relationship to disclose

DAVID M. NANUS, MD
No significant financial relationship to disclose

JOANNE MORTIMER, MD
Research funding, Novartis

ALFRED I. NEUGUT, MD, PHD
Consultant, Executive Health Group

JOSEPH O'CONNELL, MD
No significant financial relationship to disclose

THOMAS P. O'CONNOR, JR., MD
No significant financial relationship to disclose

BIMAL PATEL, MD
No significant financial relationship to disclose

DANIEL P. PETRYLAK, MD
Advisory board, Aventis, GPC Biotech, Bristol-Myers Squibb, Cell Genesys, Inc.
Honoraria, Aventis

LAWRENCE D. PIRO, MD
No significant financial relationship to disclose

W. THOMAS PURCELL, MD, MBA
Honoraria, Pfizer (no stock)

W. KIMRYN RATHMELL, MD, PHD
Honoraria, Pfizer
Research funding, Bayer

GREGORY J. RIELY, MD, PHD
Consultant, Genentech

PETER J. ROSEN, MD
Consultant, Amgen
Honoraria, Biogen Idec, Genentech, Pfizer, Amgen

JOAN H. SCHILLER, MD
Advisory board, Genentech, AstraZeneca, Pfizer, Merck, Telik, Celgene
Research funding, Genentech, Pfizer, AstraZeneca

LYNN M. SCHUCHTER, MD
No significant financial relationship to disclose

VERED STEARNS, MD
Consultant, Wyeth
Research funding, GlaxoSmithKline, Novartis, Pfizer

SHELBY TERSTRIEP, MD
No significant financial relationship to disclose

STEPHAN THOME, MD, FACP
No significant financial relationship to disclose

PIERRE L. TRIOZZI, MD
No significant financial relationship to disclose

STEVEN TUCKER, MD
No significant financial relationship to disclose

JAMES A. WALLACE, MD
No significant financial relationship to disclose

RONALD S. WALTERS, MD, MBA, MS
No significant financial relationship to disclose

JEDD WOLCHOK, MD, PHD
No significant financial relationship to disclose

RUTH T. YOUNG, MD, MA
Leader, Vanderbilt-Ingram Cancer Center
Stock ownership, Amgen, Bristol-Myers Squibb, Digene, Genentech, GlaxoSmithKline

DAN ZUCKERMAN, MD
No significant financial relationship to disclose

CONTINUING MEDICAL EDUCATION (CME) INFORMATION

Program Overview

The ASCO Self-Evaluation Program (*ASCO-SEP™*) is a comprehensive resource designed to help physicians assess their level of knowledge in the various areas of oncology and provide current understanding of cancer, its treatment, and the supportive care needed to optimize the quality of life for people with cancer. This program includes 19 chapters and a companion self-assessment tool with rationales covering the full range of topics in oncology, to include major cancer types, epidemiology and cancer prevention, strategies for geriatric cancers, molecular biology and an overview of biologic therapy.

Target Audience

The ASCO Self Evaluation Program (*ASCO-SEP™*) is targeted to fellows certifying for the subspecialty exam as well as practicing oncologists who are enrolled in a Maintenance of Certification program. *ASCO-SEP™* is also appropriate for use as a teaching tool for training and continuing education purposes.

Needs Statement

Over 1.4 million new cancer cases are expected to be diagnosed in the United States in 2007.[1] Cancer accounts for one of every four deaths in the US — more than 1,500 people a day — making it the second most common cause of death in this country.[1] Over the last three decades, however, investment in clinical cancer research, screening, and prevention has reduced cancer incidence and death rates, increased survival rates, and significantly reduced the symptoms and side effects of cancer and its treatment.[2] As an example, the number of US cancer deaths declined slightly in 2003, the first drop since 1930.[2]

The American Society of Clinical Oncology's Self Evaluation Program (*ASCO-SEP™*) seeks to reflect within its chapters the state of oncology as we know it today. It is not meant to be a textbook and it does not include future directions. Rather, this publication serves as a comprehensive overview of this subspecialty, for use in review, self-assessment and teaching activities.

A study done by the National Cancer Institute (NCI) Office of Education and Special Initiatives (OESI) in the spring of 2005 found that oncologists surveyed indicated that there is a gap between the cancer care patients receive and the care indicated by current evidence.[3] Through this publication, ASCO looks to narrow this gap by providing a vehicle to validate current knowledge as well as improve overall competency in oncology.

Learning Objectives

Upon completion of this educational activity, participants will be able to:

- Apply the basic principles of molecular biology, epidemiology and clinical pharmacology to the practice of oncology;
- Incorporate appropriate imaging and diagnostic techniques to accurately identify and stage neoplastic disease;
- Discuss current treatment options with patients diagnosed with cancer and recommend approaches based on current evidence; and
- Assess and mitigate potential symptoms impacting quality of life, relating to treatment toxicity, comorbidities, or late effects.

CME Accreditation Statement

The American Society of Clinical Oncology is accredited by the Accreditation Council for Continuing Medical Education to provide continuing medical education for physicians.

The American Society of Clinical Oncology designates this educational activity for a maximum of 43.5 *AMA PRA Category 1 Credit(s)™*. Physicians should only claim credit commensurate with the extent of their participation in the activity.

Date of Original Release

The original release date for this material is February 1, 2008. The CME credit availability expires February 31, 2010.

Method of Instruction and Participation

The enclosed chapters consist of lecture text and self-assessment items. After completing the chapter the

1. *American Cancer Society: Cancer Facts & Figures 2007.* Atlanta, GA; American Cancer Society: 2007.
2. Ozols, RF, Herbst RS, et al. *Clinical Cancer Advances 2006: Major Research Advances in Cancer Treatment, Prevention, and Screening — A Report from the American Society of Clinical Oncology.* J Clin Oncol 25:1-30, 2007.
3. National Cancer Institute's Office of Education Special Initiatives. *A Study to Determine How to Improve the Dissemination and Implementation of Evidence-Based Practices in Cancer Care: Report of Practitioner Survey Findings.* February 2006.

physician is encouraged to respond to questions about the content of the activity and complete an evaluation of the activity.

Estimated Time to Complete the Activity

It is estimated that the time to complete the activity will range from 1.0 hours to 3.5 hours for each chapter; credit is also awarded for participating in the comprehensive self assessment. It is estimated that the time to complete the entire self evaluation program and associated evaluation will be 43.5 hours.

Obtaining Continuing Medical Education Credit

To receive CME credit, please complete both the Evaluation and Request for CME Credit.

Copies of these forms are available on the *ASCO-SEP*™ website or on pages 39i - 49i in the book. Submit online, or use the information below to fax, mail or email (if scanned) the completed forms:

ASCO/CME
1900 Duke Street; Suite 200
Alexandria, VA 22314
Fax: 703-684-5482
E-mail: cme@asco.org
www.asco.org/ascosep

For ASCO members, a certificate of CME credit will be available to print within two weeks at ASCO's CME bank. Certificates for nonmembers will be emailed within two to three weeks.

Even if you are not interested in CME Credit, we encourage you to provide your feedback by completing the Evaluation.

Unlabelled Usage Statement

The information presented is that of the contributing authors and does not necessarily represent the views of the American Society of Clinical Oncology. Specific therapies discussed may not be approved and/or specified for use as indicated. Therefore, before prescribing any medication, please review the complete prescribing information including indications, contraindications, warnings, precautions and adverse effects.

CONTENTS

CHAPTER 18

CHAPTER 19

1

EPIDEMIOLOGY AND PREVENTION

Alfred I. Neugut, MD, PhD

LEARNING OBJECTIVES

After reviewing this chapter, the reader should be able to

- Analyze the relationship between study design and outcome measures
- Apply knowledge of key terms and concepts of epidemiology to evaluation of clinical trial design and reported results
- Address the effects of socioeconomic factors on cancer care and treatment outcomes
- Discuss with patients and colleagues the efficacy of various cancer prevention strategies (e.g., chemoprevention, lifestyle modification, smoking cessation) and make case-appropriate recommendations
- Use available research and resources to evaluate cancer screening tests for efficacy and clinical value

Epidemiology is the study of disease in populations, including its distribution, determinants, natural history, and survival. Rather than the individual patient, its perspective is that of public health. The traditional focus and goal of epidemiology has been disease prevention and control through primary prevention and screening interventions, but, more recently, epidemiology also has included the assessment of treatment outcomes, including survival and long-term sequelae.

Because of its emphasis on populations, epidemiology generally uses rates (with denominator populations — those rates standardized to a population — and time frames) or relative measures rather than absolute figures to measure relevant statistics. Descriptive epidemiology encompasses incidence and mortality rates, survival rates, and time trends. Incidence and mortality rates are commonly expressed as the number of newly diagnosed cases or deaths per 100,000 in the group at risk. These rates are frequently age and gender adjusted, meaning they are mathematically adjusted to a standard population to remove the effect of a population's age and gender distribution which may change over time.

The American Society of Clinical Oncology and Dr. Neugut would like to gratefully acknowledge Otis W. Brawley, MD, for his contributions to the original content of this chapter.

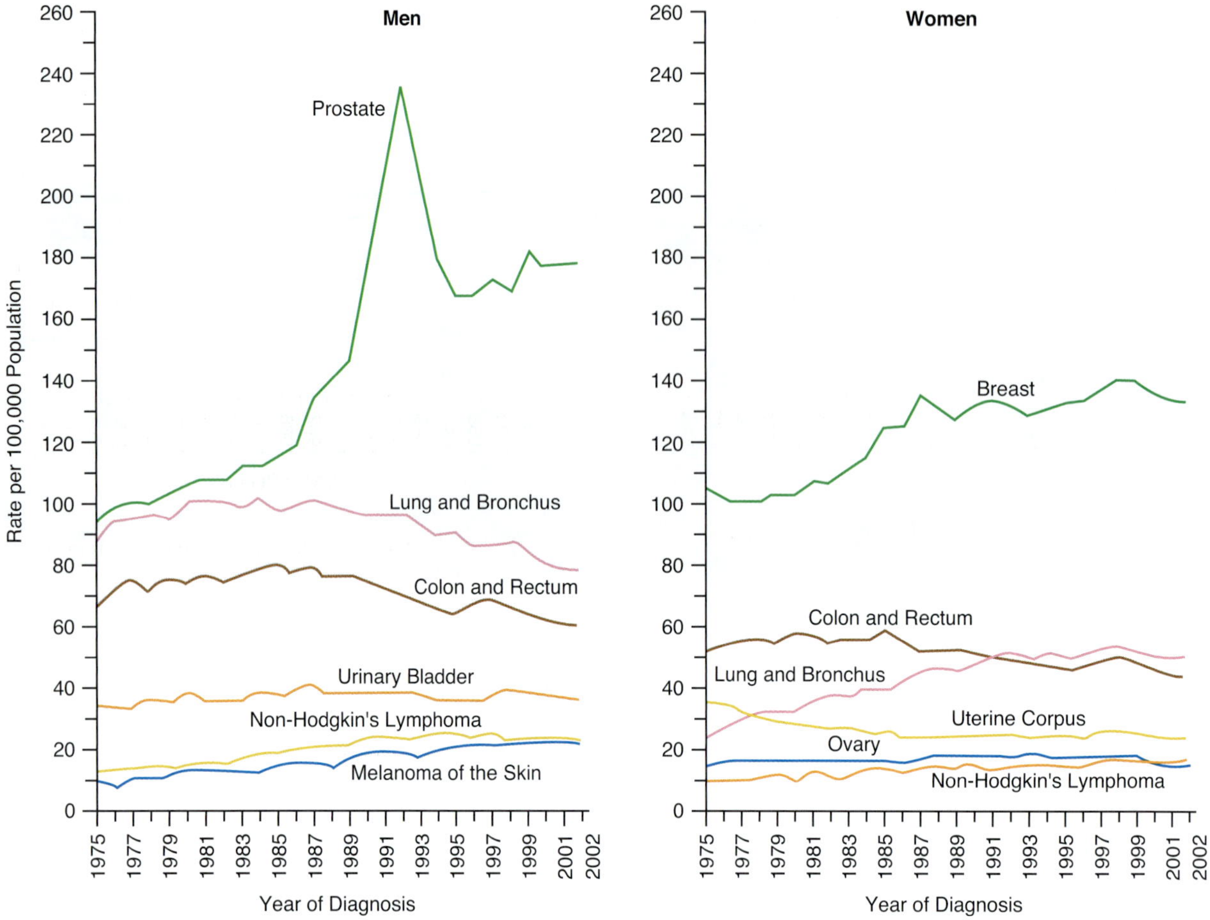

FIG. 1-1. U.S. annual age-adjusted cancer incidence rates (1975 to 2002) among men and women for selected cancers[1,2]

Cancer is primarily a disease of older people. With the extensive increase during the past 30 years in the number of individuals in the United States who are age 70 and older, the absolute number and the crude rate per 100,000 patients with cancer also has increased. Furthermore, there are substantially more older women than men, so a difference in gender distribution would magnify or diminish with age as well. Adjusting disease rates for age and gender removes the effects of gender and aging of the population. As a result, any observed increases in age- and gender-adjusted incidence and mortality rates are the result of causes other than the aging population (Fig. 1-1).[1,2]

Survival is defined as the time from diagnosis to death. A commonly used measure is the proportion of people alive at 5 years after diagnosis (Table 1-1).

The American Cancer Society publishes an annual estimate of the absolute number of new cancer cases and deaths.[2] These numbers are widely quoted, especially by the lay press. It should be emphasized that these figures are not rates and are subject to fluctuations in the age and gender distribution of the population. The American Cancer Society also publishes time trends of incidence and mortality rates for major cancers during the past 75 years; these figures can give interesting insights into the inroads made by

TABLE 1-1. Definition of Terms Related to Survival

Term	Definition
Survival time	Time from the initial diagnosis of cancer to death
Disease-free survival	Time from complete remission to relapse of disease
Five-year survival rate	Proportion of patients who are alive 5 years after the time of diagnosis
Disease-specific survival rate	Proportion of patients who have not died of the specific disease (does not take into account deaths unrelated to the disease)
Overall survival rate	Proportion of patients who are alive at a specific time after the diagnosis (takes into account all causes of death)

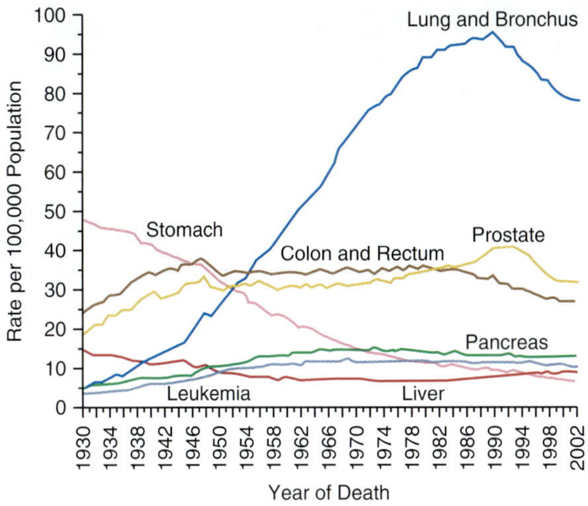

FIG. 1-2. U.S. annual age-adjusted cancer death rates (1930 to 2002) among men for selected cancers[2]

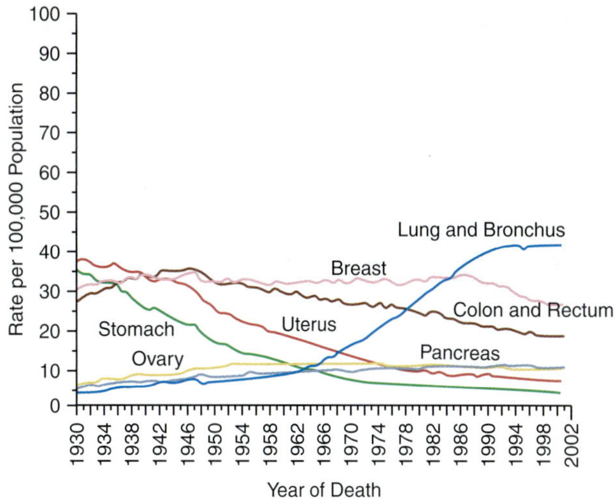

FIG. 1-3. U.S. annual age-adjusted cancer death rates (1930 to 2002) among women for selected cancers [2]

primary prevention, screening, and treatment, as well as into changes brought about by increases or decreases in risk factors (Figs. 1-1, 1-2, and 1-3).[1,2]

RISK

Much of epidemiology involves assessment of cancer risk. A person can be at increased risk of cancer because of either extrinsic or intrinsic factors, or a mix thereof.

- Extrinsic influences are factors outside of the patient's own body, such as environmental pollutants, cultural habits, infectious factors, and diet.
- Intrinsic influences are factors unique to each patient, such as genetics.
- To assess etiology, risk is usually reported relative to another population. For example, between 1996 and 2000, the breast cancer mortality rate for black women was 35.9 per 100,000, and the rate for non-Hispanic white women was 27.4 per 100,000. During that period, the relative risk of death for black women was 1.31 times that of white women (35.9 divided by 27.4).

From an epidemiologic perspective, an etiologic agent or risk factor is anything that raises the probability that an individual will develop the disease. These risk factors can include demographic characteristics (e.g., increasing age or race/ethnicity) or lifestyle and behavioral factors, such as smoking. They also include endogenous factors, such as genes, polymorphisms, and genetic mutations that have been identified as predisposing a person for a disease. Undoubtedly most cancers arise from a combination of genetic and exogenous factors that combine to define certain demographic patterns. These patterns are recognized as the populations in which a specific cancer is most likely to occur.

Certain genetic mutations occur with high frequency but convey only a slight increase in probability of the cancer occurring. These are referred to as genetic polymorphisms and are usually thought to provide increased susceptibility to an environmental carcinogen or to modify risk in some other way. For example, genetic polymorphisms for the cytochrome P450 enzyme system that metabolizes carcinogens in cigarette smoke can thus cause variability in susceptibility to its effects. Better known are the uncommon genetic mutations that convey high risk of malignancy development, such as the mutations of the *BRCA* or familial adenomatous polyposis (*FAP*) genes. *BRCA1* and *BRCA2* are genes with well-defined DNA sequences. Some *BRCA1* and *BRCA2* mutations increase the risk of breast and ovarian cancer and possibly of other malignant diseases when compared with risk for individuals without the mutations.[3] Other *BRCA* mutations have an unknown effect on breast cancer risk. Knowledge regarding genetic risk factors for a particular cancer and the ability to predict development of a particular cancer can help oncologists develop and select intervention options. Knowledge of the risk factor also may present ethical dilemmas. These factors include the conveyance of knowledge of risk to third parties in the family, selection of embryos for implantation during in vitro fertilization on the basis of genetic testing, or the use of amniocentesis for testing of known genes, the results of which could be followed by abortion. However, knowledge may allow for early interventions that could prevent disease or limit its severity.

To address risk from genetic factors, it is critical to take a good family history from patients with cancer. This is particularly important in younger patients. Such a history should include a census of all first-degree relatives (i.e., parents, siblings, and children) at a minimum, with their genders, current age or age at death, any cancers diagnosed, as well as the age at diagnosis. Suspicious histories, or early age at diagnosis for certain cancers, should lead to referral to a genetic counselor for further evaluation and testing. The results of these evaluations have implications for the patient regarding risk of further cancers, as well as implications for other members of the patient's family.

Just as for genetic information, the clinician should make an effort to collect relevant risk factor information for patients with cancer or for healthy patients who are undergoing wellness exams. Minimal information should include tobacco use, height and weight, family history, and an occupational history. Other factors should be included as relevant to a specific symptom or diagnosis. This information can be used to provide advice and guidance to the patient (e.g., regarding tobacco cessation), to identify patients at high risk for certain cancers, and to guide early detection and prevention strategies.

Chemoprevention and screening are options for certain high-risk populations. Individuals at high risk of cancer may engage in intensive screening for the cancer in question. Although such screening may be clinically prudent, it may be less effective for individuals at very high risk. In theory, a screening test might benefit those at risk for sporadic cancers and not benefit those at genetically high risk for a cancer.

Population categorization is important in epidemiology. Populations can be delineated by gender, nationality, culture, race and ethnicity, socioeconomic status, age, and other characteristics. This is the basis of descriptive epidemiology — along with time trends — and is used to provide clues as to etiology. For example, a cancer that has a strong predominance in men may have a specific occupational component to it. Differences in incidence rates for various cancers found in both Japan and the United States have suggested hypotheses regarding diet and the use of green tea.

Race and ethnicity are common ways of dividing populations in the United States. It should be remembered that race is a sociopolitical categorization.[4] The definitions used by the United States when generating population statistics are not formulated on the basis of science. Much concern has arisen in the past decade regarding disparities in outcomes, in particular for a wide range of cancers, for black as compared with white patients. In some instances, these disparities also reflect differences in incidence, but, in others, they may reflect differences in stage at diagnosis, access to treatment, or in tumor biology. Race and ethnicity can correlate with other methods of categorization, such as poverty or prosperity, both of which are capable of changing the incidence of cancer and its related mortality.

Socioeconomic status and education also can be related to the risk of disease and death. Higher rates of breast cancer among white women in the San Francisco Bay area and on Long Island were linked to a higher prevalence of professional women in those areas who, as a cohort, are less likely to have a full-term pregnancy by age 30, a known risk factor for breast cancer.[5] Socioeconomic status also has been related to type of treatment received and subsequent outcomes for various cancers, although this variable is heavily confounded with race/ethnicity and education.[6] In a classic study, Ayanian et al.[7] found that uninsured women with breast cancer and women on Medicaid had a 49% (95% CI: 20, 84) and 40% (95% CI: 4, 89) higher risk of death, respectively, than women with private insurance. A similar effect for socioeconomic status was found for survival of patients with colorectal cancer[8] and quality of life for prostate cancer survivors.[9]

KEY POINTS

- Epidemiology is the study of the distribution, etiology, and natural history of disease in populations.
- Epidemiology can include assessment of treatment outcomes, disease prevention, and disease screening.
- Epidemiology addresses these issues with a public health and public policy perspective as opposed to the perspective of an individual patient.
- Risk can be increased by both extrinsic and intrinsic influences.
- To assess etiology, a population risk is usually reported relative to another population.

In analytic epidemiology, observational studies are carried out to ascertain whether associations exist between an exposure and an outcome. Although a statistical association may exist between the two, there is always concern that this may reflect bias in the way the study was conducted or in the presence of confounding factors. Confounding factors are factors that are associated with both the exposure and the outcome and can lead to an observed association, which is not truly a relationship between the two. For example, a study may show that asbestos workers have an elevated risk of lung cancer as compared with the general population. However, one must be concerned that asbestos workers may be heavier smokers than other individuals in the general population and that cigarette smoking is associated with lung cancer risk; thus, smoking may confound the observed association. Therefore, it is mandatory in a study that looks at this exposure and outcome, to collect smoking information so that it can be statistically controlled and the individual effect of asbestos exposure can be appropriately measured.

Epidemiologic observational studies fall into two broad categories: cohort studies and case-control studies. Participants in cohort studies are categorized on the basis of their exposure and then followed to determine whether the outcome develops differently in the exposed and unexposed groups. Case-control studies enroll participants who have the outcome or disease under study, in addition to a control group of healthy participants. Both groups are then assessed for exposure. Both types, of studies have their advantages and disadvantages. In both types, one must try to avoid bias, or directional error. For example, in a case-control study, a patient with cancer may be inclined to give a positive answer more frequently than a control participant to a question regarding smoking history — this is referred to as recall bias.

Recently there has been increasing interest in molecular epidemiology — the use of sophisticated molecular markers in conjunction with the traditional tools of analytic epidemiology to investigate etiologic or other questions in cancer epidemiology. Biomarkers can be used to measure exposures or endpoints in place of the more traditional answers to questionnaires and, in some instances, biomarkers can give a more objective unbiased assessment.

Many contemporary studies in clinical oncology use epidemiologic methodology to address clinical questions in oncology. When randomized trials may be difficult to conduct, observational studies, like cohort or case-control studies, may be used to answer typical questions regarding the efficacy of a drug or the incidence of an adverse event from a drug. Therefore, an understanding of these analytic tools is imperative for the modern oncologist.

PATTERNS OF CARE AND OUTCOMES RESEARCH

Although descriptive epidemiology and the determination of etiologic risk factors have been the traditional domain of epidemiology, the assessment of treatment outcomes in populations has become an important aspect of epidemiology. A phase II clinical trial can demonstrate the efficacy of a treatment intervention (e.g., tumor shrinkage), and a phase III study compares two interventions to determine which is superior. Prevention trials usually require phase III studies to show efficacy. Clinical trials demonstrate "efficacy" of a treatment. How well the intervention works in the population as a whole in routine practice is termed "effectiveness."

The study of patterns of care or treatments used is an aspect of outcomes research. Numerous studies often demonstrate geographic and regional differences in the preferred treatment of cancers. For example, for women with localized breast cancer, the decision to treat with lumpectomy and radiation therapy or with mastectomy may vary depending on the patient's geographic location.[10] Similar regional differences have been noted for prostate cancer screening and for the types of treatment used for localized prostate cancer.[11]

Many of the disparities in outcomes among groups as defined by race and socioeconomic status have been linked to differences in patterns of care. For example, treatment is less than optimal for a substantial proportion of patients with cancer who are poor or of certain ethnic backgrounds.[12] The reasons for these variations in care are complex. Some are the result of sociocultural differences in attitudes toward therapy. Patient–physician communication also can play a major role.[13] In other cases, poverty, lack of insurance, or underinsurance can make access to care difficult.[7, 14] Logistic difficulties, such as problems with transportation to a treatment center, also may play a role. Patients with severe comorbid disease or poor performance status may justifiably not be offered aggressive cancer treatments because they are at higher risk of a treatment-related morbidity.

KEY POINT

- Most clinical trials are designed to determine "efficacy," meaning how well the treatment works in a selected environment. Some larger trials and outcomes studies are designed to show "effectiveness," meaning how well the treatment works in the population as a whole.

CANCER PREVENTION

Prevention is intended to reduce cancer incidence and mortality. Primary cancer prevention is best defined as the use of interventions to lower cancer incidence. Important to prevention is the fact that carcinogenesis is not a distinct event but rather a process that occurs over time. It is a cumulative continuum of discrete cellular changes resulting in uncontrolled growth. Primary prevention involves interventions or manipulations of the genetic, biologic, and environmental factors in the causal pathway of carcinogenesis. Smoking cessation, sun avoidance, diet modification, weight loss and physical activity, cancer virus vaccination, and chemoprevention (e.g., tamoxifen for breast cancer prevention) are primary prevention activities. Screening for asymptomatic cancers is considered secondary prevention, which is intended to reduce mortality. For some cancers, intraepithelial neoplasia is an intermediate step in carcinogenesis, and treatment of this condition is a form of cancer prevention.[15]

SMOKING CESSATION

Tobacco use is the most avoidable risk factor for cardiovascular disease, pulmonary disorders, and cancer. Smoking cessation and avoidance have the potential to save and extend more lives than any other public health activity. A smoker has a one in three lifetime risk of dying prematurely of a smoking-related disease. More human lives are lost because of cardiovascular disease caused by smoking than from smoking- related cancer. In addition to lung cancer, cigarette smoking has been linked to cancer of the larynx, oropharynx, esophagus, kidney, bladder, pancreas, and probably colon.[16]

The risk from tobacco smoke is not necessarily limited to the smoker. Epidemiologic studies strongly suggest that environmental tobacco smoke, often called secondhand or passive smoke, may cause lung cancer and other pulmonary diseases in nonsmokers. The amount of smoke exposure, as well as the degree of inhalation of cigarette smoke, is correlated with the risk of mortality associated with lung cancer. Light and low-tar cigarettes are not safer because smokers tend to inhale them more frequently and deeply. Compared with their nonfiltered counterparts, filtered cigarettes allow smaller particles to get into the peripheral parts of the lung and cause different histologic subtypes of cancer,[17-19] speci fically adenocarcinoma. Those who stop smoking almost immediately stop increasing their risk of cancer, although it takes some time before their risk of cancer declines. Some carcinogen-induced gene mutations, however, may persist for years.

More than 80% of adult American smokers begin smoking before age 18.[20] Therefore, communicating health messages to the pediatric and adolescent population is a major public health challenge. Studies show that a physician's simple advice to avoid or quit smoking can positively influence patients.

Among the most effective smoking cessation interventions are governmental actions. Tax increases on cigarettes and restrictions on venues where smoking is permitted have been very effective in reducing smoking prevalence rates.[21] Current smoker rates are down to 20% or less in the United States, and most tobacco-related cancers in this country now occur in former smokers. However, smoking remains a major factor globally, especially in Asia, and lung cancer is the leading cause of cancer mortality worldwide.

Smoking is an addiction. It is easier for light smokers — the less addicted — to quit. Experts believe that heavy smokers generally need an intensive, broad-based cessation program that includes counseling, behavioral strategies, and drug therapy, such as nicotine-replacement therapy and bupropion. Most Americans who successfully quit smoking do so on their own without participation in an organized cessation program, but such strategies can be helpful for some. Smokers who stop completely are more likely to be successful than smokers who gradually reduce the number of cigarettes smoked or change to cigarettes containing lower amounts of tar or nicotine. The smoker who is quitting goes through a process with identifiable stages that include contemplation of quitting, an action phase during which the smoker quits, and a maintenance phase.

Much of the literature focuses on the risks of cigarette smoking. Cigar smokers do not inhale, but the health risks associated with cigars are similar to those of cigarettes, especially the risks of oropharyngeal cancers.[22] Smokeless tobacco, or chewing tobacco, is the fastest growing segment of the tobacco industry and represents a serious health risk. Chewing tobacco has been linked to dental caries, gingivitis, oral leukoplakia, and oral cancer. In addition, the nitrosamines found in this product have been shown to cause lung cancer in animal studies. Esophageal cancer is linked to the carcinogens in tobacco that dissolve in saliva, are swallowed, and then come into contact with the esophagus.

SUN AVOIDANCE

Results of epidemiologic studies show a correlation between the risk of nonmelanoma skin cancers (basal and squamous cell) and cumulative exposure to ultraviolet radiation. Possible risk factors for melanoma include a propensity to sunburn, a large number of benign melanocytic nevi, and atypical nevi. A history of severe sunburns, especially in childhood and adolescence, is associated with increased risk of melanoma in adulthood. Reduction of sun exposure through the use of protective clothing and through a change in one's pattern of outdoor activities to avoid the most intense and direct sunlight have been advocated as ways to reduce the risk of skin cancer.

DIET MODIFICATION

Rates of cancers of the breast, colon, endometrium, and prostate are higher in the West than in the Far East. Immigrants from those areas and their offspring acquire a higher risk after they have been in the United States for some time. These observations are the basis for the belief that dietary modification can significantly lower cancer risk for individuals in the United States.[23] Diet is a highly complex exposure to many nutrients and chemicals. Low-fat diets, which are usually low in red meat and high in fruits and vegetables, may render some protection through anticarcinogens found in vegetables, fruits, legumes, nuts, and grains. Potentially protective substances found in foods include phenols, sulfur-containing compounds, and flavones.[24] Although the cancer-prevention benefits are theoretical and not fully demonstrated, such a diet does lower the risk of cardiac disease. However, vitamins, minerals, or nutritional supplements in amounts greater than those provided by a good diet have not been demonstrated to be of value.

Despite correlative data, the dietary fat–cancer hypothesis has not been definitively demonstrated. Case-control and cohort epidemiologic studies yield conflicting results. No prospective clinical trial has demonstrated that cancer can be prevented through lowering dietary fat or increasing fiber intake. Recent studies, including randomized trials, have been consistent in showing no effect of dietary fiber intake on colon cancer risk.[25, 26] The Women's Health Initiative, which included a randomized trial with a low-fat diet intervention, also did not support an effect on breast cancer or colon cancer risk.[27, 28]

WEIGHT LOSS AND PHYSICAL ACTIVITY

A major recent public health concern has centered on the obesity epidemic in the United States. Obesity represents the effects of an individual's net caloric intake, which is the amount consumed versus the amount expended through physical activity. Changes in either of these variables will impinge on the measure of obesity, thereby affecting cancer risk. Obesity affects cancer risk through a number of mechanisms including hormone metabolism, thereby affecting breast, endometrial, and prostate cancer risk or by increasing esophageal reflux, which affects occurrence of Barrett's metaplasia and esophageal adenocarcinoma.[29]

OCCUPATIONAL CARCINOGENS

Since Percival Pott recognized an increased risk of scrotal cancer among chimney sweeps in 18th-century London, there has been an awareness that occupational exposures can increase the risk of certain cancers. The most important of the recent occupational carcinogens has been asbestos, which is prominent among construction workers, pipefitters, and shipyard workers. It has been closely linked to the incidence of mesothelioma, lung cancer, and possibly gastroinetestinal tract malignancies. Another classic exposure has been radon inhalation, which occurs in uranium miners and increases the risk of lung cancer. Various other organic and aromatic chemicals are linked to the risks of leukemia and cancers of the urinary collecting system.

CANCER VIRUS VACCINATION

Virally induced cancer has been recognized since the early part of the 20th century with the discovery of Rous sarcoma virus in chickens. In humans, several viruses, including hepatitis B (hepatocellular carcinoma), hepatitis C (hepatocellular carcinoma), Epstein-Barr virus (Burkitt's lymphoma), and human papillomavirus ([HPV]; cervical cancer and other anogenital squamous cell malignancies) have been clearly established as carcinogenic. An understanding of retroviruses has broadened our appreciation of other viral agents, such as human herpesvirus 8 and Kaposi's sarcoma.[30,31] In addition, the bacterium, *Helicobacter pylori*, was found to be associated with gastric cancer. These are particularly exciting findings because these agents provide targets for vaccination as a means of primary prevention. This has been achieved for hepatitis B[32] and for HPV.[33] Recently, a new success has been the introduction of a vaccine for several subtypes of HPV. This will be used for vaccinating young girls prior to their becoming sexually active, which should reduce the incidence of cervical cancer by 70% or more. Because these same viruses also are involved in other anogenital cancers, incidence of anal, vaginal, and penile cancers may decline, particularly if male vaccination is introduced in the future.

CHEMOPREVENTION

Cancer chemoprevention is the use of natural or synthetic chemical agents to reverse, suppress, or prevent carcinogenesis before the development of an invasive malignant process.[34] Cancers are prevented through chemoprevention or, in certain cases, through surgical removal of the organ at risk. Although the concept that pharmacologic agents can prevent a cancer is relatively new, the idea that a compound can prevent chronic disease is not. Antihypertensive agents are used to prevent heart disease, kidney disease, and stroke. Lipid-lowering drugs are prescribed to prevent coronary artery disease.

The initial genetic changes of carcinogenesis are termed "initiation." This alteration can be inherited or acquired. Acquired genetic damage is the result of physical, infectious, or chemical carcinogens (Table 1-2). The influences that cause the initiated cell to change phenotypically are called promoters. Known promoters include androgens linked to prostate cancer and estrogen linked to breast and endometrial cancers. The distinction between the initiator and promoter can sometimes blur; some components of cigarette smoke are referred to as "complete carcinogens" and serve as both initiator and promoter. Cancer can be prevented or controlled through interference with the factors causing disease initiation, promotion, or progression.

Compounds of interest in chemoprevention include anti-inflammatory agents, antioxidants, differentiating agents, or hormone antagonists. A long-term, randomized, placebo-controlled clinical trial is generally necessary to establish the efficacy of a chemopreventive agent, and several large clinical trials have been completed.[35-37] As discussed in the following sections, tamoxifen and raloxifene have been shown to reduce the incidence of breast cancer. In addition, nonsteroidal anti-inflammatory drugs reduce the occurrence of colorectal adenomas in various circumstances, and finasteride reduces the incidence of prostate cancer. Retinoids may inhibit head and neck cancers, and selenium is under study for prostate cancer.

Cancers of the Lung, Head and Neck, and Esophagus

Tobacco smoking is the major cause of squamous cell cancers of the lung, head, neck, and esophagus. The risk of a second cancer of the lung, head, or neck is high — as great as 5% per year of smoking — for patients cured of these diseases. This is because of "field cancerization," meaning the carcinogens in tobacco smoke affect all tissues exposed to them. Even after smoking cessation, the tissues that have come in contact with smoke have residual molecular damage. For the esophagus, head, and neck, alcohol ingestion has an interactive effect with smoking. Other cancers of the lung (e.g., small cell and adenocarcinoma) also are associated with tobacco use. Very high rates of oral cancer are found in India in association with betel nut chewing.

In the United States, incidence rates for esophageal adenocarcinoma are among the most rapidly increasing. This occurs as a sequelae of Barrett's esophagus and is thought to be the result of gastroesophageal reflux disease.[38] Esophagogastroduodenoscopy often is used as regular surveillance to detect Barrett's esophagus in patients with gastroesophageal reflux disease; however, there is no convincing evidence that

TABLE 1-2. Examples of Inhibitors and Promoters of Cancer

Carcinogen	Associated Cancer or Neoplasm
Alkylating agents	Acute myelocytic leukemia, bladder
Androgens	Prostate
Aromatic amines (dyes)	Bladder
Arsenic	Lung, skin
Asbestos	Lung, pleura, peritoneum
Benzene	Acute myelocytic leukemia
Chromium	Lung
Diethylstilbestrol (prenatal)	Vaginal (clear cell)
Epstein-Barr virus	Burkitt's lymphoma, nasopharynx
Estrogens	Endometrium, breast
Ethyl alcohol	Liver, esophagus, head and neck
Helicobacter pylori	Gastric
Hepatitis B virus	Liver
Hepatitis C virus	Liver
Human T-cell leukemia (HTLV)-1 virus	Adult T-cell leukemia, lymphoma
Human immunodeficiency virus (HIV)	Non-Hodgkin's lymphoma, Kaposi's sarcoma, squamous cell cancer of cervix
Immunosuppressive agents (azathioprine, cyclosporine, corticosteroids)	Non-Hodgkin's lymphoma
Nitrogen mustard gas	Lung, head and neck, nasal sinuses
Nickel dust	Lung, nasal sinuses
Phenacetin	Renal, pelvis, bladder
Polycyclic aromatic hydrocarbons	Lung, skin (especially squamous cell)
Schistosomiasis	Bladder (squamous cell)
Sunlight (ultraviolet)	Skin (squamous cell and melanoma)
Tobacco (including smokeless)	Upper aerodigestive tract, bladder
Vinyl chloride	Liver (angiosarcoma)

These agents are thought to act as cancer initiators or promoters for the cancers with which they have been associated.

demonstrates a reduction in the subsequent incidence or mortality of esophageal adenocarcinoma.

Several large-scale studies have been launched to assess potential chemopreventive agents for patients at high risk for lung cancer. The Alpha-Tocopherol, Beta-Carotene Cancer Prevention Trial (ATBC)[39] and the Beta-Carotene and Retinol Efficacy Trial (CARET)[40] were prevention trials that showed the importance of testing even seemingly harmless chemoprevention agents, such as vitamins, before widespread use. The results of both trials are in contrast to numerous observational studies. The ATBC trial enrolled Finnish male smokers between ages 50 and 69. Participants received alpha-tocopherol, beta-carotene, both, or placebo in a randomized, two-by-two factorial design. After a median follow-up of 6 years, there was a significant increase in lung cancer incidence and mortality for the subjects who received beta-carotene. Alpha-tocopherol had no effect on lung cancer mortality. CARET enrolled 17,000 smokers and workers exposed to asbestos. Participants were randomly assigned to four arms and received beta-carotene, retinol, both, or placebo in a two-by-two factorial design. The results of the trial demonstrated a 28% increase in lung cancers and a 17% increase in deaths for the participants receiving beta-carotene. The reason for this outcome is uncertain; it occurred despite beta-carotene's role as both an antioxidant and as a precursor to retinol.

Retinoids have proven to be effective as chemopreventive agents for squamous cell malignancies of the head and neck, possibly by promoting terminal differentiation.[41]

Gastric Cancers

Heavy intake of smoked and cured meats and foods, limited consumption of fresh fruits and vegetables, and infection with *H. pylori* are associated with an increased risk of gastric cancer.[38] Gastric cancer was the most common cancer in the United States prior to World War II, but it is now much less common. This decline is thought to be because of increased consumption of fresh meats, fruits, and vegetables. Experimental evidence of causality is scarce. It remains a very common cancer in Japan, Latin America, China, and in other parts of the developing world. A randomized trial in China of eradication of *H. pylori* infection with a combination of omeprazole, amoxicillin, clavulanate, and metronidazole did not show a reduction in subsequent gastric cancer. Nonetheless, patients who had no gastric pathology at study entry did show a significant benefit.[42] There are no randomized trial data to support screening for groups at high risk (e.g., Asians) for *H. pylori,* which would lead to institution of eradication procedures to reduce the subsequent risk of gastric cancer. Studies are underway to elucidate this question further.

Colon Cancer

Findings from epidemiologic studies suggest that nonsteroidal anti-inflammatory agents, such as piroxicam, sulindac, and aspirin, have protective effects against adenomatous polyps and invasive cancer. The results of prospective intervention trials have demonstrated some positive effects on the prevention of polyps; however, randomized trials have yet to demonstrate conclusively that these agents prevent colon cancer. In a placebo-controlled trial, high-dose celecoxib, a cyclooxygenase-2 (COX-2) inhibitor, was found to reduce the occurrence of colorectal polyps for patients with familial adenomatous polyposis.[43] A prospective randomized trial of patients with a history of colorectal adenomas demonstrated a 20% reduction in recurrence of polyps for patients who received celecoxib.[44] Trials to assess COX-2 inhibitors and other non steroidal anti-inflammatory agents for the prevention of colorectal adenomas have shown preventive benefits; however, these agents are associated with increased cardiovascular risk.

The Women's Health Initiative was a prospective, randomized study involving postmenopausal women randomly assigned to either combination estrogen plus progestin or to placebo. The rate of colorectal cancer was lower for women taking the study drug compared with women taking placebo.[45] However, the effect is offset by the life-threatening cardiovascular and breast cancer risks associated with treatment with estrogen plus progestin.[46]

The results of epidemiologic studies indicate that diets high in calcium are associated with a lower risk of colon cancer. However, in the Women's Health Initiative study, calcium and vitamin D supplementation did not lower the incidence of colorectal cancer.[47] Evidence from prospective randomized studies shows that calcium supplementation decreases the risk of recurrence of adenomatous polyps by approximately 20%.[48] Calcium binds bile and fatty acids, reducing intraluminal exposure to compounds that cause hyperproliferation of the colonic epithelium.

Obesity is associated with an increased risk of colorectal cancer. However, in another Women's Health Initiative randomized controlled trial there was no difference in the incidence of colorectal cancer among women assigned to a low-fat diet as compared with controls.[28]

Colectomy is used as a preventive measure for individuals at extremely high risk of colon cancer as a result of a history of ulcerative colitis or of a genetic predisposition to the disease, such as familial adenomatous polyposis.[49]

No chemopreventive agent is recommended for prevention of colorectal cancer for individuals at average risk. The use of nonsteroidal anti-inflammatory agents for patients with familial adenomatous polyposis following colectomy may be reasonable in conjunction with endoscopic screening.

Liver Cancer

Hepatitis B-induced hepatocellular carcinoma is one of the most commonly diagnosed cancers in Asia. The hepatitis B vaccine has been advocated for its ability to prevent the disease. The reductions in the incidence of hepatocellular carcinoma in Taiwan and elsewhere suggest some success.[50] Although hepatocellular carcinoma is much less common in the United States, there has been a recent rise in incidence rates due to an epidemic of hepatitis C.

Breast Cancer

Tamoxifen has mixed estrogenic and antiestrogen activities. It acts as an estrogen agonist in the endometrium and bone and as an estrogen antagonist in breast tissue. It also upregulates transforming growth factor-beta, which decreases breast cell proliferation. In randomized, placebo-controlled trials to assess tamoxifen as adjuvant therapy for patients with early-stage breast cancer, this drug was found to prevent new cancers in the contralateral breast. The Breast Cancer Prevention Trial was a randomized, placebo-controlled study of more than 13,000 women at high risk of breast cancer. After a median treatment of 69 months, tamoxifen was found to decrease the period risk of breast cancer by 49%. It also was associated with a reduction in bone fractures and with a small increase in risk of endometrial cancer, stroke, pulmonary emboli, and deep vein thrombosis.[35] A trial to compare tamoxifen with another selective estrogen-receptor modulator, raloxifene, for postmenopausal women, was recently completed (the Study of Tamoxifen and Raloxifene [STAR] Trial). Raloxifene decreased the risk of invasive breast cancer by amounts similar to tamoxifen but did not decrease the risk of noninvasive breast cancer. Compared with tamoxifen, raloxifene was associated with less risk of endometrial cancer, as well as with lower risk of thromboembolic events and cataracts.[37]

The Women's Health Initiative was discontinued early partially because of the increased risk of breast cancer (odds ratio 1.26) among women who were postmenopausal and who were taking active hormone replacement.[45] A parallel trial of estrogen alone compared with placebo for women with a prior hysterectomy demonstrated a nonsignificantly decreased risk of breast cancer among women taking estrogen.[51]

Obesity also is associated with an increased risk of breast cancer. As was the case with colorectal cancer, a Women's Health Initiative study demonstrated that subjects who followed a low-fat diet did not have a reduced incidence of breast cancer.[27]

Prophylactic bilateral mastectomy to prevent breast cancer has not been well assessed. In a prospective series of 139 women with *BRCA1* and *BRCA2* mutations, 76 chose prophylactic bilateral mastectomy and 63 chose close surveillance. At 3 years, there was no breast cancer diagnosed in those who chose surgery; eight women in the surveillance group had been diagnosed with breast cancer. This study is small, of short duration, and, by design, prone to selection biases. However, it is fair to say that the short-term risk of breast cancer appears to be lower for women with certain *BRCA1* and *BRCA2* mutations and who choose prophylactic mastectomy. Because this surgery leaves some breast tissue behind, a patient's risk is not reduced to zero. When coupled with prophylactic bilateral salpingo-oophorectomy, ovarian cancer risk is markedly decreased, and there is an added benefit for breast cancer prevention. Retrospective analysis of mastectomies for 214 women at high risk of breast cancer because of family history suggests that prophylactic mastectomy can lead to a 90% reduction in risk.[52] The effect of this procedure on mortality for women at high risk of breast cancer is not completely known.[53]

Prostate Cancer

Androgens stimulate prostate cell proliferation and, in laboratory animals, cause prostate carcinogenesis. Finasteride decreases androgenic stimulation of the prostate by inhibiting the production of 5-alpha-reductase. This enzyme, which is found in high amounts in the prostate, converts testosterone to the more potent dihydrotestosterone. Finasteride was tested as a preventive agent for prostate cancer in the Prostate Cancer Prevention Trial, a 10-year, randomized, placebo-controlled study involving 18,000 men aged 55 and older. Results of the study showed that this drug was associated with a 24.8% reduction in the risk of prostate cancer during the treatment period. There are some concerns regarding an observed increased incidence of high-grade tumors that developed while patients were treated with finasteride.[36] However, the significance of this observation was unclear.

Findings from epidemiologic studies indicate a correlation between high intake of antioxidants, such as selenium and vitamin E, and lower risk of prostate cancer. The results of a small, randomized skin cancer prevention trial of selenium compared with placebo showed a significant decrease in the number of prostate cancers in men treated with selenium compared with men receiving placebo.[54] Eight years into the ATBC Prevention Trial, which enrolled 29,000 men, there were 99 cases of prostate cancer reported among men receiving vitamin E and 151 cases reported among men taking placebo. The cancers diagnosed were almost all detected as a result of the work-up of symptoms because there is no prostate cancer screening in Finland.[55]

The prostate cancer findings in both of these trials were incidental results of a secondary analysis. A prospective, randomized, placebo-controlled trial — the Selenium and Vitamin E Cancer Prevention Trial (SELECT) — is ongoing to properly assess these drugs in 32,400 subjects.

> **KEY POINTS**
>
> - Avoidance of carcinogens is the most efficient way to prevent cancer. Smoking is the cause of nearly one-third of all cancers in the United States. Other environmental influences, such as sun overexposure, certain chemicals, and certain infectious agents are associated with cancer causation.
> - Drugs and vitamins to be used for prevention must undergo the same rigorous assessment of efficacy and toxicity as do therapeutic agents prior to recommendation. Indeed, because they are generally administered to a healthy population, their toxicity profiles must be safer than those of average drugs.

Gynecologic Cancer

Laser ablation, conization, or hysterectomy is used to treat cervical dysplasia or intraepithelial neoplasia, both of which are precursors to cervical cancer. Vaccines for HPV have been approved and will undoubtedly lower the incidence of cervical cancer.[33] Recent studies have shown a strong protective effect against ovarian cancer for oral contraceptive hormone preparations.[56] However, there is no current recommendation for their use on a routine basis for prevention. For women at very high risk of ovarian cancer because of a *BRCA* genetic mutation, bilateral salpingo-oophorectomy remains the treatment of choice (including fallopian tube removal).[57]

CANCER SCREENING

Cancer screening is an attempt to detect cancer or its precursors early in asymptomatic individuals, with the goal of intervening and decreasing morbidity and mortality. A screening test is not typically diagnostic for cancer; rather, it determines whether cancer might be present and if additional testing, including a biopsy and staging, is necessary. To be of true benefit, screening must lead to earlier treatment that offers a better outcome compared with treatment that would occur at the onset of symptoms. Because of various biases (discussed further in the chapter), the ideal evaluation of a screening technology is through the assessment of disease-specific and overall mortality in a randomized clinical trial.

Early detection of an apparently localized cancer does not automatically confer benefit. There are screening tests for some diseases that have been found to be of no benefit, such as chest x-ray screening for lung cancer, which was used in the 1960s,[58,59] or urine screening for vanillylmandelic acid to detect neuroblastoma.[60] Alpha-fetoprotein testing to screen for hepatocellular carcinoma also has not proven to be valuable in reducing mortality. A number of common screening tests used in the United States offer undetermined benefit.

POTENTIAL BIASES

Screening is subject to several biases, including lead-time, length, and selection biases, the influences of which are lessened in a randomized trial.[61] These biases can lead one to believe that there is a benefit to a screening test when, in truth, there is none; there can even be a net harm. Screening, regardless of benefit, will increase the number of specific cancers diagnosed. It also can produce a shift in stage that will improve survival statistics without reducing mortality (i.e., the number of deaths of a given cancer per number of people at risk of the disease). In such a case, apparent duration of survival, measured from the date of diagnosis, would increase without lives being saved or life expectancy being changed.

When pure lead-time bias occurs, survival — the time from diagnosis to death — is increased, but treatment does not prolong life. Patients do not live longer, they are merely diagnosed at an earlier date. The screening test only prolongs the time the individual is aware of the disease and the time the individual is treated as a patient.

Length bias occurs when slow-growing, less aggressive cancers are detected during screening. Cancers diagnosed as the result of the onset of symptoms between scheduled screenings are, on average, more aggressive, and treatment outcomes are not as favorable. An extreme form of length bias is termed overdiagnosis, or detection of pseudodisease. Some undetected slow-growing tumors fulfill the histologic criteria for cancer but will never be clinically significant or cause death. This phenomenon is compounded by the fact that the most common cancers are most frequent among older people. Other competing causes of death, such as heart disease, become more relevant. This is particularly common in prostate cancer.

Selection bias must be considered when assessing the results of any clinical trial. The group most likely to seek entry in the study may differ from the general population to which the study result might be applied. In a screening trial, individuals may have volunteered because of a particular risk factor not found in the larger population, such as a strong family history. In general, volunteers are more health conscious and are likely to have better prognoses or lower mortality rates regardless of actually being screened; this trend is referred to as the "healthy volunteer effect."

ASSESSMENT OF SCREENING TESTS

As a result of the biases above, a screening intervention is best evaluated in a population-based, randomized, controlled screening trial with cause-specific mortality as the endpoint.[61] Because the gold-standard randomized screening trials are large (often involving thousands of people) and last for years, less definitive study designs often are used to estimate the efficacy and effectiveness of screening practices. In order of strength of evidence, efficacy can by assessed using the following:

- findings of internally controlled trials in which intervention-allocation methods other than randomization are used, such as allocation determined by birth date or by date of clinic visit;
- results of cohort or case-control analytic observational studies;
- findings of multiple time series studies, with or without the intervention; and
- opinions of respected authorities based on clinical experience, descriptive studies, or consensus reports of experts.

The latter form of evidence is the weakest, because even experts can easily be misled by the biases described.

POTENTIAL HARMFUL EFFECTS

Subjects can be harmed as a result of screening. A harmful effect can be associated with the test itself, the work up of positive results of screening tests (both true-positive and false-positive results), and injuries from the treatment of true-positive results. Screening can detect some cancers that would never have caused medical problems. The unnecessary treatment of these cancers can be harmful.

ACCURACY

The accuracy of any medical test is described using four indices: sensitivity, specificity, positive predictive value, and negative predictive value. The results of screening tests can be classified into four categories (Tables 1-3 and 1-4). Sensitivity and specificity are relatively independent of the underlying prevalence or risk of the population being screened, but the positive and negative predictive values are highly dependent on prevalence (Table 1-5). In other words, screening is most beneficial, efficient, and economical when targeting a cancer common to the general population or groups with a high prevalence (or high risk) of the specific disease being screened. Sensitivity need not be extremely high (Table 1-5). However, it is worth reiterating that the key criterion for the public health recommendation of a screening test is that it is able to reduce cancer mortality.[62]

TABLE 1-3. Indices for Describing the Accuracy of Screening Tests

Term	Definition	Ability of Test	Equation
Sensitivity	Proportion of people with the disease who have a positive result on a screening test	To detect disease when it is present	A / (A + C)
Specificity	Proportion of people who do not have the disease who have a negative result on a screening test	To correctly identify the absence of disease	D / (B + D)
Positive predictive value	Proportion of people with a positive result on a predictive value screening test who actually have the disease	To accurately predict the presence of disease	A / (A + B)
Negative predictive value	Proportion of people who have a negative result on a screening test who truly do not have the disease	To accurately predict the absence of disease	D / (C + D)

Abbreviations: A, true-positive result; B, false-positive result; C, false-negative result; D, true-negative result.

SCREENING FOR SPECIFIC CANCERS

Results from good studies are convincing that screening for cervical, colon, and breast cancers is beneficial at certain ages for people at normal risk. Although special surveillance of individuals at high risk for some specific cancers because of family history or genetic risk may be prudent, few studies have been carried out to assess its true worth.

A number of organizations have evaluated certain screening tests and considered whether to endorse routine use of such measures. The U.S. Preventive Services Task Force[63] and the Canadian Task Force on Preventive Health Care[64] published screening recommendations after a rigorous review process. Each recommendation is made with a thorough, structured evaluation of the literature by screening experts. The American Cancer Society publishes the most commonly quoted screening guidelines (Table 1-6).[65]

Breast Cancer

Studies of breast self-examination have not shown that this practice decreases mortality.[66] The results of the largest randomized, controlled study of breast self-examination reported to date showed both an increased rate of biopsy and enhanced detection of benign lesions but little or no stage shift and no reduction in breast cancer mortality.[67]

TABLE 1-4 Types of Results on Screening Tests

Term	Test Result	Disease Present
True positive (A)	Positive	Yes
False positive (B)	Positive	No
False negative (C)	Negative	Yes
True negative (D)	Negative	No

Findings from several randomized trials indicate that screening women with normal risk who are older than 50 using mammography alone or mammography and clinical breast examination every 1 to 2 years decreases mortality by 20% to 30%. Each trial has been criticized for a certain aspect of its design but there is power in the consistency of the observations.[68]

Experts disagree on whether women of average risk between the ages of 40 and 49 benefit from screening (Table 1-6). A meta-analysis of eight large randomized trials showed no benefit from mammography screening for women in this age group when assessed 5 to 7 years after trial entry.[69] There was a small benefit for women 10 to 12 years after entry, which may have been the result of screening these women after they turned 50. In randomized screening studies of women ages 50 to 69, the decline in benefits begins approximately 5 years after the initiation of screening. Nonetheless, current U.S. guidelines recommend initiating screening at age 40. There is no consensus on the age at which to cease screening.

The results from outcomes studies show that there is substantial variation among U.S. radiologists regarding recommendations for additional testing or biopsy. This disparity is especially notable among younger women. In large cohorts, nearly half of all women between the ages of 40 and 49 screened annually for 10 years will have false-positive mammograms necessitating repeat mammography, ultrasound examination, or biopsy. In addition, the diagnosis of ductal carcinoma in situ has risen dramatically since the widespread introduction of mammographic screening for women younger than 50.

TABLE 1-5 Influence of Prevalence on Predictive Value

Positive Predictive Value for a Disease with Prevalence of Five Affected Individuals per 1,000 Population			Positive Predictive Value for a Disease with Prevalence of One Affected Individual per 10,000 Population		
	Sensitivity			Sensitivity	
	0.8	0.95		0.8	0.95
Specificity			Specificity		
0.95	7%	9%	0.95	0.2%	0.2%
0.999	80%	83%	0.999	7%	9%

The positive predictive value is expressed as a percentage. It is influenced by the sensitivity and specificity of the screening test and by the prevalence of the disease for which the individual is being screened. The positive predictive value is particularly influenced by the specificity of the screening test at a given prevalence for relatively uncommon diseases, such as cancer.

Mammography may not be as sensitive for detecting breast cancers among women with *BRCA1* or *BRCA2* mutations. This weakness may be because such women tend to have cancers at a younger age, when mammography is less sensitive. Recent studies have suggested that magnetic resonance imaging (MRI) has greater sensitivity than mammography or ultrasound. Its high cost and unproven survival benefit make it undesirable for general use, but it can increase yield in a cost-effective fashion for women at high risk, especially young *BRCA* mutation carriers.[70,71]

Cervical Cancer

No randomized clinical trial has been done to determine whether cervical cancer screening with a Pap test reduces mortality, but findings from several cohort and case-control studies have shown the utility of this test. Regular Pap testing is recommended for women who are sexually active or who are older than 18. The recommended interval for Pap testing ranges from 1 to 3 years. An upper age limit at which screening ceases to be effective is not known. In the United States, Pap testing has resulted in a decrease in cervical cancer incidence because screening usually finds and eliminates the precursor lesion, cervical intraepithelial neoplasia.

In 2002, the American Cancer Society revised its screening guidelines to recommend that screening start approximately 3 years after a woman begins having vaginal intercourse, but no later than age 21.[72] The American Cancer Society recommends that cervical screening be performed annually in the case of regular Pap tests or every 2 years in the case of liquid-based cytologic tests. Women who have had normal results on three consecutive tests may be screened every 2 to 3 years. Women with certain risk factors, such as infection with the human immunodeficiency virus (HIV) or a weakened immune system, might be screened more frequently. Women age 70 and older who have had normal results on three or more Pap tests and no abnormal results within the past 10 years may choose to stop cervical cancer screening.

The association of cervical cancer with HPV has led to use of HPV screening as a means of screening for cervical neoplasia. This has been recommended for use in resource-poor environments where Pap tests are difficult to conduct properly. In addition, HPV screening also can be used to elucidate diagnosis based on Pap tests that give equivocal outcomes.[73]

Colorectal Cancer

Several methods are recommended for colorectal cancer screening.

- Fecal occult-blood testing
- Rigid and flexible sigmoidoscopy
- Colonoscopy
- Radiographic barium contrast studies

The results of randomized studies indicate that annual fecal occult-blood testing can reduce colorectal cancer mortality by one-third.[74] The rate of false-positive results for fecal occult-blood testing is 1% to 5%. Less than 10% of individuals with occult blood found in stool analysis have cancer, and approximately one-fifth to one-third have adenomas.

Findings from two case-control studies found that screening sigmoidoscopy is associated with a decrease in mortality among participants age 50 and older.[75] The results from other studies show that approximately one-half of all polyps are found with the 35-cm flexible scope and two-thirds to three-quarters are found with a 60-cm scope. Diagnosis of polyps by sigmoidoscopy should lead to evaluation of the entire colon with colonoscopy. Two randomized trials of sigmoidoscopy are in progress.

Although no study results have clearly demonstrated benefit, it is prudent to use colonoscopy as a screening tool for individuals at average risk for colorectal cancer. This rationale is an extension of the available data for sigmoidoscopy.[76] Colonoscopy should be used for those at high risk, such as those with a genetic predisposition to colorectal

TABLE 1-6 Screening Recommendations for Asymptomatic Subjects with Normal Risk*

Test or Procedure	U.S. Preventive Services Task Force	Canadian Task Force on Preventive Health Care	American Cancer Society
Fecal occult-blood testing (FOBT)	Annual home FOBT for individual age 50 or older	FOBT every 1 to 2 years for patients age 50 or older	Annually, FOBT or fecal immunochemical test (FIT) starting at age 50
Sigmoidoscopy	Every 5 years for individuals age 50 or older	Every 10 years for patients age 50 or older	Every 5 years, starting at age 50
FOBT and flexible sigmoidoscopy	Annual home FOBT and flexible sigmoidoscopy every 5 years for individual age 50 or older	Insufficient evidence	Annual FOBT and flexible sigmoidoscopy every 5 years, starting at age 50
Double contrast barium enema (DCBE)	Every 5 years for individuals age 50 or older	No recommendation	Every 5 years, starting at age 50
Colonoscopy	Every 10 years for individuals age 50 or older	Insufficient evidence	Every 10 years, starting at age 50
Digital rectal examination (DRE)	No recommendation	Poor evidence to include or exclude for men older than age 50	No recommendation
Prostate-specific antigen (PSA) and DRE	Insufficient evidence to recommend	Insufficient evidence to include PSA in periodic health exam (PHE). Poor evidence to include or exclude DRE from PHE.	Shared decision between physician and patient. Annually, starting at age 50 men with a life expectancy of at least 10 more years
Pap test	Begin 3 years after the onset of sexual activity or age 21, whichever first. Insufficient evidence to recommend the use of new technologies to screen. Routine screening is not recommended for women older than 65 who have had adequate screening with normal Pap tests and who are not at high risk for cervical cancer. No screening is recommended for women who have had a total hysterectomy for benign disease.	Annual screening to begin following initiation of sexual activity or at age 18. After two normal smears, screen every 3 years to age 69.	Begin 3 years after a woman begins vaginal intercourse, but no later than age 21. Screen annually with conventional Pap tests and every 2 years with liquid-based Pap tests. At or after age 30, women with three normal tests in a row may screen every 2 to 3 years with cervical cytology alone, or every 3 years with HPV DNA test plus cervical cytology. Women ages 70 and older who have had three or more normal Pap tests and no abnormal tests in the last 10 years and women who have had a total hysterectomy may choose to stop cervical cancer screening.
HPV DNA Test	Insufficient evidence to recommend	No recommendation	No recommendation

*Continued on next page

TABLE 1-6 Continued

Test or Procedure	U.S. Preventive Services Task Force	Canadian Task Force on Preventive Health Care	American Cancer Society
Breast self-examination (BSE)	No recommendation	Insufficient evidence to make recommendation	Beginning in their early 20s, women should be advised about the limitations and benefits of BSE. Women may choose not to do BSE or to do BSE irregularly.
Breast clinical examination (CBE)	Recommended with mammogram	Recommended with mammogram	Every 3 years for women in their 20s and 30s; Annually for women ages 40 and older
Mammography	Every 1 to 2 years for women ages 40 and older with or without CBE	Mammogram and CBE every year for women ages 50 to 69	Annually, starting at age 40. CBE should be performed prior to mammography.
Cancer-related check-up	No recommendation	No recommendation	On the occasion of a periodic health exam, cancer-related check-up should include exam for cancers of the thyroid, testicles, ovaries, lymph nodes, oral cavity, and skin. Counseling about tobacco, sun exposure diet and nutrition, risk factors, sexual practices, and environmental and occupational exposures should occur at the time of the health exam.

Abbreviations: HPV, human papillomavirus.

*These recommendations were made for the general population — asymptomatic people who have no risk factors, other than age or gender, for the targeted condition.

cancer and those with inflammatory bowel disease. Little information is available on the utility of the barium enema as a screening tool. The barium enema is insensitive for flat lesions and small polyps.[77, 78]

Recent interest has centered on virtual colonography as well. The evidence suggests that, in certain instances, it may substitute for colonoscopy, but the evidence remains too sparse for a clear-cut recommendation.

Lung Cancer

Screening for lung cancer with chest x-ray and sputum cytologic testing was evaluated in four randomized lung cancer screening trials in the 1960s and 1970s. No reduction in lung cancer mortality was seen in these studies.[79] A randomized trial of chest x-ray screening is currently underway as well to reassess its value.

Studies have shown that spiral computerized tomography (CT) can diagnose lung cancers at early stages, but it is unclear whether it will save lives. This technology is being evaluated in a large, randomized clinical trial. Spiral CT also can detect many benign processes that cause noncalcified lung radio densities; these are false-positive findings. Although it is not known whether spiral CT saves lives, it increases the number of lesions diagnosed and, thus, will increase the number of diagnostic and therapeutic procedures performed (*See Fig. 6-1 in Lung Cancer Chapter*).[80, 81]

Ovarian Cancer

Adnexal palpation, transvaginal ultrasound, and measurement of serum CA-125 have been considered for ovarian cancer screening. No randomized prospective trial of screening for ovarian cancer has shown an improvement in ovarian cancer mortality. The results of such studies could lead to futile invasive diagnostic testing that might include laparotomy. Two randomized clinical trials are in progress to evaluate screening with CA-125 and transvaginal ultrasound. There is no general consensus on screening for ovarian cancer in women with average risk.

Prostate Cancer

The digital rectal examination and measurement of serum prostate-specific antigen are commonly used in the United States, despite the fact that most professional organizations advise caution in the use of such screening tools. (Table 1-6). No well-designed, conducted, and analyzed study has been completed to test the true benefits of screening and treatment of prostate cancer, but trials are in progress.[82] Prostate cancer is prone to lead-time bias, length bias, and overdiagnosis. Whereas screening using prostate-specific antigen levels and digital rectal examination clearly detects many asymptomatic cancers, its ability to reliably distinguish tumors that could be lethal but are still curable from those that pose little or no threat to health is limited. It has been estimated that more than 30% of localized prostate cancers diagnosed during screening are indolent and clinically insignificant. Treatment of screen-detected cancers may cause morbidity, such as impotence and urinary incontinence, and it carries a small risk of death.[83]

Most expert organizations do not recommend screening for prostate cancer. In late 2002, the U.S. Preventive Services Task Force examined the evidence in support of screening and found there was insufficient evidence to recommend it. The American Cancer Society and the American Urological Association recommend that men older than 50 with normal risk be offered screening and be allowed to make a choice after being informed of its potential risks and benefits (Table 1-6).

Skin Cancer

No randomized study has been conducted to assess whether screening for skin cancer decreases mortality. Screening programs in Scotland and Australia may have caused the stage shift in diagnosed melanomas.[84] These programs also may reinforce sun avoidance and other prevention behaviors.

KEY POINTS

- Evaluation of the benefits/efficacy of a cancer screening test is far more complicated than simply the performance of the test and the location of a localized cancer.
- The biases of screening are volunteer selection, lead-time, length time, and overdiagnosis. These biases can make a screening test appear beneficial when there is actually no benefit, or even harm.
- To offset these biases, a randomized trial is the best way to assess a screening test with the endpoint of reduction in cancer-related mortality.

BARRETT'S ESOPHAGUS

The dramatic rise in the incidence of esophageal adenocarcinoma during the past 2 decades has raised concerns regarding prevention. These tumors are known to arise from Barrett's esophagus, a metaplastic change in the esophageal mucosa that later progresses to dysplasia and malignancy. The main risk factor for Barrett's esophagus is gastroesophageal reflux disease, a condition that apparently has increased dramatically, perhaps partially because of the epidemic of obesity. Thus, there has been a major effort to conduct esophagogastroduodenoscopy on patients with persistent gastroesophageal reflux disease to detect early-stage Barrett's esophagus and to intervene in this pathway with the use of proton pump inhibitors and close surveillance with endoscopy. This has become a recommendation of the American Gastroenterological Association despite the absence of any randomized trial or other high-quality evidence demonstrating a significant benefit from the point of view of cancer prevention or survival benefit.[85]

REFERENCES

1. SEER Cancer Statistics Review, 1975–2000. Bethesda, MD: National Cancer Institute. http://seer.cancer.gov/csr/1975–2000. Accessed September 27, 2007.
2. Jemal A, Siegel R, Ward E, et al. Cancer statistics, 2006. *CA Cancer J Clin.* 2006;56(2):106–130.
3. Lux MP, Fasching PA, Beckmann MW. Hereditary breast and ovarian cancer: review and future perspectives. *J Mol Med.* 2006;84(1):16–28.
4. Brawley OW. Population categorization and cancer statistics. *Cancer Metastasis Rev.* 2003;22(1):11–19.
5. Kulldorff M, Feuer EJ, Miller BA, et al. Breast cancer clusters in the northeast United States: a geographic analysis. *Am J Epidemiol.* 1997;146(2):161–170.
6. Link BG, Northridge ME, Phelan JC, et al. Social epidemiology and the fundamental cause concept: on the structuring of effective cancer screens by socioeconomics status. *Milbank Q.* 1998;76(3):375–402, 304–305.
7. Ayanian, JZ, Kohler BA, Epstein AM. The relation between health insurance coverage and clinical outcomes among women with breast cancer. *N Engl J Med.* 1993;329(5):326–331.
8. Hodgson DC, Fuchs CS, Ayanian JZ. Impact of patient and provider characteristics on the treatment and outcomes of colorectal cancer. *J Natl Cancer Inst.* 2001;93(7):501–515.
9. Penson DF, Stoddard ML, Pasta DJ, et al. The association between socioeconomic status, health insurance coverage, and quality of life in men with prostate cancer. *J Clin Epidemiol.* 2001;54(4):350–358.
10. Gilligan MA, Kneusel RT, Hoffmann RG, et al. Persistent differences in sociodemographic determinants of breast conserving treatment despite overall increased adoption. *Med Care.* 2002;40(3):181–189.
11. Lu-Yao G, Albertsen PC, Stanford JL, et al. Natural experiment examining impact of aggressive screening and treatment on prostate cancer mortality in two fixed cohorts from Seattle area and Connecticut. *BMJ.* 2002;325 (7367):740.

12. Shavers VL, Brown ML. Racial and ethnic disparities in the receipt of cancer treatment. *J Natl Cancer Inst.* 2002;94(5):334–357.

13. Liang W, Burnett CB, Rowland JH, et al. Communication between physicians and older women with localized breast cancer: implications for treatment and patient satisfaction. *J Clin Oncol.* 2002;20(4):1008–1016.

14. Gornick ME, Eggers PW, Reilly TW, et al. Effects of race and income on mortality and use of services among Medicare beneficiaries. *N Engl J Med.* 1996;335(11):791–799.

15. Greenwald P. Lifestyle and medical approaches to cancer prevention. *Recent Results Cancer Res.* 2005;166:1–15.

16. Thun MJ, Apicella LF, Henley SJ. Smoking vs other risk factors as the cause of smoking-attributable deaths: confounding in the courtroom. *JAMA.* 2000;284(6):706–712.

17. Shields PG. Tobacco smoking, harm reduction, and biomarkers. *J Natl Cancer Inst.* 2002;94(19):1435–1444.

18. Wynder EL, Muscat JE. The changing epidemiology of smoking and lung cancer histology. *Environ Health Perspect.* 1995;103 (Suppl 8):143–148.

19. Carpenter CL, Jarvik ME, Morgenstern H, et al. Mentholated cigarette smoking and lung-cancer risk. *Ann Epidemiol.* 1999;9(2):114–120.

20. Bowen DJ, Orlandi MA, Lichtenstein E, et al. Intervention effects on youth tobacco use in the Community Intervention Trial (COMMIT). *Tob Control.* 2002;11(4):382.

21. Stoner WI, Foley BX. Current tobacco control policy trends in the United States. *Clin Occup Environ Med.* 2006;5(1):85–99, ix.

22. Baker F, Ainsworth SR, Dye JT, et al. Health risks associated with cigar smoking. *JAMA.* 2000;284(6):735–740.

23. Greenwald P, Clifford CK, Milner JA. Diet and cancer prevention. *Eur J Cancer.* 2001;37(8):948–965.

24. Key TJ, Schatzkin A, Willett WC, et al. Diet, nutrition and the prevention of cancer. *Public Health Nutr.* 2004;7(1A):187–200.

25. Schatzkin A, Lanza E. Polyps and vegetables (and fat, fibre): the polyp prevention trial. *IARC Sci Publ.* 2002;156:463–466.

26. Park Y, Hunter DJ, Spiegelman D, et al. Dietary fiber intake and risk of colorectal cancer: a pooled analysis of prospective cohort studies. *JAMA.* 2005;294(22):2849–2857.

27. Prentice RL, Caan B, Chlebowski RT, et al. Low-fat dietary pattern and risk of invasive breast cancer: the Women's Health Initiative Randomized Controlled Dietary Modification Trial. *JAMA.* 2006;295(6):629–642.

28. Beresford SA, Johnson KC, Ritenbaugh C, et al. Low-fat dietary pattern and risk of colorectal cancer: the Women's Health Initiative Randomized Controlled Dietary Modification Trial. *JAMA.* 2006;295(6):643–654.

29. Bianchini F, Kaaks R, Vainio H. Weight control and physical activity in cancer prevention. *Obes Rev.* 2002;3(1):5–8.

30. Serraino D, Piselli P, Scognamiglio P. Viral infections and cancer: epidemiological aspects. *J Biol Regul Homeost Agents.* 2001;15(3): 224–228.

31. Parkin DM. The global health burden of infection-associated cancers in the year 2002. *Int J Cancer.* 2006;118(12):3030–3044.

32. Chien YC, Jan CF, Kuo HS, et al. Nationwide hepatitis B vaccination program in Taiwan: effectiveness in the 20 years after it was launched. *Epidemiol Rev.* 2006;28:126–135. Epub 2006 Jun 16.

33. Roden R, Wu TC. How will HPV vaccines affect cervical cancer? *Nat Rev Cancer.* 2006;6(10):753–763.

34. Greenwald P. Cancer chemoprevention. *BMJ.* 2002;324(7339):714–718.

35. Fisher B, Costantino JP, Wickerham DL, et al. Tamoxifen for prevention of breast cancer: report of the National Surgical Adjuvant Breast and Bowel Project P-1 Study. *J Natl Cancer Inst.* 1998;90 (18):1371–1388.

36. Thompson IM, Goodman PJ, Tangen CM, et al. The influence of finasteride on the development of prostate cancer. *N Engl J Med.* 2003; 349(3):215–224.

37. Vogel VG, Costantino JP, Wickerham DL, et al. Effects of tamoxifen vs raloxifene on the risk of developing invasive breast cancer and other disease outcomes: the NSABP Study of Tamoxifen and Raloxifene (STAR) P-2 trial. *JAMA.* 2006;295(23):2727–2741.

38. Crew KD, Neugut AI. Epidemiology of upper gastrointestinal malignancies. *Semin Oncol.* 2004;31(4):450–464.

39. Virtamo J, Pietinen P, Huttunen JK, et al. Incidence of cancer and mortality following alpha-tocopherol and beta-carotene supplementation: a postintervention follow-up. *JAMA.* 2003;290(4):476–485.

40. Omenn GS, Goodman GE, Thornquist MD, et al. Risk factors for lung cancer and for intervention effects in CARET, the Beta-Carotene and Retinol Efficacy Trial. *J Natl Cancer Inst.* 1996;88(21): 1550–1559.

41. Hong WK, Lippman SM, Itri LM, et al. Prevention of second primary tumors with isotretinoin in squamous cell carcinoma of the head and neck. *N Engl J Med.* 1990;323(12):795–801.

42. Wong BC, Lam SK, Wong WM, et al. Helicobacter pylori eradication to prevent gastric cancer in a high-risk region of China: a randomized controlled trial. *JAMA.* 2004;291(2):187–194.

43. Steinbach G, Lynch PM, Phillips RK, et al. The effect of celecoxib, a cyclooxygenase-2 inhibitor, in familial adenomatous polyposis. *N Engl J Med.* 2000;342(26):1946–1952.

44. Bertagnolli MM, Eagle CJ, Zauber AG, et al. Celecoxib for the prevention of sporadic colorectal adenomas. *N Engl J Med.* 2006;355 (9):873–884.

45. Chlebowski RT, Wactawski-Wende J, Ritenbaugh C, et al. Estrogen plus progestin and colorectal cancer in postmenopausal women. *N Engl J Med.* 2004;350(10):991–1004.

46. Nelson HD, Humphrey LL, Nygren P, et al. Postmenopausal hormone replacement therapy: scientific review. *JAMA.* 2002;288 (7):872–881.

47. Wactawski-Wende J, Kotchen JM, Anderson GL, et al. Calcium plus vitamin D supplementation and the risk of colorectal cancer. *N Engl J Med.* 2006;354(7):684–696.

48. Grau MV, Baron JA, Sandler RS, et al. Vitamin D, calcium supplementation, and colorectal adenomas: results of a randomized trial. *J Natl Cancer Inst.* 2003;95(23):1765–1771.

49. Lynch HT, Lynch JF. Hereditary cancer: family history, diagnosis, molecular genetics, ecogenetics, and management strategies. *Biochimie.* 2002;84(1):3–17.

50. Lee CL, Hsieh KS, Ko YC. Trends in the incidence of hepatocellular carcinoma in boys and girls in Taiwan after large-scale hepatitis B vaccination. *Cancer Epidemiol Biomarkers Prev.* 2003;12(1):57–59.

51. Stefanick ML, Anderson GL, Margolis KL, et al. Effects of conjugated equine estrogens on breast cancer and mammography screening in postmenopausal women with hysterectomy. *JAMA.* 2006;295(14): 1647–1657.

52. Hartmann LC, Schaid DJ, Woods JE, et al. Efficacy of bilateral prophylactic mastectomy in women with a family history of breast cancer. *N Engl J Med.* 1999;340(2):77–84.

53. Levine DA, Gemignani ML. Prophylactic surgery in hereditary breast/ovarian cancer syndrome. *Oncology* (Williston Park). 2003;17(7): 932–941.

54. Clark LC, Dalkin B, Krongrad A, et al. Decreased incidence of prostate cancer with selenium supplementation: results of a double-blind cancer prevention trial. *Br J Urol.* 1998;81(5):730–734.

55. The effect of vitamin E and beta carotene on the incidence of lung cancer and other cancers in male smokers. The Alpha-Tocopherol, Beta Carotene Cancer Prevention Study Group. *N Engl J Med.* 1994;330 (15):1029–1035.

56. Bernstein L. The risk of breast, endometrial and ovarian cancer in users of hormonal preparations. *Basic Clin Pharmacol Toxicol.* 2006;98: 288–296.

57. Sogaard M, Kjaar SK, Gayther S. Ovarian cancer and genetic susceptibility in relation to the BRCA1 and BRCA2 genes. Occurrence, clinical importance and intervention. *Acta Obstet Gynecol Scand.* 2006; 85:93–105.

58. Marcus PM. Lung cancer screening: an update. *J Clin Oncol.* 2001;19 (18 Suppl):83S–86S.

59. Marcus PM, Bergstralh EJ, Fagerstrom RM, et al. Lung cancer mortality in the Mayo Lung Project: impact of extended follow-up. *J Natl Cancer Inst.* 2000;92(16):1308–1316.

60. Woods WG, Gao RN, Shuster JJ, et al. Screening of infants and mortality due to neuroblastoma. *N Engl J Med.* 2002;346(14):1041–1046.

61. Prorok PC. Epidemiologic approach for cancer screening. Problems in design and analysis of trials. *Am J Pediatr Hematol Oncol.* 1992;14(2):117–128.

62. Kramer BS, Brawley OW. Cancer screening. *Hematol Oncol Clin North Am.* 2000;14(4):831–848.

63. U.S. Preventive Services Task Force. Agency for Healthcare Research and Quality Web site. http://www.ahrq.gov/clinic/uspstfix.htm. Updated 2006. Accessed July 11, 2007.

64. Canadian Task Force on Preventive Health Care. CTFPHC Systematic Reviews and Recommendations Web site. http://www.ctfphc.org/. Updated August 17, 2005. Accessed July 11, 2007.

65. Smith RA, Cokkinides V, Eyre HJ. American Cancer Society guidelines for the early detection of cancer, 2006. *CA Cancer J Clin.* 2006;56(1):11–25.

66. Barry H. Breast self-examination does not reduce mortality. *Am Fam Physician.* 2003;67(8):1784.

67. Thomas DB, Gao DL, Ray RM, et al. Randomized trial of breast self-examination in Shanghai: final results. *J Natl Cancer Inst.* 2002;94 (19):1445–1457.

68. Green BB, Taplin SH. Breast cancer screening controversies. *J Am Board Fam Pract.* 2003;16(3):233–241.

69. Fletcher SW, Black W, Harris R, et al. Report of the International Workshop on Screening for Breast Cancer. *J Natl Cancer Inst.* 1993;85 (20):1644–1656.

70. Le-Petross HT. Breast MRI as a screening tool: the appropriate role. *J Natl Comp Cancer Netw.* 2006;4(5):523–526.

71. Plevritis SK, Kurian AW, Sigal BM, et al. Cost-effectiveness of screening BRCA1/2 mutation carries with breast magnetic resonance imaging. *JAMA.* 2006;295(20):2374–2384.

72. Saslow D, Runowicz CD, Solomon D, et al. American Cancer Society guideline for the early detection of cervical neoplasia and cancer. *CA Cancer J Clin.* 2002;52(6):342–362.

73. Wright TC, Jr., Schiffman M, Solomon D, et al. Interim guidance for the use of human papillomavirus DNA testing as an adjunct to cervical cytology for screening. *Obstet Gynecol.* 2004;103(2):304–309.

74. Mandel JS, Church TR, Bond JH, et al. The effect of fecal occult-blood screening on the incidence of colorectal cancer. *N Engl J Med.* 2000;343 (22):1603–1607.

75. Ault MJ, Mandel SA. Screening for colorectal cancer. *N Engl J Med.* 2000;343(22):1652; author reply 1652–1654.

76. Neugut AI, Forde KA. Screening colonoscopy—Has the time come? *Am J Gastroenterol.* 1988;83:295–297.

77. McLeod RS. Screening strategies for colorectal cancer: a systematic review of the evidence. *Can J Gastroenterol.* 2001;15(10):647–660.

78. Pignone M, Rich M, Teutsch SM, et al. Screening for colorectal cancer in adults at average risk: a summary of the evidence for the U.S. Preventive Services Task Force. *Ann Intern Med.* 2002;137(2):132–141.

79. Marcus PM, Bergstralh EJ, Zweig MH, et al. Extended lung cancer incidence follow-up in the Mayo Lung Project and overdiagnosis. *J Natl Cancer Inst.* 2006;98(11):748–756.

80. Manser RL, Irving LB, Byrnes G, et al. Screening for lung cancer: a systematic review and meta-analysis of controlled trials. *Thorax.* 2003;58 (9):784–789.

81. Henschke CI, Yankelevitz DF, Libby DM, et al. Survival of patients with stage I lung cancer detected on CT screening. *N Engl J Med.* 2006;355 (17):1763–1771.

82. Andriole GL, Reding D, Hayes RB, et al. The prostate, lung, colon, and ovarian (PLCO) cancer screening trial: Status and promise. *Urol Oncol.* 2004;22(4):358–361.

83. Harris R, Lohr KN. Screening for prostate cancer: an update of the evidence for the U.S. Preventive Services Task Force. *Ann Intern Med.* 2002;137(11):917–929.

84. MacKie RM, Hole D, Hunter JA, et al. Cutaneous malignant melanoma in Scotland: incidence, survival, and mortality, 1979–94. The Scottish Melanoma Group. *BMJ.* 1997;315(7116):1117–1121.

85. Wani S, Sharma P. The rationale for screening and surveillance of Barrett's metaplasia. *Best Pract Res Clin Gastroenterol.* 2006;20(5): 829–842. Review.

2

MOLECULAR BIOLOGY

Bruce E. Clurman, MD, PhD

LEARNING OBJECTIVES

After reviewing this chapter, the reader should be able to

- Describe basic principles of molecular biology
- Discuss methods of analyzing cancer genes in tumors
- Describe the functions of dominant oncogenes and their roles in tumorigenesis
- Describe the roles and functions of tumor suppressor genes in oncogenesis
- Discuss the major cellular pathways that are mutated in cancers and the multistep nature of cancer
- Define cellular checkpoints and their role in carcinogenesis

Deoxyribonucleic acid (DNA) is a macromolecule composed of four nucleotides — two purines, adenine (A) and guanine (G), and two pyrimidines, cytosine (C) and thymine (T) (Fig. 2-1). Each nucleotide base is connected to a deoxyribose sugar, and a phosphodiester bond between the 5′carbon of one sugar and the 3′carbon of the next sugar forms the DNA strand. The nucleoside components extend along one side of the chain and form hydrogen bonds with complementary bases on another strand to create a double-stranded DNA molecule, which usually assumes the shape of a double helix. The base pairing between strands matches a purine and a pyrimidine; cytosine and guanine pair through three hydrogen bonds and adenine and thymidine pair with two hydrogen bonds. When DNA is replicated, the strands separate and each one provides a template for an exact complement to be synthesized.

The nucleotide base pairs that constitute genes are arranged in triplets, termed codons, that specify which amino acids will be incorporated into proteins. The first step in protein synthesis is transcription of the DNA template into a messenger ribonucleic acid (mRNA)

The American Society of Clinical Oncology and Dr. Clurman would like to gratefully acknowledge Edward P. Gelmann, MD, for his contributions to the original content of this chapter.

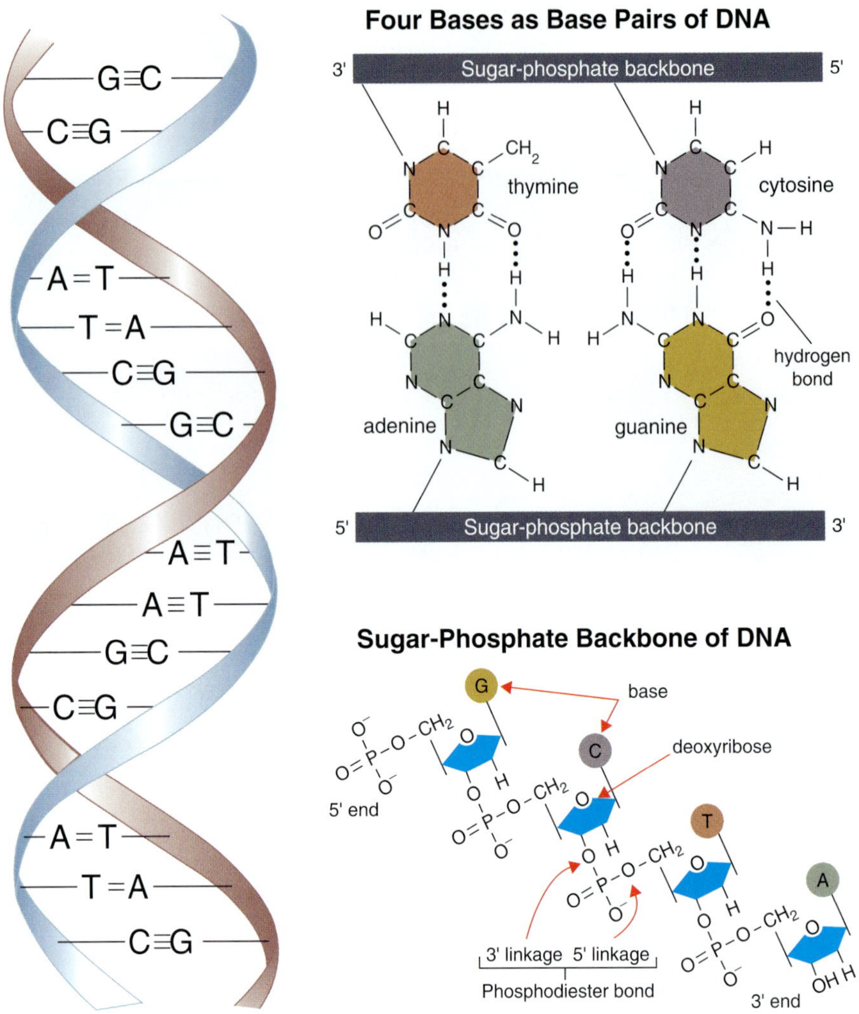

FIG. 2-1 The double helix structure of DNA includes hydrogen bonding between adenine (A) and thymine (T) bases and between guanine (G) and cytosine (C) bases.

Right top: Close-up of hydrogen bonds between the two pairs of bases. Right bottom: A single strand of DNA showing the molecular structure of the backbone made of phosphodiester bonds between sugar molecules.

copy. RNA has a fundamentally similar strand structure to DNA, except that it is composed of a single strand using ribose instead of deoxyribose, and the nucleoside uracil replaces thymine. During transcription, exact RNA copies of the DNA templates are synthesized.

The term "gene," from a molecular viewpoint, refers to a DNA sequence that encodes a functional protein or RNA. Most genes are discontinuous and arranged in segments called exons and introns. A linear RNA copy is transcribed from the DNA, and the introns are subsequently spliced out to generate an mRNA that contains a continuous coding sequence comprised of the exons (Fig. 2-2). The mRNA serves as a template for the attachment of ribosomes and the synthesis of proteins. The 5' and 3' extremities of mRNA extend beyond the coding regions and have regulatory functions, such as determining mRNA stability and translational efficiency. In addition to the exons and introns, genes contain control elements that regulate their expression (Fig. 2-2). The promoter resides immediately upstream from the coding sequence and contains nucleotide motifs that determine the site for initiating mRNA transcription. Gene expression also is controlled by regulatory elements called enhancers that may be located large distances from the genes they control. Promoters and enhancers provide elements that bind to proteins, called transcription factors, which establish the timing and tissue-specific characteristics of gene expression. Many transcription factors bind directly to DNA via specific sequence motifs, and they may subsequently recruit additional proteins into the transcription complex. Proteins that mediate the assembly of transcription complexes are termed co-activators, whereas co-repressors compete for binding to transcription factors, and repress transcription.

DNA is packaged into chromatin by tightly winding around proteins called histones, which maintain the DNA in nucleosomal complexes at intervals of approximately 120 nucleotides (Fig. 2-3A). Chromatin is in a highly dynamic state. Chromatin modifications and remodeling profoundly influence gene expression, which is known as epigenetic gene regulation.[3] Nucleosomes undergo covalent modifications (e.g. histone acetylation, phosphorylation, and methylation), changes in subunit composition (e.g. replacement of core histones by specialized histones), and repositioning (which alters DNA accessibility), and

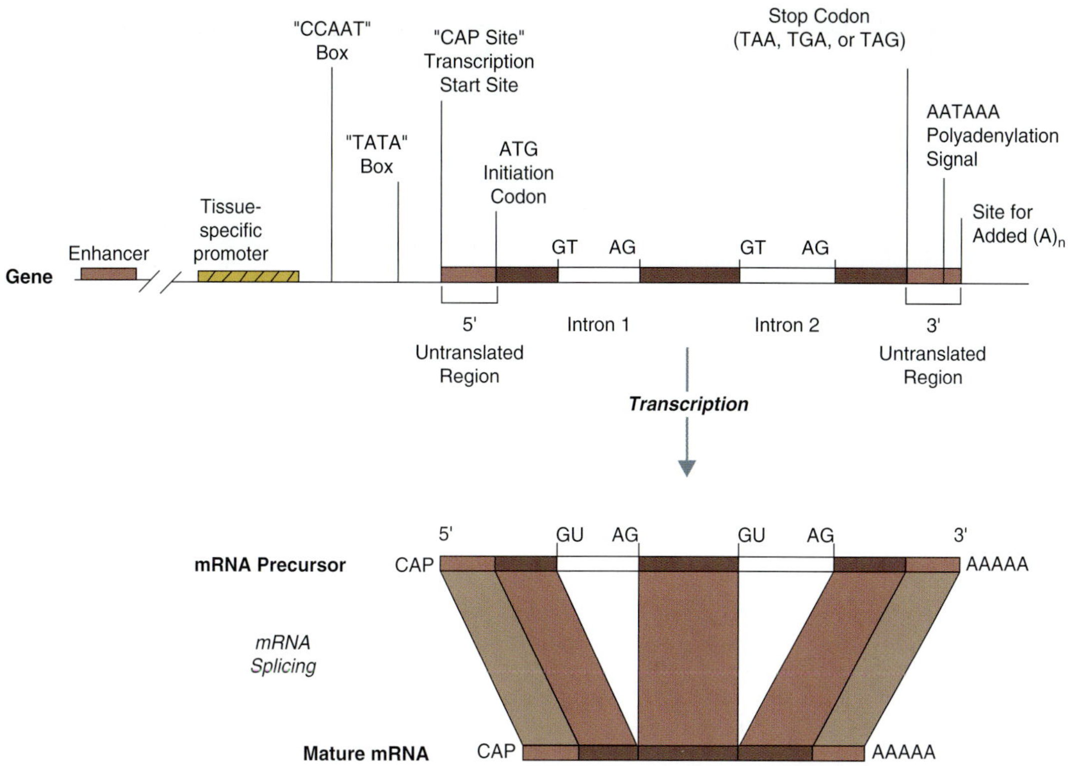

FIG. 2-2 Schematic diagram of an idealized gene, including promoter elements, an enhancer, and the transcribed region of the gene.

The gene has two introns, each beginning with GT and ending with AG; these are spliced out to generate the mature mRNA. Both promoter elements and enhancers can be tissue specific.

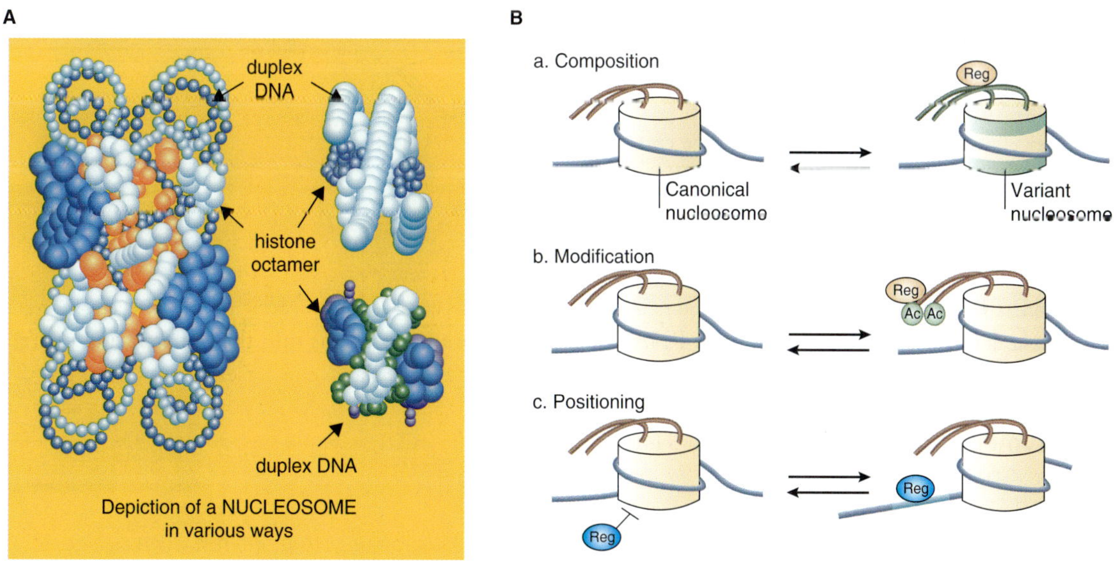

FIG. 2-3 **A.** Nucleosome structure. **B.** Nucleosome regulation.

A. *The view is down the molecular 2-fold axis; DNA is represented by a tube that almost completely occludes the protein.*
B. *a. Remodeling complexes can remove the canonical H2A–H2B dimers and replace them with variant histones (indicated in green), forming a variant nucleosome with unique tails that might bind unique regulatory proteins. b. Nucleosome modification (only acetylation [Ac] is depicted for simplicity) allows the binding of regulatory factors, which have specialized domains that recognize acetylated histone tails. c. Nucleosome repositioning allows the binding of a regulatory factor to its site on nucleosomal DNA (light-blue segment). Remedies are necessary to provide rapid access to nucleosomal DNA by sliding of the octamer along the DNA.*

Reprinted by permission from Macmillan Publishers Ltd: *Nat Rev Mol Cell Biol.* Saha A, Wittmeyer J., Cairns BR. Chromatin remodelling: the industrial revolution of DNA around histones. 2006;7(6):437–447.

these modifications ultimately make DNA more or less accessible to RNA polymerase (Fig. 2-3B).[4,5] Transcription complexes contain a few to more than a dozen proteins, including histone acetylases and deacetylases that promote or repress transcription, respectively. Because of their ability to regulate gene expression, histone deacetylase inhibitors are being intensely studied as potential therapeutic agents,[6] and the histone deacetylase inhibitor vorinostat was approved for use in management of advanced cutaneous T-cell lymphoma. Another epigenetic modification that alters DNA accessibility to RNA polymerase is DNA methylation at CpG dinucleotide pairs, and DNA methylation inhibits transcription. Indeed, promoter methylation is one way that cancer cells downregulate expression of tumor suppressor genes (discussed further). The drug 5-azacytidine, which is approved for treatment of myelodysplastic syndrome, inhibits DNA methylation, and this re-establishes expression of genes that were repressed by methylation.[7]

The human genome contains approximately 3 billion nucleotides that are partitioned among 23 chromosomes. Although the human genome sequence was completed more than 5 years ago, the exact number of human genes remains unclear; most estimates are in the range of 30,000 to 35,000 genes. Most human cells contain a complete genomic copy of DNA, but there are exceptions. For example, erythrocytes (which have lost their nuclei) contain no genomic DNA, and mature lymphocytes delete fragments of DNA that encode either immunoglobulin or T-cell receptor genes in order to generate antigen-recognition proteins. Importantly, individual cell types express only a subset of the total gene complement, and this restricted gene expression underlies cellular differentiation. Thus, the control of gene expression is a critical regulatory event during growth and development, as well as for the maintenance of tissue specificity.

ANALYZING NUCLEIC ACIDS AND DETECTING CANCER-ASSOCIATED MUTATIONS

DNA

Restriction Enzymes and Electrophoretic Analyses of DNA

Restriction endonucleases are bacterial enzymes that cleave DNA at specific short sequences. Many restriction endonucleases that recognize different DNA sequences have been identified, and the locations of these cleavage sites are used to map DNA segments, which facilitate subsequent genetic analyses.[8] When DNA fragments are placed in a gel matrix and subjected to direct electric current, the DNA fragments migrate toward the anode and separate electrophoretically according to size. When DNA separated in this manner is denatured into single strands and transferred to a membrane, the single-stranded DNA can be hybridized with labeled DNA probes that bind to complementary DNA sequences fixed to the membrane (Fig. 2-4). This technique, termed Southern blotting, allows for the identification of specific DNA fragments by virtue of their homology with the probe sequence.

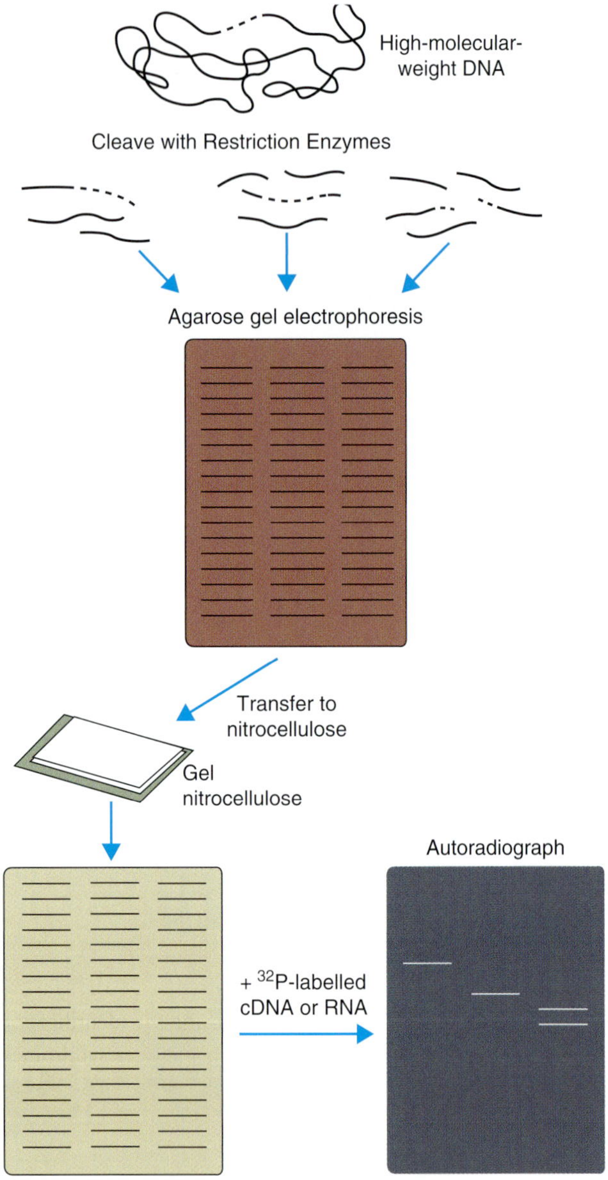

FIG. 2-4 A region of DNA of interest, such as a gene (dashed line), is shown as part of the high-molecular-weight DNA.

In this figure, DNA is cleaved with three different restriction endonucleases, generating fragments of varying length. For each endonuclease, however, the DNA sequence of interest will be contained on one or more characteristic-sized fragments. The radioactive probe will form stable base pairing and expose the x-ray film at only those positions along each lane of cleaved DNA that contain the particular fragment or fragments complementary to the probe.

KEY POINTS

- Molecular methods used to detect cancer-associated DNA mutations include extremely sensitive and versatile polymerase chain reaction (PCR)-based methods, which have revolutionized the molecular analyses of tumor DNA.
- Molecular markers that discriminate between gene alleles facilitate the mapping of genetic traits and the identification of cancer genes.

Polymerase Chain Reaction

The polymerase chain reaction (PCR) is a remarkably powerful technique that synthesizes a large quantity of a specific DNA fragment from minute amounts of template.[9] The technique relies on annealing synthetic DNA primers to DNA sequences that flank the target DNA to be amplified, as well as on DNA polymerase enzymes isolated from thermophillic bacteria that can survive high temperatures. Multiple cycles of DNA-strand synthesis, heat denaturation, and reannealing of primers allow for the repeated synthesis of the target sequence, leading to exponential amplification of the target sequence (Fig. 2-5). A wide variety of PCR-based techniques have revolutionized the methods used to manipulate, detect, and analyze nucleic acids, including methods widely employed in clinical labs to detect mutations and ascertain genotypes.

Microsatellites and Single-nucleotide Polymorphisms

PCR techniques are used to identify chromosomal regions that have a high frequency of polymorphism and can thus distinguish alleles from one another. The generation of dense maps of polymorphic markers throughout the human genome facilitated the mapping of genetic traits, such as cancer predisposition, because large family cohorts could be analyzed for polymorphic markers that segregated with the trait of interest. This general approach allowed for the identification of many genes responsible for hereditary cancer syndromes. One source of genetic polymorphisms is cytosine–adenine (CA) dinucleotide repeats called microsatellites, or short tandem repeat polymorphisms. These regions are susceptible to imperfect duplication by DNA polymerase, leading to a high degree of variability at sites throughout the genome in regions of oligomeric CA repeats. Microsatellite markers are identified by using PCR primers that are complementary to the unique regions flanking the CA repeats, and the PCR reaction will generate products of different sizes if an individual has two alleles with nucleotide-repeat regions of different lengths (Fig. 2-6). Mutations in DNA repair enzymes are found in some cancers, such as hereditary nonpolyposis colon cancer, and these result in altered microsatellite lengths that form the basis for diagnostic tests.

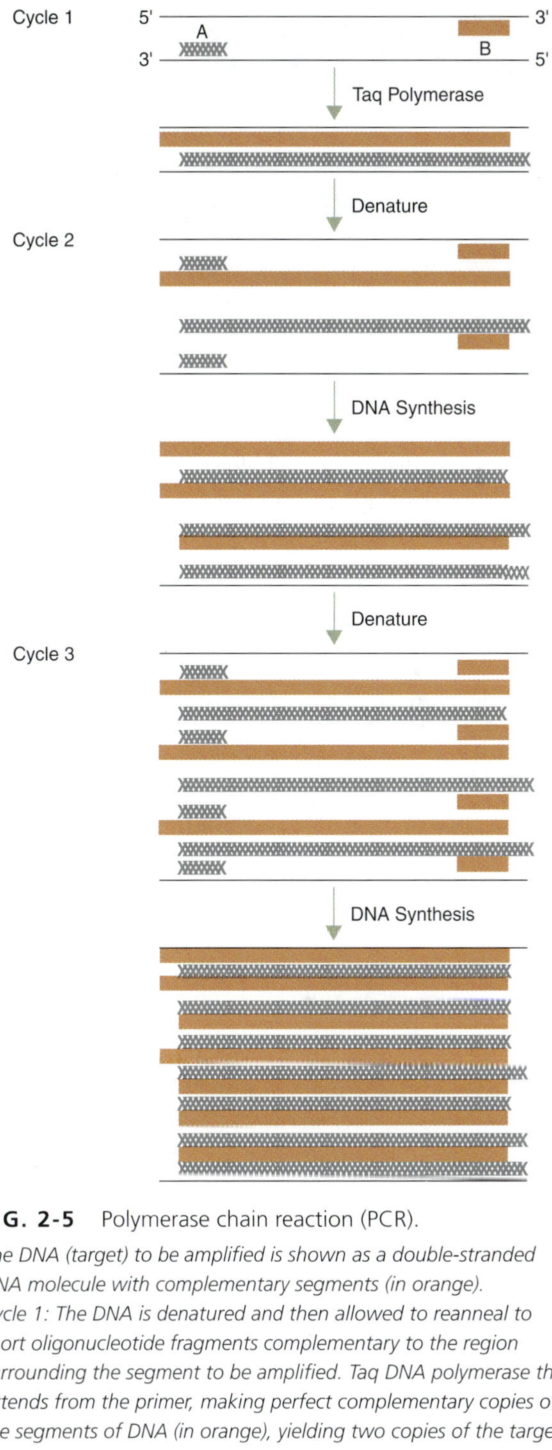

FIG. 2-5 Polymerase chain reaction (PCR).
The DNA (target) to be amplified is shown as a double-stranded DNA molecule with complementary segments (in orange). Cycle 1: The DNA is denatured and then allowed to reanneal to short oligonucleotide fragments complementary to the region surrounding the segment to be amplified. Taq DNA polymerase then extends from the primer, making perfect complementary copies of the segments of DNA (in orange), yielding two copies of the target DNA. Cycle 2: The DNA from cycle 1 is denatured and reannealed, and the steps in cycle 1 are repeated, yielding four copies of target DNA. Cycle 3: The DNA from cycle 2 is denatured, and the steps in cycle 2 are repeated, yielding eight copies of DNA. With n cycles, the amount of DNA increases exponentially as 2n.

A single-nucleotide polymorphism (SNP) in DNA on one chromosome also allows alleles to be distinguished from each other and are vital tools in mapping genetic traits, including hereditary cancer syndromes. Sometimes, an SNP will disrupt a restriction site and cause a variation in the length of the restriction fragments; this feature was initially

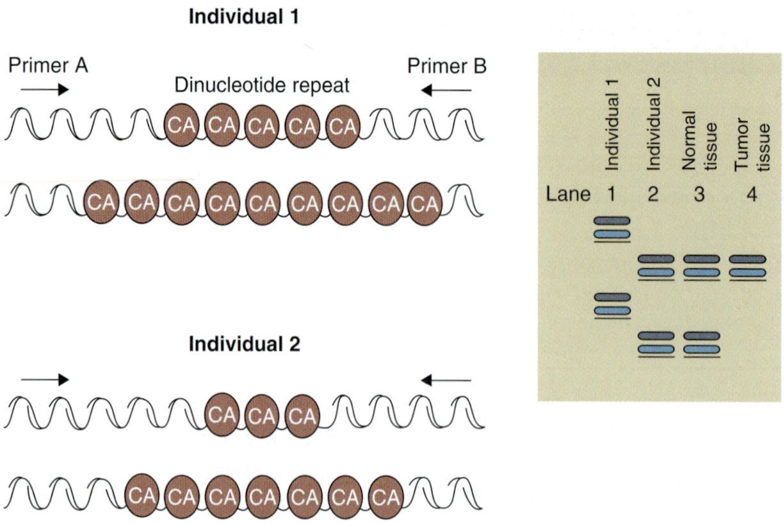

FIG. 2-6 Schematic diagram of a short tandem repeat polymorphism in humans.

The human genome contains thousands of short dinucleotide, trinucleotide, or tetranucleotide repeats dispersed along chromosomes. These repeats vary in length; for each short tandem repeat polymorphism, there are many different-sized alleles in the population, and there is a very high likelihood that any particular individual's alleles will be different. Variations in the number of repeats can be detected by using polymerase chain reaction to amplify a segment of DNA containing the polymorphic sequence, followed by electrophoresis to separate the amplified fragments. Lanes 1 and 2 show the separation of amplified alleles from individuals 1 and 2, respectively. The analysis of short tandem repeat polymorphisms can be used to detect allele loss in tumor tissue. In an individual with a polymorphism, two alleles are detected in normal tissue (individual 2; lane 3), whereas only a single allele is observed in paired tumor tissue (individual 2; lane 4).

used to discriminate between the two alleles by virtue of the restriction fragment length polymorphism (RFLP). However, current methods of SNP detection now use array-based chips that allow high-throughput and genome-wide assessment of large numbers of SNPs simultaneously.

Single-strand Chain Polymorphism. The single-strand chain polymorphism (SSCP) technique is used to detect single-nucleotide differences between otherwise identical DNA fragments. Because the electrophoretic migration of single-stranded DNA is determined by its base composition as well as by molecular weight, short DNA fragments differing at a single nucleotide can be distinguished by electrophoresis of single strands. Denaturing gel electrophoresis thus reveals the altered migration of a sequence that has been PCR-amplified from a mutated oncogene, compared with the wild-type gene. This approach can be used on genomic DNA to detect point mutations in cancer genes. However, because many genes extend over large distances, it is often more efficient to analyze mRNA, which allows for the interrogation of the entire coding sequence of a gene in fewer PCR reactions. This analysis is done by first using reverse transcriptase to convert mRNA to a DNA copy (cDNA), followed by PCR amplification (discussed further).

Sequence-specific Oligonucleotide Hybridization Some cancer genes are activated by a very limited set of mutations in tumors. In these instances, the sequence specificity of nucleic acid hybridization allowed for the development of qualitative assays that depend on the differential annealing of probes to normal or mutant DNA. A good example is the *K-RAS* gene that can be activated by mutation in the DNA encoding of one of only three specific amino acids in the K-RAS protein. Because there are a finite number of nucleotide changes that possibly can code for amino acid alterations at these sites, oligonucleotide probes can be used to identify the presence of these mutations in tumor tissues, biopsy samples, and body fluids.

RNA

Real-time PCR

RNA is very susceptible to degradation by abundant ribonucleases and is more difficult to isolate and analyze than DNA. In the pre-PCR era, RNA analyses largely relied on a technique analogous to Southern blotting, in which RNA is analyzed by blotting to a membrane and subsequent hybridization to probes (termed Northern blotting). However, Northern blotting is not quantitative and is limited by RNA degradation, as well as by the inability to detect low abundance mRNAs, many of which play key roles in cancers (e.g. transcription factors). Most current RNA analysis methods are PCR-based and use reverse transcription, in which the enzyme reverse transcriptase and DNA primers are used to first convert the mRNA to a DNA copy, called cDNA. These cDNAs are then used as templates for PCR reactions that quantitate RNA in tissue samples, or for other types of assays, such as sequencing. This general strategy is termed RT-PCR to reflect both the reverse transcription and PCR steps.

KEY POINTS

- Analyses of mRNA are used to quantitate the expression of specific genes in tumor samples. Microarray analyses can simultaneously examine the abundance of nearly all genes expressed in a cell type, and they provide important diagnostic and prognostic information for some cancers.
- The completed human genome sequence has been pivotal in enabling the development of comprehensive and high-throughput analyses of tumor DNA and RNA.

Because of their extraordinary sensitivity, developing highly quantitative real-time PCR methods was initially challenging. However, these methods are now widely used to precisely measure RNA abundance in cells and tissues. Several different types of real-time PCR assays use fluorescent dyes to measure the amount of PCR products synthesized in real-time. The amount of RNA in a sample is then determined by measuring how many amplification rounds are needed for the fluorescent signal to exceed a standardized threshold. The advantages of real-time PCR include extreme sensitivity, technical ease, and the ability to accurately quantitate DNA and RNA over a range of at least five orders of magnitude. Real-time PCR is the method of choice for analyzing the abundance of specific mRNAs in tumor samples, such as monitoring the expression of the *bcr-abl* transcript in patients undergoing therapy for chronic myeloid leukemia. Because of its capacity to discriminate 2-fold changes in nucleic acid abundance, real-time PCR assays also are used to detect allelic loss in tumors, such as the deletion of a single copy of a tumor suppressor gene.

Microarrays and Global Analyses of Transcription

The previously described methods are typically applied to studies of gene expression involving single or small numbers of genes. However, the completion of the human genome sequence, as well as technologic advances, fostered the development of global mRNA analyses that report on the expression of tens of thousands genes. Microarrays use chips, which are small slides on which either oligonucleotides or cDNAs are robotically spotted in defined arrays.[10] These arrays are interrogated by hybridizing cDNA made from tumor and control cells, each labeled with a different fluorescent dye. A computerized reader assesses the fluorescence intensity, which depends on the relative abundance of the mRNAs in two samples cells (Fig. 2-7). These methods can thus measure the relative abundance of nearly all genes that are expressed in a tissue or tumor sample (termed the transcriptome), and the enormous amount of data they generate requires sophisticated bioinformatics tools. These methods are in wide use

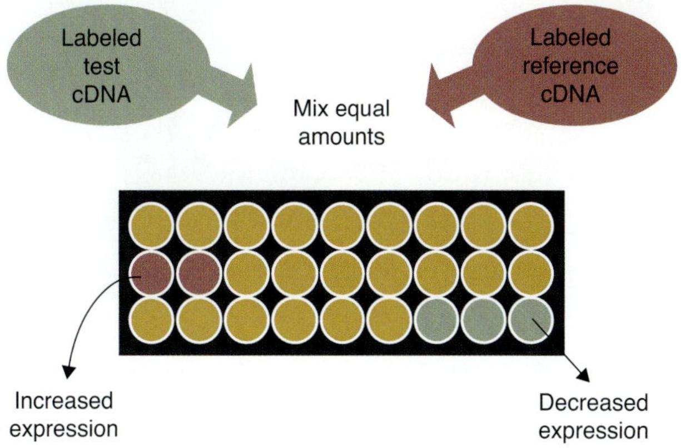

FIG. 2-7 Expression microarray.

Standard RNA and tumor RNA are converted to cDNA and labeled with different fluorescent probes. These are hybridized to arrays of microscopic dots containing DNA or oligonucleotide probes representing different genes. The resulting array of fluorescent signals is read electronically, and the output suggests differential expression of a subset of genes in the two samples.

and are essential tools in basic molecular studies of carcinogenesis. Microarray studies also are being used to define prognostic groups in clinically challenging populations. For example, microarray analyses revealed gene expression signatures that predicted time to metastases in women with node-negative breast cancer.[11] Similarly, transcriptome signatures have been used to separate morphologically indistinguishable large cell lymphomas into good and poor risk groups on the basis of their gene expression patterns (which reflect their cell of origin).[12] Whole transcriptome analyses are expensive and complex, which makes this a difficult technique to bring to the clinic. One area of research involves delineating gene subsets that can be used to accurately report prognostic or diagnostic information on smaller chips that are more easily adapted to clinical labs. For example, the expression profiles of 70 genes derived from the genome-wide profiling of breast cancers described previously are being developed into a powerful tool for predicting metastasis and survival for women with breast cancer (Fig. 2-8).[13]

MicroRNAs and siRNAs

Over the past 10 years, an entirely new class of regulatory genes, termed microRNAs (miRNAs), has been discovered and plays a fundamental role in regulating gene expression.[14] miRNAs are small RNAs (18 to 24 nucleotides) that regulate the expression of other genes by base pairing to their target mRNAs and inhibiting their expression. This is accomplished either by interfering with mRNA translation or by catalyzing mRNA destruction by cellular nuclease complexes (Fig. 2-9). miRNAS are encoded within longer primary transcripts that are cleaved by endonucleases to form the final miRNAs. Most organisms express hundreds of miRNAS — humans have more than 400 miRNA genes — that regulate many key cellular processes involved in

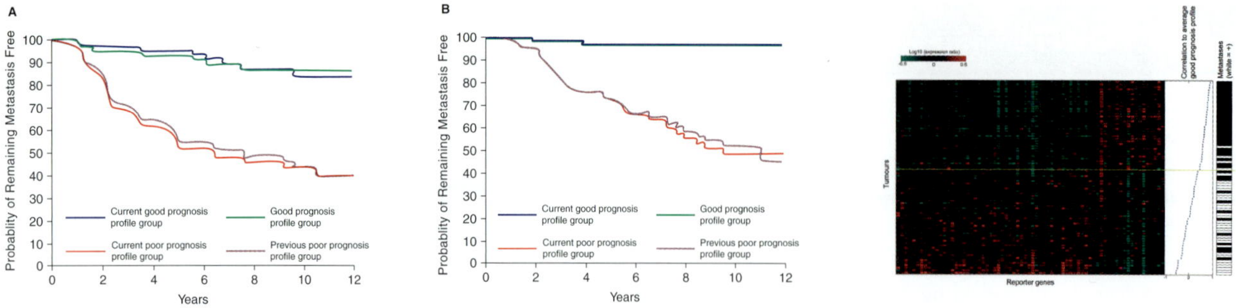

FIG. 2-8 **A.** Kaplan-Meier analysis of the probability that patients would remain free of distant metastases among 145 patients with lymphnode-negative breast cancer. **B.** Kaplan-Meier analysis of the probability of overall survival among 145 patients with lymphnode-negative breast cancer. **C.** Expression data matrix of 70 prognostic markers genes from tumors of 78 patients with breast cancer hybridized using the custom microarray. Each row represents a tumor and each column a gene. Genes are ordered according to their original ordering. Tumors are ordered by their correlation to the average profile of the good prognosis group. The metastases status for each patient is shown in the right panel. White indicates patients who developed metastases within 5 years after the initial diagnosis, black indicates patients who continued to be metastasis free for at least 5 years. Reprinted with permission from Glas AM, Floore A, Delahaye LJ, et al. Converting a breast cancer microarray signature into a high-throughput diagnostic test. *BMC Genomics*. 2006;7:278.

development, cell growth, and cell death. Although the specific target genes for individual miRNAs are just now being identified, a large number of all genes may be under miRNA control. Moreover, each individual miRNA may regulate from dozens to hundreds of genes. Thus, the complexity of the miRNA regulatory network is immense. Studies of miRNA expression patterns using PCR-, array-, and blotting-based techniques indicate that specific cancers exhibit characteristic patterns of miRNAs. Importantly, aberrant miRNA expression directly contributes to neoplasia.[15] Similar to microarray-based transcriptome analyses, global analyses of miRNA expression may soon become an important tool in cancer diagnosis and prognosis.

Small interfering RNAs (siRNAs) are a synthetic form of miRNA that play important roles in molecular oncology research. siRNAs are short, double-stranded miRNAs that efficiently catalyze the degradation of their cognate mRNAs. siRNAs are generated from longer-stranded RNAs, and this response probably first arose as a cellular defense against RNA viruses. Researchers can design siRNAs that will inhibit expression of any gene that they wish to target, and these techniques are revolutionizing studies of gene function. Indeed, genome-wide siRNA screens are being used not only to ascertain gene function but also to identify potential drug targets in cancer cells.

CHROMOSOME ANALYSIS

KARYOTYPING

Cancer cells exhibit chromosome abnormalities, which are often pathognomonic for their respective diseases. Karyotype analyses examine an individual's entire chromosome complement, either in normal cells or in tumor cells. In classical karyotype analyses, chromosomes from metaphase spreads are examined by a cytogeneticist based on their banding patterns and morphology. These classic techniques are still in wide use, particularly in the diagnosis and treatment of hematologic malignancies and in prenatal screening. However, these methods often are augmented with newer techniques that are more sensitive and/or comprehensive. Several cytogenetic methods use fluorescence in situ hybridization (FISH), in which fluorescently labeled nucleic acid probes are hybridized to their homologous sequences in either metaphase or interphase cells. A large number of chromosome and gene-specific probes facilitate the use of FISH to determine the copy number of an oncogene in cancer tissues. For example, interphase FISH analysis to detect amplified *HER2* gene copy number in breast cancer tissues is a test that, if positive, is a treatment indication for trastuzumab (Fig. 2-10). Another common use of FISH entails the use of probes that specifically detect gene fusions and chromosomal translocations, such as the *bcr-abl* fusion, in interphase tumor cells. The ability of FISH-based methods to study large numbers of cells and identify a rare cell with an abnormal karyotype makes these methods useful for detecting residual disease when malignant cells harbor a cytogenetic marker.

KEY POINTS

- Karyotyping reveals large-scale DNA anomalies in tumor cells, such as translocations and deletions.
- New methods that incorporate hybridization techniques, such as spectral karyotyping and comparative genomic hybridization, have greatly increased the sensitivity of cytogenetic analyses. In-situ hybridization techniques are used frequently to detect structural abnormalities in tumor DNA, such as translocations, and to detect residual disease in hematologic cancers.

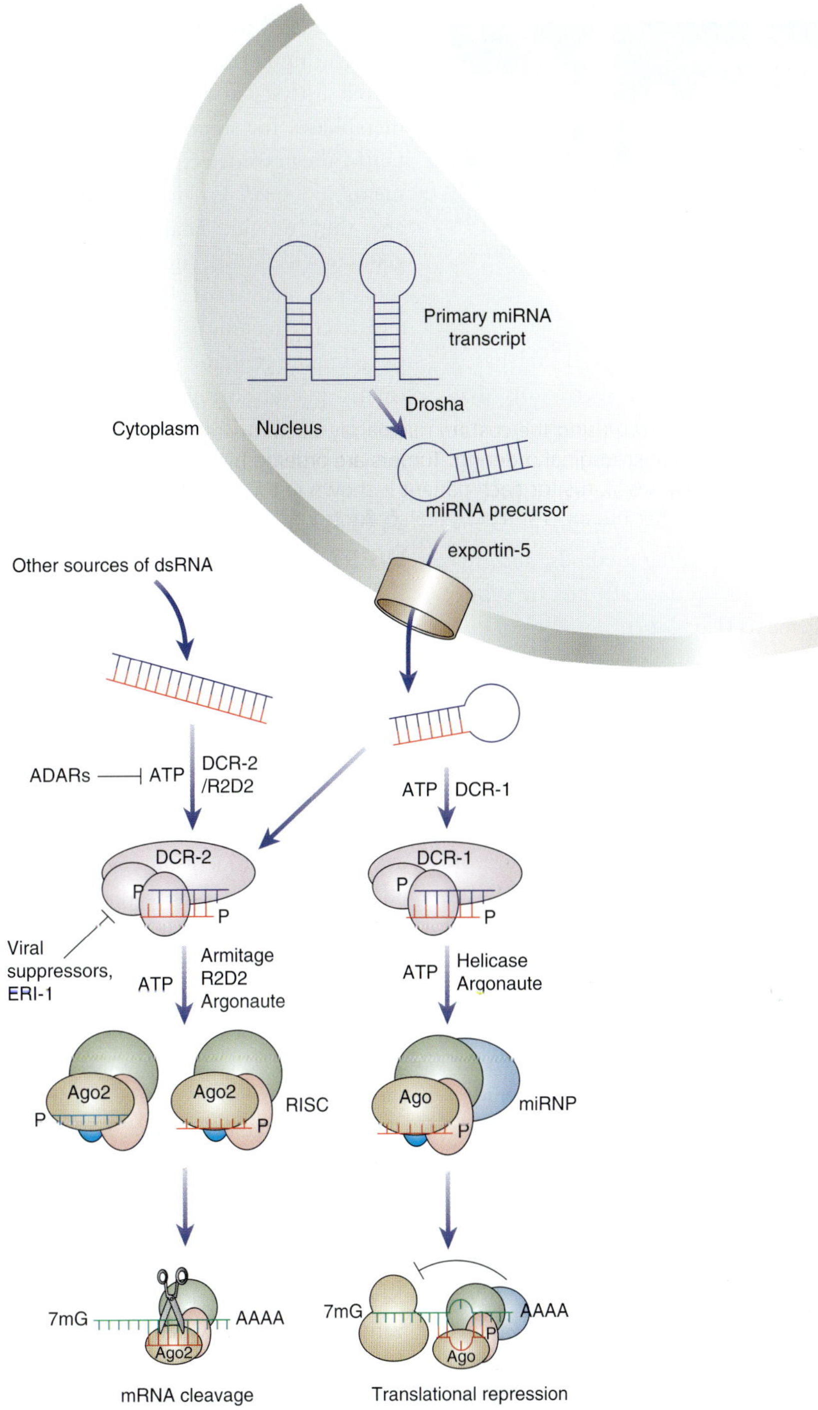

FIG. 2-9 Model of small-RNA-guided post-transcriptional regulation of gene expression.

Primary miRNA transcripts are processed to miRNA precursors in the nucleus by the RNase-III-like enzyme Drosha. The miRNA precursor is subsequently exported to the cytoplasm by means of the export receptor exportin-5. The miRNA precursor is further processed by Dicer to siRNA-duplex-like intermediates. The duplex is unwound while assembling into miRNP/RISC. Mature miRNAs bind to Ago proteins, which mediate translational repression or cleavage of target mRNAs. Other sources of long dsRNA in the cytoplasm of a cell are viral RNAs, artificially introduced dsRNA, dsRNAs generated by RdRPs, and genomic sense and antisense transcripts. Like miRNA precursors, long dsRNA is processed by the RNase III enzyme Dicer into 21 to 23 nucleotide dsRNA intermediates. Assisted by the RNA helicase Armitage and R2D2, the single-stranded siRNA-containing RISC is formed. The stability of the dsRNA and its recognition by Dicer can be regulated by specific ADARs and the exonuclease ERI-1.

Adapted by permission from Macmillan Publishers Ltd: Meister G, Tuschl T. Mechanisms of gene silencing by double-stranded RNA. *Nature*. 2004; 431(7006):343–349.

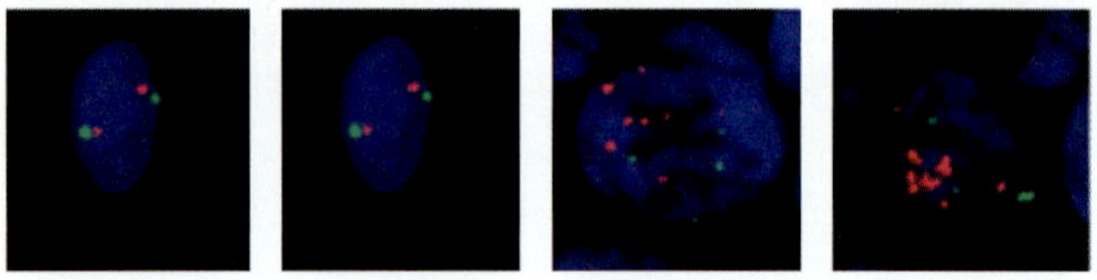

FIG. 2-10 Interphase fluorescence in situ hybridization (FISH) for HER2 showing different degrees of gene amplification in interphase tumor cells.

Spectral karyotyping is a genome-wide FISH-based method for characterizing chromosomal aberrations that might not be appreciated by classical techniques. Spectral karyotyping uses a panel of chromosome-specific probes that are labeled with different flourochromes and hybridized to metaphase chromosome spreads. Each chromosome is thus visualized by color using digital imaging methods, and this allows the identification of chromosomes affected by subtle and/or complex rearrangements (Fig. 2-11).

COMPARATIVE GENOMIC HYBRIDIZATION

Comparative genomic hybridization (CGH) is a cytogenetic technique that identifies DNA gains and losses in a tumor by using hybridization in order to compare it with a normal sample.[16] It is used to identify genomic regions that exhibit altered copy number in tumors, and it has the advantage of analyzing entire genomes in a single experiment. To perform CGH, differentially labeled tumor and normal DNA are hybridized to a reference sample, and amplifications or deletions of tumor DNA are identified by deviations in the ratio of signal provided by the normal and tumor probes. Initial CGH methods entailed hybridizing the labeled DNA to normal metaphase spreads. However, array CGH is a more recent approach, in which labeled tumor and normal DNA are hybridized to chips containing arrayed DNA fragments representing entire genomes. These methods permit karyotypic analyses of tumor cells that do not yield sufficient metaphases for standard or spectral karyotyping. Importantly, they can detect copy number changes in DNA fragments too small for detection by karyotyping techniques, and they provide analyses of DNA copy number at a genome-wide scale. Indeed, the comprehensive and high-resolution analyses of copy number provided by array CGH and related techniques are providing unique insights into the complex genomic gains and losses that drive neoplastic transformation. Array CGH can be used to analyze fresh or frozen tissues, cell lines, and archival formalin-fixed, paraffin-embedded samples.

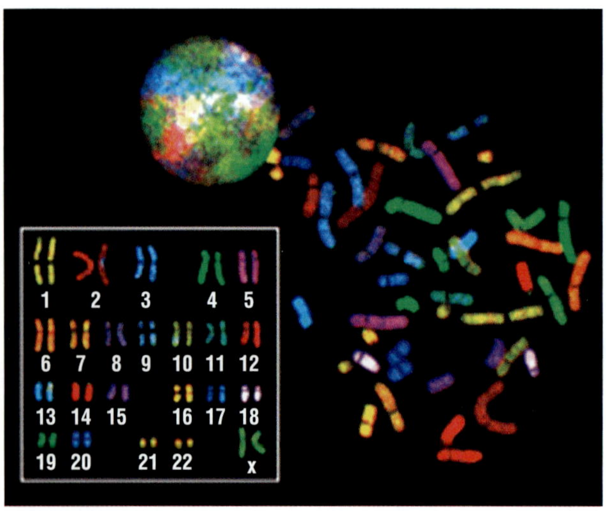

FIG. 2-11 Spectral karyotype showing different dyes characteristic for each chromosome.
This technique allows for rapid analysis of metaphase spreads for chromosomal loss and translocation.

ANALYSIS OF PROTEINS

WESTERN BLOTTING AND IMMUNOHISTOCHEMISTRY

Like nucleic acids, proteins can be separated by gel electrophoresis and transferred to membranes. The membrane can then be exposed to a variety of detection probes, most commonly antibodies (termed Western blotting). Western blotting can detect changes in protein size (e.g., caused by truncation), post-translational modifications (e.g., phosphorylation), and differences in protein abundance.[17] Pathology departments routinely employ immunohistochemical methods that use antibodies to detect the expression of specific proteins in tumor cells. In many cases these studies use paraffin-fixed or frozen tissue samples and play important diagnostic roles. Examples include antibodies to intermediate filament proteins (which are used to define the origins of poorly differentiated cancers), immunodetection of neuron-specific enolase and synaptophysin (used to distinguish neuroendocrine cancers), and studies of steroid-hormone receptor expression in breast cancer. Another important immunohistochemical diagnostic technique, particularly for hematologic cancers, is flow cytometry, which detects multiple cell surface markers in complex cell populations, such as bone marrow. Because of their high sensitivity, as well as their ability to analyze large numbers of cells, flow cytometric methods are very useful for detecting small numbers of tumor cells in a population of normal cells. For example, flow cytometric analyses of bone marrow or peripheral blood leukemia can detect residual amounts of leukemia that are below the limits of morphologic detection. Immunohistochemical detection also is used as a surrogate for certain oncogene mutations. For example, some mutations that inactivate the *p53* tumor suppressor stabilize the p53 protein and lead to increased p53 abundance that can be directly detected by anti-p53 antibodies.

MASS SPECTROMETRY AND PROTEOMICS

The methods described previously are used to study the expression of relatively small numbers of individual proteins in biologic samples. However, analogous to the effect of microarray

KEY POINTS

- Protein analyses reveal protein abundance, as well as functional modifications such as phosphorylation and acetylation.
- Mass spectrometry-based proteomics allow for large-scale analyses of protein expression and modifications in tumor tissues.

methods on large-scale genomic analyses of RNA expression, proteomic methods are rapidly being developed that allow global studies of protein expression. These sophisticated methods use mass spectrometers, differential protein labeling, and bioinformatics to quantitate and identify proteins present in complex biologic samples. The completion of the human genome sequence greatly enabled these proteomic approaches because the annotated genome sequence facilitated construction of comprehensive databases used to identify the peptides analyzed by mass spectrometry. One intense area of proteomics research involves methods for early cancer detection based on defining protein signatures indicative of early-stage cancers in tissues, such as peripheral blood.[18] Proteomic methods will likely be an important tool in cancer detection, diagnosis, and prognosis in the near future.

ONCOGENES: THE ENGINES OF CANCER

Transforming a normal cell into a malignant cell involves a series of mutations in genes, termed oncogenes, that directly contribute to neoplasia when their functions are altered.[19,20] To date, perhaps several hundred human genes have been implicated as proto-oncogenes, which are genes that have the potential to be converted into oncogenes. Oncogenes are either dominant or recessive, and they normally function in cellular processes such as cell division, apoptosis, and differentiation. Dominant oncogenes sustain gain-of-function mutations in cancers, whereas recessive oncogenes, also called tumor suppressor genes, sustain loss-of-function mutations in cancers.

IDENTIFICATION OF DOMINANT ONCOGENES

Experimental Cancer Models: Retroviruses and Transfections

Many dominant oncogenes were first discovered through studies of animal cancers induced by a subset of retroviruses, called RNA tumor viruses. One class of RNA tumor viruses carries viral oncogenes within their viral genomes, and several dozen viral oncogenes were identified in the 1970s and 1980s. The major breakthrough with respect to human cancer came with the realization that viral oncogenes represent mutated versions of host proto-oncogenes that were captured by the viral genomes during their life cycle. Many

KEY POINTS

- Proto-oncogenes are normal cellular genes that can be converted into oncogenes by mutation or by epigenetic mechanisms, which alter their normal functions or expression.
- Dominant oncogenes are activated in tumors by mechanisms such as amplification, point mutations, and translocations.
- Tumor suppressor genes are recessive oncogenes that are inactivated in tumors by diverse mechanisms including deletions, point mutations, and silencing.

viral oncogenes are the counterparts of extremely important human oncogenes, and the identification of their cellular counterparts established the framework within which we understand the role of dominant oncogenes in tumorigenesis.

The second class of RNA tumor viruses cause animal cancers by a mechanism termed insertional activation, in which the integration of a viral genome into a host chromosome activates a cellular proto-oncogene. These retroviruses have been used as powerful genetic tools for oncogene discovery, and the complete sequencing of the human and mouse genomes has led to a new generation of high-throughput insertional mutagenesis screens yielding a large number of previously unknown proto-oncogenes.[21]

The other major experimental strategy initially used to identify oncogenes is called DNA transfection. In this approach, DNA is extracted from tumor cells and introduced into recipient cells by a technique called transfection. The recipient cells used in these experiments, such as murine NIH3T3 cells, undergo morphologic and growth alterations when they are transfected with an oncogene and are said to become transformed. The transfected tumor cell DNA is subsequently isolated and sequenced from the transformed cells, allowing the identification of the transferred oncogene. Many critical human oncogenes, including *Ras* and *HER2*, were originally isolated from transfection experiments.

Chromosomal Translocations

Recurrent chromosomal translocations are frequently found in cancers. This is particularly true for hematologic malignancies, which are characterized by many chromosomal translocations that often involve immunoglobulin and T-cell receptor genes (Fig. 2-12).[22] Specific translocations have extremely important diagnostic and prognostic implications, and serve as molecular markers for the detection of residual disease and relapse. Like the sites of retroviral insertions discussed previously, the regions of DNA commonly involved with translocations usually contain proto-oncogenes that are activated by the DNA rearrangement.

Chromosomal translocations activate proto-oncogenes by two distinct mechanisms.[23] The most common mechanism involves the creation of fusion genes when the translocation joins two genes normally found on separate chromosomes. This type of translocation usually involves transcription factors or tyrosine kinases, and the protein products of these novel fusion genes have biologic activities that differ from the parental proto-oncogene. An example of this type of translocation is the *BCR-ABL* fusion that results from the reciprocal exchange of DNA between chromosomes 9 and 22, t(9; 22), known as the Philadelphia chromosome (Fig. 2-13). The translocation juxtaposes the 5' end of the *BCR* gene on chromosome 22 and the 3' end of the *c-ABL* oncogene on chromosome 9. The resultant novel gene produces a hybrid mRNA that codes for the BCR-ABL oncoprotein, which deregulates the tyrosine kinase activity normally associated with the c-ABL protein. Another chromosomal translocation that generates a fusion genes is seen in acute promyelocytic leukemia (APL). In this case, a reciprocal chromosomal translocation fuses the retinoic acid receptor-alpha (*RARalpha*) gene at 17qll.2 with the *PML* gene at 15q22, and the fusion creates a dominant inhibitory RARalpha protein that blocks expression of *RARalpha* target genes.

Translocations also may activate proto-oncogenes by deregulating their expression without altering their protein structure. An example of this type of translocation is found in Burkitt's lymphoma, which is characterized by translocations that cause the *c-myc* oncogene, located on chromosome 8, to be juxtaposed to immunoglobulin genes that are located on chromosomes 14, 2, and 22. In each case, these translocations deregulate *c-myc* expression by placing it under the control of strong transcriptional elements contained within the immunoglobulin locus. Other examples of proto-oncogenes

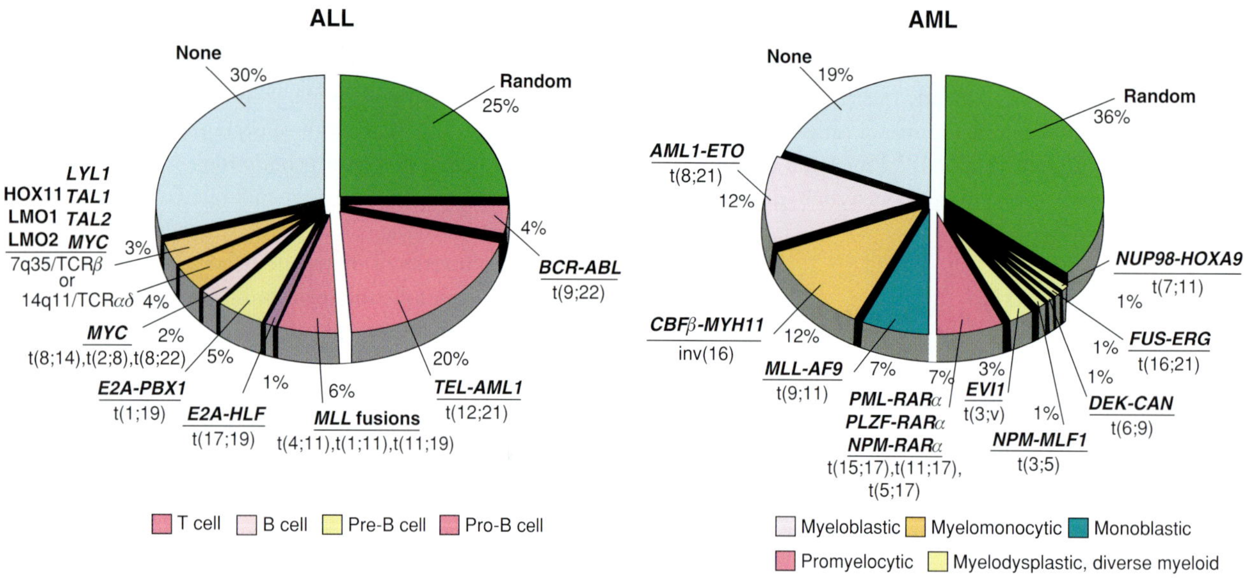

FIG. 2-12 Distribution of translocation-generated oncogenes among the acute leukemias of children and young adults.

The products of these aberrant genes are most often nuclear proteins active in transcription, with the notable exception of BCR-ABL, which encodes a cytoplasmic protein containing the activated ABL tyrosine kinase domain. In ALL, gene fusions tend to be specifically associated with one of the commonly recognized immunologic subtypes of the disease, as indicated by the color coding on the chart. The T-cell leukemias (orange) are characterized by translocations that dysregulate the expression of proto-oncogenes. The MYC *gene also is dysregulated through translocation into the vicinity of one of the Ig loci in B-cell leukemia (pink) and Burkitt's lymphoma. In the pre-B (yellow) and pro-B (magenta) immunologic subtypes of ALL, fusion genes encoding chimeric oncoproteins are produced. The* BCR-ABL *and* MLL *gene fusions have also been identified in the chronic and acute myeloid leukemias, respectively, suggesting that they arise in primitive stem cells with multilineage potential. "Random" refers to sporadic translocations that have been observed only in leukemic cells from single cases. "None" refers to leukemias that lack identifiable gene abnormalities. In AML, the genes show specific associations with disease subtypes corresponding to the morphologic stages of normal myeloid cell development. Although both the* AML1-ETO *and* CBFbeta -MYH11 *fusion genes lead to alterations in the CBF transcription complex, they appear to disrupt hematopoiesis through distinct mechanisms because they are associated with different morphologic subtypes of AML. Other rearrangements affect the* RARalpha *gene on chromosome 17 in promyelocytic progenitors, resulting in fusions with PML or, rarely, PLZF or NPM. Less frequent translocations give rise to fusion genes associated with myelodysplastic syndrome, progressing to AML (NPM-MLF1, DEK-CAN, and NUP98-HOXA9).*

From Look AT. Oncogenic transcription factors in the human acute leukemia. *Science*. 1997;278(5340):1059–1064. Reprinted with permission from AAAS.

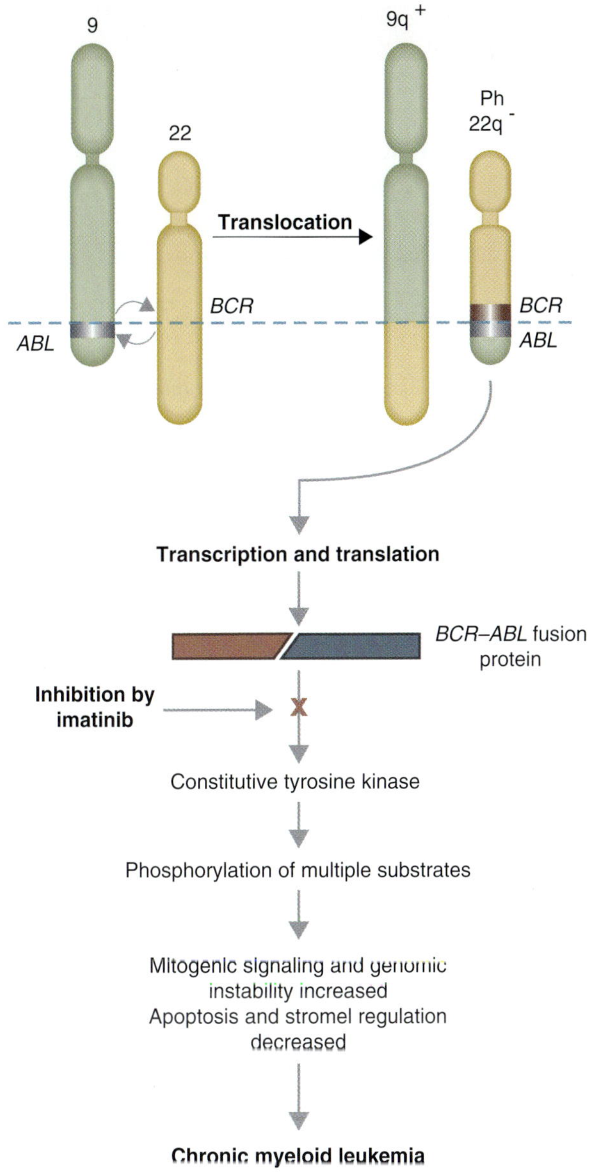

FIG. 2-13 Translocation leading to the Philadelphia (Ph) chromosome and the role of *BCR-ABL* in the pathogenesis of chronic myeloid leukemia.
The Ph chromosome is a foreshortened chromosome 22 resulting from an exchange between the long arms of chromosomes 9 and 22.

that are activated by translocations involving immunoglobulin genes include cyclin D1 (found in 11:14 translocations in mantle cell lymphoma) and *bcl-2* (found in 14:18 translocations in follicular lymphoma). Table 2-1 lists representative proto-oncogenes involved in translocations with immunoglobulin and T-cell receptor loci.

Recurrent chromosomal translocations also are found in solid tumors, most notably soft tissue sarcomas. Perhaps the most widely characterized examples are translocations involving the Ewing's sarcoma (*EWS*) gene on chromosome 22. These translocations most commonly fuse *EWS* to the *FLI-1* gene on chromosome 11 (t11:22, q24;q12) and create a transcription factor containing a DNA-binding domain derived from *FLI-1* and transcriptional activation domain from *EWS*. Variant translocations involving *EWS* also occur in Ewing's sarcoma, and these join *EWS* to several other fusion partners. Alveolar rhabdomyosarcomas also contain a pathognomonic translocation, (t2:13) (q35;q14), which fuses the *PAX3* and *FHK4* transcription factors.

DNA AMPLIFICATION

DNA amplification results in the increased copy number of a gene and is a mechanism by which cancer cells increase the expression of a gene product. Accordingly, many solid tumors exhibit amplification of known proto-oncogenes (Table 2-2).[24] Gene amplification can be detected by many methods, including karyotypic analyses (as either chromosomal or extrachromosomal amplicons), CGH, FISH, and Southern blotting. Immunohistochemical detection of the overexpressed protein product often is used as a surrogate for detection of amplified genes. For example, *HER2* amplification is detected by interphase FISH or immunohistochemical analysis. Similarly, *N-MYC* gene amplification and overexpression of its protein product, which are associated with advanced stages and poor prognosis of neuroblastoma, are most commonly identified by immunohistochemical staining.

Point Mutations

Dominant oncogenes are frequently activated by point mutations that alter their activity. For example, the *K-RAS* gene is mutated in a large number of human cancers by alterations of amino acids 12, 13, or 61. Because point mutations are more difficult to detect than structural rearrangements, finding point mutations traditionally has not been a common means of oncogene discovery. However, because some common oncogenes are activated by only a few specific point mutations, it is possible to identify these known mutations in cancer specimens by using techniques such as sequence-specific oligonucleotide hybridization and single-strand confirmation polymorphism (SSCP). Recently, the National Institutes of Health has embarked on a major initiative, called the Cancer Genome Atlas, to completely sequence the genomes of common human cancers. These efforts may reveal new insights into the role and prevalence of oncogene point mutations in cancers.[25]

DETECTION OF TUMOR SUPPRESSOR GENE INACTIVATION

Loss of tumor suppressor gene alleles occurs commonly in cancers.[26] Delineating a locus involved by allelic loss in a tumor type is often the first step toward identifying a tumor suppressor gene. Sites of allelic loss are determined by analyzing polymorphic markers in both tumor and normal DNA from an individual, and these analyses can define the smallest region of allelic loss that is common to a number of patients, thereby localizing the disease gene. Classical methods used to identify candidate tumor suppressor genes within regions of allelic loss

TABLE 2-1 The Immunoglobulin and T-Cell Receptor Gene-Associated Translocations

Translocation	Genes	Major Structures	Disease
t(8;14)(q24;q32)	*MYC*	BHLH	Acute lymphoid leukemia
t(2;8)(p12;q24)	*IGH* *IGK*	BHLH	Acute lymphoid leukemia
t(8;22)(q24;q11)	*MYC* *MYC*	BHLH	Acute lymphoid leukemia
t(14;19)(q32;q13)	*IGH* *IGL*	IkB homology	Chronic lymphoid leukemia (B-cell)
t(5;14)(q31;q32)	*BCL-3* *IL-3*	Cytokine	Chronic lymphoid leukemia (pre B-cell)
t(7;14)(q21;q32)	*IGH* *THE (CDK6)*	Cyclin- dependent kinase	Chronic lymphoid leukemia (B-cell)
t(9;14)(p21;q11)	*IGH* *p16/p19^{ARF}*	TS activity	Acute lymphoid leukemia (B-cell)
t(7;19)(q35;p13)	*TCRd* *TCRb*	BHLH	Acute lymphoid leukemia (T-cell)
t(1;14)(p32;q11)	*LYL1* *TAL1/SCL*	BHLH	Acute lymphoid leukemia (T-cell)
t(7;9)(q35;q34)	*TCRa* *TCRb*	BHLH	Acute lymphoid leukemia (T-cell)
t(11;14)(p15;q11)	*TAL2* *LMO1/rbtn1/Tgt1*	Lim domain	Acute lymphoid leukemia (T-cell)
t(11;14)(p13;q11)	*TCR* *LMO2/rbnt2/Tgt2*	Lim domain	Acute lymphoid leukemia (T-cell)
t(7;11)(q35;p13)	*TCR* *TCRb* *LMO2/rbnt2/Tgt2*	Lim domain	Acute lymphoid leukemia (T-cell)
t(7;10)(q35;q24)	*TCRb*	Homeodomain	Acute lymphoid leukemia (T-cell)
t(14;21)(q11;q22)	*HOX11* *TCRa*	BHLH	Acute lymphoid leukemia (T-cell)
t(10;14)(q24;q11)	*BHLHB1* *HOX11*	Homeodomain	Acute lymphoid leukemia (T-cell)
t(14;18)	*TCRd* *IGH*	BCL2 protein	B-cell lymphoma
(q32;q21)	*BCL2* *CCDN1*	Cyclin D1	Mantle cell lymphoma
t(11;14)(q13;q32)	*IGH*	Cyclin D1	Mantle cell lymphoma

Abbreviations: BHLH, basic helix-loop-helix; TS, thymidylate synthase.

involved positional cloning methods. This approach involves molecular methods to clone a gene on the basis of its chromosomal position without prior knowledge of the gene product and has been used to identify many tumor suppressor genes. However, the human genome sequence has given rise to bioinformatics and PCR-based methods that have largely supplanted positional cloning. Once a region of allelic loss has been sufficiently defined, all of the known genes within the region can be determined from the genomic sequence, and the candidate genes studied directly, without the need for large-scale cloning projects.

Hereditary cancer syndromes have been a rich resource for identifying tumor suppressor genes. Moreover, the effect of these studies extends far beyond hereditary cancer syndromes because the genes responsible for familial cancers are often the same tumor suppressor genes that are inactivated in sporadic cancers. In most familial cancer syndromes, a mutant copy of a recessive oncogene is inherited (most frequently this allele is deleted), followed by mutation of the remaining normal allele in cancers that develop in these individuals. Thus, the molecular signature of a classic tumor suppressor is loss of heterozygosity and intragenic inactivating mutations within the

TABLE 2-2 Oncogenes Amplified in Human Cancers.

Gene Amplified	Locus	Tumors
AKT2	19q13.2	Ovarian cancer
CCND1 (Cyclin D1)	11q13.3	HNSCC, esophageal, breast, HCC
CCNE (Cyclin E)	19q12	Gastric cancer
CDK4	12q14	Sarcoma, glioblastoma
ERBB1 (EGFR)	7p12	Glioblastoma, HNSCC
ERBB2 (EGFR2)	17q11.2–q12	Breast, ovarian, cervical cancer
FGFR1	8p11.1–p11.2	Breast cancer
FGFR2	10q25.3–q26	Breast cancer
HRAS	11p15.5	Colorectal cancer
KRAS	12p13	Colorectal, gastric cancer
MDM2	12q14	Soft tissue sarcomas, osteosarcoma, esophageal cancer
MET	7q31	Gastric cancer
MYB	6q23.3–q24	Colorectal cancer
MYC	8q24.12–q24.13	Ovarian, breast, SCLC, HNSCC, esophageal, cervical cancer
MYCN	2p24.3	Neuroblastoma

Abbreviations: HNSCC, head and neck squamous cell carcinoma; HCC, hepatocellular carcinoma; SCLC, small cell lung cancer. Reproduced with permission of The McGraw-Hill Companies. Scriver et al. *Metabolic and Molecular Basis of Inherited Disease*. 2001.

remaining allele in tumors. This is known as a two-step, or Knudson, tumor suppressor, named after classic studies that involved the loss of the *Rb* tumor suppressor in retinoblastoma. In fact, the failure to find biallelic loss in tumors was often used as evidence against the assignment of a putative locus as a tumor suppressor.

However, there are important exceptions to the Knudson model that expand our understanding of how tumor suppressor genes are mutated in cancers. For example, in some cases, loss of a single allele of a tumor suppressor is sufficient to confer cancer susceptibility or contribute to neoplastic progression, even when a normal allele persists. In the case of these haploinsufficient tumor suppressor genes, intragenic point mutations in the remaining allele will not be found, and this can initially confuse the identification of important human tumor suppressors, such as the *p27Kip1* cell cycle inhibitor. Another situation where a tumor suppressor will not conform to the Knudson model is when tumor suppressors are inactivated by epigenetic mechanisms, rather than mutation. For example, the *p16Ink4A* gene, which also functions as a cell cycle inhibitor, is deleted in many tumors but can be silenced by DNA methylation in others. In the latter cases, DNA sequence mutations do not occur, rather DNA methylation patterns implicate *p16* as a tumor suppressor.

FUNCTIONS OF ONCOGENES

MITOGENIC SIGNAL TRANSDUCTION PATHWAYS

Cell division is triggered by signal transduction pathways that are stimulated when protein growth factors bind to specific cell-surface receptors, and these pathways contain proto-oncogenes throughout the signaling chain (Table 2-3). Most growth factor receptors are anchored in the cell membrane such that an extracellular domain is available for growth factor (ligand) binding and an intracellular domain interacts with downstream signaling molecules. The intracellular portions of growth factor receptors called receptor tyrosine kinases (RTKs) contain a highly conserved tyrosine kinase domain that catalyzes the addition of phosphates to tyrosine residues. Ligand binding causes RTKs to dimerize, and this leads to autophosphorylation (Fig. 2-14). RTK tyrosine phosphorylation recruits proteins that contain SH2 domains, which recognize the phosphotyrosine motifs, then transmit the mitogenic signal down several parallel pathways, including the phosphotidylinositol-3 kinase (PI3K) and mitogen-activated kinase (MAP kinase) pathways. Many constituents of these signaling pathways were originally identified as viral oncogenes, and dominant mutations in these proto-oncogenes lead to unrestrained mitogenic signaling that may be independent of the growth factors normally needed to stimulate these pathways.

Several therapeutic strategies have been employed to target aberrant RTK activity in cancers. One approach has involved the clinical development of antibodies that bind to and inhibit RTKs. Trastuzumab is derived from a mouse monoclonal antibody that was selected for its antagonism to *HER2* activity and is an important agent in the treatment of breast cancers with *HER2* new amplification. Cetuximab is another inhibitory antibody that binds to the extracellular domain of the epidermal growth factor receptor (EGFR) that is approved for use in metastatic colon cancer and is being studied in a number of other applications. Another strategy to target RTKs in cancers involves the development of small-molecule RTK inhibitors, such as gefitinib and erlotonib. These agents bind to RTKs and inhibit their catalytic activity. Recent data demonstrate a close association between gefitinib efficacy and the presence of mutations in EGFR that are found in a small fraction of patients with lung cancers.

RAS proteins play pivotal roles in transducing mitogenic signals downstream of RTKs. One key SH2 protein that binds to phosphorylated RTKs is the adaptor protein termed Grb2 (Fig. 2-14). The GRB2/RTK complex is bound by Son of Sevenless (SOS), a guanine nucleotide-exchange factor (GEF) that activates RAS by exchanging guanosine triphosphate (GTP) with guanosine diphosphate (GDP). RAS activity also is regulated by interaction with guanosine triphosphatase-activating proteins (GAPs) that mediate hydrolysis of RAS-bound GTP to GDP. GDP-bound RAS is inactive until a GTP molecule replaces GDP in an exchange reaction mediated by a guanine exchange factor such as SOS. The amount of *Ras* activity is thus determined by the balance between GEF and GAP activity (Fig 2-15).[27] Oncogenic *RAS* mutations affect amino acids 12, 13, and 61, which are all critical for interaction with GAPs. Because reduced GAP function prolongs RAS signaling, GAPs may function as recessive oncogenes. For example, the *NF-1* gene is a GAP that acquires a loss of function mutation in neurofibromatosis. In the active GTP-bound state, RAS activates three parallel pathways: the MAP kinase pathway (which activates transcription factors), the RAL/CDC42 pathway (which regulates membrane and cytoskeletal changes), and the PI3K pathway (which affects many cellular functions, including protein synthesis and apoptosis) (Fig. 2-15). The MAP kinase pathway is stimulated by the RAF serine/threonine kinase, leading to activation of additional downstream cytoplasmic serine-threonine kinases that ultimately activate MAP kinases and other effectors. These signaling cascades promote phosphorylation and activation of nuclear proto-oncogenes that are transcription factors, such as FOS, JUN, and MYC. Each of these proteins stimulates a transcriptional program that is determined by sequence-specific DNA elements that are bound by the transcription factor. Because transcription factors regulate large numbers of genes, their oncogenic activation may have far-reaching effects on gene expression.

Because RAS pathway mutations are so frequent in cancers (e.g., 80% of pancreatic cancers, 40% of lung cancers, and 50% of colon cancers), RAS is an attractive therapeutic target. Efforts to block RAS activity have focused on the post-translational modification of all RAS proteins that adds a fatty acid moiety by covalent linkage to a C-terminal cysteine. The fatty acid is essential for the localization of RAS at the inner plasma membrane and the functioning of the molecule. Drug development of agents to block RAS prenylation have focused on farnesyl transferase, an enzyme that added a 14-carbon fatty acid to H-RAS. For example, the farnesyl transferase inhibitor tipifarnib is being studied in patients with high-risk acute myeloid leukemia (AML) and myelodysplastic syndrome. K-RAS proteins, however, are linked to 20-carbon fatty acids by one of two geranylgeranylases and, therefore, incompletely affected by the drugs with very high activity for farnesyl transferase inhibition. The fact that prenylation is an essential step in the activation of a wide range of cellular proteins, thereby presenting the potential for untoward toxicity of highly potent inhibition of prenylation, is also problematic.

KEY POINTS

- Growth factor receptors stimulate mitogenic signaling pathways that are comprised of many key proto-oncogenes, including proteins that regulate Ras activity. These pathways lead to the activation of transcription factors, such as c-myc, that stimulate complex transcriptional programs leading to cell division and cell growth.
- Tyrosine kinases play essential roles in transmitting mitogenic signaling pathways.
- Genes that regulate the cell division cycle are important dominant and recessive oncogenes.
- Many oncogenic pathways suppress programmed cell death (apoptosis).

The PI3K-AKT pathway is another crucial route of mitogenic signaling frequently mutated in cancer cells (Fig 2-16).[28,29] PI3K activation stimulates transcriptional and translation responses that promote cell growth and division. AKT is a protein kinase that is downstream of PI3K activation. AKT was first discovered as a viral oncogene, and AKT is amplified and/or overexpressed in many cancers. Moreover, a large spectrum of cancers exhibits elevated AKT activity that results from mutations in the upstream genes that regulate AKT. For example, the *PTEN* tumor suppressor opposes PI3 kinase and prevents AKT activation; *PTEN* is deleted in many cancers, including glioblastoma and melanoma, as well as prostate and endometrial cancers. AKT phosphorylates many substrates that regulate cell division, apoptosis, and protein synthesis. The PI3K-AKT pathway is widely viewed as an important therapeutic target, and both AKT and PI3K inhibitors are being studied in clinical trials.

The nonreceptor or cytoplasmic tyrosine kinases is another family of tyrosine kinases that contains important proto-oncogenes (see Table 2-3). Members of this family include SRC, FES, YES, and LCK, and these proteins normally function when bound to the plasma membrane. The c-ABL protein also is a nonreceptor tyrosine kinase, and its fusion with the *BCR* gene in chronic myeloid leukemia (CML) deregulates its tyrosine kinase activity. The

TABLE 2-3 Oncogenes

Oncogene	Lesion	Neoplasm	Proto-Oncogene
Growth factors			
v-sis		Glioma/fibrosarcoma	B-chain PDGF
int 2	Proviral insertion	Mammary carcinoma	Member of FGF family
KS3	DNA transfection	Kaposi sarcoma	Member of FGF family
HST	DNA transfection	Stomach carcinoma	Member of FGF family
int-1	Proviral insertion	Mammary carcinoma	Possible growth factor
Receptors lacking protein kinase activity			
mas	DNA transfection	Mammary carcinoma	Angiotensin receptor
Tyrosine kinases: integral membrane proteins, growth factor receptors			
EGFR	Amplification	Squamous cell carcinoma	Protein kinase (tyr) EGFR
v-fms		Sarcoma	Protein kinase (tyr) CSF-1R*
v-kit		Sarcoma	Protein kinase (tyr) stem cell factor R
v-ros		Sarcoma	Protein kinase (tyr)
MET	Rearrangement	MNNG-treated human osteocarcinoma cell line	Protein kinase (tyr) HGF/SFR
TRK	Rearrangement	Colon carcinoma	Protein kinase (tyr) NGFR
NEU	Point mutation	Neuroblastoma	Protein kinase (tyr)
	Amplification	Carcinoma of breast	
RET	Rearrangement	Carcinoma of thyroid Men 2A, Men 2B	Protein kinase (tyr) GDNFR
Tyrosine kinases: membrane associated			
SRC		Colon carcinoma	Protein kinase (tyr)
v-yes		Sarcoma	Protein kinase (tyr)
v-fgr		Sarcoma	Protein kinase (tyr)
v-fps		Sarcoma	Protein kinase (tyr)
v-fes		Sarcoma	Protein kinase (tyr)
BCR/ABL	Chromosome translocation	Chronic myelogenous leukemia	Protein kinase (tyr)
Membrane-associated G proteins			
H-RAS	Point mutation	Colon, lung, pancreas carcinoma	GTPase
K-RAS	Point mutation	Acute myelogenous leukemia	GTPase
		Thyroid carcinoma, melanoma	
N-RAS	Point mutation	Carcinoma, melanoma	GTPase
gsp	Point mutation	Carcinoma of thyroid	$G_s$alpha
gip	Point mutation	Ovary, adrenal carcinoma	G_1alpha
GEF family of proteins			
Dbl	Rearrangement	Diffuse B-cell lymphoma	GEF for Rho and Cdc42Hs
Ost		Osteosarcomas	GEF for RhoA and Cdc42Hs
Tiam-1	Metastatic and oncogenic	T lymphoma	GEF for Rac and Cdc42Hs
Vay	Rearrangement	Hematopoietic cells	GEF for Ras?
Lbc	Oncogenic	Myeloid leukemias	GEF for Rho
Serine/threonine kinases: cytoplasmic			
v-mos		Sarcoma	Protein kinase (ser/thr)
v-raf		Sarcoma	Protein kinase (ser/thr)
pim-1	Proviral insertion	T-cell lymphoma	Protein kinase (ser/thr)
Cytoplasmic regulators			
v-crk			SH-2/SH-3 adaptor
Nuclear protein family			
v-myc		Carcinoma myelocytomatosis	Transcription factor
N-MYC	Gene amplification	Neuroblastoma: lung carcinoma	Transcription factor
L-MYC	Gene amplification	Carcinoma of lung	Transcription factor
v-myb		Myeloblastosis	Transcription factor
v-fos		Osteosarcoma	Transcription factor API
v-jun		Sarcoma	Transcription factor API
v-ski		Carcinoma	Transcription factor
v-rel		Lymphatic leukemia	Mutant NFgammaB
v-ets		Myeloblastosis	Transcription factor
v-srbA		Erythroblastosis	Mutant thioredoxine receptor

Abbreviations: CSF-1R, macrophage colony-stimulating factor-1 receptor; EGFR, epidermal growth factor receptor; FGF, fibroblast growth factor; GEF, guanine nucleotide exchange factor; GDNF, glial derived neurotropic factor; HGF/SF, hepatic growth factor/scatter factor; NGF, nerve growth factor; PDGF, platelet derived growth factor.

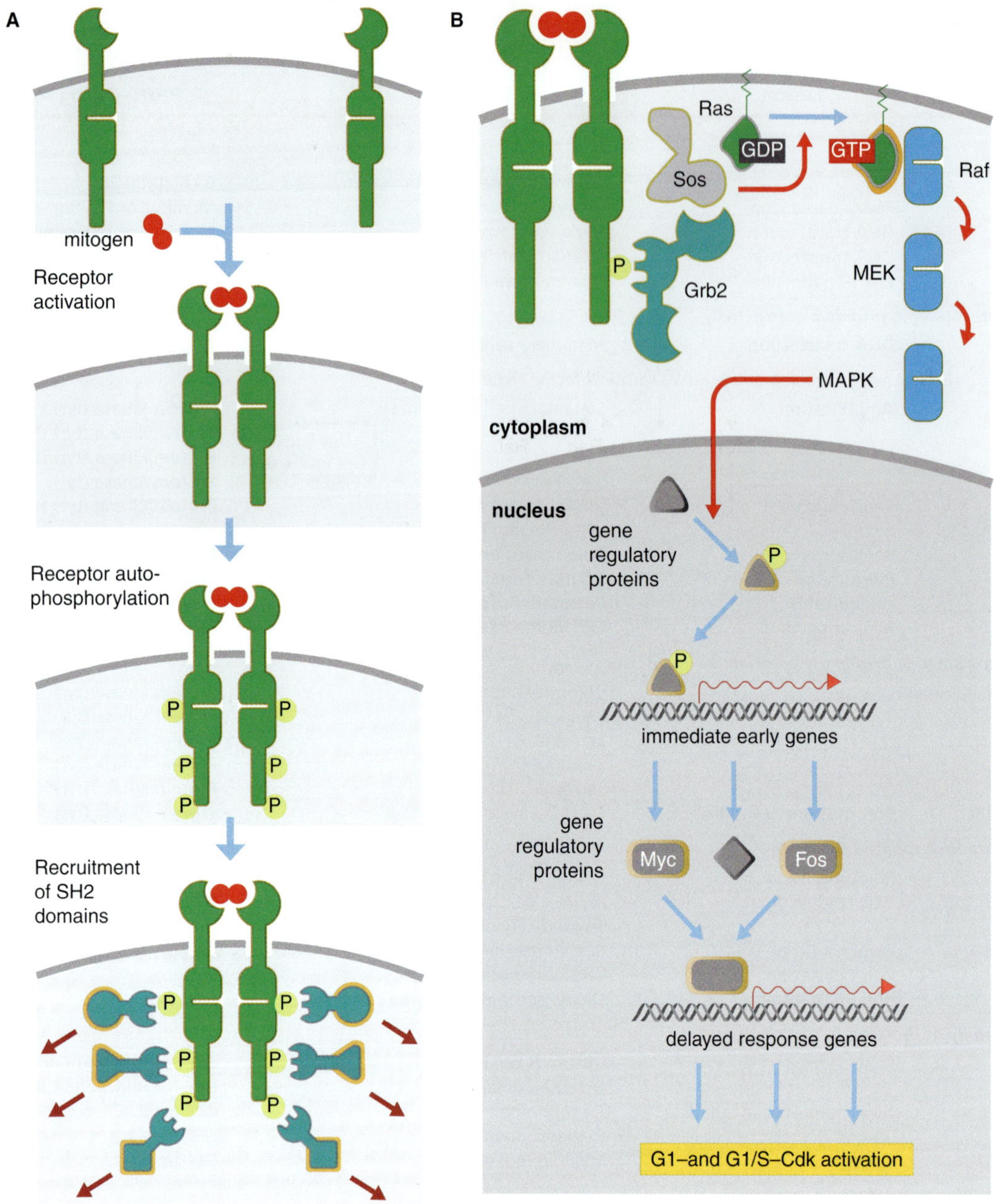

FIG. 2-14 **A.** Origin of the mitogenic signal at the cell membrane. **B.** Mitogenic signaling by the *Ras* pathway.

A. *The binding of growth factors to receptor tyrosine kinases causes receptor dimerization and autophosphorylation. The receptor tyrosine phosphorylation then recruits binding proteins that contain SH2 domains, and these transmit the mitogenic signal (see text).* ***B.*** *Ras activation stimulates the MAP kinase pathway, which leads to the activation of downstream transcription factors such as Jun and Myc (see text for details).*

Reproduced by permission of the New Science Press. From Figures 10-11 and 10-12 From Morgan, David O. *The Cell Cycle: Principles of Control* (New Science Press, 2007).

BCR-ABL kinase domain is the target for drugs like imatinib, which inhibits its kinase activity by preventing ATP from binding to the active site.[30] Imatinib and other BCR-ABL inhibitors have become a mainstay of therapy for chronic myeloid leukemia. Moreover, by virtue of the homology among tyrosine kinases, imatinib also inhibits other important kinases such as c-KIT and platelet-derived growth factor receptor (PDGFR). Indeed, inhibition of c-KIT underlies the use of imatinib in the treatment of gastrointestinal stromal cell tumors.

CELL CYCLE CONTROL

Progression through the cell division cycle is highly regulated.[31,32] The cell cycle is divided into four phases that

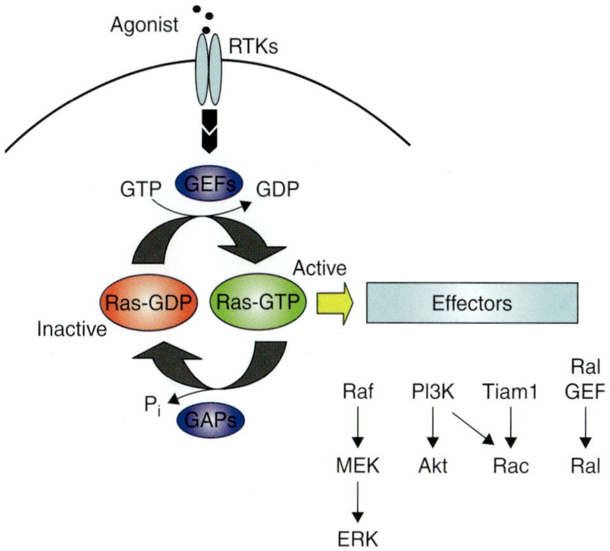

FIG. 2-15 *Ras* upstream and downstream signaling. Extracellular stimuli signal through cell surface plasma membrane receptors, for example, RTKs.

Through a variety of adaptor proteins, these signals cause guanine nucleotide exchange factors to replace the GDP-bound to inactive Ras with GTP. GAPs trigger the hydrolysis of GTP back to the inactive GDP-bound form. GTP-bound Ras binds to a plethora of downstream effector molecules to stimulate intracellular signaling of several pathways. Those with established roles in Ras oncogenesis include the Raf serine/threonine kinases, the PI3K lipid kinases, Ral GEFs, and Tiam1. Activation of these pathways and others has been shown to cause changes in many mechanisms leading to transformation, invasion, and metastasis.

Reprinted with permission from Elsevier.[27]

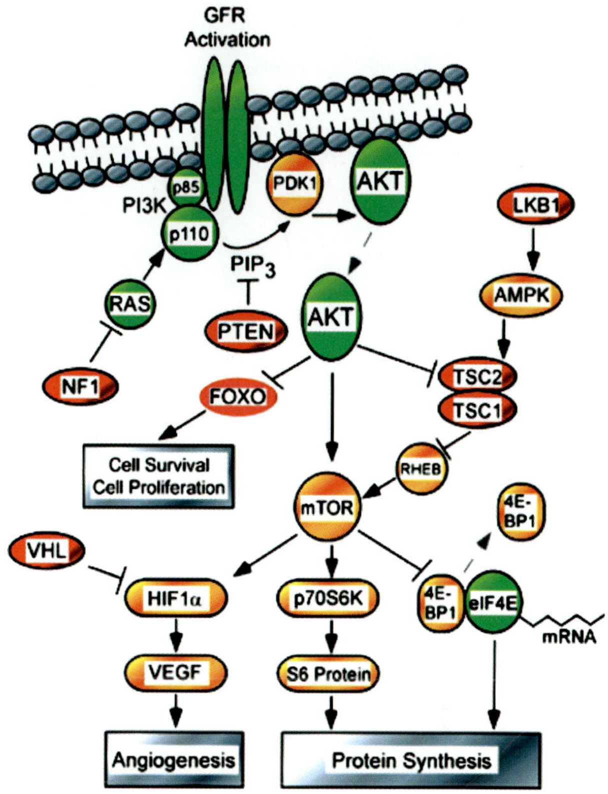

FIG. 2-16 Alterations of the AKT pathway in human cancer.

Activation of growth factor receptors (GFRs) such as the epidermal growth factor receptor, either by ligand stimulation or receptor overexpression/mutation, is one of the major mechanisms responsible for upregulation of AKT signaling. Other common mechanisms include activation of oncoproteins and inactivation of tumor suppressors intersecting the AKT signal transduction pathway. Proteins shown in green indicate oncoproteins for which overexpression and/or activating mutations have been implicated in many sporadic human cancers. Proteins in red are tumor suppressors whose loss and/or inactivation have been found to contribute to deregulation of the AKT pathway and tumor formation. FOXO transcription factors (shown in pink) have also been implicated as tumor suppressors (see text), although mutations have not been observed in any hereditary cancer syndrome to date.

Adapted by permission from Macmillan Publishers Ltd: Altomare DA, Testa JR. Pertubations of the AKT signaling pathway in human cancer. *Oncogene.* 2005;24(50):7455–7464.

coordinate cell growth, DNA replication, and cell division (Fig. 2-17).[33] G1 phase is a period of cell growth between mitosis and the onset of DNA synthesis (or between cell cycle re-entry and DNA synthesis in quiescent cells) during which cells respond to mitogenic signals and commit to the onset of DNA replication. S-phase is the period of DNA synthesis during which a cell replicates its genomic complement. G2 phase follows S-phase and is a second period of cell growth. Finally, during M phase, chromosomes are segregated and the cell divides into two daughters. Although this sequence of events describes most cell cycles, there are exceptions. For example, megakaryocytes become polyploid by undergoing repeated S-phases without mitosis. Moreover, most somatic cells at any given time have withdrawn from the cell cycle and are said to be in G0 phase, or quiescent.

It is critically important that cells execute the cell division cycle faithfully, and mutations in the genes that regulate the cell cycle are among the most common genetic changes in cancer cells.[34] A group of enzymes, termed the cyclin-dependent kinases (CDKs), orchestrates cell cycle progression. CDK holoenzymes are composed of two subunits: a catalytic subunit (the CDK) and a regulatory subunit (the cyclin) that activates the CDK. Mammalian genomes contain approximately a dozen cyclins and eight CDKs, and each cell cycle phase contains a unique profile of cyclin-CDK activities. In general, it is the cyclin subunits that are regulated during the cell cycle, and they exhibit binding preferences for specific CDKs.

In human cells, the primary cyclins during G1 phase are the D-type and E-type cyclins, and these activate CDK4/6 and CDK2, respectively. Cyclin D and cyclin E are both regulated by mitogenic signaling pathways, and they couple mitogenic signaling to the cell division machinery. Cyclin-CDKs are serine/threonine kinases that regulate cell division by phosphorylating downstream substrates. The best known of these substrates is the retinoblastoma protein (pRb),

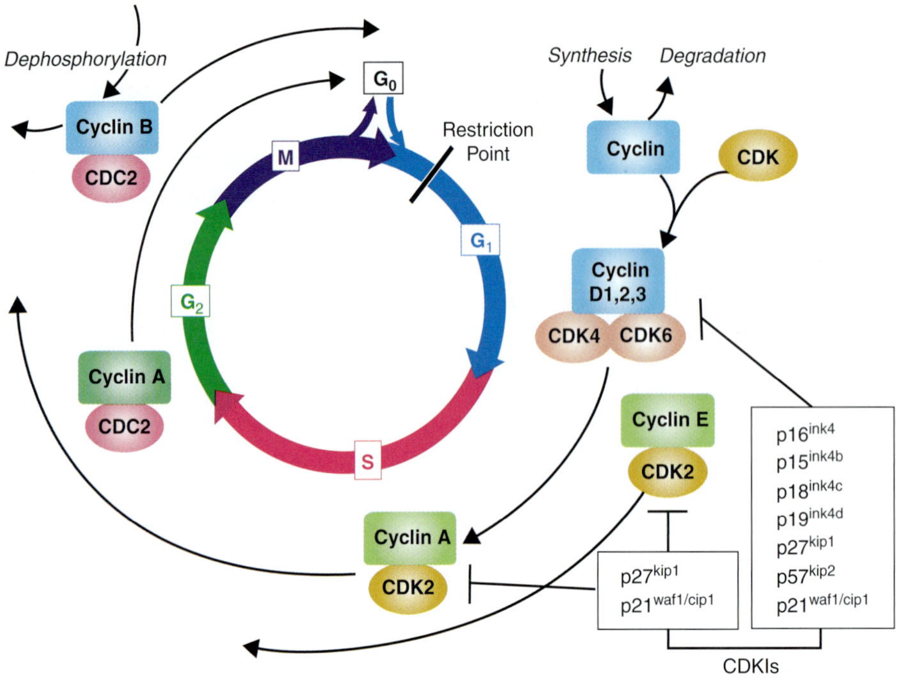

FIG. 2-17 The cell cycle.

The cell cycle is divided into four phases (G1, S, G2, and M). Progression through the cell cycle is promoted by cyclin-dependent kinases (CDKs), which are regulated positively by cyclins and negatively by CDK inhibitors (CDKIs). The restriction point is the point at which cells progress through the cell cycle independent of external stimuli.

Adapted from Schwartz G. Shah M. Targeting the cell cycle: A new approach to cancer therapy. *J Clin Oncol.* 2005; 23: 9408-9421.

which governs G1 progression; the *Rb* pathway is mutated in most cancer cells (Fig. 2-18). In resting cells, pRb is unphosphorylated and binds to E2F transcription factors, and this represses expression of *E2F* target genes. As G1 progresses, pRb is progressively phosphorylated, first by CDKs regulated by the D-type cyclins and then by cyclin E-CDK2. Ultimately, pRb phosphorylation causes it to release E2F, which then activates a transcriptional program that includes many genes involved in S-phase. Although regulation of pRb (and the related proteins p107 and p130) by the D-type cyclins is critical, cyclin E-CDK2 also phosphorylates many other proteins involved in cell processes such as histone biosynthesis, the centrosome cycle, and DNA replication.

Cyclin A and cyclin B govern cell cycle transitions beyond S-phase entry. Cyclin A associates with CDK2 and CDC2, and its activity is required for both S-phase and at the G2/M transition. Cyclin B binds to CDC2, and cyclin B-CDC2 is an essential regulator of mitotic entry and exit.

Two classes of CDK inhibitor proteins oppose cyclins and prevent CDK activity (Fig. 2-16).[35] The INK4 proteins (p15ink4b, p16ink4a, p18ink4c, and p19ink4d) inhibit only CDK4 and CDK6, whereas the Cip/Kip proteins (p21, p27, p57) are more broadly active and bind to most cyclin-CDKs. Cip/Kip proteins contain conserved regions that contain cyclin and CDK-binding motifs, as well as unique C-terminal regions that are involved in CDK-independent activities. For example, p21Cip1 binds to and regulates proliferating-cell nuclear antigen (PCNA), which is a processivity factor for DNA replication. In contrast, the p27Kip1 C-terminus regulates cell migration through its interactions with RhoA. CDK inhibitor proteins enforce cell cycle arrest in response to anti-mitogenic cues. For example, p27 is involved in cell cycle arrest after mitogen depletion, whereas p21 plays a key role in the cell cycle arrest imposed by p53 activation (discussed further).

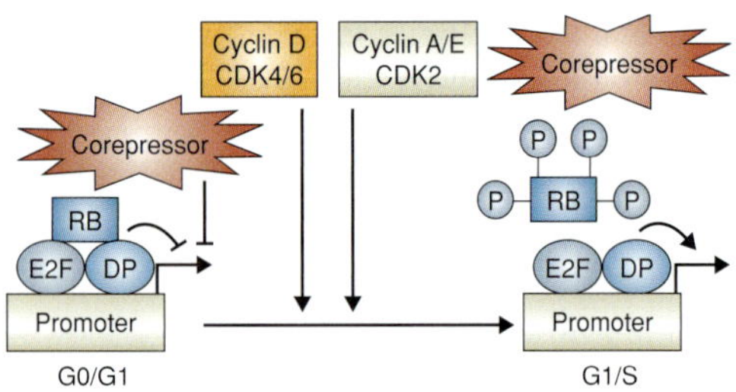

FIG. 2-18 RB and E2F function.

RB binds the transcription factor E2F and its associated subunit DP. RB represses E2F-mediated transcription by recruiting chromatin remodeling complexes to the promoter in resting cells. At the G1–S-phase transition, RB is thought to be phosphorylated by CDK2, CDK4, and CDK6. Hyperphosphorylated RB releases E2F, allowing it to activate transcription of its target genes.

Adapted by permission from Macmillan Publishers Ltd: Classon M, Harlow E. The retinoblastoma tumour suppressor in development and cancer. *Nat Rev Cancer.* 2002;2(12):910–917.

Cell cycle proteins that activate CDKs are proto-oncogenes that function as dominant oncogenes in cancers. The cyclin D1 gene is rearranged with the parathyroid hormone gene as a result of chromosome inversion in parathyroid adenomas, and it is translocated to the IgG heavy chain locus on chromosome 14 in mantle cell lymphomas, t(11;14). Both translocations render cyclin D1 expression independent of the mitogenic pathways that normally regulate its expression. The cyclin D1 gene also is amplified and overexpressed in 10% to 15% of solid tumors, such as breast and head and neck cancers. Cyclin E also is implicated as a dominant oncogene in many cancers. In some cases (e.g., breast cancer), the cyclin E gene is amplified. More commonly, however, cyclin E is oncogenically activated by disruption of its normal turnover pathway. Deregulated cyclin E activity causes genetic instability, which is thought to underlie its oncogenic activity. Cyclin E expression has been reported to function as an important indicator of outcome in some cancers, most notably early-stage breast cancer. Although less common, CDKs also can undergo oncogenic mutation. For example, a *CDK4* mutation that prevents its inhibition by INK4 proteins is involved in some cases of familial melanoma.

Genes encoding proteins that inhibit CDKs are recessive oncogenes, including CKIs and pRb itself. The INK4 proteins frequently exhibit allelic loss in cancers; *p15* and *p16* are linked and are often co-deleted, and p16 deletion occurs in many tumors including brain tumors, osteosarcoma, pediatric acute lymphoblastic leukemia, breast cancer, and head and neck cancer. Another potent tumor suppressor, termed ARF, also is contained within the p16 locus and contributes to the biologic selection for its allelic loss. In addition to deletions and point mutations, the *p16* gene also is epigenetically inactivated in tumors by promoter methylation, most notably in colon and lung cancers.

The p27Kip1 protein is an important human tumor suppressor, and p27 abundance has prognostic significance in many tumor types. p27 is an example of a tumor suppressor that is rarely mutated itself, but instead is inactivated by mutations in the pathways that regulate its degradation and/or subcellular localization. For example, p27 is mislocalized to the cytoplasm in breast cancers, and p27 degradation is accelerated in other tumors. In contrast, despite its central role in the p53 pathway, p21Cip1 is not a known tumor suppressor, highlighting the distinct biologic activities of these closely related proteins. Finally, pRb is the prototype tumor suppressor, and its role in hereditary retinoblastoma provided the basis for the Knudson's two-step model. Importantly, pRb is often mutated in sporadic cancers, such as lung cancer.

The realization that virtually all cancer cells contain mutations in the genes that regulate the cell cycle led to the widespread belief that drugs targeting cell cycle proteins, such as CDK inhibitors, would rapidly become important chemotherapeutic agents. However, this promise has not yet been fulfilled.

APOPTOSIS

Tumor growth is a consequence of both unrestrained cell division and decreased cell death, and the pathways that mediate cell death contain proto-oncogenes that are mutated in cancers. Programmed cell death, or apoptosis, is a physiologic process whereby complex biochemical pathways mediate cell death without activating inflammatory pathways (Fig. 2-19).[36] There are two distinct pathways that trigger apoptosis. Cell death via the extrinsic pathway is signaled when ligands, such as tumor necrosis factor (TNF)-alpha and FAS-ligand, bind to cell-surface death receptors, such as TNF-R1 and FAS. Ligand binding to death receptors then initiates a sequence of events leading to activation of proteases, termed caspases, that execute the apoptotic response. In contrast, the intrinsic or mitochondrial pathway results from a number of adverse stimuli, such as radiation therapy or chemotherapy, and causes changes in the mitochondrial membrane that affect the release of cytochrome C into the cytoplasm. Like the extrinsic pathways, the intrinsic pathway also activates a caspase cascade that ultimately leads to DNA fragmentation and cell death.

The Bcl-2 family contains a number of related proteins that are critical regulators of apoptosis, and these proteins can be either proapoptotic (promote cell death) or antiapoptotic (promote cell survival).[37] Bcl-2 itself is an antiapoptotic protein that was first identified as the gene activated by the 14:18 translocation found in B-cell follicular lymphomas. Although the precise mechanisms by which BCL-2 prevents cell death are not fully elucidated, they involve interaction with proapoptotic family members, as well as with mitochondrial functions. One important function of BCL-2 overexpression in tumorigenesis is that it prevents the apoptosis normally induced by dominant oncogenes, such as c-Myc. The realization that BCL-2 prevents apoptosis was pivotal in the evolution of understanding of the relationship between apoptosis and cancer. Because of their potential to induce apoptosis in tumor cells, drugs that target the BCL-2 family are being widely studied in clinical trials. Many different strategies have been evaluated, including BCL-2 inhibition by antisense oligonucleotides (oblimersen) and small-molecule inhibitors of BCL-2 proteins (e.g., ABT-737).[38]

Many oncogenes affect core apoptotic pathways. The most common mutations that impair apoptosis in tumors are those involving the *p53* tumor suppressor gene. Apoptosis is one critical outcome of p53 activation by cellular stresses, and impaired cell death is an extremely important consequence of p53 loss in tumors. Another frequently mutated cancer pathway that negatively regulates apoptosis is the PI3-kinase-AKT pathway (see Fig. 2-16). AKT interactions with apoptotic pathways are complex and include direct effects on the mitochondrial membrane, as well as on functional interactions with BCL-2 family members, FOXO transcription factors, nuclear factor-kappa B, and p53.[28,29]

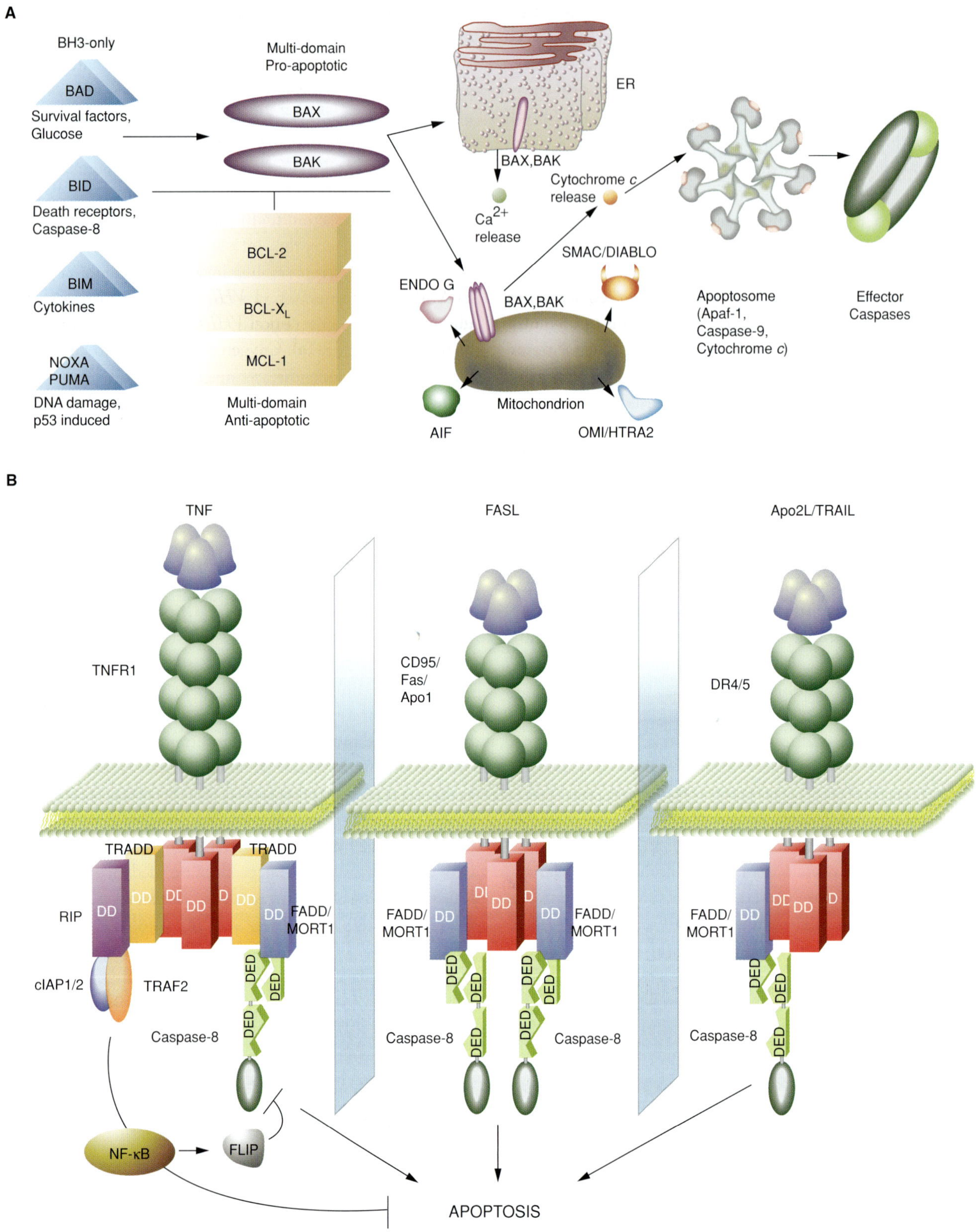

FIG. 2-19 **A.** The intrinsic apoptosis pathway. **B.** Extrinsic death receptor pathways.

The distinct composition of the Death-Inducing-Signaling Complex (DISC) downstream of the various death receptors TNFR1, CD95, and DR4/5 is illustrated.

Reprinted with permission from Elsevier.[36]

UBIQUITIN-MEDIATED PROTEOLYSIS

Many short-lived proteins are degraded in a proteolytic structure called the proteasome. Conjugation of a protein to ubiquitin is the signal for its delivery to the proteasome, and this is accomplished in a multistep reaction in which ubiquitin is ultimately transferred to lysine side chains of the target protein (Fig. 2-20).[39,40] Ubiquitin, a 76-amino acid protein, is first attached to a ubiquitin-activating enzyme, called E1, and then transferred to one of a family of carrier proteins called E2, or ubiquitin-conjugating enzymes. Each of the E2 enzymes recognizes and transfers ubiquitin only to particular proteins, thereby imposing some degree of selectivity on the process of ubiquitin-dependent proteolysis. Further selectivity arises from the fact that conjugation of many proteins to ubiquitin requires collaboration between an E2 and another enzyme called an E3, or ubiquitin ligase. Cells contain a large number of E3, and these often recognize their targets after they have been modified by specific signals (e.g., phosphorylation). The ubiquitin-proteasome system thus affords an enormous amount of regulated control over protein degradation.

E3s are classed into several groups based on shared structural motifs, which include the RING and HECT type ubiquitin ligases. Perhaps the most commonly mutated E3 ligase pathway in cancers involves Mdm2, a HECT-type ubiquitin ligase that degrades the p53 tumor suppressor. RING-finger type E3 complexes also are tumor suppressors. The Von Hippel-Lindau (VHL) syndrome is an autosomal dominant hereditary cancer syndrome in which affected individuals develop renal cell carcinoma, central nervous system hemangioblastomas, pheochromocytoma, pancreatic tumors, and other neoplasms. The *VHL* gene is located on 3p25 and was cloned in 1993. VHL disease is diagnosed by the presence of germ-line inactivating *VHL* mutations, and the remaining allele is inactivated in tumors by mutation. Importantly, the *VHL* gene also is implicated in most spontaneous renal cell carcinomas, which have allelic loss at 3p and *VHL* mutations. *VHL* functions as the substrate recognition component of an ECV RING finger E3, and *VHL* mutations inactivate this ubiquitin ligase.[41] One critical *VHL* target is hypoxia-inducible factor-1 alpha (HIF-1a). Oxygen causes HIF-1 to be hydroxylated on proline, which generates the VHL binding site and facilitates HIF-1a degradation. HIF-1a is a transcription factor that regulates genes in response to hypoxia, many of which promote angiogenesis. The angiogenic transcription program of HIF-1a may underlie the highly vascular tumors associated with VHL loss; these findings provide a rationale for trials involving agents that target angiogenesis for patients with renal cell carcinoma.

Fbw7/hCdc4 is another RING finger ubiquitin ligase that is a tumor suppressor. Fwb7 is the substrate recognition

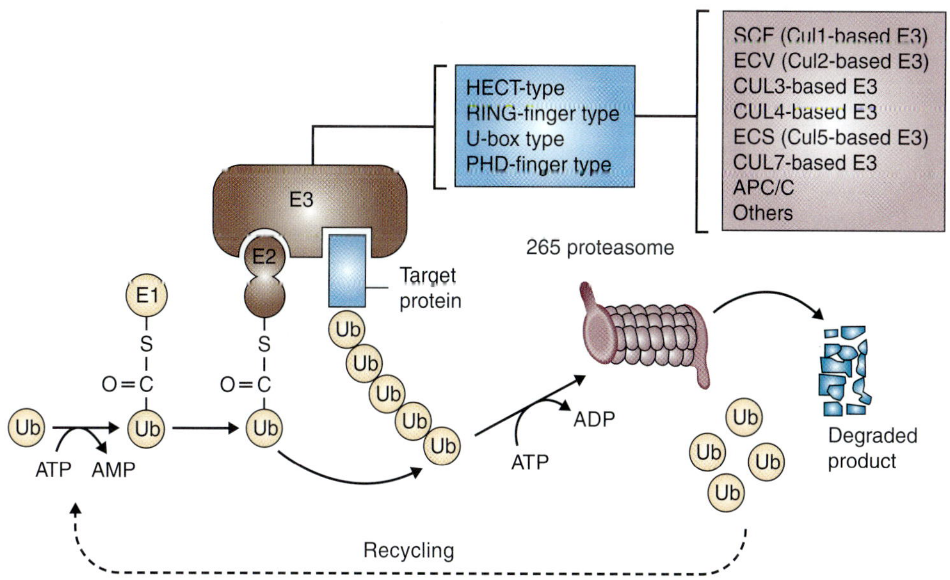

FIG. 2-20 Overview of the ubiquitin-proteasome pathway.

Ubiquitin (Ub) is a small protein that is first transferred to the ubiquitin-activating enzyme, E1, in an ATP-dependent manner. This activated ubiquitin is then transferred to the ubiquitin-conjugating enzyme, E2. Finally, the ubiquitin is covalently attached to the target protein by an E3 ubiquitin ligase, leading to formation of a polyubiquitin chain. The polyubiquitinated protein is recognized by the 26S proteasome and is destroyed in an ATP-dependent manner. There are many E3 ubiquitin ligases, which are categorized into four major classes: HECT-type, RING-finger type, U-box type, and PHD-finger type. RING-finger ligases are further divided into subfamilies, including cullin-based E3s. There are seven cullin-based E3s including the SCF-type ligases and the anaphase-promoting complex/cyclosome (APC/C).

Adapted by permission from Macmillan Publishers Ltd: Nakayama KI, Nakayama K. Ubiquitin ligases: Cell-cycle control and cancer. *Nat Rev Cancer.* 2006;6(5):369–381.

KEY POINTS

- Enzymes that promote degradation by the proteasome can function as tumor suppressors.
- Genes that regulate cellular differentiation are often mutated in hematologic cancers.
- DNA repair pathways contain many tumor suppressor genes.
- Different types of DNA repair lesions are associated with specific cancer syndromes.

component of ligase complexes that target several proto-oncogenes for degradation, including cyclin E, c-Myc, Notch, and c-Jun. In each case, these proteins are degraded after they are phosphorylated within conserved motifs called phosphodegrons, and this creates the Fbw7 binding signal. Fbw7 is located in 4q32, a region that is frequently mutated in solid tumors and in T-cell acute lymphoblastic leukemia. Fbw7 sustains both homozygous and single-allelic loss in cancers, and evidence in mice suggests that Fbw7 may function as a haploinsufficient tumor suppressor.

Pharmacologic proteasome inhibitors are in clinical trials; one compound, bortezomib, is approved for use in multiple myeloma. However, the mechanism(s) that account for the therapeutic index associated with proteasome inhibitors remains unclear because these compounds will affect a very large number of proteins normally degraded by the proteasome.

DIFFERENTIATION

Most somatic cells are in a terminally differentiated, postmitotic state, and differentiation is regulated by complex transcriptional pathways. Many proto-oncogenes affect pathways that regulate differentiation; these often are transcription factors and/or coactivators involved in leukemias and lymphomas.[42] One important proto-oncogene directly dysregulated or mutated in differentiation is the retinoic acid receptor (RAR)-alpha, which is rearranged in several translocations found in acute promyelocytic leukemia, most commonly t(15:17), which produces a PML-RAR-alpha fusion protein (Fig. 2-21). These fusion proteins act as "dominant negative" mutants that inhibit RAR-alpha target genes by recruiting co-repressors. This dominant negative RAR-alpha is targeted by all-trans retinoic acid (ATRA), which is used in conjunction with combination chemotherapy to induce remission in patients with APL. ATRA binds to the dominant negative fusion protein and prevents it from bringing co-repressors to RAR-alpha target genes. ATRA treatment thus reverses the differentiation block caused by the translocation product and allows promyelocytes to proceed down their differentiation pathway.

Core-binding factor (CBF) is another transcription factor that regulates hematopoietic differentiation and is commonly mutated by translocations in leukemias. Both components of CBF (RUNX1/AML1 and CBF-beta) are involved in translocations found in acute leukemia. Like RAR-alpha, these translocations produce dominant negative proteins that inhibit CBF target gene expression, which is thought to impair hematopoietic cell differentiation.

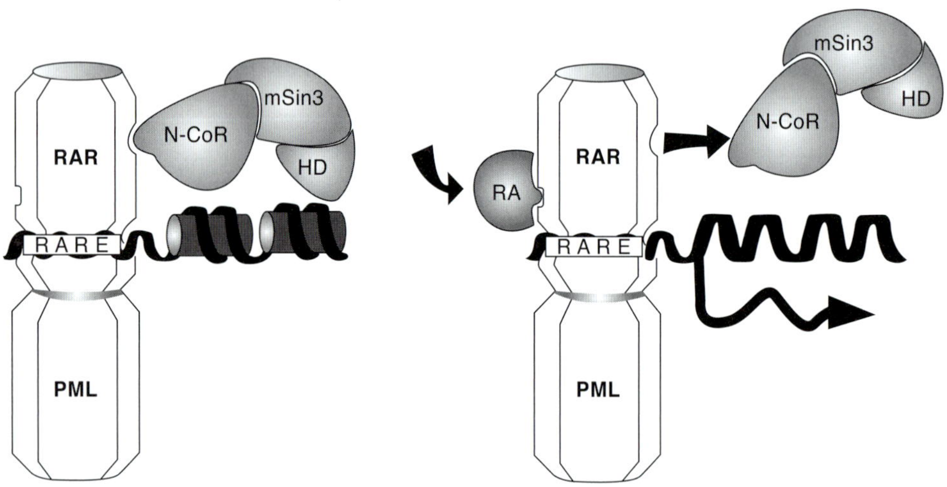

FIG. 2-21 A model for the interactions of APL fusion proteins with the N-CoR–mSin3–histone deacetylase (HD) complex.

DNA-bound PML–RARalpha interacts with N-CoR (or SMRT) and recruits the mSin3–HD complex, decreasing histone acetylation and producing repressive chromatin organization and transcriptional repression. RA induces dissociation of the N-CoR–mSin3-HD complex, recruitment of coactivators with histone acetyltransferase activity (not shown), increased levels of histone acetylation, chromatin remodeling, and transcriptional activation.

Adapted by permission from Macmillan Publishers Ltd: Grignani F, De Matteis S, Nervi C, et al. Fusion proteins of the retinoic acid receptor-alpha recruit histone deacetylase in promyelocytic leukemia. *Nature.* 1998;391(6669):815–818.

The Notch genes comprise a proto-oncogene family involved in cell-fate and differentiation pathways.[43] Notch genes encode transmembrane receptors that stimulate transcriptional programs after they bind to ligands. Ligand binding causes Notch proteins to be cleaved, forming intracellular domains that translocate to the nucleus. Notch proteins play important roles in lymphoid differentiation and are implicated in hematologic cancers. *Notch1* was first described as a oncogene by virtue of its involvement in the t(7;9) translocation found in a subset of patients with T-cell acute lymphoblastic leukemia. However, more recent studies have found *Notch1* mutations in up to 50% of patients with this disease, and these mutations are predicted to upregulate Notch activity and abundance.[44] The precise mechanisms through which Notch promotes leukemia are unknown, but they are thought to involve impaired differentiation and enhanced self-renewal. Recent data suggest that c-Myc is a critical downstream mediator of Notch activity.

DNA REPAIR PATHWAYS

Mammalian cells use three major DNA-repair pathways to maintain genomic integrity. Mutations that disrupt these pathways cause genetic instability and are associated with diseases characterized by sensitivity to DNA-damaging agents and predisposition to cancer. Ultraviolet light-induced nucleotide dimers and other DNA adducts are recognized and repaired by the nucleotide excision repair (NER) pathway. DNA-recombination repair is involved in the restoration of double-stranded breaks induced by ionizing radiation and radiomimetic agents. Finally, the DNA mismatch repair pathways correct errors during DNA replication by the removal of the mismatched strand and subsequent repair of the single-stranded patch.

NUCLEOTIDE EXCISION REPAIR PATHWAY

The nucleotide excision repair (NER) pathways correct nucleotide lesions induced by ultraviolet light and other adducts, such as those induced by chemical carcinogens.[44] There are two distinct NER pathways: a global repair pathway and a transcription-coupled repair pathway that repairs DNA damage that occurs during transcription. Mutations affecting these pathways give rise to sun-sensitive and developmental disorders, including xeroderma pigmentosum, Cockayne syndrome, and trichothiodystrophy. Xeroderma pigmentosum is an autosomal-recessive disorder with an estimated incidence rate of one out of 70,000 cases. Affected individuals have progressive neurodegeneration, extreme sensitivity to ultraviolet light, abnormalities in skin pigmentation, and a predisposition to skin cancer. Approximately one-half of affected individuals have clinical symptoms by the age of 18 months, and the average age at the time of skin cancer is 8 years. The risk of skin cancer is estimated to be 2,000 times higher than that for the general population. Eight genes have been associated with xeroderma pigmentosum. Seven of them code for excision-repair proteins, and one (xeroderma pigmentosum variant) is a DNA polymerase that is required for accurate replication of damaged DNA. In contrast, Cockayne syndrome is associated with two genes, *CSA* and *CSB*, that are involved in transcription-coupled DNA repair, and trichothiodystrophy is caused by mutation of either *ERCC2/XPD* or *ERCC3/XPB*, which encode helicase subunits of the TFIIH transcription complex. Neither Cockayne syndrome nor trichothiodystrophy is associated with an increased cancer risk.

DOUBLE-STRAND BREAK REPAIR

Damage to DNA by radiation, chemicals (such as chemotherapy), and other insults produces double-strand breaks that are recognized and repaired by a coordinated response that involves the products of many tumor suppressor genes. The loss of function of some of these genes can cause inherited syndromes that have highly variable clinical manifestations. Ataxia telangiectasia is an autosomal recessive disorder characterized by progressive cerebellar ataxia, telangiectasia, and immunodeficiency. Tumors, most commonly T-cell neoplasms, develop in more than one-third of homozygous individuals. The ataxia telangiectasia gene (*ATM*) encodes a large protein kinase with homology to phosphitidylinositol-3 kinases.[45] *ATM* is activated by serine phosphorylation in response to DNA breaks and phosphorylates a number of downstream substrates that play critical roles in DNA repair and checkpoint pathways includ ing CHK2, p53, BRCA1, and NBS1 (Fig 2-22).[46] Cells derived from patients with ataxia telangiectasia exhibit increased DNA damage after radiation therapy, as well as defects in normal cell cycle responses to DNA damage, called checkpoints.

Fanconi anemia is an autosomal-recessive disease characterized by developmental abnormalities, bone marrow failure, and susceptibility to cancers, particularly acute myeloid leukemia, squamous cell cancer of the head and neck, gynecologic cancers, and esophageal cancer. The disease is typically fatal, and the mean survival is 16 years. Similar to ataxia telangiectasia, cells derived from patients with Fanconi anemia display abnormal chromosomal breakage. However, Fanconi anemia cells are not hypersensitive to ionizing radiation, rather they are hypersensitive to DNA cross-linking by agents such as diepoxybutane (DEB) and mitomycin C. Classic studies defined many distinct FA complementation groups, and 13 FA genes have now been cloned. Remarkably, many of these proteins (A, B, C, E, F, G, L, M) form a complex that catalyzes the monoubiquitination of two FA proteins, FANCD2 and the recently discovered FANCI.[47,48] Monoubiquitinated FANCD2 and FANCI become localized to nuclear foci after DNA damage, and these foci also contain FANCD1 (identical with the BRCA2 breast cancer gene) and other proteins discussed above, including BRCA1 and NBS1 (Fig. 2-23). The FA pathway is activated by and required for the cellular response to stalled replication forks.

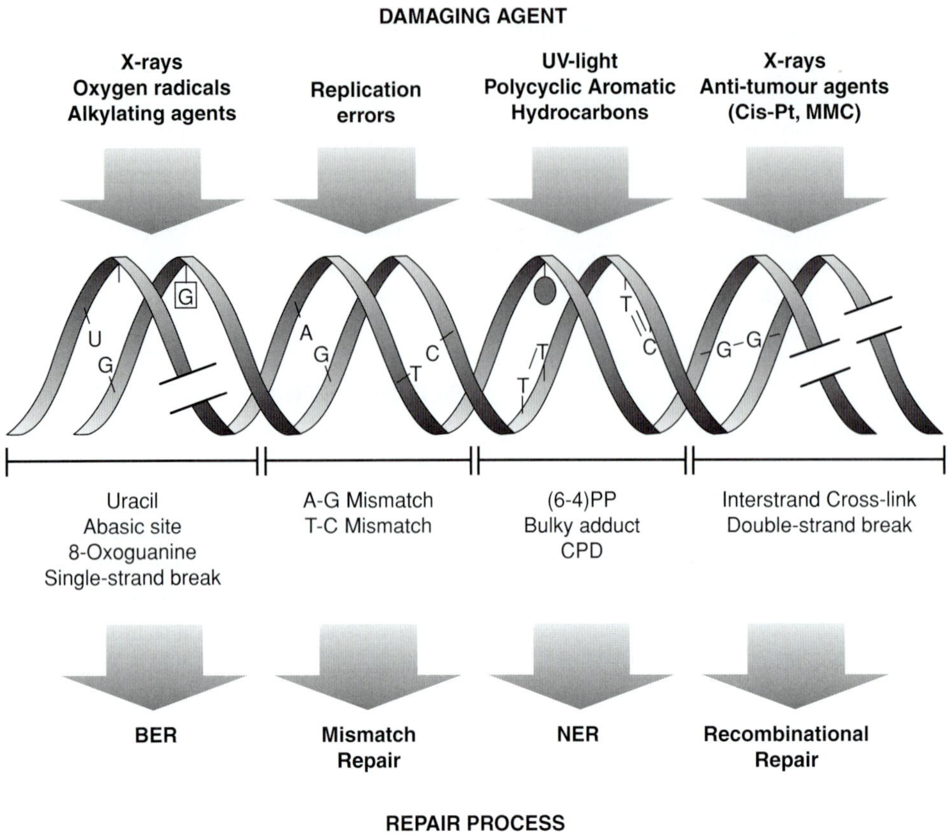

FIG. 2-22 DNA lesions and repair mechanisms.[46]

(Top) Common DNA damaging agents. (Middle) Examples of lesions that can be introduced by these agents into the DNA double helix. (Bottom) The most frequently used repair mechanisms for such lesions. Not depicted but important to realize is that distinct damaging sources can induce similar types of DNA lesions, that one agent in general induces more than one type of damage, and that the lesion spectrum of different repair pathways may overlap. DNA lesions and repair mechanisms. Abbreviations: NER, nucleotide excision repair; BER, base excision repair.

The striking intersection of the BRCA1 and FA pathways underscores the central importance of this DNA damage sensing and repair mechanism in the development of human cancers.

The Nbs1 protein is another component of nuclear repair foci implicated in a chromosomal breakage syndrome. Nijmegen breakage syndrome is an autosomal-recessive disease characterized by microcephaly, immunodeficiency, and increased frequency of hematopoietic cancers that is caused by mutations in the *NBS1* gene. NBS1 forms a complex with MRE11 and RAD50, which binds to BRCA1 in nuclear foci. Deficiency of the NBS1 protein blocks the formation of the MRE11-NBS1-RAD50 complex, and this impairs the S-phase surveillance responses triggered by ATM. Accordingly, many of the symptoms of this disease are identical to symptoms of ataxia telangiectasia.

MISMATCH REPAIR

DNA mismatch repair (MMR) corrects errors that occur during DNA replication, primarily single base mismatches, or short insertions or deletions.[49] DNA mismatches are recognized and corrected by a complex of proteins that binds to the mismatch, identify the correct DNA strand, and then excise and repair the mismatch. Several of the proteins involved in MMR are tumor suppressors that are involved in hereditary nonpolyposis colon cancer (HNPCC). Patients with HNPCC/Lynch Syndrome develop colon cancer at an early age, as well as cancers in many other organ sites. The two most commonly mutated MMR genes in Lynch syndrome are *MSH2* and *MLH1*. *MSH2* is involved with the initial recognition of the mismatch, whereas *MLH1* helps to discriminate which DNA strand contains the correct sequence. Mutations in other MMR genes are less commonly associated with HNPCC and include *MSH6*, *PMS1*, and *PMS2*. Patients with HNPCC inherit a nonfunctional MMR gene allele with subsequent loss of the remaining allele in a somatic cell that will ultimately give rise to a tumor. Importantly, the impaired MMR causes a hypermutable phenotype as evidenced by microsatellite instability (MSI). MSI is

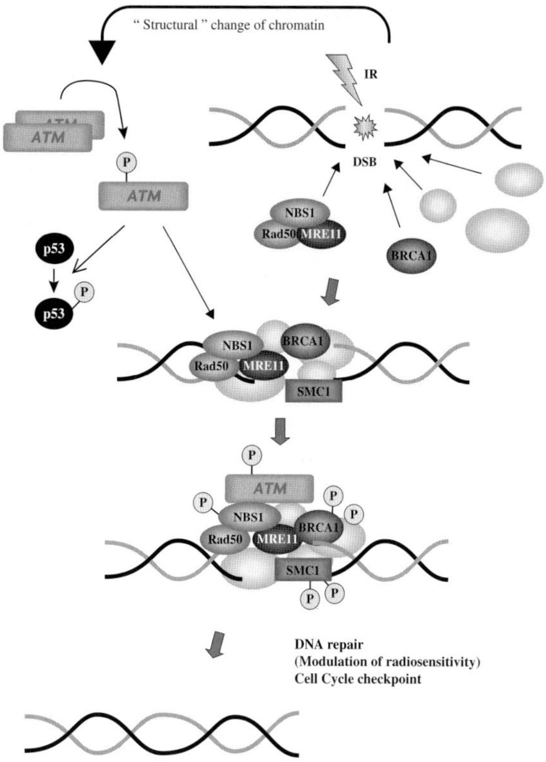

FIG. 2-23 Model for an ionizing radiation (IR)-induced signaling pathway.[45]

Chromatin structure changes caused by DNA breakage or other mechanisms lead to ATM autophosphorylation and activation. If DNA strand breaks are present, several proteins, including NBS1 and BRCA1, are recruited to the sites of the damage, independent of ATM. Activated ATM can phosphorylate substrates, such as p53, and if Nbs1 and BRCA1 are localized to the DBA breaks, activated ATM is recruited.

readily detected in tumors by PCR-based assays that reveal novel tumor-specific microsatellite fragments. Although microsatellite instability is the hallmark of HNPCC, it also is found in a subset of sporadic colon cancers. However, in these cases, *MLH1* is silenced by promoter hypermethylation rather than mutation.

CHECKPOINTS: CROSSROADS OF DNA REPAIR CELL CYCLE REGULATION AND GENETIC INSTABILITY

The fidelity of the enzymes that replicate DNA and segregate chromosomes is largely responsible for the accurate propagation of genetic information. However, these enzymes have an intrinsic error rate, and the frequency of errors is increased by genotoxic insults, such as chemical mutagens and ionizing radiation. Normal cells continually monitor DNA replication and mitosis, and stop the cell cycle if these do not occur correctly, allowing the damage to be repaired before proliferation resumes. The pathways that cause progression throughout the cell cycle to be dependent on the accurate execution of prior cell cycle events are called checkpoints.[50]

Mammalian cells have checkpoints that operate in each phase of the cell cycle, and these checkpoint pathways are intricately interwoven with the cell cycle and DNA repair machinery.[51-53] Moreover, there is substantial overlap between the components of the various checkpoint pathways. The G1 and G2 checkpoints recognize DNA damage that occurs during these cell cycle phases and initiate responses leading to either cell cycle arrest or cell death. In addition to DNA damage, the S-phase checkpoint also is activated by stresses that inhibit the proper function of the replication machinery. Enormous progress has been made in understanding the biochemistry of checkpoint pathways, although many questions still remain.

Checkpoint pathways may be broadly viewed as being composed of sensors/mediators, signal transducers, and effectors (Fig. 2-24). The sensors and mediators detect DNA damage and involve complexes (e.g., Rad9-Hus1-Rad1 and Mre1-Rad50-Nbs1), as well as proteins that accumulate in DNA repair foci (e.g., BRCA1, claspin, and FANCD2). The DNA damage signal is then transmitted by signal-transducing kinases that include ATM and ATR, and subsequently by downstream kinases, such as CHK1 and CHK2 (Fig. 2-25). Finally, the transducing kinases activate effectors, such as p53 and Cdc25, directly affect the cell cycle machinery, and block cell division through inhibition of cyclin-CDK activity.

FIG. 2-24 Schematic interaction of the FA pathway.

Protein complex 1 contains the A, B, C, E, F, G, L, M, and possibly I subunits. Protein complex 2 contains FANCD2-Ub, BRCA2, and possibly FANCJ. During S phase, when a replication fork encounters a DNA cross-link, the FA complex (complex 1) is activated. This activation leads to the monoubiquitination of FANCD2, which is then targeted to chromatin containing the cross-link. FANCD2-Ub then interacts with BRCA2 in complex 2, leading to repair of the cross-link possibly through HR and TLS. FANCD2 is deubiquitinated by USP1, thereby inactivating the pathway.

Reprinted with permission from Cold Spring Harbor Laboratory Press, 2005.[48]

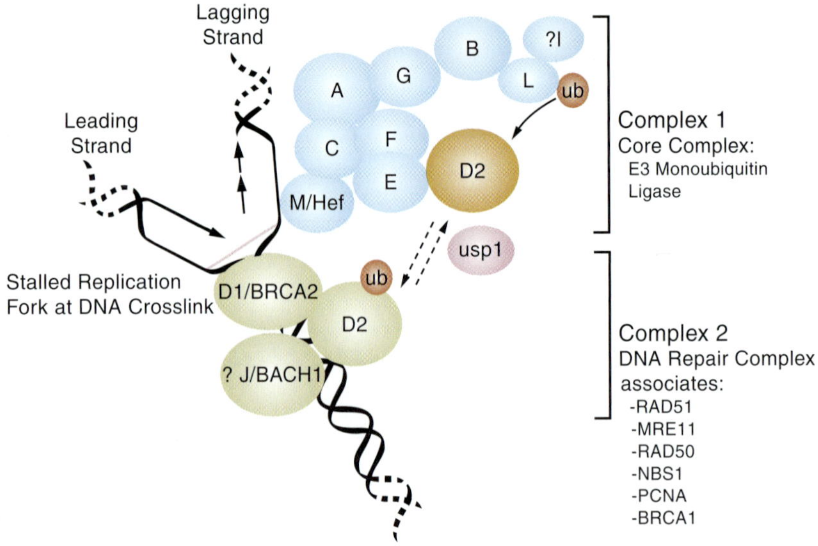

Checkpoint pathways are disrupted in most, and perhaps all, cancers. Impaired checkpoint function causes genetic instability, which drives tumor progression because the increased error rate allows mutations to accumulate in additional cancer genes. The p53 protein plays a central role in checkpoint pathways, and it is the most frequently mutated human tumor suppressor gene. Although *p53* is mutated in up to one-half of all spontaneous cancers, its role as a tumor suppressor first came to light in studies of patients with Li-Fraumeni syndrome (LFS), a rare autosomal disorder associated with the development of a wide variety of early-onset cancers, including soft tissue and bone sarcomas, as well as breast, brain, and colon cancers. p53 is a transcription factor that is activated by many triggers, including DNA damage and replication stress. When p53 is activated by signals such as DNA damage, the outcome can be cell cycle arrest, apoptosis, or cellular senescence; these alternate outcomes depend on many factors.[54–56] p53 largely accomplishes these outcomes by activating transcription of its target genes, although p53 also may play a role independent of transcription. One critical p53 target is the p21Cip CDK inhibitor; increased p21 abundance plays an essential role in G1 arrest signaled by p53 after DNA damage. Tumors most commonly inactivate p53 by loss of heterozygosity and intragenic point mutants that fall within critical p53 functional domains, and a large number of *p53* mutations have been catalogued.

Another mechanism of p53 loss in tumors involves the Mdm2 ubiquitin ligase (Fig. 2-26). Mdm2 expression is induced by p53, and it functions in a feedback loop to down-regulate p53 by catalyzing its ubiquitination. The normal Mdm2-p53 regulatory circuit is disrupted in many cancers. Mdm2 is overexpressed in a wide spectrum of neoplasms, and this leads to decreased p53 abundance and function. A second mechanism that targets this pathway involves the ARF tumor suppressor.[57] As discussed previously, ARF is encoded within the same gene as the p16Ibk44a protein and is frequently deleted in cancers. ARF normally binds to Mdm2, which prevents Mdm2 from degrading p53. However, when ARF is deleted, Mdm2 activity is unrestrained, causing p53 to be degraded. ARF expression is induced by oncogenes such as Myc and plays an important role in p53 activation by oncogenic signaling. Thus loss of ARF disables an important protective mechanism against oncogenic transformation.

There is enormous interest in developing cancer treat-

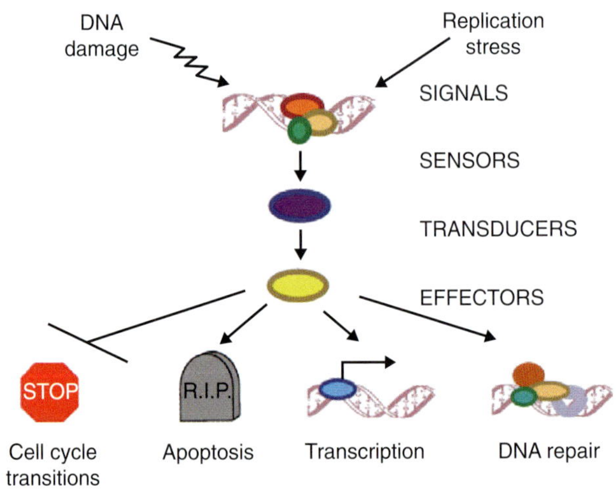

FIG. 2-25 A general outline of the DNA damage response signal-transduction pathway.

Arrowheads represent activating events and perpendicular ends represent inhibitory events. Cell-cycle arrest is depicted with a stop sign, apoptosis with a tombstone. The DNA helix with an arrow represents damage-induced transcription, while the DNA helix with several oval-shaped subunits represents damage-induced repair. For the purpose of simplicity, the network of interacting pathways are depicted as a linear pathway consisting of signals, sensors/mediators, transducers, and effectors.

Adapted by permission from Macmillan Publishers Ltd: Zhou BB, Elledge SJ. The DNA damage response: Putting checkpoints in perspective. *Nature*. 2000;408(6811):433–439.

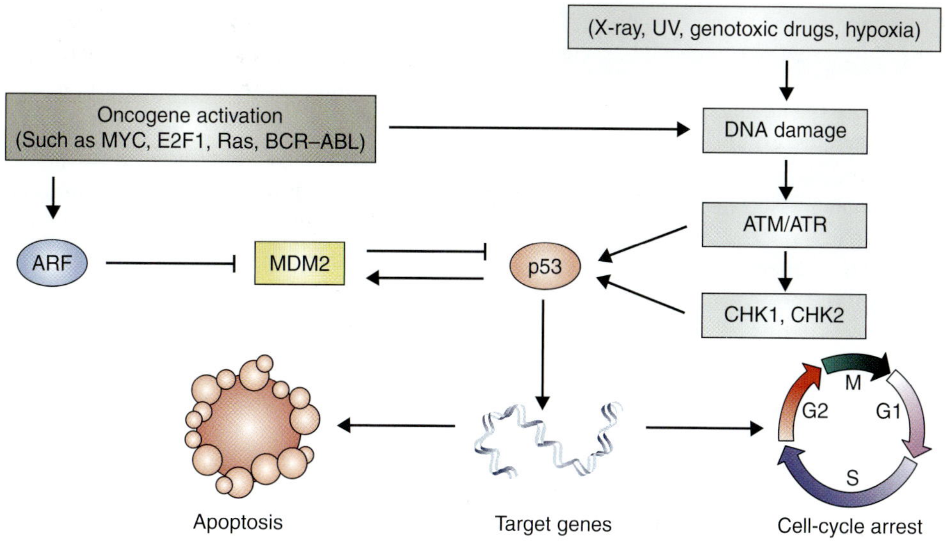

FIG. 2-26 The p53-MDM2-ARF network.

The activation of p53 classically occurs in response to many other cellular stresses that produce DNA damage, including oncogene-induced stress. Depending on the nature of the inducing signal, these DNA-damage responses activate the kinase mutated in the ataxia telangiectasia syndrome (ATM) and/or the ATM and Rad3-related kinase (ATR). These kinases phosphorylate p53 directly and also indirectly through the agency of the CHK kinases. These phosphorylations have an important role in increasing the transcriptional activity of p53. Target genes induced by p53 can generate different biologic outcomes depending on the tissue type and convergence of different activating signals. Sustained and increased signaling thresholds induced by mutated or overexpressed oncogenes activate the ARF promoter. Once expressed, the ARF protein interferes with the activity of MDM2, leading to p53 stabilization and the triggering of a complex p53-dependent transcriptional program mediated by hundreds of target genes. MDM2 is not only a negative regulator of p53-dependent transcription and turnover, but is also a canonical p53-activated gene that has a key role in negative-feedback regulation of the p53 response.

Adapted by permission from Macmillan Publishers Ltd: Sherr CJ. Divorcing ARF and p53: An unsettled case. *Nat Rev Cancer.* 2006;6(9):663–673.

ment strategies that target the p53 pathway. In fact, recent studies in model systems demonstrating the antitumor activity of p53 restoration in tumors has re-energized this active field.[58] Strategies that target the p53 pathway range from peptides that restore p53 function in cells with mutant p53 proteins to recombinant adenoviruses (e.g., Onyx-015) that selectively kill cells with *p53* mutations. However, the scope of these approaches is too great to be covered in detail here, and many reviews address this large field.[59]

The mitotic or spindle assembly checkpoint ensures that chromosomes are equally segregated to daughter cells during mitosis, and it is an extremely important safeguard against aneuploidy. The spindle apparatus is composed of tubulin and attaches to chromosomes via their kinetochores during mitosis. In a normal cell, the signal that activates the spindle checkpoint is generated by kinetochores that are unattached or have insufficient spindle tension, which delays mitosis and ensures that chromosome separation does not occur in situations where the daughter cells may receive an abnormal chromosome content because of misalignment (Fig. 2-27).[60] A number of spindle checkpoint proteins accumulate at the unattached kinetochore, including Bub1, BubR1, Mad1, and Mad2. This complex blocks mitosis by sending a poorly understood signal that inhibits the anaphase-promoting complex (APC), a RING-type E3 ubiquitin ligase that regulates mitotic entry and exit. Two critical APC targets that must be degraded for mitosis to proceed are cyclin B and securins (the latter function to hold together sister chromatids). The spindle checkpoint thus prevents mitosis in the setting of an improperly attached spindle by blocking the degradation of APC substrates. A number of chemotherapeutic agents target the spindle apparatus (e.g., taxanes and vinca alkaloids) and trigger the spindle checkpoint in normal cells. Although incompletely understood, the antitumor mechanism of these agents may involve, at least in part, defective spindle checkpoint control in tumor cells.

MULTISTEP TUMORIGENESIS

Carcinogenesis is a multistep process, and the development of fully malignant cancers requires many independent events. It is known that these steps involve the acquisition of mutations in cancer genes and that genetic instability allows these rare events to accumulate at a rate that ultimately gives rise to aggressive neoplasms. Although the specific mutations that cause human cancers vary greatly between types of cancers and individuals, the broad consequences of these mutations are abnormal phenotypes that are shared by most cancers. Weinberg and Hanahan[61] have proposed six essential

KEY POINTS

- Checkpoints ensure the fidelity of cell division and protect against genomic instability.
- Many tumor suppressor genes and DNA repair proteins are intimately associated with checkpoint pathways.
- The loss of checkpoint functions causes genomic instability and fosters the accumulation of multiple mutations in cancer cells.
- *p53* is the most commonly mutated cancer gene, and it participates in diverse checkpoint responses. *p53* senses cellular stress and signals to pathways that regulate processes such as cell cycle progression and apoptosis.
- Tumorigenesis is a multistep process that requires the accumulation of multiple mutations. All tumors share a number of attributes that contribute to their malignant phenotype, but the specific molecular events that produce these phenotypes vary greatly among tumor types and individuals.

capabilities found in tumor cells that encompass the "hallmarks of cancer." These include self-sufficiency in growth signals, insensitivity to antigrowth signals, evasion of apoptosis, limitless replicative potential, sustained angiogenesis, and tissue invasion and metastasis. These capabilities can be acquired in different sequences, and in some cases a single mutation might provide more than one capability (Fig. 2-28). Although this conceptual model is undoubtedly oversimplified, it provides an important framework with which to consider multistep carcinogenesis.

The first three of these "acquired capabilities" involve mutations within the genes that comprise the mitogenic signaling pathways, cell cycle machinery, and cell death pathways that have been outlined previously. The fourth category, limitless replicative potential, involves the acquisition of cellular immortality in tumors. Normal cells are limited in the number of times that they can divide, even when they are provided with all of the normal mitogenic stimuli required for cell division. In contrast, many cancer cells can divide with apparently limitless potential. One fundamental mechanism that limits human cell division involves the ends of chromosomes, which are called telomeres. Telomeres normally protect the ends of chromosomes, and they shorten with each cell division. Thus the length of a cell's telomeres reflects the number of divisions it has undergone. Eventually the telomeres are shortened to the point where they can no longer protect the chromosome ends, which leads to a condition termed crisis and, ultimately, to cell death. Unlike normal cells, cancer cells maintain their telomere length during cell division. This usually results from expression of the enzyme telomerase that adds DNA back to the telomere.

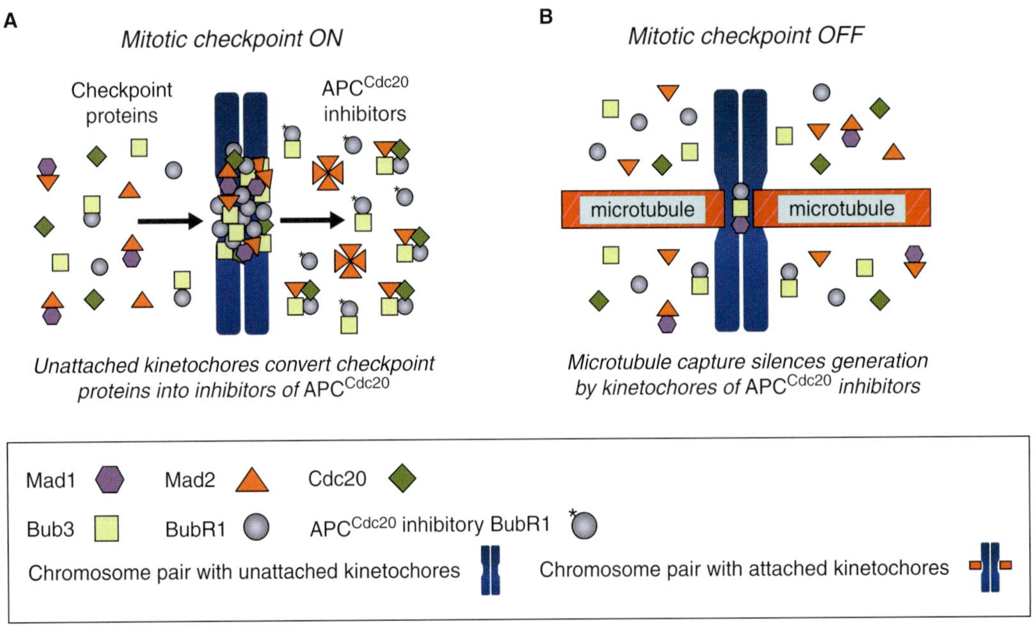

FIG. 2-27 Mitotic checkpoint signaling.

A. *Unattached kinetochores are the signal generators of the mitotic checkpoint. They recruit mitotic checkpoint proteins, including Mad1, Mad2, BubR1, and Bub3, and convert them into inhibitors of APCCdc20.*

B. *Once all kinetochores have made productive attachments to spindle microtubules, production of the APCCdc20 inhibitors is silenced.*

Reprinted with permission from Elsevier.[60]

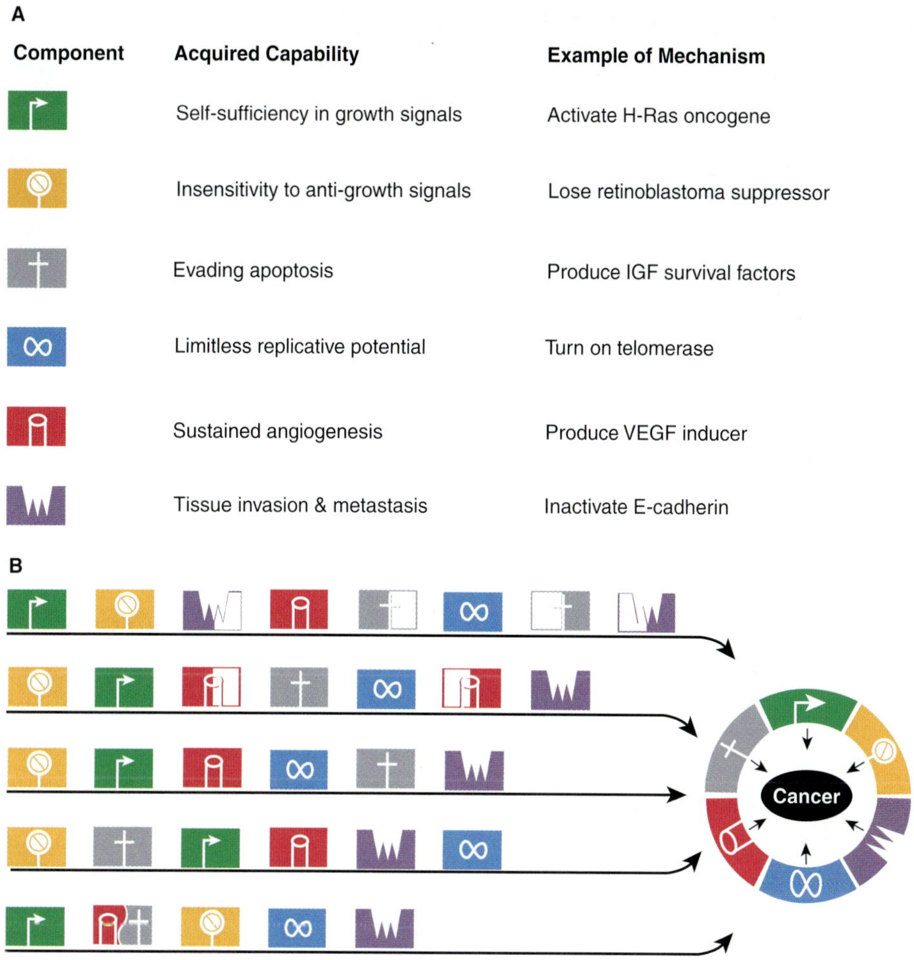

FIG. 2-28 Weinberg and Hanahan postulate that all cancers acquire the same six hallmark capabilities, but that their means of doing so may vary both mechanistically (panel A) and temporally (panel B). Thus the order in which these capabilities are acquired is highly variable across the spectrum of cancers. In some cases, a particular mutation may confer several capabilities (e.g., p53 mutation may facilitate resistance to apoptosis and angiogenesis), and thus fewer individual mutations are required to enable all six capabilities (the 5-step pathway shown). In other cases, multiple mutations may be required to enable a single capability (e.g., the 8-step pathway shown). Reprinted with permission from Elsevier

Telomerase activity can be detected in 85% to 90% of cancers, and the remainder of tumors maintain their telomeres through a different mechanism involving recombination.

The capability of sustained angiogenesis reflects the fact that tumors often outgrow their blood supply and must actively recruit vasculature in order to grow. In normal tissues, the development of new blood vessels is highly regulated by both positive and negative signals. Tumor cells promote angiogenesis by upregulating the pathways that promote blood vessel formation (e.g., increased expression of growth factors such as vascular endothelial and fibroblast growth factors) and by reducing the activity of inhibitory pathways. Some of these pathways involve transcriptional networks under the control of previously discussed genes, such as *VHL* mutations in renal cell carcinoma. The importance of these pathways in tumor cell growth has led to the development of drugs that target angiogenesis.

The last of these six capabilities, tissue invasion and metastasis, is the most heterogeneous and poorly understood. It is, however, critically important because metastasis accounts for most cancer fatalities. It is becoming clear that specific gene products are associated with the ability of tumor cells to metastasize to different organ sites. Elegant animal metastasis models, as well as transcriptional profiling of human cancers, are revealing that metastasis includes alterations in genes involved in processes such as cell adhesion, integrin signaling, growth factors, chemokine signal transduction, and extracellular proteolysis.

REFERENCES

1. Alberts B, Johnson A, Lewis J, et al. *The Molecular Biology of the Cell.* 4th ed. Oxford, United Kingdom: Garland Science Publishing; 2002.
2. Lewin B. *Genes VII.* Oxford, United Kingdom: Oxford University Press; 2000.
3. Allis CD, Jenuwein T, Reinberg D, et al. *Epigenetics.* Woodbury, NY: Cold Spring Harbor Laboratory Press; 2007:502.
4. Jenuwein T, Allis CD. Translating the histone code. *Science.* 2001;293(5532):1074–1080.
5. Saha A, Wittmeyer J, Cairns BR. Chromatin remodelling: the industrial revolution of DNA around histones. *Nat Rev Mol Cell Biol.* 2006;7(6):437–447.
6. Bolden JE, Peart MJ, Johnstone RW. Anticancer activities of histone deacetylase inhibitors. *Nat Rev Drug Discov.* 2006;5(9):769–784.
7. Karpf AR, Jones DA. Reactivating the expression of methylation silenced genes in human cancer. *Oncogene.* 2002;21(35):5496–5503.
8. Sambrook J, Russell D. *Molecular Cloning: A Laboratory Manual.* 3rd ed. Woodbury, NY: Cold Spring Harbor Laboratory Press; 2001.
9. Dieffenbach C, Dveksklar G. *PCR Primer: A Laboratory Manual.* 2nd ed. Woodbury, NY: Cold Spring Harbor Laboratory Press; 2003:519.

10. Warrington J, Todd R, Wang D. Microarrays and Cancer Research. Natick, MA: Eaton Publishing Company/Biotechniques Books; 2002:162.

11. van't Veer LJ, Dai H, van de Vijver MJ, et al. Gene expression profiling predicts clinical outcome of breast cancer. *Nature.* 2002;415(6871): 530–536.

12. Alizadeh AA, Eisen MB, Davis RE, et al. Distinct types of diffuse large B-cell lymphoma identified by gene expression profiling. *Nature.* 2000;403(6769):503–511.

13. Glas AM, Floore A, Delahaye LJ, et al. Converting a breast cancer microarray signature into a high-throughput diagnostic test. *BMC Genomics.* 2006;7:278.

14. Meister G, Tuschl T. Mechanisms of gene silencing by double-stranded RNA. *Nature.* 2004;431(7006):343–349.

15. Calin GA, Croce CM. MicroRNA signatures in human cancers. *Nat Rev Cancer.* 2006;6(11):857–866.

16. Pinkel D, Albertson DG. Comparative genomic hybridization. *Annu Rev Genomics Hum Genet.* 2005;6:331–354.

17. Walker J. *The Protein Protocols Handbook (Methods in Molecular Biology).* 2nd ed. Totowa, NJ: Humana Press; 2002:1146.

18. Srivastava S, Srivastava RG. Proteomics in the forefront of cancer biomarker discovery. *J Proteome Res.* 2005;4(4):1098–1103.

19. Weinberg R. *The Biology of Cancer.* Oxford, United Kingdom: Garland Science Publishing; 2006.

20. Vogelstein B, Kinzler, K. *The Genetic Basis of Human Cancer.* New York, NY: McGraw-Hill Education; 2002:821.

21. Suzuki T, Shen H, Akagi K, et al. New genes involved in cancer identified by retroviral tagging. *Nat Genet.* 2002;32(1):166–174.

22. Look AT. Genes altered by chromosomal translocations in leukemia and lymphomas. In: Vogelstein V, Kinzler K, eds. *The Genetic Basis of Human Cancer.* New York, NY: McGraw-Hill Education; 2002:57–92.

23. Look AT. Oncogenic transcription factors in the human acute leukemias. *Science.* 1997;278(5340):1059–1064.

24. Hogarty MD, Brodeur GM. Gene amplification in human cancers: biological and clinical significance. In: Scriver C, Beaudet A, Sly W, et al, eds. *The Metabolic and Molecular Bases of Inherited Disease.* New York, NY: McGraw-Hill Education; 2001:597–610.

25. National Cancer Institute/National Human Genome Research Institute. The Cancer Genome Atlas Web site. http://cancergenome.nih.gov/index.asp. Accessed July 11, 2007.

26. Sherr CJ. Principles of tumor suppression. *Cell.* 2004;116(2):235–246.

27. Campbell PM, Der CJ. Oncogenic Ras and its role in tumor cell invasion and metastasis. *Semin Cancer Biol.* 2004;14(2):105–114.

28. Altomare DA, Testa JR. Perturbations of the AKT signaling pathway in human cancer. *Oncogene.* 2005;24(50):7455–7464.

29. Cully M, You H, Levine AJ, et al. Beyond PTEN mutations: the PI3K pathway as an integrator of multiple inputs during tumorigenesis. *Nat Rev Cancer.* 2006;6(3):184–192.

30. Druker BJ. Imatinib as a paradigm of targeted therapies. *Adv Cancer Res.* 2004;91:1–30.

31. Clurman B, Roberts J. Cell cycle control: an overview. In: Vogelstein V, Kinzler K, eds. *The Genetic Basis of Human Cancer.* New York, NY: McGraw-Hill Education; 2002:145–157.

32. Morgan DO. *The Cell Cycle: Principles of Control (A Primer).* London, England: New Science Press; 2006.

33. Schwartz GK, Shah MA. Targeting the cell cycle: a new approach the cancer therapy. *J Clin Oncol.* 2005;23(36):9408-9421.

34. Sherr CJ. The Pezcoller lecture: cancer cell cycles revisited. *Cancer Res.* 2000;60(14):3689–3695.

35. Sherr CJ, Roberts JM. CDK inhibitors: positive and negative regulators of G1-phase progression. *Genes Dev.* 1999;13(12):1501–1512.

36. Danial NN, Korsmeyer SJ. Cell death: critical control points. *Cell.* 2004;116(2):205–219.

37. Cory S, Adams JM. The Bcl2 family: regulators of the cellular life-or-death switch. *Nat Rev Cancer.* 2002;2(9):647–656.

38. Wang S, Yang D, Lippman ME. Targeting Bcl-2 and Bcl-XL with nonpeptidic small-molecule antagonists. *Semin Oncol.* 2003;30(5) (Suppl 16):133–142.

39. Nakayama KI, Nakayama K: Ubiquitin ligases: cell-cycle control and cancer. *Nat Rev Cancer.* 2006;6(5):369–381.

40. Hershko A, Ciechanover A. The ubiquitin system. *Annu Rev Biochem.* 1998;67:425–479.

41. Kaelin WG. The von Hippel-Lindau tumor suppressor protein: roles in cancer and oxygen sensing. *Cold Spring Harb Symp Quant Biol.* 2005;70:159–166.

42. Kelly LM, Gilliland DG. Genetics of myeloid leukemias. *Annu Rev Genomics Hum Genet.* 2002;3:179–198.

43. Radtke F, Schweisguth F, Pear W. The Notch 'gospel'. *EMBO Rep.* 2005;6(12):1120–1125.

44. Weng AP, Ferrando AA, Lee W, et al. Activating mutations of NOTCH1 in human T cell acute lymphoblastic leukemia. *Science.* 2004;306(5694):269–271.

45. Kitagawa R, Kastan MB. The ATM-dependent DNA damage signaling pathway. *Cold Spring Harb Symp Quant Biol.* 2005;70:99–109.

46. de Boer J, Hoeijmakers JH. Nucleotide excision repair and human syndromes. *Carcinogenesis.* 2000;21(3):453–460.

47. Grompe M, van de Vrugt H. The Fanconi family adds a fraternal twin. *Dev Cell.* 2007;12(5):661-662.

48. Kennedy RD, D'Andrea AD. The Fanconi Anemia/BRCA pathway: new faces in the crowd. *Genes Dev.* 2005;19(24):2925–2940.

49. Jiricny J. The multifaceted mismatch-repair system. *Nat Rev Mol Cell Biol.* 2006;7(5):335–346.

50. Hartwell LH, Weinert TA. Checkpoints: controls that ensure the order of cell cycle events. *Science.* 1989;246(4930):629–634.

51. Gottifredi V, Prives C. The S phase checkpoint: when the crowd meets at the fork. *Semin Cell Dev Biol.* 2005;16(3):355–368.

52. Lukas J, Lukas C, Bartek J. Mammalian cell cycle checkpoints: signalling pathways and their organization in space and time. *DNA Repair* (Amst). 2004;3(8-9):997–1007.

53. Zhou BB, Elledge SJ. The DNA damage response: putting checkpoints in perspective. *Nature.* 2000;408(6811):433–439.

54. Poyurovsky MV, Prives C. Unleashing the power of p53: lessons from mice and men. *Genes Dev.* 2006;20(2):125–131.

55. Vogelstein B, Lane D, Levine AJ. Surfing the p53 network. *Nature.* 2000;408(6810):307–310.

56. Vousden KH, Prives C. P53 and prognosis: new insights and further complexity. *Cell.* 2005;120(1):7–10.

57. Sherr CJ. Divorcing ARF and p53: an unsettled case. *Nat Rev Cancer.* 2006;6(9):663–673.

58. Kastan MB. Wild-type p53: tumors can't stand it. *Cell.* 2007; 128(5): 837–840.

59. Wiman KG. Strategies for therapeutic targeting of the p53 pathway in cancer. *Cell Death Differ.* 2006;13(6):921–926.

60. Weaver BA, Cleveland DW. Decoding the links between mitosis, cancer, and chemotherapy: The mitotic checkpoint, adaptation, and cell death. *Cancer Cell.* 2005;8(1):7–12.

61. Hanahan D, Weinberg RA. The hallmarks of cancer. *Cell.* 2000; 100(1):57–70.

3

CLINICAL PHARMACOLOGY

Matthew P. Goetz, MD

LEARNING OBJECTIVES

After reviewing this chapter, the reader should be able to

- Apply the basic principles of clinical pharmacology to the practice of oncology
- Incorporate awareness of the effect of drug metabolism on toxicity and benefit when selecting the most appropriate treatment regimen
- Relate the principles underlying pharmacogenomics to the efficacy of commonly administered oncology drugs, toxic treatment-related events, and treatment failures
- Analyze the route of administration, recognize absorption factors, account for genetic variability in drug metabolism, and develop a plan for monitoring for outcome, toxicity, and clinical benefit when considering a drug and dosage
- Use knowledge of the three primary clinical trial phases and endpoints as they relate to pharmacology to evaluate drug efficacy study results
- Use basic principles of pharmacology and molecular biology to evaluate and appropriately incorporate emerging targeted cancer therapies

Medical oncologists are responsible for administering anticancer therapies to patients with malignancies. Many of these drugs exhibit a narrow therapeutic window, meaning the difference between the toxic and therapeutic dose is small. Traditionally, researchers have developed antineoplastic agents to be delivered at the highest maximum doses — "pushing the envelope" in the hope that the treatment will optimize the anticancer activity. Increasingly, however, the field of oncology has seen a shift toward antineoplastic therapies that "target" a specific protein or pathway regulating cell growth or function. Regardless of the agent, drug dosing requires a balance between the anticancer benefit

The American Society of Clinical Oncology and Dr. Goetz would like to gratefully acknowledge John Marshall, MD, for his contributions to the original content of this chapter.

and the known toxicities these agents cause on normal end-organ function. The purpose of this chapter is to review the fundamental principles of clinical pharmacology as they relate to the practice of oncology and to discuss the emerging area of pharmacogenomics, which refers to the relationship between specific DNA-sequence variation and drug effect.

PRINCIPLES OF CHEMOTHERAPY

Cytotoxic chemotherapy has been a relative success story. Cancers such as Hodgkin's disease, non-Hodgkin's lymphomas, testicular cancer, ovarian cancer, germ cell tumors, leukemia, Wilms' tumors, retinoblastomas, and others can be cured through the effective delivery of cytotoxic chemotherapy. There also has been an increase in the use of these agents in the adjuvant setting, in which case chemotherapy delivered after resection of the primary cancer can eliminate or suppress the growth of occult cancer cells that have already metastasized, ultimately increasing overall survival. Adjuvant chemotherapy (postoperative chemotherapy) is routinely administered for breast, colon, and lung cancers. Additionally, chemotherapy sometimes is used in combination with radiation therapy. Combined-modality approaches (chemotherapy and radiation together) are used to shrink the tumor burden in many diseases to permit surgery, to control systemic disease, or both.

Cytotoxic chemotherapy agents are active only during the cellular replication and division phases of the cell cycle. For most cancers, tumor turnover or replication is in the order of days to weeks — not hours — creating an inherent problem between cell-cycle time and the exposure obtained with most cytotoxic chemotherapy agents, which is often only hours.[1] An understanding of this principle led to the introduction of combination chemotherapy, which was developed to provide maximal cell kill within the range of tolerable toxicity for each drug, broad coverage in resistant cell lines within a heterogeneous tumor population, prevention of drug resistance, and stimulation of the cell cycle through cellular stress, thus increasing the pressure toward cell death (e.g., cisplatin and fluorouracil combinations).

However, despite tremendous advances in the optimization of current cancer chemotherapy for patients with malignancies such as lymphoma and testicular cancer, classic anticancer agents that target DNA have not led to cures in most metastatic solid tumors. Combination chemotherapy delivered to patients with metastatic disease (e.g., metastatic breast cancer) confers little or no survival advantage compared with sequential chemotherapy. In these settings, sequential single-agent chemotherapy, with or without a biologically targeted agent, is a commonly accepted approach to treatment. The balance between toxicity and efficacy is particularly important for these patients. They are at highest risk for changes in metabolism and for decreases in end-organ function, and they also are likely to take high numbers of concomitant medications.

KEY POINT

- Combination chemotherapy has become the standard of care for the majority of cancer therapy regimens.

PHARMACOKINETICS

Pharmacokinetics is the relationship between time and plasma concentration following drug administration; it has been best described as "what the body does to the drug." An understanding of the pharmacokinetics of a chemotherapy drug is critical to the optimum administration of that drug to patients. The measurement of pharmacokinetics is an outcome of most early-phase clinical trials.

From these studies, clinicians learn critical information.

- The most appropriate route of administration
- The schedule of administration
- The frequency of drug delivery
- The optimal dose

The choice of drug administration route is based primarily on pharmacokinetic assessment of bioavailability — the ability of the drug to reach its target in an active form — and the formulation of an acceptable dose preparation for oral, intravenous, intramuscular, intrathecal, or subcutaneous use. Classically, oncologic drugs have been developed using the intravenous route, particularly for water-soluble compounds, because complete absorption is guaranteed. The method of administration also is highly dependent on the ability to formulate a compound into a satisfactory pharmacologic product that can be administered by the route of choice. Several common agents (e.g., paclitaxel) are poorly soluble and must be mixed in solvents, such as cremaphore, which are associated with their own toxicities.

The difference between plasma concentrations produced by oral administration and intravenous dosing is a measure of bioavailability. (Similar calculations can be made for intramuscular or subcutaneous dosing compared with

KEY POINTS

- A broad understanding of the metabolism of cytotoxic and biologic agents is necessary.
- Bioavailability is important when using oral chemotherapy agents.
- Pharmacogenetics is increasingly recognized as an important factor influencing drug effect.
- Drug–drug interactions are an important — but often unrecognized — factor influencing drug effect.

TABLE 3-1 Selected Drug-metabolizing Enzymes of Importance in Oncology.

Reaction	Substrates	Polymorphic (Known genetic variants that influence enzyme activity)
Phase I Reactions		
Cytochrome P-450		
CYP1A1	Benzo(a)pyrene	X
CYP1A2	Theophylline, caffeine	X
CYP2B6	Cyclophosphamide	X
CYP2C8	Paclitaxel	
CYP2C9	Phenytoin, warfarin	X
CYP2C19	Omeprazole, diazepam	X
CYP2D6	Tamoxifen, codeine, granisetron, many antidepressants	X
CYP2E1	Ethanol	X
CYP3A4 / 3A5	Etoposide, vinca alkaloids, ifosfamide, docetaxel, irinotecan, bortexomib, imatinib, flutamide, exemestande, lapatanib, sunitinib, Vinca drugs (e.g., vincristine vinorelbine, vindesine, and vinblastine)	X
Ketoreductase	Anthracyclines	
Aldehyde dehydrogenases	Aldophosphamide	
Carboxylesterases	Irinotecan	
Dihydropyriminidine dehydrogenase	Fluorouracil	X
Cytosine deaminase	Cytarabine	
Phase II Reactions		
N-acetylation		
NAT2	Isoniazid	X
Glucuronidation		
UGT1A1	Bilirubin, SN-38	X
UGT2B7	Morphine, epirubicin	
Methyltransferases		
TPMT	Mercaptopurine, azathioprine	X

Modified with permission from Ratain MJ. Pharmacology of cancer chemotherapy. In: DeVita VT Jr, Hellman S, Rosenberg SA, eds. *Principles and Practice of Oncology*, 6th ed. Philadelphia, Pa: Lippincott Williams & Wilkins; 2001:337.

intravenous dosing.) Bioavailability has become more important as more cytotoxic chemotherapy agents (e.g., capecitabine), as well as biologic agents, are developed for oral dosing. The oral route has the advantage of a more prolonged exposure, thereby providing coverage throughout the cell cycle when toxicity allows. Agents with a high first-pass metabolism will, by nature, have poor oral bioavailability. Alterations in gastrointestinal tract absorptive capacity can alter oral bioavailability as well. Previous surgery, concomitant medications, malabsorption from other causes, and changes in motility, particularly with supportive-care agents, such as opiates, may alter a patient's absorption of an oral chemotherapy agent. Therefore, when considering the administration of such drugs, it is necessary to account for these possible variations within patients.

The study of pharmacokinetics is classically divided into four elements: absorption, distribution, metabolism, and excretion. Absorption is 100% when agents are administered through an intravenous route but varies when other routes of administration are used. Distribution identifies what happens to a drug after its administration. Typically, drugs distribute from the plasma into extracellular and intracellular fluids. This effect is desired, as most drugs must reach the cancer cells to have an effect. The distribution

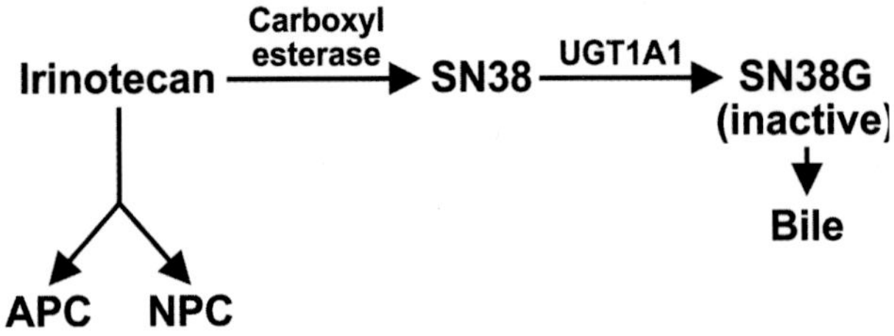

FIG. 3-1 Metabolic pathway of irinotecan, a prodrug that is activated by carboxylesterase to the active metabolite SN-38.

SN-38 is glucuronidated by uridine diphosphate glucuronosyltransferase 1A1 (UGT1A1), forming the inactive metabolite SN-38 glucuronide (SN-38G), which is eliminated in the bile. Abbreviations: APC, aminopentanecarboxylic acid; NPC, 7-ethyl-20-(4-amino-1-piperidino) carbonyloxycamptothecine.

Reprinted with permission from DeVita VT Jr, Hellman S, Rosenberg SA, eds. Principles and Practice of Oncology. Lippincott Williams & Wilkins; 2001.

phase of pharmacokinetics may be the most complicated. In the simple two-compartment model, a drug is administered to the patient and enters into the plasma compartment, followed by a distribution and redistribution of the compound to the peripheral compartment (Fig. 3-1). The drug concentration in this peripheral compartment is the critical value because this is where the drug–tumor interaction will occur. It is important to recognize that drug concentration in the peripheral compartment rarely is measured in clinical trials and is unknown for virtually all agents used today. The degree to which drugs distribute to the peripheral compartment alters their terminal half-life. Drugs that are more highly distributed to this compartment will have a longer terminal half-life.[2] This fact has important clinical ramifications for drugs such as methotrexate, which is the classic example of a drug distributing to the third space, such as pleural effusions or ascites.

Metabolism of therapeutic agents is the area in which there has been the greatest increase in research and subsequent understanding during the past several years. Specifically, there has been a dramatic increase in the understanding of the hepatic enzymes responsible for the metabolism of most agents in clinical use. In addition, cellular models have been developed that enable clinicians to define the metabolic pathways for many important chemotherapy agents. Hepatic enzymes are responsible for phase I and phase II reactions that prepare agents for their excretion by the liver or by the kidney. Hepatic and renal function is critical to the excretion of most cytotoxic chemotherapy agents. When choosing dosages for patients with cancer, clinicians have typically relied on hepatic enzyme function and serum creatinine levels as the primary means to assess end-organ function. However, other factors, such as age, gender, diet, and drug–drug interactions, can lead to clinically important variability in drug effect. Increasingly, inherited differences in the enzyme activity of phase I and phase II enzymes are recognized as one of the most important factors influencing drug effect.

EXCRETION

As stated previously, there are two major routes of excretion: the kidneys and the biliary tract. Clinicians generally use liver and renal function tests to estimate excretory function for patients. Traditionally, chemotherapy agents were administered using body surface area-adjusted doses. This method of dosing was originally used because of its relatively good correlation between creatinine clearance and glomerular filtration rate. However, for some common agents, there has been a shift away from using the traditional body surface area to using a more pharmacokinetically driven method of dosing based on the area under the curve (AUC). The classic example of this is carboplatin; well-established formulae enable oncologists to determine a more accurate dose that is reflective of renal function. Many agents in current clinical practice must be adjusted for either renal or hepatic dysfunction (Table 3-2). In particular, excretion of methotrexate and ifosfamide can be influenced by alkalization of the urine because of their weak acid nature. In addition, after biliary excretion, reabsorption of either the parent drug or its metabolites may take place in the small intestine as a result of enterohepatic circulation.

The clearance of an agent may be the most important aspect of accurate drug dosing. Clearance can be calculated by the dose divided by the AUC or dose rate divided by concentration of the steady state. Few clinicians memorize the values of clearance for agents, but it is necessary to be aware of the variability in clearance. Most of the compounds used have a variation in clearance among patients of approximately 20% to 40%, although some agents have high variability (75% to 100%). It is critical to know how to predict this variation for individual patients. The most important factors affecting this variability are genetics, drug–drug interactions, and end-organ function. Polymorphisms within the genes that encode for metabolizing enzymes are extremely common and are beginning to be recognized as accounting for a substantial portion of toxicity and clinical response in some drugs. The variability in the metabolic or excretory organs, either because of dysfunction or concomitant medications, is common and must be recognized. Many agents are highly protein bound, and variabilities within a patient's protein levels will influence drug clearance. Lastly, it is important to know which drugs form active metabolites (Table 3-3). Many agents in current use, including fluorouracil, irinotecan, and tamoxifen, must be metabolized to the actual active compound.

In summary, when choosing a medicine and a dose, clinicians must first analyze the route of administration, recognize the absorption factors that may be in play, account for any known genetic variability in drug metabolism, and develop a plan for careful outcome monitoring, namely toxicity and clinical benefit. The clinical practice of oncology requires close monitoring of toxicity and clinical benefit using traditional radiographic and clinical measures. With

TABLE 3-2 Drugs Requiring Dose Modification for Organ Dysfunction

Liver Dysfunction	Renal Insufficiency	Glomerular Filtration Rate of Less Than 25%
Doxorubicin	Cisplatin	Cyclophosphamide
Epirubicin	Hydroxyurea	Ifosfamide
Dactinomycin	Etoposide	Bleomycin
Irinotecan	Pentostatin	Streptozotocin
Paclitaxel	Fludarabine	Daunorubicin
Thiotepa	Carboplatin	Idarubacin
Vincristine	Topotecan	Epirubicin
Vinorelbine	Capecitabine	Mercaptuopurine
Vinblastine	Methotrexate	
Vindesine	Pemetrexed	
Cyclophosphamide	Bisphosphonates	
Ifosfamide		
Cytarabine		
Gemcitabine		
Etoposide		
Fluorouracil		
Docetaxel		

the introduction of biologic agents, classic toxicities, such as myelosuppression, are not commonly seen; however, other toxicities (e.g., trastuzumab-induced cardiomyopathy) will continue to require close observation and intervention as necessary.

PHARMACOGENETICS

Pharmacogenetics is the study of the role of genetic inheritance in the individual variation of drug response and toxicity. With the convergence of advances in pharmacogenetics and human genomics, the field of pharmacogenomics has blossomed during the past decade. This term is used to refer to the study of the relationship between specific DNA-sequence variation and drug effect. Much of this genetic variation is in the form of single nucleotide polymorphisms — defined as variants with frequencies of 1% or greater — which can alter the amino acid sequence of the encoded protein, alter RNA splicing, or alter transcription.

In few other disciplines of medicine are the concepts of pharmacogenetics better illustrated than in the treatment of cancer. Administration of "standard" doses of chemotherapy to patients with inherited deficiencies in enzymes responsible for their metabolism and disposition can result in marked toxicity, which can even be lethal. Conversely, patients who have increased enzymatic activity may be at risk for treatment failure — also an undesirable outcome when dealing with a potentially fatal illness. The traditional method by which individualized anticancer drug doses are developed and determined has involved the use of body surface area measurements and weight-based dosing.[3] However, multiple studies have indicated that dosing in this manner does not reliably account for the variability in clearance of most chemotherapeutic drugs.[4]

Examples of the role of pharmacogenetics have been clearly illustrated with both cytotoxic chemotherapy and with targeted therapies. Three examples illustrated in the following sections have led to recent relabeling of the individual drugs by the U.S. Food and Drug Administration (FDA) to reflect the importance of pharmacogenetics.

Thiopurines

The thiopurine drugs mercaptopurine and azathioprine (the latter of which is a prodrug that is converted to mercaptopurine in vivo), are purine antimetabolites used clinically to treat both pediatric and adult leukemias and as immunosuppressant agents.[5] Thiopurines are metabolized in part by S-methylation, catalyzed by the enzyme thiopurine S-methyltransferase (TPMT).[6,7] Dr. Weinshilboum's group first identified three groups of patients on the basis of the level of TPMT activity in their red cells and found that the level of activity was inherited in an autosomal codominant fashion.[7,8] Subsequently, it was shown that patients who received standard doses of thiopurines and who were homozygous for very low levels of TPMT activity or for no activity ($TPMT^L TPMT^L$) had greatly elevated concentrations of

TABLE 3-3 Oncology Drugs with Active Circulating Metabolites

Chemotherapy Drugs	Other Oncology Drugs
• Alkylating agents	• Analgesics
Cyclophosphamide	Morphine
Ifosfamide	Codeine
Procarbazine	Hydrocodone
Dacarbazine	
Temozolomide	
Hexamethylmelamine	
Thiotepa	
• Anthracyclines	
Doxorubicin	
Idarubicin	
Epirubicin	
• Camptothecins	
Irinotecan	
• Antimetabolites	
Tegafur, uracil, and fluorouracil (UFT)	
Methotrexate	
6-Mercaptopurine	
• Antiestrogens	
Toremifene	
Tamoxifen	
• Retinoids	
All-trans retinoic acid	

Reprinted with permission from DeVita VT Jr, Hellman S, Rosenberg SA, eds. *Principles and Practice of Oncology*. Lippincott Williams & Wilkins; 2001.

active drug metabolites, 6-thioguanine nucleotides, and a markedly increased risk of life-threatening, drug-induced myelosuppression.[9] As a result, the phenotypic test for the level of TPMT activity in red cells and, subsequently, DNA-based tests, were among the first pharmacogenetic tests to be used in clinical practice. The result of *TPMT* gene resequencing has demonstrated that the most common variant allele responsible for low levels of activity among white populations encodes a protein with two alterations in the amino acid sequence as a result of single-nucleotide polymorphisms.[10,11] These sequence changes result in a striking reduction in the quantity of TPMT,[10] at least in part because the variant protein is degraded rapidly.[12] A series of less frequent *TPMT* variant alleles also have been described.[8]

UGT1A1 and Irinotecan

Irinotecan (CPT-11) is metabolized in vivo to 7-ethyl-10-hydroxy camptothecin, SN-38 (Fig. 3-1), which is 1,000 times more potent as an inhibitor of topoisomerase I than the parent drug.[13–15] In humans, both gastrointestinal (diarrhea) and hematologic (neutropenia) toxicities are dose limiting following the administration of CPT-11. SN-38 is inactivated by glucuronidation to form the glucuronide conjugate (SN38G) in a reaction catalyzed by the polymorphic hepatic enzyme uridine diphosphate glucuronosyltransferase 1A1 (UGT1A1, Fig. 3-1).[16] A dinucleotide repeat polymorphism in the TATA box in the promoter for *UGT1A1* results in reduced hepatic *UGT1A1* expression and is thought to be the most common cause of Gilbert's syndrome (mild unconjugated hyperbilirubinemia).[17–19] Recent studies have demonstrated that patients who are homozygous for the *UGT1A1*28* polymorphism have substantially lower SN-38 glucuronidation rates and substantially higher rates of grade 4 or 5 neutropenia than those patients who do not carry this genetic variant. The importance of *UGT1A1* pharmacogenetics in mediating CPT–11-related toxicity has been recognized by the FDA. A "black-box" warning was recently applied to the CPT-11 label to recommend a dose reduction for patients homozygous for the *UGT1A1* polymorphism. However, a key area of uncertainty is what dose of irinotecan should be administered based on *UGT1A1* genotype. A Mayo Clinic prospective phase I dose-escalation trial recently demonstrated that patients homozygous for the *UGT1A1*28* polymorphism tolerate substantially lower doses of CPT–11-based chemotherapy while maintaining the same therapeutic concentration of SN38 as patients without the *28 allele (wild type), who tolerated twice the dose of irinotecan without hematologic toxicicty.[20]

Tamoxifen and CYP2D6

Tamoxifen can be considered a "prodrug" that requires metabolic activation to elicit its pharmacologic activity. Tamoxifen undergoes activation to metabolites that are 100 times more potent suppressors of estradiol-stimulated breast cancer cell growth (4-OH tamoxifen and endoxifen) compared with tamoxifen or its primary metabolite, N-desmethyl tamoxifen. Endoxifen is the most abundant active metabolite in most individuals and results from the CYP2D6 medicated oxidation of N-desmethyl tamoxifen (Fig. 3-2). In a prospective tamoxifen trial, genetic variation in *CYP2D6* and/or co-administration of CYP2D6 inhibitors were associated with a significant reduction in the mean plasma endoxifen concentrations, with the reduction in endoxifen concentrations directly related to inhibitor potency.[21,22] A recent analysis of a prospective tamoxifen trial demonstrated that genetic variation in *CYP2D6*, as measured by the *4 polymorphism, was an independent predictor of breast cancer relapse and death. Women who were homozygous for the *4 allele (*CYP2D6*-poor metabolizers) or who took potent CYP2D6 inhibitors had a 3-fold higher risk of relapse or death compared with women classified as extensive metabolizers who were not co-prescribed CYP2D6 inhibitors.[23,24] These findings led to the recommendation of an FDA advisory panel to change the tamoxifen label to reflect the importance of CYP2D6 metabolism in tamoxifen therapy.

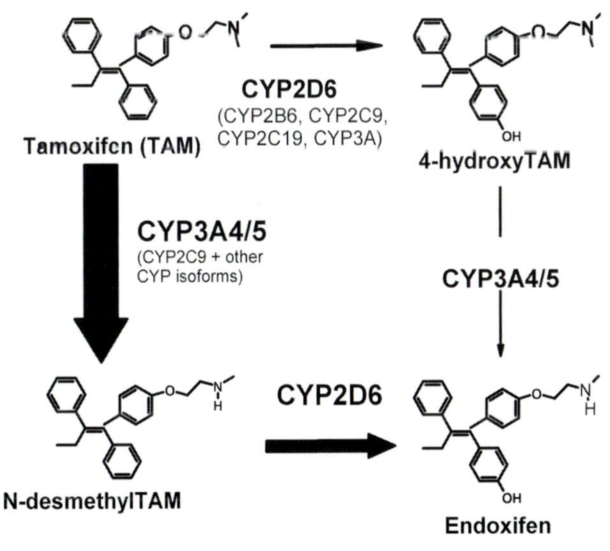

FIG. 3-2 Selected transformation pathways of tamoxifen and the main CYP enzymes involved.

The relative contribution of each pathway to the overall oxidation of tamoxifen is shown by the thickness of the arrow, and the principal P450 isoforms responsible are highlighted in larger fonts.

Modified in part from Jin Y et al. J Natl Cancer Inst. 2005;97(1): 30–39.

KEY POINT

- Pharmacogenetics is the study of the role of genetic inheritance in individual variation in drug response and toxicity. FDA-recognized examples of oncologic drugs wherein toxicity or response is influenced by pharmacogenetics includes irinotecan (*UGT1A1* and neutropenia) and tamoxifen (*CYP2D6* and relapse).

PHARMACODYNAMICS

An increased understanding of pharmacodynamics has pushed investigators to a new era of drug development and clinical research design. Specifically, in early-phase clinical research there is an increased emphasis not only on defining the pharmacokinetic parameters of a given drug but also on demonstrating some effect of the drug on the tumor or on the target endpoints. These types of studies are best done in late phase I or early phase II clinical trials, in which the dose is fixed and the variability in target modulation can be assessed more easily. One of the greatest challenges in pharmacodynamic studies is selecting the endpoint. Ideally, endpoints are tumor specific, but access to tumors is difficult. Frequently, trials are designed with the endpoint being the change in a circulating blood factor, which often is not correlated with the anticancer endpoints and must be used despite being invalid surrogate markers. However, the goal of these trials is to demonstrate a relationship between the administration of an agent and a particular pharmacodynamic parameter with a subsequent anticancer endpoint. If such a relationship is determined in early phases of clinical research, this simplifies the clinical development pathway for a particular agent. A recent example of a pharmacodynamic marker is EGFR–1-induced skin rash; a higher rate of tumor response has been observed for patients who developed skin rash compared with patients without rash.

KEY POINT

- Pharmacodynamics may become an important factor influencing drug selection, dose modifications, and outcomes predictions for some of the newer targeted therapies.

> **KEY POINT**
>
> - With few exceptions, eligible patients with cancer should be offered clinical trials as an option. An understanding of the different phases of clinical trials is necessary to best advise patients.

BIOLOGIC AGENTS

The application of pharmacodynamics has been most widely applied to novel biologic agents. Many of these agents are targeted to a particular receptor or protein within a cancer. Therefore, many clinicians believe that the expression of the target is critical when applying such an agent. The best example is the monoclonal antibody trastuzumab, which targets the receptor HER2. Extensive research with this compound has demonstrated that the expression of the HER2 receptor is critical for the activity of trastuzumab. These results have not necessarily been found in clinical trials involving other monoclonal antibodies. Without adequate pharmacodynamic measures, these relationships would never have been defined. Other examples of surrogate endpoints for biologic agents include T-cell or antibody responses (immune therapies), changes in peripheral blood lymphocytes or other changes in the blood (targeted small molecules), or the current gold standard of measuring changes in tumors themselves.

DRUG DEVELOPMENT: CLINICAL TRIAL DESIGN

The goals of clinical research are to expand knowledge about new anticancer agents through the conduct of well-designed clinical trials, to rapidly gain approval by regulatory bodies, and to obtain adequate clinical information for safe and effective drug delivery. The medical literature is focused on clinical research and clinical trial design, which makes the comprehension of trial design critical for practicing physicians.

NONCLINICAL DRUG TESTING

New compounds are discovered primarily by two means. First, there is rational design of new therapeutic agents. When a target is known, drugs can be tailored to fit the target. Second, compounds are discovered as a result of high throughput screening in which multiple compounds with unknown activity are tested against a series of cancer cell lines. Those with the best activity are selected for further development. From either source, new agents with promise are tested in vitro to determine whether the drug can kill cancer cells. If successful, in vivo testing is performed to determine whether the drug kills only cancer cells. During in vivo testing, the schedule and route of administration are investigated. Subsequently, drugs are formulated for the optimum route of administration (oral or intravenous) and the administration schedule is again optimized (e.g., daily, weekly, or via infusion). Although schedules often are based on expected toxicities, mechanisms of action, and animal studies, patient and physician convenience also is a priority.

If the agent yields positive results in nonclinical testing, clinical trials are performed. Based on toxicology studies involving animals, a starting dose is determined for phase I clinical trials using one of two standard techniques. The more common method is to take one-tenth of the lethal dose that kills 10% of the most sensitive animal species. An alternative strategy is to use one-third of the toxic dose-low (defined as the lowest dose of a substance at which any toxic effect is produced). Once the phase I dose has been selected and appropriate regulatory measures have been met, phase I clinical trials are then performed.

Phase I Trials

The primary goal of a phase I clinical trial using classic cytoxic chemotherapy has been to determine the maximum-tolerated dose. With the development of targeted therapies, most researchers focus on finding biologically active doses that modify or alter the intended target, resulting in a measurable effect. In either case, the maximally tolerated or biologically active dose is considered the recommended phase II dose. Secondary goals are to determine the optimal administration schedule, the toxicity profile of the agent, and the pharmacokinetics and pharmacodynamics, as discussed previously, as well as to observe for any clinical activity. Traditionally, patients who enter phase I clinical trials have advanced cancer. With newer nontoxic agents, phase I research now is performed more often in healthy volunteers, but ultimately, patients with cancer are enrolled. Generally, these patients have no other treatment options; clinical trials are typically a second-line or a third-line choice for patients with metastatic cancer. To be eligible, patients must have a good performance status and a relatively normal end-organ function so that adequate pharmacology can be determined. Clinical benefit is seen in approximately 35% to 45% of patients who are enrolled in studies that include at least one anticancer agent approved by the FDA, whereas the response rate to single investigational chemotherapeutic agents is less than 5%.[25]

Classic phase I design for cytotoxic chemotherapy agents has been developed largely empirically. In the classic design, three patients receive each dose level. Doses are escalated using a modified Fibonacci escalation scheme. Cohorts of three patients are expanded if toxicities occur. Pharmacokinetic measurements are typically obtained for all patients, as are toxicity and tumor assessment.

In newer trial designs, fewer patients are treated at low, theoretically inactive, doses. One popular trial design is a rapid dose-escalation scheme in which only one patient is enrolled at each dose level until a particular level of toxicity occurs. In this scheme, doses are often increased by 100%. However, one of the negative aspects of this trial design is the limited pharmacokinetic and pharmacodynamic opportunities with only one patient per dose level.

In another design, dose assignment is pharmacokinetically driven. This design is based on the immediate readout of the pharmacokinetics in an individual, and subsequent doses are chosen based on what was found in preceding patients.

Typically, phase I clinical trials are performed for patients with multiple tumor types, but there is an increasing trend to perform phase I trials for patients with single tumors, particularly when clinical efficacy is a necessary early endpoint. With agents that are not expected to be overly toxic or when clinical effects are expected before toxic effects are likely to develop, there are other designs that can be used. Recently, the phase 0 design has been introduced for some targeted therapies, in which small numbers of patients are treated with the goal of determining early on whether a given drug will affect its intended target.

Phase I clinical trials involving combination agents have the added emphasis of evaluating the interaction between the two agents. This is particularly important when there might be a pharmacologic interaction resulting in a substantial change in the toxicity profile. Phase Ib clinical trials are dose-escalation trials in which some measure of clinical outcome is included.

Following the completion of phase I clinical trials, investigators should be able to determine the existence of the following:

- acceptable drug-related toxicity,
- an appropriate administration schedule, and
- any anticancer activity.

Although investigators are discouraged from making definitive decisions regarding the efficacy of a given cancer drug tested in a phase I study, observed tumor activity in the phase I setting is usually the impetus for studying the drug in subsequent phase II studies.

Phase II Trials

The primary goal of phase II clinical trials is to determine the efficacy of an agent. Somewhat unique to oncology, the single-arm phase II trial, in which the complete and partial response rates are determined, is used to make phase III design decisions. Typically, a fixed dose and schedule of the therapy are selected, and patients have only one tumor type. The ideal setting is one in which all patients have the same characteristics and have received the same previous therapy. All patients begin receiving the study drug at the same dose level, and typically all patients have measurable disease. The primary endpoint is the response rate or the percent of participants free of progression at a certain point. Additionally, an important endpoint is to confirm the toxicity profile that was first defined in the phase I clinical trial. Phase II trials also offer an opportunity to explore molecular endpoints.

The choice of tumor type is based on preclinical and early clinical research, as well as the molecular biology of the mechanism of the agent's action. Many studies involve patients who have untreated metastatic cancer; however, some studies involve patients who have highly refractory tumors to quickly evaluate efficacy and to obtain regulatory approval. Phase II clinical research is typically the standard point at which decisions are made about the subsequent development of a given compound. If no clinical activity has been observed in phase II studies, the development of the drug is usually not continued.

Although the classic statistical design for a phase II single-arm trial has relied on drug response (complete or partial), newer targeted therapies are generally tested using time-to-disease progression endpoints. Additionally, randomized phase II trials are sometimes performed to establish proof of efficacy of a biologic agent.

Phase III Trials

The ultimate goal of phase III clinical research is either to gain approval of a new agent by a regulatory body or to displace the current standard of care. These trials are large, ranging from as few as 300 patients to as many as several thousand patients. By definition, these trials are randomized clinical studies. The design and size of each trial hinges specifically on the selected endpoints. The gold-standard endpoint is survival, recognized by all regulatory agencies. However, for breast and colorectal cancers, the FDA now recognizes disease-free survival, defined as the time to the first event, defined as relapse or death. Additionally, response rate, time to disease progression, quality of life, and other nontraditional endpoints have been incorporated into phase III clinical trial designs and have provided support to the approval process of many new agents in oncology.

NEW MEDICINES AND NOVEL MECHANISMS OF ACTION

A growing understanding of the molecular, genetic, and biochemical changes that occur during the processes of carcinogenesis, progression, and metastasis has shifted drug development toward therapeutics that act on specific molecular targets responsible for the malignant phenotype. Recent advances in drug development have included drugs that target signal transduction (the HER receptor family, Ras, Raf, and MEK kinases); oncogenic proteins, such as bcr/abl; cell-cycle regulating proteins, such as the cyclins, the cyclin-dependent kinases, and inhibitors of cyclin-dependent kinases; and proteins involved in the tumor angiogenesis, such as endothelial growth factor receptors. Although the scope of discovery is not possible to review here, there are three areas worth emphasizing.

- Targeted therapies
- Angiogenesis inhibition
- Immunotherapy

Targeted therapies may represent the most exciting new field in the treatment of cancer. An increased understanding of the molecular biology of cancer and the specific key pathways in oncogenesis have given investigators an extensive selection of new targets toward which to direct therapies. Tyrosine kinases, pathways controlling apoptosis, and cell cycling represent important cancer-specific targets. Several targeted agents recently approved for clinical use include the monoclonal antibodies trastuzumab (*HER2* positive breast cancer) and cetuximab (colon cancer and head and neck cancer), as well as small molecules targeting tyrosine kinases, such as erlotinib (lung and pancreatic cancers). Many additional drugs also are in development. The clinician should have sound knowledge about the molecular biology of cancer and, in particular, a good understanding of when these agents can be used.

Angiogenesis is a second emerging area in cancer treatment, which has been driven by the concept that drug-induced inhibition of new blood vessel growth can halt the growth, survival, and metastatic spread of cancer with few side effects. Most recently, bevacizumab, a novel vascular endothelial growth factor antagonist, has been shown to statistically significantly prolong the time to disease progression when administered with standard cytotoxic chemotherapies in colon, breast, and lung cancers. Additionally, the multityrosine kinase inhibitors sunitinib and sorafenib (which inhibit vascular endothelial growth factor receptor trysoine kinases) have demonstrated significant antitumor activity in renal cell carcinoma, leading to FDA approval for the treatment of metastatic disease.

Immunotherapy is a third area in which important research is taking place. Clinicians have known for many years that using nonspecific enhancers of the immune system, such as interleukin-2 (aldesleukin) and interferon, can generate immune responses that lead to clinical responses for patients with kidney cancer or melanoma. More recently, there has been increased interest in the development of immune-based therapy for more common solid tumors, such as cancers of the breast, lung, and gastrointestinal tract. Although no vaccine or immune therapy has been approved for clinical use in the United States, many agents in this category are in phase II and early phase III clinical trials; it is hoped that, in time, these agents will change the practice of oncology.

KEY POINT

- Substantial gains have been realized in the development of drugs for novel targeted therapies, including, but not limited to, angiogenesis, signal transduction growth pathways, and immune stimulation.

REFERENCES

1. Bartek J, Lukas J. Chk1 and Chk2 kinases in checkpoint control and cancer. *Cancer Cell.* 2003; 3(5):421–429.
2. Li J, Gwilt P. The effect of malignant effusions on methotrexate disposition. *Cancer Chemother Pharmacol.* 2000; 50(5):373–382.
3. Gurney H. Dose calculation of anticancer drugs: a review of the current practice and introduction of an alternative. *J Clin Oncol.* 1996;14(9): 2590–2611.
4. Baker SD, Verweij J, Rowinsky EK, et al. Role of body surface area in dosing of investigational anticancer agents in adults, 1991–2001. *J Natl Cancer Inst.* 2002;94(24):1883–1888.
5. Lennard L. The clinical pharmacology of 6-mercaptopurine. *Eur J Clin Pharmacol.* 1992;43(4):329–339.
6. Woodson LC, Weinshilboum RM. Human kidney thiopurine methyltransferase. Purification and biochemical properties. *Biochem Pharmacol.* 1983; 32(5):819–826.
7. Weinshilboum RM, Sladek SL. Mercaptopurine pharmacogenetics: monogenic inheritance of erythrocyte thiopurine methyltransferase activity. *Am J Hum Genet.* 1980; 32(5):651–662.
8. Raftogianis RB, Wood TC, Weinshilboum RM. Human phenol sulfotransferases SULT1A2 and SULT1A1: genetic polymorphisms, allozyme properties, and human liver genotype-phenotype correlations. *Biochem Pharmacol.* 1999;58(4):605–616.
9. Lennard L, Van Loon JA, Weinshilboum RM. Pharmacogenetics of acute azathioprine toxicity: relationship to thiopurine methyltransferase genetic polymorphism. *Clin Pharmacol Ther.* 1989;46(2):149–154.
10. Szumlanski C, Otterness D, Her C, et al. Thiopurine methyltransferase pharmacogenetics: human gene cloning and characterization of a common polymorphism. *DNA Cell Biol.* 1996;15(1):17–30.
11. Dehal SS, Kupfer D. CYP2D6 catalyzes tamoxifen 4-hydroxylation in human liver. *Cancer Res.* 1997;57(16):3402–3406.
12. Tai HL, Krynetski EY, Schuetz EG, et al. Enhanced proteolysis of thiopurine S-methyltransferase (TPMT) encoded by mutant alleles in humans (TPMT*3A, TPMT*2): mechanisms for the genetic polymorphism of TPMT activity. *Proc Natl Acad Sci U S A.* 1997;94(12): 6444–6449.
13. Kaneda N, Nagata H, Furuta T, et al. Metabolism and pharmacokinetics of the camptothecin analogue CPT-11 in the mouse. *Cancer Res.* 1990;50(6):1715–1720.
14. Kawato Y, Aonuma M, Hirota Y, et al. Intracellular roles of SN-38, a metabolite of the camptothecin derivative CPT-11, in the antitumor effect of CPT-11. *Cancer Res.* 1991;51(16):4187–4191.
15. Rivory LP, Riou JF, Haaz MC, et al. Identification and properties of a major plasma metabolite of irinotecan (CPT-11) isolated from the plasma of patients. *Cancer Res.* 1996;56:3689–94.
16. Iyer L, King CD, Whitington PF, et al. Genetic predisposition to the metabolism of irinotecan (CPT-11). Role of uridine diphosphate glucuronosyltransferase isoform 1A1 in the glucuronidation of its active metabolite (SN-38) in human liver microsomes. *J Clin Invest.* 1998;101(4):847–854.
17. Bosma PJ, Chowdhury JR, Bakker C, et al. The genetic basis of the reduced expression of bilirubin UDP-glucuronosyltransferase 1 in Gilbert's syndrome. *N Engl J Med.* 1995;333(18):1171–1175.
18. Monaghan G, Ryan M, Seddon R, et al. Genetic variation in bilirubin UPD- glucuronosyltransferase gene promoter and Gilbert's syndrome. *Lancet.* 1996;347:578–581.
19. Beutler E, Gelbart T, Demina A. Racial variability in the UDP-glucuronosyltransferase 1 (UGT1A1) promoter: a balanced polymorphism for regulation of bilirubin metabolism? *Proc Natl Acad Sci U S A.* 1998;95(14):8170–8174.

20. Goetz MP, Safgren S, Goldberg RM, et al. A phase I dose escalation study of irinotecan (CPT-11), oxaliplatin (Oxal), and capecitabine (Cap) within three UGT1A1 TA promoter cohorts (6/6, 6/7, and 7/7). *J Clin Oncol.* 2005;23, 16S:138.

21. Jin Y, Desta Z, Stearns V, et al. CYP2D6 genotype, antidepressant use, and tamoxifen metabolism during adjuvant breast cancer treatment. *J Natl Cancer Inst.* 2005;97(1):30–39.

22. Borges S, Desta Z, Li L, et al. Quantitative effect of CYP2D6 genotype and inhibitors on tamoxifen metabolism: implication for optimization of breast cancer treatment. *Clin Pharmacol Ther.* 2006;80(1):61–74.

23. Goetz MP, Rae JM, Suman VJ, et al. Pharmacogenetics of tamoxifen biotransformation is associated with clinical outcomes of efficacy and hot flashes. *J Clin Oncol.* 2005;23(36):9312–9318.

24. Goetz MP, Knox S, Suman VJ, et al. The impact of cytochrome P450 2D6 metabolism in women receiving adjuvant tamoxifen. *Breast Can Res Treat.* 2007;101(1):113–121.

25. Horstmann E, McCabe MS, Grochow L, et al. Risks and benefits of phase I oncology trials, 1991 through 2002. *N Engl J Med.* 2005;352(9):895–904.

4

BIOLOGIC THERAPY

Pierre L. Triozzi, MD

LEARNING OBJECTIVES

After reviewing this chapter, the reader should be able to

- Identify the components of the immune system and describe the effector and regulatory action of cells and cytokines
- Apply understanding of the inter-relationships between tumors and the immune system, including immune surveillance, immune escape, and immune subversion to prediction of outcomes, drug resistance, treatment failure, tumor growth, and progression
- Summarize the activities and clinical indications for cytokines, monoclonal antibodies, and adoptive cellular therapy
- Incorporate appropriate clinical use of cytokines, monoclonal antibodies, and adoptive cellular therapy into practice and manage associated toxicities
- Describe the development of cancer vaccines and strategies to inhibit negative regulatory immune responses
- Evaluate appropriate use of immunotoxins and radioimmunoconjugates in patient populations

Biologic therapy, whether for cancer, infections, or other diseases, refers to the use of biologic products, or substances that are made by living organisms, such as cells, antibodies, and cytokines. In biologic therapy for cancer, biologic products are administered primarily to generate or to restore host immune responses to tumors. The distinctions between biologic therapy and chemotherapy are, to some extent, being effaced. Biologic agents also have been exploited to mediate nonimmunologic antitumor activities; for example, in addition to activating immune effector mechanisms, antibodies may mediate antitumor effects by directly inhibiting the activity of growth factor receptors. Cytokines that are produced by nonimmune cells and that do not directly activate immune effector mechanisms, such as erythropoietin and keratinocyte growth factor, are used clinically. Biologic therapy can be limited by many of the same toxicities that limit chemotherapy. Furthermore, chemotherapy can be administered to promote antitumor immune responses.

The American Society of Clinical Oncology and Dr. Triozzi would like to gratefully acknowledge Ernest C. Borden, MD, for his contributions to the original content of this chapter.

Since the introduction of interferons as pharmaceutical agents using recombinant DNA technology more than 20 years ago, progress in biologic therapy for cancer has been rapid. Several cytokines have been approved by the U.S. Food and Drug Administration (FDA), and an increasing number of monoclonal antibodies are being used clinically. Adoptive cellular therapy is practiced in the setting of hematopoietic stem cell transplantation (HSCT). Only cancer vaccines have yet to fulfill the standards for regulatory approval. Several advances have been made in understanding the molecular mechanisms of antigen presentation, the activation of immune effectors, and immune response regulation. Advances also have been made in understanding how tumors can evade and subvert immune responses. This chapter will focus on the immunology, pharmacology, and toxicology, as well as the spectrum of antitumor activity of biologic therapy. More detailed review of the clinical application of specific agents is provided in site-specific chapters.

IMMUNE RESPONSE

The immune system functions to protect against microbial pathogens while simultaneously maintaining tolerance to "self." This innate response forms the first line of defense. Innate immune cells (e.g., macrophages, dendritic cells, and natural killer [NK] cells) express receptors (e.g., toll-like receptors) with which they recognize conserved molecular patterns, such as unmethylated CpG DNA motifs, found on microbes but not on human tissues. Stimulation via these receptors triggers a cascade of events that include the production of cytokines, activation of cellular cytotoxicity, an increase in nitric oxide synthesis, and activation of the complement system. These events promote the elimination or lysis of microbial pathogens as well as promote recruitment and activation of other immune cells.

Microbial/cellular fragments produced by the destruction affected by innate response are taken up by antigen-presenting cells, such as macrophages, dendritic cells, and B cells, which process the fragments and present these to generate "adaptive" immune effectors, namely, T cells and antibody-producing B cells. These cells express highly diverse, somatically generated, antigen-specific receptors — the T-cell antigen receptors (TCR) and the B-cell antigen receptors (BCR) — generated by random rearrangement of the TCR and immunoglobulin (Ig) gene segments, respectively. The adaptive response allows generation of extremely diverse T and B cell repertoires that, compared with the innate response, provides a more specific but also broader and more flexible repertoire of responses that includes "memory."

Innate and adaptive immune responses are under the regulation of a number of cells and cytokines. A key step in the generation of adaptive immunity is the presentation of antigens by antigen-presenting cells to T-helper cells, which promote cellular effectors including cytolytic T lymphocytes or humoral effectors known as antibodies, through the production of specific cytokines. Regulatory T cells and several cytokines also serve to suppress the immune response so as to maintain tolerance to self and limit immune-mediated damage to normal tissues.

KEY POINTS

- Cells of both the antigen-nonspecific innate and antigen-specific adaptive response have been implicated in antitumor immunity.
- Specific immunity to tumors requires uptake of tumor antigens by antigen-presenting cells and presentation to T-helper cells, which coordinate the generation of cellular and/or humoral responses.

IMMUNE CELLS

A wide variety of hematologic (and nonhematologic) cells are important in innate and adaptive immunity. The following are considered to play prominent roles in antitumor immune responses.

T CELLS

T cells play a central role in the adaptive immune responses as effectors and as regulators. The TCR is part of a signaling complex, which includes the TCR dimer, the accessory molecules CD4 or CD8, and the CD3 signal transduction module, which comprises various chains. Unlike antibodies, which can react to intact proteins, T cells via the TCR only

KEY POINTS

- T cells recognize antigen presented to the T-cell antigen receptors as peptide fragments within major histocompatibility complex molecules. T-cell activation not only requires stimulation through the T-cell antigen receptor but also through immune costimulatory receptors.
- T-helper cells promote T-helper cell type 1 (Th1)-associated cytolytic T lymphocytes through the production of cytokines, such as interferon-gamma and interleukin-2 (IL-2), and promote Th2-associated antibody through production of cytokines, such as IL-4 and IL-5.
- Cytolytic T lymphocytes kill tumors by apoptosis via granule exocytosis and fas-mediated mechanisms.
- B-cells produce antibodies, which recognize antigens in their native conformation.The two principle ways antibodies can react against tumors are by complement-mediated and antibody-dependent cellular mechanisms.
- Dendritic cells are the most efficient antigen-presenting cells.
- Cellular immune responses appear to be central in the generation of effective antitumor immunity.

react to peptide fragments of antigens that are noncovalently complexed with major histocompatibility complex (MHC) molecules, which are integral membrane glycoproteins. There are two types of MHC molecules. Class I MHC (e.g., human leukocyte antigen type A2 [HLA-A2]) is expressed on all cell types and serves as the antigen-presenting molecule for CD8+ T cells. Class II MHC (e.g., HLA-DR) is recognized by CD4+ T cells and is present primarily on antigen-presenting cells (i.e., dendritic cells, macrophages, and B cells) but also can be present on other cells, including tumor cells. Polymorphisms within MHC molecules determine whether a peptide fragment will complex with the MHC molecule and, thus, whether a T cell from an individual will respond to a specific epitope of an antigen, resulting in the phenomenon referred to as MHC-restriction. T-cell activation not only requires the presentation of antigen within the context of a MHC molecule and stimulation through the CD3 module but also "costimulatory" signals and adhesion molecules (Fig. 4-1).

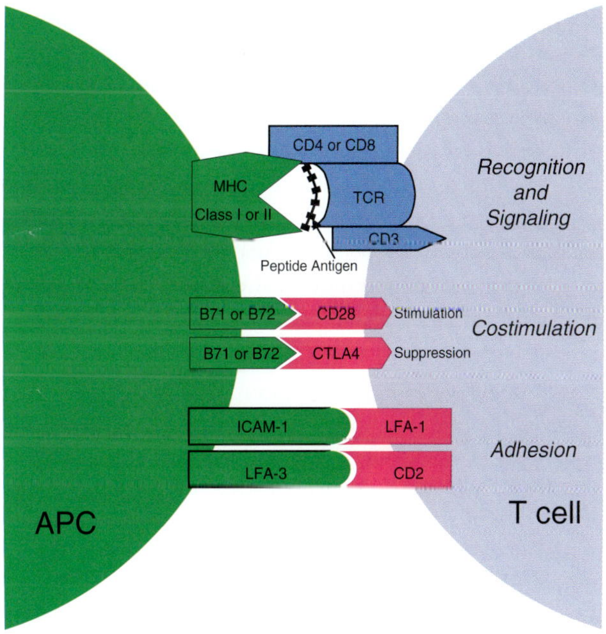

FIG. 4-1 Examples of the cell surface molecules involved in T-cell antigen recognition and activation.

T cells recognize antigen presented to the TCR as peptide fragments within MHC molecules on antigen-presenting cells. The primary costimulatory signal is delivered through the CD28 receptor on the T cell after engagement of its ligands, B7-1 (CD80) or B7-2 (CD86), on the antigen-presenting cells. Engagement of the CTLA-4 receptor (CD152) on the T cell by the same B7-1 or B7-2 ligands results in attenuation of the response. Failure of the costimulatory B7/CD28 complex to be engaged results in either a non-activating T-cell event and/or anergy. Fully effective engagement is also dependent upon the interaction of adhesion molecules on antigen-presenting cells, e.g., intercellular adhesion molecule (ICAM-1) (CD54) and leukocyte function-associated antigen (LFA-3) (CD58), bound by their corresponding receptors on T cells, e.g., LFA-1 (CD11a) and CD2, respectively. Abbreviations: FasL, Fas ligand.

Cytolytic T Lymphocytes

Cytolytic T lymphocytes (CTL) are primarily CD8+ T cells and, thus, recognize antigens presented within the context of MHC class I. Two mechanisms are involved in the cell killing mediated by these lymphocytes. The predominant mechanism is granule exocytosis and the release of perforin and granzymes. The second mechanism is mediated by the death activator, Fas ligand, which is expressed on the cell surface of CTL. Both mechanisms cause cells to undergo apoptosis (programmed cell death) (Fig. 4-2). When appropriately activated, these cells also produce cytokines, such as interferon-gamma, that also can mediate antitumor effects. CTL can move to another cell and, by reorienting their granules to another region of contact, destroy it. In this manner, these lymphocytes can kill many tumor cells, resulting in a very

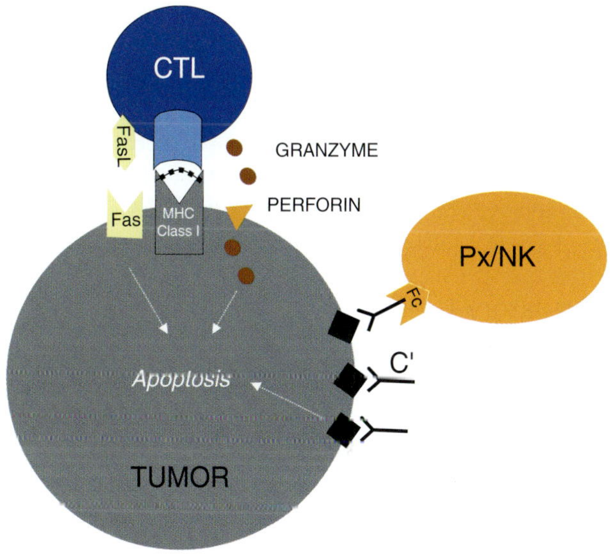

FIG. 4-2 Mechanisms of cell killing by CTL and antibody. *After attaching to the MHC-peptide complex, CTL discharge cytoplasmic granules containing perforin and granzymes by exocytosis. Perforin molecules insert themselves into the plasma membrane of target cells, which enables granzymes to enter the cell. Granzymes are serine proteases that once inside the cell activate caspases that cause the cells to undergo apoptosis.*

When CTL bind to their target, they also up-regulate Fas ligand (FasL) on their surface, which binds with the Fas receptor on the surface of the target cell leading to its death, also by apoptosis. Antibody recognizes antigen in its native conformation. After binding, a complement reactive site on the antibody is activated that sets into motion a cascade of reactions including the activation of many molecules of the complement system, which in turn, activate increasing amounts of enzymes resulting in CMC. A product of the complement cascade also strongly activates phagocytosis by macrophages and neutrophils. These phagocytes (Px) and also NK cells bind their Fc receptor (CD16) to the antibody and destroy the antibody-bound cell (antibody-dependent cellular mechanisms). Antibody-recognizing cell surface molecules that regulate cell signaling/growth can directly elicit apoptosis. Abbreviations: C', complement.

robust as well as a very specific response that is considered to play a central role in immune-mediated tumor rejection.

T-helper Cells

T-helper cells secrete cytokines that regulate all immune cells. They are essential in generating CTL, determining B-cell antibody class switching, and maximizing the activity of phagocytes. Most T-helper cells express CD4 and, thus, recognize antigens expressed by class II MHC. Depending on the nature of the peptide and the activation status of the antigen-presenting cells, either a cellular immune mediated by CTL and by macrophages, referred to as a Th1 response, or a humoral immune response mediated by antibody, referred to as a Th2 response (which also includes activation of eosinophils), is promoted. Predominant cytokines produced in a Th1-associated response are interferon-gamma and interleukin-2 (IL-2). Predominant cytokines produced in a Th2-associated response are IL-4 and IL-5. The requirement for CD4+ T cells in antitumor response has been largely attributed to providing help to naive CD8+ T cells, leading to their differentiation and activation into tumor-specific CTL. Cytokines produced by T-helper cells also may mediate antitumor effects by activating macrophages and NK cells. T-helper cytokines(e.g., interferon-gamma) also may directly suppress tumor growth.

Regulatory T cells

A variety of T cells have the capacity to control and regulate immune responses, preventing reactivity to self while allowing for appropriate responses to nonself antigens. CD4+CD25+ regulatory T (T-reg) cells actively down-regulate the activation and expansion of self-reactive lymphocytes, thus playing a central role in maintaining immune self-tolerance. T-reg cells express CTLA-4 (a glucocorticoid inducible tumor necrosis factor [TNF] receptor) and FOXP3 (a forkhead family transcriptional regulator). Although not specific, FOXP3 is useful as a marker as well as a critical factor for the differentiation of T-reg cells. The mechanism of suppression of self-reactive lymphocytes by T-reg cells is not clear but does appear to involve direct cell–cell contact. Given that many tumor-associated antigens are normal self-constituents, "naturally occurring" CD4+CD25+ T-reg cells engaged in the maintenance of self-tolerance may impede tumor-reactive T cells. What are referred to as type 1 regulatory T (Tr1) cells comprise a subset of CD4+ T cells that are generated by antigen-specific activation in the presence of IL-10. Tr1 cells can promote T-cell anergy and suppress immune responses, primarily via the production of high levels of IL-10 and of transforming growth factor (TGF)-beta. These "induced" regulatory cells also have been implicated in suppressing tumor-reactive T cells.

B CELLS

Antibody-producing B cells are involved in adaptive immunity and also serve as antigen-presenting cells. The BCR binds soluble antigens, which are then internalized by receptor-mediated endocytosis. The antigen is processed into peptide fragments that are then displayed at the cell surface within class II MHC. T-helper cells specific for this structure (i.e., with a complementary TCR) bind the B cell and secrete cytokines that stimulate the B cell to proliferate into cloned cells with identical BCR, switch from synthesizing the BCR as integral membrane proteins to synthesizing them as soluble versions, and, ultimately, differentiate into plasma cells that secrete antibodies (i.e., the soluble version of the BCR). Immunoglobulin class switching — from immunoglobin M (IgM) to immunoglobin G (IgG) — is controlled by the nature of the activating agent/antigen and the influence of cytokines produced by T-helper cells. In contrast to T cells, which recognize only processed peptide antigen, antibodies produced by B cells recognize the intact protein antigen in its native conformation. Antibodies also can recognize polysaccharides and nucleic acids. Antigen-binding specificity is encoded by three complementarity-determining regions, whereas the Fc-region is responsible for binding to serum proteins (e.g., complement) or to cells. Cytotoxicity is mediated by complement-mediated or, for IgG in particular, antibody-dependent cellular mechanisms. Antibodies also can directly mediate antitumor effects by interacting with cell surface receptors that regulate cell growth (Fig. 2). Although cellular immune responses appear to be central in the generation of effective antitumor immunity, there is a substantial body of data to indicate that antibodies also are important. Furthermore, the antitumor effects of antibodies have been validated by the clinical efficacy of monoclonal antibodies specific for tumor-associated molecules.

DENDRITIC CELLS

Dendritic cells are a widely distributed, heterogeneous population of antigen-presenting cells that are derived from bone marrow progenitors and circulate in the blood as immature precursors prior to migration into peripheral tissues. Within different tissues, dendritic cells differentiate and become active in the taking up and processing of antigens. Dendritic cells function at the intersection of the innate and adaptive immune responses. Upon stimulation provided by microbes (via TLR), cytokines, and/or T-cell signals (e.g., CD40 ligand), dendritic cells undergo further maturation and migrate to secondary lymphoid tissues where they present antigen to T cells. The nature of the immune response elicited depends on a variety of factors including the mode and duration of activation and the cytokine microenvironment. Two distinct lineages have been described in humans. CD11 c-positive dendritic cells, referred to as myeloid dendritic cells (DC1), express the receptor for granulocyte-macrophage (GM) colony-stimulating factor (CSF) and other myeloid markers. DC1 are the Langerhans and interstitial dendritic cells that reside in tissues and are the most efficient antigen-presenting cells, particularly with regard to the primary activation of naïve T cells. DC1 have been shown to stimulate tumor-reactive CTL through an IL-12–dependent mechanism. CD11c-negative dendritic cells, referred to as plasmacytoid dendritic cells (DC2), lack myeloid cell markers and express the receptor for IL-3 (CD123). They reside in peripheral blood, and following viral encounter, they secrete large amounts of interferon-alpha, a cytokine with immunomodulatory as well as antiviral properties. Their role in antitumor immunity is less clear.

MACROPHAGES

Macrophages, which derive from peripheral blood monocytes, are specialized phagocytes that are widely dispersed throughout the body. Phagocytosis is mediated through several cell surface receptors for complement and other opsonins. Macrophages engulf particles into phagosomes that then fuse with cytoplasmic lysosomes. They express Fc receptors for immunoglobin and can mediate antibody-dependent cellular mechanisms. Similar to dendritic cells, macrophages can participate in initial capture and processing of potential antigens (innate immunity) and then in activation of specific T- and B-cell effector mechanisms (adaptive immunity). Antibody-dependent cellular mechanisms mediated by macrophages have the advantage of stimulating Tcells because the digested foreign cell proteins are then presented within MHC molecules. Activated macrophages can be directly cytotoxic for cells, including tumor cells, by generating several cytotoxic mediators, such as peroxide and reactive nitrogen intermediates. How macrophage cellular cytotoxicity is triggered has not been established. In addition to their phagocytic, antigen-presenting cellular, and cytotoxic activities, macrophages also are potent secretory cells. Macrophages produce a variety of cytokines, such as TNF-beta, IL-1, IL-6, and IL-8, that regulate local and systemic immune responses.

NK CELLS

NK cells are a relatively small population (less than 10%) of circulating lymphocytes distinct from T and B cells. They are part of the innate response. Although the cytotoxic mechanisms are similar to CTL, NK cells do not require recognition of MHC molecules and, thus, killing by NK cells is designated non–MHC-restricted lysis. In fact, class I MHC molecules send a negative regulatory signal through receptors on the NK cells (killer inhibitory receptors [KIR]) that inhibit their lytic function. Conversely, loss of class I MHC on tumor cells may result in NK cell killing of cells that might otherwise escape T cell recognition. Also in contrast to CTL, NK cells also express Fc receptors and thus can mediate antibody-dependent cellular mechanisms. When activated, NK cells also produce interferon-gamma. Although NK cells do not require activation for lytic activity, the stimulation of NK cells with interferons and IL-2 markedly enhances their antitumor activity. Although CTL can kill multiple cells, there is evidence that NK cells must rearm themselves in response to IL-2 before they are effective against new targets. Furthermore, there is no memory component to the response.

KEY POINT

- Cytokines can function indirectly and can enhance the activity of antitumor immune effectors. Several cytokines also have been shown to directly inhibit tumor cell growth.

CYTOKINES

Cytokines are a diverse group of small proteins released by immune and nonimmune cells distributed throughout the body. Cytokines play integral roles in innate and adaptive immunity as effector and regulatory molecules. They also play an integral role in a variety of other biologic processes. Cytokines, which are active at very low concentrations, may act locally (autocrine or paracrine) or at a distance (endocrine). They are characterized by pleiotropy (one cytokine, multiple effects), redundancy (multiple cytokines, one effect), and synergy (the sum of the response together is greater than the sum of the individual responses). The administration of a cytokine will initiate a cascade of cytokine production and both stimulatory (amplification) and inhibitory/antagonistic effects. Cytokines act on their target cells by binding specific membrane receptors that contain cytokine-specific and signal-transducing subunits. Cytokines can be divided into groups based on function; chemokines are cytokines that have chemoattractants, or a cellular source, and lymphokines are cytokines produced by lymphocytes. Study of the structure and function of cytokine receptors, however, has led to improved understanding of cytokine action and to more useful classifications (Table 4-1). Cytokines can lead to the destruction of tumors by one of two general mechanisms. They can function indirectly and enhance the activity of antitumor cellular or humoral immune effector mechanisms. They also can interact directly with tumor cells; several cytokines, such as TNF-beta, interferon-alpha and interferon-gamma, IL-4, and IL-6, have been shown to initiate tumor cell apoptosis or cell cycle arrest.

IMMUNE SURVEILLANCE

The existence of cancer immune surveillance — that the innate/adaptive immune system continually recognizes and removes malignant cells that arise during one's life — has been difficult to prove. Immune surveillance has been demonstrated in several animal models. Studies from more than 50 years ago showed that growth of a syngeneic tumor in a mouse could be prevented by prior exposure with that same tumor but not a

TABLE 4-1 Examples of Cytokines Involved in Immune Regulation

Group	Function	Receptor	Examples
Hematopoietic	Leukocyte proliferation, differentiation, and activation	Multimers with Trp-Ser-X-Trp-Ser motif Signals primarily by receptor-associated JAK and STAT	IL-2, IL-3, IL-4, IL-6, IL-7, IL-11, IL-12, G-CSF, GM-CSF
Interferon	Inhibit virus replication	Two polypeptide chains with tandem fibronectin domains Signals primarily by JAK-STAT	Interferon-alpha, interferon-beta, interferon-gamma
TNF	Inflammation and other biologic processes	Four extracellular domains activate caspases that mediate apoptosis ("death receptor") or pathways that promote cell survival and inflammation	TNF-alpha
Chemokine	Attract leukocytes to inflammatory sites	Seven transmembrane helices interact with G proteins	MIP-1alpha, IL-8
IL-1	Inflammation and hematopoiesis	Extracellular Ig domain and cytosolic Toll-IL-1 receptor (TIR) domain TIR activates signaling pathways	IL-1beta
Growth factor	Growth and differentiation of nonimmune cells	Multimeric complexes with intrinsic tyrosine or serine/threonine kinase activities	TGF-beta, VEGF

Abbreviations: JAK, Janus tyrosine kinase; STAT, signal transducer and activator of transcription.

different tumor. Tumor resistance in these mice could be transferred to another syngeneic mouse by transplanting spleen cells, T cells in particular, from the resistant mouse. Antibodies seemed less important because much weaker resistance resulted from the transfer of serum from the resistant mouse. It also has been demonstrated that animals deficient in immune-related molecules, such as interferon-gamma, are more susceptible to the development of experimental or spontaneous cancers.

Although direct evidence is lacking, several lines of evidence support the view that immune responses can recognize and eliminate human tumors. Individuals with suppressed immune systems, such as organ transplant recipients or patients affected with primary or acquired immunodeficiency disorders, present an increased risk for developing malignancy. The rare spontaneous regression of cancer has been associated with brisk infiltrations of immune cells, suggesting a role for immune surveillance in cancer control. Brisk lymphocytic infiltrate in tumor specimens is an independent positive prognostic factor for some cancers, such as melanoma and ovarian cancer[1,2]; likewise, the natural occurrence of a humoral immune response to a tumor-associated antigen is associated with a favorable clinical outcome in cancers, such as breast cancer.[3] Human T cells that accumulate within the mass of a tumor can be shown in some instances to proliferate in response to lyse autologous tumor cells in vitro with specificities for the autologous tumors and MHC-matched tumor cells expressing the target antigen. Finally, a variety of immunotherapy modalities have produced objective tumor responses in patients. Treatment of patients with melanoma using CTL that have been expanded ex vivo can result in

KEY POINT

- Although direct evidence for immune surveillance of tumors in humans is lacking, several lines of evidence, including clinical observations, support its existence.

substantial tumor regression. Furthermore, T cells sensitized to peptide fragments of melanoma antigens also can induce tumor regressions.[4]

TUMOR ANTIGENS

Effective surveillance requires that the tumor express determinants capable of being recognized by the immune system (i.e., tumor antigens). Numerous tumor-associated antigens, such as carcinoembryonic antigen (CEA) and prostate-specific antigen (PSA), have been defined with antibodies and applied in diagnosis and in monitoring response to therapy. Whether these antigens can serve as targets for tumor rejection and for the cellular response that appears to be necessary is not clear. As outlined previously, antigens that are recognized by the T cells differ substantially from those defined by antibodies. To function as a T-cell rejection antigen, the tumor must express the associated peptide determinant in the context of MHC molecules. Failure of antigen processing or binding to MHC molecules or inadequate expression of costimulatory or adhesion molecules may lead to poor immunogenicity. Several types of antigens that can potentially serve as tumor rejection antigens have been identified by a variety of techniques (Table 4-2). Oncofetal, cancer-testis (a group of oncofetal antigens), and differentiation/lineage-specific antigens are expressed by normal adult tissues and, therefore, are not tumor specific. In contrast to those that are overexpressed and not mutated (e.g., HER2), oncogenes/tumor suppressors that are mutated (e.g., *p53*) can be considered tumor specific.

KEY POINTS

- A variety of antigens that can potentially function as tumor rejection antigens have been identified. Most are not tumor specific.
- Cancer evasion is aided by the fact that most tumor antigens are self-proteins, which impede the generation of immunity via toleragenic mechanisms, such as the elaboration of T-reg cells.
- Cancer evasion of the immune system results not only from immunosuppressive factors secreted by or expressed on the tumor but also from the ability of the tumor to modulate antigen expression and to develop mechanisms of resistance to immune effectors.

IMMUNE ESCAPE

Tumors can express properties that enable them to "escape" immune responses. Because most of the tumor antigens identified are nonmutated self-antigens, a high degree of immunologic tolerance exists that limits the generation of immune effectors. As noted, CD4+CD25+ T-reg cells engaged in the maintenance of self-tolerance may impede tumor-reactive T cells. There is evidence that the frequency of CD4+CD25+ T-reg cells is elevated in tumor sites and/or in the peripheral blood of patients with advanced tumors. In addition, it has been shown that CD4+CD25+ T reg cells can impair the induction of antigen-specific T cells as well as

TABLE 4-2 Examples of Tumor Antigens

	Example	Associated malignancies (examples)
Oncofetal	CEA	Colorectal, breast, non-small cell lung cancers
	Beta-hCG	Colorectal, pancreatic, non-small cell lung cancers
Cancer-testis	MAGE	Melanoma, lung, bladder, liver
	NY-ESO	Melanoma, lung, bladder, liver
Oncogene/tumor suppressor	HER-2	Breast cancer
	P53	Multiple
	Ras	Multiple
	Bcr-abl	Chronic myeloid leukemia
Differentiation/lineage specific	PSA	Prostate cancer
	Prostatic acid phosphatase	Prostate cancer
	gp100	Melanoma
	Tyrosinase	Melanoma
	MART/Melan-A	Melanoma
	Ig (idiotype)	B-cell malignancies
Aberrantly glycosylated molecules	MUC1 (mucin)	Pancreatic, breast
	GM2 (ganglioside)	Melanoma, neuroblastoma
	GD2 (ganglioside)	Melanoma, neuroblastoma
Viral	E6, E7 (HPV)	Cervical cancer
	EBNA (Epstein-Barr virus)	Burkitt's lymphoma, nasopharyngeal carcinoma

predict reduced survival in patients with cancer.[5] Tumors are heterogeneous, and the repertoire of tumor antigens on cells of one tumor may be variable, even within the same patient. Down-regulation of MHC class I molecules and other components of the antigen-presentation process can occur. Tumors also are considered to be able to evade immune responses because they do not normally express the ligands recognized by innate immune cells that microbes express (the "danger" hypothesis), nor do they express the costimulatory ligands necessary to stimulate adaptive T cells. Tumor cells and the surrounding stroma may release a number of suppressive cytokines and other soluble factors, such as prostaglandin E2, that create an environment that is not conducive to immunity.

Antigen-presenting cell function can be inhibited. Experimental studies have demonstrated that cancer-associated factors inhibit the production and stimulatory capacity of dendritic cells. Tumor-associated dendritic cells may actually induce tolerance, especially when presenting self-antigens. Several clinical studies have demonstrated dendritic-cell deficiencies in patients with cancer, which has been implicated in cancer progression and in the inability of patients with cancer to respond to immunotherapies.[6] The infiltration of plasmacytoid dendritic cells with T-cell suppressive activities has been implicated in cancer progression.[7]

Down-regulation of the expression of CD3 zeta-chain of the TCR complex and impairment of T-cell function have been shown for T cells isolated from patients with cancer. The T-helper cell response also may be skewed toward a Th2 phenotype, which inhibits Th1 response and the cellular immunity that is critical in mediating tumor rejection.[8] A wide variety of tumor cell types are known to secrete IL-10 directly or to induce its secretion by other cells. Increased serum levels of IL-10 have been reported in patients with cancer, which could provide conditions that would favor the induction of Tr1 cells. TGF-beta is produced not only by host cells but also by several tumors and can inhibit the differentiation of T cells into CTL and T-helper cells. By producing cytokines (e.g., GM-CSF), cancers can promote the infiltration of a population of immature myeloid cells, termed myeloid suppressor cells, that can inhibit T cell function partially through the generation of toxic nitrites.[9]

Several membrane-associated factors expressed by tumor cells also have been identified and have been shown to directly inhibit T cell function. These include PD-L1/B7-H1, which engages an inhibitory costimulatory receptor on activated T cells (PD-1). The expression of Fas ligand by some tumor cells may help to maintain a state of immune privilege by inducing apoptosis of Fas-sensitive infiltrating T (and NK)-effector cells — the "Fas counterattack." There also is evidence that the expression of anti-apoptotic molecules by the tumor that block perforin or death receptor-dependent cytotoxicity can result in escape despite the expression of the target antigen. In addition, tumor-associated factors, such as tumor-associated mucins, have been shown to reduce binding of antibodies to tumor cell surfaces.

Tumors are characterized by significant molecular instability as well as by clonal heterogeneity. As tumors develop, the immune system places cancer cells under selective pressure; it detects those that are more antigenic and susceptible to immune effectors. The resistant cells escape and, in turn, will proliferate and spread to distant sites. Loss of tumor antigens in humans following immunotherapy has been reported.[10] This phenomenon, called immune editing, has been implicated in the resistance of tumors to immunotherapies, analogous to the selective pressure induced by chemotherapy and the development of drug resistance.

IMMUNE SUBVERSION

Although effective antitumor immunity has been demonstrated in experimental systems and in some patients, immune responses are abundantly present in tumor-bearing hosts that provide no apparent protection to the host and may contribute to the oncogenic process. Not only can tumors escape immune response, they can exploit or subvert the immune response to promote their growth, invasion, and metastasis.

Local tumor growth within the stroma is promoted by angiogenesis. Immune cells, including macrophages, T cells, and neutrophils, fully participate in tumor angiogenesis by secreting cytokines, such as IL-1, IL-8, and vascular endothelial cell growth factor (VEGF), that directly affect endothelial cell functions including endothelial cell proliferation, migration, and activation. Macrophages, a prominent component of the leukocyte infiltrate in tumors, are a major source of VEGF, which is considered to play a central role in tumor angiogenesis.

Not only do macrophages produce angiogenic factors, they also produce proteases that degrade the extracellular matrix — matrix metalloproteinases. Hence, macrophages can promote tumor cell invasion and metastasis. Accumulating data show that many tumor cells express chemokine receptors and respond to chemokine gradients in vitro. Experimental studies in vivo also have indicated that certain chemokines can serve as tissue-specific attractant molecules for tumor cells, promoting tumor-cell migration/metastasis to particular sites.

Several cytokines produced by immune cells have been shown to transmit cell growth signals in several tumor cell types and directly promote tumor cell growth;

KEY POINTS

- Tumors can subvert the immune response by stimulating the production of immune cell factors that promote angiogenesis, invasion, and metastases.
- Immune cell cytokines also may function as tumor growth factors.

TGF-beta, TNF-alpha, and IL-6 are able to promote the growth of some tumors (while suppressing the growth of others).

BIOLOGIC THERAPIES

Several biologic therapies for cancer have been developed and are applied clinically (Table 4-3). An antitumor immune response can be stimulated through one of several mechanisms: modifying tumor cells to increase their susceptibility to immune effectors, increasing immune effectors, and decreasing immune suppressors. There are two general approaches. "Active" immunotherapy attempts to stimulate (in vivo) an intrinsic immune response to the tumor, either nonspecifically with cytokines or specifically with vaccine approaches. "Passive" or "adoptive" therapy involves the preparation of antibodies and immune cells outside the body (ex vivo) followed by administration to patients. Biologic agents also can mediate antitumor effects by nonimmune effector mechanisms.

CYTOKINES

Interferons

Interferons-alpha and beta (referred to as type I interferons), which are produced by many cell types, and interferon-gamma (referred to as type II interferon), which is produced primarily by lymphocytes, mediate a wide variety of biologic effects. A diversity of genes, at least a few hundred, are transcriptionally induced by interferons. Interferons, type I in particular, inhibit virus replication in infected cells. Interferons affect nearly all phases of the innate and adaptive immune responses. All enhance class I MHC and thereby promote CD8+ CTL responses, and interferon-gamma is capable of inducing class II MHC. Interferons enhance NK cell cytotoxicity, up-regulate Fc receptors, and promote antibody-dependent cellular mechanisms. They regulate the balance between Th1 and Th2 cells, promoting, for the most part, Th1 responses. In addition to affecting humoral immunity by modulating T-helper cells, interferons can have direct effects on B cells, including regulating proliferation and immunoglobin secretion and class switching. Interferon-gamma also plays an important role in macrophage activation. Again, the immune effects elicited can be antagonistic (e.g., the stimulatory effect of NK cells may be offset by the up-regulation of MHC class I molecules on the tumor). A role for immunomodulation is supported by the appearance of autoantibodies or clinical manifestations of autoimmunity in patients with melanoma manifesting improved survival with interferon-alpha treatment.[11] Interferons can directly inhibit the growth of tumor (and normal) cells. The relative sensitivity to cell-cycle arrest or to apoptosis-inducing effects varies with the cell and with the type of interferon. Interferons have anti-angiogenic activity, which is supported by the success of interferon-alpha2 in treating hemangiomas and Kaposi's sarcoma, which are angioproliferative diseases.

> **KEY POINTS**
>
> - Interferons can mediate direct and indirect antitumor effects. Clinical trials have established a number of indications for interferon-alpha, both in hematologic malignancies and in solid tumors.
> - IL-2 was approved for metastatic renal cell cancer and melanoma on the basis of experience with high-dose intravenous bolus of the agent, a regimen limited by significant toxicity.
> - Hematopoietic factors, recombinant G-CSF, and GM-CSF, are commonly used for the prophylaxis of febrile neutropenia and in hematopoietic cell transplantation. Their ability to modulate antitumor immune responses is under investigation.

Among the more than 20 different known interferons, only interferon-alpha2 has been extensively and clinically evaluated for cancer. Two recombinant interferon-alpha2 preparations have been approved for use in patients with cancer: interferon alpha-2a and interferon alpha-2b. A variety of doses have been applied. High-dose regimens apply more than 10 million international units (MIU), intermediate-dose regimens use 5 to 10 MIU, and low-dose regimens use 3 MIU or less. Interferon has been administered by a variety of routes (e.g., intravenous, subcutaneous, and intratumorally) and by a variety of schedules. The plasma half-life is approximately 4 hours, and interferons are usually administered either daily or three times per week. A pegylated form of interferon-alpha2 has resulted in higher serum levels with the advantage of once-weekly administration. Its evaluation in cancer, however, has been limited. There are four types of toxicity: constitutional, neuropsychiatric, hepatic, and hematologic. Flu-like symptoms, such as fever, chills, and myalgia, are associated with the initiation of interferon therapy. They are generally not dose-limiting and usually disappear after 1 to 2 days of therapy, at most after 1 to 2 weeks. With continued administration, neuropsychiatric side effects, such as fatigue and depression, may develop and become limiting. The latter can be occasionally partially ameliorated with the serotonin reuptake family of antidepressants. Liver function tests should be checked. Granulocyte counts and, to a much lesser extent, lymphocyte and platelet counts decline. Treatment should be temporarily suspended if hepatic transaminases rise more than 5 times normal or if granulocytes lower to less than 500 mm^3 and restart at a lower dose when recovery is evident. Changes in these laboratory values are not a cause for treatment discontinuation unless they become severely abnormal (e.g., hepatic transaminases more than 10 times normal).

Interferon-alpha has been approved for use in hairy cell leukemia, chronic myeloid leukemia (CML), follicular lymphoma, Kaposi's sarcoma, and melanoma. Several other

TABLE 4-3 Examples of Biologic Therapies for Cancer in Clinical Use

	Effects	Cancer Indications
Recombinant cytokines		
Interferon-alpha2a Interferon-alpha2b	Immune (up-regulate MHC, activate NK cells) Antiangiogenesis Direct antiproliferative	Hairy cell leukemia, CML, follicular lymphoma, Kaposi's sarcoma, melanoma
Aldesleukin (IL-2)	Activate CTL and NK cells	Renal cell carcinoma, melanoma
Sargramostim (GM-CSF)	Stimulates the development and function of neutrophils, monocyte-macrophages, and DC	Shorten chemotherapy-induced neutropenia in elderly patients with AML, promote myeloid reconstitution after HSCT, mobilize stem cells
Filgrastim (G-CSF) Pegfilgrastim (G-CSF)	Stimulates the development and function of neutrophils	Shorten chemotherapy-induced neutropenia, promote myeloid reconstitution after HSCT, mobilize stem cells
Oprelvekin (IL-11)	Stimulates thrombopoiesis	Shorten chemotherapy-induced thrombocytopenia
Monoclonal antibody (unconjugated)		
Rituximab	Binds CD20 Mediates CMC/antibody-dependent cellular mechanisms Direct antiproliferative	Follicular lymphoma, DLBCL
Trastuzumab	Binds HER-2 Mediates CMC/antibody-dependent cellular mechanisms Direct antiproliferative Antiangiogenesis	Breast
Altemtuzumab	Binds CD52 Mediates CMC/antibody-dependent cellular mechanisms	CLL
Bevacizumab	Binds VEGF Antiangiogenesis	Colorectal, non-squamous NSCLC
Cetuximab	Binds EGFR Mediates CMC/antibody-dependent cellular mechanisms Direct antiproliferative Antiangiogenesis	Colorectal, head and neck
Panitumumab	Binds EGFR Mediates CMC/antibody-dependent cellular mechanisms Direct antiproliferative Antiangiogenesis	Colorectal
Adoptive cellular therapy		
DLI	Mediates GVL effect	CML and other hematologic malignancies

Abbreviations: MHC, major histocompatibility complex; CML, chronic myeloid leukemia; AML, acute myeloid leukemia; HSCT, hematopoietic stem cell transplantation; DLBCL, diffuse large B-cell lymphoma; CLL, chronic lymphocytic leukemia; VEGF, vascular endothelial growth factor; NSCLC, non-small cell lung cancer; EGFR, growth factor receptor; DLI, donor leukocyte infusion; GVL, graft-versus-leukemia; GM-CSF, granulocyte macrophaqe-colony stimulating factor; CTL, cytotoxic T lymphocytes; NK, natural killer.

hematologic malignancies and solid tumors have therapeutic sensitivity to interferon-alpha, including cutaneous T cell lymphoma, multiple myeloma, and renal cell carcinoma.

Before the introduction of interferon-alpha, splenectomy was the standard of care for patients with hairy cell leukemia. Low-dose interferon-alpha treatment was shown to normalize blood counts within 4 to 5 months. However, the bone marrow was rarely completely cleared of hairy cells, thereby resulting in interferon-alpha being largely supplanted when more effective chemotherapeutics, such as pentostatin and cladrabine, were introduced.

Intermediate-dose interferon-alpha led to complete hematologic response for most patients with CML and partial cytogenetic response in up to 40% when treatment was started during the chronic phase of the disease. Before the use of interferon-alpha, cytogenetic responses rarely, if ever, resulted from chemotherapeutic agents. Therapy with low-dose cytarabine and interferon-alpha provided even better cytogenetic response and more prolonged disease control. The evolutionary change in therapy for CML caused by the introduction of imatinib mesylate has resulted in the general replacement of interferon-alpha, either alone or in combination with cytarabine. However, as resistance to imatinib mesylate has emerged, randomized trials comparing combinations of interferon-alpha with imatinib mesylate are in progress.

Interferon-alpha is active in follicular lymphoma. Initial studies showed a 50% objective response rate, which led to several studies, both in combination with chemotherapy and as maintenance therapy, with varying results. In most studies, interferon-alpha was associated with a prolongation of remission but not of overall survival. In a large phase III clinical trial, patients were randomly assigned to interferon-alpha or to observation following induction with an intensive anthracycline-containing regimen and, in some cases, radiotherapy. Neither progression-free survival nor overall survival was affected by post-remission therapy.[12] Although results of randomized trials and toxicities associated with interferon-alpha have led many clinicians to abandon its use altogether in follicular lymphoma, a phase III study is ongoing testing standard versus intensive dose maintenance. In addition, interferon-alpha is being studied in combination with rituximab and with fludarabine.

The response rates with interferon-alpha as a single modality in metastatic melanoma is equivalent to chemotherapy agents, such as dacarbazine, at 15%.[13] The pleiotropic effects of interferon-alpha, coupled with its activity against metastatic melanoma, resulted in its evaluation in the adjuvant setting for patients at high risk for disease recurrence after primary surgery. Randomized trials demonstrated significant improvement in disease-free survival; the effect on overall survival is less clear.[14] Because of these studies, interferon-alpha, administered intravenously at high doses for the first month followed by 11 months of intermediate doses subcutaneously, has become a standard adjuvant treatment for patients with melanoma. Interferon-alpha has been combined with chemotherapy in several studies in melanoma. These "biochemotherapy" programs yield higher response rates for metastatic disease; overall survival rates, however, were not significantly improved. Because of the substantial toxicities associated with biochemotherapy programs that often require prolonged hospitalization, the modest effects on overall outcome have led to an eclipse of this approach for metastatic melanoma. It is, however, an approach that is being evaluated in the adjuvant setting.

Initial treatment regimens for Kaposi's sarcoma associated with human immunodeficiency virus (HIV) infection employed high doses of interferon-alpha that were associated with significant response rates but also with high levels of toxicity. In subsequent studies that primarily applied intermediate doses combined with antiretroviral medications, responses were observed primarily in patients with CD4 counts greater than 400 mm^3. Although still applied to treat Kaposi's sarcoma, for more advanced disease in particular, interferon-alpha has been supplanted by chemotherapy.

Interferon-alpha as a single agent has been effective in patients with advanced cutaneous T-cell lymphoma.[15] Approximately 50% respond partially and 25% completely, although most relapse within a year. Although regimens have not been established, low and intermediate doses appear to be as effective as high doses. A number of clinical trials have demonstrated activity in multiple myeloma. Small, statistically significant increases in progression-free survival and overall survival were identified in meta-analysis, particularly for patients receiving maintenance therapy following chemotherapy or autologous HSCT.[16] Although now being supplanted by more active agents, such as sunitinib, response rates of 15% have been documented in several trials of interferon-alpha for metastatic renal cancer.[17,18] Patients with low tumor burden, good performance status, and lung and lymph node metastases respond best. When compared with chemotherapy or hormone therapy in phase III trials, interferon-alpha prolonged survival for a few to several months. Although the contribution of interferon is not entirely clear, patients with metastatic renal cell carcinoma with a good performance status who received interferon-alpha after nephrectomy showed improved survival, despite the presence of metastases.[19]

Several clinical trials testing novel applications of interferons in patients with hematologic malignancies and solid tumors are in progress. It should be noted that interferons also have had an effect in several other diseases. Interferon-alpha also is used to treat condyloma accuminata and hepatitis B and C. Interferon-beta is used to treat multiple sclerosis; interferon-gamma is used to treat chronic granulomatous disease.

IL-2

IL-2 is a T-cell growth factor. Antigen binding to the TCR stimulates the secretion of IL-2 and the expression of IL-2 receptors (CD25). The interaction between IL-2 and the IL-2 receptor stimulates the growth, differentiation, and survival of antigen-selected T cells. IL-2 is a major activator of CTL and NK cytotoxicity. Interest in IL-2 as a therapeutic agent for patients with cancer was initially driven by the observation that lymphokine-activated killer (LAK) cells (which are generated by culturing peripheral blood cells with IL-2 and which, for the most part, represent IL-2-activated NK cells) killed a broad range of tumor types. IL-2 is necessary for the development of memory T cells. It also indirectly regulates B cells and hematopoiesis. More recent studies have focused on the role of IL-2 in maintaining immunologic tolerance. IL-2 is required for the generation and maintenance of CD4+CD25+ T-reg cells, which, as noted, has been implicated in abrogating antitumor activity.[20] Furthermore, IL-2 is involved in activation-induced cell death, a process that leads to the elimination of self-reactive T cells.

Recombinant IL-2, aldesleukin, has been applied in a variety of doses, routes, and schedules. The plasma half-life is short — 1 to 2 hours. The high-dose regimen that led to FDA approval applies 600,000 to 720,000 IU/kg three times daily as an intravenous bolus. The maximum amount of doses that most patients can tolerate is 14. A rest period of 5 to 9 days between cycles is recommended. Because of toxicities, administration of high-dose aldesleukin requires particular expertise, and patients must be treated in a step-down situation or intensive care unit. These toxicities stem from a capillary-leak syndrome, which is characterized by increased vascular permeability and decreased microcirculatory perfusion and leads to interstitial edema and multiple organ failure. Administering aldesleukin in high doses is comparable to inducing a controlled state of septic shock with fever, hypotension, decreased renal function, hyperbilirubinemia, rash, and marked malaise. Lower-dose regimens administered subcutaneously are much better tolerated but are of uncertain clinical benefit. Decisions regarding the relative benefits of aldesleukin must be influenced by evaluations of toxicity and quality of life associated with the different regimens and schedules.

Aldesleukin was approved as treatment for patients with metastatic renal cell cancer on the basis of experience with the high-dose regimen. Objective responses occur in a minority of patients, approximately 15%. More importantly, in approximately 5% of all treated patients, the response is complete and sustainable for many months or even years without additional therapy. Although FDA approval was granted only to high-dose bolus aldesleukin, other regimens have efficacy for renal cell cancer. Lower-dose aldesleukin administered subcutaneously was associated with similar response rates in several small nonrandomized studies but has not been evaluated sufficiently to determine its effect on long-term outcome.

A response in approximately 15% of patients with melanoma also has been reported with high-dose bolus aldesleukin, with a long-term sustained response achieved in 3% to 5% of patients. These findings led to approval in management of metastatic melanoma. Lower-dose aldesleukin has produced disappointing response rates in melanoma. To exploit potentially synergistic antitumor effects, aldesleukin has been applied with interferon-alpha. In several studies in patients with melanoma, the response rates were generally not higher than those achieved with either agent alone. In addition, aldesleukin has been incorporated into biochemotherapy regimens for metastatic melanoma, which have, as noted previously, increased the response rate.[21]

IL-2-based programs have demonstrated activity in a variety of other solid tumors, such as colon, pancreatic, and hepatocellular cancers, as well as mesothelioma, but not at levels required for regulatory approval. Activity also has been observed in hematologic malignancies, including acute myelogenous leukemia (AML). Studies evaluating predictors of response to IL-2 and novel applications are in progress.

GM-CSF

GM-CSF is a hematopoietic factor that stimulates the development of neutrophils and monocyte-macrophages and promotes the proliferation and development of early erythroid, megakaryocytic, and eosinophilic progenitor cells. It is produced by endothelial cells and fibroblasts as well as by T cells and monocyte-macrophages. GM-CSF produces a variety of effects on cells of the neutrophil and monocyte-macrophage lineages, including augmentation of monocyte-macrophage MHC class II expression and enhancement of granulocyte and macrophage cellular cytotoxicity and antibody-dependent cellular mechanisms. GM-CSF also serves as the principal mediator of the proliferation and differentiation of myeloid dendritic cells. It enhances dendritic cell antigen-uptake, MHC, and costimulatory molecule expression, as well as the ability of dendritic cells to stimulate T cells. However, GM-CSF has been shown to stimulate myeloid suppressor cells and to promote angiogenesis by stimulating VEGF production.

Although recombinant GM-CSF (sargramostim) can be administered intravenously, subcutaneous administration is preferred. Because of the sensitivity of rapidly dividing myeloid cells, sargramostim is typically initiated 1 to 3 days after completion of chemotherapy and administered daily through post-nadir recovery, usually for 2 weeks. Sargramostim has been well tolerated. Side effects include pain and inflammation at the injection sites, bone pain, myalgia, arthralgia, and low-grade fever, which usually are not limiting. Nausea, fluid retention, dyspnea, pericarditis, pleuritis, pulmonary emboli, splenomegaly, and hypersensitivity reactions have been reported but are rare.

Sargramostim is indicated for use following induction chemotherapy in patients with AML who are ages 50 to 70 years in order to shorten the time to neutrophil recovery. It also is indicated for use in mobilization and following

TABLE 4-4 Summary of 2006 Update of ASCO Recommendations for the Use of CSFs[22]

- Reduction in febrile neutropenia is an important clinical outcome that justifies the use of colony stimulating factors (CSFs), regardless of effect on other factors, when the risk of febrile neutropenia is approximately 20% and no other equally effective regimen that does not require CSFs is available.
- Primary prophylaxis is recommended for the prevention of febrile neutropenia in patients who are at high risk based on age, medical history, disease characteristics, and myelotoxicity of the chemotherapy regimen.
- CSF use allows a modest to moderate increase in dose-density and/or dose-intensity of chemotherapy regimens. Dose-dense regimens should only be used within an appropriately designed clinical trial or if supported by convincing efficacy data.
- Prophylactic CSF for patients with diffuse aggressive lymphoma aged 65 years and older treated with curative chemotherapy (combination cyclophosphamide, doxorubicin and vincristine [CHOP] or more aggressive regimens) should be given to reduce the incidence of febrile neutropenia and infections.
- Current recommendations for the management of patients exposed to lethal doses of total body radiotherapy, but not doses high enough to lead to certain death due to injury to other organs, includes the prompt administration of CSFs.

transplantation of autologous peripheral blood progenitor cells, in myeloid reconstitution after autologous and allogeneic HSCT, and in HSCT failure or engraftment delay. As with the recombinant granulocyte (G)-CSF, sargramostim can be used for the prevention of febrile neutropenia in adults with nonmyeloid malignancies receiving myelosuppressive chemotherapy. However, there have been fewer trials of sargramostim as primary prophylaxis for febrile neutropenia in this setting. ASCO guidelines for the use of colony-stimulating factors have recently been revised (Table 4-4).[22]

Although GM-CSF can mediate other antitumor activities, such as stimulation of macrophage cytotoxicity, it is its ability to function as an immunoadjuvant and to stimulate tumor-specific T-cell responses that has led to its evaluation in a number of clinical trials. A variety of cancer vaccine approaches that incorporate GM-CSF have been tested clinically.[23] There also is evidence that administering sargramostim as monotherapy has antitumor activity in patients with melanoma and prostate cancer.[24,25]

G-CSF

G-CSF is a hematopoietic factor produced by macrophages, lymphocytes, fibroblasts, and endothelial cells. It induces the production and release of neutrophilic granulocytes in the bone marrow and enhances their functional capacity in the periphery. Moreover, G-CSF possesses essential neutrophil-activating functions, such as the oxidative burst, degranulation, phagocytosis, and chemotaxis. G-CSF markedly stimulates neutrophil antibody-dependent cellular mechanisms. As a regulator of neutrophil activity, G-CSF plays a role in innate immune responses. There is growing evidence that G-CSF also exerts immunoregulatory effects in adaptive immunity. G-CSF mediates anti-inflammatory reactions accompanied by Th2 differentiation and promotes toleragenic antigen-presenting cell/T-cell interactions.

Recombinant G-CSF (filgrastim), which has a plasma half-life of 3.5 hours, is usually administered subcutaneously daily for up to 2 weeks, until post-nadir neutrophil recovery is at normal or near-normal neutrophil levels. Because of the sensitivity of rapidly dividing myeloid cells, filgrastim should be administered no earlier than 24 hours after the administration of cytotoxic chemotherapy and no earlier than 24 hours before the administration of chemotherapy. A pegylated form of recombinant G-CSF, pegfilgrastim, has a variable plasma half life of 15 to 80 hours, which allows administration once per cycle rather than daily. Pegfilgrastim is administered as a single subcutaneous injection once per chemotherapy cycle. Pegfilgrastim should not be administered in the period between 14 days before and 24 hours after administration of cytotoxic chemotherapy. The safety data appear to be similar between filgrastim and pegfilgrastim. The most commonly observed adverse effects are mild-to-moderate bone pain after repeated administration and local skin reactions at the site of injection. Bone pain, reported in approximately 20% of patients, is rarely dose limiting and can usually be controlled with analgesics; it is not an indication to discontinue therapy. Fever, diarrhea, edema, dyspnea, skin rash, splenomegaly (with rupture), and hypersensitivity reactions also may occur.

Filgrastim and pegfilgrastim are indicated to decrease the incidence of infection, as manifested by febrile neutropenia, in patients with nonmyeloid malignancies who are receiving myelosuppressive chemotherapy associated with a significant incidence (20%) of severe neutropenia with fever (Table 4-4).[22] In addition to the chemotherapy regimens, several other factors are considered when assessing the risk of febrile neutropenia and whether to administer recombinant G-CSF in this setting. These include factors that are treatment-related (e.g., severe neutropenia with similar chemotherapy), patient-related (e.g., age older than 65 years, open wounds, and chronic lung or heart disease), and cancer-related (e.g., bone marrow involvement with tumor). Filgrastim also is used following induction or consolidation chemotherapy treatment for adults with AML, for patients with nonmyeloid malignancies who are undergoing myeloablative chemotherapy followed by HSCT, and for the mobilization of hematopoietic progenitor cells.

Recombinant G-CSF is indicated to reduce the magnitude and sequelae of neutropenia (e.g., fever, infections, and oropharyngeal ulcers) in symptomatic patients with congenital, cyclic, or idiopathic neutropenia.[26] The imunomodulatory effects of G-CSF, such as the ability to promote antibody-dependent cellular mechanisms and to promote T-cell tolerance in pathologic conditions associated with a Th1/Th2 imbalance, are under investigation.

IL-11

IL-11 is produced by eosinophils, fibroblasts, and a variety ofepithelial cells. IL-11 functions primarily as a hematopoietic factor and interacts with other early and late growth factors to stimulate various stages and lineages of hematopoiesis. Its effects on platelets are particularly prominent. IL-11 synergizes with IL-3, thrombopoietin, or stem cell factor to stimulate thrombopoiesis. Early and later stages of megakaryocytopoiesis, including proliferation and differentiation of megakaryocyte precursors and maturation of megakaryocytes, are stimulated to produce an increase in peripheral platelet count. IL-11 also regulates macrophage proliferation and differentiation.

Recombinant IL-11, oprelvekin, is indicated for the prevention of severe thrombocytopenia and the reduction of the need for platelet transfusions following myelosuppressive chemotherapy in adult patients with nonmyeloid malignancies who are at high risk of severe thrombocytopenia. Oprelvekin must be administered to patients sufficiently in advance of the platelet nadir (within 6 to 24 hours after chemotherapy) to allow adequate time for megakaryocyte maturation and platelet formation. Therefore, the maximum platelet response coincides with the time when the platelet nadir would normally be experienced. Toxicity can be limiting; more than 30% of patients will experience edema, nausea and vomiting, mouth sores, diarrhea, or shortness of breath. Edema is the result of a renal effect, resulting in plasma-volume expansion and, in some situations, a capillary leak syndrome. Because oprelvekin does not eliminate the development of thrombocytopenia and because of its toxicity, it has limited clinical application. The immunologic effects of IL-11, which include the ability to inhibit IL-2 and interferon-gamma and stimulate IL-10 production, are poorly understood. Nonhematopoietic effects of IL-11 include potential beneficial clinical effects in damaged or inflamed intestinal mucosa, including potential mitigation of mucositis.

Other cytokines

Several other recombinant and purified cytokines, including IL-1beta, IL-3, IL-4, IL-6, IL-7, IL-12, TNF-alpha, MIP-1-alpha, interferon-beta, and interferon-gamma have been tested or are currently being tested in patients with cancer. Thus far, clinical antitumor activity has been limited and/or toxicity has been limiting. These and other cytokines remain of substantial investigative interest because of effects on immune cell function and, in some instances, their ability to directly inhibit tumor cell growth. Cytokines that also influence structure and function of the microenvironment, including endothelial cells, have been identified. Currently available cytokines or other cytokines may ultimately play new roles in systemic therapies, as part of cytokine gene immunotherapy or ex vivo as modulators of immune cell function.

MONOCLONAL ANTIBODIES

Adoptive therapy with monoclonal antibodies has been one of the major advances in cancer immunotherapy. The monoclonal antibodies used in initial clinical trials were mouse and usually generated a vigorous human–anti-mouse antibody (HAMA) response. Therapeutic monoclonal antibodies are either chimeric with the mouse variable fused to human constant (65% to 90% human) chain, humanized with the mouse hypervariable/complementarity-determining regions grafted to human immunoglobin (95% human), or fully human. Many of these antibodies have been effective as monotherapy. However, effectiveness often can be enhanced by their combined application with other treatment modalities. Antibodies naturally have long serum half-lives. Several limitations, however, have been identified. Although now rare, immune responses to the artificial humanized antibody can still be problematic. The antigenic heterogeneity of most tumors presents challenges,

KEY POINTS

- The effectiveness of monoclonal antibodies to tumor-associated antigens has been established for both hematologic malignancies and solid tumors.
- Monoclonal antibodies can mediate antitumor activity via immune mechanisms (e.g. antibody-dependent and complement-mediated cellular mechanisms) and by nonimmunologic mechanisms (e.g., direct induction of apoptosis).
- Although active as single agents, monoclonal antibodies are most often applied with chemotherapy or radiation therapy.
- Most monoclonal antibodies have been well tolerated. Infusion reactions and organ toxicities can occur.

as do the small fraction of injected antibodies that actually bind to tumors and the inability of antibodies to penetrate into large tumor masses. Furthermore, binding of antibodies to circulating antigens also can limit delivery to the tumor.

Rituximab

The first monoclonal antibody to receive FDA approval for therapeutic use was rituximab, a human/mouse chimeric IgG1 directed to CD20, a transmembrane protein expressed on malignant and normal B cells. CD20 is expressed on more than 90% of cells for B-cell non-Hodgkin's lymphoma and to a lesser degree on chronic lymphocytic leukemia (CLL). CD20 function is not established. The intracellular portion of CD20 contains phosphorylation sites for several signaling kinases. It may affect cell cycle through calcium channel regulation. The cytotoxic effects of rituximab appear to involve antibody-dependent cellular mechanisms, complement-mediated cellular mechanisms, and induction of apoptosis.

The dosing of rituximab is dependent on the clinical setting. Rituximab is usually administered intravenously weekly for 4 or 8 doses. Serum concentrations double from the first to the fourth infusion, and elimination plasma half-life increases from 3 to 9 days because of elimination of circulating CD20+ B cells and reduction/saturation of CD20–binding sites. Rituximab infusions are generally well tolerated. Infusion-related reactions occur in the majority of patients, usually mild-to-moderate flu-like symptoms, and premedication with acetaminophen and diphenhydramine is recommended. Severe infusion reactions, such as bronchospasm and hypotension, are found in 10% of patients and are usually reversible with appropriate interventions. Transient hypotension may occur; therefore, withholding antihypertensives 12 hours before infusion should be considered. To address infusion reactions, the initial infusion is administered slowly. If hypersensitivity or infusion-related events do not occur, the infusion rate is increased incrementally. Subsequent infusions also are administered more slowly, initially with incremental rate increases. Rituximab can elicit a tumor lysis syndrome. It also induces lymphopenia, which lasts for approximately 6 months. Full recovery occurs in 9 to 12 months. CD20 is not expressed on hematopoietic stem cells. Patients who subsequently develop progressive disease may be safely retreated.

Rituximab is active in various lymphoid malignancies, including follicular lymphoma and diffuse large B-cell lymphoma (DLBCL). Optimal use has yet to be clarified. Initial studies in patients with relapsed or refractory follicular lymphoma demonstrated its efficacy as a single agent or in combination with chemotherapy without adding toxicity. More recent studies have demonstrated activity as first-line therapy in combination with cyclophosphamide, vincristine, and prednisolone (CVP) chemotherapy. Patients with follicular lymphoma who respond to rituximab can be retreated with rituximab at progression. Response rates for retreatment are comparable to first-line treatment, which is unique for cancer chemotherapy.[27] The magnitude of benefit of maintenance therapy versus retreatment at progression is similar.[28] Trials in elderly patients have demonstrated that the addition of rituximab to combination cyclophosphamide, doxorubicin, vincristine, and prednisone (CHOP) chemotherapy significantly improved complete remission and event-free and overall survival rates when compared with CHOP alone.[29] These positive results have been extended to younger patients. Rituximab in combination with CHOP or other anthracycline-based chemotherapy has become accepted as the new standard for the treatment of DLBCL. However, the best combination of rituximab and CVP, CHOP, or any other chemotherapy is not known.

Rituximab also is being incorporated into the therapy of other CD20+ B-cell malignancies. In addition, rituximab is being used in several immune-related diseases, such as rheumatoid arthritis, immune thrombocytopenic purpura, systemic lupus erythematosus, and myasthenia gravis, as well as for organ transplant recipients.

Alemtuzumab

Alemtuzumab is a humanized IgG1 directed against CD52, a nonmodulating glycoprotein expressed on the surface of normal and malignant B and T cells, NK cells, monocytes, macrophages, and tissues of the male reproductive system. CD52 function is unknown. The cytotoxic effects of alemtuzumab are presumed to involve antibody-dependent and complement-mediated cellular mechanisms.

Alemtuzumab is usually initiated at low, intravenous, daily doses, with gradual dose escalation until a maintenance dose is reached. The maintenance dose is administered three times a week for up to 12 weeks. There is a rise in serum concentration with repeated infusions that corresponds with the reduction in malignant lymphocytosis. If therapy is interrupted for 7 or more days, it must be reinstituted at lower doses with gradual dose escalation. The subcutaneous route of administration is gaining popularity because it is effective and has fewer side effects than intravenous infusions. Alemtuzumab administration can be limited by toxicity, which includes infusion-related toxicities such as hypotension, rigors, fever, dyspnea, bronchospasm, chills, and/or rash. Premedication with diphenhydramine and acetaminophen before infusion is recommended, as is hydrocortisone if infusion-related events occur. Alemtuzumab induces profound lymphopenia, and a variety of opportunistic infections have been reported. Severe and prolonged myelosuppression also can occur. Infection prophylaxis, trimethoprim/sulfamethoxazole, and famciclovir (or its equivalent) are necessary and must be continued for 2 months after completion of therapy or until CD4 cell counts are greater than 200, whichever occurs later.

Alemtuzumab is indicated for the treatment of B-cell CLL in patients who have been treated with alkylating agents and who have shown no response to fludarabine therapy. Response rates of approximately 30% can be achieved.[30] Comparative, randomized trials demonstrating increased survival or clinical benefits, such as improvement in disease-related symptoms, have not yet been reported.

Alemtuzumab also has demonstrated activity in T-prolymphocytic leukemia and in cutaneous T-cell lymphoma. In addition, it is being used as an immunosuppressive agent for various autoimmune diseases and as part of the conditioning regimens for allogeneic HSCT to prevent graft-versus-host disease (GVHD).

Trastuzumab

The antibody with the greatest effect in solid tumors is trastuzumab, a humanized IgG1 directed against the extracellular domain of HER2, also known as ErbB2, a member of the epidermal growth factor (EGF) family of receptor tyrosine kinases. It is overexpressed by 20% to 30% of human breast cancers. Overexpression is implicated in the malignant transformation process and is an independent, adverse prognostic factor in breast cancer, which may predict for response to both chemotherapy and hormone agents. HER2 also is overexpressed by other carcinomas. Trastuzumab exerts antitumor effects by several mechanisms that are not yet completely understood. Immune effector mechanisms, namely antibody-dependent and complement-mediated cellular mechanisms, are considered to be central. Trastuzumab has direct antiproliferative effects, which include cell-cycle arrest and/or induction of apoptosis; it markedly accelerates HER-2 endocytosis and degradation. Trastuzumab also can mediate antiangiogenic effects, including the inhibition of VEGF production.

Trastuzumab is administered intravenously, and a loading dose is administered initially followed by weekly administration. Other regimens, such as a dosing of every 3 weeks, also have been effectively applied. Trastuzumab is generally well tolerated. Infusion reactions do occur, but premedication is usually not required. Cardiac dysfunction can be problematic. It was observed in almost 30% of patients who were receiving an anthracycline and cyclophosphamide; concurrent therapy with anthracyclines is not recommended. Cardiac dysfunction also has been observed in approximately 15% of patients receiving trastuzumab plus paclitaxel and in approximately 5% of patients receiving trastuzumab alone. Cardiac myocytes (transverse tubules) express HER2. There are reports of fatalities in patients with poor performance status and lung dysfunction.

Trastuzumab has been shown to benefit patients with breast cancer whose tumors have *HER2* gene amplification as detected by fluorescence in situ hybridization (FISH), which is closely associated with immunohistochemical staining at the 3+ level. It is effective when used as first-line monotherapy for patients with advanced breast cancer, for whom it produces a response rate of approximately 25%. It improves survival by approximately 20% for patients with metastatic breast cancer when combined with paclitaxel (or anthracycline-cyclophosphamide regimen) compared with chemotherapy alone.[31] As a single agent, trastuzumab is indicated for the treatment of patients with metastatic breast cancer whose tumors overexpress *HER2* and who have received one or more chemotherapy regimens for their metastatic disease. Trastuzumab combined with paclitaxel is indicated for treatment of patients with metastatic breast cancer whose tumors overexpress *HER2* and who have not received chemotherapy for their metastatic disease. Trastuzumab also has demonstrated activity when used in other combinations, including with docetaxel, vinorelbine, capecitabine, gemcitabine, and/or platinums. The results of trials that evaluated trastuzumab in the adjuvant setting have recently been presented and have demonstrated that recurrence rate is reduced by one-half and the death rate by one-third.[32,33] As part of a treatment regimen containing doxorubicin, cyclophosphamide, and paclitaxel, trastuzumab is indicated for the adjuvant treatment of patients with *HER2*-overexpressing, node-positive breast cancer.

Trastuzumab is being evaluated in other cancers that overexpress *HER2*, such as non-small cell lung (NSCLC), ovarian, gastric, and pancreatic cancers.

Bevacizumab

Bevacizumab is humanized IgG1 directed against VEGF. Often overexpressed by tumor cells as well as by tumor-associated macrophages, VEGF has proven to be a pivotal stimulator of endothelial cell migration and proliferation. Bevacizumab binds one VEGF isoform and prevents the interaction of VEGF with its receptors (Flt-1 and KDR) on endothelial cells. Bevacizumab has been shown to inhibit endothelial cell proliferation and new blood vessel formation in in vitro models and to reduce tumor microvascular growth and metastatic disease progression in several in vivo animal tumor models.

Bevacizumab is administered intravenously every 14 days. The plasma half-life is approximately 20 days (free plus bound to circulating VEGF). After correcting for body weight, men have a higher bevacizumab clearance, as do patients with higher tumor burden. There is, however, no evidence of lesser efficacy in men or in patients with higher tumor burden. Clinical toxicities include gastrointestinal perforations, wound healing complications, and hemorrhage. At least 28 days following major surgery must pass, and the incision should be fully healed prior to administrating bevacizumab. Administration also should be suspended several weeks prior to elective surgery. In addition, hypertensive crisis, nephrotic syndrome, and congestive heart failure have been observed. Bevacizumab must be suspended in patients with gastrointestinal perforation, wound dehiscence, serious bleeding, nephrotic syndrome, or hypertensive crisis. The risk of continuation or temporary suspension in patients with moderate to severe proteinuria is unknown. Infusion reactions are relatively uncommon.

Clinical trials have suggested clinical effectiveness in several cancers. The most advanced data have emerged in metastatic colorectal carcinoma and NSCLC combined with chemotherapy. Significant improvement in response rate and significant prolongation of survival have been observed when compared with chemotherapy alone. Bevacizumab is approved for use combined with 5-flurouracil-based chemotherapy as first-line or second-line treatment of patients with metastatic colorectal cancer.[34] Bevacizumab combined with carboplatin and paclitaxel also is indicated for first-line treatment of patients with unresectable, locally advanced, recurrent or metastatic non-squamous cell NSCLC.[35] Hemorrhagic complications are more common in patients with squamous cell histology. Correlation of the antitumor activity with measures of angiogenesis inhibition has been difficult to demonstrate.

Bevacizumab has shown activity in breast, pancreatic, prostate, head and neck, and renal cell cancers, as well as in several hematologic malignancies. In addition to promoting angiogenesis, VEGF has immunosuppressive effects. The immunomodulatory effects of bevacizumab are under investigation.

Cetuximab

As with HER2, overexpression by tumors of the EGF receptor (EGFR), also known as ErbB1, confers a negative prognosis. Cetuximab is a human/mouse chimeric IgG1 to the extracellular domain of EGFR. It competitively inhibits the binding of EGF and other ligands, such as TGF-alpha. It blocks activation of receptor-associated kinases, resulting in inhibition of cell growth, apoptosis, and decreased VEGF and matrix metalloproteinases production. EGFR is expressed in many normal epithelial tissues, such as skin. Many human carcinomas overexpress EGFR. In animal studies, cetuximab inhibited tumor cells that overexpress EGFR in vitro and in vivo, and it increased activity of chemotherapy.

Cetuximab is administered intravenously; a loading dose is initially administered, followed by weekly infusions. The plasma half-life is approximately 5 days. Women have 25% lower clearance than men; response and toxicity are similar. In general, cetuximab has been well tolerated. Infusion reactions do occur, particularly with the initial infusions, and premedication with diphenhydramine is recommended. The most common side effect has been an acne-like skin rash, which develops in up to 75% of patients and which probably represents the biologic effects of blocking EGFR present in the skin. The development of a rash has been associated with greater therapeutic effectiveness. Life-threatening toxicities, such as interstitial lung disease, have been rarely observed.

Cetuximab is indicated for use in colorectal and head and neck cancers. It is indicated in combination with irinotecan for patients with EGFR-positive metastatic colorectal cancer who are refractory to irinotecan, resulting in a response rate approaching 25%. Cetuximab also is indicated for use as a single agent for patients with colorectal cancer who are unable to tolerate irinotecan-based chemotherapy, resulting in a response rate of approximately 10%.[36] The addition of cetuximab to high-dose radiation in patients with locoregionally advanced, squamous cell carcinoma of the head and neck resulted in a statistically significant improvement in overall survival (49.0 months vs. 29.3 months, $p = 0.03$),[37] leading to its treatment indication in this setting. As a single agent, cetuximab is indicated for the treatment of patients with recurrent or metastatic squamous cell carcinoma of the head and neck for whom prior platinum-based therapy has failed.

Cetuximab is being evaluated in other cancers that express EGFR, such as NSCLC and pancreatic cancer, as well as in several novel combination programs.

Panitumumab

Panitumumab is a recombinant, human IgG2 monoclonal antibody that also binds specifically to EGFR. In contrast to cetuximab, panitumumab is fully human. The theoretical advantage conferred by this agent, compared with its chimeric counterpart, is that there is less potential for an antigenic response. The mechanism of antitumor activity is considered to be identical to that of cetuximab.

Panitumumab is administered intravenously, and there is no loading dose. The elimination plasma half-life is approximately 7 days, and panitumumab is administered every 14 days. Because it is fully human, decreases in allergic reactions were predicted, and, as such, the development of human anti-human antibodies has not been detected with treatment. Approximately 1% of patients exposed to panitumumab, however, experienced a severe infusion reaction, whereas approximately 3% of patients treated with cetuximab experienced severe infusion reactions. Other toxicities appear to be similar. Skin rash with variable presentation is common. Other common adverse events include hypomagnesemia, abdominal pain, nausea, and diarrhea. Rare but serious adverse events, such as pulmonary fibrosis, also have been observed.

Panitumumab is approved for the treatment of EGFR-expressing metastatic colorectal carcinoma with disease progression on or following chemotherapy regimens containing fluoropyrimidine, oxaliplatin, and irinotecan. It was approved on the basis of a phase III trial in which patients were randomly assigned to receive either panitumumab with best supportive care or to best supportive care alone.[38] Patients receiving panitumumab had a statistically significant greater progression-free survival, median 8 weeks (95% CI, 7.9–8.4) versus 7.3 (95% CI, 7.1–7.7). A partial response rate of 8%

with panitumumab compared with 0% for best supportive care also was observed. An association between the development of rash and response was suggested. There was no difference in overall survival between the two study arms. Patients who received best supportive care alone could crossover to treatment. No patients who had been previously treated with cetuximab were included, and it is unknown if there will be cross-resistance with panitumumab. Of note, inclusion criteria within the studies included EGFR staining; however, a relationship between extent of EGFR staining and patient response could not be demonstrated.

A direct comparison of panitumumab and cetuximab will be required to truly determine if there is any difference in efficacy. Panitumumab is being studied in renal cell carcinoma and in NSCLC. Additionally, clinical trials are in progress to determine efficacy in combination with other chemotherapeutic agents and as a radiosensitizing agent.

ADOPTIVE CELLULAR THERAPY

One method of dealing with the deficiencies in immune effector cells present in cancer patients is to infuse immune cells generated ex vivo. A variety of immune effector cells have been generated for adoptive cellular therapy and tested in clinical trials (e.g., LAK cells, tumor-infiltrating lymphocytes, CTL, and monocyte/macrophages). Early efforts examined the infusion of LAK cells, which had little activity and required the coadministration of high-dose IL-2 to maintain their activity. Initial studies in patients with advanced melanoma and renal cell carcinoma demonstrated antitumor activity. Comparable results, however, were subsequently seen with IL-2 alone. Similarly, studies on the effects of the infusion of tumor-infiltrating lymphocytes, which were generated by culturing cells obtained from surgically excised tumors with IL-2 and with other cytokines ex vivo, demonstrated antitumor activity when administered with IL-2. Methods of generating antitumor CTL by culturing peripheral blood, lymph node cells, and tumor-infiltrating lymphocytes with cytokines and tumor antigens ex vivo also have been evaluated clinically, as have gene-modified CTL genetically engineered by the stable transfection of a TCR to specifically recognize MHC-tumor antigen complexes.[39] Dendritic cells also have been generated ex vivo and applied in vaccine approaches. These types of approaches are cumbersome and have not demonstrated sufficient clinical activity to warrant regulatory approval.

Cells infused in allogeneic HSCT represent an effective adoptive cellular therapy in clinical use. An allogeneic graft-versus-leukemia (GVL) effect, which is a restricted form of GVHD, has been suggested by the increased relapse rate for recipients of T cell-depleted allografts, higher relapse rates after either syngeneic or autologous transplants, and the lower frequency of relapse for patients with more severe GVHD. Given the clinical observations suggestive of important GVL activity after allogeneic transplant, it was logical to test the use of donor leukocyte infusion (DLI) in patients whose malignancies relapsed post transplant. Numerous reports have documented success of DLI in patients with CML; the majority of these patients achieved durable complete molecular remission. AML has only modest response rates, and acute lymphoblastic leukemia rarely responds. DLI also can eradicate EBV-associated post-transplant lymphoproliferative disease following allogeneic transplant. More recent studies have identified potential target antigens in patients responding to DLI. The major drawback of DLI infusion is GVHD, which is a major source of transplant-related mortality, and methods of promoting GVL over GVHD are under investigation.[40]

Non-myeloablative conditioning regimens using immunosuppressive doses of chemotherapy to allow donor engraftment and GVL effects without the toxicity of myeloablative preparative regimens are under investigation. Investigators have begun to explore the potential of allogeneic stem cell transplantation to generate analogous graft-versus-tumor (GVT) effects in patients with metastatic solid tumors. Regression of disease compatible with a GVT effect has been described in patients with metastatic renal cell and other carcinomas.[41] The response to DLI or to nonmyeloablative transplantation is usually delayed, with median time to response of 4 to 6 months, and, therefore, is not applicable to patients with advanced, rapidly progressing malignancy. Ongoing research in optimizing both the cellular product by a variety of techniques, including gene modification, and host environment will continue to improve adoptive cellular therapy approaches.

KEY POINTS

- Many cells of the immune response generated and/or modified ex vivo can be administered to an individual to augment an antitumor immune response.
- Donor leukocyte infusion in the setting of allogeneic hematopoietic cell transplantation represents an effective adoptive cellular therapy in clinical use.
- Aside from donor leukocyte infusion in the transplant setting, adoptive cellular therapy is largely conducted in the context of clinical trials.

CANCER VACCINES

Vaccines, an example of active specific immunotherapy, have been an attractive and aggressively pursued approach for the treatment of several cancers. Cancer vaccines have taken several forms, including cells, proteins, peptides, viral vectors, and plasmids. Many have specifically targeted the tumor-associated antigens outlined previously (Table 4-2). Others have applied tumor cells as a source of multiple antigens, defined and undefined.[42]

Both autologous and allogeneic tumor cell vaccines have been tested clinically. Because it remains uncertain which tumor antigens may be most important for mediating rejection and because tumor antigens may vary by patient, autologous tumor vaccines, prepared from surgical specimens, have the advantage of containing a multiplicity of relevant antigens. Allogeneic tumor cell vaccines, derived from established tumor cell lines, offer the ease of a prepackaged product with a diversity of tumor antigens as well as the immunogenicity of using an allogeneic cell. To augment the immune response, chemically defined or cytokine-immunologic adjuvants are used or the tumor is modified genetically to produce an immunostimulatory cytokine, such as GM-CSF, or an immunostimulatory molecule, such as B7. Although immunologically active, phase III clinical trials have not demonstrated significant clinical activity.[43]

Many recent studies have focused on dendritic cell-based vaccines to present tumor antigens. The clinical use of these vaccines was initially limited by cell numbers, but this problem has been overcome by the ability to generate dendritic cells ex vivo from peripheral blood cells using a variety of methods including culturing peripheral blood monocytes with GM-CSF and IL-4. Tumor antigens are provided by either pulsing the dendritic cells with tumor-associated peptides or proteins, coculturing with tumor cells, or by making genetic modifications. Intradermal, subcutaneous, intratumoral, and intralymphatic routes have all been used. Dendritic cell-based immunizations have been demonstrated to be safe and feasible. Antigen-specific immune responses have been induced, and clinical responses, although infrequent, have been observed.[44]

Tumor-associated, protein, carbohydrate, and ganglioside antigens have been tested. Lysates from primarily allogeneic but also from autologous tumor cells have been used as a source of tumor antigens for cancer vaccine approaches. These antigens often are complexed with a carrier (e.g., keyhole limpet hemocyanin) to form a hapten-carrier complex to enhance immunogenicity. A variety of chemically defined, cytokine, and dendritic cellular preparations have been applied as immunologic adjuvants. Heat shock proteins are also under investigation, which are intracellular molecules that act as chaperones for peptide antigens that can be derived from autologous tumor cells and represent a source of immunogenic tumor-derived antigens.

Tumor-derived peptides that contain the appropriate MHC class I or class II restricted amino acid sequence can be synthetically manufactured and administered together with a chemically defined cytokine or, as noted previously, dendritic cell-based adjuvants. Peptide-based vaccines require knowledge and matching of the exact human leukocyte antigen haplotype and antigen to provide the appropriate peptide epitope for each individual. This approach does allow for the assessment of the frequency of T cell responses by measuring specific production of interferon-gamma by T cells stimulated with the peptide in what is referred to as ELISPOT assays and also by flow cytometry with "tetramer" reagents, which are based on the peptide. In most clinical trials of this approach, specific T-cell responses have been induced. In addition, evidence of a broader response to tumor-antigen epitopes has occurred with some antigens that had not been present in the immunogen (epitope spreading). Clinical responses, however, have rarely been observed.

Vaccines that mimic the immunogenicity of infectious organisms may ultimately prove to be the most effective strategy. In this respect, recombinant viral and DNA vaccines have significant advantages over alternative immunization strategies. In such approaches, cDNA that encodes one or several antigens is inserted into a viral or plasmid vector and used for vaccination, with the aim of expressing the antigens with their subsequent uptake and presentation by antigen-presenting cells (i.e., "cross-priming") or by directly infecting/transducing antigen-presenting cells. Viruses have the advantage over nonviral vectors, such as plasmid DNA, because they efficiently penetrate cells, mimicking natural infection, thereby leading to more potent cell-mediated immune responses.[45] By providing the complete DNA sequence for the neoantigen, presentation is not restricted to a predefined MHC allele. Administration of vaccines based on viral vectors (e.g., adenovirus or vaccinia) may, however, generate immune responses against viral antigens, which make booster immunizations less likely to be effective and which may hamper clinical efficacy. One strategy is a diversified prime-boost approach in which a patient is immunized sequentially with the tumor antigen expressed by different viral vectors. There has been great interest in plasmid ("naked DNA" or polynucelotide) vaccines. The immunogenicity of plasmid vaccines is, in part, the result of the expression of unmethylated CpG motifs that can activate innate effectors. Although plasmid vaccines have been effective in eliciting CTL in preclinical studies, the results of the early-phase clinical trials have been disappointing.[46]

It should be noted that vaccines targeting viruses associated with the development of cancer have been effectively applied. Administration of a human papillomavirus (HPV)-16 vaccine reduced the incidence of both HPV-16 infection and HPV-16-related cervical intraepithelial neoplasia.[47] Immunization against hepatitis B has affected the incidence of hepatocellular carcinoma.[48] The focus of ongoing preclinical and clinical studies has been on identifying suitable targets, improving the capacity of cancer vaccines to stimulate cellular immunity, and dealing with tumor escape phenomena. The optimal strategy for assessing vaccine efficacy also has not been firmly identified and is under investigation.

IMMUNOTOXINS AND RADIOIMMUNOCONJUGATES

Biologic agents have been used to deliver toxins or radiation to malignant cells, as opposed to activate host antitumor mechanisms. Denileukin diftitox is a recombinant immunotoxin consisting of IL-2 fused to the enzymatically active domains of diphtheria toxin. It is internalized into IL-2 receptor-bearing cells (CD25) by endocytosis. Diphtheria toxin is activated, inhibits protein synthesis, and leads to apoptosis. Denileukin diftitox is active and approved for use in cutaneous T-cell lymphoma. Response rates of approximately 30% in refractory patients with extensive plaques and disfiguring tumors can be achieved.[49] Cytokine release may occur, the result of the killing of T cells, and can result in capillary leak syndrome. Denileukin diftitox also is active in non-Hodgkin and Hodgkin lymphoma, as well as in psoriasis, rheumatoid arthritis, and HIV infection.

Gemtuzumab ozogamicin consists of another toxin, ozogamicin, conjugated to a humanized monoclonal antibody directed at CD33 on AML cells. It has demonstrated a complete response rate of 15% to 20% in relapsed AML.[50] Its use has been complicated by the development of a sporadic veno-occlusive disease of the liver but is approved for use in patients older than 60 who have relapsed AML.

Two mouse monoclonal antibodies to CD20 conjugated to radioisotopes, ^{131}Iodine-tositumomab and ^{90}Yttrium-ibritumomab, have demonstrated substantial clinical effectiveness in patients with lymphoma. Both are indicated for the treatment of indolent B-cell lymphoma and related conditions. Clinical results are excellent with complete response rates of 20% to 40% and overall response rates of 60 to 80%. Toxicity is typically quite mild. The main side effect is reversible myelosuppression.[51,52]

INHIBITING REGULATORY RESPONSES

A major strategy for antitumor immunomodulation is to block one or more of the negative immunoregulatory host mechanisms. The elimination of cells or cytokines that inhibit immune responses may permit a more effective and persistent immune response to a tumor. This strategy does, however, carry the risk of autoimmune disease. The removal of negative immunoregulatory mechanisms cannot be effective unless there is a simultaneous positive immune response to the tumor. This may occur naturally, as is observed in select patients, such as patients with malignant melanoma. Alternatively, it may have to be induced, for example, by a cancer vaccine.

Several chemotherapy regimens, including the conditioning chemotherapy applied for HSCT, can eliminate suppressor mechanism, and this observation has led to novel treatment programs to exploit this activity.[53] Antibodies that target costimulatory or regulatory receptors on antigen-presenting and T cells, deplete T-reg cells, or neutralize immune suppressive cytokines are under investigation. One of the best studied blocking approaches targets CTLA-4. As noted, CTLA-4 functions as a coinhibitory receptor to attenuate activation during T-cell priming and limits effector cell expansion (Figure 4-1). CTLA-4 is expressed by CD4+CD25+ Treg cells. Tumor regressions associated with evidence of autoimmunity have been observed with antibody blockade of CTLA-4 in patients with melanoma.[54] As outlined previously, denileukin diftitox selectively eliminates CD25-expressing cells. Denileukin diftitox has been shown to reduce the number of CD4+CD25+ T-reg cells present in the peripheral blood of patients with renal cell carcinoma and to improve the immune response to a dendritic cell-based vaccine.[55] The use of antibodies to IL-10 and to TGF-beta is under investigation.

REFERENCES

1. Tuthill RJ, Unger JM, Liu PY, et al. Southwest Oncology Group. Risk assessment in localized primary cutaneous melanoma: a Southwest Oncology Group study evaluating nine factors and a test of the Clark logistic regression prediction model. *Am J Clin Pathol.* 2002;118(4):504–511.
2. Zhang L, Conejo-Garcia JR, Katsaros D, et al. Intratumoral T cells, recurrence, and survival in epithelial ovarian cancer. *N Engl J Med.* 2003;348(3):203–213.
3. von Mensdorff-Pouilly S, Verstraeten AA, Kenemans P, et al. Survival in early breast cancer patients is favorably influenced by a natural humoral immune response to polymorphic epithelial mucin. *J Clin Oncol.* 2000;18(3):574–583.
4. Rosenberg SA. Progress in human tumour immunology and immunotherapy. *Nature.* 2001;411(6835):380-384.
5. Curiel TJ, Coukos G, Zou L, et al. Specific recruitment of regulatory T cells in ovarian carcinoma fosters immune privilege and predicts reduced survival. *Nat Med.* 2004;10(9):942–949.
6. Almand B, Resser JR, Lindman B, et al. Clinical significance of defective dendritic cell differentiation in cancer. *Clin Cancer Res.* 2000;6(5):1755–1766.
7. Zou W, Machelon V, Coulomb-L'Hermin A, et al. Stromal-derived factor-1 in human tumors recruits and alters the function of plasmacytoid precursor dendritic cells. *Nat Med.* 2001;7(12):1339–1346.
8. Rayman P, Wesa AK, Richmond AL, et al. Effect of renal cell carcinomas on the development of type 1 T-cell responses. *Clin Cancer Res.* 2004;10(18 Pt 2):6360S–636S.
9. Almand B, Clark JI, Nikitina E, et al. Increased production of immature myeloid cells in cancer patients: a mechanism of immunosuppression in cancer. *J Immunol.* 2001;166(1):678–689.
10. Maeurer MJ, Gollin SM, Martin D, et al. Tumor escape from immune recognition: lethal recurrent melanoma in a patient associated with downregulation of the peptide transporter protein TAP-1 and loss of expression of the immunodominant MART-1/Melan-A antigen. *J Clin Invest.* 1996;98(7):1633–1641.
11. Gogas H, Ioannovich J, Dafni U, et al. Prognostic significance of autoimmunity during treatment of melanoma with interferon. *N Engl J Med.* 2006;354(7):709–718.
12. Fisher RI, Dana BW, LeBlanc M, et al. Interferon alpha consolidation after intensive chemotherapy does not prolong the progression-free survival of patients with low-grade non-Hodgkin's lymphoma: results of the Southwest Oncology Group randomized phase III study 8809. *J Clin Oncol.* 2000;18(10):2010–2016.

13. Hernberg M, Pyrhonen S, Muhonen T. Regimens with or without interferon-alpha as treatment for metastatic melanoma and renal cell carcinoma: an overview of randomized trials. *J Immunother.* 1999;22(2): 145–154.

14. Kirkwood JM, Manola J, Ibrahim J, et al. Eastern Cooperative Oncology Group. A pooled analysis of Eastern Cooperative Oncology Group and intergroup trails of adjuvant high-dose interferon for melanoma. *Clin Cancer Res.* 2004;10(5):1670–1677.

15. Jumbou O, N'Guyen JM, Tessier MH, et al. Long-term follow-up in 51 patients with mycosis fungoides and Sezary syndrome treated by interferon-alfa. *Br J Dermatol.* 1999;140(3):427–431.

16. Myeloma Trialists' Collaborative Group. Interferon as therapy for multiple myeloma: an individual patient data overview of 24 randomized trials and 4012 patients. *Br J Haematol.* 2001;113(4):1020–1034.

17. Pyrhonen S, Salminen E, Ruutu M, et al. Prospective randomized trial of interferon alfa-2a plus vinblastine versus vinblastine alone in patients with advanced renal cell cancer. *J Clin Oncol.* 1999;17(9):2859–2867.

18. Medical Research Council Renal Cancer Collaborators. Interferon-alpha and survival in metastatic renal carcinoma: early results of a randomized controlled trial. *Lancet.* 1999;353(9146):14–17.

19. Flanigan RC, Salmon SE, Blumenstein BA, et al. Nephrectomy followed by interferon alfa–2b compared with interferon alfa-2 alone for metastatic renal cell cancer. *N Engl J Med.* 2001;345(23):1655–1659.

20. Ahmadzadeh M, Rosenberg SA. IL-2 administration increases CD4+ CD25(hi) Foxp3+ regulatory T cells in cancer patients. *Blood.* 2006;107 (6):2409–2414.

21. Dutcher J. Current status of interleukin-2 therapy for metastatic renal cell carcinoma and metastatic melanoma. *Oncology* (Williston Park). 2002;16(11 Suppl 13):4–10.

22. Smith TJ, Khatcheressian J, Lyman GH, et al. 2006 update of recommendations for the use of white blood cell growth factors: an evidence-based clinical practice guideline. *J Clin Oncol.* 2006;24(19): 3187– 3205.

23. Warren TL, Weiner GJ. Uses of granulocyte-macrophage colony-stimulating factor in vaccine development. *Curr Opin Hematol.* 2000;7(3): 168–173.

24. Rini BI, Weinberg V, Bok R, et al. Prostate-specific antigen kinetics as a measure of the biologic effect of granulocyte-macrophage colony-stimulating factor in patients with serologic progression of prostate cancer. *J Clin Oncol.* 2003;21(1):99–105.

25. Spitler LE, Grossbard ML, Ernstoff MS, et al. Adjuvant therapy of stage III and IV malignant melanoma using granulocyte-macrophage colony-stimulating factor. *J Clin Oncol.* 2000;18(8):1614–1621.

26. Smith TJ, Khatcheressian J, Lyman GH, et al. 2006 update of recommendations for the use of white blood cell growth factors: an evidence-based clinical practice guideline. *J Clin Oncol.* 2006;24(19):3187– 3205.

27. Davis TA, Grillo-Lopez AJ, White CA, et al. Rituximab anti-CD20 monoclonal antibody therapy in non-Hodgkin's lymphoma: Safety and efficacy of re-treatment. *J Clin Oncol.* 2000;18(17):3135–3143.

28. Hainsworth JD, Litchy S, Shaffer DW, et al. Maximizing therapeutic benefit of rituximab: maintenance therapy versus re-treatment at progression in patients with indolent non-Hodgkin's lymphoma—a randomized phase II trial of the Minnie Pearl Cancer Research Network. *J Clin Oncol.* 2005;23(6):1088–1095.

29. Coiffier B, Lepage E, Brière J, et al. CHOP chemotherapy plus rituximab compared to CHOP alone in elderly patients with diffuse large-B-cell lymphoma. *N Engl J Med.* 2002;346(4):235–242.

30. Keating MJ, Flinn I, Jain V, et al. Therapeutic role of alemtuzumab (Campath-1H) in patients who have failed fludarabine: Results of a large international study. *Blood.* 2002;99(10):3554–3561.

31. Slamon DJ, Leyland-Jones B, Shak S, et al. Use of chemotherapy plus a monoclonal antibody against HER2 for metastatic breast cancer that overexpresses HER2. *N Engl J Med.* 2001;344(11):783–792.

32. Romond EH, Perez EA, Bryant J, et al. Trastuzumab plus adjuvant chemotherapy for operable HER2-positive breast cancer. *N Engl J Med.* 2005;353(16):1673–1684.

33. Piccart-Gebhart MJ, Procter M, Leyland-Jones B, et al; Herceptin Adjuvant (HERA) Trial Study Team. Trastuzumab after adjuvant chemotherapy in HER2-positive breast cancer. *N Engl J Med.* 2005;353(16):1659–1672.

34. Hurwitz H, Fehrenbacher L, Novotny W, et al. Bevacizumab plus irinotecan, fluorouracil, and leucovorin for metastatic colorectal cancer. *N Engl J Med.* 2004;350(23):2335–2342.

35. Sandler A, Gray R, Perry MC, et al. Paclitaxel-carboplatin alone or with bevacizumab for non-small-cell lung cancer. *N Engl J Med.* 2006;355 (24):2542–2550.

36. Cunningham D, Humblet Y, Siena S, et al. Cetuximab monotherapy and cetuximab plus irinotecan in irinotecan-refractory metastatic colorectal cancer. *N Engl J Med.* 2004;351(4):337–345.

37. Bonner JA, Harari PM, Giralt J, et al. Radiotherapy plus cetuximab for squamous-cell carcinoma of the head and neck. *N Engl J Med.* 2006; 354(6):567–578.

38. Van Cutsem E, Peeters M, Siena S, et al. Open-label phase III trial of panitumumab plus best supportive care compared with best supportive care alone in patients with chemotherapy-refractory metastatic colorectal cancer. *J Clin Oncol.* 2007;25(13):1658–1664.

39. Morgan RA, Dudley ME, Wunderlich JR, et al. Cancer regression in patients after transfer of genetically engineered lymphocytes. *Science.* 2006;314(5796):126–129.

40. Tey SK, Bollard CM, Heslop HE. Adoptive T-cell transfer in cancer immunotherapy. *Immunol Cell Biol.* 2006;84(3):281–289.

41. Childs R, Chernoff A, Contentin N, et al. Regression of metastatic renal-cell carcinoma after nonmyeloablative allogeneic peripheral-blood stem-cell transplantation. *N Engl J Med.* 2000;343(11):175–183.

42. Ribas A, Butterfield LH, Glaspy JA, et al. Current developments in cancer vaccines and cellular immunotherapy. *J Clin Oncol.* 2003;21(12): 2415–2432.

43. Sondak VK, Sabel MS, Mule JJ. Allogeneic and autologous melanoma vaccines: where have we been and where are we going? *Clin Cancer Res.* 2006;12(7 Pt 2):2337s-2341s.

44. Banchereau J, Palucka AK. Dendritic cells as therapeutic vaccines against cancer. *Nat Rev Immunol.* 2005;5(4):296–306.

45. Bonnet MC, Tartaglia J, Verdier F, et al. Recombinant viruses as a tool for therapeutic vaccination against human cancers. *Immunol Lett.* 2000;74(1):11–25.

46. Haupt K, Roggendorf M, Mann K. The potential of DNA vaccination against tumor-associated antigens for antitumor therapy. *Exp Biol Med.* 2002;227(4):227–237.

47. Koutsky LA, Ault KA, Wheeler CM, et al. Proof of Principle Study Investigators. A controlled trial of a human papillomavirus type 16 vaccine. *N Engl J Med.* 2002;347(21):1645–1651.

48. Chang MH, Chen TH, Hsu HM, et al. Taiwan Childhood HCC Study Group. Prevention of hepatocellular carcinoma by universal vaccination against hepatitis B virus: the effect and problems. *Clin Cancer Res.* 2005;11(21):7953–7957.

49. Olsen E, Duvic M, Frankel A, et al. Pivotal phase III trial of two dose levels of denileukin diftitox for the treatment of cutaneous T-cell lymphoma. *J Clin Oncol.* 2001;19(2):376–388.

50. Sievers EL, Larson RA, Stadtmauer EA, et al. Efficacy and safety of gemtuzumab ozogamicin in patients with CD33-positive acute myeloid leukaemia in first relapse. *J Clin Oncol.* 2001;19(13):3244–3254.

51. Kaminski MS, Zelenetz AD, Press OW, et al. Pivotal study of iodine I 131 tositumomab for chemotherapy-refractory low-grade or transformed low-grade B-cell non-Hodgkin's lymphomas. *J Clin Oncol.* 2001;19(19):3918–3928.

52. Witzig TE, Gordon LI, Cabanillas F, et al. Randomized controlled trial of yttrium-90-labeled ibritumomab tiuxetan radioimmunotherapy versus rituximab immunotherapy for patients with relapsed or refractory low-grade, follicular, or transformed B-cell non-Hodgkin's lymphoma. *J Clin Oncol.* 2002;20(10):2453–2463.

53. Rosenberg SA, Dudley ME. Cancer regression in patients with metastatic melanoma after the transfer of autologous antitumor lymphocytes. *Proc Natl Acad Sci USA.* 2004;101(Suppl 2):14639–14645.

54. Phan GQ, Yang JC, Sherry RM, et al. Cancer regression and autoimmunity induced by cytotoxic T lymphocyte-associated antigen 4 blockade in patients with metastatic melanoma. *Proc Natl Acad Sci USA.* 2003;100(14):8372–8377.

55. Dannull J, Su Z, Rizzieri D, et al. Enhancement of vaccine-mediated antitumor immunity in cancer patients after depletion of regulatory T cells. *J Clin Invest.* 2005;115(12):3623–3633.

5

BREAST CANCER

Lisa A. Carey, MD

LEARNING OBJECTIVES

After reviewing this chapter, the reader should be able to

- Apply the understanding of the epidemiology of breast cancer, including genetic and environmental risk factors and ethnic and geographic variability to the treatment of patients and the evaluation and design of clinical trials
- Discuss with patients both medical and surgical prevention strategies and the current consensus of the application of these results to clinical practice and recommend optimal strategies based on patient profile, risk factors, and preference
- Identify and incorporate optimal screening and diagnostic approaches
- Describe the prognostic factors associated with breast cancer
- Explain and employ state-of-the-art approaches to the multidisciplinary treatment of all stages of breast cancer
- Identify and manage the potential side effects and toxicities of local, regional, and systemic therapy for breast cancer

Breast cancer remains one of the most common cancers in the world. In western industrialized countries, it is the most prevalent cancer in women; in the United States it accounts for 31% of all cancers in this group.[1] It is estimated that breast cancer develops in one out of eight American women during her lifetime, assuming a life expectancy of 85 years. The risk is considerably higher for women with pre-existing risk factors, such as older age, a strong family history of breast cancer, known mutations in the breast cancer predisposition genes, or a personal history of histologically demonstrated precursor lesions.

The American Society of Clinical Oncology and Dr. Carey would like to gratefully acknowledge Gabriel N. Hortobagyi, MD, for his contributions to the original content of this chapter.

The American Cancer Society estimates that 178,480 women and 2,030 men will be diagnosed with breast cancer in the United States during 2007.[2] The incidence of this disease has decreased recently: the annual percent increase was 3.7% between 1980 and 1987, a far lower increase of 0.4% between 1987 and 2001, and a decrease of −3.9% between 2001 and 2004.[3] A particularly steep decline (−6.7%) was noted in 2003, possibly due to the decline in the use of hormone replacement therapy after publication of the Women's Health Initiative (discussed in detail further in this chapter).[4] It has been hypothesized that the earlier increase in incidence was temporary and was secondary to the introduction of systematic use of screening mammography and the to lead-time bias associated with earlier diagnosis. With the onset of routine use of screening mammography in the 1980s, the anatomic extent of disease decreased, with an increase in localized (node-negative) disease from 48% in 1975 to 1979 to 63% in 1998 to 2003; conversely the proportion with regional (node-positive) disease has decreased from 41% to 30% over the same time period. Those with distant disease at diagnosis, approximately 5% to 10%, has not changed and likely reflects a biologically aggressive group of tumors that are unlikely to be affected by early detection maneuvers. The incidence of breast cancer in situ, a preneoplastic condition best detected by mammography, increased 2.5% per year between 1995 and 2004.[3]

The American Cancer Society estimated 40,410 deaths related to breast cancer in 2005 — 39,950 of them among women. Breast cancer represents 15% of all cancer-related deaths, which makes it the second leading cause among women in the United States (lung cancer being the leading cause). In the United States, age-adjusted mortality from breast cancer decreased 2.3% per year from 1990 to 2002. Mathematical modeling suggests that the improved mortality from breast cancer is attributed to improved screening and to improved adjuvant therapies.[5] The recent shift in the stage at diagnosis to smaller, more node-negative tumors has real prognostic effect; the 5-year survival rates in the United States for breast cancer diagnosed in localized, regional, and disseminated stages are 98%, 81%, and 26%, respectively.

Important differences exist in the incidence of breast cancer and its related mortality rates among various ethnic groups. In 2005, there were an estimated 19,240 new cases of breast cancer and 5,640 deaths among black women in the United States. The incidence is 12% lower in black women than in white women (118 versus 134 per 100,000 women in the population), but the mortality rate is 26% higher among black women (34 versus 25 per 100,000 women). This difference may be partially because the disease is diagnosed at later stages in black women, which may be because the access to diagnosis and treatment differs between the two populations[6] and because of unfavorable biologic characteristics. Black women with breast cancer have a greater frequency of estrogen receptor (ER)-negative and poorly differentiated tumors. Recent studies have found that in young black women, the frequency of one of the more aggressive hormone receptor-negative molecular subtypes, the basal-like subtype, is more than double that of older black women or white women of any age.[7] Of black women with breast cancer, disease is diagnosed in a localized stage in 53%, regional stage in 35%, and disseminated in 9%. The improvements in breast cancer survival have been seen across all groups, however inequities still remain; between 1975 and 2002, the relative 5-year survival rates increased from 76% to 90% for white women and from 63% to 77% for black women. Both the incidence of breast cancer and the mortality rate are lower among Hispanic, American Indian, and Asian women.

KEY POINTS

- More than one million new cases of breast cancer are diagnosed worldwide each year.
- Since the early 1990s, United States national statistics suggest that there has been a gradual but persistent decline in the mortality rate related to breast cancer.

Breast cancer is a worldwide problem, with more than 1 million cases in 2002. It is the most common malignancy in women, comprising 23% of all female cancers. The incidence of breast cancer globally has been increasing. Regional variations are striking, with an approximately 3-fold higher rate of breast cancer in industrialized nations (more than 80 per 100,000 women) compared with developing nations (fewer than 30 cases per 100,000 women).[8,9] The reasons for the higher incidence are unclear. Potential contributors include the following: hormone differences, such as earlier onset of menses and later menopause, which are attributed to better nutrition; increased body weight; delayed or low parity; use of hormone replacement therapy; alcohol intake; obesity; and reduced physical activity. Breast cancer also is the primary cause of cancer death in women worldwide, with an estimated 411,000 women dying of the disease in 2002.[8] Mortality varies to a lesser degree by region; for example, even though incidence differs by 6-fold, the difference in survival between central African and the United States is far more modest, with 12.1 deaths per 100,000 women in central Africa compared with 19.4 per 100,000 in the United States. The paradox of far higher incidence but only modestly higher mortality among industrialized countries likely is because of mammography, which detects lower stage, more treatable tumors, and because of more effective and widespread use of adjuvant treatments, such as endocrine therapy and chemotherapy. Recent data suggest that global mortality, which had been increasing until the 1980s, has begun to decline, particularly among industrialized nations.

TABLE 5-1 Established Risk Factors for Breast Cancer

Risk Factor	Relative Risk
• Sex (female vs. male)	100
• *BRCA1* or *BRCA2* mutation	6.0–14.0
• Family history of breast cancer	
First-degree relative	1.4–13.6
Second-degree relative	1.5–1.8
• Age (≥ 50 vs. < 50 years)	6.5
• Benign breast disease	
Atypical hyperplasia	4.0–4.4
Hyperplasia	2.0
Breast biopsy	1.5–1.8
• Nulliparity	2.0
• Age at first live birth (> 30 vs. < 20 years)	1.3–2.2
• Age at menopause (≥ 55 vs. < 55 years)	1.5–2.0
• Age at menarche (< 12 vs. ≥ 14 years)	1.2–1.5
• Hormone-replacement therapy	1.0–1.5
• Exposure to ionizing radiation	1.4
• Alcohol consumption (12 g/day [30 mL/day] vs. none)	1.1–4.0
• Increased body mass index	
Premenopausal women	0.54
Postmenopausal women	1.26–2.52

RISK FACTORS

The incidence of breast cancer is influenced by certain well-established risk factors (Table 5-1). The two most prominent risk factors are sex and age. Breast cancer is 100 times more common among women than men. The incidence of breast cancer increases substantially with age, ranging from fewer than 10 cases per 100,000 women per year between the ages of 20 and 30, to more than 300 cases per 100,000 women per year in those women older than 60. The rate of increase in incidence declines after menopause, especially after age 80. Mortality rates parallel this pattern, although mortality from breast cancer decreases after the seventh decade of life because of the increasing frequency of other causes of death.

KEY POINTS

- Breast cancer is 100 times more common among women than men.
- Breast cancers associated with *BRCA1* mutations are frequently of a higher grade and are hormone receptor negative. Recent data suggest that most of these cancers are of the basal-like subtype.
- The lifetime risk of invasive breast cancer for individuals with *BRCA1* or *BRCA2* mutations ranges from 50% to 87%; for ovarian cancer, the risk is 15% to 65%.

FAMILIAL RISK

Having close relatives with breast or ovarian cancer increases the risk of breast cancer several-fold.[10] Individuals with a first-degree relative (i.e., mother or sister) with the disease have an approximately 2-fold increased risk compared with women without such a family history. This increase is greater (up to approximately 10-fold) if the first-degree relative had bilateral breast cancer and if the disease was diagnosed before age 50. Both the paternal and maternal sides of the family contribute to increased risk. A family history of ovarian or prostate cancer also increases the risk of breast cancer and of having one of the familial breast cancer syndromes.

GENETIC RISK

Since the identification and cloning of *BRCA1* and *BRCA2*, two genes associated with familial breast (and ovarian) cancer, much has been learned about the role of these genes in normal development and malignant transformation. *BRCA1* and *BRCA2* account for most cases of hereditary breast cancer in the United States and Europe, and are inherited in an autosomal dominant fashion.[11] *BRCA1* and *BRCA2* act as tumor-suppressor genes, and, in association with *RAD51*, operate in a common DNA damage-response pathway implicated in double-strand DNA repair.[12–15] Breast cancers associated with *BRCA1* mutations are frequently of a higher grade and are hormone receptor negative, and gene expression array studies have found that the majority are of the basal-like subtype[16]; however, cancers arising in the setting of *BRCA2* mutation are more likely to be of luminal subtype and hormone receptor positive[17] (see the section "Molecular Profiling" for detailed information). A higher proportion of cancers related to a *BRCA1* mutation have atypical or typical medullary histologic features.[18,19] Breast cancers associated with mutations in *BRCA2* do not differ appreciably from sporadic cancers. No special tumor phenotype has been ascribed to ovarian cancers associated with *BRCA1* or *BRCA2*. The lifetime cumulative risk of invasive breast cancer for individuals with *BRCA1* or *BRCA2* mutations ranges from 50% to 87%; for invasive epithelial ovarian cancer, the risk is 15% to 65%. Familial breast cancer, however, accounts for fewer than 10% of all breast cancers, and *BRCA1*-related and *BRCA2*-related familial disease constitutes only two-thirds to three-fourths of these cases. Among women with breast cancer who are younger than age 35, 10% to 15% have a *BRCA1* mutation. Women with *BRCA1* and *BRCA2* mutations already affected by the disease have a risk, to age 70, of contralateral breast cancer that ranges between 50% and 64%. The risks of cancer of the stomach, gallbladder, bile ducts, and pancreas are increased for carriers of the *BRCA2* mutation, and the risks for breast and possibly early-onset prostate cancer (diagnosis before age 55) are increased for male carriers of the mutation. Other genetic abnormalities and less common familial cancer syndromes (e.g., Li-Fraumeni syndrome, Cowden's disease, and Peutz-Jegher's syndrome) are responsible for an additional small percentage of breast cancers.[10,15,20,21] Li-Fraumeni syndrome is a rare, highly penetrant, autosomal-dominant condition caused by mutations in the *P53* gene, which plays a critical role in cell-cycle control and apoptosis. Li-Fraumeni syndrome is characterized by early-onset breast cancer (diagnosis before age 40), soft tissue sarcomas, leukemia, primary brain tumors, and adrenocortical cancers. Cowden's syndrome, or multiple hamartoma syndrome, is caused by mutations in the *PTEN* gene and accounts for fewer than 1% of hereditary breast cancers. Peutz-Jegher's syndrome is an autosomal dominant condition caused by mutations in the *STK11* gene, resulting in a predisposition to cancers of the stomach, colon, pancreas, small bowel, thyroid, breast, lung, and uterus.[22]

The cloning of *BRCA1* and *BRCA2*, and the presumed appearance of additional molecular genetic markers of risk, have brought the issue of genetic screening and counseling to the forefront. Both negative and positive test results are associated with a variety of emotional, legal, economic, and work-related issues. Ongoing clinical trials will determine who will benefit most from screening, how screening and counseling should be conducted, and what type of societal involvement is needed so that genetic screening can be used without exposing the subject to unexpected risks and consequences.

ETHNIC BACKGROUND

Variation by ethnicity can reflect either nature (genetics) or nurture (environment). Most of the current knowledge about genetic risk factors derives from women of European descent, and the understanding of genetics is much more limited in the black, Hispanic, and American Indian populations. The results of studies of *BRCA1* and *BRCA2* mutations indicate a higher incidence of such mutations among women with Ashkenazi Jewish heritage. In fact, a single *BRCA1* mutation (founder mutation) can be found in as many as 1% of Ashkenazi Jewish women. Founder mutations also have been identified in several other ethnic groups located in Hungary, Iceland, Russia, Israel, France, Belgium, and Scandinavia. Regarding environmental influences, exposure to Western lifestyles has a profound effect on breast cancer risk. Among Asian Americans immigrating from regions with traditionally low breast cancer risk, this risk increases among the immigrants themselves after arrival, and their children and grandchildren have approximately the same risk as U.S.-born white women.[23,24]

REPRODUCTIVE RISK FACTORS

The risk of breast cancer is 30% to 50% higher for nulliparous women than it is for parous women.[25] In general, the earlier the age of the first full-term pregnancy, the lower the risk. Early onset of menarche, late onset of menopause, and greater number of years with ovulatory cycles have all been associated with an increased risk of breast cancer. Findings from some studies suggest that high parity may have a protective effect above and beyond that of an early first pregnancy. It is likely that lactation, especially of longer duration, also confers some protection and reduces the risk, although there is ongoing controversy about the magnitude of the protective effect. Recent studies suggest that the traditional associations between reproductive risk factors and breast cancer are limited to the ER-positive subtypes and may be different for ER-negative subtypes.[26–28]

SOCIOECONOMIC CLASS

Breast cancer is found more frequently among women of higher economic class and educational status. This finding is probably related to lifestyle factors, such as diet and age at first childbirth.

EXOGENOUS HORMONES

Current use of estrogen-replacement therapy by women who have used estrogens for several years has been associated with a modest increase in risk; the use of combined estrogen and progestin-containing preparations increases this risk several-fold.[29–31] However, risk decreases upon discontinuation of hormone-replacement therapy, and no increase in risk can be identified 5 years after the cessation of treatment.

DIET

Many studies have attempted to establish a correlation between the risk of breast cancer and dietary intake of animal proteins, total calories, animal fat, fiber, and micronutrients.[32-34] Most of the studies used more-or-less sophisticated epidemiologic techniques, but essentially all of the earlier studies addressing this issue were retrospective in nature. Findings from some earlier studies suggested that increased caloric and saturated fat intake might be correlated with increased risk of breast cancer; the results of more recent and definitive studies have not supported this hypothesis. The Women's Health Initiative randomized trial of a low-fat dietary intervention did not significantly affect breast cancer risk.[35] The influence of dietary fiber intake on risk is the subject of several ongoing laboratory and epidemiologic studies. The Malmo prospective cohort study in postmenopausal women suggested an association of a high-fiber/low-fat diet with lower risk of breast cancer, but this has not been confirmed.[36] Confounding the issue is the potential for unmeasured variables, such as total energy intake and inherited variations in metabolism, to play a role in assessment of dietary and toxin effects in cancer risk. More than minimal alcohol intake (one or two drinks per day or 30 to 60 mL per day) is associated with an increased risk; this linear correlation has been a reproducible finding across the majority of studies and may relate to higher estrogen levels with alcohol consumption.

As suggested by the results of the Women's Health Initiative study and further discussed in this chapter, it is likely that risk factors differ among biologically distinct subtypes of breast cancer making global examinations of risk less likely to be fruitful.

OBESITY

Obesity has been associated with increased risk of postmenopausal breast cancer, the supposed mechanism via increased circulating estrogens. The risk increases with increasing body mass index (BMI) and is associated with increased mortality.[37] Obesity is felt to be responsible for approximately 15% to 20% of cancer-related deaths in the United States.

PHYSICAL ACTIVITY

Regular physical activity, especially if strenuous, has been shown to correlate with reduced rates of breast cancer in multiple epidemiologic studies.[38] The greatest effect of physical activity appears to be in early life, especially during adolescence.

IONIZING RADIATION

Repeated exposure to radiation, such as fluoroscopic chest x-rays and radiation therapy for postpartum mastitis and dermatologic or arthritic conditions, is definitely linked to a greater risk of breast cancer, and appears to be dose related. Thoracic risk is 10-fold or greater for long-term survivors of Hodgkin's disease previously treated with mantle radiation therapy. Intensive mammographic surveillance and regular physical examination of the breasts is indicated for such women. However, the risk as a result of common diagnostic radiographic procedures appears to be minimal and of theoretical import only.

ENVIRONMENTAL FACTORS

Cigarette smoking is a controversial risk factor. Some studies have found no correlation with risk whereas others have. Complicating the evaluation is the emerging understanding of the role of variations in inherited detoxifying enzymes.[39] There is much interest in determining whether other occupational and environmental exposures influence risk, and several major prospective studies are ongoing around the world. However, no definitive correlation with any environmental factors has been documented.

BENIGN AND PREMALIGNANT BREAST DISEASE

Some forms of benign breast disease are associated with an increase in risk of subsequent development of breast cancer. This increased risk is at best modest for proliferative lesions without atypia or nonproliferative lesions. The association is far stronger in patients with lesions that demonstrate atypia (atypical ductal or lobular hyperplasia), in whom the risk is increased approximately 4-fold.[40] The premalignant lesion ductal carcinoma in situ (DCIS) is managed similarly to invasive cancers because of a fairly high risk of local recurrence. However, women with a diagnosis of DCIS also have elevated risk of cancer elsewhere in the breast and in the contralateral breast. Lobular carcinoma in situ (LCIS) is considered a benign but high-risk histology, although there is some debate about high-grade LCIS overlap with DCIS. LCIS carries an approximately 1% to 2% per year risk of development of ipsilateral or contralateral DCIS or invasive breast cancer.[41]

Dense breasts on mammography also is associated with risk of breast cancer, with relative risks ranging from approximately 2-fold to 6-fold across studies.[42]

COMBINATIONS OF FACTORS

Each individual factor independently influences the risk of breast cancer. How these various risk factors interact and how to combine them for optimal assessment of risk is less well established. Using statistical methodology to group several risk factors, some investigators[43–45] have developed modeling techniques to enhance the sensitivity and predictive value of risk assessment (Table 5-2). The modified Gail model is widely used in the United States and western Europe for individual risk assessment and determination of eligibility for chemoprevention trials.[46] In that context, its clinical utility has been confirmed in white, North American populations, although its applicability to other ethnic groups and cultural environments has not been established. As other risk factors are validated and as molecular markers predictive of risk are developed, these models will need to be updated and have prospective validation.

TABLE 5-2 Risk Model and Associated Relative Risks*

Risk Factor (Code No.)	Number of Relatives with Breast Cancer	Associated Relative Risk	Number of Cases (2,852 Patients)	Number of Controls (3,146 Controls)
Age at Menarche (years)				
≥ 14 (0)	—	1.000	790	926
12 to 13 (1)	—	1.099	1,554	1,735
< 12 (2)	—	1.207	508	485
No. of Previous Breast Biopsies				
Age < 50				
0 (0)	—	1.000	635	794
1 (1)	—	1.698	113	93
> 2 (2)	—	2.882	66	24
Age ≥ 50				
0 (0)	—	1.000	1,551	1,817
1 (1)	—	1.273	312	300
> 2 (2)	—	1.620	175	118
Age at First Live Birth (years)				
< 20 (0)	0 (0)	1.000	167	285
	1 (1)	2.607	44	40
	≥ 2 (2)	6.798	8	0
20 to 24 (1)	0 (0)	1.244	708	1,042
	1 (1)	2.681	208	123
	≥ 2 (2)	5.775	25	5
25 to 29 or nulliparous (2)	0 (0)	1.548	986	1,106
	1 (1)	2.756	247	178
	≥ 2 (2)	4.907	46	20
≥ 30 (3)	0 (0)	1.927	307	291
	1 (1)	2.834	87	50
	≥ 2 (2)	4.169	19	6

*Relative risk compared with an individual of the same age without any risk factors is estimated by determining the person's associated relative risk for the age of menarche, number of previous biopsies, and the combination of age at first live birth and the number of relatives with breast cancer, and multiplying these three numbers together.

Modified with permission from Gail MH, Brinton LA, Byar DP, et al. Projecting individualized probabilities of developing breast cancer for white females who are being examined annually. *J Natl Cancer Inst.* 1989;81:1879-1886.

PREVENTION

Metastatic breast cancer is considered incurable for most patients. However, cure is highly likely with available combined-modality therapies for patients with primary breast cancer, although the frequency of treatment failure and breast cancer-specific death rate is related to the stage of disease at the time of presentation. Thus, more than 90% of patients with noninvasive (in situ) breast cancer remain without evidence of the disease 10 years after appropriate local therapy only. Conversely, approximately 50% of patients who have stage III disease at the time of initial diagnosis and who are aggressively treated remain without recurrence after 10 years. Therefore, although efforts to improve the efficacy and safety of therapeutic approaches continue, there has been increasing interest in the development of preventive strategies.

KEY POINTS

- A meta-analysis of five randomized trials confirmed that the administration of a selective estrogen-receptor modulator (SERM) to women at risk of breast cancer resulted in a significant and reproducible reduction in the incidence of the disease by approximately 38%.
- For women at highest risk, such as those with *BRCA1* or *BRCA2* mutations, prophylactic mastectomy reduces risk by more than 90%.
- Prophylactic oophorectomy in women with *BRCA1* or *BRCA2* mutations reduces the risk of ovarian cancer and, when performed in premenopausal women, reduces the risk of breast cancer.

There are multiple techniques to attempt to reduce risk, and ongoing studies are designed to explore most of these research options. Hormone interventions, chemoprevention, prophylactic surgery, dietary interventions, and behavior modifications represent the leading research directions.

CHEMOPREVENTION

Adjuvant antiestrogen therapy with tamoxifen, a selective estrogen-receptor modulator (SERM), given for 5 years to patients with hormone receptor-positive breast cancer, regardless of age or menopause status, has been shown to reduce the annual odds of recurrence by just under one-half and the annual odds of death by one-third.[47] Additional analyses of these same randomized trials also have shown that administration of adjuvant tamoxifen reduces the incidence of second primary (or contralateral) breast cancers by approximately 40%. In view of the excellent tolerance to adjuvant tamoxifen in more than 55 large randomized trials including more than 37,000 patients and follow-up periods of months to two or more decades, several controlled clinical trials were initiated to determine whether long-term antiestrogen therapy was able to reduce the incidence of breast cancer in high-risk participants.[48-52] The largest of these trials, the National Surgical Adjuvant Breast and Bowel Project (NSABP) Breast Cancer Prevention Trial (BCPT), eventually enrolled 13,388 women (Table 5-3).[49] The results of the two largest trials clearly demonstrated a highly significant reduction in risk of 30% to 50% for participants who received tamoxifen. The BCPT also indicated that tamoxifen reduced the incidence of benign breast disease, as well as the frequency of breast biopsies for premalignant lesions. No significant difference in survival was seen. However, the study was unblinded early as mandated by the independent monitoring committee for ethical reasons, many of the women on placebo crossed over to receive tamoxifen, undermining this endpoint. The findings of two other studies, the Multiple Outcomes of Raloxifene Evaluation (MORE) and Raloxifene Use for The Heart (RUTH) studies, demonstrated a highly significant reduction in breast cancer incidence for those patients treated with raloxifene (also a SERM); however, breast cancer events were secondary objectives in these studies.[53-55] Raloxifene did not have the risk of endometrial cancer associated with tamoxifen, prompting the second NSABP breast cancer prevention trial, the Study of Tamoxifen and Raloxifene (STAR) trial, in which approximately 20,000 women who were postmenopausal and at elevated risk of developing breast cancer were randomly assigned to receive tamoxifen or raloxifene for 5 years. At approximately 5 to 6 years follow-up, the women who received tamoxifen had a similar incidence of invasive breast cancer and a nonsignificantly lower risk of noninvasive breast cancer, but they had a higher risk of uterine hyperplasia and thromboembolic disease compared with those women who received raloxifene.[56] Based on the results of the hormone therapy prevention trials with tamoxifen or raloxifene, patients with a 5-year risk of developing breast cancer equal to or exceeding 1.67% (approximately the risk of a 60-year-old woman) are eligible for such interventions. The benefit-to-risk ratio for tamoxifen is greater for women who are premenopausal than for those who are postmenopausal. A meta-analysis of the older randomized trials confirmed that the administration of a SERM to women at risk resulted in a significant and reproducible 38% reduction in the incidence of breast cancer.[57] The reduction was observed in the development of ER-positive disease, with no substantial change in risk for ER-negative cancer. The intervention was particularly effective for subsets of women at high risk, such as patients with a personal history of atypical ductal hyperplasia or lobular neoplasia. These studies were not powered to detect a significant survival benefit from these interventions. Nevertheless, whereas nonsignificant reductions in deaths were observed in the Royal Marsden, Italian, and BCPT prevention trials, International Breast Cancer Intervention Study (IBIS-I) showed an increase in overall mortality. A meta-analysis of these four tamoxifen prevention trials desmonstrated an approximate 10% (statistically nonsignificant) reduction in the annual odds of death. Risk stratification techniques have been developed that can help identify those with the least risk and greatest potential for benefit.[58]

Tamoxifen received approval from the U.S. Food and Drug Administration (FDA) for use in reducing the incidence of breast cancer; a similar approval will likely be obtained for raloxifene. Tamoxifen is associated with an increased risk of endometrial cancer[52] (1.6% compared with baseline risk of 0.05% at 7 years; relative risk, 3.3) and thromboembolic phenomena; these effects are more common among women who are postmenopausal women. Conversely, both drugs are

TABLE 5-3 Overview of the Breast Cancer Chemoprevention Trials

Trial	Comparison	Participants	OR
P-1[52]	Tamoxifen vs placebo	13,388	0.57 (0.46-0.70)
IBIS-1[48]	Tamoxifen vs placebo	7,152	0.68 (0.50-0.92)
Royal Marsden[50]	Tamoxifen vs placebo	2,494	1.06 (0.7-1.7)
Italian[51]	Tamoxifen vs placebo	5,408	0.76 (0.47-1.60)
MORE[53,54]	Raloxifene vs placebo	7,705	0.76 (0.47-1.60)
RUTH[55]	Raloxifene vs placebo	10,101	0.56 (0.38-0.83)
STAR[56]	Tamoxifen vs raloxifene	19,747	1.02 (0.82-1.28)

effective antiosteoporosis drugs — raloxifene is approved for this indication, and tamoxifen significantly reduced fracture risk by 32% in the BCPT. Partially because of the rare but serious complications, there is ongoing uncertainty and controversy in the medical community about the optimal use of these agents for prevention, as well as about the selection of candidates for this intervention. It appears that women who have had a hysterectomy and for whom the risk of breast cancer is high as defined by the Gail model, would likely benefit from either raloxifene (postmenopausal only) or tamoxifen (regardless of menopausal status).[58] However, in postmenopausal women with an intact uterus, raloxifene might be preferred. Preliminary data based on a small subset of participants in BCPT suggested that chemoprevention might not affect the risk of breast cancer for carriers of the *BRCA1* mutation; the findings of other studies suggest that ovarian ablation results in risk reduction for breast cancer, even in the presence of *BRCA1* or *BRCA2* mutations.[59,60] Additional studies will be needed before these issues are resolved.

During the past decade, selective aromatase inhibitors have become the treatment of choice for first-line and second-line treatment of patients with hormone receptor-positive metastatic breast cancer who are postmenopausal.[61] The results of adjuvant clinical trials of aromatase inhibitors have demonstrated the benefit of this class of drugs in treatment of postmenopausal women with hormone receptor-positive breast cancer. Aromatase inhibition is associated with a reduction in second primary breast cancers, which has prompted initiation of the IBIS-II and MAP.3 chemoprevention trials, which were designed to compare 5 years of anastrozole and exemestane, respectively, to 5 years of placebo for high-risk patients.[62]

The only chemoprevention of known benefit is hormone manipulation as described previously. Other compounds have or are being tested. Retinoids have multiple effects on the growth factor systems involved in the development and progression of breast cancer. They bind to retinoid receptors, with the complex acting as a transcription factor that binds to the retinoid-response elements of multiple genes. Preclinical experiments have shown that various retinoids have therapeutic effects against established breast cancer and, in separate experiments, are able to reduce the frequency with which the disease develops. On the basis of these studies, Veronesi et al.[63] developed a large, prospective, randomized trial involving 3,000 patients with T1, N0 primary breast cancers. Patients were randomly assigned to receive either 200 mg of 4-hydroxyphenylretinamide (fenretinide) or a placebo for 5 years. Serial analyses of this study suggested a marginal decrease in the incidence of primary ovarian cancer; however, the study did not accomplish the primary efficacy objective, with no differences in the incidence of second breast cancer being observed. In other randomized trials, retinoids alone or in combination with tamoxifen are under evaluation in the adjuvant and the chemoprevention settings. Vitamin A, beta-carotene, and vitamin E also are being studied as adjuvant therapy for breast cancer in various trials around the world. Exploratory trials funded by the National Cancer Institute (NCI) are being conducted to assess the effects of retinoids in association with SERMs and other chemopreventive agents for patients with noninvasive breast cancer or subsets of benign breast disease thought to be markers for high-risk disease (i.e., atypical ductal hyperplasia or atypical lobular hyperplasia). A major emphasis in many of these trials is to identify intermediate (or surrogate) biologic endpoints that facilitate the evaluation of newer and potentially more promising preventive agents, such as oltipraz, dehydroepiandrosterone, genistein, and others.

PROPHYLACTIC SURGERY

Surgical removal of the breasts has been proposed for many years as a potential preventive intervention. Most early reports were based on subcutaneous mastectomies and high-risk participants were not systematically selected. During the past decade, several retrospective reviews of high-risk patients selected on the basis of family history or the presence of *BRCA1* or *BRCA2* mutations have appeared in the literature. These reports provide compelling data that suggest that prophylactic bilateral mastectomy is associated with a 90% or greater reduction in the incidence of breast cancer.[64-67] Whereas randomized, controlled trials would be preferred, such designs are difficult to conduct in high-risk populations. Epidemiologic data that link risk to certain hormone events suggest additional interventions of potentially preventive value.

In addition to decreasing the risk of ovarian cancers by more than 90%, bilateral oophorectomy also has been shown to reduce the incidence of breast cancer among women with *BRCA1* and/or *BRCA2* mutations who are premenopausal.[60]

DIETARY AND LIFESTYLE INTERVENTIONS

Epidemiologic research demonstrated broad differences in the incidence of breast cancer in different geographic regions. It is hypothesized that dietary modifications, such as reductions in caloric intake and in the fat content of the diet, might decrease breast cancer risk. Dietary interventions have been tested in preclinical animal experiments with mixed results. Depending on the model and animal species used, decreased caloric intake and a low-fat diet have been associated with either a decreased risk or no change in the incidence of breast cancer. Currently, the value of dietary interventions for the prevention of breast cancer is being tested in several large, multicenter clinical trials.[68] The Women's Health Initiative (also discussed previously) was a randomized, placebo-controlled, multicenter trial involving women between the ages of 50 and 79 who were postmenopausal. Three different interventions were built into this study, one of which was a low-fat dietary intervention. Approximately 48,000 women were randomly assigned to receive an intervention designed to result in a diet comprised of no more than 20% of calories from fat and at least five servings of fruit and vegetables per day or to no intervention.[35] There was no significant difference between the two arms in risk of invasive breast cancer development; however, the intervention arm failed to meet dietary goals, and there was a suggestion of an interaction with the hormone receptor status of the tumor. Regardless of whether a reduction in dietary fat intake can be translated into a tangible reduction in risk, the reduction in dietary fat may have salutary effects on cardiovascular disease and the prevention or control of other chronic illnesses. Because obesity in women who are postmenopausal is associated with a greater risk of breast cancer, weight-reduction strategies might reduce the incidence of the disease, although this has not been systematically tested. Even in the absence of such prevention benefits, weight reduction should be encouraged for middle-aged and older adults because its favorable effects on other health conditions can be clearly documented. The association of breast cancer with moderate to heavy alcohol intake suggests that interventions that reduce alcohol consumption might, in turn, reduce risk. However, there are no clinical trials addressing this hypothesis for the purposes of prevention.

SCREENING

In several clinical trials, screening mammography was shown to reduce the breast cancer-related mortality rates by 20% to 39% for women age 50 and older. In a meta-analysis of 13 prospective randomized trials, a 26% reduction in the relative risk of breast cancer-related mortality was found with screening mammography for women age 50 to 74.[69,70] The efficacy of screening mammography for women age 40 to 49 is more controversial.[71] The same meta-analysis demonstrated no significant decrease in the relative risk of death from breast cancer in this group, although there was a nonsignificant reduction of 13%. Considerable variability was observed in the methods used in the randomized trials; in some, mammography was the only screening method, whereas clinical breast examination was included in others. In some of the studies, mammography was obtained through a single view, whereas others involved two views. The interval between screening events ranged from 12 to 30 months.

There is no evidence of benefit from routine screening for women younger than 40 in whom the risk is average. There also is no information about the efficacy of screening mammography for women older than 74. The American Cancer Society recommends that as long as an older woman is in good health and remains a candidate for breast cancer treatment if diagnosed, she should continue to be screened for breast cancer.[72] The U.S. Preventive Services Task Force also concluded that the existing evidence can be extrapolated to women older than 70 if comorbid conditions do not compromise life expectancy.[73] Statistical criticisms have advanced the randomized trials of screening mammography[74] noting

KEY POINTS

- In a meta-analysis of 13 prospective randomized trials, a 26% reduction in the relative risk of breast cancer mortality was found with screening mammography for women between the ages of 50 and 74.
- Reports suggest that for women with high risk based on a family history of breast cancer or on *BRCA1* and/or *BRCA2* mutations, magnetic resonance imaging (MRI) detects occult disease that is undetectable by physical examination or by mammography.

that a reduction in breast cancer mortality did not necessarily decrease overall mortality particularly for patients younger than age 50.[75] Despite these considerations, published reports show that for breast cancers found during systematic screening of women between ages 40 and 49, the average tumor size is smaller and the fraction of node-negative disease is greater than for unscreened controls. These results have been advocated as reasons to propose screening even in the absence of significant reductions in the relative risk of death in randomized studies. Advocates of screening mammography for younger women have pointed out that the incidence of breast cancer is much lower among women younger than 50; therefore, the statistical power of published randomized trials of screening for women younger than 50 was insufficient. Even after pooling all of the data involving women younger than 50 who participated in randomized trials, the power of the observation would still be insufficient to detect a 15% to 30% reduction in the relative risk of death. There is no definitive information on the ideal interval between screening and the optimal combination of screening methods. However, most experts would recommend screening every 1 to 2 years for women age 50 or older and yearly for women age 40 to 49. There also is no definitive information to determine whether two screening views are more sensitive than one. The NCI and most professional societies have reiterated their strong support for systematic screening mammography for women older than 40.

Film or digital mammography continues to be the most effective method for early detection of breast cancer. The false-negative rate for mammography for women with fatty breasts who are postmenopausal is well under 10%; it is higher (more than 15%) for women with dense breasts. The lower sensitivity of screening mammography for patients younger than 50 years is partially the result of dense breast tissue in younger women. Dense breasts are not only a function of young age but also are related to hormone-replacement therapy or to familial or genetic components, and thus represent a risk factor for breast cancer. In a large international study including approximately 50,000 women who underwent both screening procedures, digital mammography was more sensitive than film mammography in women with dense breasts.[76]

The value of breast self-examination as part of a systematic screening program is another subject of controversy.[73] Proponents argue that breast self-examination is an inexpensive method that leads to the detection of smaller lesions, identifies mammographically silent lesions, and provides the patient the opportunity to participate actively in her own care. Opponents assert that there is no evidence that adding breast self-examination to mammography and physical examination by a physician increases the yield of a screening program or significantly decreases breast cancer-related mortality. In addition, opponents state that self-examination leads to anxiety and unnecessary physician visits and diagnostic interventions when patients find perceived or real changes during self-assessment of their breasts. Appropriately designed clinical trials will be the only method to determine whether this procedure is of value in reducing mortality. However, this outcome might be difficult to demonstrate in industrialized countries where screening is based on sensitive mammography that is likely to detect breast masses that are much smaller than the lower limits of detection by breast self-examination. Conversely, there are ongoing trials in developing countries where periodic screening mammography is beyond the capabilities of the public health system (because of limited financial resources) and where breast self-examination and assessment by a physician might be cost-effective methods for earlier diagnosis of breast cancer (earlier than stage III and IV disease). There is evidence that training lay people and health care professionals improves the efficacy of the physical evaluation of the breast. Few large prospective trials have been performed — one in China including more than 30,000 women and the interim analysis of another in Russia including more than 100,000 women. Neither of these studies demonstrated the clinical utility of the procedure; however, the data as currently exist are considered insufficient.[77,78]

Breast ultrasonography has improved substantially from the technical point of view; it can detect much smaller lesions than it could 10, or even 5, years ago. Sonography also can detect some lesions not detected or well defined by film mammography. However, there are no data that document the value of sonography in the absence of mammography for screening purposes. Furthermore, there are no data supporting the systematic use of both breast ultrasonography and film mammography for screening purposes. Breast ultrasonography has substantial value for the evaluation of suspicious lesions found during screening mammography and for the characterization of lesions found by physical examination but not detected by mammography. Furthermore, it is a useful, practical, and relatively inexpensive method of directing fine-needle aspiration biopsies. Unfortunately, breast sonography is not very well standardized, and its efficacy is highly operator dependent.

Newer imaging modalities are under evaluation for the diagnosis and screening of breast cancer. MRI provides excellent characterization of breast lesions. Several reports have suggested that this technology, especially with the use of an appropriate contrast material, has greater sensitivity than mammography.[79,80] Proponents present information to suggest that MRI detects multicentric lesions more effectively than mammography or sonography and that it defines the extent of disease more accurately than other imaging methods. These features could improve the ability to obtain clear surgical margins after lumpectomy and contribute to the accuracy of response evaluation after neoadjuvant systemic therapy.

In early 2007 the American Cancer Society recommended the use of screening MRI in women with high risk.[81] In women at very high risk of breast cancer, including those patients with familial breast cancer or with *BRCA1* and *BRCA2* mutations and in whom the disease tends to develop at an early age, most experts would recommend that screening should begin early, although the exact timing is not well established. Because of the issues related to dense breasts and the relative lack of sensitivity of mammography in this situation, other imaging modalities are reasonable, including digital mammography and MRI. Recently, several prospective studies, including a large international study, suggest the use of MRI for women at high risk on the basis of family history or *BRCA1* and *BRCA2* mutations. MRI detects occult disease that is undetectable by mammography or by physical examination; therefore, it may be the optimal screening choice in patients with a high prevalence of disease.[82–84] The development of MRI equipment specifically designed for breast imaging, as well as a substantial reduction in the price and duration of the examinations, will help in the definitive evaluation of the role of MRI in screening of breast cancer. MRI of the breast lacks a generally accepted standard procedure for performance and interpretation. Therefore, the results from one institution are not necessarily reproducible in another.

Positron emission tomography (PET) also has been evaluated as a diagnostic procedure for breast cancer.[85,86] Using 18-fluorodeoxyglucose, or [^{11}c]-methionine, PET detects most large primary tumors and large regional lymph node deposits. Proposed uses for PET in breast cancer are the differentiation between recurrent disease and radiation therapy-related fibrosis, identification of metastatic lesions, and the early determination of response to radiation therapy, chemotherapy, or hormone therapy. Definitive studies in support of these indications are lacking.

There is no evidence that PET has a role in screening for early breast cancer. Technical improvements in PET scanning to boost its ability to detect smaller lesions, a marked reduction in the cost and duration of examinations, and completion of prospective trials to validate these indications will be necessary for PET to become a useful and cost-effective screening method.

DIAGNOSIS

Once a suspicious abnormality is detected in the breast by physical examination or imaging, a definitive diagnosis must be made. The gold standard continues to be histopathologic examination of a biopsy specimen. Whether the abnormality is palpable or forms a mass, as well as how deep within the breast parenchyma it is located, will determine the optimal method to establish a firm diagnosis. Simple cysts detected by ultrasound can often be aspirated; often, no further histologic or cytologic evaluation is required if the cyst disappears.

Fine-needle aspiration biopsy is an excellent diagnostic method for most clinically palpable lesions in the breast and axilla that allows real-time relatively low morbidity diagnosis in order to thoughtfully plan definitive surgical interventions. The rate of false-positive results on evaluation of tissue obtained by fine-needle aspiration biopsy ranges from 0% to 0.4%. False-negative rates in recent large series have ranged from 0% to 4%, similar to the rates associated with core-needle biopsies.[87] DNA does not distinguish invasive from noninvasive carcinoma and aspirates often do not provide sufficient cells for receptor analysis.

Definitive diagnosis and receptors can be obtained from a core (cutting)-needle biopsy. Image-detected lesions are usually approached by needle-localization and stereotactic biopsies. Following the surgical excision of the suspicious lesion, specimen radiography often is often carried out to confirm that the entire mammographic abnormality has been removed. Incisional biopsies are reserved for cases in which a fine-needle aspiration or core-needle biopsy yielded insufficient amounts of tissue, results were inconclusive, or cases involving inflammatory breast cancer. The purpose of an incisional biopsy is the inclusion of a full-thickness skin sample to document the presence of dermal lymphatic invasion. If the diagnosis of cancer can be established on a core-needle or fine-needle aspiration biopsy, diagnostic excisional biopsies are discouraged.

PROGNOSTIC MARKERS

Once the diagnosis has been established and the prognosis estimated, treatment planning proceeds. To a large extent, the characteristics of the tumor and the patient's preferences will guide the initial treatment. Most early breast cancers are treated with an initial surgical intervention that is designed to remove the primary breast tumor. The axillary lymph nodes are usually staged, using either a sentinel lymph node biopsy or a level I and II axillary lymph node dissection. The size of the primary tumor in relation to the size of the breast, the presence of additional foci of cancer or mammographic abnormalities, history of chest irradiation (e.g., as in Hodgkin's disease), and the patient's preference for a total mastectomy or breast conservation (surgical removal of the affected area via excisional biopsy, lumpectomy, tumorectomy, or segmental mastectomy followed by radiation therapy to the remainder of the breast) determine which approach the oncologist will use. Conversely, larger tumors are increasingly being managed with initial chemotherapy (termed primary, preoperative, or neoadjuvant chemotherapy) followed by local therapy.

PROGNOSTIC DETERMINANTS OF LOCAL THERAPY

Tumor Size and Extent

Effective breast conservation (lumpectomy plus radiotherapy) requires the ability to excise the tumor fully with negative (tumor-free) surgical margins and acceptable cosmesis. Small tumors lend themselves to lumpectomy because removal of a small tumor leaves the shape and size of the breast almost intact, usually offering excellent cosmetic results. The size of the breast also is an important consideration; thus, even relatively small tumors in very small breasts may require the excision of a substantial portion of the gland, leaving unsatisfactory cosmetic results. A mastectomy often is preferable in these cases, especially when associated with breast reconstruction. Defining the size of the breast lesion is sometimes difficult, especially for tumors that are diffuse, stellate, and not encapsulated. In these cases, the initial excision often has positive margins that require excision of additional tissue; not uncommonly, mastectomy is required because of the inability to achieve negative margins. High-quality imaging, using mammography, sonography, and sometimes MRI, is critical for optimal preoperative assessment and treatment planning. The administration of neoadjuvant chemotherapy to patients with large breast cancers often results in a sufficient reduction in tumor size to convert a mastectomy-only candidate into a candidate for breast-conserving surgery. Locoregional extension through pectoralis into the chest wall (T4a disease) and direct extension to the skin (T4b) are generally not amenable to breast conservation unless effectively cytoreduced by neoadjuvant (preoperative) chemotherapy. Inflammatory breast cancer (T4d), which is characterized by erythema and induration of the breast and often accompanied by dermal lymphatic invasion by tumor emboli, are not considered for breast conservation.

Extensive Intraductal Component

An extensive intraductal component is defined as ductal carcinoma in situ admixed and extending beyond the invasive tumor that comprises at least 25% of the tumor volume. It often is a manifestation of multifocal disease. The presence of extensive intraductal cancer was proposed as an adverse risk factor for local recurrence following breast-conserving surgery. More recent analyses suggested that an extensive intraductal compo-

KEY POINT

- Involvement of the axillary lymph nodes remains the most reliable and reproducible prognostic indicator for primary breast cancer.

nent may have minimal or no adverse prognostic value when all margins of resection are histopathologically tumor free.

Lymphatic Invasion

Lymphatic invasion within the breast is associated with a poor outcome. However, it is not entirely clear to what extent lymphovascular invasion contributes to prognosis beyond other known prognostic factors, and it does not necessarily alter local management.

Dermal lymphatic invasion is a special circumstance. Dermal lymphatic invasion is one of the characteristics of inflammatory breast cancer, a unique subset of breast cancers that are typically high grade, rapidly growing, and carry a poor prognosis. These tumors are diffusely growing breast cancer and are not considered amenable to breast conservation.

Multiple Tumor Foci or Diffuse Microcalcifications

When mammography shows diffuse microcalcifications throughout the breast, or multiple primary lesions are found distant from each other, a total mastectomy is the preferred surgical intervention.

Age

Women younger than 35 years have an increased risk of local recurrence in the breast despite optimal breast-conservation surgery. Although breast cancer in the very young is associated with various adverse prognostic indicators (e.g., ER negativity, poorly differentiated tumors, and high proliferative fraction), and it may serve as a surrogate marker for those indicators, in multivariate analyses, young age remains as an independent adverse prognostic factor. The likelihood of *BRCA1* or *BRCA2* mutations[88] is as high as 10% in women who develop breast cancer when younger than 35; some of the "local recurrences" reported in such very young women may actually reflect new second primary tumors.

BRCA1 or *BRCA2* Mutations

There are several issues to consider in local treatment of a woman with breast cancer who is a known carrier of a *BRCA1* or *BRCA2* mutation.[89] First is whether there is an increased risk of locoregional relapse of the existing tumor; recent data are reassuring that, with well-delivered radiation therapy following lumpectomy, these rates are not significantly different from those for controls. A separate issue is the high risk of a second primary cancer in women with an inherited predisposition and a personal history of one cancer. Although the ipsilateral risk may or may not be abrogated by radiation therapy, these patients have an excess risk of contralateral breast cancer that in some series approaches 50%. Reasonable local approaches to women with *BRCA1* and/or *BRCA2* mutations is bilateral mastectomy or ipsilateral breast conservation, with a careful discussion of prevention and early detection plans for both ipsilateral and contralateral new primaries.

PROGNOSTIC DETERMINANTS OF ADJUVANT THERAPY

After definitive surgical resection and complete pathologic assessment, several tumor characteristics are used as important prognostic indicators to determine the need for additional therapy and as predictive factors to determine the specific type of therapy.

Lymph Node Involvement

Involvement of the axillary lymph nodes remains the most reliable and reproducible prognostic indicator for primary breast cancer. In general, 50% to 70% of patients with positive lymph nodes will have a relapse in the absence of systemic therapy, whereas only 20% to 35% of patients with negative lymph nodes are expected to relapse after local-regional treatments. Each additional positive lymph node identified increases the risk of recurrence and metastasis by several percentage points. Thus, the risk is greater for patients with four to 10 positive lymph nodes than for patients with one to three positive nodes, and the probability of recurrence and metastasis is more than 80% for patients with 10 or more positive nodes. Prior to the use of sentinel lymph node mapping and biopsy, the results of clinical studies had demonstrated that lymph node negativity is reliable only if at least six, but preferably 10 axillary lymph nodes were removed and examined. Both macrometastasis (greater than 2 mm) and micrometastasis (between 0.2 and 2 mm, termed "NI(mic) in American Joint Committee on Cancer staging system) in the lymph nodes have prognostic significance; micrometastases carry a risk of recurrence intermediate between node-negative and macrometastatic node-positive disease. Involvement of internal mammary lymph nodes pathologically or radiographically also is associated with poor outcome similar to multiple involved axillary lymph nodes.

The development and adoption of sentinel lymph node mapping and biopsy has changed the practice of both surgery and pathology.[90–92] Patients with clinically negative lymph nodes are candidates for sentinel lymph node biopsy. With only one to three nodes to process, the pathologist is able to perform multiple sections of each lymph node, thereby increasing the sensitivity of the test for microscopic metastatic deposits. The increased number of sections and the use of investigational procedures, such as immunohistochemistry, contribute to a higher detection rate of micrometastases within the sentinel lymph nodes. The prognostic significance of isolated metastatic cells (smaller than 0.2 mm) or metastases found only by special means, such as immunohistochemistry, in nodes considered negative by traditional processing methods is the subject of intensive investigation in several large, multicenter controlled trials. In general, if one or more sentinel lymph nodes are positive, axillary dissection is then performed. The non-sentinel nodes obtained are handled in a conventional manner, without step-sectioning. Although axillary dissection remains the standard of care, some studies are examining the role of radiotherapy for management of the axilla after positive sentinely lymphadenectomy. Sentinel lymph node biopsy is not appropriate for clinically palpable pathologic nodes and has not been validated in large (more than 5 cm) tumors.

Tumor Size

Tumor size has prognostic significance for the determination of the potential need for adjuvant therapy. The size of the tumor is directly correlated with the risk of recurrence or metastasis. Tumor size adds less to the determination of prognosis for patients with node-positive breast cancer than it does for patients with node-negative disease, for whom tumor size often is the main prognostic factor. The determination of tumor size should be on the basis of the invasive component only.

Histologic Type

Pure noninvasive breast cancers do not have any substantial systemic risk. Although tamoxifen often is administered to patients with ER-positive DCIS who were treated with breast conservation, the purpose is to reduce local recurrence and prevent new primaries.

Most invasive breast cancers are ductal type. A significant proportion of the remainder are a combination of ductal and lobular or pure lobular histology. The prognoses of ductal and lobular cancers are similar enough to prompt the same treatment modalities. Several less common types have more favorable prognosis. These histologic subtypes include pure tubular, mucinous or colloid, and papillary cancers.[93] These cancers are usually small and found in a node-negative stage. The more favorable prognosis of these histologic types supports the use of breast-conserving therapy and often justifies the omission of adjuvant systemic treatment. Thus, noninvasive breast cancers do not require adjuvant systemic treatment (although adjuvant tamoxifen may be offered to reduce the risk of a second primary breast cancer), and tubular, colloid, and papillary cancers smaller than 3 cm often are treated without systemic adjuvant therapy. When stringently defined, pure or typical medullary cancer also is considered to have a better prognosis than ductal cancer, although not as favorable as tubular or colloid types. However, atypical medullary cancers — those cancers that do not fulfill the necessary histologic criteria — or mixed medullary and ductal cancers have prognoses similar to prognoses for the common varieties of ductal and lobular breast cancers. Lastly, a relatively rare histology, metaplastic cancer has aggressive characteristics and is associated with a poor prognosis.

Histologic Grade or Differentiation

The clear definition of histologic differentiation grades led to the recognition that those grades had reproducible prognostic significance. Trained, experienced breast pathologists can recognize poorly differentiated, moderately well-differentiated, and well-differentiated tumors without much difficulty; the assessment of the histologic grade for those tumors is reasonably reproducible. Furthermore, although there is some variation among different pathologists, the concordance rate is acceptable. Reports from the Surveillance, Epidemiology, and End Results (SEER) tumor registry provided strong evidence in support of the prognostic value of histologic grade determined by average pathologists.[94] Nuclear grade is similarly useful, although histologic grade might be a more reliable prognostic indicator because it includes not only cellular, but also tissue-related, criteria. Smaller tumors are more often well differentiated, whereas larger tumors are frequently poorly differentiated. Tumor grade or differentiation also is associated with other prognostic indicators, such as ER expression, progesterone receptor (PR) expression, HER2 status, and S-phase fraction.

Lymphatic invasion

Dermal lymphatic invasion often is found as part of inflammatory breast cancer, which carries a poor prognosis. Other histologic factors, including lymphatic and vascular invasion (without dermal lymphatic invasion), tumor necrosis, and mononuclear cell infiltration, have been related to poor prognosis. However, these factors have had insufficient evaluation or have not been shown to be independent prognostic indicators in multivariate analysis.

Markers of Proliferative Capacity

Measures of the proliferation rates of malignant tissues have prognostic value for breast cancer. High proliferative index also is often associated with other negative prognostic factors such as tumor size, lymph node status, grade, and HER2 status; for this reason there is debate about the independent information provided by proliferative index alone. The proliferative capacity of the malignant cell can be assessed by several techniques including mitotic indices, the thymidine-labeling index, or S-phase fractions. The mitotic index is determined by counting mitotic figures using light microscopy on a tumor specimen stained with hematoxylin and eosin. It is a technique applicable in any surgical pathology laboratory, and it has been validated by both univariate and multivariate analyses. The mitotic index is an integral component of the Nottingham prognostic index and other successful prognostic indices of reproducible value.[95,96] The thymidine-labeling index also was shown to be effective and reproducible, but it is much more labor intensive; for this reason, it has not gained general acceptance. Ki-67, MIB1, and proliferating-cell nuclear antigen are immunohistochemical markers for the proliferation rate of malignant tumors. These tests reflect the expression of proteins involved in the control of the cell cycle or preferentially expressed during certain phases of the cell cycle. Ki-67 has been extensively evaluated and found to correlate strongly with the results of S-phase fraction. The usefulness of the proliferating-cell nuclear antigen requires additional evaluation. Cyclin D1 and E expression have been associated with adverse outcome, however their contribution to prognosis independent of other markers has yet to be verified.[97,98] Many other proteins have been proposed to serve as prognostic indicators, and some are under active evaluation. At this time, they have no role outside the context of a clinical trial.

Steroid Receptors

Both ER and PR have been extensively studied in patients with primary breast cancer.[99] The reports of the existence of two subtypes of ER, ER alpha and beta, have no known prognostic implication to date, and current methods measure ER alpha only.[100] Both ER and PR have weak prognostic value; their primary value is in predicting efficacy of endocrine therapy. There is no role for endocrine therapy in ER- and PR-negative disease, however, it is a mainstay of therapy for ER- or PR-positive disease. Whereas patients with ER-positive tumors tend to have better short-term disease-free and overall survival rates than do patients with ER-negative tumors, the differences between the two groups tend to diminish or even disappear with time. This is partially because ER-positive breast cancer, unlike ER-negative, has a persistent risk of relapse many years after diagnosis.[101] Analyses have suggested that the hazard rate for recurrence is greater for ER-negative tumors during the first 3 to 4 years, but beyond this period of time, the hazard rate of ER-positive tumors exceeds the rate for those that are ER-negative. The PR appeared in some studies to be a more valuable prognostic indicator than the ER, although this has not been validated. Evaluation of both receptors, previously carried out mostly by ligand binding assays, is done using immunohistochemical or immunocytochemical methods with a fairly high degree of reliability.

The optimal indication of steroid hormone receptors is not for determining prognosis but for predicting response to systemic therapy and, therefore, the selection of optimal adjuvant systemic treatments. Analyses of large databases derived from prospective clinical trials suggest that the expression of any estrogen receptor should be interpreted as a positive assay, because even patients with very low expression of the estrogen receptor can benefit from endocrine interventions to some extent.[102] Conversely, if receptor expression is completely absent, there is no reason to consider endocrine therapy. Emerging data from chemotherapy trials also suggest that ER-negative tumors respond more often and more completely to chemotherapy than their ER-positive counterparts.[103] Pathologic complete response to neoadjuvant therapy only rarely occurs in ER-positive tumors.

HER2/*neu*

Also identified as C-erbB-2, HER2/*neu* is a normal gene that is amplified (multiple gene copies) or overexpressed (excess production of the p185 protein) in 20% to 30% of breast cancers.[104] Gene amplification and protein overexpression correlate strongly, although single-copy overexpressors are reported in approximately 5% of patients with breast cancer who have HER2-overexpressing tumors. The HER2 protein is a transmembrane protein that has intrinsic tyrosine kinase activity and belongs to the family of type I protein tyrosine kinase growth factor receptors. HER2 amplification is defined as excess copy number of the gene, usually measured by fluorescence in situ hybridization (FISH), and HER2 overexpression is defined as excess (3+) membranous protein expression, usually measured using immunohistochemistry.[105] HER2 amplification or overexpression is associated with highly proliferative, high grade, hormone receptor-negative tumors and increased risk of relapse and shorter survival in most reported studies that did not include trastuzumab therapy. Molecular subtyping using gene expression arrays confirm a biologically distinct HER2+/ER- subtype that is characterized by expression of the proliferative and the HER2-related clusters of genes and low or no expression of ER-related genes. There also are a small proportion of luminal tumors that express both the ER and HER2 clusters of genes that is entirely distinct from the HER2+/ER- subtype. Both are clinically HER2 positive and appropriately treated with HER2-targeted therapy; there are no data suggesting a differential response to HER2-targeted therapy by ER status or subtype.

Even more than a prognostic indicator, HER2 overexpression or amplification serves as a predictor of response to HER2-directed therapies such as trastuzumab, a monoclonal antibody that targets the extracellular domain of the p-185 oncoprotein. Some studies suggest that HER2 overexpression is a marker of relative resistance to tamoxifen and sensitivity to anthracyclines, however, this is controversial. HER2 expression can be tested with immunohistochemical or cytochemical techniques, whereas amplification is usually assayed by fluorescence in situ hybridization (FISH); test kits for both approaches are commercially available.

Prognostic Indices

Several clinically useful prognostic indices that incorporate relevant clinical variables have been developed. These models include but are not limited to the following: the Nottingham Prognostic Index,[96] which includes tumor grade, involvement of the axillary lymph nodes, and hormone receptor status; the St. Gallen's risk categories for node-negative disease, which includes hormone receptor status, tumor size and grade, and patient age[106]; and a web-based tool, Adjuvant! online, which includes patient age, comorbid conditions, grade, hormone receptor status, tumor size, and the number of involved nodes.[107] This tool not only estimates risk of relapse and death from breast cancer, but it also allows modeling that includes other prognostic variables than those automatically included, and it estimates the benefit of specific adjuvant therapies.

Molecular Profiling

Clinicians have long known that ER-negative breast cancer differs in behavior from ER-positive breast cancer. With the advent of technology permitting genome-wide examination, this clinical impression has been confirmed, and it has become increasingly clear that breast cancer actually represents a group of biologically distinct diseases. Gene expression array analyses have reproducibly demonstrated several molecular subtypes of breast cancer.[108] The main ER-positive subtypes are called "luminal," termed thus because of their gross similarity in expression pattern to the luminal epithelial component of the breast. The most commonly noted luminal subtypes are Luminal A and Luminal B. Both are ER positive or PR positive, however Luminal A tumors are typically lower grade, with higher expression of estrogen receptor and related genes, lower likelihood of HER2 expression, and lower proliferative indices. As mentioned, these tumors often are appropriate for adjuvant endocrine therapy with consideration of chemotherapy if relapse risk warrants; if a patient has HER2-positive disease, adjuvant HER2-directed therapy, such as trastuzumab, also can be considered.

The two main ER-negative subtypes are the HER2-positive/ER-negative subtype, which is characterized by expression of proliferation genes and HER2, but not ER or its related genes, and the basal-like subtype. The HER2-positive/ER-negative subtype is often treated with chemotherapy and HER2-targeted therapy. The basal-like subtype is characterized by the absence of expression of both hormone receptors and HER2. Adjuvant therapy choices for basal-like breast cancer are limited to chemotherapy. Detailed molecular subtyping is not yet available for clinical purposes, however, the biologic heterogeneity suggested by current examinations may well play a role in more sophisticated treatment decision-making in the future.

Several genomic-based prognostic profiles have been developed and validated for clinical use. Among others, already validated molecular prognosticators include a 70-gene prognostic profile for node-negative disease in women age 60 and younger,[109] a 76-gene prognostic profile for node-negative disease,[110] and a 21-gene panel (the "Recurrence Score") for residual risk in node-negative/hormone receptor-positive disease managed with tamoxifen.[111] Each of these assays appears to provide independent prognostic information beyond clinical variables. Despite similar clinical utility and oftentimes similar populations, many gene profiles do not identify the same genes. Recent studies suggest that despite this discordance in specific genes, prognostic profiles give similar results when tested on biologically concordant subtypes, which suggests that they are identifying similar pathways.[112] Whether these improvements in prognostication result in more thoughtful use of adjuvant therapy and improved outcome is being examined in several large international trials from the TransBIG consortium and the Breast Intergroup.

STAGES 0 TO III DISEASE MANAGEMENT

Staging classifications were designed to identify prognostically distinct subgroups of patients and to select, on the basis of risk, the optimal therapeutic strategy. There were five or more staging classifications used by different practitioners or investigators 30 years ago. Over the past 3 decades, the tumor, node, metastasis (TNM) classification system, jointly developed and periodically updated by the American Joint Committee on Cancer and the Union Internationale Contre le Cancer, was universally adopted. The TNM staging system is based entirely on anatomic, imaging, and histopathologic measurements, as well as on evidence of dissemination, without including any of the modern prognostic factors described previously.[113] Despite this limitation, the TNM system provides reproducible prognostic information; the latest update of the TNM classification for breast cancer was implemented in January 2003 (Table 5-4).

Primary therapy for breast cancer should provide optimal local and systemic control of disease and the highest cure rate possible, as measured by disease-free and overall survival rates, while preserving the best possible quality of life. Several organizations have published online guidelines to aid in decision making regarding adjuvant therapies.[106,107,114] Although it is recognized that breast cancer may be treated using several different approaches, the following overview identifies currently accepted treatment strategies by stage. However, it is crucial to realize that decision making regarding breast cancer adjuvant therapy is heavily influenced by the biology of the tumor as indicated by the hormone receptor and HER2 statuses (Fig. 5-1).

STAGE 0 (NONINVASIVE DISEASE)

Stage 0 refers to noninvasive breast cancer or DCIS. This stage used to be diagnosed as a palpable mass, however, since the adoption of screening mammography, DCIS is usually a mammographic finding. It can be optimally treated by performing a total mastectomy; the failure rate of treatment is less than 2%. With a total mastectomy, there is a 97% to 98% long-term disease-free survival rate for patients with noninvasive breast cancer.

However, because more advanced, invasive cancers are treated with breast-conserving surgery, clinical trials were conducted to determine whether breast-conserving therapy would be appropriate for DCIS. The results of the two largest randomized studies showed that lumpectomy and radiation therapy produced long-term results identical to the results obtained after a total mastectomy. Therefore, treatment options for most cases of DCIS can reasonably include lumpectomy followed by radiation therapy to the breast, or total mastectomy.[115] Because axillary lymph node involvement is rare for patients with DCIS, an axillary dissection is not indicated. However, some experts, in the recent past, recommended an axillary dissection for larger noninvasive tumors (larger than 5 cm) because microinvasion is easier to overlook in a larger tumor unless exhaustive histologic examination of the entire specimen is carried out. Since the development and adoption of sentinel lymph node biopsy, patients with higher-risk DCIS often have a sentinel lymph node

TABLE 5-4 Tumor, Node, and Metastasis (TNM) Classifications (A) and Staging System (B) of the American Joint Committee[113] on Cancer[114]

A. T and N Classifications

Primary Tumor (clinical or pathologic)

Tx	Cannot be assessed
T0	None
Tis	Carcinoma in situ
T1	Tumor ≤ 2cm in longest dimension
T2	Tumor > 2cm but ≤ 5cm
T3	Tumor > 5cm
T4	Direct extension through chest wall (T4a), to skin (T4b), both (T4c), or inflammatory breast cancer (T4d)

Ipsilateral regional lymph nodes

Clinical	N0	No palpable lymph nodes
	N1	Palpable but movable ipsilateral axillary nodes
	N2	Matted axillary lymph nodes (N2a) or clinically apparent in internal mammary nodes without axillary involvement (N2b)
	N3	Both infraclavicular (N3a) or internal mammary (N3b) and axillary nodes; Supraclavicular nodes with or without axillary nodes (N3c)
Pathologic	pN0	No involvement greater than 0.2 mm
	pN1	1-3 positive* axillary nodes; positive internal mammary node that was not clinically apparent
	pN2	4-9 positive axillary nodes; positive, clinically apparent internal mammary node without axillary involvement
	pN3	≥10 positive axillary nodes; supraclavicular or infraclavicular nodes; positive clinically apparent internal mammary node with axillary involvement

B. Staging System

Stage	Tumor (T)	Node (N)	Metastasis (M)
0	Tis	N0	M0
I	T1*	N0	M0
IIA	T0	N1	M0
	T1	N1	M0
	T2	N0	M0
IIB	T2	N1	M0
	T3	N0	M0
IIIA	T0	N2	M0
	T1	N2	M0
	T2	N2	M0
	T3	N1	M0
	T3	N2	M0
IIIB	T4	N0	M0
	T4	N1	M0
	T4	N2	M0
IIIC	Any T	N3	M0
IV	Any T	Any N	M1

Note: If pathologic staging performed after neoadjuvant therapy, the TNM stage is preceded by a "y" designation. * positive = at least 0.2 mm on hematoxylin and eosin staining, nodal metastases measuring > 0.2 mm but ≤ 2 mm are termed "micrometastases" and can be designated "mic."
B. Staging System
*T1 – subsets include T1a (≤ 0.5 cm), T1b (0.6–1.0 cm), T1c (1.1–2.0 cm).

KEY POINTS

- With a total mastectomy, there is a 97% to 98% long-term disease-free survival rate for patients with noninvasive breast cancer.
- For many cases of DCIS, a lumpectomy followed by radiation therapy to the breast represents the optimal treatment option, with tamoxifen considered as additional local prophylaxis if the disease is ER positive.

biopsy first, and only if one or more lymph nodes are positive is an axillary lymph node dissection considered. In one large clinical trial (NSABP B-24), the value of adding adjuvant tamoxifen to lumpectomy and radiation therapy was assessed.[116] The results showed that tamoxifen reduced the risk of local recurrence and second primary breast cancer to a significant degree. Because mortality after optimally treated DCIS is rare, no effect of tamoxifen on mortality was detected. Subsequent reports suggest that the benefit of tamoxifen in DCIS is limited to the ER-positive subset.[79]

STAGE I

Most patients with stage I disease, especially patients with unifocal neoplasms, are excellent candidates for treatment with a lumpectomy combined with radiation therapy or mastectomy. For patients with specific contraindications for breast-conserving surgery, such as prior radiation to the chest region, total mastectomy is the treatment of choice. It is estimated that 50% to 80% of stage I breast cancers can be treated optimally with tumorectomy and radiation therapy.[117] However, only 30% to 60% of patients with stage I disease receive that treatment in the United States, with major geographic variations occurring throughout the country.[118–120] The rate of breast-conserving therapy is highest in the Northeast and Pacific coast regions and lowest in the South and Southeast regions, with an intermediate rate in other areas of the country.[120] There are few absolute contraindications for breast-conserving therapy, and the choice between it and a mastectomy is based on an acceptable trade-off between local control and cosmesis. The standard of care today for patients treated with breast-conserving surgery includes radiation therapy to the breast to provide optimal local-regional control. Some experts believe that breast-conserving surgery without radiation therapy might be a satisfactory alternative for patients, especially patients who are elderly, with very small, well-differentiated, and ER-positive tumors if wide (more than 10 mm) negative margins are obtained. A prospective randomized trial of women ages 70 and older with stage I, ER-positive breast cancer who were treated with lumpectomy and adjuvant tamoxifen with or without radiation found a very low recurrence rate overall, a significant difference between the arms in local recurrence (1% with radiation compared with 4% without; $p < 0.001$), and no difference in survival.[121] Another surgical option that preserves the breast is a quadrantectomy, introduced by Veronesi and colleagues. This procedure requires a wider resection of breast tissue with a more generous margin of normal tissue around the resected tumor. Although the local control rate is higher after a quadrantectomy than after a tumorectomy (both followed by radiation therapy), the cosmetic results of the former procedure are inferior. Patients receiving quadrantectomies often need partial reconstructive procedures. Quadrantectomies are more frequently performed in Europe and South America, whereas a lumpectomy is the preferred method in North America.

It is now generally agreed upon that stage I breast cancers larger than 1 cm in maximum diameter are associated with a risk of recurrence that exceeds 10% and, therefore, systemic adjuvant therapies are warranted (Figure 5-1). If the ER or PR status of the tumor is positive, endocrine therapy is indicated. Tamoxifen, when administered for 5 years to patients with hormone receptor-positive tumors, has been shown in multiple clinical trials and the Oxford meta-analysis to reduce annual odds of recurrence by 40% to 50%. Tamoxifen also reduced the odds of death by 33% for both premenopausal and postmenopausal women (Table 5-5).[122] Ovarian ablation or suppression reduces the proportional risk of relapse and death by 10% to 20% in premenopausal women; this benefit is more prominent in women who did not also receive chemotherapy. The relative roles of ovarian ablation/suppression, chemotherapy, and tamoxifen

KEY POINTS

- Mastectomy and lumpectomy plus radiation therapy provide equivalent disease control and survival in most women with breast cancer.
- Most women with stage I breast cancers can be treated optimally with lumpectomy and radiation therapy.
- Stage I breast cancers larger than 1 cm are associated with a risk of recurrence that exceeds 10% and, therefore, systemic adjuvant therapies should be considered.
- Tamoxifen, when administered for 5 years to patients with hormone receptor-positive tumors, has been shown in multiple clinical trials and in the Oxford meta-analysis to reduce the annual odds of recurrence by approximately 40% to 50%. The odds of death also were reduced by approximately 33% for both premenopausal and postmenopausal women. For postmenopausal women, use of an aromatase inhibitor instead of tamoxifen or sequentially following tamoxifen is appropriate.

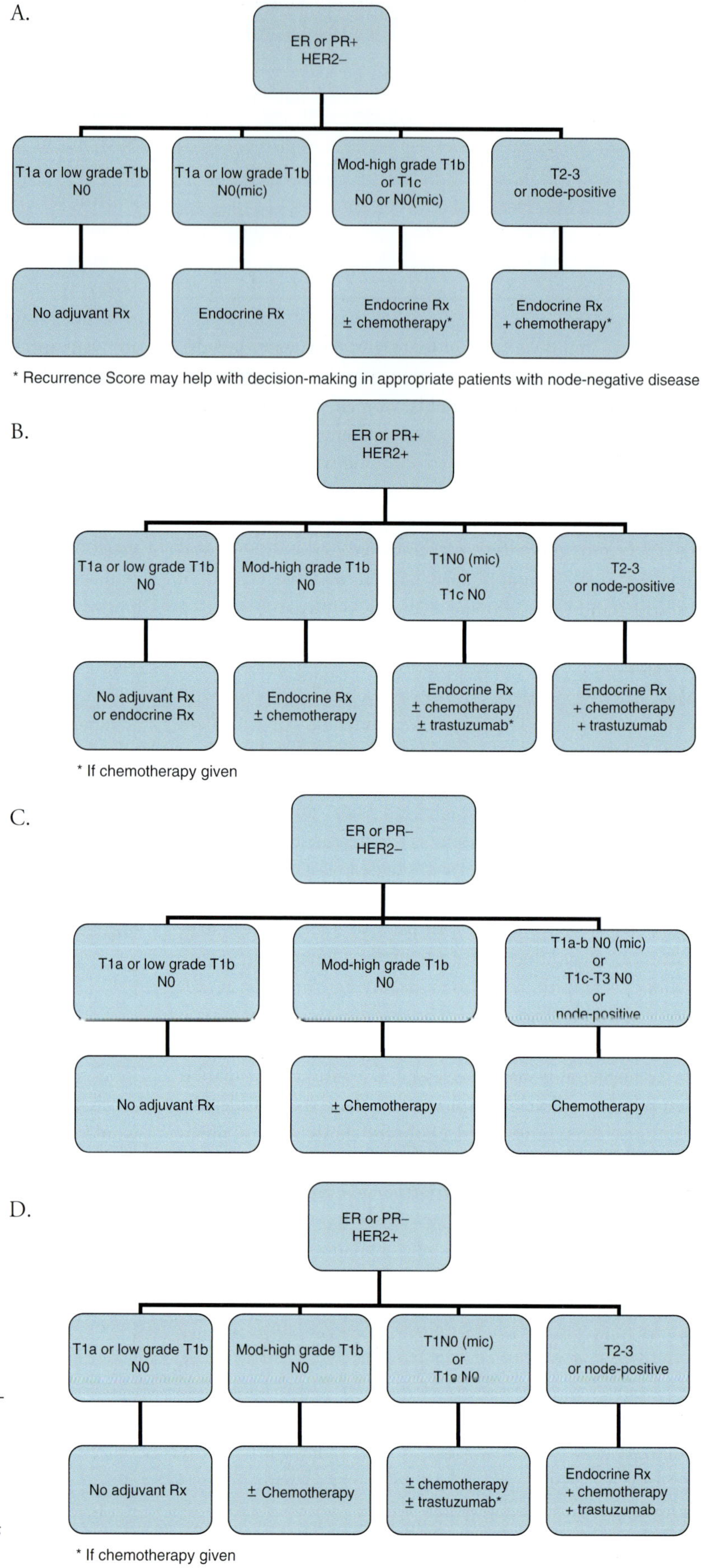

FIG. 5-1 Guidelines for adjuvant systemic therapy for hormone receptor-positive, HER2-negative (A), hormone receptor-positive, HER2-positive (B), hormone receptor-negative, HER2-negative (C), and hormone receptor-negative, HER2-positive (D).

N0 (mic) = micrometastatic disease in lymph nodes less than 0.2 mm.

in women who are premenopausal and who have hormone receptor-positive breast cancer are the subject of several large international studies. In women who are postmenopausal, adjuvant aromatase inhibitors, either instead of or subsequent to 2 to 5 years of tamoxifen, provide a small but real benefit over tamoxifen alone regarding relapse (approximately 10% to 20% fewer relapses, proportionally) and endo metrial pathology; however, the survival benefit has been more difficult to demonstrate and they are inferior regarding bone health.[123]

The addition of adjuvant chemotherapy to the endocrine treatment of patients with ER-positive invasive breast cancer larger than 1 cm in diameter is thought to increase the relative reduction in odds of recurrence by another 36% for younger women and 15% for older women.[122] Because of the strong effect of adjuvant endocrine therapy, the absolute benefit of chemotherapy is far smaller for patients with hormone receptor-positive breast cancer that is stage I or node-negative stage II than for patients with hormone receptor-negative disease. If clinical decision-making is difficult regarding the risk–benefit of adding chemotherapy to endocrine therapy, the genomics-based prognostic tool, the Recurrence Score (described previously) was developed to predict the risk of recurrence in patients with node-negative, ER-positive breast cancer, despite tamoxifen treatment status. The tool also can help distinguish those tumors with a higher or lower residual risk.[111] The systemic adjuvant therapy of choice for patients with node-negative, ER-negative tumors is combination chemotherapy.[122] The polychemotherapy regimens are discussed in the section Stage II. However, the additional benefit of more aggressive regimens is quite small in patients with a baseline low risk, such as stage I, so if chemotherapy is administered, less aggressive regimens, such as four cycles of doxorubicin and cyclophosphamide or 6 months of combination cyclophosphamide, methotrexate, and fluorouracil, may be considered. A small recently reported study suggests that combination docetaxel and cyclophosphamide may be at least as effective as combination doxorubicin and cyclophosphamide and may be considered a reasonable alternative, particularly for those patients previously exposed to anthracyclines or those who have cardiac risks.[124] Largely indirect evidence suggests that more modern, aggressive regimens, such as those described further may provide 15% to 30% superior efficacy but generally at the cost of increased toxicity. If chemotherapy is administered to patients with HER2-positive disease, adding HER2-targeted therapy with trastuzumab should be considered for those patients with particularly high risk as described in the Stage II section. However, very few stage I cancers were included in the randomized trials of trastuzumab. Trastuzumab has additional cardiac toxicity particularly if an anthracycline regimen is used, and this commits the patient to more than 1 year of adjuvant infusional therapy. There is ongoing controversy regarding the need for adjuvant systemic therapy for patients with invasive tumors smaller than 1 cm in diameter (T1a and T1b). Traditionally accepted prognostic indicators have not been validated in this subset of patients, and large, single-institution series have suggested that 10-year disease-free survival rates for these patients can exceed 90%.[93] Considering these statistics, adjuvant systemic therapy may be considered for appropriate patients if unfavorable biology exists (Fig. 5-1).[125]

STAGE II

Many patients with stage II breast cancer with a single focus of well-circumscribed tumor and a favorable tumor-to-breast size ratio are excellent candidates for either lumpectomy (or quadrantectomy) and radiation therapy or mastectomy. Most patients with stage II disease would be candidates for breast-conserving therapy, although fewer than one-half of the patients eligible have such therapy in the United States. For other patients with stage II breast cancer who are not candidates for breast-conserving therapy, a total mastectomy represents the local-regional treatment of choice. Patients with clinically suspicious palpable lymph nodes also should have an axillary lymph node dissection (levels I and II), whereas patients with clinically node-negative disease are candidates for sentinel lymph node biopsy.[90–92] Should the sentinel lymph node be negative, no axillary dissection would be indicated. Radiation therapy is not necessary after

TABLE 5-5 Efficacy of Tamoxifen Administered for 5 Years for Estrogen Receptor (ER)-positive or Unknown Breast Cancers[122]

Age (years)	Relative Reduction in Odds (%)	
	Reduction in Recurrence	Reduction in Death
< 40	44% (±10)	39% (±12)
40–49	29% (±7)	32% (±10)
50–59	34% (±5)	24% (±7)
60–69	45% (±5)	35% (±6)
> 70	51% (±12)	37% (±15)
Overall	41% (±3); $p < 0.00001$	34% (±4); $p < 0.00001$

total mastectomy for T2, N0 lesions, and it is controversial for patients who have up to three positive axillary lymph nodes. It is generally agreed upon that locoregional radiation therapy after mastectomy is indicated for patients with four or more positive lymph nodes.[126]

The proportional benefits of adjuvant systemic therapies described in the Stage I section hold true for other stages, however the absolute benefits grow larger as the absolute risk increases. There is a favorable risk-to-benefit ratio from adjuvant systemic therapy for patients with stage II disease.[106,127] All patients with stage II, hormone receptor-positive tumors should receive appropriate endocrine therapy that includes tamoxifen for 5 years for women who are premenopausal. These women should receive an aromatase inhibitor for 5 years or tamoxifen for 2 to 5 years followed by an aromatase inhibitor for 3 to 5 years. There are three aromatase inhibitors in clinical use, two nonsteroidal (letrozole and anastrozole) and one steroidal (exemestane). There are no data demonstrating superiority of one aromatase inhibitor over another. The rationale for using up-front aromatase inhibition rather than tamoxifen in women who are postmenopausal is illustrated by the approximate 20% decreased risk of relapse seen with aromatase inhibitors in two trials in women with ER-positive disease who were postmenopausal (Fig. 5-2).[128,129] The switching strategy of tamoxifen followed by aromatase inhibition also is superior to tamoxifen alone. This has been examined in several studies using different aromatase inhibitors for 2 to 3 years after 2 to 3 years of tamoxifen or 5 years of aromatase inhibitor after 5 years of tamoxifen. The optimal endocrine strategy is not known, however aromatase inhibition either instead of, or in addition to, tamoxifen should be considered in women who are postmenopausal.[123] The safety profile of aromatase inhibitors is superior to that of tamoxifen, with fewer cases of endometrial cancer, thromboembolic events, and gynecologic symptoms, although more musculoskeletal symptoms and issues related to estrogen deprivation-induced osteoporosis, including fracture.[131] This issue is the subject of ongoing trials to define the effect of aromatase inhibitors on bone-mineral density and the risk of fractures and to determine the efficacy of bisphosphonates in the prevention or reversal of this potential complication.

KEY POINTS

- Adjuvant chemotherapy should be considered for all patients with stage II breast cancer.
- For patients with stage II hormone receptor-positive disease, adjuvant endocrine therapy should be considered in addition to chemotherapy.

In women who are premenopausal, adjuvant ovarian ablation or suppression significantly lowers the annual odds of recurrence (17%) and death (13%).[122] Permanent ovarian ablation, such as by oophorectomy, does not appear necessary to obtain this beneficial effect because 2 to 3 years of ovarian suppression with a luteinizing hormone-releasing hormone analogue also produces long-term alteration of the clinical course of hormone receptor-positive breast cancer. Ovarian suppression with a luteinizing hormone-releasing hormone analogue administered for 2 years produces results similar to older chemotherapy regimens. This relationship of ovarian ablation/suppression to chemotherapy is confounded by the fact that adjuvant chemotherapy produces a chemical ovarian ablation in most patients who are premenopausal; this effect is dependent on age and cumulative dose of the alkylating agent employed.[131,132] Although generally well tolerated, menopausal symptoms and rapid loss of bone density are associated with premature menopause, which can be reversible upon discontinuation of the agent or with treatment.[133,134] Whether adding a luteinizing hormone-releasing hormone analogue to state-of-the-art chemotherapy and tamoxifen for a woman with hormone receptor-positive breast cancer who is premenopausal provides additional reduction in the odds of recurrence and death is not yet known. Conversely, the amount of incremental benefit is obtained by the addition of state-of-the-art chemotherapy to tamoxifen and a luteinizing hormone-releasing hormone analogue also is under investigation. Until the results of randomized trials are completed, adjuvant ovarian ablation or suppression is a reasonable addition to tamoxifen for patients with hormone receptor-positive tumors who are premenopausal and who will not be receiving chemotherapy; its role in concert with chemotherapy and tamoxifen remains unclear.

All patients with stage II breast cancer should consider adjuvant polychemotherapy; for hormone receptor-positive cases, polychemotherapy should be followed by sequential endocrine therapy. For node-negative, hormone receptor-positive disease, the Recurrence Score can help identify patients at elevated residual risk despite endocrine therapy. This assay is not validated in patients with higher-risk or node-positive disease and should not be used in this situation. Overall, postoperative adjuvant combination chemotherapy has been shown to decrease the annual odds of recurrence by approximately 37% and the annual odds of death by 30% for women younger than age 50; for women older than 50, the corresponding figures are 21% and 12%, respectively (Table 5-6).[122] If the chemotherapy regimen included an anthracycline, additional reductions of 11% and 16% for odds of recurrence and death, respectively, were noted — however at the additional cost of potential cardiotoxicity. If the regimen also contained a taxane, hazard reductions of 14% for recurrence and 13% for death were observed when compared with an anthracycline-containing regimen without a taxane.[135] Although precise calculations are not possible, it is probable that compared with no adjuvant chemotherapy, a regimen that contains an anthracycline plus a taxane would reduce the annual odds of recurrence by approximately 50% for women younger than 50 and by approximately 30% for patients older than 50. Similarly, the reductions in the odds of death would be approximately 40% for patients younger than 50 and approximately 20% for patients who are older. The effects of adjuvant chemotherapy appear greater for women younger than 50 who are premenopausal, regardless of hormone receptor status. However, chemotherapy appears somewhat more effective for women with hormone receptor-negative tumors than for those with hormone receptor-positive cancer.[103]

Regarding specific regimens, shorter, or less aggressive, regimens include combination doxorubicin and cyclophosphamide, combination docetaxel and cyclophosphamide, or combination cyclophosphamide, methotrexate, and fluorouracil, as described previously. Indirect comparisons suggest that six cycles of a combined regimen, such as fluorouracil, doxorubicin, and cyclophosphamide or fluorouracil, epirubicin, and cyclophosphamide, may be superior to four cycles of doxorubicin and cyclophosphamide or to epirubicin and cyclophosphamide; however, this has not been directly tested. The addition of a taxane has demonstrated improvement in relapse-free and overall survival in most of the randomized studies; modern anthracycline/taxane regimens include: dose-dense (every 2 weeks) doxorubicin and cyclophosphamide with paclitaxel; docetaxel, doxorubicin, and fluorouracil; or fluorouracil, epirubicin, and cyclophosphamide with paclitaxel.[135] There are no data demonstrating that one taxane is superior to another. The optimal schedule of paclitaxel appears to be weekly or every 2 weeks (dose dense), but docetaxel appears as efficacious and less toxic on a schedule of every 3 weeks. Both combination docetaxel, doxorubicin, and fluorouracil and dose-dense regimens require growth factor support to maintain schedule and prevent neutropenic complications.

Primary or preoperative (neoadjuvant) chemotherapy has become more commonly used in operable breast cancer during the past 2 decades based on randomized trials that suggest no difference in relapse-free or overall survival whether chemotherapy is administered before or after surgery.[136–138] Unlike postoperative chemotherapy, neoadjuvant chemotherapy has the appeal of in vivo chemosensitivity testing and provides the prognostic relevance of the extent of residual disease after neoadjuvant chemotherapy, which can serve as a moderately accurate intermediate biomarker for outcome for clinical trials. Most patients achieve substantial reductions in tumor size; this effect is observed in both the primary tumor and regional lymph nodes. This change increases the opportunity for breast-conserving surgery for patients with large primary tumors. Between 10% and 15% of patients have a complete pathologic response in the primary tumor after three to four cycles of an anthracycline-containing regimen; 20% to 30% of patients with biopsy-proven lymph node metastases before primary chemotherapy have pathologically negative lymph nodes after neoadjuvant chemotherapy.[139] The pathologic complete response rate increases to 20% to 30% if a second cytotoxic regimen with incomplete cross-resistance is administered.[136,140] If chemotherapy is to be administered neoadjuvantly, it is reasonable to use regimens similar to what would be used adjuvantly.

Recent studies in HER2-positive disease have demonstrated, unequivocally, that the addition of trastuzumab to polychemotherapy decreases the risk of recurrence by approximately 50%.[141–143] These studies were conducted mostly in node-positive disease, however the efficacy appeared maintained across clinical subsets including high-risk node-negative cases. All of these studies have short follow-up periods and the long-term benefit may differ; however, based on this profound effect on early relapse, the addition of 1 year of adjuvant trastuzumab to chemotherapy has become standard. Three of the trials (NSABP B-31, North Central Cancer Treatment Group [NCCTG] 9831, and Breast Cancer International Research Group [BCIRG] 006) administered doxorubicin and cyclophosphamide followed by a taxane, with or without trastuzumab added to the taxane, and followed by trastuzumab alone. This approach was well tolerated except for approximately 2% to

TABLE 5-6 Efficacy of Adjuvant Polychemotherapy According to Age[122]

Age (years)	Relative Reduction in Odds (%)	
	Reduction in Recurrence	Reduction in Death
< 40	40% (±6)	29% (±7)
40–49	36% (±4)	30% (±5)
50–59	23% (±3)	15% (±4)
60–69	13% (±3)	9% (±4)
> 70	12% (±11)	13% (±12)
Overall	23% (±2); $p < 0.00001$	17% (±2); $p < 0.00001$

FIG. 5-2 Hazard ratios for anastrozole and tamoxifen, as reported in the Arimidex, Tamoxifen, Alone or in Combination (ATAC) trial.[130]

The results were obtained after a median follow-up of 48 months. The vertical line indicates equivalence between anastrozole and tamoxifen. All squares to the left of the vertical line indicate an effect that favors anastrozole; all squares to the right of the vertical line indicate an effect that favors tamoxifen; the horizontal lines that traverse each square represent the 95% confidence interval for the observation. This is likely a class effect; very similar results have been reported from from BIG 1-98, which used a similar trial design but a different aromatase inhibitor, letrozole.[129]

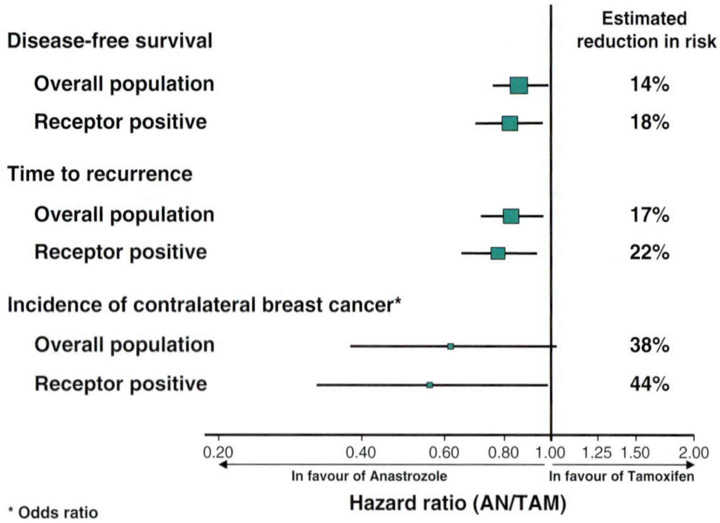

4% cardiac toxicity compared with 1% with chemotherapy alone. In BCIRG 006, a third nonanthracycline arm included docetaxel, carboplatin, and trastuzumab followed by trastuzumab alone for a total of 1 year. The patients in this third arm had less clinically significant cardiotoxicity than those who received combination chemotherapy, a taxane, and trastuzumab (1% vs. 2%, respectively). In the fourth trial, the Herceptin Adjuvant Trial (HERA), patients who were HER2 positive received any chemotherapy and were then randomly assigned to 1 year of trastuzumab or not, again with a striking improvement in outcome.[144] A second random assignment to 2 years of trastuzumab is presently immature. Therefore, 1 year of trastuzumab, administered either concurrently with chemotherapy and then after or only after chemotherapy, should be considered for patients with node-positive and high-risk, node-negative HER2-positive breast cancer.

On the basis of individual trials and the results of the Oxford overview, experts assert that the combination of chemotherapy and endocrine therapy administered sequentially represents optimal adjuvant systemic treatment for women with stage II or III breast cancer that is hormone receptor-positive. Tamoxifen added to chemotherapy and chemotherapy added to tamoxifen produces superior relapse-free and overall survival rates compared with each component used alone. For example, chemotherapy added to tamoxifen decreases the residual risk of relapse by 44% and death by 31% for women younger than 50, with far more modest benefits of 16% and 5% for older women. Randomized studies suggest that tamoxifen and chemotherapy should not be administered simultaneously; rather, chemotherapy should be completed before initiating tamoxifen.[145] Whether combinations of chemotherapy and other endocrine interventions might have adverse interactions remains to be determined. However, given that the antiproliferative effects of aromatase inhibitors also may abrogate chemotherapy effectiveness, it is reasonable to also sequence these agents after chemotherapy. Trastuzumab, at this time, should be added after anthracycline therapy; it may be given concurrent with or after taxane, and may be given concurrent with endocrine therapy.

STAGE III

Patients with stage III breast cancer can be classified into two general categories. Some have large tumors, without skin involvement or fixation to deeper tissues, which are clearly operable. Others have neoplasms that are considered inoperable because skin involvement or fixation to the underlying chest wall precludes total resection with clean margins (even after a mastectomy) or because extensive involvement of the regional lymph nodes makes the use of surgical intervention as the primary treatment futile. Patients with operable stage III breast cancer (T3, N1; some T4, N0) can be cared for in the same manner as patients with stage II breast cancer. However, primary (neoadjuvant) chemotherapy followed by surgical resection and radiation therapy is the preferred strategy.[146] Patients with inoperable stage III disease usually have primary chemotherapy using one of the more aggressive regimens detailed previously (primary hormone therapy and/or radiation therapy if the tumor is strongly steroid hormone receptor positive and there are contraindications to chemotherapy) followed by surgical resection of residual disease, postoperative systemic therapy on the basis of the characteristics of the tumor and the extent of residual disease, and radiation of the breast, chest wall, and regional lymphatic areas. Several larger, prospective randomized trials are testing the value of additional chemotherapy, both in the preoperative and postoperative setting. The results of three prospective randomized studies have shown that administering several cycles of two noncross-resistant regimens preoperatively increases the pathologic complete remission rate to 20% to 30%.[136,140,147] In the case of insufficient response to primary chemotherapy or persistently inoperable tumor, preoperative radiation

KEY POINTS

- Patients with inoperable stage III disease are usually treated with (neoadjuvant) systemic therapy, chemotherapy, or hormone therapy alone, sometimes followed by surgical resection of residual disease.
- Postoperative systemic therapy and radiation therapy are determined based on the characteristics of the tumor and on the extent of residual disease.

therapy followed by surgical resection is a reasonable alternative. These patients clearly have less-favorable prognoses with the currently available treatments, compared with patients who respond well to preoperative chemotherapy. The relationship of pathologic complete response to neoadjuvant chemotherapy and subsequent disease-free and overall survival has been demonstrated in multiple studies. Recent studies contribute that different subtypes of breast cancer respond differently to neoadjuvant chemotherapy, and, in particular, that the ER-positive subtypes have lower clinical and pathologic response rates although their long-term survival is better. This disparity between response to therapy and outcome reflects the importance of adjuvant endocrine therapy in outcome for ER-positive disease.

INFLAMMATORY BREAST CANCER

This subset of stage III disease represents the most aggressive form of breast cancer, constituting 1% to 5% of all newly diagnosed breast cancers.[148,149] It is diagnosed on the basis of a clinical triad: erythema, warmth, and edema and ridging of the skin of the breast (peau d'orange), a palpable finding on physical examination attributed to engorged dermal lymphatics. Mammography usually shows edema of the skin, especially the areola and the nipple, with architectural distortion but may not demonstrate a mass in the breast. Demonstration of dermal lymphatic invasion is ancillary evidence, but is not necessary for the diagnosis. Potential biologic markers have been studied in this variant. Most are ER negative; the data about HER2 overexpression is contradictory, with some studies showing an increased rate of overexpression, whereas others do not confirm this difference. E-cadherin expression is markedly increased and *TP53* mutations are frequent in inflammatory breast cancer, compared with noninflammatory disease. The evolution of inflammatory breast cancer is rapid; on average, fewer than 3 months elapse from the first detectable abnormality to the establishment of florid skin changes that prompt the diagnosis. Because an underlying mass is absent in more than 50% of these patients, this condition often is mistaken for a benign inflammatory or infectious condition, such as mastitis, and treated with antibiotics. Because this approach inevitably fails, a punch biopsy of skin usually provides a definitive diagnosis. Before the inclusion of systemic chemotherapy in the primary management of this disease, fewer than 5% of patients survived 5 years after surgery alone, radiation therapy alone, or a combination of the two treatment modalities. The median survival was less than 1 year, and the rapid development of multiorgan metastases was the usual clinical course. Since the introduction of primary chemotherapy into the multidisciplinary management of inflammatory breast cancer, the prognosis for this group of patients improved substantially. Most cases (60% to 90%) respond dramatically to combination chemotherapy, more than 90% of these cancers become resectable, and patients can be rendered disease free. Trimodality regimens including sequential aggressive chemotherapy using the modern regimens described previously, mastectomy, radiation therapy, and HER2-targeted and optimized endocrine therapy (for appropriate patients), result in 5-year survival rates that routinely exceed 40%. Long-term follow-up of patients treated with multidisciplinary protocols has shown 10-year progression-free survival rates of 25% or higher. Although no randomized trials have been conducted involving patients with inflammatory breast cancer, those statistics represent such a dramatic departure from the natural history following local-regional therapy only that they provide compelling evidence of therapeutic progress. Radiation therapy is considered a cornerstone of local therapy; there are indications that suggest that hyperfractionated radiation therapy may be associated with better local control rates. The role of mastectomy also is well established.

Despite improvements in both local and systemic control of locally advanced and inflammatory disease achieved with modern combined-modality treatments, many patients with this extent of disease at diagnosis still die of the disease. Therefore, multiple attempts are underway to improve the odds of eradicating micrometastases. Among those with highest promise are new drugs such as improved taxanes, vinorelbine, new endocrine agents, growth factor inhibitors, and signal transduction inhibitors.

KEY POINTS

- Inflammatory breast cancer is diagnosed on the basis of a clinical triad: erythema, warmth, and edema (peau d'orange).
- Since the introduction of multimodality management, including aggressive primary chemotherapy, radiation therapy, and surgery, the prognosis for inflammatory breast cancer has improved substantially.

MANAGEMENT OF STAGE IV DISEASE

Patients with untreated metastatic breast cancer demonstrate considerable heterogeneity in the clinical course of the disease. Some have a fulminant clinical course, with rapid development of metastases to multiple vital organs, resistance to therapy, and death within a few months after detection of the first metastasis.[150] Others have a more indolent disease course, with slow progression alternating with long periods of stability in metastasis to soft tissues or bone. Progress in our understanding of the biology of breast cancer led to the identification of distinct, biologically different subgroups that require specific therapeutic interventions for optimal results.

Metastatic disease should be considered and approached as a chronic illness. The goals of therapy are to palliate symptoms, prolong life, and, if possible, achieve a long-term, disease-free state. Recent studies suggest that survival after the diagnosis of metastatic disease has increased, most likely because of improvements in the efficacy and the number of available options for treatment.

Upon diagnosis of metastases, the extent and location of metastatic disease must be assessed and, on the basis of available clinical information, the likelihood of rapid progression, which could cause vital organ failure or other catastrophic complications, must be determined. In addition, the relevant therapeutic interventions on the basis of estrogen and progesterone receptor assays, HER2 status, and the presence of comorbid conditions must be established.[151] Patients often are classified into low-risk and high-risk groups (Fig. 5-3). People at low risk include patients who had a long disease-free interval and have limited metastatic disease, often located in soft tissues or osseous sites. Some patients with limited visceral disease also may qualify. More often than not, low-risk patients are older and postmenopausal, and the tumors are hormone receptor positive. Patients with these characteristics and positive ER or PR status are excellent candidates for hormone therapy as the first intervention for metastatic breast cancer. Patients with ER or PR receptor-negative tumors might be treated with sequential single-agent chemotherapy or trastuzumab (if HER2 positive).

Patients in the high-risk group often have the opposite characteristics: hormone receptor-negative tumors, a short (less than 24 months) disease-free interval, and visceral dissemination. High-risk patients are candidates for cytotoxic chemotherapy.

The general paradigm for treatment is as follows: patients with hormone receptor-positive breast cancer, without immediate life-threatening disease, should be offered endocrine therapy. Patients with HER2-positive breast cancer should receive trastuzumab alone or trastuzumab-containing treatments, and patients with hormone receptor-negative, HER2-negative tumors should be offered cytotoxic therapy.

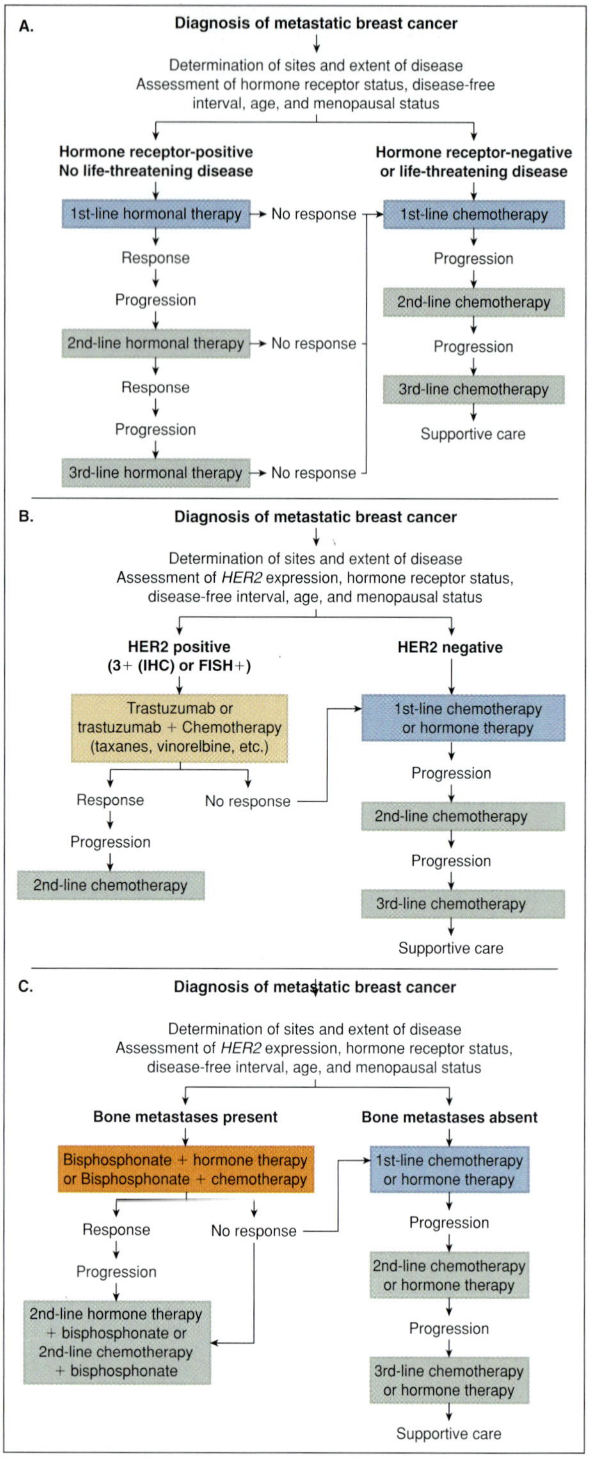

FIG. 5-3 Flow diagrams for selecting the most appropriate systemic treatment for patients with metastatic breast cancer.
A. Overall selection process based on the extent and location of metastases and the hormone receptor status. B. Selection process based on HER2 expression. C. Selection process based on the presence or absence of bone metastases.

The hormone interventions used in earlier decades have been largely replaced by modern endocrine interventions that are more specific, selective, and better tolerated (Fig. 5-4).[152]

KEY POINTS

- In general, metastatic breast cancer is incurable; however, palliation and disease control can be achieved for many years.
- Systemic therapy should take tumor phenotype into account. Patients with hormone receptor-positive disease should be considered for endocrine therapy, and those with HER2-positive disease should be considered for trastuzumab-based treatments.
- Patients with hormone receptor-negative, HER2-negative tumors should be offered chemotherapy.
- In general, single-agent chemotherapy administered sequentially is preferred over combination chemotherapy.
- Sites requiring separate consideration include bone metastases, for which bisphosphonates are routinely incorporated, and central nervous system metastases, for which local therapies, such as resection, radiosurgery, or whole-brain radiotherapy, should be considered.

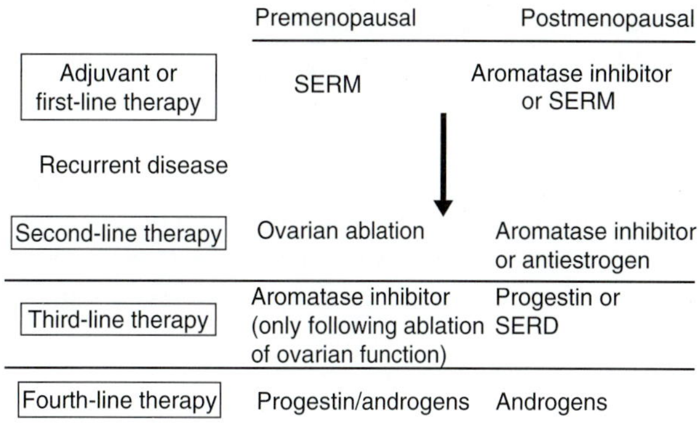

FIG. 5-4 Proposed sequence in which available endocrine agents should be used for the management of patients with breast cancer.

Patients with hormone receptor-positive breast cancer often derive benefit from multiple endocrine agents administered in sequence. Thus, although resistance to individual endocrine agents develops, the resistance can sometimes be circumvented by another endocrine agent with a different mechanism of antitumor action. Abbreviations: SERM, selective estrogen-receptor modulator; SERD, selective estrogen-receptor downregulator.

Major surgical ablative procedures to reduce the production of estrogens (adrenalectomy and hypophysectomy) are of historic interest only, having been replaced by selective aromatase inhibitors, such as anastrozole, exemestane, and letrozole for women who are postmenopausal. Although surgical oophorectomy is still a viable and effective therapeutic option, it has largely been replaced by luteinizing hormone-releasing hormone an alogues (e.g., goserelin and leuprolide), which provide an effective suppression of ovarian function, or by antiestrogens (e.g., tamoxifen, toremifene, or the pure antiestrogen fulvestrant), which compete successfully for receptor binding and, thus, interfere with estrogen-dependent signaling. Progestins, such as megestrol acetate and medroxyprogesterone acetate, also are effective and well tolerated and have displaced high-dose estrogens, androgens, and corticosteroids as third-line therapy. Assays to determine ER and PR expression serve to select patients for endocrine intervention; immunohistochemistry has been widely adopted and is considered the most reliable standard of care. Analyses of large databases have suggested that the expression of any estrogen or progesterone receptor is sufficient justification for a therapeutic trial with endocrine therapy. Conversely, tumors totally devoid of ER and PR expression are resistant to endocrine therapy. On the basis of modern, prospective randomized trials, the probability of an objective response with first-line endocrine therapy is 30% to 40% for patients with ER-positive metastatic breast cancer, although this rate may be higher in patients who were not treated with adjuvant endocrine therapy. Disease stability is achieved in an additional 20% to 30% of patients during hormone therapy, including a few minor responses.[153–155] Stable disease exceeding 6 months during endocrine therapy is associated with survival comparable to that of patients who achieve an objective response. Therefore, it is customary to express the results of endocrine therapy both in terms of objective response rate (complete and partial remissions) and clinical benefit (complete and partial remission plus stable disease exceeding 6 months).

On the basis of randomized trials, selective aromatase inhibitors have become the first-line endocrine therapy of choice for patients who are postmenopausal. These agents are not known to have antitumor activity in women with intact ovarian function so should not be used in women who are premenopausal. Another reasonable choice is a SERM, such as tamoxifen. These drugs are usually used as second-line treatment for women who are postmenopausal unless relapse occurs on an adjuvant aromatase inhibitor.

Tamoxifen and some form of ovarian suppression or ablation compete for first-line endocrine therapy of metastatic breast cancer in women who are premenopausal. Findings from a few, small randomized trials and a meta-analysis of these studies suggested that the combination of ovarian suppression or ablation with a SERM resulted in improved response rate, time to progression, and survival compared with ovarian suppression alone.[156] However, the control groups did not always receive both treatments in sequence, leaving unsettled the question of the optimal use of these two endocrine approaches.

The choice of endocrine therapy for metastatic breast cancer depends, in part, on the endocrine therapy used in the adjuvant setting and on the interval between adjuvant endocrine therapy and the detection of metastatic breast cancer. Additional endocrine agents used for second-line, third-line, and fourth-line therapies include fulvestrant, steroidal aromatase inhibitors (e.g., exemestane) if relapse occurred on nonsteroidal (e.g., letrozole and anastrozole), progestins, and synthetic androgens (e.g, fluoxymesterone). Corticosteroids have no role as primary endocrine treatment of breast cancer, although they are used as part of supportive care for patients with central nervous system (CNS) metastases, spinal cord compression, or hypercalcemia of cancer. Single-modality, sequential endocrine therapy represents the preferred approach to treatment. Combination endocrine therapies have not shown superiority over sequential use of single hormone agents in women who are postmenopausal.

As stated previously, HER2-positive disease should be treated at some point with trastuzumab-based therapy. If disease is hormone receptor positive, endocrine approaches can be used first in order to avoid committing the patient to infusional therapy. Trastuzumab as a single agent has approximately a 30% response rate in the first-line setting, and several combinations with chemotherapy have proven efficacy and safety, including paclitaxel with or without carboplatin, docetaxel, vinorelbine, capecitabine, and gemcitabine. For those patients with trastuzumab-resistant disease, the dual HER1/HER2 small molecule inhibitor lapatinib added to capecitabine provides additional benefit over capecitabine alone.[157]

Cytotoxic chemotherapy became an integral part of the management of breast cancer in the early 1970s. Several single agents produce objective responses (a 50% regression of the product of the two longest perpendicular diameters of metastatic deposits) in 20% to 60% of patients with previously untreated metastatic breast cancer. The taxanes (docetaxel, paclitaxel, and albumin-bound paclitaxel) and the anthracyclines (doxorubicin, liposomal doxorubicin, and epirubicin) are considered the most effective single agents, with platinum compounds, alkylating agents, vinca alkaloids, antimetabolites, and miscellaneous agents following. Some of the newer cytotoxic agents approved for the management of breast cancer have efficacy similar to and possibly exceeding that of doxorubicin, heretofore the most effective agent against breast cancer. Paclitaxel and docetaxel are active in previously treated patients with metastatic breast cancer, producing response rates in the 30% to 50% range for patients with anthracycline-resistant disease.[158] The activity of these agents in patients with chemotherapy-naïve metastatic breast cancer is equivalent or superior to that of the anthracyclines, and comparable to that of several older drug combinations (cyclophosphamide, methotrexate, and fluorouracil or fluorouracil, doxorubicin, and cyclophosphamide). Anthracycline and taxane combinations are somewhat more active than previously tested anthracycline-containing combinations without taxanes, producing higher overall response rates and, in some trials, longer times to disease progression. However, no survival benefit has been reported in the majority of randomized trials (Table 5-7). It should be noted that cardiac toxicity of anthracyclines is cumulative dose-related and the risk markedly increases after 350 mg/m^2; for this reason, anthracyclines for metastatic disease are often avoided for patients who received adjuvant anthracyclines. Capecitabine is active and approved for patients with anthracycline- and taxane-resistant disease.

Combination chemotherapy is associated with overall response rates ranging between 40% and 90%, whereas modern single-agent therapies produce overall response rates to first-line chemotherapy in the 20% to 50% range. Regimens that have been tested and found tolerable and superior in terms of response rate to single-agent therapy include gemcitabine added to paclitaxel, and capecitabine added to docetaxel. In general, patients with a good performance status, normal organ function, and limited extent of disease are more likely to respond than patients with the opposite characteristics. Only 15% to 20% of patients will achieve a complete remission after combination chemotherapy, and a smaller percentage after single-agent treatment. Progressive disease will develop within the subsequent 5 years for most patients who achieve a clinical complete remission, but approximately 17% of all complete remissions (fewer than 5% of all patients treated) achieved with first-line anthracycline-containing regimens last more than 10 years.[159] It is not clear that any combination chemotherapy regimen provides long-term benefit over the same drugs given in sequence, but clearly provides additional toxicity. For this reason, unless a high response rate is one of the desired objectives, single-agent sequences are preferred for patients who are candidates for chemotherapy but who are asymptomatic and have nonlife-threatening disease. In this manner, the benefit of each individual agent is used, but overlapping or additive toxicity is avoided. There are many other cytotoxic options for patients who have breast cancer that does not respond to first-line therapy and for patients in whom disease progresses after an initial response. For patients who have not been exposed to

TABLE 5-7 Some Chemotherapy Options for Metastatic Disease

- Weekly paclitaxel
- Docetaxel
- Nab (albumin-bound) paclitaxel
- Liposomal doxorubicin
- Capecitabine
- Gemcitabine
- Carboplatin
- Vinorelbine
- Weekly paclitaxel/bevacizumab
- Capecitabine/docetaxel
- Gemcitabine/paclitaxel
- Taxane/carboplatin

Most of these agents have been successfully combined with trastuzumab for HER2-postive disease.

taxanes or anthracyclines in the adjuvant setting or in first-line therapy, regimens based on these agents may be a reasonable treatment of choice. For patients who received an anthracycline-containing adjuvant chemotherapy regimen, taxanes are considered a therapeutic option for metastatic disease. For patients previously exposed to both anthracyclines and taxanes, other available choices include capecitabine, vinorelbine, and gemcitabine. In particular, capecitabine is a valuable addition to the treatment of breast cancer. Administered orally, it is well tolerated by most patients and produces lengthy responses, as well as extended periods of stability associated with excellent quality of life. Cisplatin, carboplatin, methotrexate, irinotecan, mitomycin-C, and mitoxantrone also are available. A large number of two-drug and three-drug combinations have been reported to have substantial antitumor activity, often comparable to the leading combinations. Among these, the combinations of taxanes with platinum salts have shown activity similar to other commonly used combinations, such as combination cyclophosphamide, methotrexate, and fluorouracil or the anthracycline-containing regimens. These are reasonable alternatives, but their role in the overall management of breast cancer remains to be established in controlled comparative trials.

Controversy continues regarding the optimal duration of cytotoxic therapy. Most oncologists consider it unnecessary to continue cytotoxic therapy until the onset of progressive disease. Some studies suggest that patients who received six or more cycles have a higher response rate, longer duration of response, and a better quality of life than patients treated with shorter chemotherapy programs, and that treatment until progression may be associated with longer time to progression and survival.[160] However, the likelihood of many toxicities increases with cumulative dose, and chemotherapy "holidays" or scheduled breaks from chemotherapy are reasonable. It is probable, in view of the heterogeneity of breast cancer, that there is no optimal therapy for all patients, and that different patients require different durations of treatment. Many oncologists administer chemotherapy until a maximum response is reached, and then they administer a few additional cycles before discontinuing therapy.

The combination of chemotherapy and hormone therapy for metastatic breast cancer has been evaluated. In some trials, response rates were higher and response durations may have been longer with combined therapy than with either therapy alone. However, simultaneous combinations offered no survival advantage over sequential administration of hormone therapy and chemotherapy and were often associated with additive toxicities.

Antiangiogenic strategies have been pursued in multiple tumor types with some success, including metastastic breast cancer. The most compelling evidence comes from bevacizumab studies. A randomized phase III study in pretreated patients of capecitabine with or without bevacizumab suggested a higher response rate than capecitabine alone but did not meet prespecified time to progression endpoints.[161] However, in the report from a more recent randomized phase III study of first-line therapy with weekly paclitaxel with or without bevacizumab, the time to disease progression was doubled with bevacizumab, and it was relatively well tolerated (other than causing proteinuria and hypertension). It has not been approved for this indication, but bevacizumab may become a reasonable consideration to add to chemotherapy, particularly in patients receiving weekly paclitaxel.

Multiple clinical trials have explored the contribution of high-dose chemotherapy with autologous hematopoietic stem cell support to the systemic treatment of breast cancer. Whereas uncontrolled trials suggested improved antitumor activity for high-dose chemotherapy, prospective randomized control trials have largely failed to confirm these findings.[162] Given the lack of demonstrated efficacy and the high toxicity burden, there is no demonstrated indication for high-dose chemotherapy for any stage of breast cancer.

Breast cancer commonly spreads to osseous structures; bone metastases will develop during the clinical course of the illness for up to 80% of patients with metastatic breast cancer. Bone metastases are a frequent source of morbidity and may cause substantial disability.[163] Radiation therapy is commonly employed for palliation of painful metastatic deposits or to weight-bearing bones with impending fractures. Patients with bone metastases also receive systemic treatments, including hormone therapy and chemotherapy. Several randomized clinical trials have demonstrated that the combination of bisphosphonates (clodronate, pamidronate disodium, or zoledronic acid) with chemotherapy or hormone therapy delays the appearance and reduces the severity of bone-related complications.[164] Nonetheless, the optimal time to start a bisphosphonate and the ideal duration of treatment is not clearly evident. Bisphosphonates are considered an integral part of the routine treatment of bone metastasis. Bone-seeking radionuclides (strontium-89 or samarium-159) target osseous metastases and provide temporary pain relief for some patients with systemic bone metastases. Mild but protracted myelosuppression is commonly associated with these agents, which can interfere with myelosuppressive chemotherapy. Therefore, these agents are usually reserved for third-line therapy and beyond.

The CNS is a frequent site of metastases, especially for patients with poorly differentiated, ER-negative, and HER2-positive tumors. Solitary brain metastasis is best treated with surgical removal or radiosurgery followed by radiation therapy, whereas multiple lesions usually require whole-brain radiation therapy. Leptomeningeal disease is uncommon and usually develops late in the clinical course. Despite multimodality treatment, the average survival of patients with CNS involvement is 4 to 6 months.

Pain management, prevention of chemotherapy-related nausea, dietary intervention, and psychologic support complete the multidisciplinary management of metastatic breast cancer. When used judiciously, all of these interventions contribute to the maintenance or improvement of quality of life while enhancing compliance with treatment, which, in turn, delays the progression of metastatic disease. The prudent use of hematopoietic growth factors in association with chemotherapy reduces or prevents the development of severe neutropenia and anemia, thus contributing to the prevention of complications and maintenance of quality of life.

SURVEILLANCE AFTER PRIMARY THERAPY FOR STAGES I TO III

Following completion of combined-modality treatment, it is customary to monitor the course of the disease, in part to detect and treat recurrences or metastases in a timely manner and to identify long-term sequelae of therapy. The American Society of Clinical Oncology (ASCO) recommendations are based, to a large extent, on the results of several prospective, randomized trials in which a minimalist (few tests) approach was compared with a maximalist (multiple tests and imaging studies) approach to monitoring (Table 5-8).[165] The results of these trials have not shown any survival benefit from the maximalist approach. Although recurrences were detected earlier in some cases if tests were conducted at regular intervals, there did not appear to be an effect on survival. It is likely that the lack of tangible benefit from close monitoring is the result of the noncurative nature of our treatments for metastatic disease, especially for patients already exposed to adjuvant or neoadjuvant systemic therapies.

In addition to ASCO's recommendations, it is important to emphasize other health maintenance habits: a well-balanced diet, regular exercise, and adherence to the cancer screening guidelines of proven efficacy as described by the American Cancer Society.[166] Because most breast cancers develop in women who are postmenopausal and the treatment modalities used produce estrogen deprivation, it also is important to follow the recommendations of the American College of Physicians for monitoring bone-mineral density and intervene, as appropriate, to prevent and treat osteoporosis.

GERIATRIC CONSIDERATIONS

Because half of newly diagnosed breast cancers are detected in women age 64 and older, some special considerations for the geriatric population are in order. First, the additional life expectancy of a healthy 65-year-old woman in the United States is 17.5 years, whereas that of a similarly healthy 80-year-old woman is 8.5 years. Chronologic age should not be a major determinant of treatment. Comorbid conditions increase in frequency with age and tend to be the limiting factor for survival and tolerance to treatment. Thus, the 10-year survival for patients with breast cancer with no or one comorbid condition is 97%, for patients with three comorbid conditions it is 79%, and for patients with five or more comorbidities, it is 34%. Most clinical trials, whether in the adjuvant setting or for metastatic disease, were conducted with younger women. Therefore, treatment decisions for geriatric patients are often made by extrapolation from the results in younger groups. The proportion of hormone receptor-positive tumors increases with age; thus, endocrine therapy is equally or more successful for older patients. Chemotherapy, on the other hand, tends to have greater efficacy for younger patients and for patients with ER-negative tumors. Therefore, the absolute benefit derived from chemotherapy by older patients is more modest. Older patients tend to tolerate chemotherapy well. Although myelosuppression is slightly more frequent and severe, infectious complications are no more common than for younger patients. Other toxic effects of chemotherapy tend to be more prominent for older patients, especially neurotoxicity (e.g., taxanes, platinum salts, vinca alkaloids) and renal toxicity (platinum salts, methotrexate, bisphosphonates). Cardiac dysfunction also is more frequent among older patients, which might influence the selection of drugs. In addition, older patients may have weaker social support systems, and obstacles related to transportation and lack of home caregivers are frequent. These issues are important to consider when making treatment choices.

KEY POINT

- After primary therapy for breast cancer, the cornerstones of monitoring are a complete history, physical examination, and mammography.

KEY POINT

- Chronologic age should not be a major determinant of treatment.

SIDE EFFECTS OF TREATMENT

Although clearly effective and able to produce clinical benefits, the antitumor agents used to treat patients with breast cancer can produce side effects and toxicities. Cytotoxic agents produce myelosuppression (neutropenia, thrombocytopenia, and anemia), partial or total alopecia, nausea and vomiting, oral mucositis, diarrhea, constipation, and peripheral neuropathy. Neutropenia is potentially serious because it can lead to infectious complications and death. Many of the modern adjuvant regimens, such as dose-dense doxorubicin and cyclophosphamide with paclitaxel or combination docetaxel, doxorubicin, and fluorouracil require growth factors in order to prevent infectious complications and dose delays. Another important side effect

TABLE 5-8 Recommendations of the American Society of Clinical Oncology for Follow-Up Care of Patients with Primary Breast Cancer[165]

Mode of Surveillance	Summary of Recommendations
Recommended breast cancer surveillance	
History/physical examination	Every 3 to 6 months for the first 3 years after primary therapy; every 6 to 12 months for years 4 and 5; then annually.
Patient education regarding symptoms of recurrence	Physicians should counsel patients about the symptoms of recurrence including new lumps, bone pain, chest pain, abdominal pain, dyspnea or persistent headaches. Helpful websites for patient education include www.plwc.org and www.cancer.org.
Referral for genetic counseling	Criteria include: Ashkenazi Jewish heritage; history of ovarian cancer at any age in the patient or in any first- or second-degree relatives; any first-degree relative with a history of breast cancer diagnosed before the age of 50 years; two or more first- or second-degree relatives diagnosed with breast cancer at any age; patient or relative with diagnosis of bilateral breast cancer; and history of breast cancer in a male relative.
Breast self-examination	All women should be counseled to perform monthly breast self-examination.
Mammography	First post-treatment mammogram 1 year after the initial mammogram that leads to diagnosis but no earlier than 6 months after definitive radiation therapy. Subsequent mammograms should be obtained as indicated for surveillance of abnormalities
Coordination of care	Continuity of care for patients with breast cancer is encouraged and should be performed by a physician experienced in the surveillance of patients and in breast examination, including the examination of irradiated breasts. If follow-up is transferred to a PCP, the PCP and the patient should be informed of the long-term options regarding adjuvant hormone therapy for the particular patient. This may necessitate rereferral for oncology assessment at an interval consistent with guidelines for adjuvant hormone therapy.
Pelvic examination	Regular gynecologic follow-up is recommended for all women. Patients who receive tamoxifen should be advised to report any vaginal bleeding to their physicians.
Breast cancer surveillance testing: not recommended	
Routine blood tests	CBCs and liver function tests are not recommended.
Imaging studies	Chest x-ray, bone scans, liver ultrasound, computerized tomography scans, FDG-PET scans, and breast MRI are not recommended.
Tumor markers	CA 15-3, CA 27.29, and carcinoembryonic antigen are not recommended.
FDG-PET	FDG-PET scanning is not recommended for routine breast cancer surveillance.
Breast MRI	Breast MRI is not recommended for routine breast cancer surveillance. MRI may be considered for on an individual basis in high-risk women.

Abbreviations: PCP, primary care physician; FDG-PET, [^{18}F]fluorodeoxyglucose-positron emission tomography; MRI, magnetic resonance imaging.

of chemotherapy is ovarian ablation in women who are premenopausal, with the resulting consequences of premature menopause and the development of infertility. Resumption of menses, however, can occur up to 2 years after chemotherapy. Long-term serious side effects are rare but include cardiotoxicity with anthracyclines and trastuzumab and a slight increase in the incidence of myelodysplastic syndromes and acute leukemias.[167,168] Chemotherapy-related cardiac toxicity from anthracyclines is dose-related, can be irreversible, and is associated with characteristic findings on endomyocardial biopsy. Cardiac toxicity from trastuzumab is increased in the setting of anthracycline use but is not dose-related, may be largely reversible (although this has not been definitively determined), and is not associated with characteristic pathologic findings on biopsy. Myelodysplastic syndromes and acute leukemias are of two types. The first is associated with large cumulative doses of alkylating agents; leukemias of this type develop 5 to 15 years after the initiation of chemotherapy. The second syndrome, attributed to topoisomerase II inhibitors (anthracyclines), includes myelomonocytic leukemia that develops within 2 years of initiating therapy.

Most hormone modulators can produce vasomotor instability resulting in hot flushes, irritability, and emotional problems. Other effects include mild nausea, fluid retention, and an increase in the incidence of thromboembolic phenomena. Tamoxifen has been associated with an increased risk of endometrial hyperplasia, dysplasia, and cancer, as well as the development of ovarian cysts and other benign gynecologic abnormalities.[52] Ocular toxicity also has been attributed to tamoxifen, especially when administered at high doses. Progestins cause increased appetite and weight gain, and they can occasionally cause or contribute to glucose intolerance. The third-generation selective aromatase inhibitors (anastrozole, letrozole, and exemestane) and luteinizing hormone-releasing hormone analogues (goserelin and leuprolide) also produce side effects from estrogen deprivation, including loss of bone density, increased risk of fractures, and musculoskeletal complaints.

SURVIVORSHIP

The American Cancer Society estimated in 2002 that 2.3 million women in the United States had a current or previous history of breast cancer, which illustrates the profound effect of the disease on society and the growing importance of survivorship issues.

Breast cancer survivors face several ongoing challenges. The first is physical. Long-term sequelae of breast cancer therapy can include complications of local interventions, such as postmastectomy pain syndromes, lymphedema from axillary dissection or radiation, and radiation fibrosis and cosmetic defects in the breast. Women who received chemotherapy may have complications, such as chemotherapy-induced amenorrhea, cardiac dysfunction from anthracyclines or trastuzumab, peripheral neuropathy from taxanes, or rarer and more serious complications such as myelodysplasia, or leukemia. In addition to these clinically apparent complications, it is not clear how subclinical effects from chemotherapy may interact with other comorbidities, such as diabetes, later in life. Although cognitive issues are commonly discussed in the setting of chemotherapy, patient-reported cognitive impairment does not correlate with objective findings on neurocognitive testing, and this area remains one of debate. Adjuvant hormone issues are far more common, including menopausal symptom exacerbation, such as hot flushes, vaginal dryness and atrophy, and sexual dysfunction. Hot flush amelioration may be obtained pharmacologically with agents, such as low-dose venlafaxine or gabapentin. Gynecologic issues can be difficult to manage because of the concern about use of topical estrogens in a woman if her original tumor was hormone receptor positive. These problems appear particularly prominent in women receiving aromatase inhibitors, which also cause accelerated bone loss and can cause debilitating musculoskeletal symptoms. There are an increasing armamentarium of drugs and other therapies to manage many of these long-term physical consequences of therapy; the first step is to make sure that the caregiver is aware of them and that appropriate discussions and referral to specialists is obtained.

In addition to physical issues, surviving breast cancer takes a psychologic and emotional toll on many women. Mental health scores are most affected in the first year after diagnosis, then tend to improve. Good late psychosocial function is more likely in women with fewer physical sequelae of treatment, better social support, and better relationship with their health care providers.

In addition to promoting general good health, some dietary and lifestyle interventions, such as exercise, have been associated with improved breast cancer outcome, although this requires further research. With most women surviving their breast cancer diagnosis, oncologists are challenged to find ways

KEY POINTS

- Other than an increased risk of cardiac toxicity, trastuzumab has few side effects.
- Chemotherapy will produce premature menopause, and the physician must deal with the effects of premature menopause.
- Rare long-term side effects of adjuvant chemotherapy include cardiac toxicity and acute leukemia.
- Tamoxifen can cause hot flushes, increased thromboembolic events, and endometrial cancer.
- Aromatase inhibitors are associated with bone loss problems and musculoskeletal complaints.

to personalize adjuvant therapy in order to limit unnecessary use of toxic drugs and to develop interventions and ways to provide care that will maximize long-term whole-body health.

EMERGING STRATEGIES

Many new drugs and strategies are in clinical development today. Type I topoisomerase inhibitors, novel antimetabolites, taxanes, vinca alkaloids, and other tubulin inhibitors are being tested in phase II clinical trials.

The gradual deciphering of the complex intracellular signaling pathways that modulate cell growth, differentiation, and apoptosis has led to the identification of multiple potential therapeutic targets. Given the emerging understanding of breast cancer as a group of biologically distinct diseases, it is likely that the most promising approaches will involve personalized medicine with targeting of particular weakness of an individual or group of related tumors rather than general cytotoxic approaches. Additional monoclonal antibodies targeting HER2 and other growth factors or their receptors (small molecules that target the kinase domain or other signaling steps) are under development. Attempts at genetic modification and vaccine strategies have been promising in preclinical trials and may prove fruitful in clinical trials in the future. It is expected that some of this intensive investigation will yield effective and well-tolerated anticancer drugs.

CONCLUSION

Our increased understanding of the biology, behavior, and driving-signaling pathways of breast cancer has led to the identification of specific subtypes of the disease, with distinct clinical behavior and different therapeutic requirements. Thus, for patients with hormone receptor-positive tumors, the cornerstone of treatment is endocrine therapy, supplemented by chemotherapy, radiation therapy, and symptomatic treatments. For patients with HER2-overexpressing tumors, trastuzumab is a critical part of optimal treatment, again with the addition of endocrine therapy and chemotherapy. Patients with bone metastases benefit from the inclusion of bisphosphonates in the overall treatment strategy. Much progress has been made in the treatment of breast cancer; however, there is room for improvement in the efficacy and safety and tolerance of treatments used in the management of metastatic, locally advanced, and inflammatory breast cancer.

Studies of patterns of care indicated that state-of-the-art recommendations for early diagnosis and combined-modality management are not universally applied. Guidelines developed by expert groups are not necessarily followed, leaving opportunities for improvement in the care of patients with primary and metastatic breast cancer. Evaluation of the progress achieved indicates that continued efforts at early detection and the development of more specific, more effective, and better tolerated treatments are likely to result in additional improvements in survival. Furthermore, technologic advances in such areas as genomics and proteomics, might improve selection of patients for optimal use of novel diagnostic and therapeutic interventions and further reduce the adverse reactions associated with them.

KEY POINT

- Breast cancer is biologically heterogeneous, making the need for a thoughtful and individualized approach to targeted therapy important.

REFERENCES

1. Jemal A, Siegel R, Ward E, et al. Cancer Statistics, 2006. *CA Cancer J Clin.* 2006;56(2):106–130.
2. American Cancer Society. *Cancer Facts and Figures, 2007.* Atlanta, GA: American Cancer Society; 2007.
3. Ries LAG, Melbert D, Krapcho M, et al., eds. *SEER Cancer Statistics Review, 1975–2004.* Bethesda, MD: National Cancer Institute; 2007.
4. Ravdin PM, Cronin KA, Howlader N, et al. The decrease in breast-cancer incidence in 2003 in the United States. *N Engl J Med.* 2007;356 (16):1670–1674.
5. Berry DA, Cronin KA, Plevritis SK, et al. Effect of screening and adjuvant therapy on mortality from breast cancer. *N Engl J Med.* 2005;353 (17):1784–1792.
6. Smith-Bindman R, Miglioretti DL, Lurie N, et al. Does utilization of screening mammography explain racial and ethnic differences in breast cancer? *Ann Intern Med.* 2006;144(8):541–553.
7. Carey LA, Perou CM, Livasy CA, et al. Race, breast cancer subtypes, and survival in the Carolina Breast Cancer Study. *JAMA.* 2006;295(21): 2492–2502.
8. Parkin DM, Fernandez LM. Use of statistics to assess the global burden of breast cancer. *Breast J.* 2006;12(Suppl 1):S70–S80.
9. Bray F, McCarron P, Parkin DM. The changing global patterns of female breast cancer incidence and mortality. *Breast Cancer Res.* 2004;6 (6):229–239.
10. Familial breast cancer: collaborative reanalysis of individual data from 52 epidemiological studies including 58,209 women with breast cancer and 101,986 women without the disease. *Lancet.* 2001;358(9291):1389–1399.
11. Goodwin PJ. Management of familial breast cancer risk. *Breast Cancer Res Treat.* 2000;62(1):19–33.
12. Chen JJ, Silver D, Cantor S, et al. BRCA1, BRCA2, and Rad51 operate in a common DNA damage response pathway. *Cancer Res.* 1999;59 (7 Suppl):1752s–1756s.
13. Frankish H. BRCA1 has a pivotal role in repairing DNA. *Lancet.* 2001; 357(9269):1678.
14. Le Page F, Randrianarison V, Marot D, et al. BRCA1 and BRCA2 Are Necessary for the Transcription-Coupled Repair of the Oxidative 8-Oxoguanine Lesion in Human Cells. *Cancer Res.* 2000;60(19): 5548–5552.
15. Nathanson KL, Wooster R, Weber BL. Breast cancer genetics: what we know and what we need. *Nat Med.* 2001;7(5):552–556.
16. Sorlie T, Tibshirani R, Parker J, et al. Repeated observation of breast tumor subtypes in independent gene expression data sets. *Proc Natl Acad Sci U S A.* 2003;100(14):8418–8423.
17. Bane AL, Beck JC, Bleiweiss I, et al. BRCA2 mutation-associated breast cancers exhibit a distinguishing phenotype based on morphology and molecular profiles from tissue microarrays. *Am J Surg Pathol.* 2007;31 (1):121–128.

18. Lakhani SR, Gusterson BA, Jacquemier J, et al. The pathology of familial breast cancer: histological features of cancers in families not attributable to mutations in BRCA1 or BRCA2. *Clin Cancer Res.* 2000;6(3):782–789.

19. Offit K. Are BRCA1- and BRCA2-Associated Breast Cancers Different? *J Clin Oncol.* 2000;18(21 Suppl):104s–106s.

20. Hisada M, Garber JE, Fung CY, et al. Multiple primary cancers in families with Li-Fraumeni syndrome. *J Natl Cancer Inst.* 1998;90(8):606–611.

21. Malkin D, Li FP, Strong LC, et al. Germ line p53 mutations in a familial syndrome of breast cancer, sarcomas, and other neoplasms. *Science.* 1990;250(4985):1233–1238.

22. Bignell GR, Barfoot R, Seal S, et al. Low frequency of somatic mutations in the LKB1/Peutz-Jeghers syndrome gene in sporadic breast cancer. *Cancer Res.* 1998;58(7):1384–1386.

23. Ziegler RG, Hoover RN, Pike MC, et al. Migration patterns and breast cancer risk in Asian-American women. *J Natl Cancer Inst.* 1993;85(22):1819–1827.

24. Kolonel LN, Altshuler D, Henderson BE. The multiethnic cohort study: exploring genes, lifestyle and cancer risk. *Nat Rev Cancer.* 2004;4(7):519-527.

25. Dumitrescu RG, Cotarla I. Understanding breast cancer risk—where do we stand in 2005? *J Cell Mol Med.* 2005;9(1):208–221.

26. Colditz GA, Rosner BA, Chen WY, et al. Risk factors for breast cancer according to estrogen and progesterone receptor status. *J Natl Cancer Inst.* 2004;96(3):218–228.

27. Millikan RC, Newman B, Tse CK, et al. Epidemiology of basal-like breast cancer. *Breast Cancer Res Treat.* Epub ahead of print. 2007.

28. Yang XR, Sherman ME, Rimm DL, et al. Differences in risk factors for breast cancer molecular subtypes in a population-based study. *Cancer Epidemiol Biomarkers Prev.* 2007;16(3):439–443.

29. Chen CL, Weiss NS, Newcomb P, et al. Hormone replacement therapy in relation to breast cancer. *JAMA.* 2002;287(6):734–741.

30. Ross RK, Paganini-Hill A, Wan PC, et al. Effect of hormone replacement therapy on breast cancer risk: estrogen versus estrogen plus progestin. *J Natl Cancer Inst.* 2000;92(4):328–332.

31. Rossouw JE, Anderson GL, Prentice RL, et al. Risks and benefits of estrogen plus progestin in healthy postmenopausal women: principal results From the Women's Health Initiative randomized controlled trial. *JAMA.* 2002;288(3):321–333.

32. Ballard-Barbash R, Forman MR, Kipnis V: Dietary fat, serum estrogen levels, and breast cancer risk: a multifaceted story. *J Natl Cancer Inst.* 1999;91(6):492–494.

33. Holmes MD, Hunter DJ, Colditz GA, et al. Association of dietary intake of fat and fatty acids with risk of breast cancer. *JAMA.* 1999;281(10):914–920.

34. Willett WC. Dietary fat and breast cancer. *Toxicol Sci.* 1999;52(2 Suppl):127–146.

35. Prentice RL, Caan B, Chlebowski RT, et al. Low-fat dietary pattern and risk of invasive breast cancer: the Women's Health Initiative Randomized Controlled Dietary Modification Trial. *JAMA.* 2006;295(6):629–642.

36. Mattisson I, Wirfalt E, Johansson U, et al. Intakes of plant foods, fibre and fat and risk of breast cancer—a prospective study in the Malmo Diet and Cancer cohort. *Br J Cancer.* 2004;90(1):122–127.

37. Calle EE, Rodriguez C, Walker-Thurmond K, et al. Overweight, obesity, and mortality from cancer in a prospectively studied cohort of U.S. adults. *N Engl J Med.* 2003;348(17):1625–1638.

38. Verloop J, Rookus MA, van der Kooy K, et al: Physical activity and breast cancer risk in women aged 20-54 years. *J Natl Cancer Inst.* 2000;92(2):128–135.

39. Terry PD, Goodman M. Is the association between cigarette smoking and breast cancer modified by genotype? A review of epidemiologic studies and meta-analysis. *Cancer Epidemiol Biomarkers Prev.* 2006;15(4):602–611.

40. Hartmann LC, Sellers TA, Frost MH, et al. Benign breast disease and the risk of breast cancer. *N Engl J Med.* 2005;353(3):229–237.

41. Fisher B, Costantino JP, Wickerham DL, et al. Tamoxifen for prevention of breast cancer: report of the National Surgical Adjuvant Breast and Bowel Project P-1 Study. *J Natl Cancer Inst.* 1998;90(18):1371–1388.

42. Boyd NF, Rommens JM, Vogt K, et al. Mammographic breast density as an intermediate phenotype for breast cancer. *Lancet Oncol.* 2005;6(10):798–808.

43. Claus EB, Risch N, Thompson WD. Autosomal dominant inheritance of early-onset breast cancer. Implications for risk prediction. *Cancer.* 1994;73(3):643–651.

44. Gail MH, Brinton LA, Byar DP, et al. Projecting individualized probabilities of developing breast cancer for white females who are being examined annually. *J Natl Cancer Inst.* 1989;81(24):1879–1886.

45. Gail MH, Costantino JP. Validating and improving models for projecting the absolute risk of breast cancer. *J Natl Cancer Inst.* 2001;93(5):334–335.

46. National Cancer Institute. Breast Cancer Risk Assessment Tool. http://www.cancer.gov/bcrisktool/Accessed October 17, 2007.

47. Early Breast Cancer Trialists' Collaborative Group (EBCTC). Effects of chemotherapy and hormonal therapy for early breast cancer on recurrence and 15-year survival: an overview of the randomised trials. *Lancet.* 2005;365(9472):1687–1717.

48. Cuzick J, Forbes J, Edwards R, et al. First results from the International Breast Cancer Intervention Study (IBIS-I): a randomised prevention trial. *Lancet.* 2002;360(9336):817–824.

49. Fisher B. Highlights from recent National Surgical Adjuvant Breast and Bowel Project studies in the treatment and prevention of breast cancer. *CA Cancer J Clin.* 1999;49(3):159–177.

50. Powles T, Eeles R, Ashley S, et al. Interim analysis of the incidence of breast cancer in the Royal Marsden Hospital tamoxifen randomised chemoprevention trial. *Lancet.* 1998;352(9122):98–101.

51. Veronesi U, Maisonneuve P, Costa A, et al. Prevention of breast cancer with tamoxifen: preliminary findings from the Italian randomised trial among hysterectomised women. Italian Tamoxifen Prevention Study. *Lancet.* 1998;352(9122):93–97.

52. Fisher B, Costantino JP, Wickerham DL, et al. Tamoxifen for the prevention of breast cancer: current status of the National Surgical Adjuvant Breast and Bowel Project P-1 study. *J Natl Cancer Inst.* 2005;97(9122):1652–1662.

53. Cummings SR, Eckert S, Krueger KA, et al. The effect of raloxifene on risk of breast cancer in postmenopausal women: results from the MORE randomized trial. Multiple Outcomes of Raloxifene Evaluation. *JAMA.* 1999;281(23):2189–2197.

54. Cauley JA, Norton L, Lippman ME, et al. Continued breast cancer risk reduction in postmenopausal women treated with raloxifene: 4-year results from the MORE trial. Multiple outcomes of raloxifene evaluation. *Breast Cancer Res Treat.* 2001;65(2):125–134.

55. Barrett-Connor E, Mosca L, Collins P, et al. Effects of raloxifene on cardiovascular events and breast cancer in postmenopausal women. *N Engl J Med.* 2006;355(2):125–137.

56. Vogel VG, Costantino JP, Wickerham DL, et al. Effects of tamoxifen vs raloxifene on the risk of developing invasive breast cancer and other disease outcomes: the NSABP Study of Tamoxifen and Raloxifene (STAR) P-2 trial. *JAMA.* 2006;295(23):2727–2741.

57. Cuzick J, Powles T, Veronesi U, et al. Overview of the main outcomes in breast-cancer prevention trials. *Lancet.* 2003;361(9354):296–300.

58. Gail MH, Costantino JP, Bryant J, et al. Weighing the risks and benefits of tamoxifen treatment for preventing breast cancer. *J Natl Cancer Inst.* 1999;91(21):1829–1846.

59. King MC, Wieand S, Hale K, et al. Tamoxifen and breast cancer incidence among women with inherited mutations in BRCA1 and BRCA2: National Surgical Adjuvant Breast and Bowel Project (NSABP-P1) Breast Cancer Prevention Trial. *JAMA.* 2001;286(18):2251–2256.

60. Rebbeck TR, Lynch HT, Neuhausen SL, et al. Prophylactic oophorectomy in carriers of BRCA1 or BRCA2 mutations. *N Engl J Med.* 2002;346(21):1616–1622.

61. Buzdar A, Howell A. Advances in aromatase inhibition: clinical efficacy and tolerability in the treatment of breast cancer. *Clin Cancer Res.* 2001;7(9):2620–2635.

62. Kendall A, Dowsett M. Novel concepts for the chemoprevention of breast cancer through aromatase inhibition. *Endocr Relat Cancer.* 2006;13(3):827–837.

63. Veronesi U, De Palo G, Costa A, et al. Chemoprevention of breast cancer with retinoids. *J Natl Cancer Inst Monogr.* 1992;(12):93–97.

64. Hartmann LC, Schaid DJ, Woods JE, et al. Efficacy of bilateral prophylactic mastectomy in women with a family history of breast cancer. *N Engl J Med.* 1999;340(2):77–84.

65. Hartmann LC, Sellers TA, Schaid DJ, et al. Efficacy of bilateral prophylactic mastectomy in BRCA1 and BRCA2 gene mutation carriers. *J Natl Cancer Inst.* 2001;93(21):1633–1637.

66. Meijers-Heijboer H, van Geel B, van Putten WL, et al. Breast cancer after prophylactic bilateral mastectomy in women with a BRCA1 or BRCA2 mutation. *N Engl J Med.* 2001;345(3):159–164.

67. Stoutjesdijk MJ, Boetes C, Jager GJ, et al. Magnetic resonance imaging and mammography in women with a hereditary risk of breast cancer. *J Natl Cancer Inst.* 2001;93(14):1095–1102.

68. Pierce JP, Faerber S, Wright FA, et al. A randomized trial of the effect of a plant-based dietary pattern on additional breast cancer events and survival: the Women's Healthy Eating and Living (WHEL) Study. *Control Clin Trials.* 2002;23(6):728–756.

69. Kerlikowske K. Efficacy of screening mammography among women aged 40 to 49 years and 50 to 69 years: comparison of relative and absolute benefit. *J Natl Cancer Inst Monogr.* 1997;(22):79–86.

70. Nystrom L, Andersson I, Bjurstam N, et al. Long-term effects of mammography screening: updated overview of the Swedish randomised trials. *Lancet.* 2002;359(9310):909–919.

71. Retsky M, Demicheli R, Hrushesky W. Breast cancer screening for women aged 40-49 years: screening may not be the benign process usually thought. *J Natl Cancer Inst.* 2001;93(20):1572.

72. Smith RA, Saslow D, Sawyer KA, et al. American Cancer Society guidelines for breast cancer screening: update 2003. *CA Cancer J Clin.* 2003;53(3):141–169.

73. U.S. Preventive Services Task Force. Screening for breast cancer: recommendations and rationale. *Ann Intern Med.* 2002;137(5 Part 1): 344–346.

74. Gotzsche PC, Olsen O. Is screening for breast cancer with mammography justifiable? *Lancet.* 2000;355(9198):129–134.

75. Kerlikowske K, Grady D, Barclay J, et al. Effect of age, breast density, and family history on the sensitivity of first screening mammography. *JAMA.* 1996;276(1):33–38.

76. Pisano ED, Gatsonis C, Hendrick E, et al. Diagnostic performance of digital versus film mammography for breast-cancer screening. *N Engl J Med.* 2005;353(17):1773–1783.

77. Thomas DB, Gao DL, Self SG, et al. Randomized trial of breast self-examination in Shanghai: methodology and preliminary results. *J Natl Cancer Inst.* 1997;89(5):355–365.

78. Semiglazov VF, Moiseyenko VM, Bavli JL, et al. The role of breast self-examination in early breast cancer detection (results of the 5-years USSR/WHO randomized study in Leningrad). *Eur J Epidemiol.* 1992;8(4):498–502.

79. Silverstein MJ, Lagios MD, Recht A, et al. Image-detected breast cancer: state of the art diagnosis and treatment. *J Am Coll Surg.* 2005; 201(4):586–597.

80. Tillman GF, Orel SG, Schnall MD, et al. Effect of breast magnetic resonance imaging on the clinical management of women with early-stage breast carcinoma. *J Clin Oncol.* 2002;20(16):3413–3423.

81. Saslow D, Boetes C, Burke W, et al. American Cancer Society guidelines for breast screening with MRI as an adjunct to mammography. *CA Cancer J Clin.* 2007;57(2):75–89.

82. Kriege M, Brekelmans CT, Boetes C, et al. Efficacy of MRI and mammography for breast-cancer screening in women with a familial or genetic predisposition. *N Engl J Med.* 2004;351(5):427–437.

83. Leach MO, Boggis CR, Dixon AK, et al. Screening with magnetic resonance imaging and mammography of a UK population at high familial risk of breast cancer: a prospective multicentre cohort study (MARIBS). *Lancet.* 2005;365(9473):1769–1778.

84. Lehman CD, Blume JD, Weatherall P, et al. Screening women at high risk for breast cancer with mammography and magnetic resonance imaging. *Cancer.* 2005;103(9):1898–1905.

85. Bos R, van Der Hoeven JJ, van Der Wall E, et al. Biologic correlates of (18)fluorodeoxyglucose uptake in human breast cancer measured by positron emission tomography. *J Clin Oncol.* 2002;20(2):379–387.

86. Mankoff DA, Dunnwald LK, Gralow JR, et al. Blood flow and metabolism in locally advanced breast cancer: relationship to response to therapy. *J Nucl Med.* 2002;43(4):500–509.

87. Bassett L, Winchester D, Caplan R, et al. Stereotactic core-needle biopsy of the breast: a report of the Joint Task Force of the American College of Radiology, American College of Surgeons, and College of American Pathologists. *The Breast.* 1997;47(3):317–330.

88. Langston AA, Malone KE, Thompson JD, et al. BRCA1 mutations in a population-based sample of young women with breast cancer. *N Engl J Med.* 1996;334(3):137–142.

89. Domchek SM, Weber BL. Clinical management of BRCA1 and BRCA2 mutation carriers. *Oncogene.* 2006;25(43):5825–5831.

90. Chen SL, Iddings DM, Scheri RP, et al. Lymphatic mapping and sentinel node analysis: current concepts and applications. *CA Cancer J Clin.* 2006;56(5):292–309.

91. Bonnema J, van de Velde CJ. Sentinel lymph node biopsy in breast cancer. *Ann Oncol.* 2002;13(10):1531–1537.

92. Cady B. Consensus on sentinel node biopsy. *Breast J.* 2002;8(3): 123–125.

93. Rosen PP, Groshen S, Kinne DW, et al. Factors influencing prognosis in node-negative breast carcinoma: analysis of 767 T1N0M0/T2N0M0 patients with long-term follow-up. *J Clin Oncol.* 1993;11(11):2090–2100.

94. Khan Q, Ravdin P. Data from the SEER (Surveillance, Epidemiology, and End Results) database demonstrates the validity of using routine histologic grading for prognostic assessment of patients with early breast cancer. *Breast Cancer Res Treat.* 2001;64:43.

95. Balslev I, Axelsson CK, Zedeler K, et al. The Nottingham Prognostic Index applied to 9,149 patients from the studies of the Danish Breast Cancer Cooperative Group (DBCG). *Breast Cancer Res Treat.* 1994; 32(3):281–290.

96. Haybittle JL, Blamey RW, Elston CW, et al. A prognostic index in primary breast cancer. *Br J Cancer.* 1982;45(3):361–366.

97. Keyomarsi K, Tucker SL, Buchholz TA, et al. Cyclin E and survival in patients with breast cancer. *N Engl J Med.* 2002;347(20):1566–1575.

98. Barnes DM, Gillett CE. Cyclin D1 in breast cancer. *Breast Cancer Res Treat.* 1998;52(1-3):1–15.

99. Osborne CK. Steroid hormone receptors in breast cancer management. *Breast Cancer Res Treat.* 1998;51(3):227–238.

100. Palmieri C, Cheng GJ, Saji S, et al. Estrogen receptor beta in breast cancer. *Endocr Relat Cancer.* 2002;9(1):1–13.

101. Hess KR, Pusztai L, Buzdar AU, et al. Estrogen receptors and distinct patterns of breast cancer relapse. *Breast Cancer Res Treat.* 2003;78(1):105–118.

102. Harvey JM, Clark GM, Osborne CK, et al. Estrogen receptor status by immunohistochemistry is superior to the ligand-binding assay for predicting response to adjuvant endocrine therapy in breast cancer. *J Clin Oncol.* 1999;17(5):1474–1481.

103. Berry DA, Cirrincione C, Henderson IC, et al. Estrogen-receptor status and outcomes of modern chemotherapy for patients with node-positive breast cancer. *JAMA.* 2006;295(14):1658–1667.

104. Ross JS, Fletcher JA. HER-2/neu (c-erb-B2) gene and protein in breast cancer. *Am J Clin Pathol.* 1999;112(1 Suppl 1):S53–S67.

105. Wolff AC, Hammond ME, Schwartz JN, et al. American Society of Clinical Oncology/College of American Pathologists guideline recommendations for human epidermal growth factor receptor 2 testing in breast cancer. *J Clin Oncol.* 2007;25(1):118–145.

106. Goldhirsch A, Glick JH, Gelber RD, et al. Meeting highlights: international expert consensus on the primary therapy of early breast cancer 2005. *Ann Oncol.* 2005;16(10):1569–1583.

107. Olivotto IA, Bajdik CD, Ravdin PM, et al. Population-based validation of the prognostic model ADJUVANT! for early breast cancer. *J Clin Oncol.* 2005;23(12):2716–2725.

108. Perou CM, Sorlie T, Eisen MB, et al. Molecular portraits of human breast tumours. *Nature.* 2000;406(6797):747–752.

109. Buyse M, Loi S, van't Veer L, et al. Validation and clinical utility of a 70-gene prognostic signature for women with node-negative breast cancer. *J Natl Cancer Inst.* 2006;98(17):1183–1192.

110. Foekens JA, Atkins D, Zhang Y, et al. Multicenter validation of a gene expression-based prognostic signature in lymph node-negative primary breast cancer. *J Clin Oncol.* 2006;24(11):1665–1671.

111. Paik S, Shak S, Tang G, et al. A multigene assay to predict recurrence of tamoxifen-treated, node-negative breast cancer. *N Engl J Med.*2004;351 (27): 2817–2826.

112. Fan C, Oh DS, Wessels L, et al. Concordance among gene-expression-based predictors for breast cancer. *N Engl J Med.* 2006;355(6):560–569.

113. *AJCC Cancer Staging Handbook*, 6th ed. New York, NY: Springer Publishing Company; 2002.

114. Carlson RW, Brown E, Burstein HJ, et al. NCCN Task Force Report: Adjuvant Therapy for Breast Cancer. *J Natl Compr Canc Netw.* 2006;4(Suppl 1):S1–S26.

115. Schwartz GF, Solin LJ, Olivotto IA, et al. Consensus Conference on the Treatment of In Situ Ductal Carcinoma of the Breast, April 22-25, 1999. *Cancer.* 2000;88(4):946–954.

116. Fisher B, Dignam J, Wolmark N, et al. Tamoxifen in treatment of intraductal breast cancer: National Surgical Adjuvant Breast and Bowel Project B-24 randomised controlled trial. *Lancet.* 1999;353(9169):1993–2000.

117. NIH consensus conference. Treatment of early-stage breast cancer. *JAMA.* 1991;265(3):391–395.

118. Du X, Freeman DH Jr, Syblik DA. What drove changes in the use of breast conserving surgery since the early 1980s? The role of the clinical trial, celebrity action and an NIH consensus statement. *Breast Cancer Res Treat.* 2000;62(1):71–79.

119. Legorreta AP, Liu X, Parker RG. Examining the use of breast-conserving treatment for women with breast cancer in a managed care environment. *Am J Clin Oncol.* 2000;23(5):438–441.

120. Morrow M, White J, Moughan J, et al. Factors predicting the use of breast-conserving therapy in stage I and II breast carcinoma. *J Clin Oncol.* 2001;19(8):2254–2262.

121. Hughes KS, Schnaper LA, Berry D, et al. Lumpectomy plus tamoxifen with or without irradiation in women 70 years of age or older with early breast cancer. *N Engl J Med.* 2004;351(10):971–977.

122. Early Breast Cancer Trialsists' Collaborative Group. Effects of chemotherapy and hormonal therapy for early breast cancer on recurrence and 15-year survival: an overview of the randomised trials. *Lancet.* 2005;365(9472):1687–1717.

123. Winer EP, Hudis C, Burstein HJ, et al. American Society of Clinical Oncology technology assessment on the use of aromatase inhibitors as adjuvant therapy for postmenopausal women with hormone receptor-positive breast cancer: status report 2004. *J Clin Oncol.* 2005;23(3):619–629.

124. Jones SE, Savin MA, Holmes FA, et al. Final analysis: TC (docetaxel/cyclophosphamide, 4 cycles) has a superior disease-free survival compared to standard AC (doxorubicin/cyclophosphamide) in 1016 women with early stage breast cancer. *Breast Cancer Res Treat.* 2005;94:40a.

125. Hanrahan EO, Valero V, Gonzalez-Angulo AM, et al. Prognosis and management of patients with node-negative invasive breast carcinoma that is 1 cm or smaller in size (stage 1; T1a,bN0M0): a review of the literature. *J Clin Oncol.* 2006;24(13):2113–2122.

126. Recht A, Edge SB, Solin LJ, et al. Postmastectomy radiotherapy: clinical practice guidelines of the American Society of Clinical Oncology. *J Clin Oncol.* 2001;19(5):1539–1569.

127. Eifel P, Axelson JA, Costa J, et al. National Institutes of Health Consensus Development Conference Statement: adjuvant therapy for breast cancer, November 1-3, 2000. *J Natl Cancer Inst.* 2001;93(13):979–989.

128. Howell A, Cuzick J, Baum M, et al. Results of the ATAC (Arimidex, Tamoxifen, Alone or in Combination) trial after completion of 5 years' adjuvant treatment for breast cancer. *Lancet.* 2005;365(9453):60–62.

129. Thurlimann B, Keshaviah A, Coates AS, et al. A comparison of letrozole and tamoxifen in postmenopausal women with early breast cancer. *N Engl J Med.* 2005;353(26):2747–2757.

130. Buzdar A, Howell A, Cuzick J, et al. Comprehensive side-effect profile of anastrozole and tamoxifen as adjuvant treatment for early-stage breast cancer: long-term safety analysis of the ATAC trial. *Lancet Oncol.* 2006;7(8):633–643.

131. Del Mastro L, Venturini M, Sertoli MR, et al. Amenorrhea induced by adjuvant chemotherapy in early breast cancer patients: prognostic role and clinical implications. *Breast Cancer Res Treat.* 1997;43(2):183–190.

132. Hortobagyi GN, Buzdar AU, Marcus CE, et al. Immediate and long-term toxicity of adjuvant chemotherapy regimens containing doxorubicin in trials at M.D. Anderson Hospital and Tumor Institute. *NCI Monogr.* 1986;(1):105–109.

133. Russell RG, Rogers MJ. Biphosphonates: from the laboratory to the clinic and back again. *Bone.* 1999;25(1):97–106.

134. Shapiro CL, Manola J, Leboff M. Ovarian failure after adjuvant chemotherapy is associated with rapid bone loss in women with early-stage breast cancer. *J Clin Oncol.* 2001;19(14):3306–3311.

135. Bria E, Nistico C, Cuppone F, et al. Benefit of taxanes as adjuvant chemotherapy for early breast cancer: pooled analysis of 15,500 patients. *Cancer.* 2006;106(11):2337–2244.

136. Bear HD, Anderson S, Smith RE, et al. Sequential preoperative or postoperative docetaxel added to preoperative doxorubicin plus cyclophosphamide for operable breast cancer:National Surgical Adjuvant Breast and Bowel Project Protocol B-27. *J Clin Oncol.* 2006;24(13):2019–2027.

137. Fisher B, Bryant J, Wolmark N, et al. Effect of preoperative chemotherapy on the outcome of women with operable breast cancer. *J Clin Oncol.* 1998;16(8):2672–2685.

138. van der Hage JA, van de Velde CJ, Julien JP, et al. Preoperative chemotherapy in primary operable breast cancer: results from the European Organization for Research and Treatment of Cancer trial 10902. *J Clin Oncol.* 2001;19(22):4224–4237.

139. Kuerer HM, Sahin AA, Hunt KK, et al. Incidence and impact of documented eradication of breast cancer axillary lymph node metastases before surgery in patients treated with neoadjuvant chemotherapy. *Ann Surg.* 1999;230(1):72–78.

140. Smith IC, Heys SD, Hutcheon AW, et al. Neoadjuvant chemotherapy in breast cancer: significantly enhanced response with docetaxel. *J Clin Oncol.* 2002;20(6):1456–1466.

141. Piccart-Gebhart MJ, Procter M, Leyland-Jones B, et al. Trastuzumab after adjuvant chemotherapy in HER2-positive breast cancer. *N Engl J Med.* 2005;353(16):1659–1672.

142. Romond EH, Perez EA, Bryant J, et al. Trastuzumab plus adjuvant chemotherapy for operable HER2-positive breast cancer. *N Engl J Med.* 2005;353(16):1673–1684.

143. Slamon DJ, Romond EH, Perez EA. Advances in adjuvant therapy for breast cancer. *Clin Adv Hematol Oncol.* 2006;4(3):suppl 1, 4–9.

144. Herceptin Adjuvant Trial. http://www.heratrial.com. Accessed October 17, 2007.

145. Albain KS, Green SJ, Ravdin PM, et al. Adjuvant chemohormonal therapy for primary breast cancer should be sesquential instead of concurrent: initial results from Intergroup Trial 0100 (SWOG-8814). *Proc Am Soc Clin Oncol.* 2002;21:abstract 37.

146. Giordano SH. Update on locally advanced breast cancer. *Oncologist.* 2003;8(6):521–530.

147. Gianni L, Baselga J, Eiermann W, et al. Feasibility and tolerability of sequential doxorubicin/paclitaxel followed by cyclophosphamide, methotrexate, and fluorouracil and its effects on tumor response as preoperative therapy. *Clin Cancer Res.* 2005;11(24 Pt 1):8715–8721.

148. Cristofanilli M, Buzdar AU, Hortobagyi GN. Update on the management of inflammatory breast cancer. *Oncologist.* 2003;8(2):141–148.

149. Giordano SH, Hortobagyi GN. Inflammatory breast cancer: clinical progress and the main problems that must be addressed. *Breast Cancer Res.* 2003;5(6):284–288.

150. Hortobagyi GN, Smith TL, Legha SS, et al. Multivariate analysis of prognostic factors in metastatic breast cancer. *J Clin Oncol.* 1983;1(12):776–786.

151. Cristofanilli M, Hortobagyi GN. New horizons in treating metastatic disease. *Clin Breast Cancer.* 2001;1(4):276–287.

152. Pritchard KI. Endocrine therapy for breast cancer. *Oncology* (Williston Park). 2000;14(4):483–492.

153. Bonneterre J, Buzdar A, Nabholtz JM, et al. Anastrozole is superior to tamoxifen as first-line therapy in hormone receptor positive advanced breast carcinoma. *Cancer.* 2001;92(9):2247–2258.

154. Bonneterre J, Thurlimann B, Robertson JF, et al. Anastrozole versus tamoxifen as first-line therapy for advanced breast cancer in 668 postmenopausal women: results of the Tamoxifen or Arimidex Randomized Group Efficacy and Tolerability study. *J Clin Oncol.* 2000;18(22):3748–3757.

155. Mouridsen H, Gershanovich M, Sun Y, et al. Superior efficacy of letrozole versus tamoxifen as first-line therapy for postmenopausal women with advanced breast cancer: results of a phase III study of the International Letrozole Breast Cancer Group. *J Clin Oncol.* 2001;19(13):2596–2606.

156. Klijn JG, Blamey RW, Boccardo F, et al. Combined tamoxifen and luteinizing hormone-releasing hormone (LHRH) agonist versus LHRH agonist alone in premenopausal advanced breast cancer: a meta-analysis of four randomized trials. *J Clin Oncol.* 2001;19(2):343–353.

157. Geyer CE, Forster J, Lindquist D, et al. Lapatinib plus capecitabine for HER2-positive advanced breast cancer. *N Engl J Med.* 2006;355(26):2733–2743.

158. Crown J, O'Leary M. The taxanes: an update. *Lancet.* 2000;355(9210):1176–1178.

159. Greenberg PA, Hortobagyi GN, Smith TL, et al. Long-term follow-up of patients with complete remission following combination chemotherapy for metastatic breast cancer. *J Clin Oncol.* 1996;14(8):2197–2205.

160. Stockler M, Wilcken NR, Ghersi D, et al. Systematic reviews of chemotherapy and endocrine therapy in metastatic breast cancer. *Cancer Treat Rev.* 2000;26(3):151–168.

161. Miller KD, Chap LI, Holmes FA, et al. Randomized phase III trial of capecitabine compared with bevacizumab plus capecitabine in patients with previously treated metastatic breast cancer. *J Clin Oncol.* 2005;23(4):792–799.

162. Hortobagyi GN. High-dose chemotherapy for primary breast cancer: facts versus anecdotes. *J Clin Oncol.* 1999;17(11 Suppl):25–29.

163. Lipton A. Management of bone metastases in breast cancer. *Curr Treat Options Oncol.* 2005;6(2):161–171.

164. Hillner BE, Ingle JN, Berenson JR, et al. American Society of Clinical Oncology guideline on the role of bisphosphonates in breast cancer. American Society of Clinical Oncology Bisphosphonates Expert Panel. *J Clin Oncol.* 2000;18(6):1378–1391.

165. Khatcheressian JL, Wolff AC, Smith TJ, et al. American Society of Clinical Oncology 2006 update of the breast cancer follow-up and management guidelines in the adjuvant setting. *J Clin Oncol.* 2006;24(31):5091–5097.

166. Smith RA, Cokkinides V, Eyre HJ. American Cancer Society guidelines for the early detection of cancer, 2003. *CA Cancer J Clin.* 2003;53(1):27–43.

167. Diamandidou E, Buzdar AU, Smith TL, et al. Treatment-related leukemia in breast cancer patients treated with fluorouracil-doxorubicin-cyclophosphamide combination adjuvant chemotherapy: the University of Texas M.D. Anderson Cancer Center experience. *J Clin Oncol.* 1996;14(10):2722–2730.

168. Pagano L, Pulsoni A, Mele L, et al. Acute myeloid leukemia in patients previously diagnosed with breast cancer: experience of the GIMEMA group. *Ann Oncol.* 2001;12(2):203–207.

6

LUNG CANCER

Joan H. Schiller, MD

LEARNING OBJECTIVES

After reviewing this chapter, the reader should be able to

- Recognize and classify lung cancer histology, clinical presentation, course, and prognosis
- Recommend appropriate strategies for risk reduction, prevention, and screening for lung cancer
- Identify important areas of the biology of lung cancer that may become targets for future treatment, and apply understanding of tumor biology and lung cancer genetics to the evaluation of clinical trial data
- Differentiate between small cell and non-small cell lung cancer and their respective natural histories, diagnoses, and treatments
- Preoperatively evaluate patients with lung cancer
- Incorporate both invasive and noninvasive techniques where appropriate and when indicated to stage lung cancer most effectively
- Explain to patients what they can expect from treatment for small cell and non-small cell lung cancer
- Use appropriate methods to palliate the symptoms of lung cancer, and manage lung cancer-associated paraneoplastic syndromes
- Outline the biology, natural history, and treatment of thymoma and mesothelioma

An estimated 213,000 new cases of lung cancer were expected in 2007, leading to approximately 162,000 deaths.[1] Although lung cancer accounts for approximately 13% of all cancer diagnoses, it is responsible for almost 28% of all cancer deaths. Thus, unlike breast, colon, and prostate cancers, most patients (more than 85%) who are diagnosed with lung cancer will die of the disease. Lung cancer is the leading cause of cancer deaths for both men and women.[2] More women die each year of lung cancer than of breast, cervical, and uterine cancers combined; more men die annually of lung cancer than of colorectal and prostate cancers combined. Indeed, nearly twice as many women in the United States die from lung cancer than from breast cancer. The incidence and death rates from lung cancer have been decreasing for men, although these rates continue to rise for women, presumably because of changes in cigarette smoking patterns.

The major cause of lung cancer is smoking. Numerous epidemiologic and murine studies, as well as in vitro data, have tied the present pandemic of lung cancer to the carcinogenic effects of nicotine. Some data suggest that women may be more susceptible to cigarette smoke than men, although these data are not conclusive.[2] Hypotheses include differences in the rates of carcinogen detoxification and the presence of the estrogen receptor beta in lung cancer cells.

The incidence of lung cancer, although declining for both white and black men, is approximately 50% higher for black men. Race-related variances in lung cancer, however, are complicated by differences in socioeconomic status, which are associated with disparities in smoking rates, types of cigarettes smoked, and exposures to inhaled agents in the workplace.

In the United States, the most common form of lung cancer was squamous cell cancer until approximately 1987, when it was supplanted by adenocarcinoma. Small cell lung cancer once accounted for approximately 20% of all lung cancers; its incidence appears to be declining, whereas the incidence of bronchioalveolar cancer, a subtype of adenocarcinoma found in both smokers and nonsmokers, is rising. Changing trends in cigarette composition and consequent changes in the types of carcinogens inhaled may be responsible for these patterns.

ETIOLOGY

Cigarette smoking is the most common cause of lung cancer and is responsible for approximately 85% to 90% of all cases. Other risk factors include occupational or environmental substances such as arsenic, chromium or nickel, radon, air pollution, radiation exposure, and environmental tobacco smoke.

The risk of lung cancer among cigarette smokers increases with the number of cigarettes smoked and the duration of smoking history, the latter of which is a stronger risk factor than the number of cigarettes smoked per day. This finding has a considerable implication for the many teenagers who start smoking. A tripling of the number of cigarettes smoked per day is estimated to triple the risk, whereas a tripling of the duration of smoking is estimated to increase the risk 100-fold.[3] The risk of lung cancer decreases with smoking cessation and approaches that of the nonsmoking population after 10 to 15 years of abstinence, although one study in women reported that even after 30 years, the risk was not as low as the nonsmoking population.[4] It is estimated that approximately half of all lung cancers in the United States occur in former smokers. Passive smoking also is a risk factor; the risk of developing lung cancer for nonsmoking spouses of cigarette smokers is approximately 20% to 30% higher than the risk for nonsmoking spouses of nonsmokers.[3] Approximately 25% of lung cancer cases among people who never smoked are caused by exposure to environmental tobacco smoke.[3]

Cigarette smoke contains thousands of constituents, many of which are carcinogenic. Two of the major classes of nicotine-related inhaled carcinogens include the polycyclic aromatic hydrocarbons and N-nitrosamines, which are metabolized to nitrosamine ketone and N'-nitrosonornicotine. Both compounds are activated by the p450 enzyme system and exert carcinogenic effects through the formation of DNA adducts. The distribution of benzo(a)pyrene diolepoxide adducts along the exons of the *TP53* gene occurs preferentially in codons 157, 248, and 273, which are the same mutational "hotspots" of *TP53.* Nitrosamine ketone has been postulated as one factor that leads to the increased incidence of adenocarcinomas, because it predominantly induces these tumors in mice.[3]

Smoking causes each of the four major subtypes of lung cancer, although the dose-response relationship is steepest with small cell lung cancer. Indeed, small cell lung cancer is a disease that is almost exclusively found in smokers. Although bronchioalveolar cancer is more likely to develop in nonsmokers than the other subtypes of lung cancer, smoking is still the major risk factor for this form of the disease.

Cigar smoking also is associated with an increased risk of lung cancer, although the risk is not as high as with cigarette smoking, most likely because cigar smokers do not inhale as much as cigarette smokers. Similarly, risks related to pipe smoking also are lower because of differences in smoking frequency and in depth of inhalation. Light cigarettes provide no benefit compared with other cigarettes; the lower tar and nicotine numbers on light cigarette packs and in advertisements are misleading because the low tar and nicotine levels recorded on smoking machines are artificial.

KEY POINTS

- Lung cancer is the most common cause of cancer-related deaths in the United States for both men and women, and most patients (more than 85%) will die of the disease.
- The epidemiology of lung cancer in the United States is changing somewhat, with a slight decrease in the incidence among men. There also is a decrease in large cell and small cell histologic subtypes, and an increase in adenocarcinomas for both men and women.

KEY POINTS

- Most cases of lung cancer (85% to 90%) are caused by carcinogens in tobacco smoke; a small percentage of cases are caused by passive smoking or exposure to radon, radiation, or other chemicals.
- Host differences may account for different susceptibilities to lung cancer.
- There is no role for beta-carotene, vitamin A, or any of their derivatives for the chemoprevention of lung cancer.

Radon is a naturally occurring, chemically inert gas that is a decay product of uranium. The relative risk of lung cancer is increased for underground miners who are exposed to high levels of radon. For underground miners who smoke, the risk may exceed 10 times the risk for a nonsmoking miner. The relationship between indoor residential radon exposure and lung cancer risk is less defined, although it is estimated that up to 10% of lung cancers may be caused by exposure to residential radon.

Asbestos and smoking are independent causes of lung cancer, but together they appear to act synergistically to increase the risk. For example, the relative risk of lung cancer for a nonsmoker exposed to asbestos is approximately 5, whereas the risk ratio ranges from 50 to 100 for smokers exposed to asbestos. The incidence peaks 25 to 35 years after exposure.

High doses of radiation also have been associated with an increased risk of lung cancer. For example, an increased risk has been observed for patients with breast cancer, as well as for long-term survivors of Hodgkin's disease and non-Hodgkin's lymphomas, particularly if patients continue to smoke after completing radiation therapy.

HOST FACTORS

Genetic susceptibility to lung cancer has been postulated based on the fact that cigarette smoking causes lung cancer in only a minority of people who smoke. Epidemiologic studies have shown that a family history of lung cancer is a predictor of increased risk, and familial aggregation of lung cancer has been found. Because many carcinogens in tobacco smoke are metabolized by the p450 cytochrome system, such as the polycyclic aromatic hydrocarbons, differences in subtypes or polymorphisms of these enzymes have been proposed as one mechanism of lung cancer risk. Some studies have implicated particular polymorphisms in lung cancer risk. Other enzymes that may increase risk for some individuals include differences in glutathione S-transferase, an enzyme that detoxifies reactive metabolites of polycyclic aromatic hydrocarbons, and enzymes that modulate DNA repair capacity.

Additional factors associated with increased risk include previous lung damage, such as chronic obstructive pulmonary disease, and fibrotic disorders that restrict lung capacity, such as pneumoconiosis. Diets deficient in vitamins A and C and beta-carotene intake also have been associated with increased risk, whereas fruit and vegetable consumption may be weakly protective.

Preclinical evidence suggested that higher dietary intake of retinol is associated with a decreased risk of lung cancer. Based on this evidence, three double-blind placebo-controlled chemoprevention trials were conducted involving beta-carotene, vitamin A, or one of their derivatives. A protective effect against lung cancer was not observed in any of the studies. Rather, beta-carotene supplementation was associated with an increased risk of lung cancer among high-risk populations of heavy smokers in two of the three trials.[5–7]

Familial aggregation of lung cancer has led to the hypothesis that there is a genetic susceptibility for lung cancer.[8] This may be related to inherited differences in carcinogen metabolism and activation and also to DNA repair capacity. For example, leukocyte DNA adducts were associated with a risk of lung cancer, with an odds ratio (OR) of 1.86 (95% CI; 0.88, 3.93), particularly for neversmokers (OR = 4.04; 95% CI; 1.06, 15.42).[9] Germ-line polymorphisms in genes with products that activate (cytochrome P450 1A1 [*CYP1A1*]) and detoxify (glutathione S-transferases M1 [*GSTM1*] as well as T1 [*GSTT1*]) chemical carcinogens found in tobacco smoke have been associated with a substantially greater risk of lung cancer from environmental tobacco smoke when compared with individuals who were heterozygous or homozygous carriers of the wild-type *GSTM1* allele.[10]

PATHOLOGY

More than 95% of lung cancers consist of one of the four major histologic types: squamous (or epidermoid), adenocarcinoma, large cell, or small cell. Small cell lung cancer has scant cytoplasm, small hyperchromatic nuclei with fine chromatin pattern, and indistinct nucleoli with diffuse sheets of cells, whereas non-small cell lung cancer has abundant cytoplasm, pleomorphic nuclei with coarse chromatin pattern, prominent nucleoli, and glandular or squamous architecture. Other subtypes, which are rare and therefore less well studied, include carcinoid, large cell cancer with neuroendocrine features and large cell neuroendocrine cancer.[11] Extremely rare primary tumors in the lung include sarcomas, cancers with sarcomatoid or sarcomatous elements (e.g., giant cell cancer, carcinosarcoma, and pulmonary blastoma), and cancers of salivary gland type (e.g., mucoepidermoid cancer and adenoid cystic cancer).

Adenocarcinoma, large cell cancer, and squamous cell cancer are collectively known as non-small cell cancer because of their differences in sensitivity to chemotherapy and radiation therapy when compared with small cell cancer, which is described in detail further in the chapter. Other clinical differences between small cell cancer and non-small cell cancer include the more rapid clinical course of small cell lung cancer, as well enhanced association of small cell lung cancer with paraneoplastic syndromes and neuroendocrine features on pathologic examination. Bronchioalveolar carcinoma (discussed in the following section) is a subtype of adenocarcinoma that has received considerable attention because of its tendency to occur in women and in neversmokers.

PREINVASIVE LESIONS

Squamous Dysplasia

Squamous dysplasia may be mild, moderate, or severe, depending on the severity of the atypia and the thickness of the abnormality within the bronchial epithelium. There is

KEY POINTS

- Preinvasive lung cancer lesions include squamous dysplasia and atypical adenomatous hyperplasia.
- Unlike other lung cancers, it occurs more commonly in neversmokers, and it is seen in men and women with the same frequency.
- Pulmonary neuroendocrine tumors represent a spectrum of neoplasms characterized by the presence of neurosecretory granules on electron microscopic evaluation.

increasing interest in using squamous dysplasia as an indicator of high risk when identifying patients for participation in chemoprevention studies.

Atypical Adenomatous Hyperplasia

Atypical adenomatous hyperplasia is considered a precursor to adenocarcinoma and is usually identified incidentally, often at the time of resection. The lesions are typically small (a few millimeters) and consist of discrete but ill-defined bronchioalveolar proliferation in which the alveoli are lined by monotonous, slightly atypical cuboidal to low-columnar epithelial cells. Their prognostic significance is unclear.

NON-SMALL CELL LUNG CANCER

Although the natural history of the subtypes of non-small cell lung cancer differs somewhat, when assessed on a stage-by-stage basis, histologic subtype is not a significant prognostic indicator.

Adenocarcinoma

Adenocarcinoma is the most common histologic subtype in the United States and appears to be on the rise, although the reason for this is unknown. It accounts for more than 50% of all lung cancers, has been associated with scarring, is more likely to be peripherally located than squamous cell or small cell cancer, and tends to metastasize frequently. It consists of four subtypes: acinar, papillary, bronchioalveolar, and solid with mucous formation.

Bronchioalveolar cancer is defined as an adenocarcinoma of the lung that grows in a lepidic fashion along the alveolar septae. In the 1999 World Health Organization/-International Association for the Study of Lung Cancer (WHO/IASLC) classification, the lack of invasive growth was added as an essential criterion because data suggested that surgical resection might cure disease for such patients. More than 50% of these tumors are associated with focal scars, and the tumor often grows around the edge of the scar. Histologically, pure bronchioalveolar cancer is rare; more common is adenocarcinoma, mixed subtype, with bronchioalveolar features. The tumor typically presents in one of two forms: mucinous and nonmucinous. Mucin-producing tumors are more common and tend to be multicentric, whereas nonmucinous-producing tumors tend to be solitary. A similar disease, which is caused by a retrovirus, is found in sheep; however, no viral etiology in humans has been discovered. Whereas the other histologic subtypes are predominant in men, bronchioalveolar cancer occurs in men and women in a ratio of one to one. In addition, this form of lung cancer develops in nonsmokers more than the other subtypes. Although the prognosis is excellent for patients with small, solitary nonmucinous tumors, the prognosis for patients with advanced bronchioalveolar cancer is comparable to those with other lung adenocarcinomas. However, the disease is more commonly associated with mutations in the epidermal growth factor receptor (EGFR), and thus is more responsive to EGFR tyrosine kinase inhibitors. In addition, small lesions discovered on screening computerized tomography (CT) scans, which are commonly found to have a "ground glass" histology, are often bronchioalveolar carcinomas.

Squamous Cell Cancer

Squamous cell cancers account for approximately 25% of all non-small cell lung cancers. The lesions tend to be located centrally and are more likely to cavitate than other histologic types. Squamous cell cancers, which most often arise in segmental bronchi and involve lobar and main-stem bronchi by extension, are recognized by the histologic features of intercellular bridging, squamous pearl formation, and individual cell keratizination.

Large Cell Cancer

Large cell cancers account for approximately 10% of all lung cancers, and the incidence is declining. These tumors are typically poorly differentiated and are composed of large cells with abundant cytoplasm and large nucleoli.

SMALL CELL LUNG CANCER

In the 1999 WHO/IASLC classification, small cell cancer is divided into two subtypes: so-called pure small cell lung cancer and combined histology, the latter of which consists of elements of both non-small cell and small cell lung cancers. Histologically, the tumor is characterized by small cells with scant cytoplasm, finely granular nuclear chromatin, and absent or inconspicuous nucleoli. Nuclear molding and smearing of the nuclear chromatin may be present owing to crush artifact. Mitotic figures are common and necrosis can be extensive. By electron microscopy, the cells may appear to have neuroendocrine granules. Clinically, these tumors tend to be centrally located, are often found submucosally, and are more commonly associated with paraneoplastic syndromes. In addition, because of the rapid growth and proliferation of these tumors, the clinical course tends to be more rapid. Small cell lung cancers also are more responsive to both chemotherapy and radiation therapy, although resistance usually develops.

PULMONARY NEUROENDOCRINE TUMORS

The normal lung contains neuroendocrine cells, although their significance is unclear. Neuroendocrine lung tumors represent a spectrum of pathologic entities, including typical carcinoid, atypical carcinoid, and large cell neuroendocrine cancer. Small cell lung cancer and large cell neuroendocrine cancer are high-grade neuroendocrine tumors, whereas typical carcinoid and atypical carcinoid are low and intermediate grade. Neurosecretory granules, particularly chromogranin A and synaptophism, are often seen by electron microscopy. Approximately 20% to 40% of patients with both typical and atypical carcinoids are nonsmokers, whereas virtually all patients with small cell lung cancer and large cell neuroendocrine cancer are cigarette smokers.

Carcinoid Tumors

Carcinoid tumors are low-grade malignant neoplasms of neuroendocrine cells, which are divided into typical and atypical types, with the latter possessing more malignant histologic and clinical features. Surgery is the primary treatment for typical carcinoid tumors. The prognosis is excellent for patients with typical carcinoids.

Compared with typical carcinoids, atypical carcinoids tend to be larger, have a greater number of mitoses, and are associated with necrosis. Patients are more likely to have distant metastases at presentation, and survival is significantly reduced.

Large Cell Neuroendocrine Cancer

Large cell neuroendocrine cancer is a high-grade, non-small cell neuroendocrine cancer. These tumors are characterized by histologic features similar to small cell cancer, but are formed by larger cells. Large cell neuroendocrine cancer is defined as a tumor with neuroendocrine morphologic characteristics, including organoid nesting, palisading, a trabecular pattern, and rosette-like structures. A mitotic count of 11 mitoses or more per 2 cc is the main criterion for separating large cell neuroendocrine cancers and small cell lung cancers from atypical carcinoid tumors. The mitotic rates are usually high for both large cell neuroendocrine cancers and small cell lung cancers, with an average of 70 to 80 mitoses per 2 cc. Large cell neuroendocrine cancers are separated from small cell lung cancers by using the criteria listed in Table 6-1.[12]

Large cell cancers with neuroendocrine morphology are tumors that resemble large cell neuroendocrine tumors by light microscopy but lack proof of neuroendocrine differentiation by electron microscopy or immunohistochemistry (IHC). The significance of this histology is unknown.

The prognosis for patients with large cell neuroendocrine cancer is worse than that for patients with atypical carcinoid and classic large cell cancer. Five-year survival is 21% for patients with large cell neuroendocrine cancer, 65% for atypical carcinoid, and 90% for typical carcinoid.[12]

TABLE 6-1 Characteristics of Large Cell Neuroendocrine Tumors that Distinguish Them from Small Cell Lung Cancers

- Larger cell size
- Abundant cytoplasm
- Prominent nucleoli
- Vesicular or coarse chromatin
- Polygonal rather than fusiform shape
- Less prominent nuclear molding
- Less conspicuous DNA encrustation of blood vessel walls

BIOLOGY

GROWTH FACTOR RECEPTORS

The EGFR belongs to the erbB family of growth factor receptors, which includes EGF receptor (HER1 or erbB1), HER2/neu (erbB2), HER3 (erbB3), and HER4 (erbB4). These cell-surface proteins consist of an extracellular ligand-binding domain, a transmembrane structure, and an intracellular tyrosine kinase domain. The binding of ligand to receptor activates receptor dimerization and tyrosine kinase autophosphorylation, initiating a cascade of intracellular events and leading to increased cell proliferation, angiogenesis, metastasis, and a decrease in apoptosis. Inappropriate activation of this receptor-signal transduction pathway can be caused by ligand or receptor overexpression, receptor mutation, binding of intracellular ligands, or dimerization with other receptors (heterodimerization or "receptor crosstalk").

Overexpression of EGFR has been found in as many as 70% of non-small cell lung cancers[13] and is an independent negative prognostic factor. Activating mutations have been identified[14,15] and are found most commonly in women, patients from East Asia, patients who have never smoked, and those patients with bronchioalveolar carcinoma — the group of patients who are most likely to have dramatic responses to these drugs. They are very rarely found in tumors that have *K-RAS* mutations. Somatic mutations that confer resistance to the EGFR tyrosine kinase inhibitors have also been described.[16]

The two approaches that have made the most progress in clinical development include small molecules that inhibit the tyrosine kinase domain of the receptor and monoclonal antibodies, such as trastuzumab for breast cancer, which inhibits ligand binding. The initial results of phase II studies of patients with second-line and third-line treatment of non-small cell lung cancer with gefitinib, an EGFR tyrosine kinase inhibitor, demonstrated a response rate of 10% to 20%, with rapid, dramatic, radiographic, and symptomatic improvement for some patients. However, findings from phase III trials that used concurrent chemotherapy in the first-line setting were negative.[17-19] One exception to this may be for patients who have never smoked, who seemed to derive a substantial survival benefit with the combination of chemotherapy plus erlotinib in a retrospective subset analysis.[20]

Despite the lack of benefit when combined with chemotherapy, erlotinib has been shown to prolong survival as a single agent in the second-line and third-line settings.[20] Of note, a survival benefit was observed not only for patients who are more likely to respond to these agents (i.e., women, never smokers, patients from East Asia, and those with bronchioalveolar carcinoma) as defined by classic radiographic criteria, but also for patients without these characteristics. In addition, EGFR gene and protein expression, as measured by fluorescent in-situ hybridization (FISH) or IHC, respectively, also may predict survival.[21]

This area of lung cancer biology remains an active area of investigation. As of late 2006, it was not known whether all patients should receive these drugs or if they should be reserved for patients with known clinical or biologic characteristics. Their role in first-line therapy, in the maintenance setting, or in combination with other targeted or radiation therapies also is yet to be defined. The role of tyrosine kinase inhibitors that inhibit more than just EGFR also is under active investigation.

ANGIOGENESIS

Tumor angiogenesis is a process of proliferation and migration of endothelial cells to form new blood vessels, thus nourishing the tumor and giving it access for metastasis. This process is regulated primarily by vascular endothelial growth factor (VEGF), a highly conserved, homodimeric glycoprotein. Once VEGF binds to its tyrosine kinase receptors, flt-1 and flk-1/KDR, the receptors dimerize, inducing intracellular signaling pathways and leading to endothelial cell proliferation and to the formation of new blood vessels. VEGF is overexpressed in different tumor types, including lung cancer. Both overexpression of VEGF and tumor microvessel density correlate with poor prognosis. Anti-VEGF antibodies suppress the growth of a variety of tumor cell lines in nude mice and inhibit angiogenesis in animal models of intraocular neovascularization. A number of antiangiogenic agents are undergoing clinical development, including monoclonal antibodies to the ligand, VEGF, the VEGF receptor, and to the tyrosine kinase inhibitors of the flt-1 and flk-1/KDR receptors. A phase III study in patients with non-squamous histology who received first-line treatment with combination bevacizumab plus carboplatin/paclitaxel demonstrated improved response, progression-free survival, and survival rates, compared with patients who received paclitaxel/carboplatin alone.[22]

> **KEY POINT**
>
> - A number of areas of tumor biology may be targeted for future therapeutic use, such as growth factor receptors, angiogenesis, tumor suppressor genes, and oncogenes.

TUMOR SUPPRESSOR GENES

The *TP53* tumor suppressor is the most frequently mutated gene in cancer and is found in more than 50% of tumors. In lung cancer, loss of one *TP53* allele on chromosome 17p13 and mutational inactivation of the other allele occurs in more than 75% of small cell lung cancers and in 50% of non-small cell lung cancer. Although *TP53* mutations are common in patients with lung cancer, their prognostic significance is unclear. The literature contains divergent results; some investigators report that the *TP53* mutation is a favorable prognostic factor, others consider it negative, and still others find that it has no prognostic significance.

ONCOGENES

RAS proteins are a family of guanine nucleotide-binding proteins that play an important role in the intracellular-signaling pathway. In response to the interaction between tyrosine kinase receptors and their ligands, such as growth factors, RAS becomes activated in the triphosphate form, which leads to a cascade of downstream events responsible for the regulation of cell cycle and apoptosis, including the RAF-1/mitogen-activated protein kinase pathway and the RAC/RHO pathway. If mutated, the protein products of the mutated genes remain in an active state, resulting in a continuous "on" signal that causes uncontrolled cell growth. RAS proteins are products of three proto-oncogenes: *H-RAS*, *K-RAS*, and *N-RAS*. Most mutations of the *K-RAS* oncogene in non-small cell lung cancer occur at codons 12, 61, and 63. *K-RAS* mutations are found primarily in patients with lung adenocarcinomas (approximately 30%) and in smokers; however, they very rarely are found in patients with small cell lung tumors, squamous cell carcinomas, or pate. *K-RAS* mutations are almost never present in EGFR-mutated disease.

After synthesis, RAS proteins undergo a process of post-translational modifications. One step in this process is farnesylation, induced by the enzyme farnesyltransferase. This enzyme transfers a farnesyl isoprenoid group from farnesyl diphosphate to RAS, which is necessary for incorporation into the cell membrane. This particular step is the target of a class of novel biologic agents called farnesyl transferase inhibitors.

CLINICAL PRESENTATION

Most patients with lung cancer present with symptomatic disease (Table 6-2). The most common symptoms are anorexia, fatigue, weakness, and cough. Patients with bronchioalveolar cancer can have bronchorrhea (large quantities

TABLE 6-2 Symptomatic Disease at Presentation for Patients with Lung Cancer

Typical
- Cough
- Increased production of sputum
- Shortness of breath

Common
- Fatigue
- Weight loss
- Anorexia
- Low-grade fever

Less Common
- Chest pain (usually from a pleural-based lesion)
- Hemoptysis
- Hoarseness (secondary to laryngeal nerve involvement)
- Bone pain

Infrequent
- Signs and symptoms consistent with obstruction of the superior vena cava, superior sulcus, or Pancoast tumors
- Pericardial tamponade
- Pleural effusion
- Paraneoplastic syndromes
- Signs and symptoms consistent with brain metastases

of foamy sputum) and shortness of breath out of proportion to the radiographic findings.

Metastatic disease at the time of presentation is common in small cell lung cancer (75%) and adenocarcinoma (50%), and many metastatic sites are possible. Adrenal metastases occur in roughly one-half of all patients with lung cancer. Liver and bone marrow metastases develop in approximately 20% to 30% of patients, and brain metastases occur in approximately 10% to 15%.

Paraneoplastic syndromes are caused by humeral factors produced by cancer cells that act at a distant site from both the primary site and its metastases. The two most common paraneoplastic syndromes in patients with non-small cell lung cancer are hypercalcemia and hypertrophic pulmonary osteoarthropathy. Although hypercalcemia is most often caused by diffuse skeletal metastases, it is the result of ectopic production of a parathyroid hormone-related peptide or other humoral substances in approximately 10% to 15% of patients. Humoral-associated hypercalcemia is most commonly associated with squamous cell cancers and least commonly with small cell lung cancer. Hypertrophic pulmonary osteoarthropathy is characterized by clubbing of the digits and, when severe, painful peritonitis of the long bones. Hypertrophic pulmonary osteoarthropathy is most common with adenocarcinoma, although it is not pathognomonic for cancer; it also is found with other pulmonary diseases.

In small cell lung cancer, the most common paraneoplastic syndromes are related to ectopic hormone production. Inappropriate secretion of antidiuretic hormone is observed in up to 5% of patients. The hallmark of inappropriate secretion of antidiuretic hormone is the inappropriate concentration of urine in the setting of plasma hypo-osmolarity in the absence of thyroid or adrenal dysfunction. Definitive therapy includes treatment of the underlying cancer; in the interim, however, fluid restriction or demeclocycline may be required.

Excessive production of corticotropin may result in Cushing's syndrome with excess cortisol production, resulting in muscle weakness, weight loss, hypertension, hyperglycemia, and profound hypokalemia. This syndrome is most commonly found in small cell lung cancer. As a result of the rapid tumor growth, the classical physical stigmata of Cushing's syndrome are often absent.

Small cell lung cancer also is associated with paraneoplastic neurologic abnormalities. Central nervous syndrome (CNS) paraneoplastic disorders include:

- cerebellar degeneration,
- dementia,
- limbic encephalopathy, and
- visual paraneoplastic syndrome with optic neuritis and retinopathy.

Cerebellar degeneration is characterized by progressive cerebellar dysfunction with ataxia, dysarthria, hypotonia, and dementia. This syndrome is associated with four different antineuronal antibodies, the most common being an antibody against Purkinje cell proteins. Limbic encephalopathy is characterized by progressive dementia, hallucinations, depression, agitation, anxiety, or disturbances in affect. Paraneoplastic sensory neuropathy often is caused by an anti-Hu antibody and is associated with subacute distal sensory loss and the absence of deep tendon reflexes with normal muscle strength. Anti-Hu is a circulating polyclonal immunoglobulin G that reacts with CNS neurons and the dorsal root and trigeminal ganglia. It can be associated with encephalopathy, autonomic neuropathy, and cerebellar degeneration.

KEY POINTS

- Common symptoms of lung cancer include local symptoms, such as cough and shortness of breath, and constitutional symptoms, such as fatigue, weakness, anorexia, and weight loss.
- The most common sites for metastasic disease in lung cancer are the adrenal glands, liver, bone, and brain.
- Patients with lung cancer may present with a number of paraneoplastic syndromes.

Eaton-Lambert syndrome, or the myasthenic syndrome, occurs in less than 1% of patients. It is characterized by proximal muscle weakness and, unlike with true myasthenia gravis, muscle strength tends to improve with repeated activity and successful treatment of the underlying malignant disease. Response to edrophonium is poor.

SCREENING

Most patients with lung cancer present with advanced disease, raising the question of the role of screening to detect these tumors at an earlier stage when they are theoretically more curable. The three screening interventions that have been explored for lung cancer include chest x-ray, cytologic analysis of sputum, and low-dose spiral CT. However, the role of screening patients at high risk for the development of early-stage disease has become increasingly contentious. To help evaluate the pertinent literature, useful definitions are reviewed below.

Length-time Bias. Length-time bias refers to the tendency of the screening test to detect indolent, slower-growing cancers that take longer to become symptomatic as compared with faster-growing, more aggressive tumors. Faster-growing, more aggressive cancers present with symptoms sooner, and thus are more likely to be diagnosed between screening events, leaving only the slow-growing tumors to be detected in the presymptomatic phase.

Lead-time Bias. Lead-time bias assumes that a treatment intervention is not effective (perhaps because the cancer has already metastasized) and that early detection does not result in a delay in death. Instead, the disease is simply detected earlier, before the patient became symptomatic. However, detecting a tumor earlier does not necessarily mean that the period of illness or of survival is longer, it merely indicates an earlier awareness of disease.

Over-diagnosis. Over-diagnosis is an extreme form of length bias in which the screening test detects a lung cancer that is not lethal — it behaves like a benign process and does not result in the death of the individual (e.g., the test discovers a tumor with which individual will die, not a tumor that will cause the death).

Stage Shift. In addition to identifying more earlier-stage cancers, an effective screening test also should result in fewer late-stage cancers.

Survival. Survival refers to the number of people who remain alive at a certain point in time relative to diagnosis. By definition, all screened patients will have a longer survival because they are diagnosed earlier, even if the date of death remains the same. For example, if 10 patients are diagnosed with lung cancer in 2005 because of symptoms, and if five of those patients die in the year 2010, the 5-year survival is 50% (five patients living at 5 years out of 10 patients with cancer). If the same 10 patients are screened and diagnosed with lung cancer in 2000, and if all 10 will be alive in 2005, then the 5-year survival will be 100%, even though the same five patients still die in 2010. (Fig. 6-1)

Mortality. Mortality is a reflection of how many patients died of the disease. In the example used for survival, the lung cancer mortality is 50% in both the symptom-detected and the screening-detected scenarios — 50% of patients who were screened (five of 10 patients screened) died of lung cancer, as did five of 10 patients who were diagnosed with lung cancer because they presented with symptoms. (Fig. 6-1)

Lead-time bias, length-time bias, and over-diagnosis may explain why screening could cause an improvement in survival without an improvement in mortality. If a screening test is effective, in addition to identifying more earlier-stage cancers, it also should result in fewer late-stage cancers. However, this has not been the case observed thus far with lung cancer screening.[23] In a recent updated analysis of three single-arm studies involving CT screening for more than 3,200 patients, the number of new lung cancer cases, lung cancer resections, advanced lung cancer cases, and deaths from lung cancer were compared with those numbers that would have been predicted based on validated models designed to estimate an individual's level of risk. One hundred nine patients had a lung resection compared with 10.9 expected cases. However, there was no evidence of a decline in the number of deaths from lung cancer (38 deaths from lung cancer observed and 38.8 expected; relative risk [RR], 1.0; 95% CI; 0.7, 1.3; $p = 0.90$).[24]

The other possible major disadvantage against screening is the financial and mental toll of false positives. In one study, more than 70% of patients who underwent CT scanning had a finding at some point that necessitated further testing.[25]

Results from five randomized screening studies in the 1980s of chest x-rays with or without cytologic analysis of sputum did not show any effect on lung cancer-specific mortality from screening patients at high risk, although earlier-stage cancers were detected in the screened groups.[26] These studies have since been criticized for their design and statistical analysis, but they are the only randomized screening studies conducted in lung cancer.

Since the publication of these studies, low-dose, non-contrast, thin-slice, helical or spiral CT has emerged as a possible new tool for lung cancer screening. Spiral CT is a scan in which only the pulmonary parenchyma is examined, thus negating the use of intravenous contrast medium and the necessity of a physician's presence. This type of scan can usually be done quickly (within one breath) and involves

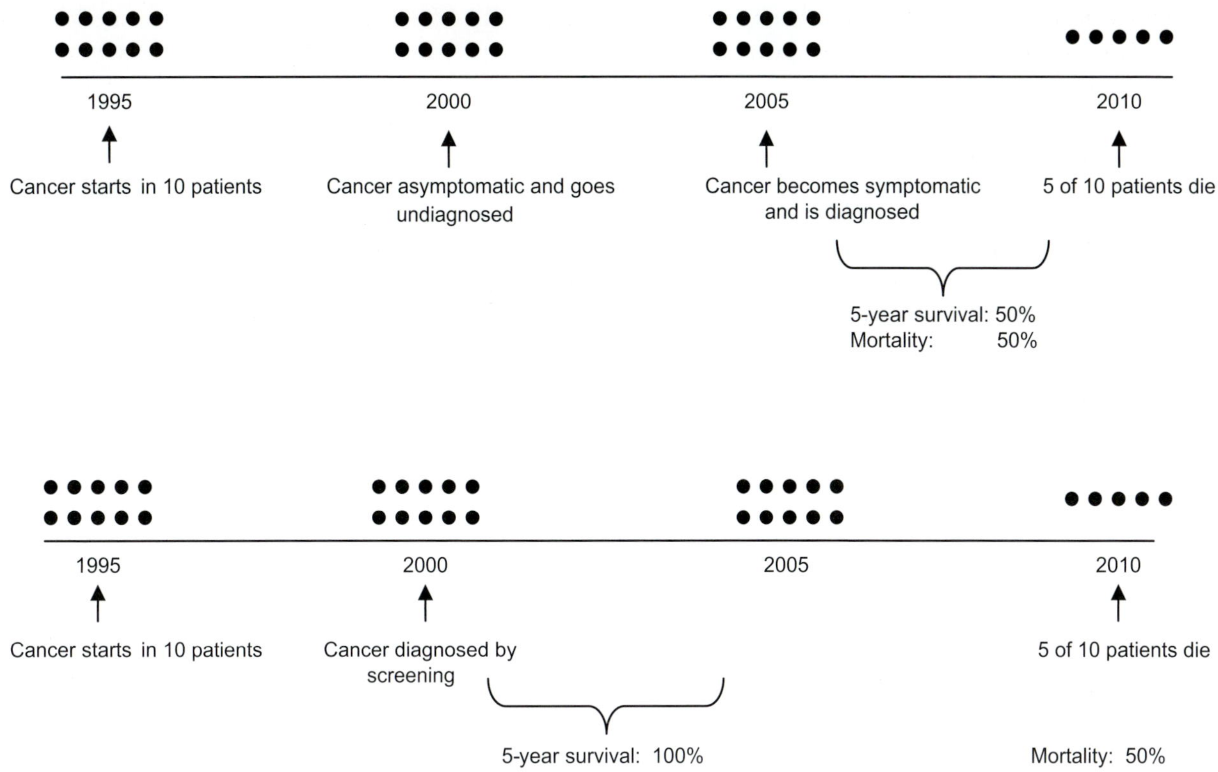

FIG. 6-1 Lead-time bias and its effects on survival and mortality rates.
• = *patient*

low doses of radiation. In a nonrandomized controlled study from the Early Lung Cancer Action Project (ELCAP), low-dose CT was shown to be more sensitive than chest x-ray for detecting lung nodules and lung cancer in early stages.[27] Survival also is longer, as demonstrated by a study published in the *New England Journal of Medicine.* In the study, the International Early Lung Cancer Action Program (I-ELCAP) found that the 10-year survival rate of 412 patients with clinical stage I lung cancer was 92%.[28] This is as would be predicted because, as discussed previously, survival is relative to the point of diagnosis.

Despite these promising results, it is unclear whether screening with spiral CT will result in a reduction of mortality rates for or related to lung cancer. Concerns include issues related to lead-time bias, length time bias, and overdiagnosis, the latter of which is based on the assumption that some tumors are more indolent than others and are never "destined" to give the patient substantial problems; however, these problems will go undetected throughout the patient's life. For example, in a Japanese study in which approximately 8,000 individuals who belonged to an insurance group were screened using CT scans, 23 of the 40 lung cancers detected were identified in neversmokers.[29] Given the low incidence of lung cancer for patients who have never smoked, presumably these are an example of overdiagnosis. In addition, many of the small "ground glass" opacities found on screening CT have subsequently been found to have very long doubling times (more than 400 days), again raising the concern of overdiagnosis. Therefore, in this scenario, it is expected that although more cancers would be detected in the screened group, the outcome would be the same.

KEY POINTS

- In randomized studies, no screening method has been demonstrated to reduce mortality from lung cancer for patients at high risk.
- Low-dose spiral computerized tomography (CT) is more sensitive in detecting smaller lesions than chest x-ray or cytologic analysis of sputum. The 10-year survival of these patients is quite good, although there are no data on lung cancer-specific mortality available for this group of patients.

In some parts of the United States, such as the Midwest, the incidence of benign nodules is extremely high, possibly making the cost of the test with subsequent follow-up scans prohibitive. For example, in a study conducted at the Mayo Clinic in which only 1.4% of patients were diagnosed with lung cancer, 51% of patients had at least one calcified nodule on initial CT, and 74% had an uncalcified lung nodule at some point during the 5-year follow-up period.[26] No stage shift was detected, and no significant difference was found in lung cancer mortality rates of cancers detected in subsequent examinations for this trial compared with the Mayo Lung Project after separation of participants into subsets (2.8 vs. 2.0 per 1,000 person-years, p = 0.43).[23]

The appropriate management of these small lesions is unknown. Unnecessary treatment may include thoracotomy and lung resection, thus adding to the cost, mortality, and morbidity of treatment. All of these issues must be discussed with individuals seeking advice regarding screening (Table 6-3).

To help resolve the issue, the National Cancer Institute has recently finished accruing more than 50,000 participants for a large randomized controlled trial of chest x-ray compared with low-dose helical CT — the National Lung Screening Trial. Until these results become available, routine screening with cytologic analysis of sputum, chest x-ray, or spiral CT cannot be recommended. Rather, physicians must discuss the possible benefits and risks of screening, the latter of which includes the chance of a false-positive test, which will result in multiple follow-up tests and in possible biopsies for a malignancy that may not be life-threatening. Potential benefits include the increased likelihood of detecting an early-stage lung cancer.

TABLE 6-3 Points about Screening for Lung Cancer to Share with Patients[30]

- Results from observational studies of CT screening among patients at high risk (i.e., those with a history of heavy smoking) indicate a high rate of diagnosis of lung cancer in stage I (a relatively curable stage).
- No data are available from randomized trials, which are ongoing; results are expected in 4 to 5 years.
- It is not clear that diagnosing a smaller lung cancer earlier results in more cures from lung cancer; because some of the tumors grow so slowly, they may never become symptomatic and may never need treatment.
- CT screening reveals many noncalcified nodules, only a small fraction of which will be found to be lung cancer. The patient must be prepared to live with this uncertainty and must be able to commit to frequent follow-up scans.
- Costly invasive procedures that are associated with serious risks may be required to evaluate some nodules.
- A diagnostic work-up should be done by physicians who are experienced in such evaluation.
- The selection of a facility with physicians who are experienced and credentialed in multidisciplinary fields (including thoracic surgery, pathology, and pulmonology) is critical to an optimal outcome.
- The most effective way for smokers to improve their health is to stop smoking.

PROGNOSTIC FACTORS

Favorable prognostic factors for both non-small cell and small cell cancers include stage, performance status, lack of substantial weight loss (less than 5%), and female sex. Age is not an independent prognostic factor; "fit" older patients tend to fare as well or as poorly as their younger counterparts. Histologic subtype also is not an independent prognostic factor, although adenocarcinoma is more likely to metastasize earlier than squamous cell; however, once metastasized, these two histologies have similar prognoses. Mutations of the *TP53* gene and the oncogene *K-RAS*, although clearly associated with non-small cell lung cancer, do not appear to have clinically significant prognostic or predictive significance. Although other biologic factors, such as the expression of the EGFR or microvessel density, have been found to be associated with unfavorable outcome in retrospective studies, these findings have yet to be confirmed prospectively.

PREOPERATIVE EVALUATION FOR NON-SMALL CELL LUNG CANCER

The suitability of the patient for a definitive resection depends on two factors: the stage of the lesion and the ability of the patient to withstand surgery. A detailed discussion of the preoperative evaluation and comorbid conditions are beyond the scope of this chapter; however, assessment of pulmonary reserve is discussed here.

MEDICAL ASSESSMENT OF PULMONARY RESERVE

Preoperative evaluation for a thoracotomy starts with spirometry. The forced vital capacity is the value that has been used most commonly to assess suitability for surgery; a predicted postoperative forced vital capacity of less than 1 L or a preoperative value of less than 2 L for a pneumonectomy or less than 1.5 L for a lobectomy usually suggests that the patient is at risk for perioperative complications. If there is concern that the forced vital capacity may not be adequate or that the patient has signs or symptoms of interstitial lung

KEY POINTS

- Good clinical prognostic factors include stage of disease, performance status, lack of substantial weight loss, and female sex.
- Biologic prognostic factors including *K-RAS* and/or *TP53* mutations, as well as microvessel density, have not been shown to be clinically useful.
- "Fit" older patients generally tolerate treatment as well as their younger counterparts and experience the same benefit.

disease, a diffusing capacity should be obtained. A diffusing capacity lower than 50% predicted suggests increased risk of postoperative morbidity or mortality. The amount of postoperative pulmonary reserve is most commonly predicted by a perfusion scan. For patients with borderline results, an oxygen consumption test can be helpful for predicting postoperative risk. Patients with predicted maximum consumption of more than 20 mL/kg per minute are generally not at increased risk; a predicted maximum consumption less than 15 mL/kg per minute indicates an increased risk of complications or death, and patients with a predicted maximum consumption less than 10 mL/kg per minute are at high risk of perioperative complications.

A quick way to assess a patient's pulmonary reserve is simply to determine their ability to climb a flight of stairs. Patients who are able to climb one flight of stairs without stopping generally will have a predicted maximum consumption of more than 20 mL/kg per minute, whereas patients who cannot climb one flight of stairs will have a value of less than 10 mL/kg per minute.

The pulmonary status should be optimized as much as possible before surgery. Treatment of bronchitis with antibiotics, bronchodilators, and/or oral corticosteroids is helpful. The patient should quit smoking, if applicable, and preoperative training with incentive spirometry and weight reduction should be considered when appropriate.

NON-SMALL CELL LUNG CANCER

DIAGNOSIS AND STAGING

The diagnosis of lung cancer is made through evaluation of specimens obtained by bronchial biopsy or percutaneous needle biopsy. Although the disease is usually discovered on chest x-ray, CT of the chest and upper abdomen is necessary to evaluate the extent of the primary disease, mediastinal extension, or lymphadenopathy, as well as the presence or absence of other parenchymal nodules for patients in whom surgical resection is a consideration. Bone scans should be obtained for patients with bone pain, chest pain, or an elevated calcium or alkaline phosphatase level. Positron emission tomography (PET) scans also are helpful in detecting bone metastases; if a PET scan is done as part of the staging work-up, a bone scan does not need to be performed. CT or magnetic resonance imaging (MRI) of the head is not routinely performed in the absence of signs or symptoms related to the CNS.

KEY POINT

- Preoperative evaluation should include determinations of forced vital capacity and a predicted postoperative value, a diffusing capacity, and the maximum oxygen consumption.

TABLE 6-4 TNM Definitions

Primary Tumor (T)	
TX	Tumor proven by the presence of malignant cells in bronchopulmonary secretions but not visualized on radiographs or by bronchoscopy, or any tumor that cannot be assessed as in a re-treatment staging.
T0	No evidence of primary tumor.
Tis	Carcinoma in situ.
T1	A tumor of no more than 3 cm in greatest dimension, surrounded by lung or visceral pleura, and without evidence of invasion proximal to a lobar bronchus at bronchoscopy.
T2	A tumor of more than 3 cm in greatest dimension, or a tumor of any size that either invades the visceral pleura or has associated atelectasis or obstructive pneumonitis extending to the hilar region. At bronchoscopy, the proximal extent of demonstrable tumor must be within a lobar bronchus or at least 2 cm distal to the carina. Any associated atelectasis or obstructive pneumonitis must involve less than an entire lung.
T3	A tumor of any size with direct extension into the chest wall (including superior sulcus tumors), diaphragm, or the mediastinal pleura or pericardium, without involving the heart, great vessels, trachea, esophagus, or vertebral body, or a tumor in the main bronchus within 2 cm of the carina without involving the carina.
T4	A tumor of any size with invasion of the mediastinum or involving the heart, great vessels, trachea, esophagus, vertebral body, or carina, or the presence of malignant pleural effusion. This category also includes any satellite nodules within the same lobe.
Node Involvement (N)	
N0	No demonstrable metastasis to regional lymph nodes.
N1	Metastasis to lymph nodes in the peribronchial, ipsilateral hilar region, or both, including direct extension.
N2	Metastasis to ipsilateral mediastinal lymph nodes, subcarinal lymph nodes, or both.
N3	Metastasis to contralateral mediastinal lymph nodes, contralateral hilar lymph nodes, ipsilateral or contralateral scalene, or supraclavicular lymph nodes.
Distant Metastasis (M)	
MX	Cannot be assessed.
M0	No distant metastasis.
M1	Distant metastasis, including pulmonary nodule not in the same lobe as the primary tumor.

KEY POINTS

- Although positron emission tomography (PET) is more sensitive and specific than CT for staging disease in the mediastinum, it probably cannot replace mediastinoscopy because of the incidence of false-positive and false-negative results (the one exception may be patients with a normal mediastinum on CT and a normal PET scan).
- PET is useful in helping direct the surgeon as to which nodes should be biopsied, as well as detecting distant metastases.
- Mediastinoscopy should be performed for all patients with enlarged nodes detected by CT or PET.

TABLE 6-5 Comparison of Sensitivity and Specificity of Positron Emission Tomography (PET) and Computerized Tomography (CT)

	Sensitivity (%)	Specificity (%)	Accuracy (%)
Detection of Mediastinal Metastases[33]*			
PET	91	86	—
CT	75	66	—
Staging of Mediastinal Disease[34]			
PET	96	93	94
CT	68	65	66

*The sensitivity and specificity of PET for detecting distant metastases were 82% and 93%, respectively.

Mediastinal nodal metastasis is a critical factor in determining tumor resectability (Table 6-4). Mediastinoscopy has long been considered the gold standard for mediastinal staging and has been recommended for mediastinal lymph nodes larger than 1 cm as detected by CT, regardless of whether they appear positive or negative on a PET scan. Patients with a normal mediastinum on CT whose lymph nodes also appear negative on a PET scan probably do not need to undergo a preoperative mediastinoscopy, although the lymph nodes still must be sampled at the time of thoracotomy.

INVASIVE STAGING: MEDIASTINOSCOPY, ENDOSCOPIC ULTRASOUND, AND TRANSTHORACIC AND TRANSBRONCHIAL BIOPSIES

Accurate staging of the mediastinum is critical for patients with non-small cell lung cancer because the treatment of stage I disease is likely to differ substantially from the treatment of stage IIIA disease. Clinical staging has been shown to differ markedly from pathologic staging at the time of resection.[31] In a review of numerous clinical trials, the performance of transthoracic, transbronchial, and endoscopic ultrasound-guided needle aspirations or biopsies was compared with mediastinoscopy for staging disease in the mediastinum.[31] Transthoracic and endoscopic needle aspirations had similar sensitivities to mediastinoscopies, although these results may have been because the transthoracic and endoscopic ultrasound needle aspirations were generally performed only in patients with enlarged nodes detected by CT, resulting in fewer false-negative results. However, mediastinoscopy has a higher negative predictive value.

POSITRON EMISSION TOMOGRAPHY

PET, a metabolic imaging scan using 18-fluorodeoxyglucose (FDG), was developed as a useful complementary tool for staging. PET is more sensitive, specific, and accurate than CT and could potentially prevent patients with advanced disease from undergoing unnecessary invasive procedures.[32]

In a prospective study, a standard approach to staging of non-small cell lung cancer (CT, ultrasound, and bone scan) was compared with PET to determine which approach could more accurately detect metastases in mediastinal lymph nodes and distant sites.[33] Mediastinal involvement was confirmed histopathologically, and distant metastases were confirmed by other imaging tests. The results of PET, CT, and histology also were compared in a study involving 168 mediastinal nodes in 54 patients.[34] PET had higher rates of sensitivity and specificity than CT in both studies (Table 6-5). However, the limitations of PET include the cost, limited availability, inability to detect lesions smaller than 8 mm, and lack of specificity, particularly for patients with inflammatory or granulomatous disease. Thus, it is not clear whether PET can replace mediastinoscopy because the scan can yield false-positive results when an inflammatory process is present and false-negative results when low-metabolic lung tumors such as bronchioalveolar cancer or carcinoid tumors are present. Despite these problems, preoperative PET, in addition to a conventional workup, has been demonstrated to reduce the number of "futile" thoracotomies, as defined by benign disease, exploratory thoracotomy, pathologic stage IIIA (N2) or IIIB disease, postoperative relapse, or death within 12 months.[35] PET also has been used to detect distant metastases; indeed, it is in this area that some investigators believe PET may have its primary role in staging.[32] Negative results of PET for patients without symptomatic disease probably obviates the need for bone imaging.[32] PET may ultimately be useful for judging response to therapy, because PET scans done early after treatment have been demonstrated to be better predictors of survival than CT.[36]

TREATMENT: NON-SMALL CELL LUNG CANCER

Treatment of non-small cell lung cancer is based on disease stage, although the performance status, comorbid conditions, and other relevant social factors of the patient must be taken into account.

OCCULT, IN SITU LESIONS

Porphyrins are naturally occurring respiratory pigments in the protoplasm of plant and animal cells, which, when exposed to 1,630 nanometers of red light in the presence of oxygen, convert to an excited state. This excitability, in turn, interacts with molecular oxygen to form singlet oxygen or oxygen-free radicals, resulting in cell death in the tissues in which they are released. Photoporphyrins are selectively retained by cancer cells, with the ratio of tumor-to-normal-tissue fluorescence being greater than one at 24 to 48 hours after injection. This makes it possible to expose tumors to photoporphyrins and red light, which results in tumor cell death. The procedure is approved for microinvasive lung cancer for patients who are not candidates for surgery.

STAGES I AND II DISEASE

Approximately one-third of all patients with lung cancer present with stages I and II disease. The treatment of choice is surgery, which can result in cure for many patients (Table 6-6). The preferred surgical procedure is lobectomy, although for patients in whom disease crosses a major fissure or involves the proximal main-stem bronchus, pneumonectomy may be required. Lobectomy has traditionally been the procedure of choice, even for patients with small, peripheral lesions, because wedge resections have been shown to be associated with increased local recurrence and decreased survival. Research is ongoing regarding the management of the small lesions discovered on low-dose, noncontrast-enhanced, thin-slice, helical CT.

Conventional high-dose radiation therapy results in a cure for approximately 15% to 35% of patients with medical contraindications to surgery but who have adequate pulmonary function. In small studies, the use of ultra-high doses of radiation in a few fractions, delivered using extracranial stereotactic techniques to small volumes, has resulted in a cause-specific survival rate approaching 80% at 2 years.

The role of adjuvant and neoadjuvant chemotherapy for patients with stage I non-small cell lung cancer is under active investigation (discussed further in the chapter). The risk of second lung cancers is high (approximately 2% to 3% annually) for patients with resected stage I non-small cell lung cancer. Vitamin A or one its derivatives (beta-carotene or cis retinoic acid) has not been found to have any chemopreventive effect and is deleterious in current smokers. Other agents are under investigation.

The subset of T3, N0 disease has a different natural history and treatment strategy than stage III N2 disease and, thus, has been moved to stage IIB. Patients with this stage disease, often including patients with superior sulcus

KEY POINTS

- Treatment of stages I and II non-small cell lung cancer involves surgery (if the patient is a candidate) or radiation therapy (if the patient is not a candidate).
- Optimal management of Pancoast tumors includes concurrent chemoradiation followed by surgical resection.
- Adjuvant chemotherapy is indicated for patients with stages II and IIIA disease; it should be discussed with patients with stage IB disease, particularly those with larger tumors (greater than 4 cm). Cisplatin is slightly more effective than carboplatin, which may be important in a potentially curative situation. Evidence from randomized trials suggests that the second drug should be vinorelbine or etoposide, although studies evaluating other drugs are ongoing.
- The role of neoadjuvant chemotherapy is unclear, although patients tend to tolerate it better than postoperative adjuvant therapy. Preliminary data suggest that the patients most likely to benefit from surgery following neoadjuvant therapy are patients whose mediastinal lymph nodes clear following treatment.
- Treatment of stage IIIA disease is in flux but involves both systemic chemotherapy and local therapy (surgery and/or radiation).
- Treatment of stage IIIB non-small cell lung cancer (without a pleural effusion) involves combined-modality treatment with chemotherapy and radiation therapy. Evidence from randomized trials suggests that concurrent chemotherapy and radiation therapy will result in the best survival, albeit at an increase in toxicity.

TABLE 6-6 International Staging Classification for Lung Cancer

		5-year Survival Rate (%)	
Stage	TNM Subset	Clinical Stage	Pathologic Stage
IA	T1, N0, M0	61	67
IB	T2, N0, M0	38	57
IIA	T1, N1, M0	34	55
IIB	T2, N1, M0	24	39
IIIA	T3, N1, M0		
	T1 to 3, N2, M0	9	25
IIIB	T4, any N, M0		
	Any T, N3, M0	13	23
IV	Any T, any N, M1	1	Negligible

tumors, have historically been treated with low-dose postoperative radiation therapy. Patients with peripheral chest wall invasion should have resection of the involved ribs and underlying lung. Most clinical data suggest that a 35% 5-year survival is obtained. Chest wall defects are then repaired with chest wall musculature or with hernia mesh and methylmethacrylate. Five-year survival rates as high as 50% have been found.

PANCOAST TUMORS

Pancoast, or superior sulcus, tumors are in the upper lobe, adjoining the brachial plexus and are frequently associated with Horner's syndrome or shoulder and arm pain; the latter is caused by rib destruction, involvement of the eighth cervical vertebra or T-1 nerve roots, or both. The Southwest Oncology Group (SWOG) has reported the best results from an Intergroup trial in which patients with superior sulcus tumors were treated with cisplatin/etoposide and concomitant radiation therapy followed by attempted surgical resection.[37] A total of 54 thoracotomy specimens (65%) showed either a complete response or minimal microscopic disease on pathologic evaluation. The 2-year survival rate was 55% for all eligible patients and 70% for patients who had a complete resection.

STAGE III DISEASE

Treatment of locally advanced non-small cell lung cancer is one of the most controversial issues in the management of lung cancer. Treatment options include surgery for less advanced disease or radiation therapy, both of which have been given with or without chemotherapy to control micrometastases. Interpretation of the results of clinical trials involving patients with locally advanced disease has been clouded by a number of issues, including changing diagnostic techniques, different staging systems, and heterogeneous patient populations with tumors that range from nonbulky stage IIIA (clinical N1 nodes with N2 nodes discovered only at the time of surgery or mediastinoscopy) to bulky N2 nodes (enlarged adenopathy clearly visible on chest x-rays or multiple nodal level involvement) to clearly inoperable stage IIIB disease.

For some subsets of stage IIB (T3, N0), IIIA (T3, N1), or IIIB (T4, N0 ± 1) tumors, the role of surgery may be less related to the potential of micrometastatic disease and more to the location of the tumor (e.g., superior sulcus, chest wall, and proximal airway). For each location, a determination must be made on the basis of the potential of surgical resectability.

NONBULKY STAGE IIIA DISEASE

The primary treatment of stages II and IIIA (clinical N0) disease is surgical resection, and cure is achieved in 25% to 50% of patients (Table 6-6). However, even with complete resection, the cure rate is disappointing. Patients with "incidental N2" disease should receive postoperative adjuvant chemotherapy.

Adjuvant Therapy

Given the high rate of recurrence for patients who have undergone reportedly curative resection for early-stage disease, there is considerable interest in postoperative adjuvant therapy to eradicate micrometastatic disease (Table 6-7).

Thoracic Radiation Therapy. Postoperative radiation therapy has been shown to reduce local recurrence after resection of stage II or III squamous cell cancer of the lung but does not prolong survival.[38]

Chemotherapy. A meta-analysis published in 1995 of more than 4,300 patients given cisplatin-based adjuvant therapy showed a trend toward an improved survival rate of approximately 5% at 5 years, which bordered on significance ($p = 0.08$).[39] Subsequently, three randomized studies, published in 2000 or later, demonstrated no significant survival advantage from the addition of more "modern" postoperative chemotherapy regimens for stages II and IIIA (N2) disease.[40–42] However, since that time, at least three additional randomized trials and two meta-analyses showed a survival benefit in response to postoperative adjuvant-based therapy.[43–45]

In the International Adjuvant Lung Trial (IALT), patients with resected stage I to IIIA disease were randomly assigned to either observation or chemotherapy (cisplatin plus either etoposide, vinorelbine, vinblastine, or vindesine).[43] Patients also were allowed to receive postoperative thoracic radiation at the discretion of the participating site. Although the study was terminated early because of poor accrual, there was a significant improvement in median survival, disease-free survival, 5-year survival, and 5-year disease-free survival in favor of the chemotherapy arm (hazard ratio [HR] = 0.86 for survival). Although the magnitude of the difference was relatively small (4% at 5 years), it was approximately the same as that reported in the meta-analysis.

A randomized trial by the National Cancer Institute of Canada randomly assigned 482 patients with stage IA or II disease to postoperative observation or to vinorelbine and cisplatin. Overall survival was significantly prolonged for the chemotherapy group as compared with the observation group (94 vs. 73 months; HR for death = 0.69; $p = 0.04$), as was relapse-free survival (not reached vs. 46.7 months; hazard ratio for recurrence = 0.60; $p < 0.001$). Five-year survival rates were 69% and 54% for the two groups, respectively ($p = 0.03$).[45] Of note, this 15% absolute benefit at 5 years is among the highest in all of oncology for adjuvant chemotherapy.

A randomized French study (Adjuvant Navelbine International Trialist Association) also examined vinorelbine and cisplatin therapy for patients with postoperative stage I

TABLE 6-7 Adjuvant Therapies

Study	Treatment	Patients	5-year Survival (%)	Median Survival	Hazard Ratio	P Value
ECOG 3590 (II–IIIA)[40]	Surgery → radiation therapy vs. postop concurrent radiation therapy plus cisplatin and etoposide	242 246		39 months vs. 38 months	0.92	0.56
ALPI (I–IIIA)[42]	Surgery vs. postop mitomycin, vindesine, and cisplatin	603 606	51 43		0.96	0.589
IALT (IB–IIIA)[43]	Surgery vs. postop cisplatin and etoposide, or vinca alkaloids	405 361	40 44.5		0.86	0.03
CALGB (IB ASCO 06)[48]	Surgery vs. postop carboplatin and paclitaxel	172 172	57 59		0.8	0.10
NCI-C (IB–II)[45]	Surgery vs. postop cisplatin and vinorelbine	241 241	54 69		0.80	0.03
ANITA (IB, II, IIIA)[46]	Surgery vs. postop cisplatin and vinorelbine	433 407	43 51	44 months 66 months	0.80	0.017

Abbreviations: ECOG, Eastern Cooperative Oncology Group; ALPI, Adjuvant Lung Project Italy; IALT, International Adjuvant Lung Cancer Trial; CALGB, Cancer and Leukemia Group B; NCI-C; National Cancer Institute of Canada; ANITA, Adjuvant Navelbine International Trialist Association; postop, postoperative.

(T2, N0), II, or IIIA disease. Eight hundred forty patients were randomly assigned. Median survival was 65.8 months in the treatment arm and 43.7 months in the observation arm (p = 0.0131; HR = 1.264 [1.05, 1.52]). Survival at 2, 5, and 7 years was 68%, 51%, and 45% in the treatment arm, respectively, and 63%, 43%, and 37% in the observation arm, respectively. Five-year survival by stage I/II/IIIA were 62%, 52%, and 42%, respectively, in the treatment arm and 63%, 39%, and 26% in the observation arm, respectively.[46]

In 2004, the Cancer and Leukemia Group B (CALGB) reported a trial of adjuvant paclitaxel and carboplatin following resection for patients with stage IB non-small cell lung cancer.[47] Although originally reported as a positive study, an update presented at the American Society of Clinical Oncology's (ASCO) 2006 Annual Meeting[48] indicated that the trial did not quite meet statistical significance (HR = 0.80; p = 0.10). It was unclear if this was because the study was confined to patients with stage IB disease, because it used carboplatin instead of cisplatin, because it used paclitaxel instead of vinorelbine, or because, with 344 patients, it was an underpowered study to detect a hazard ratio of 0.80. Given that the majority of the other positive adjuvant trials also have resulted in hazard ratios of approximately 0.80, at least one component for the "negative'" p value of 0.10 may be the small size of the trial.

There now have been two meta-analyses that have reported a benefit with adjuvant chemotherapy, in addition to the 1995 *Lancet* meta-analysis. One study examined abstracted data from 11 trials conducted with a total of 5,716 patients. Adjuvant chemotherapy yielded a survival advantage compared with surgery alone (HR = 0.872; 95% CI; 0.805, 0.944; p = 0.001). In a subset analysis, both cisplatin-based chemotherapy (HR = 0.891; 95% CI; 0.815, 0.975; p = 0.012) and single-agent therapy with tegafur and uracil (HR = 0.799; 95% CI; 0.668, 0.957; p = 0.015) were found to yield a significant survival benefit.[49] The second meta-analysis (Lung Adjuvant Cisplatin Evaluation) presented at the 2006 ASCO Annual Meeting, analyzed data from five randomized trials of more than 4,500 patients.[50] This study used individual patient data to determine the benefit of adjuvant cisplatin-based chemotherapy and found a statistical benefit with cisplatin chemotherapy (p = 0.004).

Thus, chemotherapy is clearly indicated for patients with stages II and microscopic IIIA disease. It remains to be determined whether it is a benefit for patients with stage IB disease and whether carboplatin can be substituted for cisplatin (although the majority of the data would suggest not) or if paclitaxel can be substituted for the vinca alkaloids.

Neoadjuvant Therapy

The following three potential advantages of neoadjuvant chemotherapy have been identified.

- Improved tolerability occurs when neoadjuvant therapy is administered before surgery (90% of patients will receive the planned dose preoperatively compared with 60% postoperatively).
- Micrometastases are attacked earlier rather than later.
- Downstaging with chemotherapy may allow complete resection.

Two small randomized studies published in 1994 raised considerable interest in the role of neoadjuvant chemotherapy.

In these trials, each of which involved 60 patients, surgery alone was compared with surgery plus preoperative chemotherapy for stage IIIA disease. In one study conducted in Europe, preoperative chemotherapy followed by surgery and postoperative mediastinal radiation therapy was compared with surgery and postoperative mediastinal radiation therapy for patients with stage IIIA disease. The median survival time was 26 months for the 30 patients who received neoadjuvant chemotherapy compared with 8 months for the 30 patients treated with surgery alone.[51] Investigators at the M. D. Anderson Cancer Center randomly assigned patients to either surgery alone or to three cycles of chemotherapy, followed by surgery and three cycles of postoperative chemotherapy. The median survival time for the 32 patients in the surgery-alone group was 14 months compared with 21 months for the 28 patients in the combined-modality arm.[52] Criticisms of these studies include their small size, imbalances between the two arms, and poor survival of the control arms.

In a larger randomized French trial, preoperative chemotherapy plus surgery was compared with surgery alone for 355 patients with resectable stages I (except T1, N0), II, and IIIA (including N2) disease. The findings did not show a benefit with neoadjuvant chemotherapy.[53] A subset analysis suggested a survival advantage for neoadjuvant chemotherapy for N0 and N1 disease, but not for N2 disease.

Intergroup Trial (0139) was a randomized study of patients with pathologically staged N2 disease who received 45 Gy of induction radiation therapy plus two cycles of cisplatin and etoposide.[54] The patients were subsequently randomly assigned to surgery or to boost radiation therapy plus an additional two cycles of chemotherapy. A significant improvement in progression-free survival at 5 years for the trimodality arm (22% vs. 11%; p = 0.017) was observed. Although there was a trend for improved 5-year overall survival with trimodality therapy, this was not significant (22% vs. 11%; p = 0.10). There were greater treatment-related mortalities in the surgery arm compared with the chemoradiation-alone arm (8% vs. 2%), with the majority of deaths occurring in patients undergoing pneumonectomy. This lack of improvement in overall survival was attributed in part to a crossing of the survival curves, presumably because of increased toxicity in the trimodality arm. However, the survival curves subsequently separated so that by the third year, an absolute benefit of 5% was observed in the surgical arm. More patients in the trimodality arm were alive without progression of disease (p = 0.008) but more patients died without progression (p = 0.021).

A recent meta-analysis of seven randomized clinical trials showed that preoperative chemotherapy improved survival with a hazard ratio of 0.82 (95% CI; 0.69, 0.97; p = 0.02).[55] This is equivalent to an absolute benefit of 6%, increasing overall survival across all stages of disease from 14% to 20% at 5 years.

It should be noted that, if neoadjuvant chemotherapy is used, its role is to control micrometastatic disease. Thus, patients who have persistent N2 disease following neoadjuvant chemotherapy do not have a favorable prognosis. Neoadjuvant chemotherapy generally should not be used to render inoperable disease operable.

BULKY STAGE IIIA (N2) DISEASE AND STAGE IIIB DISEASE WITH NO PLEURAL EFFUSION (DRY IIIB)

The optimal treatment for bulky stages IIIA and IIIB disease also is controversial. Investigational efforts have been directed toward identifying the optimal combined-modality approach, which involves treatments directed at local control of the disease (surgery or radiation therapy) and micrometastatic disease (chemotherapy). Possibilities for bulky stage IIIA disease include preoperative or postoperative chemotherapy plus surgery, as addressed previously, or chemotherapy plus radiation therapy. Stage IIIB disease generally is considered unresectable, with the treatment consisting of combined chemoradiation or, in the case of IIIB disease with malignant pleural effusion, chemotherapy alone.

Chemotherapy plus Radiation Therapy

Chemotherapy plus radiation therapy is the treatment of choice for patients with bulky or inoperable stage IIIA or IIIB disease without pleural effusion. The results from randomized studies have demonstrated an improvement in median and long-term survival with chemotherapy followed by radiation therapy compared with radiation therapy alone.[56,57]

The results from two randomized studies, one conducted by a Japanese group and the other by the Radiation Therapy Oncology Group (RTOG), showed a survival advantage with concurrent chemoradiation compared with a sequential approach, albeit at the expense of increased toxicity. In the Japanese trial, two cycles of mitomycin-C, vindesine, and cisplatin (MVP) were given concurrently or sequentially with 56 Gy of radiation.[58] Patients in either arm who had a response received another two cycles of MVP after radiation therapy was completed. The response rate and median survival were significantly better with concurrent chemoradiotherapy (84% vs. 66%, p = 0.0002; 17 months vs. 13 months, p = 0.04). Initial findings from a confirmatory randomized RTOG trial also showed a trend in favor of concurrent cisplatin, vinblastine, and radiation therapy compared with sequential chemoradiation (median survival, 17 months vs. 15 months; p = 0.08).[59] The final results are pending.

Chemotherapy can be administered in either full systemic doses with radiation therapy, in weekly radiosensitizing doses, or in a combination of both. Although single-agent weekly carboplatin has not resulted in a survival benefit when administered with radiation therapy, preliminary results from phase I and II studies of weekly doses of 50 mg/m^2 of paclitaxel and carboplatin (AUC 2) with concurrent radiation therapy proved promising.[60] However, a CALGB trial compared concomitant chemoradiotherapy, consisting of low-dose weekly carboplatin and paclitaxel, with induction therapy prior to the same concomitant chemoradiotherapy regimen. The median survival with chemoradiation was 11.4 months compared with 14 months for induction chemotherapy followed by chemoradiation ($p = 0.154$). One-year survival estimates are 48% for chemoradiation (range: 41% to 57%) and 54% for induction chemotherapy followed by chemoradiation (range: 47% to 62%). The median survival achieved in each of the treatment groups was low compared with other reports in the literature, possibly indicating that chemoradiation with low-dose weekly carboplatin and paclitaxel is not optimal.

Thus, major questions remain unanswered regarding the best combination and scheduling of chemotherapy and radiation therapy. Although results from the Japanese trial demonstrated a slightly superior outcome with concurrent chemoradiotherapy, the mitomycin-based approach is not widely used in the United States. The RTOG trial involved an older chemotherapy regimen, and none of the newer agents, such as carboplatin, paclitaxel, docetaxel, gemcitabine, and vinorelbine, have been tested in this context. The SWOG reported promising results with consolidation docetaxel following full-dose cisplatin/etoposide and concurrent radiation therapy, but these results were not confirmed in a randomized setting.[61] The efficacy of sensitizing doses of concurrent chemotherapy also has yet to be compared with full doses of chemotherapy in randomized trials. Newer methods, schedules, and techniques of administering radiation therapy also appear promising, such as the dose-density concept for radiation therapy, in which patients are treated with a 2-week course of continuous hyperfractionated accelerated radiation therapy administered 3 times daily and followed by chemotherapy.[62]

STAGE III, N2 DISEASE

Treatment of patients with stage III, N2 non-small cell lung cancer is in flux, as seen from the previous discussion. Although results from ongoing or recently completed randomized studies are maturing, some general guidelines for treating a patient can be identified.

- Clinical N0 disease by CT and PET — A resection should be performed. If microscopic N2 disease is detected at surgery, postoperative chemotherapy, radiation therapy, or both, should be considered.
- Nonbulky N2 by CT (e.g., one node measuring 1 to 2 cm) and/or by PET — The age, performance status, and comorbid conditions of the patient should be considered. If the patient is an excellent surgical candidate, it is not unreasonable to have a discussion regarding the use of surgery plus chemotherapy and/or radiation therapy, stressing that the optimal treatment has not been clearly identified. Options include adjuvant chemotherapy with or without postoperative radiation therapy or neoadjuvant chemotherapy. In the latter scenario, some surgeons recommend a mediastinoscopy after two cycles of the induction chemotherapy, rationalizing that if the N2 nodes remain positive following chemotherapy, a definitive resection should not be attempted, and the patient should proceed with definitive radiation therapy or with combined chemotherapy and radiation. Combined preoperative chemoradiation should be administered cautiously and only to the extremely fit patient who will be undergoing resection by an experienced thoracic surgeon (given the high incidence of postoperative deaths), particularly for patients undergoing a right-sided pneumonectomy. If the patient is a borderline surgical candidate, treatment should consist of chemotherapy plus thoracic radiation therapy.
- Bulky N2 nodes — chemotherapy plus radiation therapy is indicated. The presence of pathologically involved N2 nodes should be confirmed histologically, because enlarged nodes detected by CT will be pathologically negative for approximately 30% of patients. The age, performance status, and comorbid conditions of the patient must be considered. If the patient has an excellent performance status, concurrent chemoradiotherapy is likely to provide a small survival benefit, albeit at the expense of enhanced toxicity. Weekly, low-dose, concurrent chemotherapy has not been compared with full-dose chemotherapy in randomized trials, although it is often administered concurrently with radiation therapy if proceeded or followed by two to three cycles of standard-dose chemotherapy.

STAGE IV DISEASE

Chemotherapy improves survival for patients with metastatic non-small cell lung cancer (a 1-year survival rate of approximately 10% for untreated patients compared with 35% to 40% for treated patients). In addition, chemotherapy can reduce symptoms and improve quality of life; therefore, it is usually recommended for patients with good performance status. Because chemotherapy is not curative, goals for treatment that should be discussed with the patient include palliation of symptoms and a modest improvement in survival.

The principal factors that are predictors of response to chemotherapy and survival are performance status and extent of disease. Favorable prognostic factors include no weight loss, female sex, normal level of serum lactate dehydrogenase, and no bone or liver metastases.

First-line Chemotherapy

Chemotherapy for metastatic non-small cell lung cancer has traditionally consisted of a platinum-based regimen. Results from randomized studies also have shown an improvement in survival, symptomatology, and quality of life for patients treated with cisplatin-based therapy compared with patients treated with best supportive care. The median survival and 1-year survival rates have increasingly improved with use of second-generation and third-generation chemotherapy regimens (Table 6-8). Findings from numerous randomized studies have not shown an advantage of one new doublet regimen compared with another, although there are differences in toxicity, cost, schedule, and convenience.

Recently, an Eastern Cooperative Oncology Group (ECOG) phase III trial of 878 patients randomly assigned to chemotherapy (paclitaxel and carboplatin) or to chemotherapy plus bevacizumab has been reported.[22] Median survival for patients who received chemotherapy plus bevacizumab was 12.3 months compared with 10.3 months for those who received chemotherapy alone (HR = 0.79, $p = 0.003$). The median duration of progression-free survival for patients who received chemotherapy plus bevacizumab was 6.2 months compared with 4.5 months for those who received chemotherapy alone (HR = 0.66, $p < 0.001$), with corresponding response rates of 35% and 15%, respectively ($p < 0.001$). However, because of the grades III through V bleeding episodes observed in the phase II study that preceded this one, it should be noted that eligibility to this study was restricted to patients with non-squamous cell carcinoma, no brain metastases, and no hemoptysis, bleeding disorders, or anticoagulation requirement. Despite these restrictions, significant bleeding was more frequent for patients who received chemotherapy plus bevacizumab (4.4% vs. 0.9%, $p = 0.001$). There were 15 treatment-related deaths in the group of patients who received chemotherapy plus bevacizumab, including five as a result of pulmonary hemorrhage. Thus, it is the role of the treating physician to explain the risks and benefits of bevacizumab to their patients with advance non-small cell lung cancer.

Older Patients. Treatment of older patients (age 65 or older) tends to be complicated by comorbid conditions and multiple medications. However, studies show that fit older patients are likely to benefit as much from chemotherapy as their younger counterparts. Evidence from a phase III study in which patients older than 70 with advanced disease were randomly assigned to best supportive care or to weekly vinorelbine indicated that patients who received vinorelbine had better scores on quality-of-life scales than the control group, as well as fewer lung cancer-related symptoms; however, patients in the chemotherapy group experienced more severe toxicity-related symptoms.[63] There was a significant survival advantage for patients who received vinorelbine (median survival, 28 weeks vs. 21 weeks). Subset analyses of other randomized trials show that the response rate, toxicity, and survival for fit older patients with non-small cell lung cancer receiving platinum-based treatment appear to be similar to the same variables for younger patients; however, for patients age 70 or older, comorbidity is greater and the frequency of leukopenia and neuropsychiatric toxicity is higher. Hence, advanced age alone should not preclude appropriate treatment.

Patients with Poor Performance Status. The survival rates for patients with a poor performance status ECOG performance status of 2, 3, or 4) is significantly shorter than the rates for patients with a good performance status. Patients with a poor performance status also are less likely to tolerate treatment. Retrospective, subset analyses suggest that patients with a performance status of 2 may derive a benefit from chemotherapy. However, given the overall short survival — particularly for patients with a performance status of 3 or 4 — and the minimal benefit derived from chemotherapy, these patients probably should not be treated outside of a clinical study.

TABLE 6-8 Survival Rates for Chemotherapy for Non-small Cell Lung Cancer

	Chemotherapy Agents	Median Survival (months)	1-year Survival (%)	2-year Survival (%)
Best supportive care only		4–5	5–10	< 5
First-generation chemotherapy regimens	Cisplatin, vinblastine, mitomycin, vindesine	5–6	10–15	< 5
Second-generation chemotherapy regimens	Carboplatin, etoposide	6	20–25	< 10
Third-generation chemotherapy regimens	Paclitaxel and docetaxel, gemcitabine, vinorelbine, irinotecan	8–9	35–40	10
Non-squamous cell No brain metastases No hemoptysis No anticoagulants	Carboplatin and paclitaxel plus bevacizumab	12	50	20

TABLE 6-9 Randomized Trials of Maintenance Chemotherapy for Advanced Non-small Cell Lung Cancer*

Authors	Treatment Comparison	Median Survival (months)	1-year Survival (%)
Depierre et al.[64]	Vinorelbine vs.	13	53
	best supportive care	10	40
Socinski et al.[65]	Four cycles of carboplatin plus paclitaxel	7	28
	Carboplatin plus paclitaxel at disease progression	9	35
Smith et al.[66]	Three cycles of mitomycin-C, vindesine, and cisplatin	6	22
	Six cycles of same regimen	7	25

*None of the differences found in any study were significant.
†Random assignment was done after patients had a complete or partial response to induction chemotherapy.

Duration of Therapy. Results from three randomized studies did not show a survival difference with prolonged (more than six) cycles of chemotherapy compared with fewer (four to six) cycles (Table 6-9).[64–66] Thus, continuing chemotherapy until disease progression cannot be routinely recommended.

Number of Drugs. Although the findings from numerous phase I and II studies have demonstrated the feasibility of triplet combinations, the results of most randomized trials have not demonstrated a survival advantage and have been at the expense of enhanced toxicity and cost. Thus, three-drug regimens cannot be routinely recommended, with the exception of bevacizumab with a platinum-based doublet for patients with non-squamous non-small cell lung cancer.

In randomized studies, single-agent paclitaxel, gemcitabine, or docetaxel was compared with double-agent cisplatin plus either paclitaxel, gemcitabine, or docetaxel (Table 6-10).[67–75] The findings from all these trials showed a survival advantage for the two-drug regimens. These results can be interpreted either as demonstrating the advantages of cisplatin for the treatment of advanced non-small cell lung cancer or as evidence of the superiority of doublet compared with single-agent therapy.

Treatment with a platinum-based doublet represents the standard of care in North America for patients with advanced disease.

Cisplatin versus Carboplatin. Meta-analyses have suggested that cisplatin may have a small benefit in terms of survival compared with carboplatin for patients with advanced disease, albeit with a different toxicity profile.[76,77] Whereas this small difference may be of limited clinical consequence for patients with metastatic disease, it may be more important in the adjuvant setting, where cure is the goal.

Nonplatin-based Regimens. Given the toxicities associated with cisplatin, there is considerable interest in combining nonplatinum agents. In general, the findings from most recent randomized studies show similar outcomes with nonplatinum regimens compared with platinum-based regimens.[78]

SECOND-LINE CHEMOTHERAPY

In two randomized trials, second-line docetaxel was evaluated for patients for whom first-line therapy failed. In one trial, docetaxel at a dose of 75 mg/m^2 significantly prolonged survival compared with best supportive care.[79] Although this dose of docetaxel resulted in a response rate of 7% and had no effect on overall survival for this patient

KEY POINTS

- Cytotoxic chemotherapy improves survival and symptomatology for patients with metastatic non-small cell lung cancer. In general:
- Two drugs (or "doublets") are used for patients with good performance status.
- Of the doublets tested, no one doublet has been shown to have a major advantage in terms of efficacy. They differ in terms of cost, side effects, and schedule.
- Non-platin doublets probably have roughly the same efficacy as platin-based doublets.
- Four to six cycles are usually administered.
- Bevacizumab prolongs survival when administered with carboplatin/paclitaxel in a subset of patients (those with non-squamous cell carcinoma, no brain metastases, no significant hemoptysis, and patients not requiring anticoagulation therapy).
- The fit elderly tolerate chemotherapy and derive the same survival benefit as their younger counterparts.

TABLE 6-10 Randomized Trials of Single Drugs Compared with Cisplatin-based Doublets

Study	Therapy	Overall Response	Median Survival (months)	1-year (%)	Overall Survival (p value)
Wozniak et al.[67] (432 patients)	Cisplatin;	12	6	20	
	Cisplatin/vinorelbine	26	8	36	0.0018
Sandler et al.[68] (522 patients)	Cisplatin;	11	8	28	
	Cisplatin/gemcitabine	30	9	39	0.004
Von Pawel et al.[69] (446 patients)	Cisplatin;	14	7	23	
	Cisplatin/tirapazamine	28	9	34	0.0078
Gatzemeier et al.[70] (414 patients)	Cisplatin;	17	9	36	
	Cisplatin/paclitaxel	26	8	30	NS
LeChevalier et al.[71] (612 patients)	Vinorelbine;	14	8	30	
	Cisplatin/vinorelbine	30	10	35	0.01*
Lilenbaum et al.[72] (584 patients)	Paclitaxel;	17		33	
	Carboplatin/paclitaxel	29	9	37	< 0.05
Sederholm[73] (67 patients)	Gemcitabine;	12	9	32	
	Carboplatin/gemcitabine	30	11	44	0.0024
Gerogoulias et al.[74] (307 patients)	Docetaxel;	20	8	40	
	Cisplatin/docetaxel	36	19	45	NS
Negoro et al.[75] (398 patients)	Irinotecan;	21	12	—	NS
	Cisplatin/vindesine;	32	11	—	
	Cisplatin/irinotecan	44	13	—	

NS = not significant.
*For comparison of cisplatin/vinorelbine with vinorelbine only.

population, response to the drug included improved time to disease progression and improved 1-year survival. Moreover, response also improved quality of life. Previous exposure to paclitaxel did not affect response to docetaxel, suggesting no cross-resistance between the two agents. In the second study, docetaxel was compared with either vinorelbine or ifosfamide.[80] Although overall survival was not significantly different among the three groups, the 1-year survival associated with docetaxel was significantly better than that associated with the control treatment (32% vs. 19%; p = 0.025).

A phase III study compared pemetrexed with docetaxel.[81] Although no difference in survival was observed (1-year survival of 29.7% in both arms), patients randomly assigned to receive docetaxel were more likely to have febrile neutropenia (12.7% vs. 1.9%; p = 0.001), infections (3.3% vs. 0%; p = 0.004), and hospitalizations for neutropenic fevers (13.4% vs. 1.5%; p = 0.001) than patients who received pemetrexed, thus resulting in the U.S. Food and Drug Administration approval of pemetrexed as second-line therapy for non-small cell lung cancer.

THIRD-LINE CHEMOTHERAPY

Gefitinib and erlotinib are tyrosine kinase inhibitors of the EGF pathway. Erlotinib was approved in the United States for patients with non-small cell lung cancer for whom both a taxane and a platinum drug have failed, based in large part on a randomized, placebo-controlled, double-blinded clinical trial conducted by the National Cancer Institute of Canada, BR21. In BR21, patients with stage IIIB or IV non-small cell lung cancer and a performance status of 0 to 3 who had received one or two prior chemotherapy regimens were randomly assigned in a 2:1 ratio to receive oral erlotinib, at a dose of 150 mg daily, or to placebo.[20] Overall survival rates were 6.7 months and 4.7 months for erlotinib and placebo, respectively (HR = 0.70; p < 0.001). The interaction between erlotinib was only found in smoking status, where current or former smokers had a hazard ration of 0.9, and never-smokers had a hazard ratio of 0.4.

The prognostic and predictive value of *EGFR* mutations and expression remains an area of active investigation.[82] In BR21, in a multivariate analysis, survival was longer for patients who received erlotinib and whose disease expressed *EGFR* by fluorescent in situ hybridization (FISH) or immunochemistry (IHC) than it was among patients with EGFR-positive disease who received placebo (HR = 0.64) or among patients with EGFR-negative disease, regardless of treatment group (HR = 0.93). Mutational status had no effect on survival.[83] In another study, amplification or high polysomy of the *EGFR* and high protein expression were statistically significantly associated with better response (36% vs. 3%; mean difference, 34%; 95% CI; 16.6, 50.3; $p < 0.001$), disease control rate (67% vs. 26%; $p < 0.001$), time to progression (9.0 vs. 2.5 months, $p < 0.001$), and survival (18.7 vs. 7.0 months; $p = 0.03$).[21] Although *EGFR* mutations (seen in 15 of 89 patients) also were statistically significantly related to response and time to progression, the association with survival was not statistically significant, and 40% of the patients with mutation had progressive disease. In a multivariable analysis, only a high *EGFR* gene copy number remained statistically significantly associated with better survival (HR = 0.44; 95% CI; 0.23, 0.82). However, it should be noted that this was a retrospective subgroup analysis, and prospective randomized studies are planned or underway. Other smaller, single-arm prospective phase II studies have demonstrated high response rates for patients treated with EGFR tyrosine kinase inhibitors.[84]

Unlike what is commonly seen with standard cytotoxic drugs, no decrease in response rate with the EGFR tyrosine kinase inhibitors was found with an increase in the number of prior chemotherapy regimens. In addition to its oral route of administration, the other advantage of erlotinib is its side effect profile; the most common side effects — rash and diarrhea — are rarely severe. Although interstitial pneumonitis has been reported with gefitinib and erlotinib, this potentially severe side effect is rare in the United States.[85]

Isolated Brain Metastases. For patients with controlled disease outside of the brain who have an isolated cerebral metastasis in a resectable area, resection followed by whole-brain radiation therapy is superior to whole-brain radiation therapy alone and may improve survival. Another therapeutic option for tumors smaller than 3 cm in diameter is stereotactic radiosurgery, which uses a stereotactic fixation system and noncoplanar convergent beams that create a sharp peripheral dose falloff along the edge of the target. Stereotactic radiosurgery spares the surrounding normal tissue, enabling the use of a single, large fraction of radiation. Survival is improved when administered with whole-brain radiation therapy.

SMALL CELL LUNG CANCER

STAGING

Because of the propensity of small cell lung cancer to metastasize quickly and the fact that micrometastatic disease is presumed to be present in all patients at the time of diagnosis, the disease is usually classified into either limited or extensive stage. Limited-stage disease is typically defined as being encompassed within one radiation port, and is usually limited to the hemithorax and to regional nodes, including mediastinal and ipsilateral supraclavicular nodes. Extensive-stage disease is usually defined as disease that has spread outside those areas.

PROGNOSTIC FACTORS

As with non-small cell lung cancer, the major pretreatment prognostic factors are stage of disease, performance status, serum lactic acid dehydrogenase, and gender. If the patient's initial poor performance status is the result of the underlying malignant disease, symptoms often disappear quickly with treatment, resulting in a net improvement in quality of life. However, major organ dysfunction from nonmalignant causes often results in an inability of the patient to tolerate chemotherapy.

PRETREATMENT EVALUATION

Common sites of metastases include the brain, liver, bone marrow, bone, and the CNS. For this reason, a complete staging work-up consists of a complete blood cell count, liver function tests, CT scan of chest and upper abdomen, CT or MRI of the brain, bone scan, and evaluation of bone marrow aspirate. However, this work-up should not be undertaken unless the patient is a candidate for combined-modality treatment with chest radiation and chemotherapy, the patient is being evaluated for a clinical study, or the information is helpful for prognostic reasons. If the patient is not a candidate for combined-modality treatment or a clinical study, it is usually appropriate to stop the staging at the first evidence of extensive-stage disease. In addition, because the chance of metastases to only the bone marrow is less than 10%, biopsy of bone marrow is usually unnecessary except in certain cases of limited-stage disease, where demonstration of localized disease may be important for psychosocial reasons or for eligibility for a clinical study. A PET scan can provide useful information and can replace the bone scan.

KEY POINTS

- Etoposide with either cisplatin or carboplatin remains the standard of care for the treatment of patients with small cell lung cancer, with an optimum duration of four to six cycles.
- Concurrent chemotherapy and thoracic radiation confers a survival benefit for patients with limited-stage small cell lung cancer, as does prophylactic cranial irradiation for patients who have a complete response to therapy.
- Second-line chemotherapy for small cell lung cancer is ineffective for patients in whom first-line treatment failed within 2 to 3 months.
- Small cell lung cancer often demonstrates features of neuroendocrine differentiation, which may be identified histopathologically, and it is associated with paraneoplastic syndromes.
- Small cell lung cancer is exquisitely sensitive to both chemotherapy and radiation therapy, although resistant disease often develops.

TREATMENT

The cornerstone of treatment of patients with small cell lung cancer is combination platinum-based chemotherapy. Until recently, no clear survival advantage was demonstrated for any one regimen. With standard chemotherapy — etoposide with either cisplatin or carboplatin — an overall response rate of 75% to 90% and a complete response rate of 50% for localized disease can be anticipated. For extensive-stage disease, an overall response rate of approximately 50% and a complete response rate of approximately 25% are common. Tumor regressions usually occur quickly, often within the first two cycles of treatment, and provide rapid palliation of tumor-related symptoms. Despite these high response rates, the median survival time remains approximately 14 months for limited-stage disease and 9 months for extensive-stage disease. Less than 5% of patients with extensive-stage disease survive more than 2 years. Although initial results of irinotecan plus cisplatin showed improved survival compared with etoposide plus cisplatin in a Japanese population, these results were not confirmed in a non Asian population.[86]

Dose Intensity

Dose intensity has been evaluated in a number of randomized studies. Most — although not all — failed to show a benefit in survival, regardless of whether the chemotherapy was delivered in higher doses or more frequently (dose density). In addition, a meta-analysis of chemotherapy dose intensity for small cell lung cancer, in which doses not requiring bone marrow transplantation support were evaluated, showed no consistent correlation between dose intensity and outcome.[87] The role of marrow-ablative doses of chemotherapy with subsequent progenitor cell replacement (e.g., autologous bone marrow transplantation) was evaluated in several phase I and II clinical trials, and the results for survival were not promising. In a randomized phase III study, when high-dose chemotherapy was compared with conventional-dose chemotherapy, the high-dose regimen with stem cell support prolonged relapse-free survival but not overall survival.[88]

Duration and Maintenance of Therapy

The findings from most randomized studies do not show a survival benefit for prolonged administration of chemotherapy or for consolidation chemotherapy. The results of several randomized studies have demonstrated no survival benefit for prolonged first-line treatment when compared with treatment initiated on relapse. The optimal duration of treatment for patients with small cell lung cancer is four to six cycles.

Second-line Therapy

No curative regimens for patients with recurrent disease have been identified. The chance of response to second-line agents is related to when the relapse occurred following induction chemotherapy; patients who experience relapse more than 3 months after completing first-line chemotherapy are considered to have sensitive disease and are more likely to have a response than patients who experience disease progression during or within 2 to 3 months after receiving a first-line regimen (resistant disease). The only drug approved for second-line therapy for small cell lung cancer in the United States is topotecan, which is associated with a 20% to 40% response rate for patients with sensitive disease and with a median survival of 22 to 27 weeks.[89] For patients with refractory disease, the response rate in phase II studies has ranged from 3% to 11%. The median survival is approximately 20 weeks. Patients with sensitive disease also may have a response to repeat treatment with the first-line regimen. Other drugs that have modest activity in phase II studies in the second-line setting include combination cyclophosphamide, doxorubicin, and vincristine, as well as paclitaxel.

Older Patients

As is the case with non-small cell lung cancer, treatment of older patients is often complicated by poor performance status and comorbid conditions. However, unlike older patients with non-small cell lung cancer, older patients with small cell lung cancer do not benefit from single-agent therapy. Two randomized studies, in which single-agent etoposide was compared with standard combination chemotherapy, were stopped early because the single-agent arm was associated with a shorter median and long-term survival, greater toxicity, and decreased quality of life.[90,91] Therefore, the standard treatment of fit older patients remains combination chemotherapy administered on a 3-week schedule.

Chemotherapy plus Radiation to the Thorax

Radiation therapy to the thorax is associated with a small, significant improvement in long-term survival for patients with limited-stage disease (rates of approximately 5% at 3 years).[92] Chemotherapy given concurrently with thoracic radiation is superior to sequential chemoradiation in terms of survival; however, it is associated with substantially more esophagitis and hematologic toxicity. To decrease the morbidity associated with such treatment, as well as to improve overall outcome, investigative efforts have focused on optimizing the radiation fields, fractionation, and schedule. In one randomized study, twice-daily, hyperfractionated radiation was compared with a once-daily schedule; both were administered concurrently with four cycles of cisplatin and etoposide. Survival was significantly higher with the twice-daily regimen (median survival, 23 months vs. 19 months; 5-year survival, 26% vs. 16%), albeit at the expense of more grade 3 esophagitis.[93] In another randomized trial, early administration of thoracic radiation as part of the combined-modality therapy for limited-stage disease was superior to late or consolidative thoracic radiation.[94] These data suggest that patients with good performance status who have limited disease should receive concurrent chemoradiation, preferably administered twice daily in an accelerated, hyperfractionated approach.

Prophylactic Cranial Irradiation

Brain-only metastases is the first site of relapse for approximately one-third of all patients who have relapsing small cell lung cancers; another one-third of such patients will have both brain and systemic metastases as the first site of relapse, and the remaining one-third of patients will have systemic-only disease. Because of the morbidity associated with brain metastases, the role of prophylactic cranial irradiation has been studied in numerous randomized trials. These findings have generally demonstrated that prophylactic cranial irradiation does not enhance survival, although it does decrease the risk of brain metastases by approximately one-half without enhanced neurotoxicities, including cognitive dysfunction, ataxia, and seizures. However, in a meta-analysis of seven randomized trials, prophylactic cranial irradiation was shown to increase 3-year survival, with a net gain of 5%.[95] Typically, in the United States, patients are administered 24 Gy in 12 fractions. However, the optimal dose and schedule are not clear; the meta-analysis demonstrated a trend toward improved control with higher doses.

Although prophylactic cranial irradiation had been generally reserved for patients with limited-stage disease in whom a complete response is achieved with induction chemotherapy, a recent report from the European Organisation for Research and Treatment of Cancer also showed a survival benefit for patients with extensive-stage disease who had a response to their induction chemotherapy.[96] Thus, prophylactic cranial irradiation should be considered for all patients who have complete or very good partial remission after induction therapy.

PALLIATION

APPROACHES TO PALLIATION

Radiation Therapy

Palliative radiation therapy often is helpful for controlling pain related to bone metastases or for improving neurologic function for patients with brain metastases. Radiation therapy to the thorax may help control hemoptysis, superior vena cava syndrome, airway obstruction, laryngeal nerve compression, and other local complications.

Chemotherapy

In randomized trials involving patients with non-small cell lung cancer and patients with small cell lung cancer, chemotherapy has been shown to reduce the incidence of cancer-related symptoms such as pain, cough, hemoptysis, and shortness of breath.

Colony-stimulating Factors

Filgrastim, a granulocyte colony-stimulating factor (CSF), decreases the incidence of neutropenic fevers, the median duration of neutropenia, days of hospitalization, and days of antibiotic treatment for patients with extensive-stage small cell lung cancer. However, as discussed previously, the clinical benefit of maintaining a dose-intense approach for patients with this disease has not been established. In addition, caution must be exercised when using a CSF for patients receiving combined-modality treatment that consists of both chemotherapy and radiation therapy to the thorax, as this combination has been associated with an increase in thrombocytopenia.

Palliation for Complications

Palliative measures should be considered for potential complications, such as superior vena cava syndrome, pleural effusion, bronchial obstruction, cachexia, bone metastases, and brain metastases (Table 6-11).

Superior Vena Cava Syndrome

Superior vena cava syndrome occurs when the superior vena cava becomes obstructed either directly by a tumor or by metastases to regional lymph nodes. Common symptoms include distension of the collateral veins over the anterior chest wall and neck; swelling and puffiness of the neck, face, throat, eyes, and arms; headache; and cyanosis. Although once thought to represent a medical emergency, in almost all cases, the symptoms are mild enough that treatment can be delayed until a histologic diagnosis has been determined. Radiation therapy is used to treat patients with non-small cell lung cancer or other less chemosensitive tumors, whereas patients with extensive-stage small cell lung cancer and mild symptoms may often be treated with chemotherapy alone. Concurrent chemoradiation therapy usually is necessary for patients with both small cell and non-small cell lung cancer who present with severe symptoms. Other options include the placement of stents, although the literature regarding their role is relatively sparse.

Pleural Effusion

Palliative thoracentesis should be done for patients who are symptomatic from pleural effusions, and management with intermittent thoracentesis can frequently be effective if the effusion does not reaccumulate quickly. When reaccumulation is rapid, pleurodesis may be considered. The two most common methods of a pleurodesis are through a chest tube or thoracoscopy. Common sclerosing agents include doxycycline, talc, and bleomycin; talc is the most effective. Long-term drainage through a catheter may be helpful for patients with recurrent effusions or patients who are not

KEY POINT

- Every attempt should be made to palliate the symptoms of patients with lung cancer.

TABLE 6-11 Palliative Approaches to Complications

- Superior Vena Cava Syndrome
  - Chemotherapy alone (mild symptoms)
  - Concurrent chemoradiation therapy (severe symptoms)
  - Radiation therapy to the thorax (patients with non-small cell lung cancer)
  - Placement of stent
- Pleural Effusion
  - Intermittent thoracentesis
  - Pleurodesis
  - Long-term catheter drainage
  - Systemic chemotherapy
- Bronchial Obstruction
  - High-dose endobronchial radiation therapy
  - Placement of stent
  - Nd-YAG endobronchial laser therapy
  - Electrocautery
  - Photodynamic therapy
- Cachexia
  - Megestrol acetate (160 - 800 mg daily)
- Bone Metastases
  - Bisphosphonates (pamidronate or zoledronate)
- Brain Metastases
  - Corticosteroids
  - Resection or stereotactic radiation and whole brain radiation (for isolated brain metastases for patients with non-small cell lung cancer)
  - Whole-brain radiation therapy (for multiple metastases)

candidates for a pleurodesis. Systemic chemotherapy often reduces the effusion for patients with small cell lung cancer.

THYMOMAS

The thymus contains two major cell populations, epithelial cells and lymphocytes. A number of different tumors can arise in the thymus, including thymomas, Hodgkin's and non-Hodgkin's lymphomas, carcinoid tumors, and germ cell neoplasms. Thymomas are malignant neoplasms originating within the epithelial cells of the thymus, which often contain admixtures of lymphocytes.[97] Thymic cancers also are tumors of the thymic epithelium, but they are associated with a paucity of lymphocytes and are more aggressive.

The nomenclature for the histologic subclassification of thymic malignancies is under discussion. Although some subtypes of thymoma may have more invasive potential, prognosis is more commonly associated with the invasiveness of the tumor. Most thymomas are well encapsulated, but they are considered malignant because of their invasive potential. Cytokeratin is a useful diagnostic marker to distinguish thymomas from non-epithelial cell malignancies.

Thymomas are the most common anterior mediastinal tumors in adults, representing approximately 20% to 30% of all anterior mediastinal tumors. Although they usually present in the fourth and fifth decades of life, cases have been reported from infancy into the ninth decade. At presentation, one-third of patients have an asymptomatic anterior mediastinal mass on chest x-ray; one-third have local symptoms such as cough, superior vena cava syndrome, and dysphagia; and one-third have myasthenia gravis. Distant metastases are uncommon, with the most common metastatic site being the pleura. Staging of thymomas is based on invasion into surrounding tissue.

A number of paraneoplastic syndromes have been associated with thymomas. Myasthenia gravis, an autoimmune disorder caused by circulating acetylcholine-receptor antibodies resulting in acetylcholine-receptor deficiency at the motor end plate, occurs in approximately one-third of patients with thymoma, although it is rarely seen with thymic cancers. Approximately two-thirds of patients with myasthenia gravis will have thymic lymphoid hyperplasia, and 10% to 15% will have thymoma. This syndrome is characterized by diploplia, dysphagia, weakness of the ocular muscles, and limb muscles that are easily fatigued (the proximal muscles more so than the distal ones). Interestingly, thymomas associated with myasthenia gravis tend to be less aggressive, and histologically, they tend to have a larger lymphocyte-to-epithelial cell ratio. Other paraneoplastic syndromes include pure red cell aplasia, hypogammaglobulenemia and other autoimmune disorders, and vasculitides. Surgical removal of all thymic tissue, not just tumor tissue, usually results in an attenuation of the severity of myasthenia gravis, although complete disappearance of all symptoms of the disorder is uncommon. Thymectomy may result in normalization of the bone marrow for up to 40% of patients with pure red cell aplasia, although the procedure rarely results in return of normal immunoglobulin levels for patients with immunodeficiency.

The treatment of choice for thymomas is resection. Long-term survival for patients with encapsulated, noninvasive

KEY POINTS

- Thymomas are often encapsulated, well differentiated, and associated with paraneoplastic syndromes such as myasthenia gravis.
- The optimal treatment of thymomas is thymectomy and complete surgical resection, in which case the survival is excellent.
- Thymic carcinomas are more aggressive than thymomas.

(stage I) tumors is excellent, approaching 90% to 95% at 10 years. The negative prognostic factors include:

- tumor size greater than 10 cm,
- tracheal or vascular compromise,
- age younger than 30 years,
- presence of hematologic paraneoplastic syndromes, and
- extent of the surgical resection.

Some oncologists recommend postoperative radiation for all patients with thymoma regardless of stage, although for patients with encapsulated tumors (stage I), the risk of recurrence is low. Adjuvant postoperative radiation therapy is recommended for all patients with invasive disease. For patients in whom complete resection is not possible because of extensive invasion, debulking with a subtotal resection followed by radiation therapy may result in improved survival.

The optimal management of incompletely resected or unresectable thymomas is controversial. Thymomas are chemosensitive tumors, and thus debulking with chemotherapy for inoperable tumors is being investigated. In one small series, combination cyclophosphamide, doxorubicin, and cisplatin yielded a response rate of 70%.[98]

Thymic cancers are aggressive and characterized by a high degree of histologic anaplasia and architectural atypia. A number of different subtypes have been described, although more than half are undifferentiated.

MALIGNANT MESOTHELIOMA

Mesotheliomas arise from mesothelial cells, the cells that form the serosal lining of the pleura, pericardium, and peritoneal cavities. Although benign mesotheliomas have been described, most are malignant neoplasms with an aggressive clinical course.[99]

Malignant mesotheliomas are rare, with approximately 2,500 new cases diagnosed annually in the United States. Although approximately 80% are associated with exposure to asbestos, only approximately 5% of asbestos workers are diagnosed with mesothelioma. In contrast to lung cancer and asbestosis, smoking does not increase the risk of mesothelioma. Unlike asbestosis, in which there is a dose-response relationship, this association does not exist for mesothelioma, with the exception of chrysotile asbestos, which may be oncogenic only at high doses.

The various types of asbestos are divided into two major groups: serpentine, represented by chrysotile, the most common form of asbestos in the Western world; and rod-like amphiboles, which include crocidolite, the most oncogenic type of asbestos.

Carcinogenic effects of asbestos appear to result from its physical properties rather than from its chemical structure, with long, rod-like fibers of narrow diameter being more likely to induce tumors in laboratory animals. It is postulated that chrysotile asbestos fibers are less carcinogenic because the fibers can be partially digested and removed from the lung, whereas amphibole asbestos is more resistant to solubalization by cellular enzymes and accumulates in the lungs. The fibers cause mutagenic changes by several different mechanisms, including direct physical effects on chromosomes; the production of hydroxyl radicals and superoxide anions leading to DNA-strand breaks and deletions; stimulation of the autophosphorylation of the EGFR, leading to a cascade of mutagenic signaling; and increased production of inflammatory cytokines. The expression of the Simian virus 40 large-tumor antigen in mesothelioma cells and not nearby normal cells, and the capacity of antisense T-antigen treatment to arrest mesothelioma cell growth in vitro, suggest that Simian virus 40 also may be a contributing factor to the development of mesothelioma, particularly for patients exposed to asbestos. Mesothelioma also has been associated with Thorotrast exposure and radiation.

Three histologic variants of mesothelioma have been described: epithelial, which is the most common form and is associated with the best prognosis; sarcomatoid; and mixed. To distinguish mesotheliomas from metastatic adenocarcinomas, the periodic acid-Schiff stain is frequently used before and after diastase digestion. Neutral mucopolysaccharides that are strongly positive to periodic acid-Schiff stain are found in intracellular secretory vacuoles and in intra-acinar vacuoles in most adenocarcinomas but are rarely found in most mesotheliomas. Immunoperoxidase staining for Leu M1, Mayer's mucicarmine stain, and carcinoembryonic antigen are usually absent in mesotheliomas but positive in most adenocarcinomas.

Mesothelioma most commonly develops in the fifth to seventh decade, and it affects men and women in a ratio of 5:1. The onset of disease occurs 20 to 50 years after exposure. Family members also are at higher risk of mesothelioma, presumably because of exposure to asbestos fibers brought home on the clothing and bodies of individuals who work with asbestos.

The typical presentation consists of dyspnea or chest wall pain secondary to a pleural effusion. A total of 60% of mesotheliomas occur on the right side, and bilateral involvement of the chest wall is present at the time of diagnosis in less than 5% of cases. Repeated cytologic examination of pleural fluid may be negative, necessitating either a thoracoscopy or thoracotomy, despite the risk of seeding the biopsy site or surgical scar with tumor.

Mesotheliomas tend to be locally invasive. For approximately 20% of patients, a chest wall mass develops over tracts resulting from thoracentesis, chest tubes, or thoracotomy. Direct involvement of the ribs, diaphragm, pericardium, and vertebrae is common. Although various staging classifications have been described, the most recent staging system proposed by the International Mesothelioma Interest Group emphasizes the importance of local extent of the tumor and nodal involvement.[100]

Extrapleural pneumonectomy should be considered for stage I disease (tumor confined within the capsule of the parietal pleura, e.g., involving only the ipsilateral lung, pericardium, and diaphragm). Extrapleural pneumonectomy includes en bloc resection of the parietal pleura, lung pericardium, and diaphragm. Given the extent of the resection and long duration of anesthesia needed, this procedure should be reserved for patients younger than 65 who are in good health. The entire hemithorax is at risk of recurrence because mesotheliomas arise from the pleura; thus, curative radiation would necessitate exposing large volumes of normal tissue, and as such, this treatment is limited by the tumor volume and normal tissue toxicities. The best results have been described in a retrospective series reported by Sugarbaker et al,[101] in which the median survival was 21 months for 120 patients treated with extrapleural pneumonectomy, four to six cycles of adjuvant chemotherapy, and adjuvant radiation therapy to the ipsilateral hemithorax and mediastinum. Patients with pure epithelial type and no nodal involvement had a significantly better outcome than patients with sarcomatous/mixed histology or nodal involvement. The 2-year and 5-year survival rates for the 39 patients with epithelial tumors and negative lymph nodes were 74% and 39%, respectively, compared with 52% and 10% for the 28 patients with epithelial histology and positive lymph nodes, and 20% and 0% for patients with a sarcomatous/ mixed histology.

For patients with unresectable disease, effusions may be controlled by thoracoscopy with talc pleurodesis. Pleurectomy with decortication — which involves resection of the parietal, mediastinal, and diaphragmatic pleura and involved viscera, but the lung remains in place — although rarely curative, also can be used to control effusions. Smaller doses of radiation (21 Gy in three fractions) prevent seeding of the surgical wound by mesothelioma cells.

The prognosis is poor for patients who have unresectable disease at the time of presentation, with a median survival of approximately 12 months. Single-agent chemotherapy yields response rates of 5% to 20%, with the most active agents being doxorubicin and cisplatin.[86,102,103] Combination chemotherapy, which is usually cisplatin based, typically yields a response rate of 15% to 20%. Although single-agent gemcitabine is associated with a response rate of 12% or less, findings from a phase II study of gemcitabine plus cisplatin showed a 48% response rate.[104,105] The best results have been reported with pemetrexed and cisplatin. Pemetrexed inhibits intracellular folate-responsive enzymes, including thymidylate synthase, dihydrofolate reductase, and glycinamide ribonucleotide formyltransferase. Findings from a phase III study, in which cisplatin was compared with cisplatin plus pemetrexed, demonstrated a 9-month median survival for patients treated with cisplatin alone and a 12-month survival for patients treated with the combination ($p = 0.02$), making this regimen the standard of care for patients with advanced mesothelioma.[105]

KEY POINTS

- Approximately 80% of mesotheliomas are associated with exposure to asbestos, including indirect exposure.
- The epithelial histologic form of mesothelioma is associated with a better prognosis than the sarcomatoid or mixed forms.
- A trimodality approach consisting of extrapleural pneumonectomy, chemotherapy, and postoperative radiation therapy should be considered for younger patients with good performance status, particularly patients with negative mediastinal nodes and the epithelial variant.

REFERENCES

1. Jemal A, Siegel R, Ward E, et al. Cancer Statistics, 2006. *CA Cancer J Clin.* 2006;56(2):106–30.
2. Brownson RC, Chang JC, Davis JR. Gender and histologic type variations in smoking-related risk of lung cancer. *Epidemiology.* 1992;3(1):61–64.
3. Alberg A, Samet J. Epidemiology of lung cancer. *Chest.* 2003;123 (1 Suppl):21S–49S.
4. Ebbert JO, Yang P, Vachon CM, et al. Lung cancer risk reduction after smoking cessation: observations from a prospective cohort of women. *J Clin Oncol.* 2003;21(5):921–926.
5. Omenn G, Goodman G, Thornquist M, et al. Effects of a combination of beta carotene and vitamin A on lung cancer and cardiovascular disease. *N Engl J Med.* 1996;334(18):1150–1155.
6. The Alpha-Tocopherol, Beta Carotene Cancer Prevention Study Group. The effect of vitamin E and beta carotene on the incidence of lung cancer and other cancers in male smokers. *N Engl J Med.* 1994;330(15):1029–1035.
7. Menkes MS, Comstock GW, Vuilleumier JP, et al. Serum beta-carotene, vitamins A and E, selenium, and the risk of lung cancer. *N Engl J Med.* 1986;315(20):1250–1254.
8. Gorlova OY, Weng SF, Zhang Y, et al. Aggregation of cancer among relatives of never-smoking lung cancer patients. *Int J Cancer.* 2007;121(1):111–118.
9. Peluso M, Munnia A, Hoek G, et al. DNA adducts and lung cancer risk: a prospective study. *Cancer Res.* 2005;65(17):8042–8048.
10. Bennett WP, Alavanja MC, Blomeke B, et al. Environmental tobacco smoke, genetic susceptibility, and risk of lung cancer in never-smoking women. *J Natl Cancer Inst.* 1999;91(23):2009–2014.
11. Travis W. Pathology of lung cancer. *Clin Chest Med.* 2002;23(1):65–81.
12. Travis W. High-grade neuroendocrine (NE) tumors: what we know and important unanswered questions. *Lung Cancer.* 2003;41:S101.
13. Rusch VD, Klimstra E, Venkatraman P, et al. Overexpression of the epidermal growth factor receptor and its ligand transforming growth factor alpha is frequent in resectable non-small cell lung cancer but does not predict tumor progression. *Clin Cancer Res.* 1997;3:515–522.

14. Lynch TJ, Bell DW, Sordella R, et al. Activating mutations in the epidermal growth factor receptor underlying responsiveness of non-small-cell lung cancer to gefitinib. *N Engl J Med.* 2004;350(21): 2129–2139.
15. Johnson BE, Janne PA. Epidermal growth factor receptor mutations in patients with non-small cell lung cancer. *Cancer Res.* 2005;65(17): 7525–7529.
16. Kobayashi S, Boggon TJ, Dayaram T, et al. EGFR mutation and resistance of non-small-cell lung cancer to gefitnib. *N Engl Med.* 2005;352(8):786–792.
17. Kris MG, Natale RB, Herbst RS, et al. Efficacy of gefitinib, an inhibitor of the epidermal growth factor receptor tyrosine kinase, in symptomatic patients with non-small cell lung cancer: a randomized trial. *JAMA.* 2003;290(16):2149–2158.
18. Fukuoka M, Yano S, Giaccone G, et al. Multi-institutional randomized phase II trial of gefitinib for previously treated patients with advanced non-small-cell lung cancer (The IDEAL 1 Trial) [corrected]. *J Clin Oncol.* 2003;21(12):2237–2246.
19. Bell DW, Lynch TJ, Haserlat SM, et al. Epidermal Growth Factor Receptor Mutations and Gene Amplification in Non-Small-Cell Lung Cancer: Molecular Analysis of the IDEAL/INTACT Gefitinib Trials. *J Clin Oncol.* 2005; 23(31):8081–8092.
20. Shepherd FA, Rodrigues Pereira J, Ciuleanu T, et al. Erlotinib in previously treated non-small-cell lung cancer. *N Engl J Med.* 2005;353(2):123–132.
21. Cappuzzo F, Hirsch FR, Rossi E, et al. Epidermal growth factor receptor gene and protein and gefitinib sensitivity in non-small-cell lung cancer. *J Natl Cancer Inst.* 2005;97(9):643–655.
22. Sandler A, Gray R, Perry MC, et al. Paclitaxel-carboplatin alone or with bevacizumab for non-small-cell lung cancer. *N Engl J Med.* 2006;355(24):2542–2550.
23. Marcus PM, Bergstralh EJ, Zweig MH, et al. Extended lung cancer incidence follow-up in the Mayo Lung Project and overdiagnosis. *J Natl Cancer Inst.* 2006;98(11):748–756.
24. Bach PB, Jett JR, Pastorino U, et al. Computed tomography screening and lung cancer outcomes. *JAMA.* 2007;297(9):953–961.
25. Swensen SJ, Jett JR, Hartman TE, et al. CT Screening for Lung Cancer: Five-year Prospective Experience. *Radiology.* 2005;235(1):259–265.
26. Bach PB, Kelley MJ, Tate RC, et al. Screening for lung cancer: a review of the literature. *Chest.* 2003;123(1 Suppl):72S–82S.
27. Henschke CI, McCauley DI, Yankelevitz DF, et al. Early Lung Cancer Action Project: overall design and findings from baseline screening. *Lancet.* 1999;354(9173):99–105.
28. Henschke CI, Yankelevitz DF, Libby DM, et al. Survival of patients with stage I lung cancer detected on CT screening. *N Engl J Med.* 2006;355(17):1763–1771.
29. Nawa T, Kusano S, Kawasaki Y, et al. Lung cancer screening using low-dose spiral CT: results of baseline and 1-year follow-up studies. *Chest.* 2002;122(1):15–20.
30. Mulshine JL, Sullivan DC. Clinical practice. Lung cancer screening. *N Engl J Med.* 2005;352(26):2714–20.
31. Toloza E, Harpole L, Detterbeck F, et al. Invasive staging on non-small cell lung cancer: a review of the current evidence. *Chest.* 2003;123 (1 Suppl):157S–166S.
32. Toloza E, Harpole L, McCrory DC. Non-invasive staging on non-small cell lung cancer: a review of the literature. *Chest.* 2003;123 (1 Suppl):137S–146S.
33. Pieterman RM, van Putten JW, Meuzelaar JJ, et al. Preoperative staging of non-small-cell lung cancer with positron-emission tomography. *N Engl J Med.* 2000;343(4):254–261.
34. Gupta N, Graeber G, Bishop H. Comparative efficacy of positron emission tomography with fluorodeoxyglucose in evaluation of small (<1 cm), intermediate (1 to 3 cm), and large (>3 cm) lymph node lesions. *Chest.* 2000;117(3):773–778.
35. van Tinteren H, Hoekstra O, Smit E, et al. Effectiveness of positron emission tomography in the preoperative assessment of patients with suspected non-small-cell lung cancer: the PLUS multicentre randomised trial. *Lancet.* 2002;359(9315):1388–1392.
36. MacManus MP, Hicks RJ, Matthews JP, et al. Positron emission tomography is superior to computed tomographic scanning for response-assessment after radical radiotherapy or chemoradiotherapy in patients with non-small cell lung cancer. *J Clin Oncol.* 2003;21: 1285–1292.
37. Rusch V, Diroux D, Kraut M, et al. Induction chemoradiation and surgical resection for non-small cell lung carcinomas of the superior sulcus: initial results of Southwest Oncology Group Trial 9416 (Intergroup Trial 0160). *J Thorac Cardiovasc Surg.* 2001;121(7): 472–483.
38. PORT Meta-analysis Trialists Group. Postoperative radiotherapy in non-small cell lung cancer: systematic review and meta-analysis of individual patient data from nine randomized controlled trials. *Lancet.* 1998;352(9124):257–263.
39. Non-small Cell Lung Cancer Collaborative Group. Chemotherapy in non-small cell lung cancer: a meta-analysis using updated data on individual patients from 52 randomized clinical trials. *BMJ.* 1995; 311(7010):899–909.
40. Keller SM, Adak S, Wagner H, et al. A randomized trial of postoperative adjuvant therapy in patients with completely resected stage II or IIIA non-small-cell lung cancer. Eastern Cooperative Oncology Group. *N Engl J Med.* 2000;343(17):1217–1222.
41. Ichinose Y, Tada H, Koike T, et al. A randomized phase III trial of postoperative adjuvant chemotherapy in patients with completely resected stage IIIa N2 non small cell lung cancer: Japan Clinical Oncology Group (JCOG 9304) Trial. *Proc Am Soc Clin Oncol.* 2001;20:211a.
42. Scagliotti GV, Fossati R, Torri V, et al. Adjuvant Lung Project Italy/European Organisation for Research and Treatment of Cancer-Lung Cancer Cooperative Group Investigators. Randomized study of adjuvant chemotherapy for completely resected stage I, II, or IIIA Non-Small-Cell Lung Cancer. *J Natl Cancer Inst.* 2003;95(19):1453–1461.
43. Arriagada R, Bergman B, Dunant A, et al. Cisplatin-based adjuvant chemotherapy in patients with completely resected non-small-cell lung cancer. *N Engl J Med.* 2004;350(4):351–360.
44. Kato H, Ichinose Y, Ohta M, et al. A randomized trail of adjuvant chemotherapy with uracil-tegafur for adenocarcinoma of the lung. *N Engl J Med.* 2004;350(17):1713–1721.
45. Winton T, Livingston R, Johnson D, et al. Vinorelbine plus cisplatin vx. Observation in resected non-small-cell lung cancer. *N Engl J Med.* 2005;352(25):2589–2597.
46. Douillard JY, Rosell R, De Lena M, et al. Adjuvant vinorelbine plus cisplatin versus ovservation in patients with completely resected stage IB-IIIA non-small-cell lung cnacer (Adjuvant Navelbine International Trialist Association [ANITA]): a randomised controlled trial. *Lancet Oncol.* 2006;7(9):719–727.
47. Strauss G, Herndon J, Maddaus M, et al. Randomized clincial trail of adjuvant chemotherapy with paclitaxel and carboplatin follwiong resection in Stage IB non-small-cell lung cancer INSCLC: Report of Cancer and Leukemia Group B (CALGB) Protocol 9633. *ASCO Annual Meeting Proceedings. Part II.* 2004;22:7019.

48. *Journal of Clinical Oncology. 2006 ASCO Annual Meeting Proceedings Part I.* Vol 24, No. 18S (June 20 Supplement), 2006:7007.

49. Hotta K, Matsuo K, Ueoka H, et al. Meta-analysis of randomized clinical trials comparing Cisplatin to Carboplatin in patients with advanced non-small-cell lung cancer. *J Clin Oncol.* 2004;22(19):3852–3859.

50. *Journal of Clinical Oncology. 2006 ASCO Annual Meeting Proceedings Part I.* Vol 24, No. 18S (June 20 Supplement), 2006:7008.

51. Rosell R, Gomez-Codina J, Camps C, et al. A randomized trial comparing preoperative chemotherapy plus surgery with surgery alone in patients with non-small-cell lung cancer. *N Engl J Med.* 1994;330(3):153–158.

52. Roth J, Fossella F, Komaki R, et al. A randomized trial comparing perioperative chemotherapy and surgery with surgery alone in resectable stage IIIA non-small-cell lung cancer. *J Natl Cancer Inst.* 1994;86(9):673–680.

53. Depierre A, Milleron B, Moro-Sibilot D, et al. the French Thoracic Cooperative Group. Preoperative chemotherapy followed by surgery compared with primary surgery in resectable stage I (except T1N0), II, and IIIa non-small cell lung cancer. *J Clin Oncol.* 2002;20(1):247–253.

54. *Journal of Clinical Oncology. 2005 ASCO Annual Meeting Proceedings Part I.* Vol 23, No. 18S (June 20 Supplement), 2005:7014.

55. Burdett S, Stewart L, Rydzewska L. A Systematic Review and Meta-analysis of the Literature: Chemotherapy and Surgery versus Surgery Alone in Non-small Cell Lung Cancer. *J Thorac Oncol.* 2006;1(7):1611–1621.

56. Dillman RO, Seagren SL, Propert KJ, et al. A randomized trial of induction chemotherapy plus high-dose radiation versus radiation alone in stage III non-small cell lung cancer. *N Engl J Med.* 1990;323(14):940–945.

57. Sause WT, Scott C, Taylor S, et al. Radiation Therapy Oncology Group (RTOG) 88–08 and Eastern Cooperative Oncology Group (ECOG) 4588: preliminary results of a phase III trial in regionally advanced, unresectable non-small-cell lung cancer. *J Natl Cancer Inst.* 1995;87(3):198–205.

58. Furuse K, Fukuoka M, Kawahara M, et al. Phase III study of concurrent versus sequential thoracic radiotherapy in combination with mitomycin, vindesine, and cisplatin in unresectable stage III non-small-cell lung cancer. *J Clin Oncol.* 1999;17(9):2692–2699.

59. *Journal of Clinical Oncology. 2000 ASCO Annual Meeting Proceedings Part I.* Vol 18, No. 18S (June 20 Supplement), 2000:484.

60. Choy H, Akerley W, Safran H, et al. Multiinstitutional phase II trial of paclitaxel, carboplatin, and concurrent radiation therapy for locally advanced non-small-cell lung cancer. *J Clin Oncol.* 1998;16(10):3316–3322.

61. *Journal of Clinical Oncology. 2007 ASCO Annual Meeting Proceedings Part I.* Vol 25, No. 18S (June 20 Supplement), 2007:7512.

62. Saunders M, Dische S, Barrett A, et al. Randomised multicentre trials of CHART vs. conventional radiotherapy in head and neck and non-small-cell lung cancer: an interim report. *Br J Cancer.* 1996;73(12):1455–1462.

63. Effects of vinorelbine on quality of life and survival of elderly patients with advanced non-small-cell lung cancer. The Elderly Lung Cancer Vinorelbine Italian Study Group. *J Natl Cancer Inst.* 1999;91(1):66–72.

64. *Journal of Clinical Oncology. 2001 ASCO Annual Meeting Proceedings Part I.* Vol 19, No. 18S (June 20 Supplement), 2001:309.

65. Socinski MA, Schell MJ, Peterman A, et al. Phase III trial comparing a defined duration of therapy versus continuous therapy followed by second-line therapy in advanced-stage IIIB/IV non-small-cell lung cancer. Screening for lung cancer with low-dose helical computed tomography: Anti-lung Cancer Association Project. *J Clin Oncol.* 2002;20(5):1335–1343.

66. *Journal of Clinical Oncology.* 1998 *ASCO Annual Meeting Proceedings Part I.* Vol 16, No. 18S (June 20 Supplement), 1998:457.

67. Wozniak AJ, Crowley JJ, Balcerzak SP, et al. Randomized trial comparing cisplatin with cisplatin plus vinorelbine in the treatment of advanced non-small-cell lung cancer: a Southwest Oncology Group study. *J Clin Oncol.* 1998;16(7):2459–2465.

68. Sandler A, Nemunaitis J, Denham C, et al. Phase III trial of gemcitabine plus cisplatin versus cisplatin alone in patients with locally advanced or metastatic non-small cell lung cancer. *J Clin Oncol.* 2000;18(1):122–130.

69. von Pawel J, von Roemeling R, Gatzemeier U, et al. Tirapazamine plus cisplatin versus cisplatin in advanced non-small-cell lung cancer: a report of the international CATAPULT I study group. Cisplatin and tirapazamine in subjects with advanced previously untreated non-small-cell lung tumors. *J Clin Oncol.* 2000;18(6):1351–1359.

70. Gatzemeier U, von Pawel J, Gottfried M, et al. Phase III comparative study of high-dose cisplatin versus a combination of paclitaxel and cisplatin in patients with advanced non-small-cell lung cancer. *J Clin Oncol.* 2000;18(19):3390–3399.

71. Le Chevalier T, Brisgand D, Douillard J, et al. Randomized study of vinorelbine and cisplatin versus vindesine and cisplatin versus vinorelbine alone in advanced non-small-cell lung cancer: results of a European multicenter trial including 612 patients. *J Clin Oncol.* 1994;12(2):360–367.

72. Lilenbaum RC, Herndon JE, 2nd, List MA, et al. Single-agent versus combination chemotherapy in advanced non-small-cell lung cancer: the cancer and leukemia group B (study 9730). *J Clin Oncol.* 2005;23(1):190-196.

73. *Journal of Clinical Oncology.* 2002 *ASCO Annual Meeting Proceedings Part I.* Vol 21, No. 18S (June 20 Supplement), 2002:291.

74. *Journal of Clinical Oncology.* 2002 *ASCO Annual Meeting Proceedings Part I.* Vol 21, No. 18S (June 20 Supplement), 2002:291 Georgoulias V, Ardavanis A, Agelidou M, et al. Preliminary analysis of a multicenter phase III trial comparing docetaxel (D) versus docetaxel/cisplatin (DC) in patients with inoperable advanced and metastatic non-small cell lung cancer (NSCLC). *Proc Am Soc Clin Oncol.* 2002;21:291a.

75. Negoro S, Masuda N, Takada Y, et al. Randomised phase III trial of irinotecan combined with cisplatin for advanced non-small-cell lung cancer. *Br J Cancer.* 2003;88(3):335–341.

76. Ardizzoni A, Boni L, Tiseo M, et al. Cisplatin- versus carboplatin-based chemotherapy in first-line treatment of advanced non-small-cell lung cancer: an individual patient data meta-analysis. *J Natl Cancer Inst.* 2007;99(11):847–857.

77. Hotta K, Matsuo K, Ueoka H, et al. Meta-analysis of randomized clinical trials comparing cisplatin to carboplatin in patients with advanced non-small-cell lung cancer. *J Clin Oncol.* 2004;22(19):3852–3859.

78. D'Addario G, Pintilie M, Leighl NB, et al. Platinum-based versus non-platinum-based chemotherapy in advanced non-small-cell lung cancer: a meta-analysis of the published literature. *J Clin Oncol.* 2005;23(13):2926–2936.

79. Shepherd F, Dancey J, Ramlau R, et al. Prospective randomized trial of docetaxel versus best supportive care in patients with non-small-cell lung cancer previously treated with platinum-based chemotherapy. *J Clin Oncol.* 2000;18(10):2095–2103.

80. Fossella FV, DeVore R, Kerr RN, et al. Randomized phase III trial of docetaxel versus vinorelbine or ifosfamide in patients with advanced non-small-cell lung cancer previously treated with platinum-containing chemotherapy regimens. The TAX 320 Non-Small Cell Lung Cancer Study Group. *J Clin Oncol.* 2000;18(12):2354–2362.

81. Hanna N, Shepherd FA, Fossella FV, et al. Randomized phase III trail of pemetrexed versus docetaxel in patients with non-small-cell lung cancer previously treated with chemotherapy. *J Clin Oncol.* 2004;22(9):1589–1597.

82. Takano T, Ohe Y, Sakamoto H, et al. Epidermal Growth Factor Receptor Gene Mutations and Increased Copy Numbers Predict Gefitinib Sensitivity in Patients with Recurrent Non-Small-Cell Lung Cancer. *J Clin Oncol.* 2005;23(28):6829–6837.

83. Tsao MS, Sakurada A, Cutz JC, et al. Erlotinib in lung cancer– molecular and clinical predictors of outcome. *N Engl J Med.* 2005;353(2):133–144.

84. Inoue A, Suzuki T, Fukuhara T, et al. Prospective phase II study of gefitinib for chemotherapy-naive patients with advanced non-small-cell lung cancer with epidermal growth factor receptor gene mutations. *J Clin Oncol.* 2006;24(21):3340–3346.

85. Inoue A, Saijo Y, Maemondo M, et al. Severe acute interstitial pneumonia and gefitinib. *Lancet.* 2003;361(9352):137–139.

86. Noda K, Nishiwaki Y, Kawahara M, et al. Irinotecan plus cisplatin compared with etoposide plus cisplatin for extensive small-cell lung cancer. *N Engl J Med.* 2002;346(2):85–91.

87. Klasa R, Murray N, Coldman A. Dose-intensity meta-analysis of chemotherapy regimens in small-cell carcinoma of the lung. *J Clin Oncol.* 1991;9(3):499–508.

88. Elias AD, Ayash L, Frei E 3rd, et al. Intensive combined modality therapy for limited-stage small-cell lung cancer. *J Natl Cancer Inst.* 1993;85(7):559–566.

89. von Pawel J, Schiller J, Shepherd F, et al. Topotecan versus CAV for the treatment of recurrent small cell lung cancer. *J Clin Oncol.* 1999;17(2):658–667.

90. *Journal of Clinical Oncology.* 1996 *ASCO Annual Meeting Proceedings Part I.* Vol 15, No. 18S (June 20 Supplement), 1996:2019.

91. Girling DJ. Comparison of oral etoposide and standard intravenous multidrug chemotherapy for small-cell cancer: a stopped multicentre randomized trial. Medical Research Council Lung Cancer Working Party. *Lancet.* 1996;348(9027):563–566.

92. Warde P, Payne D. Does thoracic irradiation improve survival and local control in limited-stage small-cell carcinoma of the lung? A meta-analysis. *J Clin Oncol.* 1992;10(6):890–895.

93. Turrisi AT, Kim K, Blum R, et al. Twice-daily compared with once-daily thoracic radiotherapy in limited small-cell lung cancer treated concurrently with cisplatin and etoposide. *N Engl J Med.* 1999;340(4):265–271.

94. Murray N, Coy P, Pater J, et al. Importance of timing for thoracic irradiation in the combined modality treatment of limited-stage small-cell lung cancer. *J Clin Oncol.* 1993;11(2):336–344.

95. Auperin A, Arriagada R, Pignon J, et al. Prophylactic cranial irradiation for patients with small cell lung cancer in complete remission. *N Engl J Med.* 1999;341(7):476–484.

96. Noda K, Nishiwaki Y, Kawahara M, et al. Irinotecan plus cisplatin compared with etoposide plus cisplatin for extensive small-cell lung cancer. *N Engl J Med.* 2002;346(2):85–91.

97. Thomas CR, Wright C, Loehrer PJ. Thymoma: state of the art. *J Clin Oncol.* 1999;17(7):2280–2289.

98. Loehrer PJ, Perez CA, Roth LM, et al. Chemotherapy for advanced thymoma. Preliminary results of an intergroup study. *Ann Intern Med.* 1990;113(7):520–524.

99. Carbone M, Kratzke RA, Testa JR. The pathogenesis of mesothelioma. *Semin Oncol.* 2002;29(1):2–17.

100. Rusch VW. A proposed new international TNM staging system for malignant pleural mesothelioma from the International Mesothelioma Interest Group. *Lung Cancer.* 1996;14(1):1–12.

101. Sugarbaker D, Norberto JJ, Swanson S. Extrapleural pneumonectomy in the setting of multimodality therapy for diffuse malignant pleural mesothelioma. *Semin Thorac Cardiovasc Surg.* 1997;9(4):373–382.

102. Ong ST, Vogelzang NJ. Chemotherapy in malignant pleural mesothelioma: a review. *J Clin Oncol.* 1996;14(3):1007–1017.

103. Vogelzang NJ. Emerging insights into the biology and therapy of malignant mesothelioma. *Semin Oncol.* 2002;29(6 Suppl 18):35–42.

104. Byrne MJ, Davidson JA, Musk AW, et al. Cisplatin and gemcitabine treatment for malignant mesothelioma: a phase II study. *J Clin Oncol.* 1999;17(1):25–30.

105. Vogelzang NJ, Rusthoven JJ, Symanowski J, et al. Phase III study of pemetrexed in combination with cisplatin versus cisplatin alone in patients with malignant pleural mesothelioma. *J Clin Oncol.* 2003;21(14):2636–2644.

7

HEAD AND NECK CANCER

Arlene A. Forastiere, MD

LEARNING OBJECTIVES

After reviewing this chapter, the reader should be able to

- Recognize clinical presentation of head and neck cancers and apply appropriate examination, imaging, and diagnostic modalities to make an accurate diagnosis and effectively stage identified disease
- Appropriately employ each treatment modality in the management of early-stage and locally advanced disease and associated toxicities
- Describe the indications for using concurrent chemoradiotherapy as primary curative treatment without surgery and in the adjuvant setting
- Appropriately use chemotherapy with palliative intent and understand the current role of biologic therapies
- Address the differences in natural history, management, and indications for systemic therapy for differentiated thyroid cancers, anaplastic thyroid cancer, and medullary thyroid cancer
- Summarize key issues that are the focus of current investigation in head and neck cancer

The term head and neck cancer refers to a heterogenous group of malignant tumors arising from the epithelial lining of the upper aerodigestive tract. The specific primary sites are subdivided by anatomic boundries: the lip and oral cavity, pharynx (nasopharynx, oropharynx, and hypopharynx), larynx, and the nasal cavity and paranasal sinuses (Table 7-1, Fig. 7-1). Squamous cell cancer or a variant is the most common histologic type, accounting for 85% to 95% of cancers. Etiologic factors include tobacco and alcohol use and viruses, such as the human papilloma virus (HPV) and the Epstein-Barr virus (Table 7-2). The other two anatomic sites included in the head and neck region are the thyroid gland and salivary glands. These cancers are most commonly histologic variants of adenocarcinoma.

The American Society of Clinical Oncology and Dr. Forastiere would like to gratefully acknowledge David G. Pfister, MD, for his contributions to the original content of this chapter.

EPIDEMIOLOGY AND RISK FACTORS

INCIDENCE RATES

Head and neck cancer constitutes approximately 3% of all new cases of cancer in the United States and accounts for 2% of all cancer deaths. Worldwide, this cancer is a significant public health concern, with an estimated 664,000 new cases diagnosed in 2002 and 350,000 deaths.[1] Head and neck cancer affects men and women in a ratio of 2.5:1, although the ratio varies according to the primary site (e.g., 7:1 for cancer of the larynx). The median age of incidence is approximately 60 years. The age-adjusted incidence and mortality are highest among black men, who generally present at a more advanced stage, compared with white individuals. In addition, stage-specific survival rates also are lower for this racial group.

EPIDEMIOLOGY—ROLE OF TOBACCO AND ALCOHOL

Epidemiologic data document a multiplicative risk relationship between tobacco and alcohol. For example, the relative risk of oral and pharyngeal cancer is increased nearly 40-fold for patients with more than a 40 pack-year history of smoking who consume 30 or more alcoholic drinks per week.[2] Overall, an estimated 75% of head and neck cancers can be attributed to tobacco and alcohol use, highlighting the importance of tobacco and alcohol counseling in medical practice and as part of prevention strategies. The type of tobacco product used affects the distribution of observed primary sites. Smokeless tobacco and other oral chewed carcinogens — betel quid, a combination of betel leaf, lime, and areca nut, which commonly is used in India and parts of Asia — are associated with the development of cancers of the oral cavity. Black, air-cured tobacco (as commonly found in cigars and pipe tobacco) is more irritating to the respiratory mucosa than blonde or flue-cured tobacco (more commonly found in cigarettes) and is associated with a higher risk of head and neck cancer.

Because many patients with head and neck cancer are malnourished at the time of diagnosis, dietary deficiencies have been postulated as risk factors, and both laboratory and epidemiologic data suggest that vitamin A and its analogues may be protective. The Plummer-Vinson syndrome, which is most commonly seen in women younger than 50, is associated with iron-deficiency anemia, hypopharyngeal webs, dysphagia, and a higher risk of cancers of the postcricoid and hypopharynx.

The majority of tumors of the sinonasal tract originate in the maxillary sinus, and only 50% are of squamous cell histology. These cancers are associated with certain occupational exposures (e.g., nickel, radium, mustard gas, chromium, and byproducts of leather tanning and woodworking).

KEY POINTS

- Tobacco and alcohol use are the major risk factors for squamous cell cancer of the head and neck, and the use of both results in a multiplicative increase in risk.
- There is evidence for a causal association between high-risk oncogenic human papilloma virus (HPV) and cancers of the lingual and palatine tonsils, and these cancers are increasing in incidence in the United States.
- The survival prognosis is substantially better for HPV-positive cancers compared with HPV-negative cancers.
- The incidence of second primary cancers for patients with a history of squamous cell cancer of the head and neck is 3% to 7% annually, particularly for other sites of the head and neck, lung, and esophagus.

TABLE 7-1 Head and Neck Cancer: Primary Sites

Primary Sites
Oral Cavity and Lip
Floor of mouth
Oral tongue
Buccal mucosa
Alveolar ridges
Hard palate
Retromolar trigone
Pharynx
Nasopharynx (includes superior surface of soft palate)
Oropharynx (includes inferior surface of soft palate, uvula, base of tongue, tonsil, posterior pharyngeal wall)
Hypopharynx (pyriform sinus, postcricoid, posterior wall)
Larynx
Supraglottic larynx (false cords, arytenoids, epiglottis)
Glottic larynx (includes commissures)
Subglottic larynx
Nasal Cavity and Paranasal Sinuses
Nasal cavity
Maxillary sinuses
Ethmoid sinuses
Frontal sinuses
Sphenoid sinuses

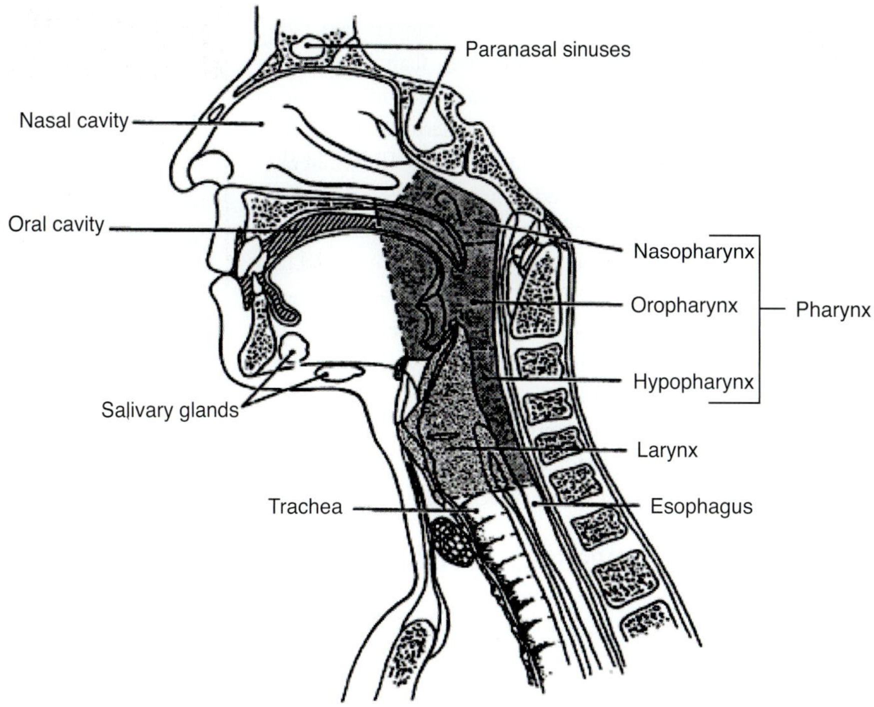

FIG. 7-1 Saggital section showing head and neck cancer primary tumor sites.
Reprinted with permission from BC Decker.

TABLE 7-2 Characteristics of Virus-Associated Head and Neck Cancers

	Human Papillomavirus	Epstein-Barr Virus
Anatomic site	Oropharynx	Nasopharynx
Anatomic sub-site	Lingual & palatine tonsils	Fossae of Rosenmuller
Percent virus associated	60%–70%	WHO I: 70%–80% WHO II–III: 100%
Associated histopathology	Basaloid	Lymphoepithelioma
Viral transmission	Sexual	Oral
Viral genome	Episomal/integrated	Episomal/integrated
Viral oncogenes	E6 and E7	LMP-1 and EBNA1
Cofactors	Tobacco & alcohol	Diet and genetics
Clinical presentation	Unknown primary	Distant metastases
Prognosis controlled for stage	Improved	Improved

EPIDEMIOLOGY—ROLE OF VIRUSES

There is a rising incidence of oral cancers in the United States in individuals younger than 45 who do not report a history of alcohol or tobacco abuse,[3] which has focused attention on the roles of both viral infection (e.g., HPV) and genetic susceptibility.[4,5] The verrucous cancer subtype of squamous cell cancer is strongly associated with HPV. Genetic material from high-risk oncogenic strains (most commonly HPV types 16 and 18) is found in approximately 60% of oropharyngeal cancers arising from the palatine and lingual tonsils.[4] The transforming potential results from viral proteins E6 and E7 that inactivate the tumor suppressor proteins p53 and pRb, which results in loss of cell cycle regulation, cellular proliferation, and chromosomal instability.[5] The histology of HPV-associated cancers frequently is basaloid or poorly differentiated squamous cell cancer, and the initial presentation often is as an unknown primary site with a large cystic neck node(s). These patients tend to be younger and have a history of minimal tobacco and alcohol exposure. Multiple investigators report an improved prognosis of a 59% reduction in risk of death from HPV-positive cancer compared with HPV-negative cancers (HR = 0.41; 95% CI; 0.20, 0.88).[4] In situ hybridization, which is available at a limited number of referral centers, is the only useful test to confirm the diagnosis.[5]

Nasopharyngeal and paranasal sinus cancers are not associated with tobacco or alcohol use. Cancer of the nasopharynx is especially common among individuals from endemic areas in southern China and northern Africa, where World Health Organization (WHO) subtypes II (nonkeratinizing) and III (undifferentiated cancer), rather than type I (keratinizing), predominate. Epstein-Barr virus is associated with cancer of this site, and the viral genome can be found in nasopharyngeal cancer tissues and dysplastic lesions that progress to invasive disease. However, the exact role this virus plays in etiology is still being defined, and evidence of the Epstein-Barr virus can be found in nonmalignant nasopharyngeal tissue as well. Some environmental factors, such as consumption of salted fish, also may be important. The peak incidence occurs during the sixth and seventh decades of life.

MOLECULAR PROGRESSION MODEL

A molecular progression model for the transformation of normal mucosa to invasive squamous cell cancer has been in development for more than a decade. The most common genetic alteration in these tumors is the loss of chromosomal region 9p21 and is an early event. Mutations of *p53* occur in approximately one-half of patients and are particularly common among patients with substantial exposure to tobacco and alcohol. The histologic evolution through the interval steps of hyperplasia, dysplasia, and carcinoma in situ is associated with accumulating molecular events.[6]

SECOND PRIMARY TUMORS OF THE AERODIGESTIVE TRACT

Given the central role of tobacco in the genesis of many head and neck cancers, medical comorbidity and synchronous or metachronous second primary tumors (3% to 7% per year, depending on whether tobacco use continues) are common among these patients.[7] Within the aerodigestive tract, the most frequent site of a second primary tumor is the lung, followed by the esophagus. A solitary pulmonary nodule is not rare in the work-up of a new pharyngeal or laryngeal cancer and should not be assumed to be a metastasis, particularly in the patient with an early-stage cancer. For example, a patient with early glottic cancer, no involved neck nodes, and a lung nodule is much more likely to have a second primary tumor than metastatic cancer, mandating a curative treatment approach for both primaries.

PREVENTION AND CHEMOPREVENTION

Stopping the use of tobacco and alcohol (the two primary risk factors for squamous cell cancer of the head and neck) is central to any prevention program. Counseling combined with the use of a pharmacologic intervention, such as a tapering nicotine patch, doubles success rates; however, only a minority of smokers succeed in quitting on their first attempt. Important reasons for smoking cessation that clinicians can discuss with their patients include the fact that the rate of second primary tumors is higher among patients who continue to smoke and that continuing to smoke adversely influences the effectiveness and tolerance of cancer treatment.

> **KEY POINTS**
>
> - Stopping the use of tobacco and alcohol, the two primary risk factors for squamous cell cancer of the head and neck, is central to any prevention program.
> - Chemopreventive agents currently are not part of standard clinical practice but remain an area of active investigation.

ORAL PREMALIGNANCY

Patients with head and neck cancer, specifically oral cancers, often have diffuse mucosal abnormalities related to tobacco (including marijuana) and alcohol use and betal quid chewing. Oral premalignancy, or intraepithelial neoplasia (IEN), is the precursor to invasive oral cancer. Understanding the stepwise molecular events to define risk of progression to invasive disease and potential targets for intervention is an area of intense research interest. The loss of genomic material containing tumor suppressor genes (loss of heterozygosity [LOH] or allelic imbalance) of regions on chromosomes 3p and 9p, *p16* promoter hypermethylation and *p53* mutation are steps in the progression of IEN to invasive cancer. Histologically, the most frequent IEN lesion is leukoplakia. Understanding the molecular events in the transformation of leukoplakia to invasive cancer may allow for stratification of patients by risk and the testing of novel therapies in this population. There is no safe, effective systemic therapy for long-term use.

Testing of retinoids to halt or reverse the processes that ultimately lead to epithelial carcinogenesis began in the mid-1980s. Trials investigating 13-*cis*-retinoic acid (13cRA) in high and low doses showed that high-dose 13cRA was able to reverse oral IEN in approximately two-thirds of premalignant lesions and maintain the effect for as long as treatment was continued. However, intolerable side effects preclude chronic, long-term dosing.[8]

PREVENTION TRIALS USING RETINOIDS

The results of other randomized studies do not show a clear improvement in outcome. No reduction in second primary tumors was found in a study of etretinate (50 mg daily for 1 month, followed by 25 mg daily for 24 months) in patients with early-stage disease, but there were concerns regarding patient compliance and follow-up assessments for second primary tumors.[9] In a placebo-controlled Intergroup trial of a tolerable, low dose of isotretinoin in patients with curatively-treated stage I or II squamous cell cancer of the head and neck, isotretinoin had no significant effect on the rate of second primary tumors (HR = 1.06; 95% CI; 0.83, 1.35) or on overall survival (HR = 1.03; 95% CI; 0.81, 1.32).[10]

The European Organization for Research and Treatment of Cancer (EORTC) found no significant benefit in the rate of second primary tumors, event-free survival, or overall survival when vitamin A and antioxidant therapy (N-acetylcysteine) were used for patients with head and neck or lung cancer who had been treated with curative intent.[11] Patients in this study were randomly assigned to receive vitamin A for 2 years, N-acetylcysteine for 2 years, both treatments, or no treatment.

Thus, no systemic therapy can be recommended, and patients with oral premalignant mucosal changes should be enrolled in clinical trials. Bioadjuvant therapy, in which drug combinations (e.g., 13cRA plus interferon-alpha2a plus vitamin E) are used to address the risk of both primary tumor recurrence and the risk of second primary lesions, is being explored.

Targeting the epidermal growth factor receptor (EGFR) is another area of investigation for reversal of IEN. Studies show that EGFR activation (phosphoryation) is present in 30% to 50% of dysplastic oral lesions and in nearly all invasive carcicnoma; however, EGFR activation is not present in normal oral mucosa. This pathway mediates cell proliferation and inhibition of apoptosis and leads to enhanced survival and invasion. Clinical trials are being initiated to evaluate EGFR pathway inhibition with EGFR antibodies or small molecule EGFR tyrosine kinase inhibitors.

KEY POINTS

- Many presenting signs and symptoms are referable to a particular primary site (e.g., hoarseness can refer to the larynx or hypopharynx and unilateral otitis media, to the nasopharynx).
- The location of pathologic lymph nodes in the neck may suggest the primary site.
- The initial staging evaluation for head and neck cancer includes comprehensive examination of the head and neck, imaging (computerized tomography or magnetic resonance imaging) of the primary site and neck, chest x-ray, and routine lab screenings.
- Uniformly accepted criteria for unresectability include: base of skull involvement, fixation to the prevertebral fascia, carotid encasement, and involvement of the pterygoid musculature.
- Early-stage disease is defined as disease limited to a small primary tumor (T1 or T2) and either no regional node involvement or a single ipsilateral node smaller than 3 cm in diameter (N0 or N1). Locally advanced disease is defined as the presence of a large primary tumor (T3 or T4) or the presence of large, multiple, or contralateral regional node involvement (N2 or N3).

CLINICAL PRESENTATION, DIAGNOSIS, AND STAGING

In general, cancers of the oral cavity, oropharynx, larynx, and hypopharynx are characterized by disease confined to the primary site with or without spread to regional nodes at the time of diagnosis and late metastatic spread. Less than 10% of patients have distant disease at presentation. Thus, initial staging and management focus on the extent of local-regional involvement and the effect of the choice of treatment on speech and swallowing function, as well as on the risk of recurrence.

PRESENTING SIGNS AND SYMPTOMS

Clinical signs and symptoms vary with the anatomic site affected. For example, patients with hypopharyngeal or laryngeal cancer often seek medical attention because of sore throat, hoarseness, or difficulty swallowing. Tumors of the glottic larynx tend to be diagnosed at an earlier stage than those of the supraglottic larynx or hypopharynx because hoarseness is an early symptom at the former subsite. The eustachian tubes are frequently invaded by nasopharyngeal disease, leading to otitis media that, in an adult, mandates careful assessment of the nasopharynx. With more advanced tumors at this site, double vision may be the presenting symptom because of invasion of the cavernous sinuses and the branches of the third, fourth, and, particularly, the sixth cranial nerves, which track with these vascular structures.

The discovery of a painless lump in the neck is not an uncommon presenting complaint of a patient with head and neck cancer. The location of cervical adenopathy, denoted by dividing the neck into levels (Fig. 7-2), may direct the physician to the primary site. For example, cancers of the oral cavity typically spread to lymph nodes in the submental and submandibular areas (level I), laryngeal cancer spreads to the upper part of the neck (levels II and III), nasopharyngeal cancer spreads to the upper part of the neck and posterior triangle (levels II and V), and disease confined to the lower part of the neck or supraclavicular area should raise suspicion about a primary lesion below the clavicles or possibly disease in the thyroid (levels IV and V). Spread to the neck is uncommon for patients with primary cancers of the glottic larynx or paranasal sinus. Involvement of the neck nodes is prognostically significant, reducing the cure proportion for a given T stage by 50%.

DIAGNOSTIC EVALUATION

A comprehensive examination of the head and neck with the assistance of mirrors or fiberoptic scopes is central to the evaluation. Because lymph nodes track along the internal jugular vein, examination of the neck for enlarged lymph nodes is facilitated by rotating the head toward the side being examined to promote relaxation of the sternocleidomastoid muscle on that side.

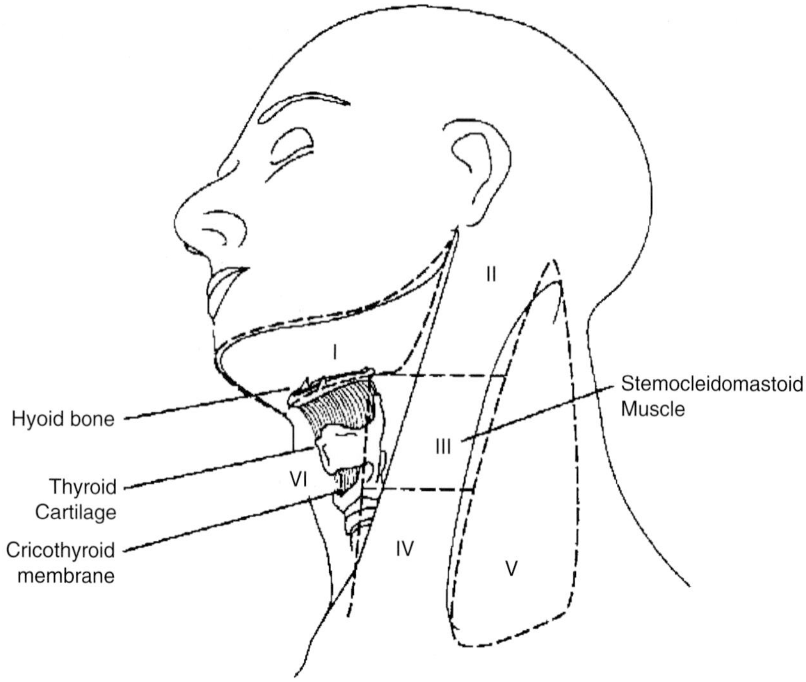

FIG. 7-2 Cervical lymph node levels.
Reprinted with permission from BC Decker.

A commonly found mucosal lesion is leukoplakia, a white, hyperkeratotic patch, distinguishable from thrush in that it does not scrape off. The majority (approximately 80%) are benign lesions that can be observed without treatment. By contrast, erythroplakia appears as a red, velvety patch and is associated with a 90% incidence of severe dysplasia, carcinoma in situ, or invasive disease on microscopic examination

Examination under anesthesia often is necessary and important, especially for patients with tumors of the larynx or pharynx. The routine application of so-called triple endoscopy (laryngoscopy or pharyngoscopy with bronchoscopy and esophagoscopy added) to rule out synchronous tumors is controversial. If the primary site is known, the yield of bronchoscopy or esophagoscopy is generally low. However, most clinicians would agree that these procedures are indicated for patients who have evidence of diffuse mucosal abnormalities in the setting of a malignant neck node without a clear primary site, particularly when the lymph node is located in the lower part of the neck, thus increasing the likelihood of a lung or esophageal primary tumor. This recommendation for triple endoscopy may change, however, with the widespread use of positron emission tomography (PET)/computerized tomography (CT) imaging.

The current recommendations for imaging of the primary site and neck specify CT or magnetic resonance imaging (MRI) for demarcating the extent of disease. A high-quality CT scan performed with contrast medium is less expensive than MRI and is sufficient for most cases. An extensive search for distant metastases in patients with head and neck cancer without suspicious symptoms is not routinely done because the overall incidence of spread below the clavicles at the time of presentation is low (10% or less), particularly in the absence of involvement of the lymph nodes. Hence, performing PET/CT or other body imaging is not cost-effective and should not be done routinely. A chest x-ray is done as much to rule out a second primary lung cancer or to document chronic obstructive pulmonary disease as to find lung metastases. A high resolution CT scan is more sensitive than a chest x-ray for the identification of a new primary site or metastases and could have specific indication in the patient presenting with bulky N2 or N3 neck disease or a primary site of the hypopharynx, both of which are risk factors for metastatic spread. Formal imaging of the liver and bones should only be done if clinically indicated based on symptoms or a biochemical abnormality. By contrast, the evaluation for metastatic disease with a body CT scan and bone scan, or 18-fluorodeoxyglucose (FDG)-PET/CT, is an appropriate part of the work-up for patients with nasopharyngeal cancer with lymph node involvement. In this setting, the incidence of distant metastases approaches 60%, and bone is the most common site of metastasis.

FDG-PET is appropriate when the primary site is unknown or to evaluate an equivocal finding on cross-sectional imaging, but routine application of this test, particularly if management will not be affected, is expensive and not indicated. FDG-PET does not displace cross-sectional imaging of the primary site and neck and is best interpreted in the context of a separate or fused cross-sectional study performed with contrast. As with any diagnostic test, FDG-PET is not perfect. False-positive results can be related to dental disease or an inflammatory process in the neck or elsewhere, and uptake by lesions smaller than 1 cm is inconsistent. FDG-PET with a fused contrast-enhanced CT scan may be useful in identifying spread to regional nodes in the N0 neck, the knowledge of which would alter radiation portals or the choice of neck dissection to be performed.[12–14] Additionally, PET imaging may prove useful in the post-treatment assessment of patients with node-positive disease who were treated with chemoradiotherapy and for whom a planned neck dissection is being considered.[15] Although the number of institutional case series in the literature is increasing, no clear guidelines have been established for these particular clinical situations.

Histologic proof of cancer typically is obtained from a biopsy of the primary site, a neck node, or both. At least initially, needle aspiration of a lymph node is preferred to excisional biopsy, especially for an apparently malignant node with an occult primary lesion. This approach is both safe and feasible, and the theoretical risk of seeding malignant cells along the needle track has not been a problem clinically. Straightforward squamous cell cancers should pose few challenges to the cytopathologist; poorly differentiated tumors or lymphomas are more problematic. If an excisional biopsy is necessary, it ideally should be done to facilitate its incorporation into the definitive treatment of the patient. A surgeon capable of performing a neck dissection should be involved if squamous cell cancer is suspected.

STAGE CLASSIFICATION

The stage groupings for all primary sites are based on the tumor, node, and metastasis (TNM) classification of the American Joint Committee on Cancer (AJCC) and the International Union Against Cancer (UICC). The TNM system is based on both clinical examination and radiographic information (Tables 7-3 and 7-4, Fig. 7-3). A few general rules of the clinical staging may be identified.

TABLE 7-3 American Joint Committee on Cancer Staging: Lip and Oral Cavity, Oropharynx, Hypopharynx, and Larynx

Primary Tumor (T)	
Tx	Primary tumor cannot be assessed
T0	No evidence of primary tumor
Tis	Carcinoma *in situ*
Lip and Oral Cavity	
T1	Tumor 2 cm or less in greatest dimension
T2	Tumor greater than 2 cm but less than 4 cm in greatest dimension
T3	Tumor greater than 4 cm in greatest dimension
T4 (lip)	Tumor invades through cortical bone, inferior alveolar nerve, floor of mouth, or skin of face, i.e., chin or nose
T4a	(oral cavity) Tumor invades adjacent structures (e.g., through cortical bone, into deep [extrinsic] muscle of tongue [genioglossus, hyoglossus, palatoglossus, and styloglossus], maxillary sinus, skin of face)
T4b	Tumor invades masticator space, pterygoid plates, or skull base and/or encases internal carotid artery
Oropharynx	
T1	Tumor 2 cm or less in greatest dimension
T2	Tumor greater than 2 cm but less than 4 cm in greatest dimension
T3	Tumor greater than 4 cm in greatest dimension
T4a	Tumor invades the larynx, deep/extrinsic muscle of tongue, medial pterygoid, hard palate, or mandible
T4b	Tumor invades lateral pterygoid muscle, pterygoid plates, lateral nasopharynx, or skull base or encases carotid artery
Hypopharynx	
T1	Tumor limited to one subsite of hypopharynx and 2 m or less in greatest dimension
T2	Tumor invades more than one subsite of hypopharynx or an adjacent site, or measures greater than 2 cm but less than 4 cm in greatest diameter without fixation of hemilarynx
T3	Tumor greater than 4 cm in greatest dimension or fixation of hemilarynx
T4a	Tumor invades thyroid/carcoid cartilage, hyoid bone, thyroid gland, esophagus, or central compartment soft tissue
T4b	Tumor invades prevertebral fascia, encases carotid artery, or involves mediastinal structures

TABLE 7-3 (Continued)

Larynx—Supraglottis	
T1	Tumor limited to one subsite of supraglottis with normal vocal cord mobility
T2	Tumor invades mucosa of more than one adjacent subsite of supraglottis or glottis or region outside the supraglottis (e.g., mucosa of base of tongue, vallecula, medial wall of pyriform sinus) without fixation of the larynx
T3	Tumor limited to larynx with vocal cord fixation and/or invades any of the following: postcricoid area, pre-epiglottic tissues, paraglottic space, and/or minor thyroid cartilage erosion (e.g., inner cortex)
T4a	Tumor invades through the thyroid cartilage and/or invades tissues beyond the larynx (e.g., trachea, soft tissues of neck including deep extrinsic muscle of the tongue, strap muscles, thyroid, or esophagus)
T4b	Tumor invades prevertebral space, encases carotid artery, or invades mediastinal structures
Glottis	
T1	Tumor limited to the vocal cord(s) with normal mobility
T2	Tumor extends to supraglottis and/or subglottis, and/or with impaired vocal cord mobility
T3	Tumor limited to the larynx with vocal cord fixation and/or invades paraglottic space, and or minor thyroid cartilage erosion
T4a	Tumor invades through the thyroid cartilage and/or invades tissues beyond the larynx (e.g., trachea, soft tissues of neck including deep extrinsic muscle of the tongue, strap muscles, thyroid, or esophagus)
T4b	Tumor invades prevertebral space, encases carotid artery, or invades mediastinal structures
Regional Lymph Nodes (N)	
NX	Regional lymph nodes cannot be assessed
N0	No regional lymph node metastasis
N1	Metastasis in a single ipsilateral lymph node, 3 cm or less in greatest dimension
N2	Metastasis in a single ipsilateral lymph node, greater than 3 cm but less than 6 cm in greatest dimension, or in multiple ipsilateral lymph nodes, none greater than 6 cm in greatest dimension, or in bilateral or contralateral lymph nodes, none greater than 6 cm in greatest dimension
N2a	Metastasis in a single ipsilateral lymph node, greater than 3 cm but less than 6 cm in greatest dimension
N2b	Metastasis in multiple ipsilateral lymph nodes, none greater than 6 cm in greatest dimension
N2c	Metastasis in bilateral or contralateral lymph nodes, none more than 6 cm in greatest dimension
N3	Metastasis in a lymph node, greater than 6 cm in greatest dimension
Distant Metastasis (M)	
MX	Distant metastasis cannot be assessed
M0	No distant metastasis
M1	Distant mestasis

Stage Grouping

Stage 0	Tis	N0	M0
Stage I	T1	N0	M0
Stage II	T2	N0	M0
Stage III	T3	N0	M0
	T1	N1	M0
	T2	N1	M0
	T3	N1	M0
Stage IVA	T4a	N0	M0
	T4a	N1	M0
	T1	N2	M0
	T2	N2	M0
	T3	N2	M0
	T4a	N2	M0
Stage IVB	T4b	Any N	M0
	Any T	N3	M0
Stage IVC	Any T	Any N	M1

Used with permission of the American Joint Committee on Cancer (AJCC), Chicago, Illinois. The original source for this material is the AJCC Cancer Staging Manual, Sixth Edition (2002) published by Springer Science and Business Media LLC, www.springerlink.com

TABLE 7-4 Nasopharyngeal Carcinoma: Classification and TNM Staging

Classification of Nasopharyngeal Carcinoma

WHO Classification	*Former Terminology*
Type 1. Squamous cell carcinoma	Squamous cell carcinoma
Type 2. Nonkeratinizing carcinoma	Transitional cell carcinoma
Without lymphoid stroma	Intermediate cell carcinoma
With lymphoid stroma	Lymphepithelial carcinoma (Regaud)
Type 3. Undifferentiated carcinoma	Anaplastic carcinoma,
Without lymphoid stroma	Clear cell carcinoma
With lymphoid stroma	Lymphoepithelial carcinoma (Schminke)

Primary Tumor (T)

TX	Primary tumor cannot be assessed
T0	No evidence of primary tumor
Tis	Carcinoma *in situ*
T1	Tumor confined to the nasopharynx
T2	Tumor extends to soft tissues
T2a	Tumor extends to the oropharynx and/or nasal cavity without parapharyngeal extension
T2b	Any tumor with parapharyngeal extension
T3	Tumor involves bony structures and/or paranasal sinuses
T4	Tumor with intracranial extension and/or involvement of cradial nerves, infratemporal fossa, hypopharynx, orbit, or masticator space

Regional Lymph Nodes (N)

NX	Regional lymph nodes cannot be assessed
N0	No regional lymph node metastasis
N1	Unilateral metastasis in lymph node(s), 6 cm or less in greatest dimension, above the supraclavicular fossa
N2	Bilateral metastasis in lymph node(s), 6 cm or less in greatest dimension, above the supraclavicular fossa
N3	Metastasis in a lymph node(s) 6 cm or greater and/or to supraclavicular fossa
N3a	Greater than 6 cm in dimension
N3b	Extension to the supraclavicular fossa

Distant Metastasis (M)

MX	Distant metastasis cannot be assessed
M0	No distant metastasis
M1	Distant metastasis

Stage Grouping

Stage 0	Tis	N0	M0
Stage I	T1	N0	M0
Stage IIA	T2a	N0	M0
Stage IIB	T1	N1	M0
	T2	N1	M0
	T2a	N1	M0
	T2b	N0	M0
	T2b	N1	M0
Stage III	T1	N2	M0
	T2a	N2	M0
	T2b	N2	M0
	T3	N0	M0
	T3	N1	M0
	T3	N2	M0
Stage IVA	T4	N0	M0
	T4	N1	M0
	T4	N2	M0
Stage IVB	Any T	N3	M0
Stage IVC	Any T	Any N	M1

Used with permission of the American Joint Committee on Cancer (AJCC), Chicago, Illinois. The original source for this material is the AJCC Cancer Staging Manual, Sixth Edition (2002) published by Springer Science and Business Media LLC, www.springerlink.com.

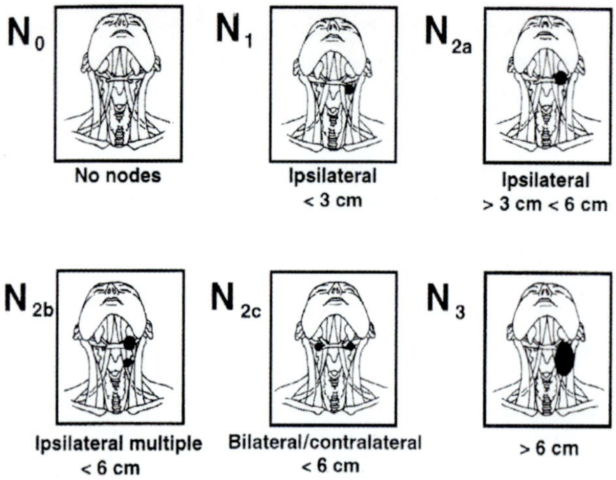

FIG. 7-3 TNM Staging of cervical nodes for all primaries except nasopharynx.

Reprinted with permission from BC Decker.

- Primary tumors of the oral cavity and oropharynx that are 4 cm or larger are T3, and those with massive local invasion of adjacent structures are T4.
- Vocal cord paralysis in the setting of a primary tumor of the larynx or hypopharynx indicates a T stage no less than T3.
- For all primary sites except the nasopharynx, the nodal classifications are the same. In addition, the nasopharynx is one primary site for which an alternative staging system — the Ho staging system — is commonly used, particularly in Asia. Because definitions for component stages vary between the TNM/UICC and Ho systems, these differences must be considered when reviewing the results of therapy.
- For all primary sites except the nasopharynx, the TNM stage grouping is the same; clinical lymph node involvement indicates an overall stage of at least stage III; the presence of distant metastases indicates stage IVc disease, and locally-advanced resectable and unresectable stage IV disease (without distant metastases) are designated as IVa and IVb, respectively.
- The term early-stage disease refers to stages I and II disease and low-volume stage III disease (e.g., T1 or T2 and N0 or N1); the term locally advanced disease refers to stages III and IV disease, specifically a large primary tumor (T3 or T4) or the presence of multiple or bulky neck nodes (N2 or N3). These designations correlate with the efficacy of single or multimodality management.

A major modification to the 2003 version of the AJCC TNM staging system is the division of stage T4 into T4a and T4b categories, which distinguishes a deeply invasive primary lesion that is resectable from one that is unresectable for cure. There is general agreement among surgeons regarding the following criteria for unresectability: base of skull involvement, fixation to the prevertebral fascia, carotid encasement, and involvement of the pterygoid musculature. Additional criteria that many would consider appropriate are the inability to perform an adequate reconstruction for a functional result, a low likelihood of achieving negative margins, and a requirement for total glossectomy. Assignment to the stage IVb category has implications for prognosis (i.e., worse) and treatment (i.e., primary surgical management not planned). For these primary sites, stage IVb disease now includes patients with T4b, any N category, and no metastasis (M0), or any T category and N3 (any neck node larger than 6 cm in greatest diameter). Stage IVc includes any T and N category, as well as M1 disease.

PRINCIPLES OF MANAGEMENT

Historically, surgery and radiation therapy have been the central treatment modalities because they have curative potential. Management of the primary site and neck are separate but related concerns, affecting which modality is used or how to integrate combined-modality therapy when such treatment is necessary. Although chemotherapy may enhance the effects of radiation therapy, chemotherapy by itself is not a curative modality. TNM stage groupings are helpful for defining prognosis and treatment options. Management of head and neck cancer is best served by multidisciplinary treatment planning that involves not only a surgeon, medical oncologist, and radiation oncologist but also dentists, prosthodontists, nutritionists, audiologists, speech and swallowing therapists, physical and occupational therapists, and psychiatrists, as necessary. Plans for rehabilitation are an integral part of this process.

NEWLY DIAGNOSED T1 TO T2, N0 TO N1, AND M0 (STAGES I, II, AND LOW-BULK III) DISEASE

Single-modality treatment with surgery or radiation is typically used for patients with previously untreated stage I, II, or low-bulk stage III disease, essentially a small primary tumor with or without a single ipsilateral node measuring 3 cm or less in diameter. Cure rates for this group are quite good, ranging from 52% to 100%, depending on the

KEY POINTS

- Single-modality treatment with surgery or radiation therapy is typically used with curative intent for previously untreated patients with stage I, II, and low-bulk stage III disease.
- Combined-modality treatment with surgery and radiation or chemoradiotherapy is typically used with curative intent for previously untreated patients with bulky stages III and IV disease without distant metastases.
- Metastatic disease below the clavicles and local-regional recurrent disease without a surgical or radiation option are generally incurable and treated with palliative intent.

TABLE 7-5 Concurrent Chemoradiotherapy Standard of Care

	Regimen
Organ Preservation	
• Larynx	RT/cisplatin[17,18]
• Oropharynx	RT/carboplatin/5-FU[19,20]
Nasopharynx	RT/cisplatin plus cisplatin/5-FU[21]
Unresectable disease	RT/cisplatin[22]
Postoperative adjuvant	RT/cisplatin[23–26]

Abbreviations: RT, radiotherapy; 5-FU, fluorouracil.

primary site. Strategies to decrease the morbidity associated with treatment and prevent second primary tumors have been research priorities. The chosen modality depends on local expertise, anticipated functional outcome, and patient preference. For example, a T1, N0, M0 tumor of the glottic larynx can be managed with surgery or radiation. The 5-year overall survival rates associated with primary surgery (e.g., cordectomy and hemilaryngectomy) and primary radiation therapy with salvage surgery as necessary have been comparable (approximately 90%).[16] A cordectomy requires less time than radiation therapy and initially is cheaper, but repeat procedures may be necessary and lead to a related decrease in function. Radiation therapy is associated with excellent control rates and voice function outcome, but it requires a 6-week course and initially may be more expensive.

NEWLY DIAGNOSED T3, T4 OR N2, N3, AND M0 (HIGHER-BULK STAGE III AND STAGES IVA AND IVB) DISEASE

If a higher-bulk stage III or a stage IV tumor is resectable, the standard approach is surgery followed by adjuvant radiation therapy with or without concurrent chemotherapy based on pathologic risk features (see Principles of Surgery) or combined chemotherapy and radiotherapy if organ preservation is desireable. If unresectable, the approach is radiation and concomitant chemotherapy. Cure rates are more disappointing for this group, ranging from 10% to 65%, depending on the primary site and disease extent. Data from randomized trials support integrated chemotherapy and radiation as standard treatment options for patients with advanced, resectable cancers of the larynx and hypopharynx, with the intent of avoiding total laryngectomy, and for patients with cancers of the oropharynx when a nonsurgical approach is chosen. For patients with advanced tumors of the oropharynx, nasopharynx, or unresectable squamous cell cancers of the upper aerodigestive tract, combined-modality therapy improves survival compared with radiation alone (Table 7-5).[17–26] When primary chemotherapy and radiation therapy are used, surgery is reserved for persistence or recurrence of resectable disease. For locally advanced, resectable cancers of the oral cavity, primary surgical management with appropriate reconstruction and postoperative radiation therapy is the mainstay of treatment because anticipated functional outcomes are favorable.

RECURRENT DISEASE WITHOUT A SURGICAL OR RADIATION OPTION, OR M1 DISEASE

For patients without a surgical or radiation option for whom chemotherapy is used, including patients with distant metastases, such disease is generally not curable and the median survival ranges from 5 to 9 months for various available standard drugs. The identification of more effective chemotherapy has been a priority for this group of patients.

PRINCIPLES OF SURGERY

Complete removal of the tumor with negative margins defines an oncologically adequate surgical resection. Depending on the primary site and the size of the tumor, complete surgical extirpation may necessitate removal of key structures, such as the larynx, eye, or mandible. The potential adverse effect on cosmesis and function underscores the importance of rehabilitation as part of the treatment strategy. A variety of skin and bone flaps, as well as customized obturators and prosthetics, successfully address many defects that arise from surgery. Function-preserving procedures are applicable for selected patients in whom negative margins are achieved while uninvolved structures necessary for function are preserved. Examples include various subtotal laryngectomy procedures for which adding a postoperative course of radiation therapy often compromises the functional outcome. Thus, all of these factors must be considered when deciding the best therapeutic option for each patient.

As the spectrum of reconstructive options increases, defining precise, reproducible criteria for tumor unresectability remains a challenge and complicates interpretation of the

KEY POINTS

- Function-conserving procedures are applicable to selected patients in whom negative margins can be achieved with preservation of structures important for function.
- Conservative or debulking surgery is not part of routine clinical practice for head and neck cancer.
- Comprehensive neck dissections involve removal of all five lymph node levels and are usually performed with therapeutic intent. Selective neck dissections involve removal of fewer than all five levels and are generally done electively to improve staging precision.

literature. A patient with an unresectable tumor should be distinguished from a patient with disease that is clearly resectable, but for whom there are medical contraindications to surgery (i.e., medically inoperable).

Different types of neck surgery or dissection are used to address suspected or proven disease in the cervical lymph nodes. A comprehensive neck dissection involves the en bloc removal of all five lymph node levels (Fig. 7-2). Three important structures are potentially jeopardized by this procedure: the sternocleidomastoid muscle, the internal jugular vein, and the spinal accessory nerve. If none of these structures is spared, the procedure is considered a radical neck dissection, which also is associated with the highest likelihood of postoperative shoulder pain and weakness. Different types of comprehensive neck procedures that spare one, two, or three of these structures (so-called modified-radical neck dissections) may be performed for selected patients without compromise in disease control. Comprehensive neck dissections generally are done with therapeutic intent, such as when cancerous lymph nodes are suspected or known to be present. In other settings, selective neck dissections are used, whereby fewer than five lymph node levels are removed. Selective procedures usually are performed electively in part to improve staging precision, such as when there are no palpable lymph nodes, but the estimated risk of occult metastases exceeds 15% to 20%, and negative findings on specimen analysis may obviate the need for postoperative radiation therapy.

PRINCIPLES OF RADIATION THERAPY

The curability of head and neck cancer with radiation therapy is inversely related to tumor bulk. The rate of disease control with radiation alone decreases with increasing T stage. This finding explains why radiation can be used as a single modality to treat early-stage disease but is generally applied as an adjunct to surgery or combined with chemotherapy for more advanced tumors.

RADIATION DOSE AND FRACTIONATION

The dose of radiation necessary to sterilize squamous cell cancer varies, with the fractionation size and schedule used. Standard, once-daily fractionation consists of 2.0 Gy per day with a total dose of 70 Gy or greater to the primary site and gross adenopathy and 50 Gy or greater to uninvolved nodal stations at risk. When given postoperatively, the total dose to the primary site and involved nodal stations is 60 Gy or greater, and the dose to uninvolved nodal stations at risk is 50 Gy or greater. Postoperative radiation generally begins 4 to 6 weeks after surgery. The delivery of radiation requires careful treatment planning. In particular, the spinal cord must be blocked to prevent radiation-induced cervical myelopathy.

Potential improvements in the therapeutic index of radiation for head and neck cancer may be achieved by altering the radiation fractionation (more than one fraction per day, often with change in the fraction size). The results

> **KEY POINTS**
>
> - Compared with standard schedules, altered-fractionation radiotherapy improves local-regional control of advanced tumors, albeit with increased acute local toxicity.
> - Head and neck radiation commonly causes acute toxicities including mucositis, edema, and xerostomia. Other potential toxicities include hypothyroidism, Lhermitte's syndrome, long-term induration and fibrosis, and osteoradionecrosis of the mandible.
> - Pilocarpine and amifostine may ameliorate radiation-induced xerostomia.

of randomized trials have established the therapeutic benefits of an altered-fractionation strategy, particularly with regard to local-regional control. In one seminal study by the Radiation Therapy Oncology Group (RTOG),[27] more than 1,000 previously untreated patients with stage II, III, or IV squamous cell cancer of the head and neck were randomly assigned to four different radiation-only treatment arms: standard fractionation, 2 Gy daily, and 70 Gy over 7 weeks; hyperfractionation, 1.2 Gy twice daily, and 81.6 Gy over 7 weeks; accelerated fractionation with a split, 1.6 Gy twice daily, 67.2 Gy over 6 weeks; and accelerated fractionation with a concomitant boost, 1.8 Gy daily, 1.5 Gy daily as a boost for the last 12 days only, and 72 Gy over 6 weeks.

With a median follow-up of 41.2 months among surviving patients, the hyperfractionation and concomitant boost arms yielded significantly improved local-regional control ($p = 0.045$ and $p = 0.050$, respectively), as well as a trend toward improvement in disease-free survival ($p = 0.067$ and $p = 0.054$, respectively). More acute toxicity, but not late effects, was seen in the three altered-fractionation groups. Although no significant differences in overall survival were demonstrated, a recent meta-analysis indicated a significant improvement in absolute survival at 5 years (3.4%; HR = 0.92; 95% CI; 0.86, 0.97; $p = 0.003$) with altered-fractionation approaches. This assessment included 15 randomized trials involving 6,515 patients that compared conventional radiotherapy with hyperfractionated, accelerated radiotherapy, or both.[28] The benefit was significantly higher with hyperfractionated radiotherapy than with accelerated radiotherapy (8% and 2% at 5 years, respectively). Altered-fractionation programs are increasingly being incorporated into standard practice for patients who can tolerate the added local-regional toxicity and also are being investigated in combination with concurrent chemotherapy.

RADIATION-RELATED TOXICITY

Radiation at the doses outlined previously is associated with predictable acute mucosal and skin toxicities. Pain management, nutritional support, swallowing evaluation and therapy, and aggressive oral care are required. More aggressive dosing and fractionation schedules, and the addition of concurrent chemotherapy, generally increase the severity of these acute toxicities. Depending on the amount of salivary tissue included in the radiation portal, xerostomia and loss of taste are common. Because adequate saliva is an important component of oral hygiene, careful dental assessment is necessary before the start of radiation therapy, followed by ongoing dental prophylaxis and fluoride treatments. Other potential complications include hypothyroidism, especially for patients receiving treatment to the larynx and pharynx; Lhermitte's syndrome, a self-limited, shock-like sensation extending down the spine and extremities with neck flexion; long-term induration and fibrosis; and osteoradionecrosis of the mandible.

Some degree of xerostomia is a frequently occurring long-term sequelae. Pilocarpine (a cholinomimetic, muscarinic agent) and amifostine (a thiol with chemoprotectant and radioprotectant properties) are both approved for this indication. Amifostine is only approved for use with postoperative adjuvant radiotherapy and not in the definitive setting.

More effective therapies are needed. In a prospective, randomized, double-blind, placebo-controlled trial of patients who received at least 40 Gy of radiation to the head and neck, oral pilocarpine (5 mg three times a day), improved salivary production, and symptoms of dry mouth compared with placebo.[29] Amifostine was evaluated in a multicenter, open-label, randomized trial of patients who received definitive radiotherapy or postoperative adjuvant radiotherapy and total radiotherapy doses of at least 40 Gy.[30] Patients were assigned to either radiation alone (cumulative dose of 50 to 70 Gy) or to the same radiation dose with amifostine (200 mg/m^2 intravenously daily 15 to 30 minutes before radiation).[30] The incidence of grade 2 or higher acute and chronic xerostomia (RTOG Acute/Late Morbidity Scoring Criteria) was significantly reduced in the amifostine arm (acute, 78% vs. 51%, $p < 0.0001$; chronic, 57% vs. 34%, $p = 0.002$), and median salivary production was significantly improved (0.10g vs. 0.26 g., $p < 0.04$). However, the frequency of mucositis was not significantly different between the two groups. Nausea, vomiting, hypotension, and allergic reactions were significantly more common among patients treated with amifostine ($p < 0.05$), although grade 3 toxicities were infrequent (3% to 5% of patients). More convenient and better-tolerated ways to administer this drug (e.g., subcutaneous dosing) are under study.

Conformal-intensity modulated radiation therapy (IMRT) also offers promise as a way to decrease the incidence and severity of xerostomia without compromising antitumor efficacy. The amount of salivary gland tissue included within the radiation portal can be reduced (so-called salivary gland sparing). Whether there is incremental benefit from the use of amifostine when IMRT is used is not known.

Newer strategies in various stages of clinical development include the use of growth factors, cytokine-like agents, small molecules, and anti-inflammatory drugs. The most developed of these classes of drugs is palifermin, a recombinant human keratinocyte growth factor (KGF1). In animal studies, recombinant KGF1 reverses chemotherapy-induced epithelial atrophy and stimulates oral epithelial cell differentiation and proliferation.[31] Palifermin significantly shortened both the median duration of grade 3-4 mucositis (3 vs. 9 days, $p < 0.001$) and the incidence of severe oral mucositis (20% vs. 62%, $p < 0.001$) compared with placebo in patients treated with chemotherapy- and radiotherapy-conditioning regimens in

KEY POINTS

- For patients with unresectable squamous cell cancer of the head and neck, concomitant cisplatin and radiotherapy significantly improves survival, compared with radiotherapy alone, and is the standard of care.
- Concomitant cisplatin and radiotherapy is the standard of care for postoperative adjuvant treatment for patients with positive resection margins or extracapsular extension of nodal disease.
- To preserve the larynx of patients with locally advanced, resectable cancer of the larynx, concomitant cisplatin and radiotherapy or radiotherapy alone is the standard of care. Survival rates are the same, but the need for salvage laryngectomy is significantly greater with radiotherapy alone (30% vs. 15%).
- To preserve oropharyngeal functions of speech and swallowing, concomitant chemotherapy and radiotherapy is the standard of care for T3 to T4 or N2 to N3 cancers of the oropharynx (especially the tongue base and tonsil).
- To preserve the larynx of patients with locally advanced, resectable (T2 to T4a, N0 to N2c) cancer of the hypopharynx, induction chemotherapy and radiotherapy is the standard of care based on randomized controlled trials. However, concomitant chemotherapy and radiotherapy is often used by extrapolation of results from other primary sites.
- A randomized controlled trial of cetuximab added to radiotherapy for definitive treatment of locally advanced cancer showed significantly improved survival compared with radiotherapy alone. However, no indications for using cetuximab plus radiotherapy in place of standard platinum-based chemotherapy plus radiotherapy have been established.
- There is promising data for induction chemotherapy using a taxane with cisplatin plus 5-FU regimen followed by concomitant chemoradiation (termed sequential therapy), but this is not standard of care. Trials comparing chemoradiation with or without induction chemotherapy in high-risk populations are in progress.

preparation for stem cell transplantation; it was on this basis that it was approved by the U.S. Food and Drug Administration (FDA).[32,33] A phase III multicenter study of head and neck cancer is in progress.

PRINCIPLES OF CHEMOTHERAPY

A number of drugs have activity against squamous cell cancer of the head and neck, including methotrexate, cisplatin, carboplatin, fluorouracil (5-FU), paclitaxel, docetaxel, and ifosfamide. Gemcitabine, vinorelbine, bleomycin, topotecan, and irinotecan also are active but are used less frequently in current clinical practice. The reported response proportions vary with the setting (untreated or pretreated) and the drugs used (single agent or combination). The best established and arguably most widely used treatment is a combination of cisplatin and infusional 5-FU that will cause a complete plus partial response in 60% to 90% of previously untreated, advanced, local-regional tumors; clinical complete responses are common (20% to 50%). By contrast, the activity of the same drug combination for recurrent disease is 30% to 40%, and complete responses are very infrequent. Rates of complete and partial responses from single-agent therapy are generally approximately one-half of those observed with combination chemotherapy and range from 13% to 31% for the previously listed drugs.

The use of chemotherapy for patients with potentially curable, advanced, local-regional disease is generally distinguished from the treatment of patients with incurable, recurrent, metastatic disease. For patients with potentially curable cancer, the chemotherapy literature can be divided into the following four groups:

- induction or neoadjuvant chemotherapy administered for several cycles prior to definitive local therapy (surgery or radiation therapy);
- concomitant chemotherapy and radiotherapy in the setting of locally advanced, unresectable disease;
- organ-preservation techniques for patients with resectable cancers of the oropharynx, larynx, and hypopharynx; and
- local curative therapy (surgery) followed by adjuvant chemotherapy and radiotherapy.

The goals of these multimodality approaches are to improve survival by reducing rates of local-regional recurrence and metastases, as well as to achieve preservation of the organ and its function without a decrement in the survival rates achieveable with primary surgery. The latter specifically refers to preservation of the larynx for patients with primary cancers of the larynx or hypopharynx and preservation of structures in the oropharynx for speech and swallowing function, such as the tongue.

INDUCTION CHEMOTHERAPY

Studies evaluating the integration of induction chemotherapy with local-regional treatment dominated the literature of head and neck cancer during the 1980s and early 1990s. Based on resectability status, the control arm of phase III trials was either radiation alone for those with unresectable

TABLE 7-6 Selected Randomized Trials of Induction Chemotherapy Followed by Local Treatment Versus Local Treatment Alone

Author	Year	Patients	Chemotherapy	Survival and LRC
HNCP[34]	1987	462	PB	No difference
Schuller[35]	1988	158	PBV	No difference
Jortay*[36]	1990	187	VBM	No difference
VALCSG*[64]	1991	332	PF	No difference
Jaulerry[37]	1992	100	PBVds mito	No difference
Jaulerry[37]	1992	108	PFVds	No difference
Mazeron[38]	1992	131	PFBM	No difference
Depondt[39]	1993	324	CbF	No difference
Paccagnella[41]	1994	221	PF	Improved: Induction (unresectable pts)
Dalley[40]	1995	280	PF	No difference
Lefebvre*[44]	1996	202	PF	No difference
Domenge*[42]	2000	318	PF	Improved: Induction (survival only)
Forastiere*[17]	2003	346	PF	No difference
Licitra*[43]	2003	195	PF	No difference

*Site specific trial.
Abbreviations: LRC, local-regional control; HNPC, Head and Neck Contracts Program; P, cisplatin; BM, bleomycin; V, vinblastine; VALCSG, Veterans Affairs Laryngeal Cancer Study Group; F, fluorouracil; Vds, vindesine; M, methotrexate; Cb, carboplatin; Mito, mitomycin.

disease or surgery plus adjuvant radiation for those patients whose tumors were considered resectable. The results of randomized controlled trials evaluating two to four courses of cisplatin-based combination chemotherapy as induction followed by local therapy demonstrated a decrease in distant metastases in some trials, but no significant differences were observed in either local-regional control or overall survival when compared with the standard of care in the vast majority of trials and multiple meta-analyses. This result was found despite the high level of antitumor activity for cisplatin and infusional 5-FU and the 85% complete and partial response rate. The largest randomized trials (enrollment of at least 100 patients) are described in Table 7-6.[17,34–44] Several of these trials are noteworthy.

The Head and Neck Contracts Program (HNCP) was the first and largest randomized trial to test the induction chemotherapy question.[34] A total of 462 patients with locally advanced, resectable head and neck cancer without metastasis were randomly assigned to one of three treatment groups: standard, induction, or maintenance. Standard therapy consisted of surgery and postoperative radiotherapy, induction therapy consisted of one cycle of cisplatin and bleomycin infusion followed by standard treatment, and maintenance therapy consisted of one cycle of cisplatin and bleomycin infusion followed by standard treatment followed by six planned cycles of cisplatin (80 mg/m^2). There was no significant difference in local-regional control or survival among the three groups; however, the maintenance arm had a lower rate of distant failure as site of first relapse. A subsequent multivariate analysis suggested that maintenance chemotherapy was of greatest benefit to patients with N2 disease.[45]

In another randomized controlled trial, 237 patients with stages III and IV cancer of the oral cavity, oropharynx, hypopharynx, or paranasal sinus were randomly assigned to receive standard treatment or four cycles of a cisplatin and 5-FU infusion followed by standard treatment.[41] The trial included patients with resectable or unresectable disease. The control arm, or standard local-regional treatment, was prospectively determined for each patient based on their resectability status. There was no difference in overall survival or local-regional control between the two groups, although there was a significant reduction in the incidence of distant metastases with the addition of chemotherapy. Of interest, on subset analysis, all outcomes improved for the patients with unresectable disease (3-year survival of 10% for those patients treated with radiation compared with 24% for those receiving induction chemotherapy; $p = 0.04$); only distant control improved for resectable disease with chemotherapy. These results were maintained with long-term follow-up.[46]

More than 30 randomized controlled trials were published using this induction chemotherapy design, and all but two trials found no survival advantage for induction chemotherapy. The most commonly used chemotherapy regimen was 100 mg/m^2 of cisplatin on day 1 and 1,000mg/m^2 of 5-FU every 24 hours by continuous infusion for 120 hours.

A meta-analysis of 63 randomized trials of local-regional treatment with or without chemotherapy was performed using updated patient data and was published in 2000.[47] In this comprehensive review, there was no significant survival benefit from the addition of induction chemotherapy (31 trials; 5,269 patients; HR = 0.95; 95% CI; 0.88, 1.01; $p = 0.10$). A subgroup analysis focusing on trials in which induction cisplatin and 5-FU was used showed a significant survival benefit for this regimen (HR = 0.88; 95% CI; 0.79, 0.97, $p = 0.05$).

In a more recent randomized trial, the effect of three cycles of cisplatin and 5-FU before planned surgery was evaluated in 195 patients with category T2 to T4 (greater than 3 cm; N0 to N2; M0) squamous cell cancer of the oral cavity.[43] The design of this study allowed modification of the surgical procedure based on the proximity of the tumor to the mandible. The 5-year survival rate was identical for patients who received chemotherapy before surgery and patients who did not (55%), but postoperative radiation therapy (33% compared with 46% for no preoperative chemotherapy) and mandible resection (31% compared with 52% for no preoperative chemotherapy) were used less frequently for those patients who received chemotherapy followed by surgery. Ensuring that the same operation is performed after induction chemotherapy, particularly if there is a response, is a methodologic design challenge for such studies and may, in part, explain why the approach has not yielded clear improvements in overall survival.

Taken collectively, these data did not support a role in standard clinical practice for induction chemotherapy in the setting of planned surgery and radiation with improvement in overall survival as the endpoint. However, recent trials that investigated the addition of a taxane (docetaxel or paclitaxel) to cisplatin and infusional 5-FU have stimulated much interest in the re-evaluation of induction chemotherapy. The approach likely will be of greatest research interest for patient populations at increased risk for distant metastatic disease (e.g., disease categories N2 to N3 and in selected primary sites) and for those in whom initial primary surgical treatment is not planned or feasible (i.e., unresectable disease or resectable disease with an organ-preservation endpoint).

INDUCTION CHEMOTHERAPY USING CISPLATIN AND 5-FU PLUS A TAXANE

The results from three randomized controlled trials directly comparing three or four cycles of induction combination docetaxel, cisplatin, and 5-FU to standard 100 mg/m^2 of cisplatin plus 1,000 mg/m^2 continuous infusion of 5-FU daily for 5 days) have been published and presented at international meetings.[48–50] The TAX 323 trial enrolled more than 300 patients with locally advanced unresectable disease. The control arm consisted of four cycles of the two-drug combination followed by radiotherapy, and the experimental arm consisted of four cycles of the three-drug combination (docetaxel, 75 mg/m^2; cisplatin, 75 mg/m^2; 5-FU, 750 mg/m^2 per day continuous infusion for 5 days) followed by radiotherapy.[48] The response rate to induction of the three-drug regimen was significantly higher compared with that of the two-drug regimen (68% vs 54%, p = 0.006) as was overall survival (HR = 0.73 (0.57, 0.94); p = 0.016). There also was less toxicity with the three-drug combination than with the two-drug combination.

Similarly, the TAX 324 trial randomly assigned 501 patients with unresectable or resectable disease (all sites) to three cycles of standard cisplatin and 5-FU or to combination docetaxel, cisplatin, and 5-FU (docetaxel, 75 mg/m^2; cisplatin, 100 mg/m^2; 5-FU, 1,000 mg/m^2 per day continuous infusion for 4 days).[49] Definitive local therapy in both arms consisted of standard radiotherapy plus weekly carboplatin (area under the curve [AUC] = 1.5). Overall survival was significantly improved for patients who received the three-drug therapy (HR = 0.70 (0.54, 0.90); p = 0.0058).

The third trial was conducted by the European GORTEC study group for organ preservation in patients with either cancer of the larynx or cancer of the hypopharynx.[50] A total of 220 patients were randomly assigned, and of those, just more than one-half had a hypopharynx primary tumor. The stage of the primary tumor was T3 in the majority of patients. The two treatment arms were standard cisplatin and 5-FU for three cycles (control) or combination docetaxel, cisplatin, and 5-FU for three cycles (dosing same as TAX 323). Following induction of both therapies, responding patients received 70 Gy of standard radiation or surgery for inadequate response. The three-drug therapy was shown to be statistically superior for the endpoints of response to the induction regimen (83% vs. 61%) and preservation of a functional larynx at 3 years (63% vs. 41%). More details of the patient population and outcomes are needed for interpretation of the results in the context of other larynx preservation trials for these two primary sites.

These three trials demonstrate that combination docetaxel, cisplatin, and 5-FU followed by radiotherapy alone or radiotherapy and concurrent carboplatin is superior to cisplatin and 5-FU followed by the same definitive local therapy. Also, the three-drug regimen administered in the TAX 323 seems to have an acceptable toxicity profile with lower rates of severe and life-threatening myelosuppression than observed with the two-drug regimen.[48] A fourth phase III trial has been published in final form.[51] This trial compared induction combination paclitaxel, cisplatin, and 5-FU to induction cisplatin and 5-FU in a heterogeneous population of patients with resectable and unresectable cancer. Chemoradiation was planned following induction chemotherapy but the actual treatment was not uniform. The taxane-containing treatment group had a higher overall response rate (80% vs. 68%); however, the difference in overall survival was not significant.

These trials indicate that treatment with a taxane plus cisplatin and 5-FU is more effective than cisplatin and 5-FU alone when using response rate as the measure. They do not indicate that induction combination docetaxel, cisplatin, and 5-FU is the standard of care but provide support for a prospective, randomized controlled trial that compares induction chemotherapy followed by chemoradiation (termed sequential treatment) against the standard of care of chemoradiation for nonsurgical management of resectable disease or for management of unresectable disease. Several of such trial designs are in progress in the United States. Combination docetaxel, cisplatin, and 5-FU should replace cisplatin and 5-FU as a new standard regimen for induction chemotherapy and is being used in ongoing trials.

CONCOMITANT CHEMOTHERAPY AND RADIATION

Since the early 1990s, concomitant chemotherapy and radiation has progressively displaced induction chemotherapy followed by radiation in therapeutic investigations for patients with locally advanced squamous cell cancer of the head and neck. The approach is not a new one, with the first randomized trial in which a concurrent regimen was evaluated dating back to the 1970s. Taken collectively, the results of these early randomized studies were much more encouraging than induction designs with regard to improvement in overall survival. The focus has been on drugs that show both activity against the disease and radiation-enhancement properties (e.g., cisplatin and 5-FU). The three general strategies that can be identified amidst a broad spectrum of approaches are

- concomitant, single-agent, or combination chemotherapy with continuous-course radiation;
- combination chemotherapy with planned split-course radiation; and
- rapidly alternating chemotherapy and radiation.

More recently, altered-fractionation approaches have become an added variable. Historically, the use of chemotherapy in this manner was applied to patients with unresectable disease and generally increased the severity of acute mucosal and skin toxicities but also improved local-regional control when compared with treatment using radiation alone. These encouraging efficacy results led to studies of other patient groups (e.g., resectable, organ-preservation intent, and poor-risk adjuvant).

A study first reported in 1992 was the turning point for the growing interest in concomitant chemoradiotherapy for advanced head and neck cancer.[52] In this study, the investigators randomly assigned 157 patients with unresectable squamous cell cancer of the head and neck to radiation alone (up to 70 Gy, conventional fractionation) or to a cisplatin and 5-FU combination alternating with radiation (up to 60 Gy). The complete response rate (43%) and the survival rate (41%) in the group treated with chemoradiotherapy were significantly superior to those in the radiation alone group (22% and 23%, respectively, $p = 0.01$).

The trial that led to the current standard of care for locally advanced, unresectable squamous cancers of the head and neck was Eastern Cooperative Oncology Group (ECOG) 1392.[22] Based on encouraging phase II trial data from the RTOG and the ECOG, a three-arm trial was designed. A total of 295 patients with unresectable squamous cell cancer of the head and neck were randomly assigned to one of three treatment groups: radiation alone (70 Gy, 2 Gy daily); the same radiation with concurrent cisplatin (100 mg/m^2) on days 1, 22, and 43; or split-course radiation (60 to 70 Gy, 2 Gy daily) with three cycles of concurrent bolus cisplatin and infusional 5-FU. In the third arm, the option existed to pursue surgical resection after the second cycle of chemotherapy, if possible; resection was available for all three groups if feasible after the completion of treatment.[22] With a median follow-up of 41 months, there was a significant survival advantage at 3 years associated with concurrent cisplatin and radiation compared with radiation alone (37% and 23%; $p = 0.014$). The split-course concurrent regimen offered no survival advantage compared with the control groups (27%). Toxicity of grade 3 or higher was significantly more common with concurrent therapy (52% with radiotherapy alone vs. 89% with concurrent [$p < 0.0001$]). This trial established radiation with concurrent high-dose cisplatin as the standard of care for locally advanced unresectable head and neck cancer.

The meta-analysis by Pignon et al.,[47] which included the 1992 study and others, highlights the favorable results seen with a concurrent approach in these early trials. Although significant heterogeneity among designs was noted, the concurrent chemoradiotherapy regimen was associated with an 8% absolute benefit in survival at 5 years compared with radiation alone (HR = 0.81; 95% CI; 0.76, 0.88; $p < 0.0001$). An updated analysis of 87 trials and more than 16,000 patients showed the same absolute benefit for survival with concomitant treatment (HR = 0.81; $p < 0.0001$).[53]

Some clinicians assert that using an altered-fractionation schedule would potentially negate any added benefit of chemotherapy. In one study, 122 patients with advanced squamous cell cancer of the head and neck, including both resectable and unresectable disease, were randomly assigned to continuous hyperfractionated radiation alone (75 Gy, 1.25 Gy in twice-daily fractions) or a split-course hyperfractionated radiation (70 Gy, 1.25 Gy in twice-daily fractions) with concurrent daily doses of cisplatin (12 mg/m^2) and 5-FU (600 mg/m^2) during weeks 1 and 6 of radiation therapy.[54] Two cycles of adjuvant cisplatin and 5-FU were planned in this latter study group and were administered to 57% of patients. Local-regional control was significantly better for the combined-modality group (70%) than for the radiation-alone group (44%; $p = 0.01$). The 3-year relapse-free survival rate was 41% for the radiation-alone group compared with 61% for the combined-modality group ($p = 0.08$); the 3-year overall survival rate for the radiation-alone group was 34% and 55% for the combined-modality group ($p = 0.07$). These results were not statistically significant. With multivariate adjustment for a prognostic imbalance, the latter two p values became 0.12 and 0.11, respectively. Mucositis was slower to heal, and feeding tubes were more often necessary with the addition of chemotherapy.

In a study addressing a similar question, 130 patients with stage III or IV head and neck cancer were randomly assigned to hyperfractionated radiation (77 Gy, 1.1 Gy in twice-daily fractions for 35 treatment days) with or without daily concurrent low-dose cisplatin (6 mg/m^2).[55] There was a significant improvement in overall survival at 5 years in the combined modality group (46% compared with 25% for the radiation alone group; $p = 0.0075$), as well as significant improvements in progression-free, local-regional progression-free, and distant metastasis-free survival rates. The results of these studies and others suggest that concurrent chemotherapy adds benefit in tumor control even when an altered-fractionation radiation program is used.

There is little data to determine the best option among different concurrent regimens because most studies of concurrent chemoradiotherapy include radiation alone as the control group. In a three-arm, randomized study, treatment with daily doses of cisplatin (6 mg/m^2) or carboplatin (25 mg/m^2) concurrent with radiation were compared with radiation alone.[56] Both concurrent arms yielded a significant and comparable advantage in survival compared with radiation alone. A randomized phase II study done within the RTOG (protocol 97-03) evaluated the following three different concurrent chemotherapy/radiation programs: cisplatin and 5-FU, hydroxyurea and 5-FU (split-course radiation), and paclitaxel and cisplatin.[57] The results indicated that the 2-year survival rates were comparable among the treatment arms and were collectively superior to historic RTOG results in a similar population of patients treated with concurrent high-dose cisplatin and radiation, although such a comparison must be interpreted cautiously, particularly given concerns about potential stage migration.

A meta-analysis of randomized concurrent chemoradiotherapy studies for patients with locally advanced squamous cell cancer of the head and neck, the Meta-Analysis of Chemotherapy in Head and Neck Cancer (MACH-NC), was conducted with the intent of developing clinical recommendations.[58] With data from 1,514 patients in nine trials, the investigators found that platinum-based concurrent programs offered the greatest survival advantage compared with radiation alone (odds ratio [OR] = 0.57; 95% CI; 0.46, 0.71; $p < 0.00001$). They recommended that, if concurrent therapy is pursued, a platinum-based regimen associated with a positive trial and a more favorable side-effect profile should be used. The MACH-NC analysis also confirmed that cisplatin-based chemoradiotherapy provided the most significant benefit in terms of survival and local-regional control.[59]

The use of targeted therapies concurrent with radiotherapy is an area of great interest. EGFR is highly expressed in virtually all squamous cell cancers of the head and neck, and expression is inversely associated with prognosis. Therefore, inhibitors of the EGFR have been the focus of most targeted therapy trials in head and neck cancer. Cetuximab (C225) is a chimeric immunoglobulin G antibody that binds the EGFR with affinity comparable to that observed with natural ligands. Preclinical data demonstrated at least additive effects of cetuximab combined with radiotherapy or with cisplatin, paclitaxel, and other cytotoxics. Cetuximab was approved by the FDA for use in combination with radiotherapy in patients with advanced head and neck cancer based on a multicenter trial published by Bonner and colleagues.[60] This important proof of principle trial randomly assigned patients with locally advanced squamous cell cancers of the oropharynx, larynx, and hypopharynx to treatment with radiotherapy alone (standard or altered fractionation schedules) or the same radiotherapy with concurrent weekly cetuximab. Local-regional failure-free survival and overall survival rates were significantly improved with the addition of cetuximab. The median duration of local-regional failure-free survival was 24.4 months with cetuximab and 14.89 months with RT alone ($p = 0.005$). The 3-year survival rates were 57% with cetuximab versus 44% with radiotherapy alone ($p = 0.02$). Cetuximab had no effect on distant metastases; the effect on local-regional control using standard definition (death censored, events defined as local and/or regional recurrence) was not reported. Whether this combination of radiotherapy and a biologic therapy is as effective as the standard of chemoradiation is unknown; therefore, the exact role and indications for cetuximab with radiotherapy are not clear. The patient population was heterogeneous relative to resectability, primary site, and radiation schedule. Exploratory subset analyses suggested that benefit was limited to primary sites of the oropharynx and to treatment with altered fractionation radiotherapy schedules, but the sample size was small and these analyses were unplanned.

At present, the only indication for cetuximab with radiotherapy in lieu of platinum-based chemotherapy is for the treatment of patients whose age, performance status, and/or extent of comorbid disease would preclude cisplatin or carboplatin. Numerous trials are currently testing the addition of cetuximab or small-molecule tyrosine kinase inhibitors to chemoradiation in various disease settings. One such trial, RTOG 0522, directly compares cisplatin and radiation with or without cetuximab.

In summary, concurrent chemoradiotherapy leads to improved disease control compared with radiation alone for patients with unresectable squamous cell cancer of the head and neck and represents standard treatment for patients who are able to tolerate the anticipated added treatment-related toxicity. There also is a role for this approach in the organ-preservation and larynx-preservation setting and for advanced local-regional nasopharyngeal cancer. The data showing improvement are best established for platinum-based concurrent regimens; an

TABLE 7-7 Randomized Trials Of Radiotherapy vs. Concurrent Chemotherapy or a Biologic Plus Radiotherapy

Study	Patients	Chemotherapy	RT (Gy)	Outcome Estimate (years)	RT vs. RT + Chemo (% of patients)	
					L/R Control	Survival
Merlano (1996)[52]	157	5-FU, DDP (Alt)	60–70	5	35 vs. 68	10 vs. 24
Wendt (1998)[61]	270	5-FU, DDP, LV	70.2 (bid, split)	3	17 vs. 36	24 vs. 48
Brizel (1998)[54]	116	5-FU, DDP	70–75 (Bid)	3	44 vs. 70	34 vs. 55 (NS)
Adelstein (1998)[62,63]	100	5-FU, DDP	66–72	5	45 vs. 77	48 vs. 50 (NS)
Calais (1999)[19]	226+	5-FU, Combo	70	5^	25 vs. 48	16 vs. 22
Jeremic (2000)[55]	130	DDP 6mg/m^2/d	77 (Bid)	6	36 vs. 50##	25 vs. 46
Starr (2001)	240	5-FU, DDP	70.2 (Bid, CB)	2	40 vs. 60 ++	57 vs. 68^
Adelstein (2003)[22]	271	DDP 100 m^2 x3	70	3	NR	23 vs. 37
Forastiere (2003)[17,18]	345#	DDP 100/M^2 X3	70	5	51 vs. 69	54 vs. 55 (Ns)
Bonner (2006)[60]	424	Cetuximab	70-72 (Std, Bid, Cb)	3	NR	45 vs. 55

+ Oropharynx only. # Larynx only. ## Local-regional (L/R) progression-free survival. ^ OP. ++ OP survival with local-regional control. Abbreviations: 5-FU, fluorouracil; DDP, cisplatin; LV, leucovorin; NS, not statistically significant; NR, not reported; OP, oropharynx; CB, concomitant boost.

advantage persists even when newer altered-fractionation approaches are employed. The results of randomized trials comparing concurrent chemoradiation or biologic therapy plus radiation are outlined in Table 7-7. Unless indicated, all outcome improvements were statistically signifcant.[18–20,22,52,54,55,60–62]

ADJUVANT CHEMORADIATION

The results of two randomized controlled trials have clarified the role of chemoradiation in the postoperative adjuvant setting when compared with radiotherapy alone. These studies conducted by EORTC[23] and the trial by the RTOG[24] addressed the question of whether the addition of cisplatin to standard postoperative radiotherapy based on pathologic criteria would improve the outcome of patients. The experimental arms of both studies consisted of standard fractionation radiation with concurrent cisplatin (100 mg/m^2) on days 1, 22, and 43. The 5-year results of the EORTC study indicated significant improvement in progression-free survival (47% compared with 36%, $p = 0.04$), and overall survival (53% compared with 40%, $p = 0.02$) in favor of concurrent cisplatin plus radiation. The findings of the RTOG study initially demonstrated a significant advantage with combined-modality adjuvant therapy for the first two outcomes, but not for overall survival (3-year survival was 56% compared with 47%; $p = 0.09$). In both studies, toxicity was greater with concurrent chemoradiotherapy.

Although the treatment was very similar, the high-risk pathologic features were not uniform, and the study populations differed. The entry criteria for the RTOG study were the presence of multiple positive nodes, extracapsular extension of tumor, or a positive margin. In contrast, the EORTC trial defined high risk as positive margin, extra capsular extension of nodal disease, vascular embolisms, or perineural disease; for oral cavity or oropharynx primary sites, high risk was defined as positive nodes at level IV or V. These differences may in part explain the variable outcome of the two trials. In an effort to reconcile these two trial results, a pooled analysis was performed that showed that the subsets of patients in both trials with significant benefit from cisplatin added to radiotherapy had either microscopically involved margins or extracapsular extension of disease in neck nodes.[25] The presence of either or both of these risk factors is, therefore, considered a definite indication for adjuvant chemoradiation. Since these analyses were performed, the RTOG trial data have been reanalyzed with longer follow-up and now demonstrate a significant advantage for chemoradiation regarding improvement of local-regional control. The difference in disease-free survival is no longer significant.[26] These results underscore the importance of reporting mature outcome data but do not change current treatment recommendations.

ORGAN AND LARYNX PRESERVATION

Initial organ preservation studies were developed around the use of induction chemotherapy for patients with resectable disease and subsequently have focused on concomitant chemoradiotherapy. A number of pilot studies established the feasibility of treatment with chemotherapy followed by radiation therapy, with surgery reserved for patients who had disease at the primary site that did not respond to chemotherapy, who had persistent disease after radiation, or who had local-regional recurrence. These trials yielded survival results comparable to historical controls and led to successful organ preservation for a substantial proportion of patients. Avoidance of total laryngectomy received the greatest attention in these early studies, and preservation of the larynx was the focus of three subsequent randomized trials.[44,64–66]

The Department of Veterans Affairs Laryngeal Cancer Study Group (VALCSG) conducted a seminal randomized trial in which induction cisplatin and 5-FU infusion (three cycles) followed by radiation therapy (with surgery reserved for patients who had an inadequate response, disease persistence, or relapse) was compared with total laryngectomy followed by radiation therapy.[64,65] The 332 patients had advanced, resectable, category T2 to T4 laryngeal cancer. There was no significant difference in survival between the groups with more than 10 years of follow-up subsequent to the original publication; total laryngectomy was avoided in approximately two-thirds of survivors who received combined chemotherapy and radiation. On multivariate analysis, T4 or N2 disease were both significant predictors of treatment failure, with 56% of T4 cases eventually requiring laryngectomy. The pattern of failure differed between the two treatment groups, with a significant reduction in distant failure but a higher rate of local failure for the patients randomly assigned to induction chemotherapy compared with those in the surgery control arm. Long-term quality-of-life outcomes also were assessed. Among the 46 long-term survivors surveyed, those who received induction chemotherapy plus radiation had significantly better quality-of-life scores ($p < 0.05$), better pain scores, and less depression. After 2 years, communication (speech) scores favored the induction chemotherapy group, but at longer follow-up the two treatment groups had similar speech scores.[67]

The EORTC performed a similar study in patients with advanced, resectable (T2 to T4) cancer of the hypopharynx.[44] There was no difference in survival between the two groups; the 5-year estimate of successful larynx preservation (i.e., local control and no tracheostomy or feeding tube) was 35%. These two studies established induction cisplatin and infusional 5-FU followed by radiation in the responders as an alternative to initial surgical management. This combined modality approach became a standard treatment option for patients with locally advanced, resectable laryngeal or hypopharyngeal cancer seeking to avoid total laryngectomy. Close monitoring for recurrence and timely integration of salvage surgery is an important part of these combined approaches and is necessary for survival to remain comparable to that associated with primary surgical management.

During the 1990s, interest shifted from induction chemotherapy to concomitant chemotherapy and radiation not only as definitive treatment for unresectable squamous cell cancers but also in patients with resectable disease who chose organ preservation rather than initial surgery. Available data suggested that concomitant chemotherapy with radiation was more effective than the sequential administration of these modalities because of improvement in local-regional control. In one randomized study, primary radiation therapy (68 to 72 Gy, 1.8 to 2 Gy daily) was compared with the same radiation regimen plus concurrent daily cisplatin (20 mg/m^2/day) and 5-FU (1,000 mg/m^2/day) for 4 days starting on days 1 and 22. Enrolled patients had resectable, stage III or IV squamous cell cancer of the head and neck.[62] Surgery was recommended for both groups if no response was evident at 50 to 55 Gy or for disease persistence or recurrence at the completion of treatment. Most of the 100 patients enrolled had primary lesions of the larynx, hypopharynx, or oropharynx. With a median follow-up of 5 years, overall survival was not significantly different between the two groups, but survival with successful primary-site preservation was superior in the chemoradiation group (5-year rates were 34% compared with 42%, respectively; $p = 0.004$), albeit at the expense of greater acute hematologic toxicity, mucositis, cutaneous reaction, weight loss, and the need for a feeding tube during treatment. There was no significant difference in overall survival, which was attributed to effective salvage surgery and competing causes of death.[63]

A follow-up study to the VALCSG, Intergroup R91-11, directly addressesd two questions unresolved in the prior trial, including[17] the optimal sequencing of chemotherapy and radiotherapy (induction followed by radiation or concomitant chemoradiation) and the precise contribution of chemotherapy added to radiotherapy. A total of 547 patients with category T2 to low-volume T4, nonmetastatic, squamous cell cancer of the larynx were randomly assigned to one of three treatment arms: radiation alone (70 Gy, 35 fractions); concomitant cisplatin (100 mg/m^2), administered intravenously on days 1, 22, and 43 with the same radiation dose; or induction cisplatin and 5-FU, followed by radiation for patients who had a complete or partial response of the primary site.

In all groups, laryngectomy was reserved for patients with insufficient response, suspected disease persistence, or local recurrence. A planned neck dissection was performed at approximately 8 weeks after completion of radiation in patients who had category N2 or N3 disease at initial staging.

The results at 2 years showed significant improvement in the larynx preservation rate for the concomitant-treatment arm (88%) compared with the induction arm (75%, $p = 0.005$) and the radiation-alone arm (70%, $p < 0.001$). Local-regional control also was significantly better with concomitant treatment compared with the other two treatments (78% compared with 61% and 56%, respectively). Chemotherapy suppressed distant metastases, with rates of 8%, 9%, and 16% for concomitant, induction, and radiation-alone arms, respectively. Disease-free survival was significantly better in both the concomitant (61%) and the induction (52%) arms compared with the radiation-alone arm (44%); however, the overall survival rates did not differ among the three groups. Chemotherapy-related toxicities (grades 3 to 4 mucositis in the concomitant arm and grades 3 to 4 myelosuppression in the induction arm) were more common in the combination treatment groups than in the radiation alone group, although rates for possible treatment-related deaths were not significantly different. Mature data reported after a minimum follow-up of nearly 5 years for all patients confirmed these results.[18] Laryngectomy-free survival is an endpoint that combines survival and a quality-of-life parameter and does not account for patients dying from other causes with an intact larynx. Although this would not be chosen as the primary endpoint today, laryngectomy-free survival was the endpoint used to generate the statistical hypothesis in 1990. In the initial 2-year data analysis of this endpoint, only the concomitant arm showed significant improvement when compared with radiation alone; however, in the mature analysis both induction and concomitant arms reached statistical significance when compared with radiation alone for the endpoint of laryngectomy-free survival. The importance of this finding for clinical practice is unclear because the larynx preservation and local-control results were not different for patients treated with induction chemotherapy followed by radiotherapy or with radiotherapy alone; these results were significantly inferior to the results with concomitant cisplatin and radiotherapy.

In summary, the INT R91-11 trial showed that the optimal sequencing of chemotherapy and radiotherapy to achieve larynx preservation, improve local-regional control, and reduce distant metastases is concomitant administration. Furthermore, induction chemotherapy did not improve the local-regional control or larynx preservation rates over those achievable with radiotherapy alone, but it did add substantial toxicity. For patients who wish to preserve their larynx, 100 mg/m^2 of daily cisplatin administered on days 1, 22, 43 during radiotherapy is the standard of care with surgery reserved for those patients who have persistent or recurrent disease following treatment completion.

A randomized larynx preservation trial for patients with locally advanced, resectable cancer of the larynx or the hypopharynx is in progress within the EORTC. This trial compares induction chemotherapy followed by radiotherapy with an alternating schedule of chemotherapy and radiotherapy. The preliminary results show no significant difference in rates for preservation of a functional larynx at 3 years[68] and no difference in survival. Until further details of the trial are known, induction cisplatin and 5-FU, as previously evaluated by the EORTC, remains the evidence-based recommendation for standard of care for locally advanced cancers of the hypopharynx. However, based on the data for combination docetaxel, cisplatin, and 5-FU, it would be appropriate to substitute cisplaint and 5-FU with this triple-drug regimen in this treatment sequence.

Given the results of these larynx-preservation studies, the concomitant chemoradiation approach also has been of investigational interest for locally advanced, resectable tumors of other primary sites for which surgical management may lead to substantial cosmetic or functional morbidity. An important site-specific trial was reported by the Groupe d'Oncologie Radiotherapie Tete et Cou (GORTEC).[19,20] A total of 226 patients with stage III or IV squamous cell cancer of the oropharynx were randomly assigned to either radiotherapy alone (70 Gy, 35 fractions) or the same radiation program with concomitant bolus doses of carboplatin (70 mg/m^2 daily for 4 days) and 5-FU (600 mg/m^2 as a daily 24-hour infusion for 4 days) starting on days 1, 22, and 43. Concomitant treatment yielded a better 3-year survival rate (51% compared with 31%; $p = 0.02$) and disease-free survival (42% compared with 20%; $p = 0.04$), albeit at the expense of greater toxicity. Mucositis, related weight loss and need for a feeding tube, and hematologic toxicity occurred more frequently in the chemoradiotherapy group. This treatment approach, therefore, is considered an evidence-based standard treatment option and is particularly applicable to the management of stage category T3 to T4 or N2 to N3 disease located at the base of tongue or tonsils.

Available data indicate that concomitant chemoradiation is feasible for oropharynx cancer, and disease-control outcomes compare favorably with those obtained historically with primary surgical management. However, a series of site-specific, direct, randomized comparisons to standard surgery and postoperative radiation therapy are lacking for oropharynx cancer. Nonetheless, most head and neck oncologists believe that the evidence is sufficiently compelling to support the use of concomitant chemoradiation in standard practice as initial management for advanced oropharyngeal cancer, even if resectable. For other sites of advanced resectable disease, especially the oral cavity for which good reconstructive options exist, primary surgical management is better established and remains the standard of care.

In general, for patients with locally advanced squamous cell cancer of the larynx, hypopharynx, or oropharynx, concomitant chemoradiation yields better disease control compared with radiation alone, albeit at the expense of greater acute toxicity. This is the preferred organ preservation approach for cancer of the larynx and oropharynx. It must be emphasized that successful application of a chemoradiation strategy for organ preservation requires a team approach that includes not only the head and neck surgeon, radiation oncologist, and medical oncologist but also a nutritionist, oncology nurse, and social worker. Close monitoring with comprehensive head and neck examinations and timely integration of salvage surgery, when necessary, are part of the treatment plan and are required in order for survival not to be compromised. The evaluation of functional and quality-of-life outcomes is another parameter for assessing the overall benefit of organ preservation therapies and will be an important factor in comparing therapeutic approaches.

Survivorship is an important area that needs attention. Studies of survivors of head and neck cancer have mainly focused on the relationships between social supports, tobacco and alcohol use, functional status and depression, and the influence of these factors on quality of life.[69–71] Chronic pain, xerostomia, impairments of speech and swallowing, alterations of taste and smell, and poor comesis are some of the sequelae of the treatments for head and neck cancer. These variable long-term effects can have a profound psychosocial effect on cancer survivors and their families. Fortunately, advances in reconstructive techniques and organ preservation strategies are having a positive effect on quality of life relative to the functional and cosmetic consequences of radical local therapies of the past. Nevertheless, quality-of-life and survivorship issues must be a focus of future research and an integral component of those efforts.[72]

INCURABLE RECURRENT OR DISTANT METASTATIC DISEASE

Systemic therapy

Disease that cannot be resected and has been previously irradiated or involves distant organs is considered incurable.

KEY POINTS

- Combination chemotherapy in the palliative setting leads to increased response rates as well as increased toxicity but does not significantly improve survival compared with single-agent methotrexate, a platinum-based agent, or 5-FU.
- Various biologic agents that target the EGFR pathway are under study in combination with chemotherapy, as single agents, and as multiple targeted agents. Antibodies to the EGFR and small molecule tyrosine kinase inhibitors cause major response in approximately 10% of patients who are platinum refractory. Cetuximab is the only biologic agent in its class approved for use in head and neck cancer.
- Significantly improved survival has been demonstrated for the combination of cetuximab, cisplatin, and 5-FU compared with cisplatin and 5-FU in a preliminary report.
- Reirradiation and concurrent chemotherapy may provide long-term survival for a selected subset of patients but is not standard of care.

The most commonly used cytotoxics to treat recurrent or metastatic squamous cell cancers of the head and neck are cisplatin, carboplatin, docetaxel, paclitaxel, 5-FU, and methotrexate. Activity also has been demonstrated for bleomycin, irinotecan, gemcitabine, capecitabine, oxaliplatin, cyclophosphamide, ifosfamide, and pemetrexed. Randomized trials comparing combination chemotherapy and single-agent therapy show approximately a doubling of the response rate with platinum-based combinations, but unless a clinical complete response is achieved, the duration of response is brief (2 to 4 months) and without a significant effect on overall survival.[73–75]

Toxicity is generally greater when combination chemotherapy is used. As an example, one meta-analysis included all studies in which cisplatin and 5-FU, the historical gold-standard combination regimen, was compared with single-agent therapy.[76] A significant improvement in response OR = 0.43 (95% CI 0.29 to 0.63) was documented, which translated into only a 2-week difference in the median survival. No formal quality-of-life data were available, but toxicity was greater for patients who received combination therapy. Numerous single agents have activity and can be used, but weekly methotrexate is the historical gold standard because of its ease of administration, toxicity profile, and relative low cost.[77] Combination chemotherapy should be limited to patients who have a good performance status (e.g. ECOG performance status of 0 to 1) and are thus better able to tolerate the added toxicity; for these individuals, the higher response rate may translate into better palliation, although there is no objective quality of life data to support this notion. Factors associated with poor response in this population are well known and include poor performance status, the presence of co-morbidities, bulky local-regional disease or high tumor volume, and prior treatment for recurrence.

The introduction of the taxanes in the 1990s would hopefully result in improved survival for patients with recurrent disease, but unfortunately, this has not occurred. Two different weekly schedules of paclitaxel offered no advantage compared with weekly single-agent methotrexate.[78] Results from another study showed that paclitaxel plus cisplatin did not differ significantly from standard cisplatin plus 5-FU regarding the median survival rate (9 months compared with 8 months, respectively) and the 1-year survival rate (30% compared with 41%, respectively), although the paclitaxel regimen was, on average, better tolerated.[79]

Cetuximab is the the only molecularly targeted drug to be approved for use in head and neck cancer; its indication is in patients who are platinum refractory. Phase II trials of cetuximab alone or combined with cisplatin tested in patients who had either stable or progressive disease as their best response to a standard platinum-based doublet were in the range of 10% to 13%. [80–82] In a randomized trial in which the combination of cisplatin and placebo was compared with cisplatin plus cetuximab in 123 patients, no significant difference was found in the median progression-free survival (2.7 months compared with 4.2 months, respectively; $p = 0.27$), although the rate of major response (complete plus partial) was significantly higher for patients who received cisplatin plus cetuximab (10% compared with 26%, respectively; $p = 0.03$).[83]

The small molecule tyrosine kinase inhibitors gefitinib and erlotinib have modest activity in this setting (including responses in patients who received prior chemotherapy). In a phase II trial of 52 patients, administration of 500 mg per day of gefitinib resulted in an 11% major response rate.[84] For erlotinib, administration of 150 mg per day resulted in a 4% major response rate in a phase II trial of 115 patients.[85] Disease stabilization was common at approximately 50%. Combination trials with other agents directed at EGFR pathway downstream targets, such as the vascular endothelial growth factor (VEGF) inibitor, are ongoing.[86] One phase II trial of the combination of erlotinib and bevacizumab resulted in a 17% response rate and median survival of 7.5 months in patients previously treated for recurrent disease.[87] A number of other multitargeted agents are entering clinical trials in head and neck cancer.

REIRRADIATION

Repeat radiation therapy is increasingly feasible with the greater availability of conformal technology. Building on the improved disease control seen with concurrent chemoradiotherapy for untreated patients, this approach also has been investigated in the recurrent disease setting. Phase II trials suggest that for a proportion of patients (up to 25% in some studies), disease control will be more durable than would be anticipated with chemotherapy alone. This reirradiation approach may represent a good option for selected patients but remains investigational. In one study, investigators reported the results with full-dose repeat radiation therapy with or without chemotherapy for 169 patients; complete remissions ranging from 12 to 111 months occurred in 13 patients.[88] Two successive phase II trials performed by the RTOG used split course radiation and twice-daily fractionation at a total dose of 60 Gy.[89,90] The concurrent chemotherapy in the first trial (R96-10) was 5-FU and hydro xyurea, and in the second trial (R96-11) the chemotherapy regimen was cisplatin and paclitaxel. At median follow-up of just under 2 years, the 2-year overall survival rates were 17%[89] and 25%,[90] respectively, suggesting that for a subset of patients, reirradiation might provide a survival advantage over palliative chemotherapy alone. The two studies demonstrated feasibility of the approach when analyzed for factors that predicted a favorable survival outcome; an interval of at least 3 years from the original radiation was seen in R96-10 but not in R96-11. Unfortunately, a phase III trial (R04-21) directly comparing reirradiation and concurrent chemotherapy with chemotherapy alone was terminated because of poor accrual.[89] Quality-of-life and function data in addition to close attention

KEY POINTS

- WHO type I (squamous cell cancer) is more commonly found in the United States, whereas WHO types II (nonkeratinizing cancer) and III (undifferentiated cancer) overwhelmingly predominate in endemic areas, such as southern China and northern Africa, and are associated with the Epstein-Barr virus. Types II and III are more responsive to chemotherapy and radiation therapy than type I.
- The standard of care according to stage is radiotherapy alone for stages I and IIa, and concurrent cisplatin and radiotherapy followed by three cycles of adjuvant cisplatin and 5-FU for stages IIb, III, IVA and IVB nasopharyngeal cancer.

to capturing serious late effects, including complications from vascular damage (stenosis and thromboembolism), osteoradionecrosis, and soft tissue necrosis, are critical assessments that were planned in addition to measurement of survival. Alternative phase II trials will likely be planned.

NASOPHARYNGEAL CANCER

Cisplatin-based concurrent chemoradiotherapy is the cornerstone of therapy for newly diagnosed, advanced, local-regional nasopharyngeal cancer. Although this treatment is widely used, there is more disagreement surrounding the precise role of adjuvant chemotherapy in this setting. The clinical behavior of nasopharyngeal cancer varies somewhat according to its histologic subtype. WHO type I (squamous cell cancer) is more common in the United States than in endemic areas and has a local-regional behavior more similar to that of other head and neck cancers. WHO types II (nonkeratinizing cancer) and III (undifferentiated cancer), both of which can occur with lymphoid stroma (so-called lymphoepithelioma), predominate in endemic areas, such as southern China and northern Africa, and have a higher propensity for distant metastases. WHO types II and III also are more responsive to radiotherapy and chemotherapy than is differentiated squamous histology, and more than 90% of cases are associated with the Epstein-Barr virus. Radiation is the historic mainstay of treatment for disease above the clavicles. The same drugs used in the management of squamous cell cancers arising from other sites in the head and neck, such as cisplatin, 5-FU, and the taxanes, also are active against nasopharyngeal cancer.

The management of locally advanced nasopharyngeal cancer was dramatically changed a decade ago after publication of the results of the Intergroup nasopharynx study.[20] In this trial, patients with stage III or IV nasopharyngeal cancer were randomly assigned to either radiation alone (70 Gy, 35 fractions for 7 weeks) or the same radiation schedule with three planned doses of concomitant cisplatin (100 mg/m^2) administered every 21 days, followed by three cycles of adjuvant cisplatin (80 mg/m^2) and 5-FU (1,000mg/m^2 per day for 4 days). Most patients (91%) had stage IV disease, and WHO type I histology was more common compared with series from endemic areas. Overall survival with a minimum follow-up of 5 years was significantly improved for patients who received combined-modality therapy (67% vs. 37%, $p < 0.001$), as was progression-free survival (58% vs. 29%, $p < 0.001$). This occured even though only 63% of patients received all three planned cycles of cisplatin during radiation and only 55% received all three cycles of adjuvant cisplatin and 5-FU.

The Intergroup study was criticized because the relative contributions of the concurrent and the adjuvant therapies could not be determined, and the trial results may be less applicable to endemic areas where WHO type I histologic subtypes are infrequent. However, subsequent randomized trials[92–94] in endemic areas and two meta-analyses[96,97] have confirmed the significant survival advantage afforded by concurrent platinum chemotherapy and radiation over radiation alone. By contrast, randomized trials of induction chemotherapy followed by radiation compared with radiation alone have shown no significant improvement in overall survival,[98–101] although some reported improved relapse-free survival. Two meta-analyses of trials that compared any sequence of chemotherapy and radiotherapy with radiotherapy alone have been published. The meta-analysis reported by Huncharek et al.[96] was a pooled analysis of the published results of six randomized trials comprising 1,500 patients. They reported that at 4 years chemotherapy improved progression-free survival by 34% and overall survival by 20%. The second meta-analysis used updated individual patient data from eight randomized trials (1,753 patients) with locally advanced disease, covering 1966 to 2003.[97] The effect of adding chemotherapy to radiotherapy on overall survival was an absolute survival benefit of 6% (56% to 62%) at 5 years (HR of death = 0.82; 95% CI; 0.71, 0.94; $p = 0.006$). The effect observed on event-free survival was an absolute benefit of 10% (42% to 52%) at 5 years (HR of tumor failure [local, regional, or distant] or death = 0.76; 95% CI; 0.67, 0.86; $p < 0.0001$). A significant interaction between the timing of chemotherapy and overall survival was observed with the highest benefit resulting from concomitant administration of chemotherapy and radiotherapy ($p = 0.005$).

Based on these data as a whole, the survival benefit from cisplatin-based chemotherapy and radiation administered concomitantly seems clear and is the accepted standard of care within and outside of the United States. The benefit of adjuvant chemotherapy, theoretically to suppress distant metastases common in nasopharyngeal cancer, is less widely accepted. In the United States, the standard of care for treatment of patients with nasopharyngeal cancer stages IIB, III, IVA (T4, N0 to N2, M0), and IVB (any T, N3, M0) is radiotherapy (70 Gy) with concurrent high-dose cisplatin on days 1, 22, and 43, followed by three courses of adjuvant cisplatin and infusional 5-FU — dosing and schedule per the Intergroup trial published by Al-Sarraf.[20] Radiotherapy alone is indicated for stages I and IIA (N0 and no parapharyngeal space involvement).

Current areas of investigation in the management of nasopharyngeal cancer include the potential benefit of changing the sequencing of the three cycles of chemotherapy from adjuvant (after chemoradiation) to sequential (prior to chemoradiation) and the exploration of alternative cytotoxic regimens. The high risk of distant spread coupled with the ability to successfully deliver all three cycles of adjuvant chemotherapy in only 55% of patients in the Intergroup trial has motivated the investigation of sequential chemotherapy and chemoradiation. However, there is concern that this sequence of treatment might compromise the delivery of chemoradiation, the critical curative component of the treatment. The early results from several single-institution trials of sequential therapy have shown feasibility and encouraging response and survival data. Rischin and colleagues[102] tested three cycles of induction epirubicin, cisplatin, and 5-FU followed by 60 Gy of radiotherapy and concurrent cisplatin (20 mg/m^2 daily for 5 days, administered weeks 1 and 6) in 35 patients with stage III/IV nasopharyngeal cancer. All patients completed the induction phase, and 97% completed radiotherapy and cisplatin. It is noteworthy that the total dose of radiotherapy was lower than standard and that two rather than three courses of cisplatin were administered concurrently with the radiotherapy. The overall survival at 4 years was 94%, and progression-free survival was 81%. Chan and colleagues[103] evaluated induction carboplatin and paclitaxel followed by cisplatin (40mg/m^2 per week) in 31 patients with stage III/IV nasopharyngeal cancer. All patients completed the induction phase, and 71% tolerated at least six weekly doses of cisplatin during radiotherapy. A preliminary report of the results at 2 years gave an overall survival rate of 92% and a progression-free survival rate of 78.5%. The preliminary results of a randomized phase II trial conducted by the same investigators were reported in 2005.[104] The two treatments were radiotherapy and cisplatin (40 mg/m^2 per week) with or without induction docetaxel and cisplatin. In 53 randomly assigned patients, major response to induction was observed in 86% of nasopharyngeal primary tumors and 80% of neck nodes; the complete response rate after cisplatin and radiotherapy was 96% at the primary site and 80% in regional nodes. In the chemoradiation arm, complete response was achieved in 84% at the primary site and 64% of regional nodes. The numbers of patients in these trials is small, the enrolled population is from endemic areas, and the concurrent chemoradiation regimen that is used in the United States was not evaluated. However, the results appear promising and this sequential approach warrants further study.

CANCER OF UNKNOWN PRIMARY SITE

Although for most patients the primary site will be found after comprehensive examination of the head and neck, assessment under anesthesia, and diagnostic imaging, a malignant neck lymph node without a clear primary tumor occurs regularly in the head and neck. The location of the lymph node in the neck directs the examiner toward the likely potential primary sites, and PET scanning may be helpful. A needle aspiration of the lymph node is the first choice for initial biopsy. If negative, repeat fine-needle aspiration with consideration of a core-needle biopsy, if feasible, is appropriate. If the histologic diagnosis remains inconclusive, subsequent excisional biopsy should be performed in such a way that the incision can be incorporated into an appropriate neck dissection. Open biopsy done inappropriately may contaminate the surgical field and create a larger problem.

If pathologic findings from the neck indicate a diagnosis of squamous cell cancer and a primary lesion above the clavicles is suggested, especially if the lymph node is high in the neck, a comprehensive head and neck examination under anesthesia is the next step. Directed biopsies should be performed for suspicious mucosal areas and locations known to be a source of occult tumors, namely, the hypopharynx, base of the tongue, and nasopharynx. In addition, an ipsilateral tonsillectomy is recommended based on the increasing incidence of tonsillar cancers associated with HPV.[3] Preliminary data indicate that clonal genetic changes found in benign biopsy specimens identical to those present in the malignant lymph node may prove helpful in the future for the identification of the primary site.[105] Of note, the skin, upper part of the esophagus, and lung would be other potential sources of squamous cell cancer spread to the neck. If the findings on biopsy of the lymph node indicate an adenocarcinoma, a thyroid, salivary gland, or primary lesions below the clavicles should be considered. Lymphoma is another important diagnostic possibility and may require a core-needle biopsy for diagnostic purposes. Similarly, distinguishing lymphoma from anaplastic and undifferentiated or poorly differentiated cancers can be difficult based on cytologic analysis alone and may require additional immunohistochemical studies or more tissue.

The treatment of patients with squamous cell cancer in a neck node of unknown primary site is controversial and evolving. Historically, either surgery or radiation was used to

KEY POINTS

- The search for the primary site should include fused FDG-PET/CT imaging and an examination under anesthesia with directed biopsies of the base of tongue, nasopharynx, hypopharynx, and ipsilateral tonsillectomy.
- Standard treatment consists of neck dissection followed by radiotherapy to include the likely primary sites and concurrent chemotherapy if extracapsular extension of nodal disease is present.

KEY POINTS

- Metastatic adenoid cystic cancer and adenocarcicnoma are often characterized by an indolent natural history. Systemic treatment should be delayed until substantial tumor growth can be appreciated on serial imaging studies within a 6-month timeframe.
- High-grade mucoepidermoid carcinoma responds to the same regimens used for squamous cell cancers from other sites.

treat patients with low-bulk disease in a single lymph node, whereas both modalities were necessary for patients with more advanced disease. The extent of radiation to the putative primary sites requires clinical judgment regarding the likely source of the tumor because a larger portal will increase the morbidity associated with treatment. Findings from clinical series indicate that with longitudinal follow-up, the primary site will ultimately be found for approximately 30% of patients. Long-term survival is better for patients in whom the primary lesion remains occult than for those in whom it does not. The mainstay of treatment is still a neck dissection followed by radiation with concomitant cisplatin when extracapsular extension of nodal disease is present. However, integrated concomitant chemoradiotherapy is increasingly used for these patients based on the physician's impression of the likely primary site(s).

MALIGNANT LESIONS OF THE SALIVARY GLANDS

Cancers of the major salivary glands (parotid, submandibular, sublingual) and the minor salivary glands are uncommon, accounting for fewer than 10% of epithelial head and neck tumors. Tobacco and alcohol are not risk factors for tumors of the salivary glands but there may be an association with prior exposure to radiation. The WHO classification lists 24 different histologic subtypes of malignant epithelial salivary tumors. Their small numbers and histologic and prognostic heterogeneity make them difficult to study; therefore, there are few adequately tested regimens in any one histology to guide the medical oncologist.

The most common types of salivary gland cancers are adenoid cystic carcinoma and adenocarcinoma, which originate from the intercalated ducts, and mucoepidermoid carcinoma, which originates from the secretory ducts. A histologic reading of high-grade mucoepidermoid or adenocarcinoma correlates with aggressive behavior and greater likelihood of eventual metastasis, whereas low-grade cancers of these histologies are more likely to be cured with initial local therapies. Adenoid cystic cancer is the most common tumor found in the minor salivary glands, is prone to neurotropic spread, and has the highest propensity of the different histologic subtypes for distant metastases, yet it can grow in a very indolent manner. Salivary duct carcinoma is an aggressive subtype of adenocarcinoma arising in the parotid with rapid appearance of metastases.

Surgery is the mainstay of treatment for all primary and recurrent disease above the clavicles with adjuvant radiation, as indicated by the presence of adverse pathologic features.[106] There is a tendency among medical oncologists to recommend the addition of cisplatin or other chemotherapy as a radiosensitizer to improve local-regional control, but there is no data to support this extrapolation of the results of studies of adjuvant chemoradiation of squamous cancers. The role of systemic therapy is limited to the palliative management of metastases or locally recurrent disease that is no longer treatable by surgery or radiation.

Radiation-based therapy is used for unresectable tumors. Neutron beam therapy has shown promise in this setting, especially for adenoid cystic cancer. Concurrent chemotherapy with radiation is feasible — given the data from the management of squamous cell cancers of the upper aerodigestive tract — and not uncommonly applied for unresectable disease, although there is no data of improved efficacy of this approach compared with radiation alone.

The available data regarding the activity of different chemotherapy agents are limited and commonly include mixed histologic subtypes; most older reports are case series rather than true clinical trials. A recent trial of single-agent paclitaxel showed activity in patients with mucoepidermoid carcinoma and adenocarcinoma but not in adenoid cystic carcinoma emphasizing the importance of histology specific trials.[107] The available data for other single agents and combinations of standard cytotoxics were recently reviewed by Laurie and Licitra.[108] The most commonly used regimens include cyclophosphamide, adriamycin, cisplatin, and 5-FU in various two-drug and three-drug combinations. Responses are reported for all three histologic types, but no one trial or case series includes enough patients with a given histology for statistical confidence.

As a general rule, mucoepidermoid cancer appears sensitive to the drugs used for squamous cell cancer of the head and neck. Adenocarcinoma and adenoid cystic carcinoma may be more indolent and, therefore, palliative chemotherapy should only be attempted in the symptomatic patient or when substantial tumor growth can be appreciated on serial imaging within a 6-month timeframe. In this setting, doxorubicin, cisplatin, and 5-FU are often tried as single agents; the combination of cyclophosphamide, doxorubicin, and cisplatin is a frequently used regimen.[109] Even with combination chemotherapy, the rate of complete and partial response will be low, and it is appropriate to consider investigational therapy. Epirubicin, mitoxantrone, and vinorelbine have demonstrated activity in adenoid cystic cancer[110–112] but not paclitaxel.[107]

The search for molecular targets to which there are available therapies has become the focus of recent investigations. It is reasonable to obtain a panel of immunohistochemical stains that might direct treatment.

These markers may include c-kit, EGFR, bcl-2, HER2/*neu*, and hormone receptors. The c-kit target is expressed in approximately 80% of adenoid cystic cancers, whereas EGFR expression is quite variable, and the hormone receptors and HER2/*neu* are rarely expressed. Imatinib has been evaluated in adenoid cystic carcinoma in two phase II trials with no objective responses observed despite anecdotal reports of response.[109–112] However, progressive disease was not an eligibility requirement, nor was the presence of c-kit mutations or high expression levels. Thus, further evaluation of imatinib may be warranted, but the data are insufficient to support a role for its use in adenoid cystic carcinoma. Overexpression of EGFR is commonly seen in mucoepidermoid carcinoma, whereas c-kit, HER2, and hormone receptors are rarely expressed. In adenocarcinoma, c-kit is variably expressed depending on the histologic subtype; hormone receptor expression is rare, and EGFR expression is uncommon. With the proliferation of targeted agents, there is considerable interest in evaluating multitargeted agents, such as lapatinib (dual inhibitor of EGFR and HER2),[117] and agents that affect vascular endothelial cell proliferation, such as sorafenib and axitinab. Investigational agents for adenoid cystic carcinoma and the other salivary gland histologies are best evaluated in multicenter collaborations.

Microscopically, salivary duct carcinoma looks identical to ductal breast cancer, is commonly androgen receptor positive, and may also overexpress her-2 and EGFR by immunohistochemistry. Responses have been reported to anti-androgen therapy.[118] A trial of trastuzumab in patients with HER-2 positive tumors is underway in the cooperative groups.

THYROID CANCER

The American Cancer Society estimated 30,180 new cases of thyroid cancer in the United States and 1,500 deaths from the disease in 2006.[119] The incidence of this cancer continues to rise in the United States with a 2.4-fold increase noted in incidence between 1973 (3.6 cases per 100,000 people) and 2002 (8.7 cases per 100,000 people); however, the mortality rate is stable at 0.5 deaths per 100,000 people.[120] This change in incidence is accounted for by an increase in papillary thyroid cancer but not other histologic types. Nearly 90% of these cancers are subclinical or smaller than 2 cm in size, which suggests that earlier diagnosis may account for most of the observed change in incidence.

Thyroid cancers are classified based on the two main parenchymal cells of origin — the follicular cells involved in thyroid hormone production and the parafollicular cells that produce calcitonin. The former give rise to well-differentiated thyroid cancer, which constitutes 90% of thyroid malignancies and to anaplastic thyroid cancer (1% to 2% of thyroid cancers); the latter in turn gives rise to medullary

KEY POINTS

- For differentiated thyroid cancers, poor prognostic features include age older than 45 years, male sex, poorly differentiated histology, tumor size, and extrathyroid extension at diagnosis. In contrast, involvement of the regional lymph nodes does not confer a worse prognosis for survival.
- Radioactive iodine is the treatment of choice for metastatic disease. Standard chemotherapy has disappointing activity. Radioactive iodine generally plays no role for the treatment of anaplastic or medullary thyroid cancers.
- Medullary thyroid cancer occurs as part of one form of multiple endocrine neoplasia, as well as in the familial type. Screening for germline *RET* gene mutation should be considered because total thyroidectomy, based on the results of genetic testing, often results in complete cures for young, at-risk family members.
- Identification of molecular targets is leading to trials of agents that affect the RAS/RAF/MAPK pathway.

thyroid cancer (5% to 9% of thyroid cancers). The histologic subtypes within the well-differentiated thyroid cancer classification are papillary, mixed tumors with areas of papillary and follicular histologic features, follicular, follicular variant of papillary, and Hurthle cell.

The only well-documented etiologic factor for thyroid cancer is radiation with an inverse relationship between age of exposure and risk of developing a thyroid malignancy. The risk of developing thyroid cancer is much higher for individuals who have been exposed to radioactive iodine isotopes from nuclear reactor accidents, atomic bomb development testing, and for children and young adults who have received external radiotherapy for other cancers (e.g., Hodgkin's disease, neuroblastoma, or Wilm's tumor) in contrast to individuals irradiated during childhood for benign conditions (as was common until 1960). Data from Chernobyl show that nearly all thyroid cancers developing in exposed children were well-differentiated papillary type but with a higher rate of local invasion and lymph node involvement than usually observed for this histology. More than 90% of well-differentiated thyroid cancers, however, are unrelated to radiation exposure. Papillary thyroid cancer and its variants tend to recur locally in the regional lymph nodes, whereas follicular and Hurthle cell cancers tend to recur distantly, especially in bone and lung.

A variety of prognostic systems have been developed to assist in the risk classification of patients with differentiated thyroid cancer, with potential implications for management based on risk group. Several factors have been widely accepted as being associated with a poor prognosis: age older than 45 years, male sex, poorly differentiated histology, tumor size, and extrathyroid extension at diagnosis. In contrast, involvement of the regional lymph nodes is associated with greater risk of nodal recucrrence but does not confer a worse prognosis for survival.[121] Overall, the 10-year survival rate for differentiated thyroid cancer is excellent (90%). The median age at the time of diagnosis is 45 years, and the median age at death is 75 years.[122]

The majority of thyroid cancers are detected as incidental thyroid nodules found on physical exam or by the patient presenting to the physician with a neck mass. The diagnostic evaluation should include a high-resolution ultrasound to assess the number and characteristics of nodules, including whether solid or cystic, and to aid in performing a fine-needle aspiration biopsy. Fine-needle aspiration has high sensitivity and specificity and is the test of choice when evaluating solitary thyroid nodules.[123] Routine thyroid scanning with iodine-123 or technetium-99 is not recommended. This test provides information on whether a nodule is functional; however, the majority of benign and malignant nodules are "cold" or nonfunctioning, meaning that the test is nonspecific and not cost effective. All patients with a thyroid nodule and suspected familial medullary thyroid cancer should have calcitonin level testing.

The mainstay of treatment is thyroid surgery; for differentiated thyroid cancer, levothyroxine suppression and administration of radioactive iodine are the standards. External-beam radiotherapy and chemotherapy are reserved for palliation of refractory metastatic disease. The extent of initial surgical therapy is controversial. Many experts recommend removal of the entire thyroid, with the caveats that removal of only the affected lobe and the isthmus is necessary in patients with better risk (e.g., young patients with small tumors) and that total thyroidectomy is associated with a greater risk of complications, such as vocal cord paralysis and hypocalcemia.[124]

Although controversial, most U.S. physicians will administer a single dose of radioactive iodine to ablate any normal thyroid remnant and destroy any microscopic deposits of the remaining thyroid cancer following a total thyroidectomy. It should be emphasized that use of iodinated contrast, an iodine-rich diet, and inadequate elevation of the level of thyroid-stimulating hormone (thyrotropin) can all undermine the effectiveness of treatment with radioactive iodine. Human recombinant thyrotropin has replaced the need for a patient to be put into a hypothyroid state. Dosing strategies for radioactive iodine — ablative compared with higher therapeutic doses — are determined by the patient's prognostic risk and range from 50 to 75 mCi for ablation of remnants following total thyroidectomy for low-risk patients, 100 to 150 mCi for the treatment of local-regional lymph nodes, and 150 to 250 mCi for the treatment of lung and bone metastases.

Ablation of remnants enables improved surveillance because normal thyroid cells are also removed, which could cause false-positive results on whole-body scans or false-positive elevations of serum thyroglobulin. In the absence of all normal thyroid tissue, the serum thyroglobulin is a highly sensitive and specific tumor marker.[125] After total thyroidectomy and ablation of remnants, the serum thyrotropin level generally should be suppressed with thyroxine to below-normal levels because this hormone is a potential growth factor for microscopic cancer deposits.

Six to 12 months after initial therapy, measurement of the serum thyroglobulin while the patient is on suppressive doses of thyroxine should be performed. If the serum thyroglobulin is undetectable and the findings of ultrasound imaging of the neck are negative, annual thyroglobulin levels and physical examination are sufficient for most low-risk patients. At 1 year after surgery and ablation, if there is no detectable level of serum thyroglobulin during treatment with suppressive doses of thyroxine, the thyroglobulin level should be determined after two doses of recombinant human thyrotropin. If the level rises above 2 ng/mL, a search for remaining disease is warranted. Diagnostic whole-body imaging with iodine scanning should be performed. If this is negative, FDG-PET scanning has been shown to be helpful for localizing disease in more than 60% of such cases.[126]

If metastases develop and concentrate, radioactive iodine is the treatment of choice. Complete response to treatment has been observed for 45% of patients with distant metastases, although a higher complete response rate has been noted for younger patients and those with small pulmonary metastases.[127] Chemotherapy is reserved for disease that is refractory to radioactive iodine. Some thyroid tumors grow very slowly, so a period of careful observation is reasonable before committing to treatment.

The best-studied single agent is doxorubicin, which has a 17% major response rate; when in combination with cisplatin, a 26% response rate was reported in one trial.[128] Defects in the genes involving the RAS-RAF-MAP kinase signaling pathway occur in approximately 60% of papillary thyroid cancers. Recent interest in targeted therapies has been stimulated by the discovery of activating point mutations of the *BRAF* gene that occur early and are associated with more advanced disease at diagnosis[129] and independently predict for recurrence. Clinical trials of inhibitors of *BRAF*, such as the agent sorafenib, are ongoing and show significant clinical activity for papillary thyroid cancers.[130] Small molecule inhibitors of receptor tyrosine kinases also are under evaluation in differentiated thyroid cancer. One drug with activity in preliminary reports is axitinib (AG-013736), which targets VEGF receptors 1 through 3, platelet-derived growth factor (PDGF) receptor B, and kit.[131]

ANAPLASTIC THYROID CANCER

Unlike the case with differentiated thyroid cancer, the anaplastic, or giant cell, variant is associated with an extremely poor prognosis, with the best available therapy producing a median survival of less than 1 year. An association with prior well-differentiated thyroid cancer or benign thyroid nodule disease is not uncommon. Patients are older, generally in their 60s or 70s, and the distribution between the sexes is more balanced. Distinguishing the tumor from a large cell lymphoma of the thyroid is of fundamental importance. Clinically, anaplastic thyroid cancer is characterized by a rapidly growing mass in the thyroid that invades the trachea or larynx and causes symptoms of dysphagia, hoarseness, or hemoptysis. Twenty percent to 50% of patients have distant metastases at the time of presentation (most often pulmonary), and the remainder usually manifest metastases within 1 or 2 months of diagnosis. However, most deaths are a consequence of aggressive local-regional spread and upper airway respiratory failure.

If resection is feasible, it should be pursued, although these tumors are typically unresectable at presentation and the patient often requires an urgent tracheostomy. Initial external-beam radiation-based therapy, both for definitive treatment and as an adjuvant, often with doxorubicin sensitization or doxorubicin and cisplatin, is commonly used and considered the standard of care. Chemotherapy alone has limited efficacy. Doxorubicin plus cisplatin is probably the most widely used combination.[132] Radioactive iodine generally plays no role in the treatment of these tumors.

MEDULLARY THYROID CANCER

Medullary thyroid cancer is a neoplasm of the calcitonin-producing cells that reside in the thyroid. It constitutes approximately 5% to 9% of all thyroid cancers and is associated with a mutation in the *RET* proto-oncogene. Both sporadic and familial types occur. The sporadic form is more common (60% to 70% of cases) and tends to occur in an older age group than does the familial form (40 to 45 years compared with 15 to 25 years). Three distinct familial syndromes account for the remaining 30% to 40% of cases. The *RET* mutation is transmitted in the germline, and familial medullary thyroid cancer may be part of multiple endocrine neoplasia (MEN) type 2A (medullary thyroid cancer, pheochromocytoma, and parathyroid hyperplasia) or type 2B (medullary thyroid cancer, pheochromocytoma, and intestinal and mucosal ganglioneuromatosis with characteristic marfanoid habitus) or as a familial form of medullary thyroid cancer not associated with MEN.

The clinical presentation of the sporatic type is usually a painless thyroid mass; however, high calcitonin levels may result in a watery secretory diarrhea as the primary symptom. The diagnosis is made based on a constellation of a thyroid mass, high calcitonin level, and a fine-needle aspiration specimen that stains positive for calcitonin. Screening for pheochromocytoma (catecholamine excess) is important to the exclusion of a familial syndrome in a patient otherwise believed to have the sporadic type. CT and PET imaging are useful to detect metastases, but radioactive iodine scans are of no use. For the familial syndromes, a dominant inheritance pattern is recognized, and family members of patients with newly diagnosed cases of the disease should be screened for *RET* mutations because germline mutations are substantially higher than might be expected on the basis of family history alone. Total thyroidectomy often results in complete cures for young, at-risk family members based on *RET* gene testing, even in the absence of clinically detectable thyroid abnormalities. Studies show that a minority of family members undergoing prophylactic thyroidectomy actually have histologically normal thyroid glands. More often there is evidence of C-cell hyperplasia and microscopic or macroscopic medullary thyroid cancer, which underscores the importance of operating early.

The treatment of choice for medullary thyroid cancer is a total thyroidectomy with bilateral central compartment node dissection and at least unilateral neck dissection. The risk of multifocal disease is high for both familial and sporadic types. Radiation has disappointing efficacy for macroscopic disease, and postoperative radiation therapy is not routinely used. After resection of all disease in the neck, patients should be monitored with two tumor markers: calcitonin and carcinoembryonic antigen. The survival outcome has improved with genetic testing and prophylactic surgery. Ten-year survival rates are between 70% and 80% for combined series of familial and sporadic types.

Local recurrences are usually treated surgically. Metastatic disease (commonly to the mediastinum, lung, bone, and liver) often follows an indolent course, and in this case, observation is reasonable. Palliative surgery, including tumor debulking, or radiotherapy may be used as indicated for symptom control or to manage tumor encroachment on critical structures. Diphenoxylate, octreotide, and interferon-alpha 2a may palliate the diarrhea that can occur. Doxorubicin, cisplatin, dacarbazine, 5-FU, streptozocin, and somatostatin analogues have some reported activity; however, in general, medullary thyroid cancer is resistant to standard cytotoxics making investigational therapy appropriate.[133] Multifunctional tyrosine kinase inhibitors that target *RET* plus VEGF receptors are under evaluation in phase II clinical trials, and[134] responses have been observed with ZD6474.[135] Another multitargeted small molecule inhibitor with activity in thyroid cancer is AMG 706, which is a selective inhibitor of VEGF, PDGF, and kit receptors. In one preliminary report of this compound, partial responses were observed in patients with medullary, papillary, and follicular thyroid cancers.[136]

REFERENCES

1. Parkin DM, Bray F, Ferlay J, Pisani P. Global cancer statistics, 2002 *CA Cancer J Clin.* 2005;55(2):74–108.
2. Blot WJ, McLaughlin JK, Winn DM, et al. Smoking and drinking in relation to oral and pharyngeal cancer. *Cancer Res.* 1988;48(11): 3282–3287.
3. Shiboski CH, Schmidt BL, Jordan RC. Tongue and tonsil carcinoma: increasing trends in the U.S. population ages 20–44 years. *Cancer.* 2005;103(9):1843–1849.

4. Gillison ML, Koch WM, Capone RB, et al. Evidence for a causal association between human papillomavirus and a subset of head and neck cancers. *J Natl Cancer Inst.* 2000;92(9):709–720.

5. Fakhry C, Gillison ML. Clinical implications of human papillomavirus in head and neck cancers. *J Clin Oncol.* 2006;24(17):2606–2611.

6. Forastiere A, Koch W, Trotti A, et al. Head and neck cancer. *N Engl J Med.* (2001);345(26):1890–1900.

7. Yamamoto E, Shibuya H, Yoshimura R, et al. Site specific dependency of second primary cancer in early stage head and neck squamous cell carcinoma. *Cancer.* 2002;94(7):2007–2014.

8. Hong WK, Lippman SM, Itri LM, et al. Prevention of second primary tumors with isotretinoin in squamous-cell carcinoma of the head and neck. *N Engl J Med.* 1990;323(12):795–801.

9. Bolla M, Lefur R, Ton Van J, et al. Prevention of second primary tumours with etretinate in squamous cell carcinoma of the oral cavity and oropharynx. Results of a multicentric double-blind randomised study. *Eur J Cancer.* 1994;30A(6):767–772.

10. Khuri FR, Lee JJ, Lippman SM, et al. Randomized phase III trial of low-dose isotretinoin for prevention of second primary tumors in stage I and II head and neck cancer patients. *J Natl Cancer Inst.* 2006;98(7):441–450.

11. van Zandwijk N, Dalesio O, Pastorino U, et al. EUROSCAN, a randomized trial of vitamin A and N-acetylcysteine in patients with head and neck cancer or lung cancer. For the European Organization for Research and Treatment of Cancer Head and Neck and Lung Cancer Cooperative Groups. *J Natl Cancer Inst.*2000;92(12): 977–986.

12. Ng SH, Yen TC, Chang JT, et al. Prospective study of [18F]fluorodeoxyglucose positron emission tomography and computed tomography and magnetic resonance imaging in oral cavity squamous cell carcinoma with palpably negative neck. *J Clin Oncol.* 2006;24(27): 4371–4376.

13. Waldron JN. Fluorodeoxyglucose positron emission tomography for the preoperative staging of oral cavity cancers: only one piece of the puzzle. *J Clin Oncol.* 2006;24(27):4367–4368.

14. Kovacs AF, Dobert N, Gaa J, et al. Positron emission tomography in combination with sentinel node biopsy reduces the rate of elective neck dissections in the treatment of oral and oropharyngeal cancer. *J Clin Oncol.* 2004;22(19):3973–3980.

15. Yao M, Smith RB, Graham MM, et al. The role of FDG PET in management of neck metastasis from head-and-neck cancer after definitive radiation treatment. *Int J Radiat Oncol Biol Phys.* 2005;63(4):991–999.

16. Hinerman RW, Mendenhall WM, Amdur RJ, et al. Early laryngeal cancer. *Curr Treat Options Oncol.* 2002;3(1):3–9.

17. Forastiere AA, Goepfert H, Maor M, et al. Concurrent chemotherapy and radiotherapy for organ preservation in advanced laryngeal cancer. *N Engl J Med.* 2003;349(22):2091–2098.

18. Forastiere A, Maor M, Weber R, et al. Long-term results of intergroup RTOG 91-11: A phase III trial to preserve the larynx-induction cisplatin/5-FU and radiation therapy versus concurrent cisplatin and radiation therapy versus radiation therapy. *Proc Am Soc Clin Oncol.* 24:284s,2006.

19. Calais G, Alfonsi M, Bardet E, et al. Randomized trial of radiation therapy versus concomitant chemotherapy and radiation therapy for advanced-stage oropharynx carcinoma. *J Natl Cancer Inst.* 1999;91 (24):2081–2086.

20. Denis F, Garaud P, Bardet E, et al. Late toxicity results of the GORTEC 94-01 randomized trial comparing radiotherapy with concomitant radiochemotherapy for advanced-stage oropharynx carcinoma: comparison of LENT/SOMA, RTOG/EORTC, and NCI-CTC scoring systems. *Int J Radiat Oncol Biol Phys.* 2003;55(1):93–98.

21. Al-Sarraf M, LeBlanc M, Giri PG, et al. Chemoradiotherapy versus radiotherapy in patients with advanced nasopharyngeal cancer: phase III randomized Intergroup study 0099. *J Clin Oncol.* 1998;16(4): 1310–1317.

22. Adelstein DJ, Li Y, Adams GL, et al. An intergroup phase III comparison of standard radiation therapy and two schedules of concurrent chemoradiotherapy in patients with unresectable squamous cell head and neck cancer. *J Clin Oncol.* 2003;21(1):92–98.

23. Bernier J, Domenge C, Ozsahin M, et al. Postoperative irradiation with or without concomitant chemotherapy for locally advanced head and neck cancer. *N Engl J Med.* 2004;350(19):1945–1952.

24. Cooper JS, Pajak TF, Forastiere AA, et al. Postoperative concurrent radiotherapy and chemotherapy for high-risk squamous-cell carcinoma of the head and neck. *N Engl J Med.* 2004;350(19):1937–1944.

25. Bernier J, Cooper JS, Pajak TF, et al. Defining risk levels in locally advanced head and neck cancers: a comparative analysis of concurrent postoperative radiation plus chemotherapy trials of the EORTC (#22931) and RTOG (# 9501). *Head Neck.* 2005;27(10):843–850.

26. Cooper JS, Pajak TF, Forastiere A, et al. Long-term survival results of a phase III intergroup trial (RTOG 95-01) of surgery followed by radiotherapy vs. radiochemotherapy for resectable high risk squamous cell carcinoma of the Head and Neck. *Int J Radiat Oncol Biol Phys.* 66:S14, 2006.

27. Fu KK, Pajak TF, Trotti A, et al. A Radiation Therapy Oncology Group (RTOG) phase III randomized study to compare hyperfractionation and two variants of accelerated fractionation to standard fractionation radiotherapy for head and neck squamous cell carcinomas: first report of RTOG 9003. *Int J Radiat Oncol Biol Phys.* 2000;48(1):7–16.

28. Bourhis J, Overgaard J, Audry H, et al. Hyperfractionated or accelerated radiotherapy in head and neck cancer: a meta-analysis. *Lancet.* 2006;368(9538):843–854.

29. Johnson JT, Ferretti GA, Nethery WJ, et al. Oral pilocarpine for post-irradiation xerostomia in patients with head and neck cancer. *N Engl J Med.* 1993;329(6):390–395.

30. Brizel DM, Wasserman TH, Henke M, et al. Phase III randomized trial of amifostine as a radioprotector in head and neck cancer. *J Clin Oncol.* 2000;18(19):3339–3345.

31. Borges L, Rex KL, Chen JN, et al. A protective role for keratinocyte growth factor in a murine model of chemotherapy and radiotherapy-induced mucositis. *Int J Radiat Oncol Biol Phys.* 2006;66(1):254–262.

32. Spielberger R, Stiff P, Bensinger W, et al. Palifermin for oral mucositis after intensive therapy for hematologic cancers. *N Engl J Med.* 2004;351(25):2590–2598.

33. Stiff PJ, Emmanouilides C, Bensinger WI, et al. Palifermin reduces patient-reported mouth and throat soreness and improves patient functioning in the hematopoietic stem-cell transplantation setting. *J Clin Oncol.* 2006;24(33):5186–5193.

34. Adjuvant chemotherapy for advanced head and neck squamous carcinoma. Final report of the Head and Neck Contracts Program. *Cancer.* 1987;60:301–311.

35. Schuller DE, Metch B, Stein DW, et al. Preoperative chemotherapy in advanced resectable head and neck cancer: final report of the Southwest Oncology Group. *Laryngoscope.* 1998;98(11):1205–1211.

36. Jortay A, Demard F, Dalesio O, et al. A randomized EORTC study on the effect of preoperative polychemotherapy in pyriform sinus carcinoma treated by pharyngolaryngectomy and irradiation. Results from 5 to 10 years. *Acta Chir Belg.* 1990;90(3):115–122.

37. Jaulerry C, Rodriguez J, Brunin F, et al. Induction chemotherapy in advanced head and neck tumors: results of two randomized trials. *Int J Radiat Oncol Biol Phys.* 1992;23(3):483–489.

38. Mazeron JJ, Martin M, Brun B, et al. Induction chemotherapy in head and neck cancer: results of a phase III trial. *Head Neck.* 1992;14(2): 85–91.

39. Depondt J, Gehanno P, Martin M, et al. Neoadjuvant chemotherapy with carboplatin/5-fluorouracil in head and neck cancer. *Oncology.* 1993;50 Suppl 2:23–27.

40. Dalley D, Beller E, Aroney R, et al. The value of chemotherapy (CT) prior to definitive local therapy (DLT) in patients with locally advanced squamous cell carcinoma (SCC) of the head and neck (HN). *Proc Am Soc Clin Oncol.* 1995;14:297.

41. Paccagnella A, Orlando A, Marchiori C, et al. Phase III trial of initial chemotherapy in stage III or IV head and neck cancers: a study by the Gruppo di Studio sui Tumori della Testa e del Collo. *J Natl Cancer Inst.* 1994;86(4):265–272.

42. Domenge C, Hill C, Lefebvre JL, et al. Randomized trial of neoadjuvant chemotherapy in oropharyngeal carcinoma. French Groupe d'Etude des Tumeurs de la Tete et du Cou (GETTEC). *Br J Cancer.* 2000;83(12):1594–1598.

43. Licitra L, Grandi C, Guzzo M, et al. Primary chemotherapy in resectable oral cavity squamous cell cancer: a randomized controlled trial. *J Clin Oncol.* 2003;21(2):327–333.

44. Lefebvre JL, Chevalier D, Luboinski B, et al. Larynx preservation in pyriform sinus cancer: preliminary results of a European Organization for Research and Treatment of Cancer phase III trial. EORTC Head and Neck Cancer Cooperative Group. *J Natl Cancer Inst.* 1996;88 (13):890–899.

45. Jacobs C, Makuch R. Efficacy of adjuvant chemotherapy for patients with resectable head and neck cancer: a subset analysis of the Head and Neck Contracts Program. *J Clin Oncol.* 1990;8(5):838– 847.

46. Zorat PL, Paccagnella A, Cavaniglia G, et al. Randomized phase III trial of neoadjuvant chemotherapy in head and neck cancer: 10-year follow-up. *J Natl Cancer Inst.* 2004;96(22):1714–1717.

47. Pignon JP, Bourhis J, Domenge C, et al. Chemotherapy added to locoregional treatment for head and neck squamous-cell carcinoma: three meta-analyses of updated individual data. MACH-NC Collaborative Group. Meta-Analysis of Chemotherapy on Head and Neck Cancer. *Lancet.* 2000;355(9208):949–955.

48. Vermorken JB, Remenar E, van Herpen C, et al. Cisplatin, fluorouracil, and docetaxel in unresectable head and neck cancer. *N Engl J Med.* 2007;357(17):1695-1704.

49. Posner MR, Hershock DM, Blajman CR, et al. Cisplatin and fluorouracil alone or with docetaxel in head and neck cancer. *N Engl J Med.* 2007;357(17):1705-1715.

50. Calais G, Pointreau Y, Alfonsi M, et al. Randomized phase III trial comparing induction chemotherapy using cisplatin (P) fluorouracil (F) with or without docetaxel (T) for organ preservation in hypopharynx and larynx cancer. Preliminary results of GORTEC 2000–01. *J Clin Oncol.* 24, 2006.

51. Hitt R, Lopez-Pousa A, Martinez-Trufero J, et al. Phase III study comparing cisplatin plus fluorouracil to paclitaxel, cisplatin, and fluorouracil induction chemotherapy followed by chemoradiotherapy in locally advanced head and neck cancer. *J Clin Oncol.* 2005;23 (34):8636–8645.

52. Merlano M, Benasso M, Corvo R, et al. Five-year update of a randomized trial of alternating radiotherapy and chemotherapy compared with radiotherapy alone in treatment of unresectable squamous cell carcinoma of the head and neck. *J Natl Cancer Inst.* 1996;88(9):583–589.

53. Bourhis J, Armand C, Pignon J-P Update of MACH-NC database focused on concomitant chemoradiotherapy. *Proc Am Soc Clin Oncol.* 2004;22:488.

54. Brizel DM, Albers ME, Fisher SR, et al. Hyperfractionated irradiation with or without concurrent chemotherapy for locally advanced head and neck cancer. *N Engl J Med.* 1998;338(25):1798–1804.

55. Jeremic B, Shibamoto Y, Milicic B, et al. Hyperfractionated radiation therapy with or without concurrent low-dose daily cisplatin in locally advanced squamous cell carcinoma of the head and neck: a prospective randomized trial. *J Clin Oncol.* 2000;18(7):1458–1464.

56. Jeremic B, Shibamoto Y, Stanisavljevic B, et al. Radiation therapy alone or with concurrent low-dose daily either cisplatin or carboplatin in locally advanced unresectable squamous cell carcinoma of the head and neck: a prospective randomized trial. *Radiother Oncol.* 1997;43(1): 29–37.

57. Garden AS, Pajak TF, Vokes EE, et al. Preliminary results of RTOG 9703-a phase II randomized trial of concurrent radiation (RT) and chemotherapy for advanced squamous cell carcinomas (SCC) of the head and neck. *Proc Am Soc Clin Oncol.* 2001;20:891.

58. Browman GP, Hodson DI, Mackenzie RJ, et al. Choosing a concomitant chemotherapy and radiotherapy regimen for squamous cell head and neck cancer: A systematic review of the published literature with subgroup analysis. *Head Neck.* 2001;23(7):579–589.

59. Bourhis J, Le Maitre A, Baujat B, et al. Individual patients' data meta-analyses in head and neck cancer. *Curr Opin Oncol.* 2007;19(3): 188–194.

60. Bonner JA, Harari PM, Giralt J, et al. Radiotherapy plus cetuximab for squamous-cell carcinoma of the head and neck. *N Engl J Med.* 2006;354(6):567–578.

61. Wendt TG, Grabenbauer GG, Rodel CM, et al. Simultaneous radiochemotherapy versus radiotherapy alone in advanced head and neck cancer: a randomized multicenter study. *J Clin Oncol.* 1998;16(4): 1318–1324.

62. Adelstein DJ, Saxton JP, Lavertu P, et al. A phase III randomized trial comparing concurrent chemotherapy and radiotherapy with radiotherapy alone in resectable stage III and IV squamous cell head and neck cancer: preliminary results. *Head Neck.* 1997;19(7):567–575.

63. Adelstein DJ, Lavertu P, Saxton JP, et al. Mature results of a phase III randomized trial comparing concurrent chemoradiotherapy with radiation therapy alone in patients with stage III and IV squamous cell carcinoma of the head and neck. *Cancer.* 2000;88(4):876–883.

64. Induction chemotherapy plus radiation compared with surgery plus radiation in patients with advanced laryngeal cancer. The Department of Veterans Administration Laryngeal Cancer Study Group. *N Engl J Med.* 1991;324(24):1685–1690.

65. Spaulding MB, Fischer SG, Wolf GT. Tumor response, toxicity, and survival after neoadjuvant organ-preserving chemotherapy for advanced laryngeal carcinoma. The Department of Veterans Affairs Cooperative Laryngeal Cancer Study Group. *J Clin Oncol.* 1994;12(8): 1592–1599.

66. Richard JM, Sancho-Garnier H, Pessey JJ, et al. Randomized trial of induction chemotherapy in larynx carcinoma. *Oral Oncol.* 1998;34(3): 224–228.

67. Terrell JE, Fisher SG, Wolf GT. Long-term quality of life after treatment of laryngeal cancer. The Veterans Affairs Laryngeal Cancer Study Group. *Arch Otolaryngol Head Neck Surg.* 1998;124(9):964–971.

68. Lefebvre JL, Horiot JC, Rolland F, et al. Phase III study on larynx preservation comparing induction chemotherapy and radiotherapy versus alternating chemoradiotherapy in resectable hypopharynx and larynx cancers. EORTC protocol 24954–22950. *Proc Am Soc Clin Oncol.* 2007;25:966s.

69. Hassanein KA, Musgrove BT, Bradbury E. Psychological outcome of patients following treatment of oral cancer and its relation with functional status and coping mechanisms. *J Craniomaxillofac Surg.* 2005;33 (6):404–409.

70. Duffy SA, Ronis DL, Valenstein M, et al. Depressive symptoms, smoking, drinking, and quality of life among head and neck cancer patients. *Psychosomatics.* 2007;48(2):142–148.

71. Karnell LH, Christensen AJ, Rosenthal EL, et al. Influence of social support on health-related quality of life outcomes in head and neck cancer. *Head Neck.* 2007;29(2):143–146.

72. Murphy BA, Ridner S, Wells N, et al. Quality of life research in head and neck cancer: a review of the current state of the science. *Crit Rev Oncol Hematol.* 2007;62(3):251–267.

73. Forastiere AA, Metch B, Schuller DE, et al. Randomized comparison of cisplatin plus fluorouracil and carboplatin plus fluorouracil versus methotrexate in advanced squamous-cell carcinoma of the head and neck: a Southwest Oncology Group study. *J Clin Oncol.* 1992;10(8): 1245–1251.

74. Jacobs C, Lyman G, Velez-Garcia E, et al. A phase III randomized study comparing cisplatin and fluorouracil as single agents and in combination for advanced squamous cell carcinoma of the head and neck. *J Clin Oncol.* 1992;10(2):257–263.

75. Clavel M, Vermorken JB, Cognetti F, et al. Randomized comparison of cisplatin, methotrexate, bleomycin and vincristine (CABO) versus cisplatin and 5-fluorouracil (CF) versus cisplatin (C) in recurrent or metastatic squamous cell carcinoma of the head and neck. A phase III study of the EORTC Head and Neck Cancer Cooperative Group. *Ann Oncol.* 1994;5(6):521–526.

76. Browman GP, Cronin L. Standard chemotherapy in squamous cell head and neck cancer: what we have learned from randomized trials. *Semin Oncol.* 1994;21(2):311–319.

77. Colevas AD. Chemotherapy options for patients with metastatic or recurrent squamous cell carcinoma of the head and neck. *J Clin Oncol.* 2006;24(17):2644–2652.

78. Vermorken JB, Catimel G, Mulder PD, et al. Randomized phase II trial of weekly methotrexate (MTX) versus two schedules of triweekly paclitaxel (Taxol) in patients with metastatic or recurrent squamous cell carcinoma of the head and neck (SCCHN). *Proc Am Soc Clin Oncol.* 1999;18.

79. Gibson MK, Li Y, Murphy B, et al. Randomized phase III evaluation of cisplatin plus fluorouracil versus cisplatin plus paclitaxel in advanced head and neck cancer (E1395): an intergroup trial of the Eastern Cooperative Oncology Group. *J Clin Oncol.* 2005;23(15):3562–3567.

80. Herbst RS, Arquette M, Shin DM, et al. Phase II multicenter study of the epidermal growth factor receptor antibody cetuximab and cisplatin for recurrent and refractory squamous cell carcinoma of the head and neck. *J Clin Oncol.* 2005;23(24):5578–5587.

81. Baselga J, Trigo JM, Bourhis J, et al. Phase II multicenter study of the antiepidermal growth factor receptor monoclonal antibody cetuximab in combination with platinum-based chemotherapy in patients with platinum-refractory metastatic and/or recurrent squamous cell carcinoma of the head and neck. *J Clin Oncol.* 2005;23(24):5568–5577.

82. Vermorken JB, Trigo J, Hitt R, et al. Open-label, uncontrolled, multicenter phase II study to evaluate the efficacy and toxicity of cetuximab as a single agent in patients with recurrent and/or metastatic squamous cell carcinoma of the head and neck who failed to respond to platinum-based therapy. *J Clin Oncol.* 2007;25(16):2171–2177.

83. Burtness B, Goldwasser MA, Flood W, et al. Phase III randomized trial of cisplatin plus placebo compared with cisplatin plus cetuximab in metastatic/recurrent head and neck cancer: an Eastern Cooperative Oncology Group study. *J Clin Oncol.* 2005;23(34):8646–8654.

84. Cohen EE, Rosen F, Stadler WM, et al. Phase II trial of ZD1839 in recurrent or metastatic squamous cell carcinoma of the head and neck. *J Clin Oncol.* 2003;21(10):1980–1987.

85. Cohen EE. Role of epidermal growth factor receptor pathway-targeted therapy in patients with recurrent and/or metastatic squamous cell carcinoma of the head and neck. *J Clin Oncol.* 2006;24(17): 2659–2665.

86. Seiwert TY, Haraf DJ, Cohen EE, et al. A phase I study of bevacizumab (B) with fluorouracil (F) and hydroxyurea (H) with concomitant radiotherapy (X) (B-FHX) for poor prognosis head and neck cancer (HNC). *Proc Am Soc Clin Oncol.* 2006;24.

87. Vokes EE, Cohen EE, Mauer AM, et al. A phase I study of erlotinib and bevacizumab for recurrent or metastatic squamous cell carcinoma of the head and neck (HNC). *Proc Am Soc Clin Oncol.* 2005;23.

88. De Crevoisier R, Bourhis J, Domenge C, et al. Full-dose reirradiation for unresectable head and neck carcinoma: experience at the Gustave-Roussy Institute in a series of 169 patients. *J Clin Oncol.* 1998;16(11): 3556–3562.

89. Spencer SA, Harris J, Wheeler RH, et al. RTOG 96-10: reirradiation with concurrent hydroxyurea and 5-fluorouracil in patients with squamous cell cancer of the head and neck. *Int J Radiat Oncol Biol Phys.* 2001;51:1299–1304.

90. Horwitz EM, Harris J, Langer CJ, et al. Concurrent split course hyperfractionated radiotherapy (Hfx RT), cisplatin (DDP) and paclitaxel (P) in patients with recurrent previously irradiated squamous cell carcinoma of the head and neck (SCCHN): Update of RTOG 91-11. *Proc Am Soc Clin Oncol.* 2005;23 Supplement:519s.

91. Wong SJ, Machtay M, Li Y. Locally recurrent, previously irradiated head and neck cancer: concurrent re-irradiation and chemotherapy, or chemotherapy alone? *J Clin Oncol.* 2006;24(17):2653–2658.

92. Chan AT, Teo PM, Ngan RK, et al. Concurrent chemotherapy-radiotherapy compared with radiotherapy alone in locoregionally advanced nasopharyngeal carcinoma: progression-free survival analysis of a phase III randomized trial. *J Clin Oncol.* 2002;20:2038–2044.

93. Chan AT, Leung SF, Ngan RK, et al. Overall survival after concurrent cisplatin-radiotherapy compared with radiotherapy alone in locoregionally advanced nasopharyngeal carcinoma. *J Natl Cancer Inst.* 2005;97 (7):536–539.

94. Lin JC, Jan JS, Hsu CY, et al. Phase III study of concurrent chemoradiotherapy versus radiotherapy alone for advanced nasopharyngeal carcinoma: positive effect on overall and progression-free survival. *J Clin Oncol.* 2003;21(4):631–637.

95. Wee J, Tan EH, Tai BC, et al. Randomized trial of radiotherapy versus concurrent chemoradiotherapy followed by adjuvant chemotherapy in patients with American Joint Committee on Cancer/International Union against cancer stage III and IV nasopharyngeal cancer of the endemic variety. *J Clin Oncol.* 2005;23(27):6730–6738.

96. Huncharek M, Kupelnick B. Combined chemoradiation versus radiation therapy alone in locally advanced nasopharyngeal carcinoma: results of a meta-analysis of 1,528 patients from six randomized trials. *Am J Clin Oncol.* 2002;25(3):219–223.

97. Baujat B, Audry H, Bourhis J, et al. Chemotherapy in locally advanced nasopharyngeal carcinoma: an individual patient data meta-analysis of eight randomized trials and 1753 patients. *Int J Radiat Oncol Biol Phys.* 2006;64(1):47–56.

98. Chua DT, Ma J, Sham JS, et al. Long-term survival after cisplatin-based induction chemotherapy and radiotherapy for nasopharyngeal carcinoma: a pooled data analysis of two phase III trials. *J Clin Oncol.* 2005;23(6):1118–1124.

99. Chan AT, Teo PM, Leung TW, et al. A prospective randomized study of chemotherapy adjunctive to definitive radiotherapy in advanced nasopharyngeal carcinoma. *Int J Radiat Oncol Biol Phys.* 1995;33(3): 569–577.

100. Roussy IG. Preliminary results of a randomized trial comparing neoadjuvant chemotherapy (cisplatin, epirubicin, bleomycin) plus radiotherapy vs. radiotherapy alone in stage IV (>or=N2, M0) undifferentiated nasopharyngeal carcinoma: a positive effect on progression-free survival. International Nasopharynx Cancer Study Group. VUMCA I trial. *Int J Radiat Oncol Biol Phys.* 1996;35:463–469.

101. Ma J, Mai HQ, Hong MH, et al. Results of a prospective randomized trial comparing neoadjuvant chemotherapy plus radiotherapy with radiotherapy alone in patients with locoregionally advanced nasopharyngeal carcinoma. *J Clin Oncol.* 2001;19(5):1350–1357.

102. Rischin D, Corry J, Smith J, et al. Excellent disease control and survival in patients with advanced nasopharyngeal cancer treated with chemoradiation. *J Clin Oncol.* 2002;20(7):1845–1852.

103. Chan AT, Ma BB, Lo YM, et al. Phase II study of neoadjuvant carboplatin and paclitaxel followed by radiotherapy and concurrent cisplatin in patients with locoregionally advanced nasopharyngeal carcinoma: therapeutic monitoring with plasma Epstein-Barr virus DNA. *J Clin Oncol.* 2004;22(15):3053–3060.

104. Chan AT, Hui EP, Ma BB, et al. A randomized phase II study of concurrent cisplatin-radiotherapy (RT) with or without neoadjuvant chemotherapy using docetaxel and cisplatin in advanced nasopharyngeal carcinoma (NPC). *Proc Am Soc Clin Oncol.* 2005;23.

105. Califano J, Westra WH, Koch W, et al. Unknown primary head and neck squamous cell carcinoma: molecular identification of the site of origin. *J Natl Cancer Inst.* 1999;91(7):599–604.

106. Spiro RH. Management of malignant tumors of the salivary glands. *Oncology (Williston Park).* 1998;12(5):671–680; discussion 683.

107. Gilbert J, Li Y, Pinto HA, et al. Phase II trial of taxol in salivary gland malignancies (E1394): a trial of the Eastern Cooperative Oncology Group. *Head Neck.* 2006;28(3):197–204.

108. Laurie SA, Licitra L. Systemic therapy in the palliative management of advanced salivary gland cancers. *J Clin Oncol.* 2006;24(17): 2673–2678.

109. Licitra L, Cavina R, Grandi C, et al. Cisplatin, doxorubicin and cyclophosphamide in advanced salivary gland carcinoma. A phase II trial of 22 patients. *Ann Oncol.* 1996;7(6):640–642.

110. Jones AS, Phillips DE, Cook JA, et al. A randomised phase II trial of epirubicin and 5-fluorouracil versus cisplatinum in the palliation of advanced and recurrent malignant tumour of the salivary glands. *Br J Cancer.* 1993;67(1):112–114.

111. Gedlicka C, Schull B, Formanek M, et al. Mitoxantrone and cisplatin in recurrent and/or metastatic salivary gland malignancies. *Anticancer Drugs.* 2002;13(5):491–495.

112. Airoldi M, Pedani F, Succo G, et al. Phase II randomized trial comparing vinorelbine versus vinorelbine plus cisplatin in patients with recurrent salivary gland malignancies. *Cancer.* 2001;91(3):541–547.

113. Hotte SJ, Winquist EW, Lamont E, et al. Imatinib mesylate in patients with adenoid cystic cancers of the salivary glands expressing c-kit: a Princess Margaret Hospital phase II consortium study. *J Clin Oncol.* 2005;23(3):585–590.

114. Slevin NJ, Mais KL, Bruce I, et al. Imatinib with cisplatin in recurrent and/or metastatic salivary adenoid cystic carcinoma: Response assessed by FDG-PET scanning. *Proc Am Soc Clin Oncol.* 2004; 22:514s.

115. Alcedo JC, Fabrega JM, Arosemena JR, et al. Imatinib mesylate as treatment for adenoid cystic carcinoma of the salivary glands: report of two successfully treated cases. *Head Neck.* 2004;26(9):829–831.

116. Faivre S, Raymond E, Casiraghi O, et al. Imatinib mesylate can induce objective response in progressing, highly expressing KIT adenoid cystic carcinoma of the salivary glands. *J Clin Oncol.* 2005;23(25): 6271–6273; author reply 6273–6274.

117. Agulnik M, Cohen EE, Cohen RB, et al. A phase II study of Lapatinib in recurrent or metastatic EGFR and/or ErbB2 expressing adenoid cystic (ACC) and non-ACC malignant tumors of the salivary glands (MSGT). *Proc Am Soc Clin Oncol.* 2006;24.

118. Locati LD, Bossi P, Rinaldi GR, et al. Anti-androgen therapy in recurrent and/or metastatic salivary glands carcinoma (RSGC). *Ann Oncol.* 2005;(suppl 3)16.

119. American Cancer Society. Cancer Facts and Figures 2005. Atlanta: American Cancer Society. 2005.

120. Davies L, Welch HG. Increasing incidence of thyroid cancer in the United States, 1973–2002. *JAMA.* 295(18):2164–2167.

121. Dean DS, Hay ID. Prognostic indicators in differentiated thyroid carcinoma. *Cancer Control.* 2000;7(3):229–239.

122. Mazzaferri EL, Kloos RT. Clinical review 128: Current approaches to primary therapy for papillary and follicular thyroid cancer. *J Clin Endocrinol Metab.* 2001;86(4):1447–1463.

123. Oertel YC, Oertel JE. Diagnosis of malignant epithelial thyroid lesions: fine needle aspiration and histopathologic correlation. *Ann Diagn Pathol.* 1998;2(6):377–400.

124. Shah JP, Loree TR, Dharker D, et al. Lobectomy versus total thyroidectomy for differentiated carcinoma of the thyroid: a matched-pair analysis. *Am J Surg.* 1993;166(4):331–335.

125. Mazzaferri EL, Robbins RJ, Spencer CA, et al. A consensus report of the role of serum thyroglobulin as a monitoring method for low-risk patients with papillary thyroid carcinoma. *J Clin Endocrinol Metab.* 2003;88(4):1433–1441.

126. Larson SM, Robbins R: Positron emission tomography in thyroid cancer management. *Semin Roentgenol.* 2002;37(2):169–174.

127. Schlumberger M, Challeton C, De Vathaire F, et al. Radioactive iodine treatment and external radiotherapy for lung and bone metastases from thyroid carcinoma. *J Nucl Med.* 1996;37(4):598–605.

128. Shimaoka K, Schoenfeld DA, DeWys WD, et al. A randomized trial of doxorubicin versus doxorubicin plus cisplatin in patients with advanced thyroid carcinoma. *Cancer.* 1985;56(9):2155–2160.

129. Xing M, Westra WH, Tufano RP, et al. BRAF mutation predicts a poorer clinical prognosis for papillary thyroid cancer. *J Clin Endocrinol Metab.* 2005;90(12):6373–6379.

130. Kloos RT, Ringel M, Knopp M, et al. Significant clinical and biologic activity of RAF/VEGF-R kinase inhibitor Bay 43–9006 in patients with metastatic papillary thyroid carcinoma (PTC): Updated results of a phase II study. *Proc Am Soc Clin Oncol.* 2006;24.

131. Kim S, Rosen LS, Cohen EE, et al. A phase II study of axitinib (AG-013736), a potent inhibitor of VEGFRs, in patients with advanced thyroid cancer. *Proc Am Soc Clin Oncol.* 2006;24.

132. Tennvall J, Lundell G, Hallquist A, et al. Combined doxorubicin, hyperfractionated radiotherapy, and surgery in anaplastic thyroid carcinoma. Report on two protocols. The Swedish Anaplastic Thyroid Cancer Group. *Cancer.* 1994;74(4):1348–1354.

133. Kebebew E, Clark OH. Medullary thyroid cancer. *Curr Treat Options Oncol.* 2000;1(4):359–367.

134. Ball DW. Medullary thyroid cancer: therapeutic targets and molecular markers. *Curr Opin Oncol.* 2007;19(1):18–23.

135. Wells S, You YN, Lakhani V, et al. A phase II trial of ZD6474 in patients with hereditary metastatic medullary thyroid cancer. *Proc Am Soc Clin Oncol.* 2006;24.

136. Boughton D, Rosen L, Van Vugt A, et al. Safety and antitumor activity of AMG 706 in patients (pts) with thyroid cancer (TC): A subset analysis from a phase I dose-finding study. *Proc Am Soc Clin Oncol.* 2006;24.

8

GASTROINTESTINAL CANCERS

Axel Grothey, MD

LEARNING OBJECTIVES

After reviewing this chapter, the reader should be able to

- Apply the latest information about the epidemiology of cancers of the gastrointestinal system to the treatment of patients and the conduct clinical trials
- Use appropriate prognostic factors for the development of treatment strategies for patients with cancers of the gastrointestinal system
- Based on clinical presentation, recommend appropriate imaging and diagnostic studies to accurately diagnose and stage gastrointestinal cancers
- Incorporate evidence-based standards of care into the treatment of various types of gastrointestinal cancer
- Explain to patients the current strategies for the management of cancers of the gastrointestinal system
- Examine current data that address controversies regarding pancreatic cancer treatment and make informed recommendations for care

Esophageal cancers are somewhat unique tumors that exhibit great variation in histology, geographic distribution, and incidence over time. When first described, the most common type of esophageal cancer was a squamous cell cancer of the middle to upper esophagus. However, during the past 2 decades, the incidence of squamous cell cancers has decreased and the incidence of adenocarcinomas of the esophagus and gastroesophageal junction has increased rapidly. Esophageal cancers represent the fourth most common gastrointestinal cancer (after colon, gastric, and liver cancers) and rank among the 10 most common cancers worldwide.[1] The incidence of esophageal cancers shows remarkable variation in the world, with a 60-fold difference between high- and low-incidence regions. Areas of high

The American Society of Clinical Oncology and Dr. Grothey would like to gratefully acknowledge John Marshall, MD, for his contributions to the original content of this chapter.

incidence include portions of Iran, Russia, and northern China; in the United States, squamous cell cancers dominate. The disease is less common in Japan, Europe, the United States, and Canada. In the United States, carcinoma of the esophagus is infrequent, constituting approximately 1% of all cancers and approximately 6% of gastrointestinal malignancies. During the past few years, the incidence of adenocarcinomas of the distal esophagus and gastroesophageal junction has increased, parallel to the rise of gastroesophageal reflux disease (GERD) in the general population, most notably for patients with a high body mass index. Squamous cell tumors are more likely to occur in patients who are black, and these tumors are associated with achalasia, caustic injury, tylosis, Plummer-Vinson syndrome, cigarette smoking, and excessive alcohol consumption. There also is a high frequency of secondary aerodigestive tumors among patients with squamous cell cancers of the esophagus, most certainly as a result of tobacco exposure.

Adenocarcinomas of the distal esophagus and gastroesophageal junction more typically arise in metaplastic epithelium, a condition known as Barrett's esophagus. This premalignant condition is characterized by the presence of columnar epithelium lining involving 3 cm or more of the distal tubular esophagus in the presence or absence of hiatal hernia. The incidence of Barrett's esophagus is 10% to 20% among symptomatic patients who have endoscopy, and 30% to 50% for patients with peptic strictures. Barrett's esophagus is twice as prevalent in men than in women and its frequency increases with age. The disease is less likely to occur in nonwhite populations. Although it is associated with chronic reflux disease, the true cause is unknown. Approximately 62% of cases of distal esophageal or gastroesophageal adenocarcinomas have evidence of Barrett's esophagus. It is unclear if rigorous medical management of reflux disease with long-term proton-pump inhibitors can affect the natural history of the disease or the development of the subsequent malignant process. The typical treatment for patients with Barrett's esophagus is surveillance using upper endoscopy and biopsy to examine tissue for evidence of dysplasia. High-grade dysplasia is an indication for more aggressive management, including surgical resection. Tumor markers, such as *TP53,* may be predictors of potential progression to malignant disease. There is an association between *Helicobacter pylori* and adenocarcinomas of the lower esophagus and between human papillomavirus (HPV) and squamous cell cancers of the upper esophagus.

KEY POINTS

- In the United States, esophageal squamous cell carcinoma is decreasing, and the incidence of adenociranomas is rising rapidly.
- Combined-modality chemotherapy and radiation are increasing in their importance as a neoadjuvant approach to the treatment of esophageal cancer.
- Definitive radiochemotherapy (without surgery) can be a valid treatment option for patients with squamous cell cancers of the esophagus.

ESOPHAGEAL CANCER

CLINICAL PRESENTATION AND DIAGNOSIS

The most common clinical presentation of esophageal cancer is dysphagia. Cachexia and substantial weight loss are complications of this presenting symptom, which cause many patients to be debilitated at the time of the diagnosis. Bleeding often is present as well.

Esophageal cancer should be suspected when a patient presents with dysphagia and weight loss. The history and physical examination are important elements to the diagnosis, and computerized tomography (CT) of the thorax as well as an upper endoscopy remain vital to the evaluation. The CT of the thorax should be performed with tomographic slices through the liver to evaluate the extent of disease in the upper abdomen. To diagnose and carry out clinical staging of esophageal tumors, an upper endoscopy should be performed, as well as a thorough clinical examination with careful attention to the lymph nodes in the supraclavicular and axillary regions. If needed, high-resolution ultrasound can help assess supraclavicular and axillar lymph nodes. Endoscopy enables a minimally invasive biopsy to be performed.

Newer techniques, such as endoscopic ultrasound, have become more important in the evaluation and staging of esophageal cancer. Endoscopic ultrasound can accurately assess the depth of penetration in up to 90% of tumors and determine involvement of mediastinal lymph nodes in nearly all patients, depending on the skill of the sonographer. Particularly in the era of preoperative chemotherapy and radiation, obtaining accurate staging with use of endoscopic ultrasound and CT has become a more standard component when evaluating patients with esophageal cancer. Positron emission tomography (PET), preferably as a PET/CT scan, also has been demonstrated to be useful in determining node status and detecting occult sites of distant metastatic spread, which would spare the patient the morbidity of an aggressive surgical approach. Thus, PET/CT scans have become part of the routine pretreatment diagnostic work-up for patients with esophageal cancers, especially patients with locally advanced disease (evaluating the depth of tumor penetration and lymph node metastasis according to endoscopic ultrasound).

TREATMENT

The treatment of choice for patients with esophageal cancer is controversial, but accumulating evidence from meta-analyses and clinical trials has recently led to the establishment of a relative consensus in the practical management of esophageal cancers. The standard of care had long been primary surgical resection. However, the results of surgical resection alone have been discouraging, spawning a series of clinical trials to determine the efficacy of chemotherapy and radiation. The two most commonly used surgical techniques are transhiatal esophagectomy, which is generally reserved for patients with tumors of the lower esophagus, and the Ivor-Lewis resection, which utilizes a combination of thoracotomy and laparotomy. The latter procedure is a more traditional operation for esophageal cancer, but the results associated with both approaches are similar. Operative mortality rates should be less than 5% when the operation is performed by an experienced surgeon. The results are poor for patients who have been treated with operation only shortly after disease presentation, with fewer than 10% to 15% of patients surviving 5 years. Given the morbidity associated with the surgical procedure itself, there has been a shift away from primary surgical resection in favor of newer techniques designed to control local swallowing dysfunction. These techniques are all palliative in nature and can, in select cases, be helpful before or at time of chemoradiation, include esophageal stents, laser therapy, endoscopic dilation, or intravenous or gastric/jejunal tube feeding. It is important to monitor and maintain patients' nutritional status because of the predisposition to weight loss before diagnosis and the continued difficulty with alimentation following intervention.

Because of the poor surgical outcome and the relatively advanced nature of disease at the time of diagnosis (stage II and III in most cases), there has been an increased interest in using combined-modality approaches for the treatment of patients with esophageal cancer. Initially, these approaches included only chemotherapy, but the improvement in outcome was not substantial. Similarly, radiation therapy alone for the treatment of esophageal cancer failed to yield a positive survival benefit. Radiation therapy, administered either before or after surgery, has been associated with shrinkage of the tumor, improvement in swallowing, and local-regional tumor control, but it has not been associated with better survival.

Combined-modality Treatment

Combined-modality treatment involves both chemotherapy and radiation therapy and has been the focus of most of the research for esophageal cancer during the past decade. The addition of chemotherapy is designed to treat micrometastasis and enhance the effects of radiation. The original landmark clinical trial performed by Herskovic was the first to demonstrate the benefit of combined-modality therapy.[2] In this trial, patients were randomly assigned to receive either radiation therapy alone or combined-modality radiation therapy and chemotherapy. More than 25% of patients were alive at 5 years in the group that received combined-modality therapy; none of the patients who received radiation therapy only were alive at 5 years. The median survival was 14 months for combined-modality therapy and 9 months for radiation therapy alone. The results of the study led to a series of trials designed to confirm this positive result. The purpose of these early studies was to determine if chemoradiation could be used to replace surgery for patients who were not candidates for operation or to improve surgical results with preoperative chemoradiation. The chemotherapy agents typically administered with radiation were fluorouracil, cisplatin, or mitomycin-C. With these combinations, the pathologic complete response rate was approximately 25%.[3,4] With newer chemotherapy agents, such as taxanes, the pathologic complete response rate has increased, and this finding is believed to be a good intermediate endpoint for efficacy in this clinical setting. Therefore, chemoradiation alone can be considered a viable option both for patients with localized esophageal cancer regardless of whether they are candidates for surgery. This treatment option may be particularly useful for patients who are older and patients who have poor performance status. In addition, squamous cancers (mainly found in the middle and upper esophagus) appear to be more sensitive to chemoradiation than adenocarcinomas; therefore, subsequent esophagectomy might not improve overall outcome after chemoradiation in these cancers.[5] This is especially important for cancers of the cervical esophagus, which can provide a surgical challenge.

Perioperative chemotherapy alone, without radiation, has not been shown to have any benefit for patients with local esophageal cancer. However, the Medical Research Council Adjuvant Gastric Infusional Chemotherapy trial, which compared perioperative chemotherapy using epirubicin, cisplatin, and 5-fluorouracil with surgery alone for patients with gastric and gastroesophageal cancers yielded a significant improvement in overall survival for patients who received perioperative chemotherapy (*See the section on gastric cancer for more on gastric and gastroesophageal junction cancers*).[6] Twenty-six percent of patients in this trial had esophageal and gastroesophageal junction cancers, and multivariate subgroup analyses indicated a survival benefit from perioperative chemotherapy at least for gastroesophageal junction cancers. Thus, perioperative chemotherapy should be considered for patients with gastroesophageal junction cancers who are not optimal candidates for chemoradiation. Trials comparing optimized perioperative chemotherapy with neoadjuvant chemoradiation are highly warranted, but not planned at this point.

Most commonly, chemotherapy will be reserved for patients with metastatic disease for whom palliative therapy is appropriate, which is discussed in detail further in this chapter. In contrast, preoperative neoadjuvant chemoradiation has increasingly become a standard therapy for patients with this disease. Patients are most commonly treated with either chemoradiation alone, chemoradiation followed by surgery (trimodality therapy), or continuous intensification of chemotherapy by using novel combinations of chemotherapeutic agents. The precise treatment algorithm is not well defined, and attempts to determine the optimum treatment method in randomized clinical trials have proven difficult. Various randomized trials were conducted to compare preoperative chemoradiation therapy with surgery alone, but results were conflicting. A meta-analysis, which included 18 randomized controlled trials with approximately 3,000 patients, found that trimodality therapy significantly improved 2-year survival (hazard ratio [HR] = 0.81; p = 0.002; 13% absolute difference) and reduced loco-regional recurrence when compared with surgery alone.[7] In the absence of medical contraindications, most patients in the United States with localized esophageal cancers are receiving neoadjuvant combined-modality therapy followed by surgery. This practice is so prevalent that clinical trials that try to enrollment patients to a surgery-alone arm have had major enrollment problems. Most recently, the Cancer and Leukemia Group B 9781 trial was closed after only 56 of 500 planned patients were randomly assigned to surgery alone or to surgery and combination fluorouracil and cisplatin as radiosensitizing chemotherapy.[8] However, it should be noted that the 5-year survival rate of patients receiving trimodality therapy was 39% compared with 16% for surgery alone. Median overall survival rates for the two groups were 4.5 years and 1.8 years, respectively. These results add further evidence to the use of trimodality therapy as standard of care for patients with localized esophageal cancers.

There are no convincing data that justify the routine use of adjuvant chemotherapy following surgery. Similarly, radiation therapy has no role as the sole postoperative modality. However, no data support or refute combined-modality chemotherapy and radiation therapy following initial surgical resection, although this technique is frequently employed in academic medical centers (D. Ilson. Personal communication, 2007).

In most academic medical centers, patients with stage II and stage III esophageal cancers are treated primarily with chemotherapy and radiation therapy. Chemotherapy frequently includes fluorouracil, a platinum agent, or a taxane. Following this initial treatment, patients are assessed for potential surgical intervention, or the decision is made to continue with nonoperative therapy. As stated previously, the outcomes of these two approaches — with versus without surgery — are hard to distinguish because of the lack of data.

The intent of treatment for metastatic esophageal cancer is palliation. Many agents have demonstrated some activity in esophageal cancer, including fluoropyrimidines (fluorouracil and capecitabine), platinum agents, taxanes, irinotecan, mitomycin-C, anthracyclines, and, to a lesser extent, methotrexate and gemcitabine. Treatment commonly is administered as a combination of two or three drugs or, less frequently, as single-agent therapy, depending on the patient's performance status. In most clinical trials with single-agent therapy, the response rate has ranged from 10% to 40%. Combination regimens have yielded response rates as high as 50%. Palliation of dysphagia and bleeding is important and difficult to achieve. The liberal use of esophageal stents and local therapies, such as laser therapy and brachytherapy, as well as palliative radiation with or without chemotherapy can be very useful in this setting. The activity of novel targeted agents, such as epidermal growth factor receptor (EGFR) inhibitors and vascular endothelial growth factor (VEGF) inhibitors in combination with chemotherapy and/or with radiotherapy, is being investigated in ongoing clinical trials.

GASTRIC CANCER

EPIDEMIOLOGY AND ETIOLOGY

The incidence of gastric cancer has varied considerably during the past century. In the United States, where the incidence of gastric cancer has decreased approximately 75% during the past few decades, the incidence of gastroesophageal tumors has concomitantly increased. Although gastric cancer rates have experienced a significant decline in incidence worldwide, it is still common in regions of the world where the storage of fresh foods and the quality of water are poor. Gastric cancer is a major health issue in Japan and has resulted in a unique effort to screen this population for early-stage disease. In Japan, gastric cancer is associated with a distinctly better prognosis than in Western cultures. The improved prognosis in Japan often is attributed to improvements in surgical techniques, but this hypothesis has not been universally accepted. The endoscopic screening programs in Japan also have conceivably contributed to an improved outcome through the detecting of gastric cancer lesions at an earlier — possibly more curable — stage. The lowest incidences for gastric cancer are in Western cultures and in people of higher socioeconomic status. Studies of migrant populations have supported evidence for the effect of environmental influences on the development of gastric cancer. Together, these data support the concept that gastric cancer is strongly influenced by nutritional, socioeconomic, and medical factors rather than dominated by genetic predisposition. In the United States, gastric cancer develops twice as often in men than in women, is more frequent in black men than in white men, and its incidence increases with age starting in the fifth decade. The mortality rate associated with gastric cancer has decreased for white men, but this decrease reflects a decline in the overall incidence of the disease. As mentioned previously, determining the reason for the considerable rise in the incidence of adenocarcinoma of the proximal stomach and distal esophagus remains a challenge for epidemiologists. Possible reasons for this rise include the prevalence of obesity, elevated body mass index with increased incidence of GERD, and increased calorie consumption. Aspirin and other nonsteroidal anti-inflammatory agents have been associated with a lower risk of cancer of the gastroesophageal junction.

Factors associated with an increased risk of gastric cancer include nutritional factors such as high salt and nitrate intake, a diet low in vitamins A and C, the consumption of large amounts of smoked or cured foods, lack of refrigerated foods, and poor-quality drinking water. Occupational exposure to rubber and coal also increases the risk. Cigarette smoking, *H. pylori* infection, Epstein-Barr virus, radiation

KEY POINTS

- The incidence of gastric cancer correlates with socioeconomic status and is clearly dependent on environmental factors.
- The worldwide incidence of gastric cancer is in decline; however, there is an increase in more proximal and gastroesophageal cancers.
- Controversy surrounding the best operation for gastric cancer still exists, with data from Japanese studies suggesting a better result using a more aggressive, extensive dissection.
- Randomized trials have demonstrated a benefit for adjuvant chemoradiotherapy as well as for preoperative and postoperative chemotherapy without radiation for stages I to III gastric cancer, resulting in two competing standards of care.
- Combination chemotherapy regimens have become more widely used for advanced disease, with some evidence to support benefit.

exposure, and prior gastric surgery for benign ulcer disease also have been implicated as risk factors. Genetic risk factors include type A blood, pernicious anemia, a family history of gastric cancer, hereditary nonpolyposis colon cancer (HNPCC), and Li-Fraumeni syndrome. Gastric cancer does have precursor lesions consisting of adenomatous gastric polyps, dysplasia, chronic atrophic gastritis, and intestinal metaplasia. Results from several studies have demonstrated an increased likelihood of *H. pylori* infection in patients with gastric cancer, particularly cancer of the distal stomach. Although cancer does not develop in most people with *H. pylori* infections, the increased risk for patients who are infected raises the issue of whether treatment of *H. pylori* might decrease the risk of gastric cancer. At the present time, treatment of patients with this infection should be reserved for patients with demonstrated ulcer disease, because no clear decrease in the rate of gastric cancer has been associated with such treatment.

CLINICAL PRESENTATION AND DIAGNOSIS

The common presenting symptoms for gastric cancer are bleeding, hematemesis, pain, anorexia, and dyspepsia. The first clinical symptoms often are a result of metastatic spread inside the peritoneal cavity. The disease is most often diagnosed by upper endoscopy and direct biopsy or, less commonly, by CT. It is important that a biopsy is performed for samples from any gastric ulcer because it is difficult to distinguish benign from malignant ulcers. In areas of high cancer incidence, such as Japan, mass screening programs have been successful to detect gastric cancers in an early stage, with higher cure rates observed after resection. Staging includes chest x-ray, chest CT scans, and abdominal imaging to rule out metastasis and to determine surgical resectability. The role of endoscopic ultrasound is less clear in gastric cancer than in esophageal and gastrointestinal junction cancers.

TREATMENT

The treatment of choice for patients with gastric cancer is surgical resection. Unless the tumor is at an advanced, unresectable stage at diagnosis, surgical exploration and resection are the standards of care. The type of surgery performed in Asia differs substantially from the type of resection performed in the United States. D2 resection, the standard surgery in Japan, involves the meticulous resection of all regional lymph nodes, whereas in the United States, D1 resection (removal of only perigastric lymph nodes) is standard. Data suggest that the outcome for D2 resection is better than the outcome for D1 resections; however, the disparity is thought to be caused by a fundamental difference in the disease process itself, rather than the surgical technique. Randomized trials have not clearly demonstrated a survival benefit for patients undergoing a D2, versus a D1, dissection.

Early-stage Disease

Patients with operable gastric cancer have a reasonable chance of being cured with surgery alone. Surgery cures 75% to 80% of patients with early-stage disease who have no evidence of disease in the lymph nodes. However, for patients with stage III disease, the reported 5-year survival rates are 25% or less. There is extensive literature evaluating the use of postoperative chemotherapy for the adjuvant treatment of gastric cancer. Many phase III randomized clinical trials, the majority of which used "outdated" chemotherapy regimens, have shown no clear trends toward a benefit for chemotherapy alone (without concomitant radiation). The postoperative nihilism was abandoned when a randomized trial was presented in which adjuvant chemotherapy was combined with radiation therapy.[9] Patients with stages I to III gastroesophageal or gastric cancers were randomly assigned to receive either surgery alone or surgery followed by bolus fluorouracil–based chemotherapy in combination with radiation therapy. The results showed an approximate 20% improvement in survival outcome for the group receiving the combined-modality therapy, establishing a new standard of care for patients with this disease.

More recently, perioperative chemotherapy with combination epirubicin, cisplatin, and fluorouracil administered before and after surgery for resectable gastric cancer also has shown a significant overall survival benefit compared with surgery alone.[3] As compared with the surgery group, the perioperative chemotherapy group had an increased likelihood of overall survival (HR for death = 0.75; p = 0.009; 5-year survival rate = 36% vs. 23%). Thus, either postoperative chemoradiotherapy or perioperative chemotherapy alone can be regarded as standards of care for the management of early-stage gastric cancer.

Neoadjuvant chemotherapy has been shown to shrink primary tumors and regional lymph nodes in phase II clinical trials with reproducible results; however, given the small size of these studies, the definitive role of preoperative neoadjuvant chemotherapy with or without radiation, as a means of facilitating the resection of initially unresectable tumors, is not yet established.

Advanced Disease

The treatment of metastatic cancer of the stomach is primarily palliative and confers a minimal effect on overall survival. Multiple agents are active, including fluoropyrimidines (fluorouracil, capecitabine, and S1), anthracyclines, platinum agents, taxanes (paclitaxel and docetaxel), irinotecan, and others. Combination regimens are associated with higher response rates and, according to a recent meta-analysis, also are associated with increased overall survival when compared with single-agent therapies.[10] Combinations including cisplatin and fluorouracil in various schedules were long considered the standard of care, with epirubicin commonly added to form the triple-drug regimen. A phase III trial demonstrated superiority of the addition of docetaxel to cisplatin and fluorouracil compared with cisplatin and fluorouracil alone, in terms of response rate, progression-free survival, and overall survival.[11] However, the addition of docetaxel is associated with significant toxicities, most notably, a high rate of febrile neutropenia (30%); therefore, it is not feasible for patients with gastric cancer who have a reduced performance status. Recently, a large randomized phase III trial tried to improve the regimen of epirubicin, cisplatin, and fluorouracil by substituting oral capecitabine for continuous infusion fluorouracil and by using the non-nephrotoxic compound oxaliplatin instead of cisplatin.[12] Combination capecitabine and oxaliplatin was found to be less toxic and at least as active as combination epirubicin, cisplatin, and fluorouracil, with all efficacy parameters trending toward superiority. The addition of docetaxel or epirubicin to cisplatin and fluorouracil, fluorouracil and cisplatin alone, and combination capecitabine and oxaliplatin can all be regarded accepted standards of care in the palliative therapy of advanced gastric and gastroesophageal cancers.

Radiation therapy can be effective for metastatic disease (e.g., metastasis to bony structures for symptomatic control) and perhaps for unresectable, bleeding tumors in conjuction with chemotherapy, but beyond the adjuvant setting (in conjunction with chemotherapy), it is rarely used to treat primary advanced unresectable gastric cancer.

PANCREATIC CANCER

EPIDEMIOLOGY AND ETIOLOGY

Cancer of the exocrine pancreas is a substantial health problem in the United States, with an annual incidence of 33,700 patients and an annual mortality of 33,200 cases in the United States, with virtually all of those patients dying within 2 years of diagnosis.[13] It is estimated that more than 200,000 patients die of pancreatic cancer each year worldwide.[14] The incidence of pancreatic cancer increased until the late 1970s and then reached a plateau. The risk factors for pancreatic cancer are largely unknown, although there is some suggestion of a link to tobacco exposure. Data regarding coffee and excess alcohol consumptions are conflicting; therefore, they cannot be considered true etiologic factors. There is an association between pancreatic cancer and diabetes; however, it is more likely that diabetes is an early manifestation of cancer and not necessarily a predisposing factor. Chronic pancreatitis also may be a predisposing factor. There are newly recognized inherited genetic syndromes that have been linked to pancreatic cancer, but the numbers of patients affected are limited, making the utility of this finding relatively small. There is no standard surveillance or screening for this disease.

KEY POINTS

- Pancreatic cancer has the highest lethal rate of all the gastrointestinal malignancies.
- Diagnostic tests, such as PET and endoscopic ultrasound, do not replace the need for a biopsy to prove the diagnosis.
- To date, gemicitabine, as a single agent, is the standard of care for patients with advanced pancreatic cancer.
- The best approach to adjuvant therapy is controversial.

CLINICAL PRESENTATION AND DIAGNOSIS

Symptoms associated with pancreatic cancer at the time of presentation include either abdominal pain or jaundice. The disease typically is not diagnosed for several months after the initial presentation of vague abdominal symptoms or, quite commonly, back pain. Ultimately, the diagnosis is most often made with a CT scan. When evaluating patients with adult-onset diabetes without other risk factors, physicians should consider pancreatic cancer as a possible diagnosis. The most common diagnostic tests used for pancreatic cancer are CT, magnetic resonance imaging (MRI), endoscopic ultrasound, and endoscopic retrograde cholangiopancreatography. Diagnostic tests, such as PET and endoscopic ultrasound, may play a role in distinguishing cancer from other abnormalities but do not replace a biopsy as a definitive diagnostic test.

TREATMENT

The treatment for pancreatic cancer is primarily surgical resection, which should be performed by an experienced surgeon. For patients with tumors that appear resectable, which includes only approximately 25% of all pancreatic cancers, surgery remains the only potentially curative treatment option. Tools such as endoscopic ultrasound, MRI, and PET have improved the ability to determine which patients are candidates for surgery. However, most patients with pancreatic cancer are found to have unresectable disease either because of a locally advanced disease (involvement of critical vascular structures) or obvious metastatic disease (liver, peritoneal involvement) at the time of diagnosis. The 5-year survival rate for the minority of patients who are able to undergo resection is 5% to 25%.[15]

Adjuvant Therapy

The role of adjuvant therapy after pancreatic cancer resection is controversial. Based on a small randomized study (43 patients) conducted in the United States approximately 30 years ago in which a significantly larger number of patients in the combined-modality group were alive at 1 year compared with the surgery-alone group, postoperative radiochemotherapy with bolus fluorouracil became the standard of care in the United States. Since then, the role of radiation in this context has been repeatedly challenged by European investigators, culminating in a trial suggesting that the use of radiation conferred an adverse outcome compared with patients who received adjuvant chemotherapy alone.[16,17] The complex study design, concerns about the radiation protocol, and the questionable randomization strategy used in the study have long prevented chemotherapy without radiation from becoming an accepted standard of care in the United States. Most recently, two clinical trails have set somewhat competing standards for the adjuvant therapy of pancreatic cancer. A German phase III trial demonstrated the superiority of adjuvant chemotherapy with gemcitabine compared with surgery alone for patients with resected pancreatic cancer, regardless of whether a tumor-free resection margin could be obtained.[18] An American trial documented an improved outcome for patients who received adjuvant gemcitabine followed by radiochemotherapy with fluorouracil and subsequent gemcitabine monotherapy compared with postoperative fluorouracil–based radiochemotherapy.[19] Thus, for the foreseeable future, the standards of care will differ between the United States and Europe, with adjuvant gemcitabine-based chemotherapy without radiation favored in Europe and combined-modality approaches favored in the United States.

Preoperative Chemotherapy and Radiation

Preoperative chemotherapy and radiation are used in some centers in a neoadjuvant fashion, and the results of small pilot trials regarding this treatment approach have been published. The findings suggest that this approach is tolerable with occasional tumor responses allowing subsequent surgical resection, although no survival advantage has been demonstrated.

For patients with locally advanced, unresectable disease, there are two treatment strategies. Most patients in the United States are treated with a combination of radiation therapy and chemotherapy. The standard regimen is infusion fluorouracil and radiation therapy, but the role of contemporary chemotherapy agents, including gemcitabine, oral capecitabine (a fluorouracil substitute), and targeted agents in combination with radiation therapy is now being explored. This approach may improve symptoms of pain and prevent gastric or biliary obstruction. The other feasible strategy is to initiate systemic chemotherapy as primary therapy because the clinical benefit of gemcitabine-based therapy in this setting is well documented, even in the absence of significant tumor shrinkage.

Other palliative means to treat patients in this setting include biliary stenting, intraoperative or external beam radiation therapy, and celiac axis nerve blocks. Aggressive management of symptoms, such as pain, anorexia, and obstruction, should be the primary focus.

Regarding advanced metastatic disease, several agents, such as fluoropyrimidines, gemcitabine, irinotecan, platinum compounds, and taxanes, have minor to moderate single-agent activity in pancreatic cancer. In the mid-1990s, gemcitabine was tested in a randomized clinical trial against single-agent intravenous fluorouracil.[20] Gemcitabine was found to be superior to fluorouracil regarding clinical benefit, with patients experiencing a reduction of pain as well as improvements in appetite and weight. There were few clinical responses in either arm, and the median survival (6 months compared with 4 months, respectively), as well as the 1-year survival rate, were better for patients treated with gemcitabine. Subsequently, a plethora of clinical trials have tried to outperform gemcitabine monotherapy, with all studies using the following study design: gemcitabine compared with gemcitabine plus another agent. In phase III trials, the agent used was one of several conventional chemotherapy drugs, such as fluorouracil, cisplatin, oxaliplatin, irinotecan, or pemetrexed. Novel biologic agents also were used, such as or matrixmetalloprotease inhibitors, farnesyl-transferase inhibitors, or the VEGF-inhibitor bevacizumab. All of these trials failed to lead to improvements in overall survival.

However, two recent phase III trials showed a small but significant survival benefit of similar magnitude when another agent was used in combination with gemcitabine. In the first trial, the combination of gemcitabine with erlotinib, an EGFR tyrosine kinase inhibitor was found to significantly increase progression-free (HR 0.77, 95% CI 0.64, 0.92; $p = 0.004$) and overall survival (HR 0.82, 95% CI 0.69, 0.99; $p = 0.038$), albeit with a median overall survival improvement of 2 weeks.[21] No increase in response rate was noted. Nevertheless, based on these data, erlotinib obtained approval from the U.S. Food and Drug Administration (FDA) for the treatment of advanced pancreatic cancer in conjunction with gemcitabine. The second trial, a phase III trial comparing gemcitabine with or without capecitabine, demonstrated moderate benefits regarding response rates as well as progression-free and overall survivals.[22]

Therefore, the standard of care for patients with advanced pancreatic cancer is single-agent gemcitabine or gemcitabine combined with either erlotinib or capecitabine if a more aggressive approach is warranted. The role of second-line therapies after failure of gemcitabine–based first-line approaches is unclear.

These data indicate that although pancreatic cancer has been a fertile ground for testing novel chemotherapeutic and biologic agents, no clinically relevant improvement has been made beyond gemcitabine monotherapy for the palliative treatment of this disease. Ongoing trials continue to examine the integration of targeted agents in conjunction with gemcitabine, with or without concomitant radiation for patients with locally advanced disease.

CANCERS OF THE LIVER AND BILIARY TREE

EPIDEMIOLOGY AND ETIOLOGY

Primary hepatobiliary cancers are the most common solid organ cancers and include hepatocellular cancers, cholangiocarcinomas, and gallbladder cancers. Although uncommon in Western cultures, these cancers (particularly hepatocellular cancers) represent the highest global incidence of solid organ tumors and are responsible for more than 1 million deaths annually. The risk factors for hepatocellular cancer are well known (Table 8-1). Globally, hepatitis infection is responsible for most of the disease.

HEPATOCELLULAR CANCER

Clinical Presentation and Diagnosis

Hepatocellular carcinoma is graded as well differentiated, moderately well differentiated, and poorly differentiated. The most important pathologic issue is the distinction between the fibrolamellar variant and the more traditional hepatocellular cancer. Fibrolamellar cancer is generally seen in younger patients, is much more likely to be resectable, and is less commonly associated with infection or cirrhosis. In contrast, hepatocellular cancer is found more often in men older than 65, and fewer than 25% of the tumors are resectable, often because of underlying liver disease and inadequate hepatic reserve. The predominant reason for non-resectability is the multifocal nature of the disease in the liver and detection late in the disease course, the latter of which is because of the long asymptomatic latency until diagnosis. Patients at high risk for the disease, such as patients with chronic hepatitis, are monitored with imaging tests, which are often not useful because of the similarity in appearance between cirrhotic and cancerous livers. Frequently, biopsies are required to distinguish cancer from cirrhosis. Likewise, alpha-fetoprotein tumor markers are not always helpful to distinguish between the two diseases.

TABLE 8-1 Risk Factors for Hepatocellular Cancer

Hepatitis B and C
Excessive alcohol consumption
Autoimmune hepatitis
Primary biliary cirrhosis
Androgenic steroids
Aflatoxins
Tobacco
Nitrosylated compounds
Thorotrast
Hemochromatosis
Alpha-1 antitrypsin deficiency
Wilson's disease
Porphyria
Glycogen storage disease

KEY POINTS

- Hepatocellular cancer remains a global issue, with very little progress in its treatment.
- Resection is the mainstay of treatment for this family of tumors.

Treatment

The treatment of choice for patients with hepatocellular cancer is surgical resection. However, resection is not possible in most cases. Attempts at administration of systemic chemotherapy have been unsuccessful at generating radiographic responses, with virtually no improvement in survival. Nonetheless, hepatic arterial infusions of chemotherapy as well as chemoembolization (transcatheter arterial chemoembolization) have proved to be somewhat useful. Liver-directed treatments are generally reserved for unresectable, localized disease. These approaches include alcohol injection and radiofrequency ablation. Although response rates are high, it is unclear whether these techniques result in a survival benefit.

Liver transplantation represents the ultimate local therapy for unresectable hepatocellular cancer. For patients with substantial cirrhosis, liver transplantation provides an excellent option for early-stage tumors because the procedure is therapeutic for both the cancer and for the underlying pathology. Once patients have passed the high-risk peritransplant phase, the prognosis is similar to that for patients who have had resection of more localized disease. Patients with known extrahepatic disease are not candidates for liver transplantation.

Based on repeated unfavorable results, no standard chemotherapy has emerged for advanced unresectable disease. Single-agent anthracyclines and fluoropyrimidines have been most widely used in clinical trials and clinical practice, but reported response rates and times to tumor progression vary considerably. Combination regimens are associated with higher response rates but do not necessarily translate into better overall outcome. Current trials are focusing on targeted therapies, such as angiogenesis and signal transduction inhibitors, either as single agents or in combination with chemotherapy or with other biologic agents. Most recently, a phase III trial (presented in abstract form at the 2007 ASCO Annual Meeting) of 602 patients with unresectable hepatocellular cancer compared sorafenib, an oral inhibitor of vascular endothelial growth factor receptor (VEGFR) and Raf, with placebo. In this trial, the use of sorafenib was associated with significant prolongation of progression-free (24.0 weeks vs. 12.3 weeks, $p = 0.000007$) and overall survival (46.3 weeks vs. 34.4 weeks, $p = 0.00058$). Sorafenib could emerge as new standard therapy for advanced, unresectable hepatocellular carcinoma.[23] It is unclear at this point, if the observed efficacy of sorafenib is more related to its VEGFR- or Raf-inhibitory capacity. Clinical trials using VEGF inhibitors for hepatocellular cancer are underway that could help answer this question. A potential treatment algorithm for hepatocellular cancer is outlined in Fig. 8-1.[24]

CHOLANGIOCARCINOMA

Cancers of the bile duct and gallbladder are rare, with only 9,200 cases diagnosed annually in the United States, resulting in approximately 3,300 annual deaths.[25] Because of the location of these tumors, they are frequently difficult to resect; therefore, specialized surgical intervention should always be sought. Cholangiocarcinoma is most common in female patients older than 50, and long-term survival is highly dependent on the effectiveness of surgical therapy. Conditions that are associated with an increased risk include primary sclerosing cholangitis (increased risk for patients with Crohn's disease), choledochal cysts, and other hepatic infections. Gallstones also increase the risk of cancers of the gallbladder.

Clinical Presentation, Diagnosis, and Treatment

Cholangiocarcinomas typically present with jaundice, with a mass evident on CT, ultrasound, or visualized endoscopically. The primary treatment is surgical resection. The survival rate for patients with early-stage disease ranges from 60% to 70%; however, for patients with more advanced disease, the 5-year survival rate is only 10% to 25%. Thus, the role of either preoperative or postoperative radiation and chemo therapy may be important. Although the role of radiation therapy — either alone or in combination with chemotherapy — has been evaluated in several studies, a substantial benefit has not been seen. Adjuvant therapy is used for patients with positive margins or for patients with positive lymph nodes, but there is no clear standard of care in this area. Similarly, the effectiveness of systemic chemotherapy is poor, with response rates ranging from 10% to 40% for both single-agent and combination chemotherapy regimens. Most of these regimens are gemcitabine–based or fluoropyrimidines–based and follow treatment strategies established in pancreatic cancer. The role of photodynamic therapy for superficial cholangiocarcinoma is not defined.

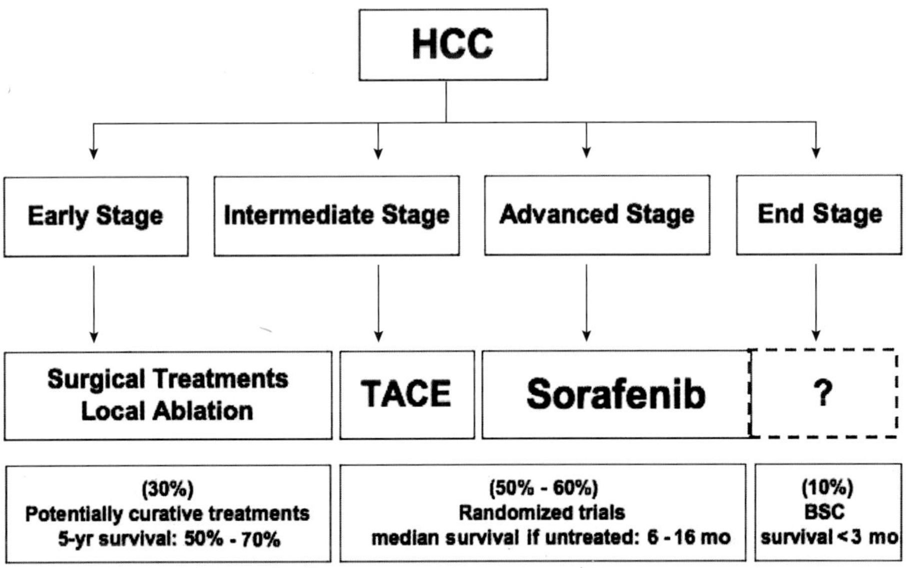

FIG. 8-1 Hepatocellular cancer (HCC) treatment algorithm.

Abbreviations: TACE, transcatheter arterial chemoembolization; yr, year; mo, months; BSC, best supportive care. Reprinted from The Lancet. with permission from Elsevier.

COLORECTAL CANCER

EPIDEMIOLOGY AND ETIOLOGY

Colorectal cancer affects approximately 150,000 patients in the United States every year. Among all cancers, it is the second leading cause of death in the United States, with more than 52,000 deaths and affecting both men and women equally.[25] Colorectal cancer is both sporadic and familial. The incidence of colorectal cancer is higher in developed countries than in developing countries. In the past decade, there has been a decrease in the incidence of colorectal cancer in the United States. Findings from epidemiologic studies indicate that during the past decade, the anatomic distribution of colorectal cancer may have shifted from the distal colon to the proximal end. These results indicate strong environmental associations for colorectal cancer. The amount of fat intake relative to dietary fiber has long been believed to have an effect. Findings from case-controlled studies demonstrate that intake of fiber-rich foods (at least 13 g per day of dietary fiber) is strongly associated with a low risk of colorectal cancer. Other etiologic factors include the content and quality of bile acids, as well as vitamin and mineral intake, with calcium appearing to play a critical role. Folate may likewise offer protection against colorectal cancer. However, data from prospective, interventional studies, indicate that the association among dietary fiber, calcium, fat intake, and colorectal cancer is less meaningful.[26,27] Additional environmental factors include intake of alcohol and tobacco, hormone replacement in women (protective), total calorie consumption, and physical activity as it relates to obesity. Interestingly, there has been an increased recognition that regular use of nonsteroidal anti-inflammatory agents including aspirin and cyclooxygenase-2 inhibitors, such as celecoxib, may have a protective effect against colorectal cancer.[28]

KEY POINTS

- Screening for colorectal cancer, which can conceivably reduce the mortality of this disease, is largely underutilized.
- Specific genetic mutations have been identified that characterize familial and sporadic colorectal cancers.
- Various conventional cytotoxic drugs (e.g., fluoropyrimidines, oxaliplatin and irinotecan), as well as targeted agents (e.g., bevacizumab, cetuximab and panitumumab) have shown proof-of-efficacy in metastatic colorectal cancer.
- Adjuvant chemotherapy with an oxaliplatin–based regimen is the standard of care for stage III colon cancer; the role of adjuvant therapy in stage II colon cancer is controversial.
- Neoadjuvant chemoradiotherapy followed by total mesorectal excision has become the standard approach for stages II and III rectal cancer.
- Patients with stage IV disease have a curative chance if their metastases are amendable for complete surgical resection.

FAMILIAL SYNDROMES — FAP AND HNPCC

There are two common inherited forms of colorectal cancer, hereditary nonpolyposis colorectal cancer (HNPCC, or Lynch I and Lynch II syndromes) and the familial adenomatous polyposis (FAP) syndrome (Table 8-2). These two recognized genetic syndromes are distinct in molecular biology and in clinical characteristics.

The first syndrome to be recognized was FAP, which is caused by an inherited mutation in the FAP coli (*APC*) gene, a key regulator of the *wnt*-signaling pathway. Mutations of the *APC* gene lead to the formation a dysfunctional protein, which prevents it from binding beta-catenin and from activating the transcription of various oncogenes. Patients with mutated *APC* have hundreds to thousands of colonic polyps, predisposing them to malignant tumors at a young age. Although FAP represents a small percentage (approximately 0.5% to 1%) of the overall number of cases of colorectal cancer, *APC* (or beta-catenin) mutations activating the *wnt*-signaling pathway have been found in the vast majority (80% to 85%) of sporadic colorectal cancers. Further gene expression studies along the adenoma-carcinoma sequence have provided an important genetic model in which specific genetic mutations leading to invasive colorectal cancers have been clearly elucidated (Fig. 8-2).[29]

HNPCC is an inherited autosomal-dominant disease with high penetrance. Patients who inherit a mutant of this gene class develop colorectal cancers at young ages. In addition, for patients with type II HNPCC (Lynch II syndrome), other cancers develop including ovarian,

TABLE 8-2 Factors that Increase the Risk of Colon Cancer

Polyposis Syndromes

- Familial polyposis
- Peutz-Jeghers syndrome
- Juvenile polyposis

Nonpolyposis Syndromes

- Hereditary nonpolyposis colorectal cancer (HNPCC)

Other

- Inflammatory bowel disease
- Prior colon cancer
- Prior polyps
- First degree relative diagnosed when younger than age 50

FIG. 8-2 Specific genetic mutations responsible for colorectal cancer.[29]

The development of approximately 80% of all colorectal cancers are dependent on the accumulation of specific genetic mutations. Reprinted from Cell, *with permission from Elsevier.*

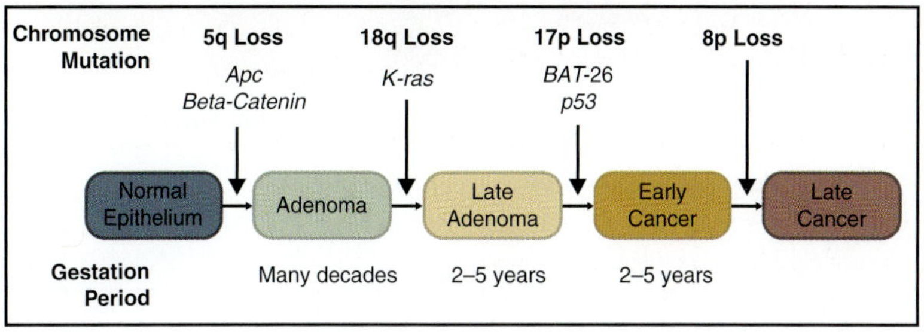

pancreatic, breast, biliary, endometrial, gastric, genitourinary, and small bowel. Approximately 5% of all colorectal cancers are attributed to this inherited syndrome. The Amsterdam Criteria and Bethesda Criteria are used to classify patients with this disease (Table 8-3). The genetic abnormality of microsatellite instability (MSI) is caused by mutations in a group of genes that code for DNA mismatch repair enzymes, including *MSH-2, MLH-1, PMS-1, PMS-2*, and *MSH-6*. The defect in mismatch repair allows spontaneous genetic mutations to accumulate in colonic mucosa, which predisposes for the development of dysplasia, and eventually, for invasive cancers. The term "microsatellite instability" denotes that with reduced or absent DNA repair activity, the length of repetitive DNA sequences varies (becomes instable) upon DNA replication. Apart from the hereditary HNPCC forms, approximately 10% to 15% of sporadic colon cancers also carry mutations (or gene promoter methylations) in the mismatch repair enzymes and are thus characterized as MSI. Depending on how much the DNA repair capacity is affected, MSI-high or MSI-low, as well as microsatellite-stable tumors, are distinguished. Clinically, patients with these tumors do not present with premalignant polyps; rather, cancers quickly develop from macroscopically normal mucosa. This issue is critical because the screening used for patients with HNPCC must be different. HNPCC is clinically associated with an early onset age, a proximal tumor location, mucinous histology, and a higher grade at the time of diagnosis. Interestingly, the prognosis for patients with this type of cancer is better, independent of stage, when compared with that for patients with microsatellite-stable tumors. The improvement is seen despite the lower responsiveness to fluorouracil–based chemotherapy, although definitive data in this regard are not yet available. Other polyposis and colorectal cancer syndromes also exist (Table 8-4).

TABLE 8-3 Criteria to Determine Predisposition to Hereditary Nonpolyposis Colorectal Cancer (HNPCC)

Amsterdam Criteria (All criteria must be met)

- Three or more family members with colorectal cancer, at least two of whom must be first-degree relatives (e.g., parent, sibling, or child)
- Family members from at least two successive generations are affected
- Development of colorectal cancer occurred before age 50 in at least one family member
- Familial adenomatous polyposis is excluded

Bethesda Criteria (Any criterion is sufficient)

- Cancer in a family that fulfills the Amsterdam Criteria
- Development of two HNPCC-related (extracolonic) cancers in one individual (i.e., endometrial, small intestine, ovarian, and gastric cancer)
- Development of colorectal cancer in an individual who has a first-degree relative with colorectal cancer and/or HNPCC-related extracolonic cancer and/or colorectal adenoma, with one of the cancers diagnosed before age 45 and the adenoma diagnosed before age 40
- Colorectal or endometrial cancer diagnosed before the age of 45
- Right-sided colorectal cancer with an undifferentiated pattern on histopathologic evaluation, diagnosed before age 45
- Signet ring cell-type colorectal cancer diagnosed before age 45
- Adenoma diagnosed before age 40

TABLE 8-4 Polyposis and Colorectal Cancer Syndromes

Syndrome	Number of Colon Polyps	Extracolonic Manifestations
Familial adenomatous polyposis	> 100, diffuse	Small-bowel adenoma and adenocarcinoma, gastric adenoma and cancer, fundic gland polyps, adrenal adenomas and cancers, thyroid cancer, and desmoid tumor
Gardner's syndrome	> 100, diffuse	Epidermoid cysts, desmoid tumors, osteomas, and fibromas
Turcot's syndrome	> 100, diffuse	Brain tumors
Flat adenoma syndrome	1 to 100, right-sided	Fundic gland polyps and periampullary cancer
Discrete adenomas	1 to 10	None
Hereditary nonpolyposis	1 to 10	Cancers of the endometrium, stomach, biliary tree, and small bowel; transitional cell cancer of the ureter and renal pelvis
Puetz-Jeghers syndrome	1 to hundreds, diffuse	Ovarian and testicular tumors

Modified with permission from Cheson BD, ed. Oncology MKSAP, 2nd ed. Philadelphia, Pa: American College of Physicians; 1999:160.

Inflammatory bowel disease, particularly ulcerative colitis, is associated with an increased risk for colon cancer, estimated to be 5% to 10% at 20 years after the time of diagnosis; it also is associated with a high incidence of synchronous cancers in 10% to 20% of cases. Crohn's disease also may have a role in colorectal cancer, particularly cancer in the ileocolic region. However, in the absence of colonic involvement by Crohn's disease, there is no increased risk of colon cancer. The risk for the development of a subsequent cancer is 3% for patients with a history of adenomatous polyps. This group of patients should be screened more frequently. Screening for familial cancers and those at otherwise high risk is more intense than that for the standard population.

SCREENING

The screening tests for colorectal cancer include digital rectal examination, fecal occult blood testing (FOBT), sigmoidoscopy, colonoscopy, air-contrast barium enema, and the most recent technique, virtual CT-colonography. Each of these tools, with the exceptions of digital rectal examinations and virtual CT-colonography (for paucity of prospective data), has been shown to have a positive effect on colorectal cancer-related mortality. However, there is still a poor compliance rate with these tests, with fewer than 30% of patients ever undergoing any screening procedures. The guidelines for standard screening options vary according to different medical societies. For example, the American Medical Association emphasizes the need for any type of testing, whereas the American Gastroenterology Association and the U.S. Preventive Services Task Force strongly recommend that clinicians screen men and women 50 years of age or older for colorectal cancer by colonoscopy. There has been a shift away from emphasizing sigmoidoscopy in favor of colonoscopy, particularly in light of the observed shift toward more proximal colon cancers in recent years. The obvious advantages of colonoscopic screening are that the entire large bowel and distal ileum can be assessed and that immediate intervention, such as biopsy and polypectomy, is possible. The results of recent studies have demonstrated that although sigmoidoscopy in conjunction with annual FOBT is an effective means of reducing the mortality related to colon cancer, approximately 8% of distal cancers and all proximal cancers (approximately 40% to 50% of all colorectal cancers) will be missed. Therefore, the most common recommendation from various organizations is for colonoscopy to be performed every 5 to 10 years for a patient with average risk starting at age 50. (*See the "Epidemiology and Prevention" chapter for more information.*)

Screening should be more regular for patients at high risk, including those with inherited syndromes, inflammatory bowel disease, and previous adenomatous polyps or colorectal cancer. Individuals with HNPCC should have screening by total colonoscopy every 1 to 3 years beginning between ages 20 and 25 because of the lack of a visible premalignant lesion in this population and the higher risk for right-sided colon cancers. If a colon cancer or severe dysplasia is found in patients with inflammatory bowel disease, the general recommendation is for a near-total or a subtotal colectomy because of the high incidence of synchronous and metachronous cancers in this population. Surgery can be less extensive for patients with sporadic cancers. For patients with type II HNPCC, a more extensive surgery can be recommended, particularly for women beyond child-bearing age, for whom hysterectomy and oophorectomy should be offered.

TREATMENT

Early-stage Disease (Stages I, II, and III)

Nearly all patients with stage 0 disease (carcinoma in situ or intramucosal cancer) are cured by endoscopic resection alone, recognizing that the lymph nodes are not adequately assessed

TABLE 8-5 Staging, Incidence per Stage and Treatment Recommendations for Invasive Colon Cancer[30]

	Stage I	Stage II	Stage III	Stage IV
Staging	T1, N0, M0 T2, N0, M0	A: T3, N0, M0 B: T4, N0, M0	A: T1-2, N1, M0 B: T3-4, N1, M0 C: Any T, N2, M0	Any T, Any N, M1
Definition	Invades submucosa (T1) or muscular propria (T2)	Invades subserosa, nonperitonealized pericolic/perirectal tissues (T3) or invades other organs/structures/ visceral peritoneum (T4)	Involves 1 to 3 (N1) or more (N2) lymph nodes	Involves distant metastases
Incidence	15%	25%	35%	25%
Usual treatment	Surgery	Surgery with or without chemotherapy	Surgery with chemotherapy	Chemotherapy with or without surgery

Used with the permission of the American Joint Committee on Cancer (AJCC). Chicago, Illinois. AJCC Cancer Staging Manual, Sixth Edition (2002) published by Springer Science and Business Media.

by this technique. The primary treatment for virtually all invasive nonmetastatic colorectal cancers is surgery. Recent studies indicate that laparoscopic-assisted surgery for colon cancer provides the same outcomes for overall survival and rate of recurrence as open laparotomy. Surgery alone is curative for more than 85% of patients who have stage I or early stage II disease. For patients with more advanced stage II disease (T4, N0), the 5-year survival rate is approximately 70% to 75%; for stage III disease (positive lymph nodes), the 5-year survival rate is 30% to 50% with surgical resection alone.

Prognostic Factors. Other factors beyond stage (Table 8-5) that adversely affect outcome include male sex, extent of local invasion (T4), undifferentiated histology, mucinous features, signet-ring features, lymphovascular invasion, and elevated levels of carcinoembryonic antigen preoperatively[30]. Another important prognostic factor is the number of lymph nodes identified in the resected specimen, with a minimum number of 12 lymph nodes necessary for adequate staging. The prognosis for colon cancer for patients with HNPCC is better than the prognosis for patients with sporadic tumors, perhaps because the accumulation of mutations do not allow for metastatic spread. Findings from retrospective studies indicate that tumor aneuploidy and S phase determined by flow cytometry are associated with a less favorable outcome, but these results have not reached a point where the techniques are applied routinely in clinical practice. Similarly, testing for microsatellite instability, *TP53* expression, mutations in the *DCC* gene, K-ras, p16, loss of heterozygosity (LOH) at 18q, thymidylate synthase, and dihydropyrimidine dehydrogenase expression eventually may play a role when treating patients. Findings have shown that high tumor concentrations of thymidylate synthase may be predictive of a poor outcome. The *DCC* gene mutation/LOH18q may distinguish patients at higher risk for metastatic disease; therefore, candidates for adjuvant therapy may be identified. These issues are being addressed in large adjuvant clinical trials.

Adjuvant Chemotherapy. The initial trial presented in the early 1990s that established adjuvant chemotherapy as standard of care in stage III colon cancer used a combination of fluorouracil and levamisole administered for 12 months. A 10% to 20% improvement in 5-year survival was documented for patients receiving postoperative adjuvant fluorouracil–based chemotherapy. Evidence from newer trials demonstrated that fluorouracil combined with leucovorin provides a superior outcome, with 6 months of therapy being adequate to achieve this survival benefit.[31] For more than a decade, the standard in adjuvant therapy remained unchanged because of the lack of novel agents with relevant activity in colorectal cancer. This changed when oxaliplatin, irinotecan, and the oral fluorouracil prodrug capecitabine were utilized for the treatment of advanced colorectal cancer, with combination regimens of infusional fluorouracil plus either irinotecan and oxaliplatin demonstrating high antitumor efficacy.

Worldwide, six phase III trials were conducted to evaluate the value of the novel chemotherapeutic agents irinotecan, oxaliplatin, and capecitabine in the adjuvant setting. To set the stage for the conduct and interpretation of these trials and their results, a large retrospective meta-analysis confirmed that for adjuvant colon cancer, 3-year disease-free survival can serve as an definitive surrogate marker for 5-year overall survival.[32] This finding had a major effect on clinical trial design and endpoint definition in subsequent studies regarding adjuvant colon cancer. Based on these findings, the FDA recognized 3-year disease free survival as an appropriate endpoint for full approval of a regimen for adjuvant colon cancer. Consequently, oxaliplatin was approved as part of adjuvant treatment for stage III colon cancer in November 2004. One trial established 6 months of oral capecitabine as a safe and at least equally effective alternative to conventional intravenous bolus fluorouracil with leucovorin for stage III colon cancer.[33] Two other trials confirmed the value of oxaliplatin as component of adjuvant chemotherapy for stage II and III colon cancer. The results of the pivotal Multicenter International Study of Oxaliplatin/5-Fluorouracil/Leucovorin in the Adjuvant Treatment of Colon Cancer trial clearly demonstrated that oxaliplatin plus infusional fluorouracil and leucovorin (FOLFOX) is superior to fluorouracil with leucovorin in terms of 3-year disease-free survival. In a subgroup analysis, only the rise in disease-free survival rates for patients with stage III disease was statistically significant, providing an absolute benefit of approximately 8% to 10% (HR 0.76, 95% CI 0.62, 0.92).[34] In unselected patients with stage II disease, the disease-free survival benefit for FOLFOX compared with fluorouracil and leucovorin alone was approximately 3.5%, but it exceeded 5% for patients with stage II tumors with clinical high-risk features (undifferentiated tumors, T4, perforation, obstruction, fewer than 10 lymph nodes identified, and angiolymphatic invasion). Results of the National Surgical Adjuvant Breast and Bowel Project C-07 trial further strengthened the role of oxaliplatin–based regimens in the adjuvant therapy of colon cancer.[35] Although irinotecan–based and oxaliplatin–based regimens are thought to be as effective as palliative therapy for advanced colorectal cancer, none of the three phase III trials using combination irinotecan, fluorouracil, and leucovorin (IFL) regimen demonstrated significantly superior efficacy regarding 3-year disease-free survival when compared with fluorouracil and leucovorin alone.

Based on these results, the standard adjuvant chemotherapy for stage III colon cancer is an oxaliplatin–containing regimen (FOLFOX or bolus fluorouracil, folinic acid, and oxaliplatin [FLOX]) administered for 6 months. Capecitabine or fluorouracil and leucovorin should be reserved for patients who are not considered optimal candidates for oxaliplatin. Of note, the efficacy and tolerability of FOLFOX is largely identical both for patients younger and older than age 70.

For patients with stage II disease, the role of adjuvant chemotherapy remains controversial; the results from a series of clinical trials demonstrated a trend toward improved recurrence-free survival and overall survival (HR 0.80, 95% CI 0.56, 1.15). Findings from two pooled retrospective analyses showed conflicting results.[36,37] One analysis suggested a 30% risk reduction, translating into an approximate 8% absolute reduction in mortality, whereas a similar pooled data set showed no benefit from adjuvant chemotherapy. An analysis of Medicare data revealed that more than 50% of patients in the United States with stage II colon cancer receive postoperative adjuvant chemotherapy.[38] It appears that patients with stage II colon cancer will have a 3% benefit in 3-year disease-free and overall survivals with fluorouracil and leucovorin as adjuvant chemotherapy. The improvement is conceivably larger with an oxaliplatin–based treatment regimen, but not all patients with stage II tumors should receive adjuvant chemotherapy.[39] Efforts have been made to individualize the baseline prognosis and to predict the benefits of chemotherapy for patients with resected colon cancer.[40] Resultantly, there are two Web-based tools available to provide data of this type (an adjuvant therapy calculator developed by the Mayo Clinic[41] and Adjuvant! Online[42]). Although neither of these tools is infallible, they can provide helpful information. The identification of prognostic factors might help distinguish patients at high risk for relapse and enrich the patient population with stage II disease, who will more likely benefit from adjuvant treatment. Apart from the clinical risk factors listed previously, molecular determinants of poor prognosis, such as microsatellite stability and LOH18q, are being evaluated in prospective clinical trials.

The role of novel targeted agents with clear efficacy in advanced colorectal cancer, such as bevacizumab, an antibody against VEGF, and cetuximab, an antibody against EGFR, are being investigated in the adjuvant setting in several large phase III trials.

Advanced Colorectal Cancer

The prognosis for patients with stage IV disease without specific therapy is poor, with a median survival of 5 to 6 months. However, a subset of patients with isolated sites of metastases is potentially curable with surgery. Nevertheless, for the majority of patients with metastatic disease, the goal of therapy is palliation using systemic chemotherapy. For decades, standard first-line therapy consisted of fluorouracil plus leucovorin, with response rates of approximately 20% and a median survival of approximately 1 year. In the late 1990s and early 2000s the addition of oxaliplatin and irinotecan to the backbone of fluorouracil and leucovorin resulted in a dramatic improvement in median survival to nearly 24 months when patients received active first-line and second-line therapy. Most recently, biologic agents, such as bevacizumab, cetuximab, and panitumumab, have further enhanced the efficacy of systemic medical therapy

The availability of various active agents for the treatment of metastatic colorectal cancer has resulted in an abundance of therapeutic options that now demands a goal-oriented, strategic approach to therapy to maximize patient benefit. When treating a patient with metastatic colon cancer, the first determination is whether a patient with stage IV disease is potentially curable by a surgical resection of metastases either at the time of diagnosis or after downsizing initially unresectable metastases by neoadjuvant chemotherapy. This will guide the choice and timing of chemotherapy because, in this scenario, the most appropriate treatment is conceivably the one that generates the highest response rates and carries the greatest potential to downsize metastases. If the patient does not appear curable, then the main goals of systemic chemotherapy are to extend the duration of a patient's life and to maintain quality of life as long as possible. In this scenario, treatment regimens that offer the longest progression-free and overall survivals as well as a favorable toxicity profile are preferred.

Fluorouracil. Until recently, standard first-line therapy for metastatic colon cancer was the fluoropyrimidine analog fluorouracil plus leucovorin as biomodulator and activator. Leucovorin forms a complex with fluorouracil that permits prolonged inhibition of the enzyme thymidylate synthase, a key factor in the DNA synthesis. Response rates of fluorouracil with leucovorin are in the range of 15% to 25%. Over time, fluorouracil has been given with leucovorin in varying schedules and doses. The most commonly used regimens in the United States included the Mayo Clinic regimen (425 mg/m^2 of fluorouracil and 20 mg/m^2 for leucovorin on days 1 to 5 every 4 to 5 weeks) and the Roswell-Park regimen (500mg/m^2 of fluorouracil and 500mg/m^2 of leucovorin administered weekly for 6 out of 8 weeks). Although these regimens used fluorouracil as bolus administration, European protocols preferred to use fluorouracil in the form of protracted infusions (e.g., for 46 hours in the French biweekly LV5FU2 regimen or for 24 hours in the German weekly Arbeitsgemeinschaft Internistische Onkologie regimen. More recently, the incorporation of the novel cytotoxic agents irinotecan and oxaliplatin into fluorouracil–based regimens has resulted in significantly improved efficacy. This has shifted the paradigm for front-line treatment from fluorouracil and leucovorin alone to combination regimens incorporating these newer agents.

Capecitabine. Capecitabine is an oral fluoropyrimidine, a prodrug of fluorouracil, which is metabolized to its active form in three enzymatic steps. Its efficacy is similar to bolus fluorouracil and leucovorin, with slightly higher response rates. Common side effects of this drug include diarrhea and hand-foot syndrome. Capecitabine has been used as backbone of combination regimens with both oxaliplatin and irinotecan, but overlapping toxicities (diarrhea) make a combination with irinotecan more difficult to tolerate than oxaliplatin. Other oral fluoropyrimidines, which have not been approved in the United States, include tegafur-uracil, S1 (a prodrug of 5-FU), gimeracil (5-chloro-2,4 dihydropyridine), which inhibits dihydropyrimidine dehydrogenase enzyme activity, and oteracil (potassium oxonate).

Irinotecan. The first chemotherapy agent other than fluorouracil that improved survival for metastatic colon cancer was irinotecan. This compound has single-agent activity, which yields a 15% response rate for patients with metastatic colon cancer refractory to fluorouracil. In a landmark clinical trial, patients with fluorouracil–refractory metastatic colon cancer were randomly selected to receive either best supportive care or single-agent irinotecan. The results of the trial demonstrated that irinotecan offers an approximate 3-month survival advantage as well as an improvement in quality of life.[43] Following this, three key trials were conducted to test the role of irinotecan in the front-line setting. In the United States, a three-arm trial was conducted to compare three treatment regimens: weekly bolus fluorouracil and leucovorin (Roswell Park regimen); IFL; and irinotecan alone.[44] The results of the trial demonstrated a survival improvement of 2 months, as well as a doubling of the response rate to nearly 40% for patients receiving the three-drug regimen. This study established the three-drug regimen as the then standard of care in the United States.

In Europe, two phase III trials were conducted, in which fluorouracil was given as an infusion in combination with irinotecan, to form the FOLFIRI regimen. The results demonstrated a similar significant increase in response rate and time to disease progression for the three-drug regimen.[45,46] However, only the trial reported by Douillard et al.,[45] demonstrated significant prolongation of overall survival, likely because of the limited availability of active second-line and third-line treatment options. The main side effects of irinotecan are diarrhea, myelosuppression, and alopecia.

Oxaliplatin. Although oxaliplatin has very limited activity in colorectal cancer as a single agent, it shows enhanced clinical efficacy in combination with fluoropyrimidines, in particular with infusional fluorouracil and leucovorin. In three European phase III trials, combination protocols of infusional fluorouracil and leucovorin plus oxaliplatin (biweekly FOLFOX or weekly FUFOX) were compared with fluorouracil and leucovorin as first-line therapy for patients with advanced colorectal cancer.[47–49] In all three studies, a higher antitumor activity was noted for the combination regimens, with response rates of approximately 50% and progression-free survival in the range of 8 to 9 months. However, this higher efficacy did not translate into a significantly improved overall survival, most likely because of the availability of active salvage therapies for both treatment arms, which blurred the effects of the first-line chemotherapy on overall survival in the trials. Of note, the median overall survival achieved with fluorouracil, leucovorin, and oxaliplatin was in the range of 17.5 to 20 months, the longest overall survival reported in phase III trials for advanced colorectal cancer up to that time. Because no overall survival benefit was achieved in these first-line trials, in 2000 the FDA did not approve oxaliplatin for colorectal cancer. The FDA approval of oxaliplatin in combination with fluorouracil and leucovorin in 2002 was based on the results of a second-line study that showed prolonged progression-free survival and increased response rates compared with infusional fluorouracil and leucovorin for patients who experienced disease progression while receiving IFL as first-line therapy. The key side effect and dose-limiting toxicity of oxaliplatin is neurotoxicity, which comes in two distinct in the forms: an acute, cold-triggered sensory neuropathy, which is temporary, rapidly reversible, and does not appear to cause structural nerve damage; and a chronic cumulative sensory neurotoxicity, which is related to the cumulative dose of oxaliplatin administered over time and constitutes the dose-limiting side effect of oxaliplatin.

Comparison of Combination Regimens.
With its FDA approval in 2000, combination IFL had emerged as standard first-line therapy for patients with advanced colorectal cancer in the United States. The encouraging results of trials conducted in Europe using oxaliplatin formed the rationale for the North Central Cancer Treatment Group/Intergroup trial N9741.[50] This pivotal and practice-changing trial compared FOLFOX and the non–fluorouracil-containing combination of irinotecan and oxaliplatin (IROX), as well as with standard combination IFL. The results of N9741 clearly demonstrated the superiority of FOLFOX compared with IFL as first-line therapy for colorectal cancer regarding response rate (45% vs. 31%, $p = 0.002$), progression-free survival (8.7 months vs. 6.9 months, $p = 0.0014$), and overall survival (19.5 months vs. 15.0 months, $p = 0.0001$). The toxicity profile likewise favored FOLFOX compared with IFL with only neurotoxicity being more prevalent for patients receiving the oxaliplatin–based combination. Results for IROX were in between the two other arms (response rate, 35%; progression-free survival, 6.5 months; overall survival, 17.4 months), and as such, FOLFOX emerged as new standard first-line therapy with rapid and widespread adaptation in the United States. It should be emphasized that N9741 did not directly compare oxaliplatin and irinotecan; rather, it compared two different combination regimens with different fluorouracil and leucovorin backbones. The higher efficacy and better tolerability observed with infusional fluorouracil and leucovorin may have contributed to the differences in efficacy between IFL and FOLFOX. Two smaller trials comparing FOLFOX and FOLFIRI with the same fluorouracil and leucovorin backbone failed to show significant differences in activity.[51,52] Although the small sample size of these trials might preclude wide-reaching conclusions, the choice between FOLFOX and FOLFIRI in the clinic should mainly be based on the expected side-effect pattern. Because the benefit of second-line therapy in colorectal cancer has been well established, patients should receive all active cytotoxic drugs in the course of their therapy to optimize outcome.

Bevacizumab.
An adequate blood supply is necessary for the rapid growth and development of tumors beyond the micrometastatic state of 1 to 2 mm in diameter. VEGF contributes to tumor growth by stimulating new tumor blood vessel growth (angiogenesis) and maintaining immature tumor vasculature. VEGF was initially characterized for its ability to induce vascular leakage and permeability (vascular permeability factor) and to induce vascular endothelial proliferation. VEGF is a member of a family of structurally related proteins. These proteins bind to the family of receptors related to VEGF, thereby stimulating various biologic processes. Antibodies directed at VEGF block VEGF interactions with its receptors, thus preventing VEGF signaling through both VEGFR-1 and VEGFR-2. Bevacizumab, a recombinant humanized monoclonal antibody to VEGF has recently demonstrated clinical efficacy for the treatment of metastatic colorectal cancer. In a large phase III placebo-controlled trial with 813 patients, irinotecan plus bolus fluorouracil and leucovorin (IFL protocol) was compared with IFL plus bevacizumab (5 mg/kg every 2 weeks) as first-line therapy for advanced colorectal cancer.[53] The addition of the anti-VEGF antibody led to significantly increased response rate (45% vs. 35%, $p = 0.0036$), progression-free survival (10.6 months vs. 6.2 months, $p < 0.00001$), and median overall survival (20.3 months vs. 15.6 months, $p = 0.00004$). This trial was the first phase III validation of an anti-angiogenic agent serving as an effective treatment option in a human malignancy. Subsequently, bevacizumab also has been shown to enhance the efficacy of oxaliplatin–based regimens in first-line and second-line settings, as well as in combination with fluorouracil and leucovorin alone or with cetuximab in a salvage therapy setting. It is important to note that bevacizumab does not appear to have significant single-agent activity in metastatic colorectal cancer. The main side effects observed with bevacizumab consist of hypertension (a class-effect of all agents targeting VEGF signaling), bleeding, gastrointestinal perforations (1.5% to 2% of patients), as well as arterial thrombotic events in approximately 4% to 5% of patients. Based on these findings, bevacizumab has emerged as standard component of first-line chemotherapy for advanced colorectal cancer. Studies are ongoing to assess the efficacy of dual antibody combinations (bevacizumab plus anti-EGFR antibody) given in conjunction with standard chemotherapy regimens. Several other agents targeting various components of the VEGF-mediated signal transduction cascade have been developed and are in clinical testing.

Anti-EGFR Antibodies: Cetuximab and Panitumumab.
Both monoclonal antibodies against the EGFR, cetuximab and panitumumab, have single-agent efficacy in advanced

colorectal cancer. Two U.S. phase II trials presented in 2001 and 2002 confirmed the activity of cetuximab for the treatment of patients who had experienced disease progression on prior irinotecan–based therapy. The single-agent response rate of approximately 10% noted with cetuximab alone was in the same range as previously noted with FOLFOX in the same setting. A large international randomized phase II trial confirmed the findings with almost identical results.[54] For patients who experienced progressive disease while receiving irinotecan–based therapy (with approximately two-thirds of patients also refractory to oxaliplatin), cetuximab monotherapy induced responses for approximately 11% of patients. When irinotecan was added, response rate and time to progression were significantly increased (HR 0.54, 95% CI 0.42, 0.71; $p < 0.001$). These data served as the basis for the approval of cetuximab as a treatment option for patients with metastatic colorectal cancer who were pretreated with irinotecan–based regimens. Single-agent panitumumab was tested against best supportive care in a large international phase III trial in a extensively pretreated population; crossover was optional upon progression.[55] Panitumumab demonstrated similar single-agent activity to cetuximab, with an approximate 10% response rate when used as salvage therapy after failure of standard chemotherapy. In comparison with best supportive care, it significantly prolonged progression-free survival (HR 0.54, 95% CI 0.44, 0.66; $p < 0.0001$). Based on these data, it was approved as a single-agent salvage therapy option in the United States in 2006. Both antibodies are being tested as components of first-line therapy in combination with modern chemotherapy regimens, such as FOLFOX and FOLFIRI. The main toxicities of anti-EGFR antibodies are skin rash, hypomagnesemia, and hypersensitivity reactions, which is particularly relevant for the chimeric antibody cetuximab.

Limited Hepatic or Pulmonary Metastasis

For the subgroup of patients with recurrent metastatic colon cancer confined to the liver, the roles of hepatic-directed chemotherapy and hepatic resection have become better defined. There is only one multicenter evaluation of potentially resectable liver metastases; the results showed an improved survival for patients undergoing resection compared with those who either had unresectable disease or had noncurative resection.[56] The survival advantage is clinically significant, with a near doubling of survival to nearly 37 months.[57] When pooling data for all patients who have a hepatic resection, the average 5-year survival rate is approximately 30%, with a less favorable prognosis for patients with multiple lesions, a short interval between the diagnosis of the primary tumor and recurrence, and presence of stage III disease at the time of initial diagnosis. Neoadjuvant chemotherapy can be used to downsize initially unresectable metastases to make them amendable for a surgical approach. It has been shown that the overall survival of patients who undergo successful neoadjuvant therapy with subsequent R0 resection of liver metastases is similar for those patients with initially resectable metastases.[58] Thus, the initial therapeutic approach for a patient with limited metastatic disease should always include consideration of a potentially curative option.

Following the resection of hepatic or pulmonary metastasis, it is unclear whether further chemotherapy should be administered. In one randomized clinical trial, half of the patients who had successful hepatic resection received both systemic and intrahepatic chemotherapy; the other half received only systemic chemotherapy.[59] The results demonstrated a survival advantage at 2 years for patients who received the intrahepatic chemotherapy combination. This approach has not gained widespread use worldwide because of its difficult drug-delivery process and its associated hepatic toxicities. A pooled analysis of two small trials that utilized adjuvant therapy after liver resection and a fluorouracil and leucovorin regimen demonstrated a strong trend toward improved outcome with systemic adjuvant chemotherapy in this setting.[60] More recent approaches have begun to examine the effects of new chemotherapy protocols that include irinotecan and oxaliplatin combinations for this patient population. It is important to note that there are substantial data to support disease resection outside of the liver, with the lung being the next most common site for secondary resection.

NEOADJUVANT AND ADJUVANT THERAPY FOR RECTAL CANCER

Cancers arising in the rectum are associated with a higher overall risk of recurrence than the recurrence risk associated with similar stages of colon cancer. In particular, local regional failures occur in 25% to 50% of patients who undergo potentially curative surgery, most likely because of close surgical margins. The reason for local recurrence in rectal cancer is believed to be the anatomic location of the rectum and the challenge this presents to the surgeon, particularly surgeons practicing in low-volume hospitals. During the past decade, total mesorectal excision has emerged as the preferred surgical technique. This technique honors natural tissue planes and decreases the chance for local seeding and for subsequent recurrence. In combination with preoperative or postoperative chemoradiation, local recurrence rates of less than 10% at 5 years can be achieved.

The recognition of the morbidity and the potential mortality associated with local relapse led to the use of both preoperative and postoperative radiation therapy as additional regional treatment options designed to reduce local recurrence. Two different approaches have been used in this regard: short-term, high-dose radiation commonly delivered as daily 5 Gy for 5 days (5 x 5) immediately before surgery, or prolonged combined-modality therapy with radiosensitizing chemotherapy administered parallel to radiation to a total dose of 50.4 Gy (45 + 5.4 Gy local boost) over

5 to 6 weeks. Both treatment approaches have been associated with a decrease in local-regional failure, but prevention of local recurrence has not uniformly been associated with improved overall survival. However, the results of one trial in which patients were randomly assigned to either 5 days of high-dose radiation therapy in the week just before surgery or to surgery alone demonstrated a survival advantage for preoperative radiation therapy.[61] A subsequent trial using the same radiation technique in combination with quality controlled surgery confirmed a low rate of local recurrence, but failed to demonstrate a survival benefit.[62] Although the shorter, high-dose preoperative radiation strategy is most commonly used in Scandinavia and in other European countries, U.S. oncologists have historically preferred combined-modality therapy as preoperative or postoperative chemoradiation. Findings from two studies of postoperative adjuvant chemoradiation demonstrated that fluorouracil–based chemotherapy plus radiation was more effective than radiation or surgery alone in preventing both local and distant recurrence.[63,64] Results from another trial showed that prolonged infusion of fluorouracil was superior to bolus administration during radiation therapy, providing a 3-year disease-free survival advantage.[65] This finding confirms that protracted delivery of chemosensitizing agents concomitant with radiation is the best way to deliver combined-modality therapy. In clinical practice, capecitabine administered twice daily parallel to radiation has become a widely used substitute for continuous infusion of fluorouracil, although definitive results of trials comparing capecitabine with fluorouracil as radiosensitizers are not available yet.

The long-standing question about whether preoperative or postoperative chemoradiation delivers improved outcome was definitively answered by the results of a large German randomized trial that compared standard continuously infused fluorouracil plus radiation either before or after quality controlled total mesorectal excision surgery.[66] Patients undergoing preoperative combined-modality therapy had a lower rate of local recurrence (at 5 years: 6% vs. 13%), lower rate of acute and chronic toxicities, and a significantly higher rate of sphincter preservation compared with postoperative chemoradiation ($p = 0.006$). This trial established preoperative neoadjuvant radiochemotherapy as new standard of care for stage II and III rectal cancers. Subsequent studies are trying to further improve the local control rate by incorporating additional radiosensitizing agents, such as oxaliplatin, and biologic agents into the preoperative treatment phase. Studies also are seeking to enhance the activity of the postoperative adjuvant therapy by using regimens effective against colon cancer, such as FOLFOX with or without the addition of novel biologic agents.

ANAL CANCERS

EPIDEMIOLOGY AND ETIOLOGY

Cancers of the anus are relatively uncommon in the United States; however, there is an increased incidence in certain populations, such as young men in whom genital infections with viral agents have been implicated. The most clear causal relationship for anal cancer is infection with HPV. One large study found a strong positive correlation between the amount of sexual activity and the risk of anal cancer.[67] In addition, an association between venereal infection in both men and women was noted. Infection with HPV was presumed to be the etiologic cause. Although earlier studies suggested that anal-receptive intercourse was directly linked to an increased risk of anal cancer, this finding has not been confirmed in more recent larger scale trials. Cancers of the anal canal also have been associated with condylomata in both the general population and in gay men. In women with a history of genital warts, anal cancer was associated with seropositivity for herpes simplex virus type 1 and *Chlamydia trachomatis.* In men with no history of genital warts, there was an association with gonorrhea. The association between acquired immunodeficiency syndrome and anal cancer has been known for some time, but the exact etiologic relationship has not been elucidated.

Most anal cancers are squamous cell cancers or cloacogenic cancers, with a few being adenocarcinomas. In addition, melanoma accounts for a small percentage of cancers found in the anal canal. Tumors tend to spread by local extension but have the potential to metastasize. Involvement of the inguinal lymph nodes is found in as many as 63% of cases. The most important prognostic factors are the T stage (T1 is less than 2 cm, T2 is 2 to 5 cm, T3 is greater than 5 cm, and T4 is invasion into adjacent organs) and the lymph node status.

TREATMENT

Initially, treatment for patients with anal cancers was surgical resection using an anterior-posterior approach. This treatment option was curative for only approximately 50% of patients and was associated with a high morbidity rate. Today, the standard approach to treatment of anal cancers is combined-modality chemotherapy and radiation. Local excision is reserved for patients with small tumors that are well differentiated or are removed incidentally at the time of hemorrhoidectomy.

In initial chemoradiation trials, combinations of fluorouracil and mitomycin-C with radiation yielded a high rate of response and of complete pathologic response.[68] Eventually, it was recognized that surgical resection was not necessary, and it is used today only as salvage therapy for patients with local recurrences following radiation. The expectation for patients is that the complete response rate with combined-modality therapy will be between 70% and 80%, with an overall 5-year

KEY POINT

- Anal cancers are often cured by chemoradiotherapy.

survival rate of more than 65%. However, a substantial number of patients will still experience either local relapse or metastatic disease. Treatment of disease in such patients is much more difficult. A phase III clinical trial that compared the role of mitomycin-C and fluorouracil with cisplatin and fluorouracil during radiation therapy did not show superiority of the experimental arm.[69] Thus, in clinical practice, the well-established combined modality approach using fluorouracil and mitomycin-C plus radiation remains the standard of care.

For patients in whom disease is present in the inguinal lymph nodes at the time of diagnosis or in whom disease develops in those nodes metachronously, additional radiation therapy, or node dissection may be beneficial, although the latter is used less frequently. Salvage radiation therapy may result in a cure for up to 50% of patients who have an incomplete response to initial combined-modality therapy or for those who have a local relapse. For patients who have metastatic disease, chemotherapy regimens used for other squamous cell cancers, such as fluorouracil, mitomycin-C, cisplatin, paclitaxel, and others should be considered, but such treatment is palliative at best.

The treatment of anal cancer in patients infected with the human immunodeficiency virus (HIV) is somewhat more complex. Standard aggressive combined-modality therapies should be used for patients with a CD4 count of more than 200/mm^3 x 10^9/L who have no signs or symptoms of other HIV-related diseases. For patients with more severe HIV-related problems, reduced doses of radiation, chemotherapy, or both, should be considered to maintain local disease control.

PANCREATIC ENDOCRINE TUMORS AND NEUROENDOCRINE TUMORS INCLUDING CARCINOIDS

Pancreatic endocrine tumors are a group of uncommon neoplasms that histologically share several key cytochemical features with melanoma, pheochromocytoma, carcinoid tumors, and medullary thyroid cancers. All amine precursor uptake and decarboxylation neoplasms have the capacity to synthesize and secrete polypeptide products that have specific endocrine hormone activity. Most behave in a malignant fashion. The types of tumors are characterized by the hormones they secrete, including gastrinomas, insulinomas, vipomas, glucagonomas, somatostatinomas, growth hormone-releasing factor tumors, and adrenocorticotropic hormone tumors. Pancreatic endocrine tumors are considered either functional if they are associated with a clinical syndrome because of the production of hormones or nonfunctional if hormones are not a substantial element of the presentation.

PANCREATIC ISLET CELL TUMORS

The diverse clinical presentation of pancreatic islet cell tumors and their frequently silent and benign pathologic presences make an accurate determination of their true incidence difficult. Many islet cell tumors remain asymptomatic and undiagnosed. Most of these tumors appear in sporadic cases without substantial personal or family history. However, certain groups of patients have clear evidence of an inherited predisposition to multiple neoplasias of the endocrine system that is manifested in an autosomal-dominant fashion. The syndrome first described (multiple endocrine neoplasia type 1) is characterized by the presence of tumors of the pituitary gland and parathyroid gland, as well as islet cell tumors of the pancreas. Multiple endocrine neoplasia type 2 typically does not involve pancreatic islet cell tumors; rather, it expresses tumors of the parathyroid, pheochromocytoma, and medullary thyroid cancer.

CARCINOID TUMORS

Most carcinoid tumors arise within the gastrointestinal system, with the appendix being the most common primary location. However, carcinoid tumors may arise throughout the body, including in the chest. Carcinoid tumors are members of the neuroendocrine tumor family and share cytochemical features with melanomas, pheochromocytomas, medullary thyroid cancers, and pancreatic endocrine tumors. Some carcinoids behave like small cell cancers and have a much more aggressive clinical behavior than common carcinoids. The determination of cancer can be made only if invasion or distant metastases is found. The disease is most commonly diagnosed during routine appendectomy. Carcinoid tumors synthesize bioactive amine and peptides, including neuron-specific enolase, 5-hydroxytryptamine, synaptophysin, chromogranin A, and other peptides such as insulin, growth hormone, neurotensin, corticotropin, gastrin, pancreatic polypeptide, and calcitonin. More than 80% of patients with resectable primary tumors are disease free at 20 years with similar overall survival rates for an age-matched and gender-matched cohort. Of those tumors with regional node metastasis, as many as 50% will recur more than 10 years after diagnosis. Typically, the prognosis for patients with resectable carcinoid tumors is good. It is important to recognize the long disease-free interval that can occur, which requires patients to have a longer period of follow-up than patients with other tumor types. It is important to note that appendectomy is inadequate surgery if the carcinoid tumor is larger than 2 cm and/or if lymphovascular invasion or involvement of the mesoappendix is present. In these cases, right hemicolectomy is indicated as definitive oncologic surgery.[70]

Carcinoid Syndrome

Just as with islet cell tumors, carcinoid tumors can manifest themselves with signs and symptoms of abnormal hormone production, namely the malignant carcinoid syndrome. Flushing is the most common sign, followed by diarrhea, heart disease (valvular abnormalities), and bronchoconstriction. Diarrhea is not necessarily related to the flushing but appears to be caused by increased gastrointestinal motility as a direct consequence of hormone secretion. For intestinal carcinoids, the characteristic carcinoid syndrome only appears when liver metastases have been established and the biogenic amines can bypass the hepatic metabolic activity. When carcinoid syndrome is suspected, serologic testing should be done to measure 5-hydroxyindoleacetic acid, serotonin levels, and/or chromogranin A. The cardiac disease associated with this condition typically involves abnormalities of the valves on the right side of the heart. Therefore, an echocardiogram is an important element in the evaluation of patients with prolonged disease courses. Novel imaging techniques, including octreotide scanning — a nuclear medicine test specifically designed for the detection of carcinoid tumors — have become more common. Individuals with positive findings on an octreotide scan are more likely to benefit from therapy with octreotide. The most common imaging techniques are CT and MRI, with the latter showing the greatest sensitivity for detection of intrahepatic metastases. PET scans commonly are ineffective because of the low proliferative and low metabolic activity of differentiated carcinoids. Selective sampling of blood through venous catheterization sometimes can be helpful, but this technique is rarely used.

Treatment of Carcinoid and Islet Cell Tumors

Surgery is the main treatment for these tumors. Most tumors are easily resectable or are found incidentally during operations for other indications. Even when the lymph nodes are involved, patients may live for long periods of time without apparent recurrence, but long-term follow-up typically shows continuing disease relapse over many years. In contrast to the situation for other tumor types, cytoreductive surgery (debulking) for palliative purposes (decreasing the amount of hormone-producing tissue) should be considered for these tumors. Such surgery includes hepatic resection or resection of other intra-abdominal and thoracic metastases. Surgical palliation of bowel obstruction from tumor masses or mesenteric fibrosis associated with carcinoid tumors may substantially improve quality of life for patients. Hepatic surgery for liver metastasis may allow patients to remain disease free for prolonged periods and may reduce hormone production.

Liver-directed therapy, such as embolization, high-frequency radioablation, or surgical resection, commonly is used for these tumor types. These techniques are particularly useful for reducing symptoms caused by local growth of the tumor or by hormone production and should be regarded as nonsurgical debulking. These procedures also are associated with a greater likelihood of prolonged tumor regression.

Radiation therapy may offer relief for local recurrence or for symptomatic metastasis, such as bone metastases, which are relatively common for patients with advanced carcinoids. An emerging area of research involves the use of radiolabeled octreotide as treatment. The results of ongoing clinical trials may highlight substantial benefits from this approach; however, radioactive octreotide therapy is not approved. Octreotide and its analogues have been used for some time to control the secretion of 5-hydroxyindoleacetic acid and other peptides. More recently, the analogues have been assessed for their antitumor activity, despite their poor tumoricidal effect resulting in few regressions. There is substantial evidence from small phase II clinical studies that these agents have cystostatic effects and may prolong survival, but these data have not been replicated in larger clinical trials. Another biologic agent that may have benefit is interferon-alpha, which has been shown to decrease the tumor size for a few patients with metastatic disease. Similar to octreotide, interferon appears to have a tumorstatic effect rather than a tumoricidal one. One trial demonstrated a survival advantage for interferon compared with the combination of streptozotocin and fluorouracil;[71] however, the role of interferon for the treatment of differentiated carcinoid tumors is being debated.

Traditional chemotherapy has been tested extensively for the treatment of patients with carcinoid cancers. Agents commonly used include fluorouracil and its oral analogue, capecitabine; streptozotocin; and anthracyclines, such as doxorubicin and liposomal doxorubicin. Unfortunately, response rates for chemotherapeutic agents in combination regimens have been poor — typically less than 20%. Therefore, for most patients, the use of systemic chemotherapy is either reserved for end-of-life care or should not be considered at all. It is important to recognize that the slow-growing nature of carcinoid tumors may allow patients to be followed for a long period of time without any considerable intervention. Patients should be monitored closely to determine if the disease is slow growing. If so, simple observation often is sufficient.

The outcome with systemic chemotherapy may be better for patients with islet cell tumors. One trial in which streptozotocin plus doxorubicin was compared with streptozotocin plus fluorouracil demonstrated that the doxorubicin–containing regimen was superior, with a 69% objective response rate and a significantly superior median survival (response rate 69% vs. 45%, $p = 0.05$; overall survival 2.2 years vs. 1.4 years, $p = 0.004$).[72] For patients who have poorly differentiated gut neuroendocrine tumors, the selection of chemotherapy is similar to that for small cell lung cancer, using most consistent regression observed using combination etoposide and cisplatin. This distinction is important and emphasizes the need for pathologic evaluation to distinguish between the small cell variant and the more slow-growing islet cell/carcinoid tumors.

Most recently, novel biologics including VEGF inhibitors, such as bevacizumab, and signal transduction inhibitors, such as mTOR inhibitors, have showed promising activity in neuroendocrine tumors. The results of definitive phase III trials are pending.

REFERENCES

1. Devesa SS, Blot WJ, Fraumeni JF Jr. Changing patterns in the incidence of esophageal and gastric carcinoma in the United States. *Cancer.* 1998;83(10):2049-2053.

2. Herskovic A, Martz K, al-Sarraf M, et al. Combined chemotherapy and radiotherapy compared with radiotherapy alone in patients with cancer of the esophagus. *N Engl J Med.* 1992;326(24):1593–1598.

3. Meluch AA, Greco FA, Gray JR, et al. Preoperative therapy with concurrent paclitaxel/ carboplatin/infusional 5-FU and radiation therapy in locoregional esophageal cancer: final results of a Minnie Pearl Cancer Research Network phase II trial. *Cancer J.* 2003;9(4):251-260.

4. Jatoi A, Martenson JA, Foster NR, et al. Paclitaxel, carboplatin, 5-fluorouracil, and radiation for locally advanced esophageal cancer: phase II results of preliminary pharmacologic and molecular efforts to mitigate toxicity and predict outcomes: North Central Cancer Treatment Group (N0044). *Am J Clin Oncol.* 2007;30(5):507-513.

5. Cooper JS, Guo MD, Herskovic A, et al. Chemoradiotherapy of locally advanced esophageal cancer: long-term follow-up of a prospective randomized trial (RTOG 85-01). Radiation Therapy Oncology Group. *JAMA.* 1999;281(17):1623–1627.

6. Cunningham D, Allum WH, Stenning SP, et al. Perioperative chemotherapy versus surgery alone for resectable gastroesophageal cancer. *N Engl J Med.* 2006;355(1):11-20.

7. Gebski V, Burmeister B, Smithers BM, et al. Survival benefits from neoadjuvant chemoradiotherapy or chemotherapy in oesophageal carcinoma: a meta-analysis. *Lancet Oncol.* 2007;8(3):226–234.

8. Tepper JE, Krasna M, Niedzwiecki D, et al. Superiority of trimodality therapy to surgery alone in esophageal cancer: Results of CALGB 9781. *Proc Am Soc Clin Oncol.* 2006; 24:18s (abstr 4012).

9. Macdonald JS, Smalley SR, Benedetti J, et al. Chemoradiotherapy after surgery compared with surgery alone for adenocarcinoma of the stomach or gastroesophageal junction. *N Engl J Med.* 2001;345(10):725–730.

10. Wagner AD, Grothe W, Haerting J, et al. Chemotherapy in advanced gastric cancer: a systematic review and meta-analysis based on aggregate data. *J Clin Oncol.* 2006;24(18):2903-2909.

11. Van Cutsem E, Moiseyenko VM, Tjulandin S,et al. Phase III study of docetaxel and cisplatin plus fluorouracil compared with cisplatin and fluorouracil as first-line therapy for advanced gastric cancer: a report of the V325 Study Group. *J Clin Oncol.* 2006;24(31):4991–4997.

12. Cunningham D, Rao S, Starling N, et al. Randomised multicentre phase III study comparing capecitabine with fluorouracil and oxaliplatin with cisplatin in patients with advanced oesophagogastric (OG) cancer: The REAL 2 trial. *Proc Am Soc Clin Oncol.* 2006; 24: 18s (abstr LBA4017).

13. Kleeff J, Michalski C, Friess H, et al. Pancreatic cancer: from bench to 5-year survival. *Pancreas.* 2006;33(2):111-118.

14. Parkin DM, Bray F, Ferlay J, et al. Global cancer statistics, 2002. *CA Cancer J Clin.* 2005;55(2):74-108.

15. Beger HG, Rau B, Gansauge F, et al. Treatment of pancreatic cancer: challenge of the facts. *World J Surg.* 2003;27(10):1075-1084.

16. Neoptolemos JP, Stocken DD, Friess H, et al. A randomized trial of chemoradiotherapy and chemotherapy after resection of pancreatic cancer. *N Engl J Med.* 2004;350(12):1200–1210.

17. Neoptolemos JP, Dunn JA, Stocken DD, et al. Adjuvant chemoradiotherapy and chemotherapy in resectable pancreatic cancer: a randomised controlled trial. *Lancet.* 2001;358(9293):1576–1585.

18. Oettle H, Post S, Neuhaus P, et al. Adjuvant chemotherapy with gemcitabine vs observation in patients undergoing curative-intent resection of pancreatic cancer: a randomized controlled trial. *JAMA.* 2007;297(3): 267–277.

19. Regine WF, Winter KW, Abrams R,et al. RTOG 9704 a phase III study of adjuvant pre and post chemoradiation (CRT) fluorouracil vs. gemcitabine (G) for resected pancreatic adenocarcinoma. *Proc Am Soc Clin Oncol.* 2006; 24:18s (abstr 4007).

20. Burris HA 3rd, Moore MJ, Andersen J, et al. Improvements in survival and clinical benefit with gemcitabine as first-line therapy for patients with advanced pancreas cancer: a randomized trial. *J Clin Oncol.* 1997; 15(6):2403–2413.

21. Hochster HS, Haller DG, de Gramont A, et al. Consensus report of the International Society of Gastrointestinal Oncology on therapeutic progress in advanced pancreatic cancer. *Cancer.* 2006;107(4): 676–685.

22. Cunningham D. Final results of a phase III trial of gemcitabine (GEM) versus gemcitabine plus capecitabine (GEM-CAP) in patients with advanced pancreatic cancer. Paper presented at: ECCO 13: The European Cancer Conference; November 2005; Paris, France.

23. Llovet J, Ricci S, Mazzaferro V, et al. Randomized phase III trial of sorafenib versus placebo in patients with advanced hepatocellular carcinoma (HCC). *Proc Am Soc Clin Oncol.* 2007; 25:18s (abstr LBA1).

24. Llovet JM, Burroughs A, Bruix J. Hepatocellular carcinoma. *Lancet.* 2003;362(9399):1907–1917.

25. American Cancer Society. *Cancer Facts & Figures.* 2007 Atlanta: American Cancer Society; 2007.

26. Park Y, Hunter DJ, Spiegelman D, et al. Dietary fiber intake and risk of colorectal cancer: a pooled analysis of prospective cohort studies. *JAMA.* 2005;294(22):2849–2857.

27. Wactawski-Wende J, Kotchen JM, Anderson GL, et al. Calcium plus vitamin D supplementation and the risk of colorectal cancer. *N Engl J Med.* 2006;354(7):684–696.

28. Koehne CH, Dubois RN. COX-2 inhibition and colorectal cancer. *Semin Oncol.* 2004;31(2 Suppl 7):12–21.

29. Kinzler KW, Vogelstein B. Lessons from hereditary colorectal cancer. *Cell.* 1996;87(2):159-170.

30. American Joint Committee on Cancer (AJCC). Chicago, Illinois. AJCC Cancer Staging Manual, Sixth Edition (2002). Published by Springer Science and Business Media.

31. Haller DG, Catalano PJ, Macdonald JS, et al. Phase III study of fluorouracil, leucovorin, and levamisole in high-risk stage II and III colon cancer: final report of Intergroup 0089. *J Clin Oncol.* 2005;23(34): 8671–8678.

32. Sargent DJ, Wieand HS, Haller DG, et al. Disease-free survival versus overall survival as a primary end point for adjuvant colon cancer studies: individual patient data from 20,898 patients on 18 randomized trials. *J Clin Oncol.* 2005;23(34):8664–8670.

33. Twelves C, Wong A, Nowacki MP, et al.Capecitabine as adjuvant treatment for stage III colon cancer. *N Engl J Med.* 2005;352(26):2696–2704.

34. Andre T, Boni C, Mounedji-Boudiaf L, et al. Oxaliplatin, fluorouracil, and leucovorin as adjuvant treatment for colon cancer. *N Engl J Med.* 2004;350(23):2343–2351.

35. Wolmark N, Wieand S, Kuebler JP, et al. A phase III trial comparing FULV to FULV + oxaliplatin in stage II or III carcinoma of the colon: Results of NSABP Protocol C-07. *Proc Am Soc Clin Oncol.* 2005; 23: 16s (abstr 3500).

36. Efficacy of adjuvant fluorouracil and folinic acid in B2 colon cancer. International Multicentre Pooled Analysis of B2 Colon Cancer Trials (IMPACT B2) Investigators. *J Clin Oncol.* 1999;17:1356–1363.

37. Mamounas E, Wieand S, Wolmark N, et al. Comparative efficacy of adjuvant chemotherapy in patients with Dukes' B versus Dukes' C colon cancer: results from four National Surgical Adjuvant Breast and Bowel Project adjuvant studies (C-01, C-02, C-03, and C-04). *J Clin Oncol.* 1999;17(5):1349–1355.

38. Schrag D, Rifas-Shiman S, Saltz L, et al. Adjuvant chemotherapy use for Medicare beneficiaries with stage II colon cancer. *J Clin Oncol.* 2002;20(19):3999–4005.

39. Benson AB, Schrag D, Somerfield MR, et al. American Society of Clinical Oncology recommendations on adjuvant chemotherapy for stage II colon cancer. *J Clin Oncol.* 2004;22(16):3408–3419.

40. Gill S, Loprinzi CL, Sargent DJ, et al. Pooled analysis of fluorouracil-based adjuvant therapy for stage II and III colon cancer: who benefits and by how much? *J Clin Oncol.* 2004;22(10):1797–1806.

41. Mayo Clinic Web site. http://www.mayoclinic.com/calcs. Accessed November 13, 2007.

42. Adjuvant! Online Web site. http://www.adjuvantonline.com. Accessed November 13, 2007.

43. Cunningham D, Pyrhonen S, James RD, et al. Randomised trial of irinotecan plus supportive care versus supportive care alone after fluorouracil failure for patients with metastatic colorectal cancer. *Lancet* 1998;352(9138):1413-1418.

44. Saltz LB, Cox JV, Blanke C, et al. Irinotecan plus fluorouracil and leucovorin for metastatic colorectal cancer. Irinotecan Study Group. *N Engl J Med.* 2000;343(13):905–914.

45. Douillard JY, Cunningham D, Roth AD, et al. Irinotecan combined with fluorouracil compared with fluorouracil alone as first-line treatment for metastatic colorectal cancer: a multicentre randomised trial. *Lancet.* 2000;355:1041–1047.

46. Kohne CH, van Cutsem E, Wils J, et al. Phase III study of weekly high-dose infusional fluorouracil plus folinic acid with or without irinotecan in patients with metastatic colorectal cancer: European Organisation for Research and Treatment of Cancer Gastrointestinal Group Study 40986. *J Clin Oncol.* 2005;23(22):4856–4865.

47. de Gramont A, Figer A, Seymour M, et al. Leucovorin and fluorouracil with or without oxaliplatin as first-line treatment in advanced colorectal cancer. *J Clin Oncol.* 2000;18(16):2938–2947.

48. Giacchetti S, Perpoint B, Zidani R, et al. Phase III multicenter randomized trial of oxaliplatin added to chronomodulated fluorouracil-leucovorin as first-line treatment of metastatic colorectal cancer. *J Clin Oncol.* 2000;18(1):136–147.

49. Grothey A, Deschler B, Kroening H, et al. Phase III study of bolus 5-fluorouracil (fluorouracil)/ folinic acid (FA) (Mayo) vs. weekly high-dose 24h fluorouracil infusion/ FA + oxaliplatin (OXA) in advanced colorectal cancer (ACRC). *Proc Am Soc Clin Oncol.* 2002;21:129a, Abstr. 512.

50. Goldberg RM, Sargent DJ, Morton RF, et al. A randomized controlled trial of fluorouracil plus leucovorin, irinotecan, and oxaliplatin combinations in patients with previously untreated metastatic colorectal cancer. *J Clin Oncol.* 2004;22(1):23–30.

51. Tournigand C, Andre T, Achille E, et al. FOLFIRI followed by FOLFOX6 or the reverse sequence in advanced colorectal cancer: a randomized GERCOR study. *J Clin Oncol.* 2004;22(2):229–237.

52. Colucci G, Gebbia V, Paoletti G, et al. Phase III randomized trial of FOLFIRI versus FOLFOX4 in the treatment of advanced colorectal cancer: a multicenter study of the Gruppo Oncologico Dell'Italia Meridionale. *J Clin Oncol.* 2005;23(22):4866–4875.

53. Hurwitz H, Fehrenbacher L, Novotny W, et al. Bevacizumab plus irinotecan, fluorouracil, and leucovorin for metastatic colorectal cancer. *N Engl J Med.* 2004;350(23):2335–2342.

54. Cunningham D, Humblet Y, Siena S, et al. Cetuximab monotherapy and cetuximab plus irinotecan in irinotecan-refractory metastatic colorectal cancer. *N Engl J Med.* 2004;351(4):337–345.

55. Peeters M, Van Cutsem E, Siena S, et al. A phase III, multicenter, randomized controlled trial (RCT) of panitumumab plus best supportive care (BSC) versus BSC alone in patients with metastatic colorectal cancer. Paper presented at: 97th Annual Meeting of the American Association for Cancer Research; April 2006; Washington, DC. Abstract CP–1.

56. Poston GJ, Adam R, Alberts S, et al. OncoSurge: a strategy for improving resectability with curative intent in metastatic colorectal cancer. *J Clin Oncol.* 2005;23(28):7125-7134.

57. Scheele J, Altendorf-Hofmann A. Resection of colorectal liver metastases. *Langenbecks Arch Surg.* 1999;384(4):313-327.

58. Bismuth H, Adam R, Levi F, et al. Resection of nonresectable liver metastases from colorectal cancer after neoadjuvant chemotherapy. *Ann Surg.* 1996;224(4):509-520; discussion 520–522.

59. Kemeny N, Huang Y, Cohen AM, et al. Hepatic arterial infusion of chemotherapy after resection of hepatic metastases from colorectal cancer. *N Engl J Med.* 1999;341(27):2039–2048.

60. Mitry E, Fields A, Bleiberg H, et al. Adjuvant chemotherapy after potentially curative resection of metastases from colorectal cancer. A meta-analysis of two randomized trials. *Proc Am Soc Clin Oncol.* 2006;24:18s, (abstr 3524).

61. Improved survival with preoperative radiotherapy in resectable rectal cancer. Swedish Rectal Cancer Trial. *N Engl J Med.* 1997;336(14):980–987.

62. Kapiteijn E, Marijnen CA, Nagtegaal ID, et al. Preoperative radiotherapy combined with total mesorectal excision for resectable rectal cancer. *N Engl J Med.* 2001;345(9):638–646.

63. Krook JE, Moertel CG, Gunderson LL, et al. Effective surgical adjuvant therapy for high-risk rectal carcinoma. *N Engl J Med.* 1991;324(11): 709–715.

64. Fisher B, Wolmark N, Rockette H, et al. Postoperative adjuvant chemotherapy or radiation therapy for rectal cancer: results from NSABP protocol R-01. *J Natl Cancer Inst.* 1998;80(1):21–29.

65. O'Connell MJ, Martenson JA, Wieand HS, et al. Improving adjuvant therapy for rectal cancer by combining protracted-infusion fluorouracil with radiation therapy after curative surgery. *N Engl J Med.* 1994; 331(8):502–507.

66. Sauer R, Becker H, Hohenberger W, et al. Preoperative versus postoperative chemoradiotherapy for rectal cancer. *N Engl J Med.* 2004; 351(17):1731–1740.

67 Frisch M, Glimelius B, van den Brule AJ, et al. Sexually transmitted infection as a cause of anal cancer. *N Engl J Med.* 1997;337(19):1350-1358.

68. Sischy B, Doggett RL, Krall JM, et al. Definitive irradiation and chemotherapy for radiosensitization in management of anal carcinoma: interim report on Radiation Therapy Oncology Group study no. 8314. *J Natl Cancer Inst.* 1989;81(11):850–856.

69. Ajani JA, Winter KA, Gunderson LL, et al. Intergroup RTOG 98-11: A phase III randomized study of 5-fluorouracil (fluorouracil), mitomycin, and radiotherapy versus 5-fluorouracil, cisplatin and radiotherapy in carcinoma of the anal canal. *Proc Am Soc Clin Oncol.* 2006;24: 18s (abstr 4009).

70. Moertel CG, Weiland LH, Nagorney DM, Dockerty MB. Carcinoid tumor of the appendix: treatment and prognosis. *N Engl J Med.* 1987;317(27):1699–1701.

71. Oberg K, Eriksson B. The role of interferons in the management of carcinoid tumors. *Acta Oncol.* 1991;30(4):519–522.

72. Moertel CG, Lefkopoulo M, Lipsitz S, et al. Streptozocin-doxorubicin, streptozocin-fluorouracil or chlorozotocin in the treatment of advanced islet-cell carcinoma. *N Engl J Med.* 1992;326(8):519–523.

9

GENITOURINARY CANCERS

David M. Nanus, MD, and Matthew I. Milowsky, MD

LEARNING OBJECTIVES

After reviewing this chapter, the reader should be able to

- Diagnose and treat germ cell tumors with an understanding of their epidemiology, pathology, and use of a risk-adapted staging system
- Understand the risk factors for and epidemiology of urothelial carcinoma and incorporate prognosis and the role for perioperative chemotherapy into management
- Implement appropriate treatment regimens for renal cell cancer based on its biology, including immunotherapy and targeted therapies
- Understand the epidemiology, biology, and management of all stages of prostate cancer
- Advise patients regarding quality of life and the late effects of treatment

Germ cell tumors are the most common neoplasms among men between the ages of 15 and 35. Approximately 8,250 cases and 370 deaths were estimated to occur in the United States in 2006, with the incidence increasing worldwide.[1] Germ cell tumors most frequently originate in the gonads (testis or ovary) and less commonly in the retroperitoneum or mediastinum. (*For a discussion of germ cell tumors in women, please see Chapter 10: Gynecologic Cancers.*) Retroperitoneal tumors often are associated with an invasive tumor or carcinoma in situ within the testis, even in the absence of a palpable mass. Primary mediastinal germ cell tumors are not associated with testicular involvement. Extragonadal germ cell neoplasms also rarely arise in the sacrum, pineal gland, paranasal sinuses, and liver. Regardless of the stage or extent of disease, the therapeutic objective is cure, which requires an integrated multidisciplinary approach.

The American Society of Clinical Oncology and Drs. Nanus and Milowsky would like to gratefully acknowledge Howard I. Scher, MD, for his contributions to the original content of this chapter.

Germ cell tumors are primarily seen in white patients. Risk factors include both abdominal and inguinal cryptorchidism, spermatic or testicular dysgenesis, and a family history that confers a 4-fold to 10-fold increase in risk.[2] Orchiopexy or surgical correction of abdominal cryptorchidism reduces the risk of germ cell tumors and results in improved ability to monitor the testis. Testicular seminoma occurs at an increased frequency in men with human immunodeficiency virus (HIV), and the treatment by stage is the same as for the HIV-negative population.[3] Klinefelter's syndrome is a risk factor for the development of mediastinal germ cell tumors. Carcinoma in situ (intratubular germ cell neoplasia [ITGCN]) is found in virtually all cases of testicular germ cell tumors. Men in whom in situ disease is identified during a testicular biopsy as part of an infertility evaluation have a 50% risk of an invasive tumor over a 5-year period. In such cases, in situ disease often is identified in the contralateral testis.[4] A metachronous or synchronous testicular primary germ cell tumor occurs in 2% of patients, with seminoma as the most common histology.[5] Serial self-examination of the remaining testis is recommended.

KEY POINTS

- Germ cell tumors are staged with a risk-adapted staging classification system that includes tumor markers.
- The different histologic subtypes of germ cell tumors have biologic significance.
- Combined-modality treatment approaches are used to achieve the highest probability of cure with the least morbidity.
- Survivorship issues are an important component of the treatment of patients with germ cell tumors.

GERM CELL TUMORS

BIOLOGY

Germ cell tumors are derived from the malignant transformation of premeiotic germ cells. In order to create a pluripotential tumor, these transformed germ cells must be able to differentiate in a manner similar to the totipotential zygote without the reciprocal genetic information that results from fertilization.[6] An isochromosome of the short arm of chromosome 12 — i(12p) — is present in 80% of all cell types, including carcinoma in situ and extragonadal tumors. The remaining cases have excess 12p genetic material as an increase in copy number, tandem duplication, or transposition, which indicates that one or more genes on 12p are involved in malignant transformation. Although the 12p target genes have not been clearly defined, several candidate genes include *CCND2* at 12p13 as well as *SOX5*, *JAW1*, and *K-RAS* mapped to an amplified region at 12p11.2-12.1.[7] Most germ cell tumors are hyperdiploid, and often triploid or tetraploid, implying that endoreduplication is important in the early steps of malignant transformation.

DIAGNOSIS

A painless testicular mass is pathognomonic of a testicular tumor; however, the majority of patients present with diffuse testicular swelling, hardness, pain, or some combination of these findings.[8] In patients who present with pain, the initial therapy often is antibiotics for infectious epididymitis or orchitis, but if symptoms do not resolve within 2 weeks, an ultrasound of the testis is indicated. If the ultrasound is abnormal and a testicular tumor is suspected, a radical inguinal orchiectomy with removal of the testis and ligation of the spermatic cord at the level of the internal ring is performed. Because the testes originate in the genital ridge and migrate through the abdomen and inguinal canal into the scrotum, the vascular and lymphatic drainage of the testes is to the renal or great vessels and the retroperitoneal nodes, respectively. A testicular biopsy or transscrotal orchiectomy is contraindicated because the normal vascular and lymphatic drainage is disturbed. Levels of alpha-fetoprotein, human chorionic gonadotropin (HCG) and lactate dehydrogenase also should be determined. Less common presentations include gynecomastia (as a result of elevated levels of HCG), back pain related to retroperitoneal nodal disease, superior vena cava syndrome from primary mediastinal tumors, and hemoptysis from extensive pulmonary metastases.

PATHOLOGY

Germ cell tumors are classified histologically into seminomas and nonseminomas. Seminomas, which account for approximately one-half of testicular germ cell tumors, retain totipotentiality and are exquisitely sensitive to radiation and chemotherapy. Nonseminomas are composed of the following cell types: embryonal carcinoma, teratoma, choriocarcinoma, and yolk-sac carcinoma (endodermal-sinus tumor, Table 9-1). Embryonal carcinoma is the most undifferentiated with totipotential capacity to differentiate into extraembryonic malignant cell types, such as yolk sac tumors and choriocarcinoma, and somatic cell types, such as teratoma. Teratoma is composed of somatic cells from two or more germ-cell layers (e.g., ectoderm, mesoderm, or endoderm), and thus differentiates into tissue types such as cartilage, muscle, mucinous glandular epithelium, and others. The presence of any component of nonseminoma with seminoma is managed as a nonseminomatous germ cell tumor. Most nonseminomas show mixed histologies including embryonal carcinoma, yolk sac tumors, teratoma, and choriocarcinoma. When reporting histology, all subtypes present must be noted, starting with the most prevalent and ending with the least common component.

Seminomas are positive for placental alkaline phosphatase and negative for low–molecular-weight keratins, whereas embryonal carcinoma almost universally expresses low–molecular-weight keratins and blood group-associated

TABLE 9-1 Histologic Classification of Germ Cell Neoplasms[8]

Germ Cell Tumors
Seminoma
Classical (typical)
Spermatocytic (present in elderly and associated with indolent course)
Nonseminoma
Teratoma
Mature
Immature
With malignant transformation
Choriocarcinoma
Yolk Sac tumor (endodermal-sinus tumor)
Embryonal carcinoma

glycoproteins; approximately 50% express placental alkaline phosphatase. Immunohistochemical analysis may be useful in the evaluation of patients with midline tumors of uncertain histiogenesis.

PATTERNS OF SPREAD

The primary lymphatic drainage for testicular germ cell tumors is to the retroperitoneal lymph nodes (primary landing zones). The right testicular artery originates from the aorta and the right testicular vein drains into the inferior vena cava, whereas the left testicular artery originates near the left renal artery and the left testicular vein terminates in the left renal vein. Right-sided tumors spread to the interaortocaval lymph nodes immediately below the renal blood vessels, and left-sided tumors spread to the para-aortic lymph nodes immediately below the left renal artery and vein. Cross metastases are more commonly seen from right to left. Invasion of the epididymis or spermatic cord may be associated with iliac nodal involvement and inguinal metastases may be seen with scrotal invasion or if there has been disturbance of the normal lymphatic drainage related to prior surgery. Additional metastatic sites include retrocrural, mediastinal, and supraclavicular lymph node involvement, lung, and, less commonly, liver, central nervous system and bone.

STAGING

The extent of disease evaluation for patients with newly diagnosed germ cell tumors includes a chest x-ray, computerized tomography (CT) of the abdomen and pelvis, and tumor markers. Indications for a CT scan of the chest include an abnormal chest x-ray, known mediastinal disease, and risk for pulmonary metastases. A bone scan and magnetic resonance imaging (MRI) of the brain are indicated only if related symptoms are present. Sperm banking should be recommended before treatment is pursued.

Measurement of tumor markers including alpha-fetoprotein, HCG, and lactate dehydrogenase are included in the staging system and used to establish the diagnosis, determine histologic subtypes, and assess treatment effects.[8] Tumor markers are measured before, during, and after treatment. The serum half-lives of alpha-fetoprotein and HCG are 5 to 7 days and 30 hours, respectively, and a slow marker decline after orchiectomy or during chemotherapy implies residual active disease. Elevated or rising alpha-fetoprotein and/or HCG levels that occur without radiologic or clinical findings imply active disease and must be managed accordingly. Other conditions associated with elevated alpha-fetoprotein levels include hepatocellular carcinoma, liver damage, and other gastrointestinal malignancies. HCG elevations may occur as a result of treatment-related hypogonadism or cross reactivity with pituitary hormones, including luteinizing hormone. This cross reactivity is generally less of an issue with current assays specific for the beta subunit of HCG. A spurious elevation in HCG also has been associated with marijuana use.[9] With these exceptions, increased levels of alpha-fetoprotein are pathognomonic of a nonseminoma, whereas elevated levels of HCG may be seen in both seminoma and nonseminoma. Lactate dehydrogenase levels can rise in patients with advanced seminoma or nonseminoma and are used for staging and assessment of outcome. Elevations in any one marker or combination are found in approximately 20% of patients with stage I disease, 40% of patients with stage II disease, and 60% or more of patients with stage III disease.

STAGE GROUPINGS

A tumor, node, metastasis (TNM) staging classification system was developed based on the International Germ Cell Cancer Collaborative Group (IGCCCG) classification.[10, 11] The adverse factors identified included mediastinal primary site, degree of elevation of alpha-fetoprotein, HCG and lactate dehydrogenase, and presence of nonpulmonary visceral metastases. Based on these findings, germ cell tumors are characterized as the following: good risk, accounting for 60% of germ cell tumors with a 91% 5-year survival rate; intermediate risk, accounting for 26% of germ cell tumors with a 79% 5-year survival rate; and poor risk, accounting for 14% of germ cell tumors with a 48% 5-year survival rate. A unique feature of this system is that it incorporates serum tumor markers as well as components of histopathology (Tables 9-2 and 9-3).

NONSEMINOMATOUS GERM CELL TUMORS

Stage I Disease

The majority of patients with clinical stage I disease have normal findings on imaging and normalization of serum tumor markers after radical inguinal orchiectomy. Approximately 30% to 40% of patients with nonseminomatous germ cell tumors present with stage I disease. The management options include surveillance and retroperitoneal lymph node dissection.

TABLE 9-2 1997 Staging Criteria[8]

Primary Tumor (T)	
pTx:	Primary tumor cannot be assessed (if no radical orchiectomy has been performed)
pTo:	No evidence of primary tumor (e.g., histologic scar in testis)
pTis:	Intratubular germ cell neoplasia (carcinoma in situ)
pTl:	Tumor limited to testis and epididymis; no vascular or lymphatic invasion Tumor may invade into the tunica albuginea but not the tunica vaginalis
pT2:	Tumor limited to testis and epididymis with vascular or lymphatic invasion or tumor extending through the tunica albuginea with involvement of tunica vaginalis
pT3:	Tumor invades the spermatic cord with or without vascular or lymphatic invasion.
pT4:	Tumor invades the scrotum with or without vascular or lymphatic invasion
Regional Lymph Nodes (N) Clinical	
Nx:	Regional lymph nodes cannot be assessed
N0:	No regional lymph node metastases
N1:	Metastasis with a lymph node mass 2 cm or less in greatest dimension; or multiple lymph nodes, none greater than 2 cm in greatest dimension
N2:	Metastasis with a lymph node mass greater than 2 cm but not more than 5 cm in greatest dimension; or multiple lymph nodes, any one mass greater than 2 cm but not greater than 5 cm in greatest dimension
N3:	Metastasis with a lymph node mass greater than 5 cm in greatest dimension
Pathologic (pN)	
pNx:	Regional lymph nodes cannot be assessed
pN0:	No regional lymph node metastases
pN1:	Metastasis with a lymph node mass 2 cm or less in greatest dimension and less than or equal to 5 nodes positive, none greater than 2 cm in greatest dimension
pN2:	Metastasis with a lymph node mass greater than 2 cm but not greater than 5 cm in greatest dimension; or greater than 5 nodes positive, none greater than 5 cm; or evidence of extranodal extension of tumor
pN3:	Metastasis with a lymph node mass greater than 5 cm in greatest dimension
Distant Metastases (M)	
Mx:	Distant metastasis cannot be assessed
M0:	No evidence of distant metastases
Ml:	Nonregional nodal or pulmonary metastases
MIB:	Nonpulmonary visceral metastases
Serum Tumor Markers (S)	
Sx:	Marker studies are not available or not performed
S0:	Levels of LDH, HCG, and AFP are within normal limits
S1 (Good):	Level of LDH is $<$ 1.5 times the normal value, and the HCG (mIu/mL) level is $<$ 5,000, and the AFP (ng/mL) level is $<$ 1,000
S2 (Intermediate):	Level of LDH is 1.5 to 10 times normal, or the HCG level is 5,000 to 50,000, or the AFP level is 1,000 to 10,000
S3 (Poor):	Level of LDH is $>$ 10 times normal, or the HCG level is $>$ 50,000, or the AFP level is $>$ 10,000
Stage Groupings	
Stage I:	Tumors limited to testis, epididymis, or spermatic cord
Stage II:	Metastatic disease limited to retroperitoneal lymph nodes
Stage IIA:	Retroperitoneal lymph nodes less than 2 cm in diameter
Stage IIB:	Retroperitoneal lymph nodes between 2 and 5 cm in diameter
Stage IIC:	Retroperitoneal lymph nodes greater than 5 cm in diameter
Stage III:	Metastatic disease above the diaphragm and all visceral sites

Abbreviations: LDH, lactate dehydrogenase; HCG, human chorionic gonadotropin; AFP, alpha-fetoprotein.

TABLE 9-3 Risk Stratification According to the International Germ Cell Consensus Classification[9]

Nonseminoma	
Good risk	Testis or retroperitoneal primary AND good markers AND no nonpulmonary visceral metastases
Intermediate risk	Testis/retroperitoneal primary AND intermediate markers AND no nonpulmonary visceral metastases
Poor risk	Mediastinal primary site OR testis or retroperitoneal primary with either nonpulmonary visceral metastases OR poor markers
Seminoma	
Good risk	Any primary AND any markers AND no nonpulmonary visceral metastases
Intermediate risk	Any primary AND any markers AND nonpulmonary visceral metastase

Surveillance is an option for compliant patients with a low risk for recurrence including T1 tumors with no vascular/lymphatic invasion or invasion into the tunica albuginea, spermatic cord, or scrotum. Absence of embryonal carcinoma in the primary tumor and presence of teratoma also are considered favorable features. Approximately 20% of patients will relapse, most commonly in the retroperitoneum, and will need chemotherapy. Most recurrences of germ cell tumors will occur in the first 2 years after therapy, and these patients must have meticulous follow-up that includes a history, physical examination, chest x ray, and measurement of serum tumor markers monthly, as well as an abdominal CT scan every 3 months during the first year.[12] During the second year, the history, physical examination, tumor markers, and chest x-ray are performed at 2-month intervals, and CT scan occurs every 3 months. Although the intervals for follow-up increase during subsequent years, it is important to remember that late recurrences can occur.[13] Compliance with this surveillance schedule, with salvage therapy as indicated, produces cure rates of 98% to 99% and spares the 75% to 80% of patients without micrometastatic disease from additional therapy.

Patients with stage I disease who have normal findings on imaging studies and normal levels of tumor markers for whom the risk of disease recurrence is high (more than 50%) based on pathologic features, including embryonal carcinoma predominant and/or the presence of lymphatic, vascular, scrotal, or spermatic-cord invasion, should be considered for a nerve-sparing retroperitoneal lymph node dissection by a surgeon experienced in the procedure. Surveillence in a compliant patient still remains an accepted option. The decision to recommend adjuvant chemotherapy is made on the basis of pathologic findings, as described for patients with pathologic stage II disease. Although there are reports using chemotherapy for clinical stage I tumors, there is limited follow-up, and many men will be exposed to unnecessary chemotherapy with the potential for long-term adverse effects.

Patients without evidence of clinical disease and persistently elevated tumor markers, including HCG, alpha-fetoprotein or both after orchiectomy (stage IS), should receive standard chemotherapy rather than surgery.

Stage II Disease

The standard treatment for a patient with stage IIA (nodes less than or equal to 2 cm) disease is a modified, bilateral retroperitoneal lymph node dissection. In this procedure, the dissection becomes unilateral at the level of the inferior mesenteric artery. Experience with the technique is essential because depending on the location of the tumor, a nerve-sparing procedure can be performed.

Approximately 20% to 25% of patients will have pathologic stage I disease (metastases with node 2 cm or less or 5 or fewer involved nodes) with an approximate 20% risk of relapse such that observation can be considered in a compliant patient. The likelihood of micrometastatic disease is 50% or more for patients with an involved node more than 2 cm in diameter, greater than 5 involved nodes, or any extranodal extension (pathologic stage II disease). Assuming that serum tumor marker levels return to normal after surgery, these patients should receive two cycles of adjuvant chemotherapy, which results in a 98% to 99% likelihood of cure.[14,15] If disease relapses or if the serum tumor markers do not decline by half-life, indicating residual active disease, then three to four cycles of therapy and subsequent surgical excision of residual macroscopically documented disease, if present, are indicated, as is required for any patient with disseminated disease.

In contrast, the majority of patients with clinical stage IIB (nodes greater than 2 cm but not more than 5 cm) disease are generally advised to have primary chemotherapy. In addition, patients with back pain related to psoas invasion, bilateral retroperitoneal involvement, suprahilar or retrocrural adenopathy, or other signs that the disease may be unresectable should undergo primary chemotherapy. Clinical stage IIC tumors (nodes larger than 5 cm) also are treated with initial chemotherapy.

Stage III Disease

Approximately 70% to 80% of patients with metastatic disease will be cured with cisplatin-based chemotherapy combined with surgery to resect residual disease as an integral part of management. The therapeutic objective is cure, with distinct approaches for disease deemed good risk (i.e., high probability of cure) and poor risk (i.e., low probability of cure). For patients with good-risk disease, the goal is to minimize toxicities without compromising cure, whereas management of poor-risk disease focuses less on toxicity and more on increasing the probability of cure.

MANAGEMENT BY RISK CLASSIFICATION

The treatment of germ cell tumors is based on the "International Germ Cell Consensus Classification," developed in 1996 (Tables 9-2 and 9-3).[9,10]

Good Risk

Approximately 60% of patients with nonseminomatous germ cell tumors present with good-risk disease. Patients with good risk include those with stage II or III disease with testis/retroperitoneal primary tumors, no nonpulmonary visceral metastases, and good-risk tumor markers. Based on the results of clinical trials, more than 90% of these patients will be cured with the use of combination chemotherapy, including cisplatin and etoposide with or without bleomycin.[16-19] Summaries of the trials are shown here.

- Four cycles of etoposide (500 mg/m^2) plus cisplatin and three cycles of bleomycin, etoposide (500 mg/m^2), and cisplatin (BEP) achieve a durable complete response in approximately 90% of patients with good-risk disease.
- The elimination of bleomycin can compromise cure if only three cycles of therapy with etoposide and cisplatin are given or adequate doses of etoposide (500 mg/m^2) are not administered.[20,21]
- Although carboplatin has less toxicity, it cannot be substituted for cisplatin because it is less effective.[22,23]

Thus, three cycles of BEP or four cycles of etoposide plus cisplatin are the standard regimens for the treatment of patients with good-risk germ cell tumors. One additional cycle of treatment is required with the regimen of etoposide plus cisplatin, but the nine bleomycin treatments are avoided. Bleomycin is associated with Raynaud's phenomenon and pulmonary toxicity, although clinically significant pulmonary toxicity is rare.[24]

The lower limit of dose for bleomycin and etoposide were addressed in a trial comparing three cycles of standard BEP (cisplatin, 20 mg/m^2 on days 1 to 5; etoposide, 100 mg/m^2 on days 1 to 5; and bleomycin, 30 kU on days 1, 8, and 15 repeated every 21 days) with four cycles of the same combination at different dosages (cisplatin, 100 mg/m^2 on day 1; etoposide, 120 mg/m^2 on days 1 to 3; and bleomycin 30 kU on day 1, repeated every 21 days). The trial was stopped when an interim analysis attributed a higher cancer death rate to the alternative regimen felt to be related to the lower total dose and dose intensity of bleomycin and to the lower dose intensity of etoposide.[25]

In an attempt to decrease toxicity, the substitution of carboplatin for cisplatin was addressed in a randomized trial in which etoposide plus cisplatin was compared with etoposide plus carboplatin (500 mg/m^2 on day 1 of each cycle) for four cycles.[22] There was a significantly inferior event-free and relapse-free survival rate for those patients who received etoposide plus carboplatin. Therefore, carboplatin should not be substituted for cisplatin in the treatment of patients with germ cell tumors.

Intermediate Risk

The intermediate-risk group includes patients with nonseminomatous tumors with intermediate-risk tumor markers and patients with seminoma who have nonpulmonary visceral metastases. A regimen that includes four cycles of BEP is the standard treatment.

Poor Risk

Patients with poor-risk disease include mediastinal primary tumors, nonpulmonary visceral metastases, or poor-risk tumor markers. These patients comprise 10% to 20% of nonseminomas and have a 5-year survival of approximately 50%. For patients with poor risk, the standard of care remains four cycles of conventional-dose BEP. A randomized trial showed that the substitution of ifosfamide for bleomycin has similar efficacy but significantly greater toxicity.[26] Additionally, the use of high-dose cisplatin (200 mg/m^2) is not superior to standard-dose cisplatin (100 mg/m^2) when administered in combination with etoposide and bleomycin.[27] A recently reported randomized phase III trial in 219 patients with intermediate-risk or poor-risk germ cell tumors compared first-line high-dose chemotherapy with two cycles of standard BEP followed by two cycles of high-dose chemotherapy (cyclophosphamide, etoposide, and carboplatin) plus stem cell rescue to four cycles of conventional-dose BEP.[28] The primary endpoint was the percentage of patients with complete response at 1 year. Final analysis showed that there was not a significant difference with a complete response at 1 year of 52% for BEP plus high-dose chemotherapy and 48% for BEP alone (p = 0.53).

SALVAGE THERAPY

Between 20% and 30% of patients with advanced germ cell tumors fail to achieve a durable response to chemotherapy regimens, including cisplatin and etoposide with or without bleomycin. Approximately 25% of patients will achieve a durable complete response using vinblastine plus ifosfamide plus cisplatin as initial salvage therapy.[29] Patients who do not achieve a durable complete response to induction chemotherapy have a particularly poor prognosis.[30] In addition, patients with a mediastinal primary tumor site rarely achieve a durable complete response to cisplatin plus ifosfamide-based salvage chemotherapy. The timing of relapse also is important with late relapse beyond 2 years associated with a high degree of resistance to standard salvage chemotherapy and an overall poor prognosis.[13] The combination of paclitaxel, ifosfamide, and cisplatin (TIP) was evaluated as second-line therapy in patients with favorable prognostic features for response, including testis primary tumor site and a prior complete response to a first-line chemotherapy program.[31] Four cycles of TIP as second-line therapy resulted in a 70% complete response rate to treatment with a 63% durable complete response rate and a 2-year progression-free survival rate of 65%. The high level of activity with TIP as salvage therapy is, in part, related to the patient selection criteria used to identify patients more likely to benefit from conventional-dose second-line therapy. A retrospective study demonstrated that the TIP regimen followed by surgery may be effective in patients with late-relapse germ cell tumors who are not candidates for primary surgery.[32] Ifosfamide-based therapy has been associated with significant hematologic, renal, and neurologic toxicities, and the use of hematopoietic growth factors is considered standard. A phase II study of cisplatin plus epirubicin also has demonstrated activity in the salvage setting.[33] Additional regimens, such as those incorporating gemcitabine and oxaliplatin, have demonstrated antitumor activity in heavily pretreated patients.[34]

HIGH-DOSE CHEMOTHERAPY WITH PERIPHERAL STEM CELL RESCUE

The use of high-dose chemotherapy with peripheral stem cell rescue should be considered for patients who do not have an initial complete response to induction chemotherapy or who relapse after first-line salvage therapy. Critical to the success of high-dose therapy is the identification of potential candidates early, as the period of myelosuppression following high-dose therapy is shorter for less heavily pretreated patients. The use of high-dose carboplatin and etoposide followed by peripheral blood stem cell transplantation or autologous bone marrow transplantation rescue with a repeat course of therapy given after hematopoietic reconstitution was evaluated as initial salvage therapy in 65 patients with testicular cancer.[35] Postchemotherapy resection of residual disease was performed in selected patients. At a median follow-up of 39 months, 37 of the 65 patients (57%) were continuously disease free and three additional patients were rendered disease free with surgery. The use of sequential, dose-intensive combination paclitaxel, ifosfamide, carboplatin, and etoposide with stem cell rescue was evaluated in 37 patients with germ cell tumors who were resistant to cisplatin and who had unfavorable prognostic features for response to conventional-dose salvage therapy.[36] Twenty-one patients (57%) achieved a complete response, and two additional patients achieved a partial response with normal tumor markers; 23 (62%) achieved a favorable response. Fifteen (41%) of the favorable responses remained durable at a median follow-up of 30 months. The major toxicity was myelosuppression with 58% of the carboplatin and etoposide cycles associated with hospitalization for nadir fever. Tandem peripheral stem cell rescue has replaced autologous bone marrow transplantation. Results for patients with primary mediastinal germ cell tumors treated with high-dose chemotherapy and stem cell rescue demonstrate worse outcome, and these patients should be enrolled in clinical trials at specialized centers.[37] Treatment-related morbidity following high-dose therapy can be significant, and all patients should be referred to major treatment centers specializing in this approach.[38]

SURGERY AFTER CHEMOTHERAPY

Surgery after chemotherapy is an integral part of the treatment of patients with germ cell tumors and should be considered for individuals with residual radiographic abnormalities but with normal serum tumor markers after treatment. A retroperitoneal lymph node dissection is the standard surgery for patients with evidence of disease in the retroperitoneum. All residual masses at all sites should be excised, as the histology at one site does not adequately predict the histology at other sites. Approximately 45% of residual masses will consist of necrotic debris or fibrosis, 40% will consist of mature teratoma, and 15% will harbor viable germ cell tumor. If viable germ cell tumor has been completely resected, two additional cycles of chemotherapy are administered. Although histologically benign, teratoma arises from malignant germ cells and may grow over time. Surgical removal is recommended. Additionally, a minority of resected teratomas will have malignant transformation to cell types including rhabdomyosarcoma, adenocarcinoma, and others. Surgical resection is the mainstay of treatment; however, chemotherapy for a particular cell type may result in major responses and long-term survival in select patients.[39]

Whether patients who initially present with visible disease on CT scan and have normalization or minimal residual disease on repeat imaging after chemotherapy should undergo surgery is controversial. CT scans of the chest can identify small residual masses in the pulmonary parenchyma. The sensitivity of this technique in the retroperitoneum remains uncertain, leading to controversy over the definition of residual retroperitoneal masses. In 87 patients with minimal residual tumor masses (largest diameter of the residual mass on transaxial plane was 20 mm or less) after chemotherapy, 58 patients (67%) had complete fibrosis or necrosis, 23 patients (26%) had teratoma, and six patients (7%) had viable malignant germ cell tumor. Thus, approximately one-third of patients had vital tumor tissue with teratoma at risk for growth and/or malignant transformation and viable germ cell tumor at risk for progression.[40] An additional concern was the poor outcome associated with late relapses and the finding that an inadequately controlled retroperitoneum is a major predisposing factor.[13,41] With nonseminomatous germ cell tumors, 18-fluorodeoxyglucose positron emission tomography (FDG-PET) scans are unable to distinguish fibrosis from teratoma, therefore limiting the utility of PET imaging in determining the histology of residual masses after chemotherapy.

An exception to the requirement for normal tumor markers is the patient with elevated serum tumor markers in whom disease did not respond to salvage chemotherapy. This clinical scenario is rare because fewer than 5% of patients who do not have normal marker status are candidates for surgical excision of a solitary residual mass. Surgery in the setting of elevated markers should only be considered by specialists with experience in the management of these cases.

SEMINOMA

Stage I

Approximately 70% of patients with seminoma have stage I disease. After radical inguinal orchiectomy, standard treatment includes adjuvant radiotherapy to the retroperitoneal lymph nodes (para-aortic field) with or without the ipsilateral pelvic lymph nodes (dogleg field), recognizing that approximately 80% of these patients do not need radiation therapy. Findings from observational studies of patients with clinical stage I seminoma indicate a 15% to 20% likelihood of disease relapse, mostly in the retroperitoneum. However, the median time to relapse exceeds 15 months, which is twice as long as for clinical stage I nonseminomatous tumors and may occur as late as 8 to 10 years. Therefore, radiation therapy remains the standard treatment in the United States for clinical stage I disease. It is contraindicated in the setting of inflammatory bowel disease or a horseshoe kidney. Radiotherapy using a para-aortic field as compared with a dogleg field is associated with reduced toxicity and a low rate of recurrence.[42] Although surveillance represents an alternative to radiotherapy, because of the low morbidity associated with radiation, surveillance is not standardly recommended in the United States. A randomized trial comparing adjuvant radiotherapy with single-dose carboplatin in the adjuvant treatment of stage I seminoma has shown noninferiority of carboplatin to radiotherapy.[43] This approach cannot be considered a standard or alternative treatment for stage I seminoma because of several issues, including the short follow-up and unknown late consequences of therapy.[44]

All patients with stage IIA and IIB disease are treated with radiotherapy to the retroperitoneal and ipsilateral pelvic lymph nodes with doses of up to 25 Gy, with a boost to gross disease of up to 30 to 35 Gy. Prophylactic mediastinal radiation is not advised because few patients relapse in the mediastinum. Chemotherapy will cure more than 90% of the patients who relapse after radiotherapy; approximately 99% of patients with early seminoma are cured.

Advanced Seminoma

Approximately 10% of patients with seminoma require chemotherapy; 15% to 20% of patients with advanced seminoma present with an elevated HCG. An elevated alpha-fetoprotein indicates a nonseminomatous tumor, and the patient should be treated accordingly. Patients with retroperitoneal masses larger than 5 cm (stage IIC), supradiaphragmatic lymphadenopathy, visceral disease, bulky retroperitoneal tumors, tumor-related back pain, elevated tumor markers, and mediastinal extragonadal presentations are treated with primary chemotherapy. Approximately 90% of patients with advanced seminoma will be classified as good prognosis and receive treatment with good-risk chemotherapy with an 86% 5-year survival.[10] Prophylactic radiation therapy to sites of initial bulky disease after chemotherapy is not indicated as it does not alter the probability of relapse or survival.

Surgery after chemotherapy is technically more difficult for patients with seminomas than for patients with nonseminomas. A classical retroperitoneal lymph node dissection is typically not carried out in this setting because of fibrosis and because of an increased likelihood of damage to the great vessels. Fortunately, surgery after chemotherapy is generally not necessary. Postchemotherapy residual masses usually represent fibrosis rather than persistent seminoma. Options have included surgery for postchemotherapy masses larger than 3 cm or close observation with CT imaging and intervention if evidence of disease progression. More recently, FDG-PET has been shown to be a reliable predictor for viable tumors in postchemotherapy seminoma.[45]

ASSOCIATED MALIGNANT DISEASE

Malignant transformation of a somatic teratomatous component of a nonseminoma to somatic malignancies including rhabdomyosarcoma, adenocarcinoma, primitive neuroectodermal tumor, and leukemia, as well as others, has been well described.[39] The presence of i(12p) or excess 12p copy number in these tumors establishes the clonal germ cell tumor origin. The finding of i(12p) or excess 12p genetic material by either molecular or cytogenetic studies correlates with response to cisplatin therapy.[46] Mediastinal nonseminomatous germ cell tumors also are associated with the presence of myeloproliferative disorders, including acute nonlymphocytic leukemia and acute megakaryocytic leukemia. A minority of patients with poorly differentiated carcinomas of unknown primary origin have a complete response to cisplatin-based chemotherapy. Presence of additional clinical features including male sex, predominant midline tumor, relatively young age, and elevated serum tumor markers has suggested that the minority of patients with poorly differentiated carcinomas of unknown primary origin may have germ cell tumors. Clinical features as well as molecular and cytogenetic studies are important in the management of carcinomas of unknown primary or midline tumors of uncertain histiogenesis.

SURVIVORSHIP AND LATE EFFECTS

An evaluation of the long-term risk of cardiovascular disease in survivors of testicular cancer demonstrated a moderately increased myocardial infarction risk at young ages in patients with nonseminomatous germ cell tumors.[47] Increased risk was associated with prior chemotherapy regimens including cisplatin, vinblastine, and bleomycin (PVB), as well as BEP, previous mediastinal irradiation, and recent tobacco use. Acute chemotherapy-induced cardiovascular changes have been shown in patients treated with cisplatin-based chemotherapy including an increase in plasma von Willebrand factor levels and an increased intima-media thickness of the carotid artery.[48] In addition to chemotherapy-induced endothelial damage, cardiovascular toxicity also is likely related to the metabolic syndrome and gonadal dysfunction.[49]

Newly-diagnosed patients with testicular cancer are at risk for decreased sperm counts or impaired sperm motility. With treatment, infertility can result from retrograde ejaculation after retroperitoneal lymph node dissection or as a result of radiation or chemotherapy. Although some patients will have long-standing chemotherapy-induced oligospermia or azospermia, normal or near-normal spermatogenesis resumes in most patients. As such, patients who are scheduled to have retroperitoneal lymph node dissection, radiation therapy, or chemotherapy are advised to bank sperm.

There is an increased risk of secondary malignancies in patients with testicular cancer that is related to prior radiotherapy or chemotherapy for at least 35 years after treatment.[50] Increased risks have been seen for cancers of the stomach, gallbladder and bile ducts, pancreas, bladder, kidney, thyroid, soft-tissue sarcoma, nonmelanoma skin cancer, and myeloid leukemia.[51] Other late effects include ototoxicity, chronic neurotoxicity, renal impairment, pulmonary toxicity, and anxiety disorder.[52,53] In light of a young age at diagnosis and high cure rates, patients with testicular cancer require specialized follow-up care with close attention to monitoring for late effects of cancer and cancer therapy.[54]

BLADDER CANCER

An estimated 61,420 (44,690 men and 16,730 women) new cases of bladder cancer and 13,060 (8,990 men and 4,070 women) related deaths were estimated to occur in the United States in 2006.[1] The incidence of bladder cancer is 3 to 4 times higher in men than in women and occurs predominantly in patients older than age 50, with a median age of 68 at diagnosis. The approximate 5:1 ratio of incidence to mortality reflects the frequency of superficial tumors compared with invasive and metastatic disease. Although white Americans have a 2-fold higher incidence of bladder cancer, black Americans have a higher mortality rate with similar grade and stage tumors.[55] Risk factors for bladder cancer include tobacco use, occupational exposures, urinary tract diseases, and pharmaceutical drug use.[56] Cigarette smoking is associated with a relative risk of developing bladder cancer that is 2 to 4 times that of nonsmokers. This risk increases in proportion to the amount and duration of cigarette exposure with heavy smokers (more than 20 cigarettes per day and/or more than 40 years), resulting in up to a 5-fold higher relative risk compared with nonsmokers. Although cessation of smoking lowers the risk, a higher risk than that of nonsmokers remains for at least 25 years. Occupational exposure to aromatic amines (particularly 2-naphthylamine, benzidine, and polycyclic aromatic hydrocarbons) is associated with an increased incidence of bladder cancer (e.g., workers in dyestuff manufacturing and rubber and aluminum industries). Infection with the trematode *schistosoma haema tobium* leads to chronic irritation of the urothelium and an increased risk of both squamous and urothelial carcinomas. Other chronic urinary tract infections, including stones and cystitis, also may lead to chronic inflammation and an

KEY POINTS

- Urothelial tumorigenesis results in three general categories of urothelial tract tumors — superficial, invasive, and metastatic — that differ with respect to tumor biology, clinical phenotype, prognosis, and management.
- The staging of urothelial tract tumors requires a transurethral resection specimen that includes muscle to ensure that an invasive tumor is not missed.
- Although the role of neoadjuvant chemotherapy has been established for the treatment of patients with invasive disease, it is not known whether chemotherapy is best applied as neoadjuvant or adjuvant therapy and whether the results in one setting can be extrapolated to the other.
- Bladder preservation may be considered in select patients using combined modality protocols with chemotherapy and radiation therapy.

increased risk of bladder cancer. Heavy use of phenacetin-containing analgesics is associated with tumors of the renal pelvis and ureter, and cyclophosphamide also has been associated with an increased risk of urothelial carcinoma. These myriad risk factors lead to field changes within the urothelium that predispose individuals to the development of recurrent tumors as well as to involvement of new locations in the urothelial tract (polychronotropism).

The three general categories of disease — superficial, invasive, and metastatic — differ in tumor biology, clinical phenotype, prognosis, and management. For superficial tumors, the goal is to prevent recurrence and progression to an incurable stage. For invasive disease, the goal is maximize the chance for cure using multimodality therapy including chemotherapy with surgery or radiation therapy.

The management of metastatic disease requires the use of established prognostic and predictive factors to determine the therapeutic objectives and potential for treatment-related toxicity. The main goals are palliation of symptoms and prolongation of survival.

PATHOLOGY

Urothelial carcinoma may occur throughout the urinary tract (i.e., in any structure lined by the urothelium), with greater than 90% originating in the bladder. Upper urinary tract tumors including the renal pelvis and ureter, account for 5% to 7% of urothelial carcinomas, with renal pelvis tumors comprising the majority. In the United States, 92% of lower urinary tract tumors are urothelial carcinomas, 5% are squamous cell cancers, 2% are adenocarcinomas, and 1% are small cell carcinomas. Lesions of mixed histology are generally variants of urothelial carcinoma. Adenocarcinomas may be of urachal origin, occurring at the junction of the urachal ligament and bladder dome. In Northern Africa and other parts of the world where there is a high prevalence of infection with *S. haematbium*, up to 75% of tumors are pure squamous cell carcinomas.

BIOLOGY

Molecular profiling has demonstrated that urothelial tumors evolve through divergent pathways corresponding to the clinical phenotypes of nonlethal, recurrent superficial lesions and lethal, invasive, and metastatic variants.[57] Deletions of both arms of chromosome 9 are seen during the earliest stages of urothelial tumorigenesis. Overexpression of *HRAS*, the first human oncogene identified in urothelial carcinoma, is seen in the majority of human urothelial cancers. The Ras signaling pathway appears to have a major role in the development of low-grade, noninvasive lesions based on the fact that 30% to 40% are characterized by activating mutations in the *HRAS* gene and 70% have mutations in *FGFR3*, an upstream tyrosine kinase receptor involved in cellular proliferation and angiogenesis. Although approximately 70% of these low-grade lesions will recur, only 10% to 15% will progress to invasive lesions. Progression of low-grade lesions to invasive disease is characterized by structural and functional alterations in the tumor suppressors, p53, and the retinoblastoma protein (Rb) in addition to chromosomal aberrations including deletions in chromosome 8p, 11p, 13q, and 14q. Approximately 20% to 30% of patients will present with high-grade muscle invasive tumors with greater than 50% of these tumors containing alterations in p53 and Rb. Despite radical cystectomy and the use of perioperative chemotherapy, up to 50% of invasive tumors will progress to local and distant metastases. This ability to invade and metastasize is not only a function of alterations in the tumor cells, but also involves the interactions of the tumor cells with the local environment. The following are specifically seen in urothelial carcinoma: defects in cell–cell adhesion, with loss or reduced expression of E-cadherin; increased levels of matrix metalloproteinases, such as MMP9 and MMP2, which lead to degradation of the extracellular matrix; and increaseed angiogenic factors, such as vascular endothelial growth factor (VEGF).

Regarding prognosis, p53 nuclear overexpression is an independent predictor of progression and decreased survival.[58] Immunohistochemical staining for p53, p21, pRB, and p16 in a series of patients with bladder cancer who underwent radical cystectomy and bilateral pelvic lymphadenectomy demonstrated that altered expression of each of the four cell cycle regulators was associated with bladder cancer outcome, with p53 as the strongest predictor.[59] Using oligonucleotide microarrays, a genetic profile consisting of 174 probes has identified patients with lymph node metastases and poor survival.[60]

DIAGNOSIS AND STAGING

The most common presenting symptom is hematuria, and patients with carcinoma in situ or invasive disease may present with irritative urinary symptoms. Less frequently, patients may present with symptoms related to distant metastases. The diagnosis is established by cystoscopy and biopsy. The TNM classification for urothelial tumors was revised in 1997 as follows:

- Ta tumors are noninvasive papillary lesions that tend to recur but not invade;
- Tis, or carcinoma in situ, is the precursor of a more aggressive and lethal invasive variant;
- T1 tumors invade the subepithelial connective tissue, including lamina propria or muscularis mucosa;
- T2 tumors invade the muscle;
- pT2a tumors invade superficial muscle;
- pT2b tumors invade deep muscle;
- T3 tumors invade perivesical tissue;
- pT3a are evident microscopically;
- pT3b are evident macroscopically (extravesical mass); and
- T4 tumors invade the prostate, uterus, vagina, pelvic, and/or abdominal wall.

The major problem with staging is that the correlation of depth of invasion determined by cystoscopy and biopsy with the results of cystectomy is only 50% to 60%. Noninvasive imaging with CT or MRI can identify extravesical or nodal disease and is more reliable if done prior to the transurethral resection with a distended bladder. The histologic grading system of well differentiated (G1), moderately differentiated (G2), and poorly differentiated (G3) is more relevant for superficial tumors because virtually all invasive neoplasms are poorly differentiated (G3).

THERAPY

Superficial Disease

Seventy percent of patients with newly diagnosed bladder cancer will present with superficial disease, with 70% confined to the mucosa (Ta or Tis) and 30% involving the submucosa (T1). The treatment involves complete removal of the lesion by transurethral resection (TUR) followed by rigorous surveillance with cystoscopy and urine cytology at 3-month intervals for recurrence and/or progression to a more advanced stage. The sensitivity of urine cytology ranges from 13% to 75%, and the limitations of cystoscopy include impaired visualization related to bleeding and difficulty distinguishing flat carcinoma in situ from benign lesions; however, urine markers under investigation, such as nuclear matrix protein, NMP22, may complement cystoscopy and urine cytology in the detection of recurrence.[61,62] Approximately 70% of patients with superficial bladder cancer will have a recurrence or a new occurrence within 5 years, and approximately 15% will progress to a more advanced stage. When urinary cytology is positive but cystoscopy reveals no visible lesions in the bladder or urethra, selective catheterization and visualization of the upper urinary tracts is warranted. Intravesical therapy has two uses: as prophylaxis, to prevent or delay tumor recurrence and/or progression, and as therapy for residual tumor or carcinoma in situ. The latter approach rarely eliminates the disease, partially because of the limited penetration of most intravesical agents. Although the indications for prophylaxis vary, intravesical therapy is generally recommended for multifocal or recurrent Ta lesions, carcinoma in situ, and T1 disease. Randomized trials have established Bacille Calmette-Guérin (BCG) with six weekly installations, including a maintenance schedule, as the intravesical treatment of choice to limit recurrence and reduce the incidence of progression.[63] Salvage intravesical therapy with BCG and interferon-alpha 2b may be effective for patients who have not responded to BCG alone. Alternative intravesical agents including mitomycin C, gemcitabine, doxorubicin, valrubicin, and thiotepa have been shown to prevent recurrence with minimal effect on progression. For disease that does not respond to BCG, these alternative agents may be considered. In some cases, cystectomy is indicated.[64]

Invasive Disease

Although the majority of patients present with superficial disease, approximately 20% to 40% of patients either present with more advanced disease or progress after therapy for superficial disease. Staging for patients with invasive disease includes a CT scan of the abdomen and pelvis, chest x-ray, and, if clinically indicated, a bone scan. The standard treatment for a muscle-invasive tumor is a radical cystectomy with bilateral pelvic lymphadenectomy that includes removal of the bladder, prostate, seminal vesicles, and proximal urethra in the man, and removal of the bladder, urethra, and uterus (including bilateral salpingo-oophorectomy), as well as excision of a portion of the anterior vaginal wall, in the woman. The pelvic lymph node dissection is a necessary part of the radical cystectomy surgery with a more extended lymph node dissection associated with an improvement in outcome.[65,66] The three main types of urinary diversions include an ileal conduit that drains to an appliance on the anterior abdominal wall, a continent cutaneous reservoir constructed from detubularized bowel segments, and an orthotopic neobladder. More men are candidates for continent urethral reservoirs than women because of anatomic considerations. It is not clear that continent reconstruction after radical cystectomy is associated with an improvement in quality of life as compared with conduit diversion.[67] In fact, most patients have a good quality of life regardless of the type of diversion used.

Prognosis varies inversely with higher T stage, lymphatic or vascular invasion in the primary tumor, and lymph node involvement. In addition, extracapsular extension of lymph node metastases is associated with a worse outcome.[68] In a series of 1,054 patients undergoing radical cystectomy and pelvic lymphadenectomy, the overall recurrence free survival rates at 5 and 10 years were 68% and 66%, respectively.[69] Patients with nonorgan-confined, lymph node-negative tumors had a significantly higher ($p < 0.001$) probability of recurrence compared with those who had organ-confined bladder cancers (Table 9-4). The 5-year and 10-year recurrence-free survival rates for the 246 patients with lymph node involvement were 35% and 34%, respectively. Patients with organ-confined tumors and fewer than five involved lymph nodes had improved survival rates. The median time to recurrence among the 311 patients in whom the cancer recurred was 12 months (range, approximately 5 months to 11 years).

TABLE 9-4 Survival Rates for Bladder Cancer According to Stage[69]

	5-year Survival (%)	10-year Survival (%)
Node-negative disease		
P2	77	57
P3a	64	44
P3b	49	29
P4	44	23
Lymph node involvement	31	23

Multivariate nomograms have been developed to predict outcome after radical cystectomy.[70,71] A partial cystectomy can provide adequate local control of invasive bladder cancer in select patients.[72] Less invasive surgical techniques, including laparoscopic and robotic radical cystectomy, are being evaluated. The use of bladder sparing protocols as alternatives to surgery in the management of invasive bladder cancer will be reviewed in the section *Bladder Preservation.*

Metastatic Disease

Urothelial tumors are sensitive to several chemotherapy agents with different mechanisms of action including methotrexate, vinblastine, doxorubicin, cisplatin, the taxanes, ifosfamide, and gemcitabine. Two-, three-, and four-drug combinations are used with the combination of methotrexate, vinblastine, doxorubicin, and cisplatin (MVAC) and with gemcitabine plus cisplatin, representing the standard regimens.[73,74] Randomized trials comparing MVAC to single-agent cisplatin and to the three-drug combination of doxorubicin, cyclophosphamide, and cisplatin demonstrated superior response rates, prolongation of time to progression, and improved overall survival for patients treated with MVAC. Increasing the dose intensity of MVAC in a 2-week schedule with growth factor support compared with classic MVAC on a 4-week schedule did not significantly improve outcome.[75]

MVAC was compared with gemcitabine and cisplatin in patients with locally advanced or metastatic urothelial carcinoma.[76] Although this trial was not designed as a noninferiority study, the results demonstrated a similar response rate (GC, 49%; MVAC, 46%; $p = 0.51$), progression-free survival (GC, 7.7 months; MVAC, 8.3 months; $p = 0.63$), and median survival (GC, 14 months; MVAC, 15.2 months; $p = 0.66$), as well as less toxicity for gemcitabine and cisplatin compared with MVAC. Specifically, treatment with gemcitabine plus cisplatin produced less neutropenia, neutropenic fever, sepsis, and mucositis, but more anemia and thrombocytopenia compared with MVAC. The combination of docetaxel and cisplatin plus granulocyte colony-stimulating factor (G-CSF) has been compared with MVAC plus G-CSF in advanced urothelial carcinoma.[77] Treatment with MVAC resulted in a superior response rate (54.2% vs. 37.4%; $p = 0.17$), median time to progression (9.4 vs. 6.1 months; $p = 0.003$), and median survival (14.2 vs. 9.3 months; $p = 0.026$). Several trials using taxanes have demonstrated promising results with the following combinations:[78]

- ifosfamide, paclitaxel, and cisplatin;
- gemcitabine, paclitaxel, and cisplatin; and
- gemcitabine, paclitaxel, and carboplatin.

The superiority of the triplet regimens, however, has not been established. A sequential regimen using gemcitabine and doxorubicin followed by the combination of ifosfamide, paclitaxel, and cisplatin demonstrated a high overall response rate.[79] In patients with renal insufficiency who are not candidates for cisplatin, alternative regimens that do not contain cisplatin, such as gemcitabine or paclitaxel with carboplatin, may be used.

An evaluation of the prognostic factors predicting long-term survival of patients with metastatic urothelial carcinoma receiving MVAC chemotherapy included Karnofsky performance status (less than or greater than 80%) and presence or absence of visceral metastases (lung, liver, or bone).[80] The median survival times for patients who had zero, one, or two risk factors were 33, 13.4, and 9.3 months, respectively. Toxicity varies as a function of risk group. For patients with poor-risk disease, treatment-related mortality has been reported for 3% to 4% of cases. Although the frequency of these events may be reduced with the use of hematopoietic growth factors, MVAC is generally not recommended for patients with poor-risk disease.

There is no accepted standard of care for second-line chemotherapy in advanced bladder cancer. Evaluations of single agents, such as ifosfamide, docetaxel, gemcitabine, paclitaxel, and pemetrexed, have demonstrated response rates between 9% and 27% with no documented improvement in survival. Although multidrug regimens have been associated with higher response rates, this does not appear to translate into an improvement in survival.

Metastatectomy is routinely performed in the management of advanced testicular germ cell tumors and may be considered in the management of other advanced urological malignancies.[81] In highly select patients with metastatic urothelial carcinoma, resection of metastatic disease can result in long-term disease control.[82,83]

PERIOPERATIVE CHEMOTHERAPY FOR INVASIVE AND LOCALLY ADVANCED DISEASE

The use of perioperative chemotherapy in the management of invasive and locally advanced bladder cancer has been studied in the neoadjuvant (preoperative) and adjuvant (postoperative) settings. The potential advantages for neoadjuvant chemotherapy include evaluation of response to therapy in vivo, with continuation of effective chemotherapy, discontinuation of chemotherapy and early cystectomy in the setting of no response or progression, tumor downstaging to allow for a less complicated surgery, and the delivery of full-dose chemotherapy without the problems associated with postoperative recovery.[78] The major advantages for the use of adjuvant chemotherapy include treatment based on pathologic criteria with the ability to select those patients at high risk who are most likely to benefit from chemotherapy and to avoid the unnecessary treatment of patients with low risk disease.

ADJUVANT CHEMOTHERAPY

Although many physicians favor the use of adjuvant chemotherapy for patients with nodal involvement and extravesical tumor extension, definitive trials are lacking.

Unfortunately, the adjuvant studies that have been performed have major limitations, including flawed statistical methodology with underpowered trials and early termination, as well as the use of suboptimal chemotherapy with non–cisplatin-containing regimens. For example, in one study, 91 patients with P3, P4, or node-positive disease were randomly assigned to receive either four cycles of adjuvant cisplatin, cyclophosphamide, and doxorubicin or observation. Although the trial demonstrated a significant delay in time to disease progression in patients who received chemotherapy, with 70% disease free at 3 years compared with 46% of untreated patients, the 5-year overall survival was not significantly different. Several methodological problems with this trial include the small sample size, premature closure, and the fact that 25% of patients assigned to chemotherapy never actually received it.[84] A German study randomly assigned patients with pT3b, pT4a, and/or lymph node involvement to observation after cystectomy or to three cycles of adjuvant MVAC or methotrexate, vinblastine, epirubicin, and cisplatin. The trial was terminated early when an interim analysis indicated an inferior disease-free survival rate and a significantly higher relapse rate (18 [82%] of 22) among untreated patients compared with patients who received chemotherapy (three [17%] of 18) ($p = 0.0012$).[85] In patients with nodal involvement, disease progressed in 92% of patients on observation compared with 73% of patients who received adjuvant chemotherapy ($p < 0.002$). A survival difference was subsequently shown; however, patients did not receive chemotherapy at the time of relapse.[86]

NEOADJUVANT CHEMOTHERAPY

Several of the initial prospective randomized trials of neoadjuvant chemotherapy using single agents and combination chemotherapy failed to demonstrate a benefit. The largest phase III neoadjuvant chemotherapy trial performed to date randomly assigned 976 patients with T2 G3, T3, T4a, N0 to NX, or M0 bladder cancer undergoing cystectomy or radiotherapy to three cycles of neoadjuvant chemotherapy with cisplatin, methotrexate, and vinblastine (CMV) or to no chemotherapy. At a median follow-up of 4 years, chemotherapy-associated mortality was 1% and cystectomy-associated mortality was 3.7%. At 7.4 years, a statistically significant ($p = 0.05$) 6% absolute survival benefit was observed for patients treated with chemotherapy. The chemotherapy regimen was associated with a higher pathologic complete-response rate.[87] A U.S. phase III intergroup trial randomly assigned patients with T2 to T4a, N0, M0 bladder cancer to neoadjuvant MVAC plus cystectomy (153 patients) or to cystectomy alone (154 patients).[88] At a median follow-up of 8.7 years, the estimated risk of death was reduced by 25% in the patients who received MVAC and cystectomy. The median survival of patients assigned to surgery alone was 46 months, compared with 77 months among patients assigned to MVAC plus cystectomy. The survival benefit of neoadjuvant MVAC was associated with tumor downstaging to pT0 (38% in those patients who received MVAC compared with 15% of those who received cystectomy), with an 85% 5-year survival for patients who experienced a pathologic complete response to neoadjuvant chemotherapy. A meta-analysis of neoadjuvant chemotherapy in invasive bladder cancer performed with data from

TABLE 9-5 Randomized Trials of Neoadjuvant Cisplatin-based Combination Chemotherapy for Invasive Bladder Cancer[87,88]

Clinical Trial	Eligible Disease	Comparison	Median Survival (years)	pT0 rate (%)	Survival Rates (%)
Grossman et al.	T2-4a, N0, M0	Three cycle of MVAC plus cystectomy	6.4	38	57 (5 years)*
		Cystectomy alone	3.8	15	42 (5 years)*
Hall et al.	T2(G3), T3-T4a, N0/NX, M0	Three cycles of CMV plus cystectomy or radiotherapy or both	NA	33	55, 50, 43** (3, 5, 7 years)
		Cystectomy or radiotherapy or both	NA	12	50, 44, 37** (3, 5, 7 years)

*$p = 0.06$ by a stratified log-rank test
**$p = 0.048$, HR = 0.85 (95% CI 0.72-1.00)
Abbreviations: MVAC, methotrexate, vinblastine, doxorubicin, and cisplatin; NA, not available CMV, cisplatin, methotrexate, and vinblastine.

2,688 patients on 10 randomized trials showed a significant overall survival benefit for platinum-based combination chemotherapy, with a 13% reduction in the risk of death and 5% absolute survival benefit at 5 years, with overall survival increasing from 45% to 50%.[89] This effect did not vary between subgroups of patients or type of local treatment. Based on these data, neoadjuvant cisplatin combination chemotherapy represents a standard of care in the management of invasive bladder cancer (Table 9-5). Although not formally evaluated in a randomized trial in the neoadjuvant setting, the most widely used regimen is the combination of gemcitabine and cisplatin. There is insufficient data to support the use of non-cisplatin chemotherapy regimens in the neoadjuvant setting. Thus, renal insufficiency may limit the ability to use perioperative chemotherapy.

BLADDER PRESERVATION

Bladder preservation can be accomplished by transurethral resection alone, radiation therapy alone, chemotherapy alone, or the combination of chemotherapy and radiation therapy. A bladder-sparing approach is only justified when the treatment can completely eradicate the tumor in the bladder, the risk of recurrence is low, and there is not substantial compromise of bladder function. It is estimated that this approach is applicable to 15% to 20% of patients who present with invasive disease, although select series suggest that this rate may be higher.

Although neoadjuvant chemotherapy in combination with local therapy has been shown to improve overall survival, the role of chemotherapy alone in bladder preservation is problematic because of the inability to definitively determine which bladders are truly without residual tumor. In addition, pathologic complete response rates after neoadjuvant chemotherapy at the time of cystectomy are only 20% to 40%. At a minimum, chemotherapy alone cannot replace definitive treatment of the bladder by surgery or radiation.

In past randomized trials, radiation therapy alone has been shown to be inferior to cystectomy with respect to survival, particularly for patients with T3 or T4 disease. Although radical cystectomy has not been formally compared with a multimodality bladder-sparing protocol, multiple studies have evaluated trimodality treatment consisting of transurethral resection (as complete as safely possible), as well as chemotherapy plus radiation therapy in select patients with long-term disease-free and overall survival rates approaching those seen in radical cystectomy series. Five-year survival rates in the range of 49% to 62% have been reported. An important component of bladder-sparing protocols includes an evaluation of early response of the primary tumor to treatment with less than a complete response requiring cystectomy. Approximately one-third of patients initiated on a bladder-sparing protocol will ultimately require cystectomy for a less-than-complete response or for recurrent invasive tumors.[90] Quality of life is another important consideration. Radiation therapy can induce disturbances in the function of the bladder, anal sphincter, and large bowel. The morbidity of radiation therapy has decreased with the availability of better imaging, allowing for a boost to the primary tumor and the reduction in fraction size. The main disadvantage for bladder preservation is the requirement for lifelong surveillance because of the risk of recurrence or development of a new bladder cancer. However, many of these new or recurrent tumors are superficial and can be managed endoscopically. In a series of 121 patients treated with sequential chemotherapy followed by concurrent chemotherapy and radiation therapy, 48 patients had a recurrence, of which 32 (66%) were superficial, occurring 2 years after treatment. Of these, 21 were treated conservatively. Thus, even when a complete remission is accomplished, continued endoscopic monitoring is essential.[91]

OTHER UROTHELIAL TRACT CANCERS

Cancers of the renal pelvis, ureter, and proximal urethra also are of urothelial origin and should be treated on the basis of primary histology. Urothelial carcinomas at any of these sites have similar response rates to multiagent chemotherapy as those for bladder tumors. Because approximately 20% to 50% of patients with urothelial carcinomas of the upper urinary tract will develop bladder cancer, surveillance cystoscopy is necessary. The two theories for the multifocal nature of urothelial carcinoma include the field cancerization effect and monoclonality (i.e., tumor cells spreading from their orgin to multiple sites). Thus, simultaneous or metachronous primary tumors of the urothelium at multiple sites may occur, and monitoring is required including follow-up cystoscopies and CT or MRI scans of the upper tracts.

Regarding the management of superficial bladder cancer with intravesical BCG, it is not uncommon for relapse to occur at the ureteral orifices, ureter, or urethra — areas that are less accessible to intravesical treatment. As such, monitoring must include periodic evaluations of the remaining urothelium with cytology and imaging to ensure that relapses or new primary tumors are identified and treated early.

With respect to non-urothelial histology, the chemotherapy used for urothelial carcinoma is not as effective. The use of chemotherapy regimens demonstrating activity in other sites with similar histology is typically used (e.g., etoposide and cisplatin for small cell carcinoma of the lung may be used for the management of small cell carcinoma of the bladder).

RENAL CANCER

Renal cell carcinomas (RCC) account for 90% of all malignant neoplasms of the kidney, with an estimated 38,890 newly diagnosed cases (24,650 men and 14,240 women) and 12,840 deaths (8,130 men and 4,710 women) in 2006.[1] Between 1975 and 1995, the incidence of RCC rose by

KEY POINTS

- The pathologic classification of renal cell cancer is based on morphology, histology, and genetic abnormalities.
- The role of surgery (the only curative modality for renal cell cancer) is changing with the advent of nephron-sparing approaches and cytoreductive surgery.
- A number of angiogenesis-directed vascular endothelial growth factor (VEGF) inhibitors have demonstrated improvement in progression-free survival in both patients who are untreated and those who are cytokine refractory.

2.3% and 3.1%, respectively, among white patients and 3.9% and 4.3%, respectively, among black patients. Renal cancers were historically called the "internist's tumor" because of the variable modes of clinical presentation, including fatigue, weight loss, or anemia. Today, only 10% of cases present with the classic triad of hematuria, abdominal pain, and a palpable mass. From 25% to 50% of patients are diagnosed because a renal mass is detected on radiographic testing done for other diagnostic purposes. Twenty-five percent of patients present with advanced disease, including locally invasive or metastatic renal-cell carcinoma, and one-third who undergo resection of localized disease will demonstrate recurrence. Risk factors for RCC include smoking, obesity, and hypertension,[92] as well as acquired cystic kidney disease associated with end-stage renal disease. Approximately 2% of cases are associated with inherited syndromes.

CT scan with contrast media is the most reliable method for detecting and staging renal cancers. MRI is useful when renal function is poor and is used to evaluate for local invasion or to assess the renal vein and inferior vena cava for thrombus. The role of PET imaging is undefined, but may be useful in evaluating for local recurrence and distant metastases.

Surgical excision is the primary treatment for patients with localized disease, either by radical nephrectomy or nephron-sparing partial nephrectomy for small tumors. Laparoscopic nephrectomy also is an effective treatment. Tumor extension into the renal vein or inferior vena cava, indicating stage III disease, does not preclude resection even if cardiopulmonary bypass is required; approximately 50% of such patients have prolonged survival if the resection is successful. There is no benefit to postoperative radiation therapy for patients with locally advanced disease. Stauffer's syndrome describes the situation of a patient with no detectable metastatic disease who has biochemical evidence of hepatic dysfunction. Although rare, patients with this disorder also are candidates for resection because the hepatopathy is often reversible after the primary tumor is removed.[93]

Cytoreductive nephrectomy should be considered as initial treatment for suitable patients with metastatic disease or to relieve symptoms or control bleeding. Two prospective randomized studies demonstrated improved survival in patients subsequently treated with interferon, with a combined analysis showing a median survival of 13.6 months for patients who received nephrectomy plus interferon compared with 7.8 months for patients who received interferon alone, despite similar low response rates to interferon.[94] Surgical excision of solitary metastases may be appropriate, especially following prolonged disease free intervals. For primary tumors and metastases, embolization is recommended preoperatively because of the highly vascular nature of these lesions.

PATHOLOGY AND MOLECULAR PATHOGENESIS

The Heidelberg classification of renal tumors introduced in 1997 correlates histopathologic features with genetic abnormalities.[95] The five main histopathologic subtypes of renal

TABLE 9-6 Pathologic Classification of Renal Epithelial Neoplasms

Type of Cancer	Growth Pattern	Cytogenetics	Familial Syndrome
Clear cell (conventional)	Acinar or sarcomatoid	3p–	von Hippel-Lindau
Papillary	Papillary or sarcomatoid	+7, +17, –Y	Hereditary papillary renal cell carcinoma (HPRC) Hereditary leiomyomatosis renal cell carcinoma (HLRCC)
Chromophobe	Solid, tubular	–1, –Y hypodiploid	Birt-Hogg-Dube syndrome (BHD)
Oncocytoma	Tumor nests	–1, –Y	Birt-Hogg-Dube syndrome (BHD)
Collecting-duct carcinoma	Papillary or sarcomatoid	Not defined	

carcinomas, based on tumor morphology, histochemistry, cytogenetics, and molecular studies, are conventional (clear-cell), papillary, chromophobe, oncocytoma, and collecting-duct or Bellini duct tumors.[96] Sarcomatoid differentiation, which is associated with a worse prognosis, can occur in any major histologic subtype. Specific cytogenetic and molecular abnormalities are associated with each histologic subtype (Table 9-6).[97]

Von Hippel-Lindau (VHL) disease is an autosomal dominant, familial cancer syndrome that predisposes individuals to RCC, retinal angiomas, hemangioblastomas of the spinal cord and cerebellum, and pheochromocytomas. Frequent loss of at least one allele on chromosome 3p in renal tumors from patients with VHL led to the identification of the *VHL* tumor-suppressor gene. This gene encodes a protein that promotes the ubiquitination and destruction of hypoxia-inducible factor (HIF)-alpha (Fig. 9-1).[98] Several proteins encoded by HIF-alpha are involved in angiogenesis, such as VEGF and platelet-derived growth factor B chain (PDGF-B). When the VHL protein is lost in renal cancers, VEGF, PDGF-B, and other proteins are overexpressed, thereby promoting angiogenesis and tumor cell growth. Defects in the *VHL* gene, including mutation or gene silencing through methylation, also occur in most tumors of patients with sporadic clear cell carcinomas. Tumor angiogenesis also is stimulated by other growth factors that activate Akt and mammalian target of rapamycin (mTOR) signaling, which also increases HIF-alpha expression.[99] Therapies that target VHL-regulated and Akt-signaling pathways have demonstrated significant antitumor activity.

Activating mutations in the MET receptor tyrosine kinase located on chromosome 7 occur in hereditary papillary renal carcinoma and in occasional sporadic papillary tumors.[100] Patients with the syndrome of hereditary leiomyomatosis and renal cancers are at risk for cutaneous and uterine leiomyomas and solitary papillary renal carcinomas.[101] This syndrome is associated with loss of function mutations in the Krebs cycle enzyme fumarate hydratase. Sporadic cases of papillary (or clear cell) renal carcinomas containing chromosomal translocations involving the *TFE3* gene at chromosome Xp11.2 are rare, more commonly occurring in children and young adults. The Birt-Hogg-Dubé syndrome is another rare autosomal dominant disorder characterized by hair-follicle hamartomas of the face and neck and, in some patients, multiple chromophobe or mixed chromophobe–oncocytoma renal tumors.[102] Collecting-duct carcinomas are more similar to transitional-cell carcinoma. Medullary carcinoma, a variant of the collecting-duct subtype, is associated with sickle cell trait or disease.

BIOLOGY

RCC can have a variable natural history that reflects the biology of the histologic tumor type. Oncocytomas are considered benign. Chromophobe carcinomas also are typically indolent and uncommonly result in metastases and cancer-related death.[103] The clinical course of clear cell carcinomas, which compromise the majority of renal tumors, is typically aggressive, although some patients can have an indolent course with stable metastases for years or metastases occurring decades after complete resection of a primary tumor. Molecular studies are attempting to identify markers that may predict prognosis.[104,105] The prognosis for papillary renal cancers is more favorable than clear cell tumors.[106] Papillary tumors have been divided into type 1

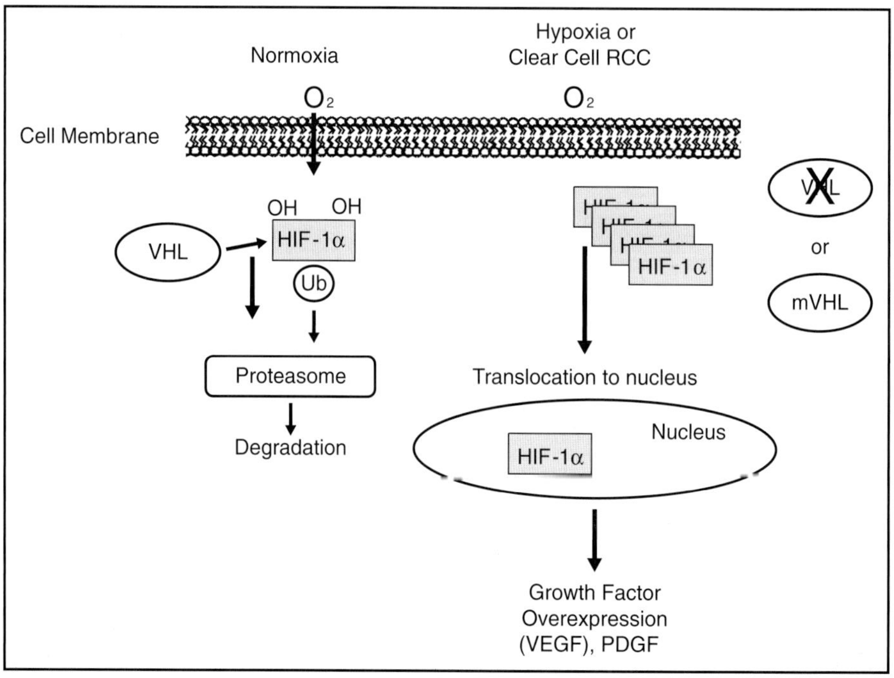

FIG. 9-1 VHL pathway in clear cell renal cancer.

Under normoxic conditions, HIF-1alpha is hydroxylated, allowing VHL to bind and target HIF-1 alpha for ubiquitination and degradation via the 26S proteasome pathway. Under hypoxic conditions, HIF-1 alpha is not hydroxylated or marked by VHL for degradation, resulting in HIF-1 alpha accumulation which translocates into the nucleus to form a complex with HIF-1 beta, which then functions to induce transcription of growth stimulatory genes such as VEGF, PDGF, TGF-alpha, and erythropoietin. Similarly, in clear cell carcinomas where VHL is lost or mutated (mVHL), HIF-1 alpha accumulates, tranlocates to the nucleus, and stimulates growth factor expression which promotes angiogenesis and tumor cell growth. (Abbreviations: VEGF, vascular endothelial growth factor; PDGF, platelet derived growth factor).

and type 2 lesions according to architectural, cytologic, and genetic features, but the biologic relevance of the different subtypes is unclear.[107] Collecting-duct carcinomas have a very aggressive clinical course with more than one-half of patients presenting with metastases[108] and a median survival of a few months for patients with metastatic disease.

SYSTEMIC THERAPIES

Patients with metastatic renal cancer may have a varied, unpredictable, and, in some cases, protracted clinical course. Thus, an important consideration for initiating systemic therapy is the documentation of clinical progression. One nomogram used to predict survival includes no prior nephrectomy, Karnofsky performance status below 80, low hemoglobin level, high corrected level of calcium, and an abnormally high level of serum lactate dehydrogenase as poor prognostic variables. The median survival was 24 months (good risk), 12 months (intermediate risk), and 5 months (poor risk) for patients with no, one or two, or three or more factors, respectively.[109]

RCC is generally highly resistant to single-agent and combination chemotherapy, except in patients with sarcomatoid or collecting-duct carcinomas for whom chemotherapy may be beneficial.[110] The combination of weekly gemcitabine with continuous infusional 5-fluorouracil or oral capecitabine has shown modest activity in clear cell renal cancers.[111] Until 2006, immunotherapy represented the primary treatment for patients with advanced renal cancer. The most extensively studied agents are interferon-alpha and aldesleukin (IL-2). Interferon-alpha has demonstrated low but reproducible response rates of 10% to 20% with occasional durable responses. Response rates greater than 30% have been reported for patients with small-volume disease that is primarily limited to the lung. Two randomized trials showed that patients treated with interferon-alpha compared with those treated with vinblastine or medroxyprogesterone achieved a small survival advantage.[112,113] A dose-response is suggested, as few responses are associated with a dose of less than 3 million units per day, with maximal benefit seen in the dose range of 5 to 20 million units daily. In randomized trials, no consistent survival benefit has been demonstrated with the addition of vinblastine, aldesleukin, 13-cis retinoic acid, or floxuridine to interferon therapy.[114]

Therapy with aldesleukin results in major responses in 10% to 15% of patients with clear cell histology, with complete responses in 4% to 5% of cases. High-dose regimens appear to be more effective than low-dose regimens.[115] Prolonged and durable responses occur more commonly in patients with a good performance status and young age, and in patients whose tumors express carbonic anhydrase IX.[116] Toxicity associated with high-dose bolus interleukin-2 related to increased vascular permeability often necessitates treating patients in an intensive-care setting and has been associated with a 4% incidence of treatment-related death. Aldesleukin has been combined in a variety of doses and schedules with autologous lymphokine-activated killer cells. These cells are obtained by leukapheresis following aldesleukin priming, expanded ex vivo, and then infused again in combination with aldesleukin. Promising early results were not confirmed in randomized comparisons.[117]

Increased expression of VEGF in clear cell renal carcinomas led to a phase II randomized trial of bevacizumab, a humanized VEGF-neutralizing antibody, in patients with cytokine-refractory disease, which demonstrated a 10% response proportion and a prolonged progression-free survival of 4.8 months compared with 2.5 months for patients who received placebo.[118] Hypertension and asymptomatic proteinuria were the most common adverse events. The addition of the epidermal growth factor receptor tyrosine kinase inhibitor erlotinib to bevacizumab improved the response proportion to 25% and the median progression-free survival to 11 months[119]; however, a subsequent randomized study suggested that the addition of erlotinib to bevacizumab was no better than bevacizumab alone.[120] A recent multicenter phase III study compared bevacizumab plus interferon-alpha with placebo plus interferon-alpha as first-line treatment for patients with metastatic RCC. The addition of bevacizumab significantly increased progression-free survival (10.2 vs. 5.4 months; HR = 0.63; $p < 0.0001$) and objective tumor response rate (30.6% vs. 12.4%; $p < 0.0001$). The contribution of adding interferon to bevacizumab therapy is unclear and will require further study.[121]

Sunitinib malate (SU11248) is an oral broad-spectrum receptor tyrosine kinase inhibitor that targets VEGF receptor, PDGF receptor, the Fms-like tyrosine kinase (FLT3), and the c-KIT receptor tyrosine kinase. Two phase II trials in patients who were cytokine refractory demonstrated a response proportion of 41% and progression-free survival of 8.2 months[122,123] and led to U.S. Food and Drug Administration (FDA) approval in 2006 of sunitinib for second-line therapy. A randomized phase III trial of sunitinib compared with interferon in previously untreated patients with clear cell carcinoma demonstrated a 31% objective response rate and a median progression-free survival of 11 months in patients treated with sunitinib compared with a 6% objective response rate and 5-month median progression-free survival for patients treated with interferon.[124] In this study, 90% of patients had undergone nephrectomy, and 93% of patients had good- or intermediate-risk disease. Sorafenib tosylate (BAY 43-9006) is another multikinase inhibitor designed as a c-Raf and b-Raf kinase inhibitor but also inhibits VEGF receptor, PDGF receptor, FLT3, and KIT. Encouraging results from a phase II randomized discontinuation trial of sorafenib in patients with renal cancer[125] led to a phase III randomized study — Treatment Approaches in RCC Global Evaluation Trial (TARGET) — of sorafenib versus placebo for second-line therapy in patients who were cytokine refractory. Based on the results of this study showing that patients receiving sorafenib had a significantly prolonged median progression-free survival compared with placebo (24 vs. 12 weeks), sorafenib was FDA approved for second-line therapy.[126] Similar to studies with sunitinib, patients had clear cell histology, an excellent performance status, good or intermediate-risk disease, and the majority had undergone nephrectomy. Toxicity from this class of drugs includes fatigue, hypertension, diarrhea, hand-foot syndrome, and myelosuppression.

The mTOR inhibitor temsirolimus demonstrated evidence of improved survival in a phase II study of patients with cytokine-refractory RCC,[127] resulting in a phase III, multicentered study in previously untreated patients with advanced RCC. Patients with three or more of the following six poor prognostic factors were randomly assigned to one of three treatment groups: a serum LDH greater than 1.5 times the upper limit of normal, a hemoglobin level below the lower limit of the normal range, a corrected serum calcium level of more than 10 mg/dL (2.5 mmol/L), a time from initial diagnosis of RCC to random assignment of less than 1 year, a Karnofsky performance score of 60 or 70, or metastases in multiple organs. Treatment consisted of 25 mg of temsirolimus weekly, interferon alone, or the combination of 15 mg of temsirolimus weekly plus interferon.[128] Single-agent temsirolimus was associated with an improvement in overall survival compared with interferon (hazard ratio [HR] = 0.73; 95% CI; 0.58, 0.92; p = 0.0078), with a median overall survival of 10.9 months compared with 7.3 months for patients receiving interferon alone. Progression-free survival was 5.5 months for the patients who received temsirolimus and 3.1 months for those who received interferon (HR = 0.66; 95% CI; 0.53, 0.81). The combination treatment did not increase survival. The most common adverse reactions were rash, asthenia, mucositis, nausea, edema, and anorexia. These data led to FDA approval of temsirolimus in May 2007.

The choice of therapy for patients with metastatic renal cancer has significantly increased with three FDA-approved drugs. Variability in trial design and eligibility criteria for the multiple studies make it difficult to compare results and to determine if one agent is superior as a first-line or second-line therapy. Table 9-7 provides the general guidelines suggested at the 2007 Annual Meeting of the American Society of Clinical Oncology. These recommendations will be revised as additional studies are completed and the results reported. There is no proven role for adjuvant cytokine therapy for patients who undergo nephrectomy and who are at high risk for recurrence. Studies examining the potential benefit of multikinase inhibitors as adjuvant therapy are underway. Renal cancer that metastasizes to the bone is typically osteolytic. Treatment with bisphosphonate therapy, such as zoledronic acid, has been shown to decrease the risk of fracture in patients with bone metastases.[129]

PROSTATE CANCER

Prostate cancer represents one-third of all newly diagnosed cancers in men and 10% of cancer deaths. It was estimated that in 2006, 234,460 men would be diagnosed with the disease, of whom 27,350 would die.[1] The 8.5:1 ratio of incidence to mortality indicates that although the disease is lethal for some, most men with prostate cancer die of other causes. Autopsy series show that nearly 70% of men older than 80 have occult prostate cancer. These facts highlight the variable clinical course of prostate cancer. Some prostate cancers may not require immediate intervention because the risk of death from noncancer-related causes may exceed that of the cancer, whereas other cancers may require combined-modality approaches, both to eradicate the tumor locally and to eliminate micrometastases.

TABLE 9-7 Therapeutic Options for Patients with Metastatic Renal Cell Carcinoma

Regimen	Setting	Therapy	Options
Treatment-naïve patient	Good or intermediate risk	Sunitinib ? Bevacizumab with or without IFN	High-dose IL-2 ? Sorafenib
	Poor risk	Temsirolimus Sunitinib	? Sorafenib
Treatment-refractory patient (Second-line therapy or greater)	Cytokine refractory	Sorafenib	Sunitinib
	Refactory to VEGF/VEGFR or mTOR Inhibitors	? Investigational	? Sequential TKI or VEGF Inhibitor

Adapted from presentation by Dr. Ronald Bukowski, ASCO 2007 Annual Meeting.
Risk defined as described in the text.
? Indicates that the stadard of care has not yet been established.
Abbreviations: IFN, interferon; IL-2, interleukin-2; VEGF, vascular endothelial growth factor; VEGFR, vascular endothelial growth factor receptor; TKI, tyrosine kinase inhibitor.

A dynamic, risk-adapted approach helps categorize prostate cancer as a series of states from prediagnosis to death for which the therapeutic objectives are distinct (Fig. 9-2). Each state represents a clinically important milestone for which interventions may be needed based on the risk of developing the disease or, for patients with a prostate cancer diagnosis, the risk of developing or the existence of symptoms, metastases, or death from prostate cancer in a given time frame. Using this framework, it is possible to understand why, in some patients, the risk of developing metastases or symptoms may be years — meaning that the risk of death from noncancer-related causes may exceed that of prostate cancer — while, in others, an immediate intervention may be indicated. Until a patient has progressive castration-resistant disease, he is unlikely to die of his illness. There are several examples of the distinct therapeutic objectives for each state.

- For men who do not have a diagnosis but who may be at high risk for the disease, prevention is the objective.
- For patients with localized disease, the objectives are to identify patients who can be cured by modalities directed at the prostate alone, patients who have tumors of such low biologic potential that they can be safely observed, and patients who have aggressive disease that will require combined-modality approaches aimed at eradicating the tumor locally and eliminating micrometastases.
- For patients with castration-resistant disease, the goal is to eliminate or prevent symptoms of disease and prolong life.

ANATOMY

The prostate is composed of branching tubuloalveolar glands that are arranged in lobules and surrounded by a stroma. Prostatic fluid is secreted through ducts to the urethra and comprises the bulk of seminal emissions. Associated structures are the dorsal vein complex, which is responsible for passive urinary control, and the pelvic plexus, which provides innervation to the pelvic organs and corpora cavernosa through the neurovascular bundle and is responsible for erectile function. Protection of these fibers is essential to preserve potency. The peripheral zone is palpable by digital rectal examination and is the site of origin of 70% of cancers. The transition zone surrounds the urethra and cannot be assessed in this manner. Up to 20% of all cancers develop here, although benign prostatic hypertrophy is more common than prostate cancer in the transition zone.

EPIDEMIOLOGY

One in six men in the United States will develop prostate cancer. Individuals with one first-degree relative diagnosed with prostate cancer have a 2-fold increased lifetime risk, which increases to 4-fold if two or more relatives are affected. Current estimates show that 5% to 10% of all cases of prostate cancer and 40% of cancers occurring at a young age are hereditary and follow a Mendelian inheritance pattern.

Whereas the frequency of histologic cancers at autopsy is similar throughout the world, the clinical incidence is substantially higher in Western countries, which suggests a role for environmental factors. High consumption of dietary fats, in particular the fatty acid a-linoleic acid, is believed to increase risk by 2-fold to 3-fold. Several potential protective dietary factors for prostate cancer incidence have been proposed, including tomatoes (lycopenes), cruciferous vegetables, carotenoids, vitamin E, selenium, fish, long-chain marine omega-3 fatty acids, soy, and polyphenols.[130] Prostate cancer affects ethnic groups differently. Matched for age, the prostates of black men have a greater number of precursor prostatic intraepithelial neoplasia lesions and larger tumors than those of white men.

PATHOLOGY AND MOLECULAR PATHOGENESIS

Prostatic intraepithelial neoplasia is cellular proliferation within glands and acini that appear architecturally benign. Autopsy studies suggest that high-grade disease precedes the development of cancer by 10 years or more; 50% of men with prostatic intraepithelial neoplasia as demonstrated on biopsy results will have cancer in 5 years.[131] More than 99% of the cancers are adenocarcinomas; fewer than 1% are pure ductal and mucinous variants. In atypical prostatic lesions, expression of alpha-methylacyl-coenzyme-A racemase (AMACR) is useful to confirm adenocarcinoma. Other histologic subtypes include small cell tumors and rare mesenchymal tumors (e.g., rhabdomyosarcomas in younger patients and leiomyosarcomas in older patients). Transitional cell cancers of the prostate are confined to periurethral ducts and are more common among patients who have been treated for superficial bladder cancer. Lymphomas and leukemias are the most frequent metastatic tumors to the prostate gland. Gleason grading is the most commonly used system to describe the morphology of prostate adenocarcinomas. Using this system, a score of 1 to 5 for the primary

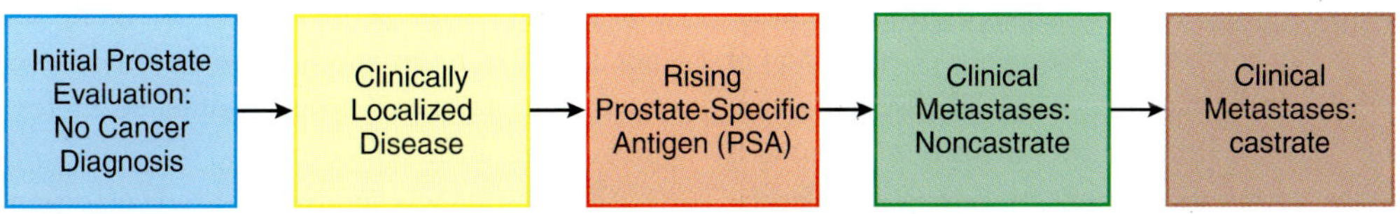

FIG. 9-2 Clinical states of prostate cancer.

Reprinted from Scher HI, Heller G. Clinical states in prostate cancer: toward a dynamic model of disease progression. Urology. 2000; 55(3):323–327, with permission from Elsevier.

and secondary growth patterns of a tumor is described. Pattern 1 tumors are the most differentiated, with discrete glandular formation, whereas pattern 5 lesions are the most undifferentiated, with virtually complete loss of the glandular architecture. The Gleason's score is determined by adding the Gleason's grade of the two most predominant histologies. The higher the Gleasons's score, the more aggressive the tumor and the greater the probability of extracapsular spread, nodal involvement, and the development of subsequent metastases.

The development of prostate cancer involves a multistep process, and specific genetic changes have been identified in tumors representing different clinical stages. Loss of function of genes that detoxify carcinogens may contribute to hypermethylation, which leads to loss of function of multiple genes including the PI-class glutathione S-transferase (*GSTPI*).[132] Gene-expression profiling has identified numerous differentially expressed genes in benign prostatic hypertrophy, as well as in malignant and progressive prostate cancer, but their clinical utility has not been confirmed.[133,134] Recently, a common gene fusion in prostate cancer was identified that brings the androgen regulated gene *TMPRSS2* (21q22.3) and an ETS transcription factor family member together — ERG (21q22.2), ETV1 (7p21.2), or ETV4 (17q21).[135] Among these, the *TMPRSS2-ERG* fusion is the most prevalent, occurring in up to 50% of clinically localized prostate cancers, suggesting that the *TMPRSS2-ERG* fusion may be one of the most common somatic genomic alterations identified in any human malignancy. The clinical and therapeutic implications of this abnormality are under investigation.

Androgens are the primary regulators of prostate cancer cell growth and proliferation. Prostate cancer rarely develops in men who are castrated or who become hypopituitary before age 40. The androgen receptor, located on chromosome Xq11-13, is a member of a super-family of ligand-dependent transcription factors that have a similar structure with different functional domains. Evidence suggests that androgen receptor signaling is important in both the development and progression of non-castrate and castrate-resistant prostate cancer.[136,137]

The molecular abnormalities may differ among primary, metastatic, and castrate-resistant prostate cancers. As such, the targets relevant for the treatment of early-stage disease may not be the same as those targets for late-stage tumors.[138] For example, the frequency of expression of HER2 and BCL-2 is higher in castrate metastatic lesions than in untreated localized tumors.[139,140] In contrast, the frequency of expression of prostate-specific membrane antigen is relatively constant across all clinical stages, although the intensity of staining is higher in castrate metastatic tumors.[141] Potential molecular targets under clinical investigation include HER2, BCL-2, VEGF, the endothelin receptor, inteleukin-6, and prostate-specific membrane antigen.

TUMOR STAGING

The TNM system describes the extent of the primary tumor, status of the regional nodes, and presence or absence of distant metastases. The clinical studies used to assess the primary tumor, including digital rectal examination, transrectal ultrasound, CT, or MRI, are not accurate for determining whether a tumor is organ confined. To improve diagnostic precision, nomograms based on the findings of the digital rectal examination, PSA level, and Gleason score of the tumor are frequently used to predict the probability of capsular penetration and seminal vesicle involvement.

Tumors detected on the basis of an abnormal level of PSA and no palpable disease on digital rectal examination are designated T1c. With the widespread use of PSA testing, stage T1c is the most frequent stage classification at the time of diagnosis. A 1997 modification to the staging system is the requirement that T1c disease be reclassified in the appropriate T category for palpable disease, if a tumor is visible on an imaging study.[142]

EARLY DETECTION AND PROSTATE CANCER SCREENING

Prostate cancer-detection strategies are applied because there is a recognized early stage that can be cured and a later stage that cannot, and the diagnostic tests used — digital rectal examination and measurement of PSA — are convenient and inexpensive. Early detection must be distinguished from screening as the use of a test on select populations who seek an evaluation after being informed of the issues surrounding the assessment.[143] In contrast, screening is the application of a diagnostic procedure on a general population. Individuals considered for screening include patients with nonmalignant enlarged prostates and patients who warrant studies to detect disease on the basis of a family history, an elevated PSA level, or urologic symptoms. They are evaluated to ensure that no cancer is present and are followed to confirm that a cancer does not develop over time.

The need to pursue a diagnosis of prostate cancer is on the basis of symptoms, an abnormal digital rectal examination, or an elevated serum PSA. Obstructive outflow symptoms are the most common. PSA is a single-chain glycoprotein with a molecular weight of 34 kD that functions as a kallikrein-like serine protease that causes liquefaction of seminal coagulum. It is prostate specific but not prostate cancer specific, and elevations may occur as a result of prostatitis, nonmalignant enlargement of the gland, prostate cancer, and biopsy of the prostate. Digital rectal examinations do not alter PSA levels appreciably. The half-life is estimated to be 2 to 3 days, and levels should be undetectable if the prostate has been removed.

PSA testing was approved for early detection in 1994. The American Cancer Society, National Comprehensive Cancer Center Network, the American Urological Association, and the American College of Radiology recommended its use, along

TABLE 9-8 Tests for Screening and Early Detection of Prostate Cancer from the National Comprehensive Cancer Network Guidelines [144]

Diagnostic Modality	Comments
Digital rectal examination	Recommended to be done yearly beginning at age 50 Recommended to be done yearly beginning at age 45 for men at high risk (black men and men with a positive family history)
Prostate-specific antigen (PSA)	Recommended to be determined yearly beginning at age 49 Recommended to be determined yearly beginning at age 45 for men at high risk
PSA density	Ratio of PSA to gland volume (ng/mL/cm^3) May help to distinguish enlargement from cancer, determining PSA density requires ultrasound or an imaging study of the prostate Ratio of more than 0.10 is considered elevated
PSA velocity	Rate of change in PSA level Rate is substantially higher for men with cancer (> 0.75 ng/mL per year), even when the PSA level is within normal limits
Age-specific PSA	PSA usually increases with age, mainly because of benign prostatic hypertrophy Age-specific upper limits of normal for white men: 2.5 ng/mL (age 40 to 49) 3.5 ng/mL (age 50 to 59) 4.5 ng/mL (age 60 to 69) 6.5 ng/mL (age 70 to 79)
Percent free PSA	Most PSA in circulation is complexed to the protease inhibitor ACT Percent free (uncomplexed) to total PSA may discriminate between 4 and 10 ng/mL Cancer is more likely when the free PSA is less than 25% of the total PSA
Transrectal ultrasound	Perform when results of digital rectal examination, PSA, or both, are abnormal Provides helpful information about the prostate volume and suspicious areas for malignant disease Aids in obtaining systematic and directed biopsy specimens

Adapted with permission from Bahnson RR, Hanks GE, Huben RP, et al. NCCN Practice Guidelines for Prostate Cancer. *Oncology* (Huntingt). 2004;14:111–119.
Abbreviation: ACT, alpha-antichymotrypsin.

with a digital rectal examination, on an annual basis for men older than 50 who have an anticipated survival of more than 10 years. It also is advised for men at age 45 who have a family history of the disease, as well as for black men (Table 9-8).[144]

In general, additional diagnostic testing is advised if the PSA level is higher than 4 ng/mL or if the digital rectal examination is abnormal. Abnormal results should be repeated for confirmation.[145] However, the data from the Prostate Cancer Prevention Trial focused on the large number of prostate cancers that can be detected with needle biopsy among men with PSA levels less than the traditional 4.0 ng/mL cutoff, with 21.1% of cancers found in men with PSA levels between 2.6 and 3.9 ng/mL.[146] The diagnosis is established by use of a transrectal ultrasound-guided needle biopsy using a biopsy gun. A minimum of 10 to 12 biopsy cores are advised,[147] and additional biopsies may be warranted if clinically indicated.

The sensitivity, specificity, and positive predictive value have been determined for digital rectal examination and PSA (using a cutoff of 4 ng/mL, Table 9-9).[148] The positive predictive value of an abnormal digital rectal examination is 21%, whereas 25% of men with an elevated PSA level and abnormal digital rectal examination have cancer. Of men with a normal digital rectal examination and a PSA level of 2.5 to 4.0 ng/mL, 17% have cancer. The sensitivity of a serum PSA level of greater than 4 ng/mL is 80% and specificity is 15% to 20%; one man in five or six will have cancer.[149] Conditions that mimic prostate cancer on digital rectal examination include acute and granulomatous prostatitis and a prostatic calculus. When trying to establish a diagnosis, transrectal ultrasound is used to ensure that biopsy specimens encompass all portions of the gland and to estimate prostate volumes for calculation of PSA density. It has no role in screening.

TABLE 9-9 Representative Sensitivity, Specificity, Positive Predictive Value, and Detection Rates of DRE, Serum PSA, and TRUS

Method	Sensitivity (%)	Specificity (%)	PPV (%)	Detection Rate (%)
Digital rectal examination (DRE)	69–89	84–98	26–35	1.3–1.7
Prostate-specific antigen (PSA)	57–79	59–68	40–49	2.2–2.6
Transrectal ultrasound (TRUS)	36–85	41–79	27–36	2.6

Adapted from Cupp MR, Oesterling JE. Prostate-specific antigen, digital rectal examination, and transrectal ultrasonography: their roles in diagnosing early prostate cancer. Mayo Clin Proc. 1993;68(3):297–306, with permission.

PSA testing has produced a shift in the frequency and proportion of men with early-stage disease.[150] Currently, 95% to 99% of PSA-detected tumors are clinically localized, 40% are not palpable, and, of these, 70% are confined to the organ according to pathologic findings. It remains controversial whether prostate cancer screening of the general population will improve prostate cancer mortality. Many clinicians attribute the decrease in the number of deaths from prostate cancer over the past decade to the widespread use of PSA testing. Others assert that the time interval over which PSA testing has been available is too short to have had an effect on death rates. Two large randomized trials of PSA screening for prostate cancer (the Prostate, Lung, Colorectal, and Ovary Cancer trial of the National Cancer Institute and the European Randomized Screening for Prostate Cancer Trial) with the common endpoint of prostate cancer-specific mortality are assessing the effectiveness of screening in men ages 50 to 74 with PSA and digital rectal examination.[151] With the recognition that no randomized trial has indicated a benefit for screening in terms of reducing mortality from prostate cancer, several national groups, including the American College of Physicians and the American Academy of Family Practitioners, modified their positions on screening and recommend that a patient be informed of the implications before PSA is measured.

Improving Specificity and Sensitivity of PSA Testing

PSA testing should be considered as a continuum, particularly as more men are diagnosed on the basis of a change in the measurement. A number of modifications to PSA testing may increase the sensitivity of PSA testing. PSA density is based on the concept that cancers produce less PSA than nonmalignant prostatic tissues; it is determined by dividing the serum PSA concentration by the volume of the prostate gland measured by transrectal ultrasound. Values of 0.15 or less are associated with a higher incidence of cancer.[152] Age-specific normal upper limits were developed to account for the normal enlargement of the gland that occurs with aging, independent of whether a cancer is present.[153]

- Ages 40 to 49: Less than 2.5 ng/mL
- Ages 50 to 59: Less than 3.5 ng/mL
- Ages 60 to 69: Less than 4.5 ng/mL
- Ages 70 to 79: Less than 6.5 ng/mL

Other modifications include PSA velocity, which is the change in the serum PSA level over time. This was developed from the Baltimore Longitudinal Study of Aging in which a rate of rise of more than 0.75 ng/mL per year, even when the PSA level was in the normal range, was associated with a higher frequency of cancer.[154]

PSA exists in serum in a complexed form bound to either alpha-l-antichymotrypsin or beta-2-macroglobulin, two extracellular protease inhibitors. When bound to these elements, the enzyme is inactive but still detectable using conventional immunoassays. For men with total PSA levels of 4 to 10 ng/mL, cancer is more likely if the percent free is less than 25%.[155]

PREVENTION

Depending on the risk of prostate cancer, a prevention approach may be considered. The Prostate Cancer Prevention Trial was a randomized, double-blind, multicenter study designed to investigate the ability of finasteride, a 5 alpha-reductase inhibitor, to prevent prostate cancer in men ages 55 and older. A total of 18,000 men were enrolled, of whom one-half received 5 mg of finasteride daily for 7 years and one-half received placebo. The results indicated a 24.8% reduction in prostate cancer risk among patients treated with finasteride, with a higher frequency of high-grade lesions for this same cohort.[146] It is unclear if the high-grade disease is clinically significant; because follow-up is short with no difference in survival between the two groups, it is difficult to formulate a specific practice policy on the basis of the outcomes. A complementary trial, the Reduction by Dutasteride of Prostate Cancer Events (REDUCE) trial in high-risk men (PSA values between 2 and 10 ng/mL and one prior negative prostate biopsy), has completed accrual.[156]

The Selenium and Vitamin E Cancer Prevention Trial (SELECT) is studying 32,400 men in a double-blind, 2 × 2, factorial design study of selenium and vitamin E alone and in combination for men with PSA levels less than or equal to 4 ng/mL. The endpoint is clinical incidence of prostate cancer.[157] Several large randomized clinical trials studying the utility of vitamin E and selenium in prostate cancer prevention are underway.

MANAGEMENT

Localized Disease

Localized prostate cancers are those confined to the prostate gland without nodal involvement or metastases. Treatment selection is based on the predicted prognosis that considers whether the disease can be eradicated by a treatment directed solely at the prostate, a combined local and systemic approach is necessary for cure, or therapy can be deferred because of a low risk of progression. In general, therapy is aimed at complete local control to decrease future spread while preserving optimal bowel, bladder, and sexual function.

Within each T category are tumors with a range of prognoses, especially for men with T1c disease, mandating the consideration of other factors to assess outcomes and select treatment. Many groups have developed prognostic models based on the combination of the initial T stage, Gleason score, and baseline PSA level. Some prognostic models use discrete cut points; others are nomograms that use PSA level and Gleason score as continuous variables. These algorithms are used to predict disease extent (i.e., organ confined or nonorgan confined and node status), and the probability of success using a PSA-based definition of failure specific to the local therapy under consideration. Specific nomograms have been developed for radical prostatectomy, external beam radiation therapy, and brachytherapy (seed implantation).[158]

Pelvic Lymph Node Involvement

The same probability plots also have been used to determine the yield of diagnostic imaging studies. Most physicians do not advise CT scans unless the PSA level exceeds 20 ng/mL or the tumor is high grade (Gleason 7 or greater). Both MRI and CT scans are used to image the pelvic lymph nodes for local staging of prostatic cancer, although MRI using novel contrast agents may improve sensitivity.[159,160] The FDA approved the radioimmunoconjugate capromab pendetide that recognizes the prostate-specific membrane antigen for the detection of prostate cancer.[161,162] If pelvic disease is documented, systemic hormone treatments are typically recommended.

Distant Metastases

Prostate cancers spread by local extension through the capsule and seminal vesicles, through the lymphatics to regional nodes, or hematogenously to bone and, rarely, visceral sites. Bone metastases are predominantly osteoblastic rather than osteolytic, although both types probably coexist in most cases. Radionuclide bone scans are a cost-effective modality to detect metastases to the skeleton. The yield of a bone scan is low for patients with tumors that are T2 or less, with a Gleason score of less than 7 and a PSA level of less than 10 ng/mL. False-negative results on scans occur in fewer than 1% of patients.[163] CT scans are useful for evaluating focal areas of the skeleton and identifying healing fractures, arthritis, Paget's disease, bone infections, and other inflammatory bone conditions.

THERAPY

Tumors that are confined to the prostate, clinical stage T1a, T1b, T1c, T2a, and T2b, and N0, are generally managed by radical surgery, radiation therapy, or, in some cases, watchful waiting. All are considered options by The American Urological Association Prostate Cancer Clinical Guidelines Panel because data reported in the literature data do not provide clear-cut evidence for the superiority of any one treatment (Table 9-10).[164] In the absence of randomized trials, comparisons between treatments have been limited by selection bias and differences in outcomes reporting, both with respect to cancer control and quality of life. Differences in selection bias relative to cancer control are being addressed with the use of nomograms and other prognostic models, although quality-of-life assessments have become more standardized.

Reported complication rates for each modality vary widely in the literature. For radical prostatectomy, impotence rates range from 25% to 89%, and incontinence figures range from 2% to 47%. The differences are related to the differences in the definitions used, whether the patient or physician is reporting, and the time from the actual treatment to the assessment of symptoms. For example, following surgery, impotence is immediate but patients may recover over time. With radiation therapy, impotence may not be immediate but instead develops over time.

Radical Retropubic Prostatectomy

The goal of radical retropubic prostatectomy is to completely excise the cancer while maintaining urinary control and preserving potency. After the prostate has been removed, PSA levels should decline to undetectable levels. Cancer control is assessed by PSA relapse-free survival, time to objective progression (local or systemic), cancer-specific survival, and overall survival. The procedure continues to evolve as clinicians use biopsy algorithms that include more extensive sampling and imaging to determine both the extent and location of the tumor within the prostate. This approach has resulted in refined selection of cases and surgical planning, which, in turn, has led to more rapid recovery, higher rates of continence, and improved potency. In a large series, continence returned in 2 months and was predicted by younger age and preservation of both neurovascular bundles. Overall, 6% of patients had mild-stress urinary incontinence (requiring one pad daily), 2% had moderate incontinence (more than one pad daily), and 0.3% had severe incontinence that required an

TABLE 9-10 Cumulative Outcomes following Treatment of Clinically Localized (T2) Prostate Cancers

	Radical Prostatectomy	External Beam Radiation Therapy	Brachytherapy	Deferred Therapy
Overall survival (%)				
5-year	68–95	51–93	57–93	67–92
10-year	44–88	41–70	—	34–70
15-year	22–75	31–33	—	—
Disease progression* (%)				
5-year	81–92	32–93	38–90	68
10-year	82	40–64	50–90	53
15-year	70	31–33	—	—
Disease-specific survival (%)				
5-year	90–97	63–96	92–100	83–99
10-year	88–93	66–86	—	84–85
15-year	—	—	—	—

*Many of the reports that included a progression endpoint were not based on measurements of prostate-specific antigen levels.
Modified with permission from Middleton RG, Thompson TM, Austenfeld MS, et al. Prostate Cancer Clinical Guidelines Panel Summary report on the management of clinically localized prostate cancer. The American Urological Association. J Urol. 1995;154(6):2144–2148.

artificial urinary sphincter, with 92% having complete continence at 1 year. With preservation of both neurovascular bundles, erectile function returns in a median of 4 to 6 months. Sacrificing one nerve bundle decreases recovery by 50%. For patients in whom removal of one or both neurovascular bundles is essential to completely excise the cancer, nerve grafts and intraoperative mapping are being explored.[165] Conventional laparoscopic and robotic radical prostatectomy has emerged as a minimally invasive alternative to open surgery for patients with clinically localized prostate cancer.[166]

Radiation Therapy

Radiation can be administered using external beam techniques, an implant or radioactive seeds, or a combination of both. Hormones may or may not be administered. As is the case with surgery, the reported outcomes vary, but most trials consider the proportion of patients who have a decline in PSA levels to less than 0.5 or 1 ng/mL, the proportion with nonrising PSA values, and the proportion with negative findings on biopsy of the prostate 2 years after the completion of treatment. Contemporary external beam radiation therapy incorporates three-dimensional conformal treatment planning with intensity modulation to maximize the administered dose to the tumor while minimizing the exposure of surrounding normal structures. These techniques allow the safe administration of higher doses, which, in turn, have resulted in improved outcomes. Compared with surgery, radiation therapy is associated with a higher frequency of bowel complications, mainly diarrhea and loose stools.

The use of interstitial radiation or implantation of radioactive seeds is based on the principle that deposition of radiation energy in tissues decreases exponentially as a square function of the distance from the radiation source. Older techniques relied on digital placement of the seeds, whereas modern techniques use computer-generated templates to place the seeds more accurately under direct visualization. The result is better cancer control and reduced toxicity. An acute toxicity associated with implantation is substantial urinary frequency. Incontinence is rare, and potency is similar to that observed with radical surgery if age-matched patients are considered.

Four prospective randomized trials have demonstrated that radiotherapy doses less than 70 Gy are inadequate for the curative treatment of clinically localized prostate cancer.[167] It is not clear if doses exceeding 78 to 79 Gy render additional benefit, although higher doses in patients at intermediate and high risk may result in improved biochemical control. The relative efficacy of external beam radiation therapy compared with permanent prostate implants remains controversial. Stage for stage, implants and high-dose radiation appear to achieve similar tumor control rates. Table 9-11 shows a risk-adapted strategy for the management of localized prostate cancer with radiation therapy.[167]

Cryosurgical Ablation and High-Intensity Focused Ultrasound

Cryosurgery and high-intensity focused ultrasound (HIFU) are minimally invasive procedures aimed at local control with low complication rates and favorable functional outcomes. These approaches often are considered for patients who are not suitable for radical surgery or who have local recurrences. Sufficient long-term follow-up is lacking to estimate efficacy regarding prostate cancer-specific mortality.

TABLE 9-11 Risk Adapted Strategy for the Management of Localized Prostate Cancer

	Low Risk	Intermediate Risk*	High Risk
EBRT Field	PORT	WPRT	WPRT
AD: timing and duration	Not Indicated	NCAD (3-6 months)	NCAD and AAD (≥ 2 years)
Brachytherapy	Monotherapy (PPI)	Combined WPRT + BT boost	Combined WPRT + BT boost
Exceptions/Considerations			
Clinical ECE	WPRT + NCAD with or without BT boost	Combined WPRT + HDR boost	Combined WPRT + HDR boost
≥ 50% positive biopsies	Treat like intermediate or high risk	Treat like high risk	
Rapid PSA DT	Consider more aggressive treatment	Consider more aggressive treatment	Consider more aggressive treatment

NOTE: Low risk, T1-T2b, GS ≤ 6 and PSA ≤ 10 ng/mL; intermediate risk, T2b and/or GS 7 and/or PSA 10 to 20 ng/mL; high risk, ≥T2c or GS 8 to 10 or PSA > 20 ng/mL.

Abbreviations: RT, radiotherapy; AD, androgen deprivation; PORT, prostate-only radiotherapy; WPRT, whole-pelvis radiotherapy; NCAD, neoadjuvant and concurrent AD; AAD, adjuvant AD; BT, brachytherapy; PPI, permanent prostate implant; HDR, high dose rate brachytherapy; ECE, extracapsular extension; PSA DT, prostate-specific antigen doubling time; GS, Gleason score.

*For GS 4 + 3 and intermediate-risk patients, consider treating like GS 4 + 4; for GS 3 + 4 with > 90% grade 3, consider treating like low risk.

Adapted from Speight JL, Roach M 3rd. Radiotherapy in the management of clinically localized prostate cancer: evolving standards, consensus, controversies and new directions. *J Clin Oncol.* 2005;23(32):8176–85.

Neoadjuvant and Adjuvant Androgen Deprivation

Neoadjuvant hormone therapy before surgery produces a reduction in the rate of positive surgical margins, from an average of 47% (range, 38% to 64%) to an average of 22% (range, 13% to 34%); however, it has not had an effect on relapse-free survival and is not recommended. The benefit of immediate adjuvant hormonal therapy following surgery in men at high risk for relapse is not proven and is under investigation in randomized trials. Limited studies suggest that perioperative chemotherapy with or without hormone therapy may improve outcomes, but this approach should be considered investigational.

In contrast to surgery, the role of neoadjuvant and concurrent hormone therapy in patients receiving radiation is established. Results of numerous randomized trials suggest that neoadjuvant and concurrent androgen deprivation is beneficial for patients with intermediate risk receiving external beam radiation therapy with an optimal duration of 3 to 4 months;[167] however, 6 months of hormone therapy was associated with a longer time to PSA recurrence and decreased mortality in men with a pretreatment PSA velocity more than 2 ng/mL per year.[168] Patients with high risk also should receive long-term adjuvant hormone therapy for at least 2 years. Pelvic nodal irradiation with concurrent androgen deprivation in patients with intermediate and high risk of nodal involvement remains controversial.

The role for immediate long-term androgen suppression in patients with pathologically documented lymph node involvement is supported by subset analysis of patients with lymph node-positive disease in RTOG 85-31. In this study, patients were randomly assigned to immediate androgen suppression in conjunction with standard external beam radiation therapy and had significantly improved outcomes ($p < 0.0001$) compared with patients who received radiation alone.[169] In another study of patients undergoing radical prostatectomy, patients with lymph node-positive disease at surgery were randomly assigned to undergo castration (surgically or medically) or observation. PSA testing was not in wide use during the conduct of this study, therefore, objective progression was defined as the development of metastases on imaging tests in 89% of patients. At median follow-up of 11.9 years, men assigned immediate hormone therapy had a significant improvement in progression-free survival (HR 3.42 [1.96-5.98], $p = 0.0001$), prostate cancer-specific survival (HR 4.09 [1.76-9.49], $p = 0.0004$), and overall survival (HR 1.84 [95% CI 1.01 3.35], $p = 0.04$).[170] Thus, there is evidence that early (adjuvant) androgen deprivation will benefit patients with node-positive disease.

Watchful Waiting and Active Surveillance

Watchful waiting or deferred therapy is a policy of no therapeutic intervention after a diagnosis has been established until disease progression is evidenced by changes in the PSA level, local tumor growth, or the development of metastases. The approach evolved from studies of predominantly older men with well-differentiated tumors in whom tumor progression was found to occur over a protracted period of time, and in which, during the follow-up interval, a substantial proportion of men died of intercurrent disease. In a structured literature review of patients treated with a deferred approach, radical prostatectomy, or external beam radiation, the 10-year mean weighted survivals were 93% for patients who received radical prostatectomy, 84% for patients treated with a deferred approach, and 74% for patients who received external beam radiation.[171] A recent retrospective population-based cohort study using the Connecticut Tumor Registry indicated that the 20-year prostate cancer-specific survival for men with a Gleason score of 6 or less managed with watchful waiting was 80% to 90%.[172] Active surveillance identifies patients with good risk (defined as a Gleason score of 6 or less, PSA level of less than 10 ng/mL, and T1c to T2a tumors) for delayed intervention who are actively monitored by serial PSA and periodic prostate rebiopsies. Therapy is offered if PSA doubling time becomes less than 3 years or the Gleason score increases to 7.[173] This approach is being evaluated in the randomized Standard Treatment Against Restricted Treatment (START) trial.

Randomized trials to establish the utility of watchful waiting are lacking. A retrospective study of 44,630 men aged 65 to 80 who were diagnosed between 1991 and 1999 with organ-confined, well- or moderately-differentiated prostate cancer stratified according to whether treatment or observation was received found a statistically significant survival advantage associated with treatment (HR = 0.69; 95% CI; 0.66, 0.72).[174] A benefit associated with treatment was seen in all subgroups examined, including older men (aged 75 to 80 at diagnosis), black men, and men with low-risk disease. In a prospective trial of 695 men randomly assigned to watchful waiting or radical prostatectomy, death from prostate cancer occurred in 14% of men assigned to watchful waiting compared with 8.6% of patients who had radical surgery, a reduction in relative hazard of 0.56 (95% CI; 0.36, 0.88). The frequency of distant metastases (relative hazard = 0.60; 95% CI; 0.42, 0.86) and local tumor progression (relative hazard = 0.33; 95% CI; 0.25, 0.44) also was lower.[175] However, the mean PSA value was 12.3 ng/mL, and 74% of patients in the observation arm had T2 disease, making it unclear if these results are applicable to the current U.S. population where nearly one-half of newly diagnosed patients have T1c prostate cancer.

RISING PSA LEVEL

The condition of rising PSA level refers to men in whom the PSA level increases after radical prostatectomy, radiation therapy, or both, with or without hormones, who have no detectable metastases on a scan. It does not refer to increases in PSA levels in patients in whom disease is managed by watchful waiting. Issues in management are whether the rising PSA value represents a local recurrence that could be eliminated with additional treatment to the prostate or prostate bed or whether it represents metastatic disease or both.

LOCAL FAILURE

For men treated with radical surgery, a local recurrence is more likely if the PSA first became detectable more than 1 year after surgery, a PSA doubling time greater than 10 months, the radical prostatectomy specimen contained a cancer of low Gleason sum (less than 7), and there was no seminal vesicle invasion or lymph node metastases in the pathologic specimen.[176] In a retrospective review of 501 patients who received salvage radiotherapy at five U.S. academic tertiary referral centers, predictors of progression were Gleason scores of 8 to 10, preradiotherapy PSA level greater than 2.0 ng/mL, negative surgical margins, PSA doubling time of 10 months or less, and seminal vesicle invasion.[177] Patients with no adverse features had a 4-year progression-free survival of 77%; however, select patients with multiple adverse features previously thought to be destined to develop progressive metastatic disease achieved a durable response to salvage radiotherapy. Other studies suggest that PSA kinetics, and specifically a pretreatment PSA velocity of greater than 2 ng/mL per year, an interval to PSA failure of less than 3 years, and a post-treatment PSA doubling time of less than 3 months, increase the risk for metastases and subsequent prostate cancer-specific mortality, making these men poor candidates for salvage radiation therapy.[178]

Patients treated initially with radiation therapy can be considered for salvage prostatectomy if they were surgical candidates at the time of diagnosis, have a life expectancy of more than 10 years, and have no metastatic disease. Biopsy confirmation of persistent disease in the gland and no evidence of spread are essential before surgery is considered. Despite refinements in case selection, incontinence rates remain high, and virtually all patients are impotent after the procedure.

SYSTEMIC RELAPSE

In most cases, the rising PSA levels represent metastatic disease that has not yet been detected. The time to development of metastases is highly variable. In one series, the median time to metastatic progression was 8 years, and 63% of the patients with rising PSA levels remained free of metastases at 5 years.[176] An issue for these patients is the role of early or deferred androgen ablation when the serum PSA level continues to rise. Guidelines for evaluating and treating men in this state recently have been updated.[179]

CLINICAL METASTASES

Noncastrate

Noncastrate metastatic prostate cancer refers to patients with metastases on an imaging study (either at the time of diagnosis or following local therapy) who have noncastrate levels of testosterone. At this point, the risk of death from prostate cancer exceeds that of noncancer-related mortality. Hormone therapy that negates androgen effects is the standard approach. More than 90% of male hormones originate in the testicles; the remainder are synthesized in the adrenal gland and may contribute up to 40% of the active androgens in the prostate. Surgical orchiectomy is the gold standard but is the least preferred by patients.

HORMONE THERAPY OPTIONS

Hormone options can be divided into those options that lower serum testosterone levels (such as gonadotropin-releasing hormone agonists or antagonists, and estrogens) and antiandrogens that do not lower testosterone but block androgen action. Response to hormone therapy can be measured by decline in PSA values, decrease in the size of nodal or visceral metastases, or improvement in cancer-related symptoms. Overall, 60% to 70% of patients with abnormal PSA levels will have normalization of the value to below 4 ng/mL after castration, 30% to 50% of measurable tumor masses will regress by 50% or more, and approximately 60% of patients will have palliation of symptoms (either urinary or osseous symptoms). Serial bone scans will show improvement in only 30% to 40% of patients. Castration is associated with gynecomastia, impotence, weakness, fatigue, hot flashes, loss of muscle masses, changes in personality, anemia, depression, and loss of bone mass over time. Prolonged time on hormone therapies that lower testosterone can result in osteoporosis. Annual dual-energy x-ray absorptiometry (DEXA) scans are frequently used to screen for the development of osteopenia and/or osteoporosis.[180] Coadministration of bisphosphonates has been demonstrated to reduce the risk of bone loss, but no guidelines currently exist for the frequency of bisphosphonate administration for patients without castration-resistant disease and bone metastases who are receiving hormone therapy.[180,181]

Nonsteroidal antiandrogens, such as flutamide, bicalutamide, and nilutamide, block the binding of androgens to the androgen receptor. They have been evaluated for the following purposes:

- to block the flare secondary to the initial rise in testosterone that results following administration of gonadotropin-releasing hormone,
- to simultaneously inhibit testicular and adrenal androgens as part of a combined androgen-blockade approach, and
- to preserve potency as monotherapy.

The initial rise in testosterone after treatment with a gonadotropin-releasing hormone agonist or antagonist can result in a clinical flare of the disease. These agents are relatively contraindicated as monotherapy for patients with severe pain, urinary symptoms, or spinal cord compromise. Antiandrogens are approved to block the flare. The combination of an antiandrogen and a gonadotropin-releasing hormone analogue also has the additional potential to block the effects of adrenal androgens, which can contribute anywhere from 5% to 45% of the residual androgens present in tumors following surgical castration alone. Whether the antitumor effects of a combined or maximal androgen-blockade approach was superior to castration alone or to gonadotropin-releasing hormone monotherapy was in question for many years. Ultimately, several thousand patients were enrolled in trials with the results showing that antiandrogens do not add to the antitumor effects of surgical castration, but provide a modest improvement for patients treated with gonadotropin-releasing hormone agonists or antagonists. Whether this superiority reflects a true effect on adrenal androgens as postulated, or results from blockade of the potentially negative effect of unopposed androgens following the initial surge of luteinizing hormone, is unclear. In addition, whether the duration of antiandrogen therapy should be short (1 to 3 months) or continuous remains controversial.

Other hormone approaches that have been investigated include high-dose bicalutamide (150 mg), which is associated with fewer hot flashes, less effect on libido, less muscle wasting, fewer personality changes, and less bone loss. Gynecomastia remains a substantial problem, but it can be partially alleviated with prophylactic breast irradiation or the addition of tamoxifen. Whether this approach is equivalent to more traditional therapies that lower testosterone levels is questionable because the results of clinical trials have been conflicting. For patients with established metastatic disease, however, antiandrogen monotherapy was inferior to testosterone-lowering therapy.[182]

EARLY VERSUS DELAYED HORMONE THERAPY

A continuing controversy is the question of early or delayed hormone therapy.[183] Data in support of early hormone therapy date back to the findings from early randomized studies in which diethylstilbestrol or orchiectomy was found to delay the development of metastases in patients with stage T3 disease. In a study conducted by the Medical Research Council, 938 patients with locally advanced or asymptomatic metastatic prostate cancer were randomly assigned to either immediate treatment (orchiectomy or medical castration) or to the same treatment deferred until an indication occurred. Treatment was commenced for local progression almost as frequently as for metastatic disease. Compared with patients treated with deferred therapy, patients treated with early therapy were less likely to have progression from M0 to M1 disease ($p < 0.001$), have pain ($p < 0.001$), and die from prostate cancer.[184]

Several randomized trials provide support for early hormone therapy in conjunction with local therapy in patients with high-risk disease. In one study conducted by Bolla et al.,[185] patients with localized disease were randomly assigned to receive radiotherapy alone or radiation therapy and 3 years of androgen ablation. Although the results showed a survival benefit, the trial was criticized for the poor outcomes in the control group. Ten-year follow-up data of RTOG 8531, which tested whether the use of lifelong hormone therapy after radiation therapy improved outcomes, showed that patients treated with early hormone therapy, when compared with those treated at relapse, respectively, had superior local, biochemical, and distant disease control rates (all $p < 0.0001$) as well as improved disease-specific survival (83% vs. 78%; $p = 0.0053$) and overall survival (47% vs. 38%; $p = 0.0043$).[183,186] Use of early hormone therapy also is supported by the trials previously described in which patients with pathologically confirmed lymph node involvement who received immediate hormone therapy had improved survival.[169,170]

In the Early Prostate Cancer Program, patients with localized disease were randomly assigned to receive 150 mg of bicalutamide or placebo. The primary endpoint was objective clinical progression that included detectable disease in soft tissue or the documentation of bone metastases at 2 years. Early combined results of three trials showed that the proportion of patients in whom osseous metastases developed within 2 years was 9% for patients who received bicalutamide and 14% for patients who received placebo. This finding represented a hazard ratio reduction of 0.58 (95% CI; 0.51, 0.66; $p < 0.001$).[187] No effect on survival was demonstrated. Subgroup analysis showed the greatest benefit in patients with nodal disease.[188] A recent update, however, showed no benefit for early bicalutamide therapy in patients with localized disease at low risk for recurrence.[189]

No prospective randomized study has evaluated the utility of initiating hormone therapy for patients with only PSA progression after definitive local therapy.

Castrate

The treatment of patients with disease that progresses during hormone therapy first requires documentation that the patient is indeed medically castrate (serum testosterone levels less than 50 ng/mL) and then a determination of disease extent. Some patients will have disease that relapses with rising PSA levels alone, others with increasing bone metastases, and still others with soft tissue spread. Disease that relapses is not necessarily refractory to additional hormone treatment. Patients who are taking an antiandrogen are first given a trial of antiandrogen withdrawal, based on the observation that these agents can contribute to the growth of the cancer in its later stages. Thereafter, a second hormone therapy, such as ketoconazole plus hydrocortisone, may be considered, but responses, when they occur, are frequently of short duration (median, 2 to 4 months), and most patients require cytotoxic therapy.

In contrast, for patients with overt symptomatic metastatic disease at the time of hormone initiation, disease typically relapses first with rising PSA levels, followed by progression on a radionuclide bone scan evaluation, then by symptoms. The presence of back pain warrants the exclusion of epidural or cauda equina disease, and, if clinically indicated, an MRI should be done. For approximately 10% to 15% of patients, disease will relapse with aggressive disease locally or in a visceral site, with or without bone disease, where the level of PSA appears to be disproportionately low for the tumor burden present. The results on repeat biopsy may indicate a neuroendocrine phenotype.

> **KEY POINTS**
>
> - A dynamic, risk-adapted approach to prostate cancer progression classifies the disease as a series of states from prediagnosis to death for which the therapeutic objectives are distinct.
> - Prostate-specific antigen (PSA) has an integral role in the diagnosis and management of prostate cancer; however, limitations in PSA sensitivity, specificity, and positive predictive value must be considered when making treatment decisions.
> - Management of the prostate cancer states are sometimes controversial; risks and benefits associated with different treatment modalities should be considered in choosing therapeutic options.
> - Chemotherapy improves survival in men with castrate-resistant metastatic prostate cancer.

Prostate cancers are sensitive to chemotherapy, with overall response rates that are similar to those associated with other tumors for which a survival benefit has been demonstrated. Chemotherapeutic regimens demonstrated antitumor activity as determined by changes in measurable disease, a greater than 50% decline in the PSA level, and objective improvements in bone scan, but had not demonstrated to affect survival.[190,191] In 2004, two randomized trials (Southwest Oncology Group 9916 and TAX 327) were reported that compared docetaxel-based therapy with mitoxantrone and prednisone in patients with castrate-resistant metastatic prostate cancer. These trials demonstrated a significant improvement in overall survival, with a median survival of more than 18 months for patients receiving docetaxel ($p = 0.02$ and $p = 0.009$, respetively).[192,193] Docetaxel also was superior to mitoxantrone with respect to pain response rate, PSA response rate, and quality-of-life indicies.[194] Based on these studies, the FDA approved the use of docetaxel (75 mg/m^2 every 21 days) together with prednisone as front-line therapy. Ongoing randomized trials are assessing whether the addition of a targeted therapy to docetaxel will improve efficacy. The benefit of chemotherapy in patients with castrate, nonmetastatic prostate cancer has not been established.

The lack of a standard effective second-line chemotherapy in castrate-resistant metastatic prostate cancer often has resulted in the use of mitoxantrone as second-line chemotherapy. Other regimens have demonstrated activity as second-line therapy and potentially may be beneficial as third-line therapy in patients with a good performance status.[195,196,197] In patients with neuroendocrine or small cell histologies, use of chemotherapy with platinum-containing regimens also may be beneficial.[198,199]

PALLIATION

An important endpoint for clinical trials is the palliation of pain. Durable relief in selected sites can be achieved with external beam radiation therapy delivered in a focal or hemibody technique. Systemic therapies also can provide palliation. The combination of mitoxantrone and prednisone is FDA approved for the palliation of pain of osseous metastases.[200] Two bone-seeking radiopharmaceutical agents, strontium-89 and samarium-153, have been shown to reduce the pain of skeletal metastases despite the lack of a survival benefit. Zoledronate has been shown to palliate symptoms and reduce the frequency of serious skeletal events, such as new pain, need for radiation therapy, and microfractures.[201] Renal insufficiency has been reported with zoledronate and other bisphosphonate use, and serum creatinines should be monitored and the dose adjusted accordingly. A rare complication of bisphosphonate therapy is osteonecrosis of the jaw, the incidence of which increases with treatment duration and is associated with dental procedures.[202]

SURVIVORSHIP

With early detection and treatment, significant numbers of men will be cured of prostate cancer by radiation or surgery. These patients may have a variety of adverse effects related to therapy, including urinary incontinence, erectile dysfunction, and post-treatment psychosocial issues. Men on hormone therapy suffer from numerous adverse effects, including decreased libido, impotence, decreased lean body mass and muscle strength, increased fat mass, decreased quality of life, and osteoporosis.[203] More recently, it has been recognized that patients on long-term androgen deprivation therapy (12 months or longer) also may develop metabolic complications, such as insulin resistance, hyperglycemia, and metabolic syndrome, which may be responsible for an increased risk of cardiovascular mortality.[204] Men receiving long-term androgen deprivation therapy should be monitored for the development of diabetes, and those who develop an adverse lipid profile should be treated according to the established guidelines for hyperlipidemia.

REFERENCES

1. Jemal A, Siegel R, Ward E, et al. Cancer statistics, 2006. *CA Cancer J Clin.* 2006;56(2):106–130.
2. Lutke Holzik MF, Rapley EA, Hoekstra HJ, et al. Genetic predisposition to testicular germ-cell tumours. *Lancet Oncol.* 2004;5(6):363–371.
3. Powles T, Bower M, Daugaard G, et al. Multicenter study of human immunodeficiency virus-related germ cell tumors. *J Clin Oncol.* 2003; 21(10):1922–1927.
4. Rajpert-De Meyts E, Bartkova J, Samson M, et al. The emerging phenotype of the testicular carcinoma in situ germ cell. *APMIS.* 2003;111(1):267–278; discussion 278–279.
5. Holzbeierlein JM, Sogani PC, Sheinfeld J. Histology and clinical outcomes in patients with bilateral testicular germ cell tumors: the Memorial Sloan Kettering Cancer Center experience 1950 to 2001. *J Urol.* 2003;169(6):2122–2125.
6. Chaganti RS, Houldsworth J. Genetics and biology of adult human male germ cell tumors. *Cancer Res.* 2000;60(6):1475–1482.
7. Reuter VE. Origins and molecular biology of testicular germ cell tumors. *Mod Pathol.* 2005;18 Suppl 2:S51–S60.
8. Bosl GJ, Motzer RJ. Testicular germ-cell cancer. *N Engl J Med.* 1997;337(4):242–253.
9. Garnick MB. Spurious rise in human chorionic gonadotropin induced by marihuana in patients with testicular cancer. *N Engl J Med.* 1980;303(20):1177.
10. International Germ Cell Consensus Classification: a prognostic factor-based staging system for metastatic germ cell cancers. International Germ Cell Cancer Collaborative Group. *J Clin Oncol.* 1997;15(2):594–603.
11. Bosl GJ. Germ cell tumors: there is still plenty to learn. *J Clin Oncol.* 1998;16(4):1244–1247.
12. Kondagunta GV, Sheinfeld J, Motzer RJ. Recommendations of follow-up after treatment of germ cell tumors. *Semin Oncol.* 2003;30(3): 382–389.
13. Carver BS, Motzer RJ, Kondagunta GV, et al. Late relapse of testicular germ cell tumors. *Urol Oncol.* 2005;23(6):441–445.
14. Motzer RJ, Sheinfeld J, Mazumdar M, et al. Etoposide and cisplatin adjuvant therapy for patients with pathologic stage II germ cell tumors. *J Clin Oncol.* 1995;13(11):2700–2704.
15. Kondagunta GV, Motzer RJ. Adjuvant chemotherapy for stage II non-seminomatous germ-cell tumors. *Semin Urol Oncol.* 2002;20(4): 239–243.
16. Bosl GJ, Gluckman R, Geller NL, et al. VAB-6: an effective chemotherapy regimen for patients with germ-cell tumors. *J Clin Oncol.* 1986;4(10):1493–1499.
17. Williams SD, Birch R, Einhorn LH, et al. Treatment of disseminated germ-cell tumors with cisplatin, bleomycin, and either vinblastine or etoposide. *N Engl J Med.* 1987;316(23):1435–1440.
18. Bosl GJ, Geller NL, Bajorin D, et al. A randomized trial of etoposide + cisplatin versus vinblastine + bleomycin + cisplatin + cyclophosphamide + dactinomycin in patients with good-prognosis germ cell tumors. *J Clin Oncol.* 1988;6(8):1231–1238.
19. Kondagunta GV, Bacik J, Bajorin D, et al. Etoposide and cisplatin chemotherapy for metastatic good-risk germ cell tumors. *J Clin Oncol.* 2005;23(36):9290–9294.
20. Loehrer PJ, Johnson D, Elson P, et al. Importance of bleomycin in favorable-prognosis disseminated germ cell tumors: an Eastern Cooperative Oncology Group trial. *J Clin Oncol.* 1995;13(2):470–476.
21. de Wit R, Stoter G, Kaye SB, et al. Importance of bleomycin in combination chemotherapy for good-prognosis testicular nonseminoma: a randomized study of the European Organization for Research and Treatment of Cancer Genitourinary Tract Cancer Cooperative Group. *J Clin Oncol.* 1997;15(5):1837–1843.
22. Bajorin DF, Sarosdy MF, Pfister DG, et al. Randomized trial of etoposide and cisplatin versus etoposide and carboplatin in patients with good-risk germ cell tumors: a multiinstitutional study. *J Clin Oncol.* 1993;11(4):598–606.
23. Horwich A, Sleijfer DT, Fossa SD, et al. Randomized trial of bleomycin, etoposide, and cisplatin compared with bleomycin, etoposide, and carboplatin in good-prognosis metastatic nonseminomatous germ cell cancer: a Multiinstitutional Medical Research Council/European Organization for Research and Treatment of Cancer Trial. *J Clin Oncol.* 1997;15(5):1844–1852.
24. Einhorn LH, Foster RS. Bleomycin, etoposide, and cisplatin for three cycles compared with etoposide and cisplatin for four cycles in good-risk germ cell tumors: is there a preferred regimen? *J Clin Oncol.* 2006;24(16):2597–2598; author reply 2598–2599.

25. Toner GC, Stockler MR, Boyer MJ, et al. Comparison of two standard chemotherapy regimens for good-prognosis germ-cell tumours: a randomised trial. Australian and New Zealand Germ Cell Trial Group. *Lancet.* 2001;357(9258):739–745.

26. Nichols CR, Catalano PJ, Crawford ED, et al. Randomized comparison of cisplatin and etoposide and either bleomycin or ifosfamide in treatment of advanced disseminated germ cell tumors: an Eastern Cooperative Oncology Group, Southwest Oncology Group, and Cancer and Leukemia Group B Study. *J Clin Oncol.* 1998;16(4):1287–1293.

27. Ozols RF, Ihde DC, Linehan WM, et al. A randomized trial of standard chemotherapy v a high-dose chemotherapy regimen in the treatment of poor prognosis nonseminomatous germ-cell tumors. *J Clin Oncol.* 1988;6(6):1031–1040.

28. Motzer RJ, Nichols CJ, Margolin KA, et al. Phase III randomized trial of conventional-dose chemotherapy with or without high-dose chemotherapy and autologous hematopoietic stem-cell rescue as first-line treatment for patients with poor-prognosis metastatic germ cell tumors. *J Clin Oncol.* 2007;25(3):247–256.

29. Loehrer PJ, Gonin R, Nichols CR, et al. Vinblastine plus ifosfamide plus cisplatin as initial salvage therapy in recurrent germ cell tumor. *J Clin Oncol.* 1998;16(7):2500–2504.

30. Motzer RJ, Geller NL, Tan CC, et al. Salvage chemotherapy for patients with germ cell tumors. The Memorial Sloan-Kettering Cancer Center experience (1979–1989). *Cancer.* 1991;67(5):1305–1310.

31. Kondagunta GV, Bacik J, Donadio A, et al. Combination of paclitaxel, ifosfamide, and cisplatin is an effective second-line therapy for patients with relapsed testicular germ cell tumors. *J Clin Oncol.* 2005;23(27):6549–6555.

32. Ronnen EA, Kondagunta GV, Bacik J, et al. Incidence of late-relapse germ cell tumor and outcome to salvage chemotherapy. *J Clin Oncol.* 2005;23(28):6999–7004.

33. Bedano PM, Brames MJ, Williams SD, et al. Phase II Study of Cisplatin Plus Epirubicin Salvage Chemotherapy in Refractory Germ Cell Tumors. *J Clin Oncol.* 2006;24(34):5403–5407.

34. Kollmannsberger C, Beyer J, Liersch R, et al. Combination chemotherapy with gemcitabine plus oxaliplatin in patients with intensively pretreated or refractory germ cell cancer: a study of the German Testicular Cancer Study Group. *J Clin Oncol.* 2004;22(1):108–114.

35. Bhatia S, Abonour R, Porcu P, et al. High-dose chemotherapy as initial salvage chemotherapy in patients with relapsed testicular cancer. *J Clin Oncol.* 2000;18(19):3346–3351.

36. Motzer RJ, Mazumdar M, Sheinfeld J, et al. Sequential dose-intensive paclitaxel, ifosfamide, carboplatin, and etoposide salvage therapy for germ cell tumor patients. *J Clin Oncol.* 2000;18(6):1173–1180.

37. Vaena DA, Abonour R, Einhorn LH. Long-term survival after high-dose salvage chemotherapy for germ cell malignancies with adverse prognostic variables. *J Clin Oncol.* 2003;21(22):4100–4104.

38. Collette L, Sylvester RJ, Stenning SP, et al. Impact of the treating institution on survival of patients with "poor-prognosis" metastatic nonseminoma. European Organization for Research and Treatment of Cancer Genito-Urinary Tract Cancer Collaborative Group and the Medical Research Council Testicular Cancer Working Party. *J Natl Cancer Inst.* 1999;91(10):839–846.

39. Donadio AC, Motzer RJ, Bajorin DF, et al. Chemotherapy for teratoma with malignant transformation. *J Clin Oncol.* 2003;21(23):4285–4291.

40. Oldenburg J, Alfsen GC, Lien HH, et al. Postchemotherapy retroperitoneal surgery remains necessary in patients with nonseminomatous testicular cancer and minimal residual tumor masses. *J Clin Oncol.* 2003;21(17):3310–3317.

41. Oldenburg J, Alfsen GC, Waehre H, et al. Late recurrences of germ cell malignancies: a population-based experience over three decades. *Br J Cancer.* 2006;94(6):820–827.

42. Fossa SD, Horwich A, Russell JM, et al. Optimal planning target volume for stage I testicular seminoma: A Medical Research Council randomized trial. Medical Research Council Testicular Tumor Working Group. *J Clin Oncol.* 1999;17(4):1146.

43. Oliver RT, Mason MD, Mead GM, et al. Radiotherapy versus single-dose carboplatin in adjuvant treatment of stage I seminoma: a randomised trial. *Lancet.* 2005;366(9482):293–300.

44. Loehrer PJ, Bosl GJ. Carboplatin for stage I seminoma and the sword of Damocles. *J Clin Oncol.* 2005;23(34):8566–8569.

45. De Santis M, Becherer A, Bokemeyer C, et al. 2-18fluoro-deoxy-D-glucose positron emission tomography is a reliable predictor for viable tumor in postchemotherapy seminoma: an update of the prospective multicentric SEMPET trial. *J Clin Oncol.* 2004;22(6):1034–1039.

46. Motzer RJ, Rodriguez E, Reuter VE, et al. Molecular and cytogenetic studies in the diagnosis of patients with poorly differentiated carcinomas of unknown primary site. *J Clin Oncol.* 1995;13(1):274–282.

47. van den Belt-Dusebout AW, Nuver J, de Wit R, et al. Long-term risk of cardiovascular disease in 5-year survivors of testicular cancer. *J Clin Oncol.* 2006;24(3):467–475.

48. Nuver J, Smit AJ, van der Meer J, et al. Acute chemotherapy-induced cardiovascular changes in patients with testicular cancer. *J Clin Oncol.* 2005;23(36):9130–9137.

49. Nuver J, Smit AJ, Wolffenbuttel BH, et al. The metabolic syndrome and disturbances in hormone levels in long-term survivors of disseminated testicular cancer. *J Clin Oncol.* 2005;23(16):3718–3725.

50. Travis LB, Fossa SD, Schonfeld SJ, et al. Second cancers among 40,576 testicular cancer patients: focus on long-term survivors. *J Natl Cancer Inst.* 2005;97(18):1354–1365.

51. Richiardi L, Scelo G, Boffetta P, et al. Second malignancies among survivors of germ-cell testicular cancer: A pooled analysis between 13 cancer registries. *Int J Cancer.* 2006;120(3):623–631.

52. Efstathiou E, Logothetis CJ. Review of late complications of treatment and late relapse in testicular cancer. *J Natl Compr Canc Netw.* 2006;4(10):1059–1070.

53. Dahl AA, Haaland CF, Mykletun A, et al. Study of anxiety disorder and depression in long-term survivors of testicular cancer. *J Clin Oncol.* 2005;23(10):2389–2395.

54. Ganz PA. Monitoring the physical health of cancer survivors: a survivorship-focused medical history. *J Clin Oncol.* 2006;24(32):5105–5111.

55. Lee CT, Dunn RL, Williams C, et al. Racial disparity in bladder cancer: trends in tumor presentation at diagnosis. *J Urol.* 2006;176(3):927–933; discussion 933–934.

56. Pelucchi C, Bosetti C, Negri E, et al. Mechanisms of disease: The epidemiology of bladder cancer. *Nat Clin Pract Urol.* 2006;3(6):327–340.

57. Wu XR. Urothelial tumorigenesis: a tale of divergent pathways. *Nat Rev Cancer.* 2005;5(9):713–725.

58. Smith ND, Rubenstein JN, Eggener SE, et al. The p53 tumor suppressor gene and nuclear protein: basic science review and relevance in the management of bladder cancer. *J Urol.* 2003;169(4):1219–1228.

59. Shariat SF, Tokunaga H, Zhou J, et al. p53, p21, pRB, and p16 expression predict clinical outcome in cystectomy with bladder cancer. *J Clin Oncol.* 2004;22(6):1014–1024.

60. Sanchez-Carbayo M, Socci ND, Lozano J, et al. Defining molecular profiles of poor outcome in patients with invasive bladder cancer using oligonucleotide microarrays. *J Clin Oncol.* 2006;24(5):778–789.

61. van Rhijn BW, van der Poel HG, van der Kwast TH. Urine markers for bladder cancer surveillance: a systematic review. *Eur Urol.* 2005;47(6):736–748.

62. Grossman HB, Soloway M, Messing E, et al. Surveillance for recurrent bladder cancer using a point-of-care proteomic assay. *JAMA.* 2006; 295(3):299–305.

63. Brassell SA, Kamat AM. Contemporary intravesical treatment options for urothelial carcinoma of the bladder. *J Natl Compr Canc Netw.* 2006;4(10):1027–1036.

64. Herr HW, Sogani PC. Does early cystectomy improve the survival of patients with high risk superficial bladder tumors? *J Urol.* 2001;166(4): 1296–1299.

65. Herr HW, Bochner BH, Dalbagni G, et al. Impact of the number of lymph nodes retrieved on outcome in patients with muscle invasive bladder cancer. *J Urol.* 2002;167(3):1295–1298.

66. Kassouf W, Leibovici D, Munsell MF, et al. Evaluation of the relevance of lymph node density in a contemporary series of patients undergoing radical cystectomy. *J Urol.* 2006;176(1):53–57; discussion 57.

67. Gerharz EW, Mansson A, Hunt S, et al. Quality of life after cystectomy and urinary diversion: an evidence based analysis. *J Urol.* 2005;174(5): 1729–1736.

68. Fleischmann A, Thalmann GN, Markwalder R, et al. Extracapsular extension of pelvic lymph node metastases from urothelial carcinoma of the bladder is an independent prognostic factor. *J Clin Oncol.* 2005;23(10):2358–2365.

69. Stein JP, Lieskovsky G, Cote R, et al. Radical cystectomy in the treatment of invasive bladder cancer: long-term results in 1,054 patients. *J Clin Oncol.* 2001;19(3):666–675.

70. Bochner BH, Kattan MW, Vora KC. Postoperative nomogram predicting risk of recurrence after radical cystectomy for bladder cancer. *J Clin Oncol.* 2006;24(24):3967–3972.

71. Shariat SF, Karakiewicz PI, Palapattu GS, et al. Nomograms provide improved accuracy for predicting survival after radical cystectomy. *Clin Cancer Res.* 2006;12(22):6663–6676.

72. Kassouf W, Swanson D, Kamat AM, et al. Partial cystectomy for muscle invasive urothelial carcinoma of the bladder: a contemporary review of the M. D. Anderson Cancer Center experience. *J Urol.* 2006;175(6): 2058–2062.

73. Sternberg CN, Yagoda A, Scher HI, et al. M-VAC (methotrexate, vinblastine, doxorubicin and cisplatin) for advanced transitional cell carcinoma of the urothelium. *J Urol.* 1988;139(3):461–469

74. von der Maase H, Sengelov L, Roberts JT, et al. Long-term survival results of a randomized trial comparing gemcitabine plus cisplatin, with methotrexate, vinblastine, doxorubicin, plus cisplatin in patients with bladder cancer. *J Clin Oncol.* 2005;23(21):4602–4608.

75. Sternberg CN, de Mulder P, Schornagel JH, et al. Seven year update of an EORTC phase III trial of high-dose intensity M-VAC chemotherapy and G-CSF versus classic M-VAC in advanced urothelial tract tumours. *Eur J Cancer.* 2006;42(1):50–54.

76. von der Maase H, Hansen SW, Roberts JT, et al. Gemcitabine and cisplatin versus methotrexate, vinblastine, doxorubicin, and cisplatin in advanced or metastatic bladder cancer: results of a large, randomized, multinational, multicenter, phase III study. *J Clin Oncol.* 2000;18(17): 3068–3077.

77. Bamias A, Aravantinos G, Deliveliotis C, et al. Docetaxel and cisplatin with granulocyte colony-stimulating factor (G-CSF) versus MVAC with G-CSF in advanced urothelial carcinoma: a multicenter, randomized, phase III study from the Hellenic Cooperative Oncology Group. *J Clin Oncol.* 2004;22(2):220–228.

78. Rosenberg JE, Carroll PR, Small EJ. Update on chemotherapy for advanced bladder cancer. *J Urol.* 2005;174(1):14–20.

79. Dodd PM, McCaffrey JA, Hilton S, et al. Phase I evaluation of sequential doxorubicin gemcitabine then ifosfamide paclitaxel cisplatin for patients with unresectable or metastatic transitional-cell carcinoma of the urothelial tract. *J Clin Oncol.* 2000;18(4):840–846.

80. Bajorin DF, Dodd PM, Mazumdar M, et al. Long-term survival in metastatic transitional-cell carcinoma and prognostic factors predicting outcome of therapy. *J Clin Oncol.* 1999;17(10):3173–3181.

81. Rasco DW, Assikis V, Marshall F. Integrating metastasectomy in the management of advanced urological malignancies-where are we in 2005? *J Urol.* 2006;176(5):1921–1926.

82. Siefker-Radtke AO, Walsh GL, Pisters LL, et al. Is there a role for surgery in the management of metastatic urothelial cancer? The M. D. Anderson experience. *J Urol.* 2004;171(1):145–148.

83. Herr HW, Donat SM, Bajorin DF. Post-chemotherapy surgery in patients with unresectable or regionally metastatic bladder cancer. *J Urol.* 2001;165(3):811–814.

84. Skinner DG, Daniels JR, Russell CA, et al. The role of adjuvant chemotherapy following cystectomy for invasive bladder cancer: a prospective comparative trial. *J Urol.* 1991;145(3):459–464; discussion 464–467.

85. Stockle M, Meyenburg W, Wellek S, et al. Advanced bladder cancer (stages pT3b, pT4a, pN1 and pN2): improved survival after radical cystectomy and 3 adjuvant cycles of chemotherapy. Results of a controlled prospective study. *J Urol.* 1992;148(2 Pt 1):302–306; discussion 306–307.

86. Stockle M, Meyenburg W, Wellek S, et al. Adjuvant polychemotherapy of nonorgan-confined bladder cancer after radical cystectomy revisited: long-term results of a controlled prospective study and further clinical experience. *J Urol.* 1995;153(1):47–52.

87. Hall RR et al. The Intl Collaboration of Trialists of the MRC Advanced Bladder Cancer Group, MRC Clinical Trials Unit. ASCO Annual Meeting. *Proc Am Soc Clin Oncol.* 2002:21:Abstract 710, No. 18S.

88. Grossman HB, Natale RB, Tangen CM, et al. Neoadjuvant chemotherapy plus cystectomy compared with cystectomy alone for locally advanced bladder cancer. *N Engl J Med.* 2003;349(9): 859–866.

89. Advanced Bladder Cancer Meta-analysis Collaboration. Neoadjuvant chemotherapy in invasive bladder cancer: a systematic review and meta-analysis. *Lancet.* 2003;361(9373):1927–1934.

90. Shipley WU, Kaufman DS, Zehr E, et al. Selective bladder preservation by combined modality protocol treatment: long-term outcomes of 190 patients with invasive bladder cancer. *Urology.* 2002;60(1):62–67; discussion 67–68.

91. Shipley WU, Winter KA, Kaufman DS, et al. Phase III trial of neoadjuvant chemotherapy in patients with invasive bladder cancer treated with selective bladder preservation by combined radiation therapy and chemotherapy: initial results of Radiation Therapy Oncology Group 89–03. *J Clin Oncol.* 1998;16(11):3576–3583.

92. Chow WH, Gridley G, Fraumeni JF Jr., et al. Obesity, hypertension, and the risk of kidney cancer in men. *N Engl J Med.* 2000;343(18): 1305–1311.

93. Delpre G, Ilie B, Papo J, et al. Hypernephroma with nonmetastatic liver dysfunction (Stauffer's syndrome) and hypercalcemia. Case report and review of the literature. *Am J Gastroenterol.* 1979;72(3): 239–247.

94. Flanigan RC, Mickisch G, Sylvester R, et al. Cytoreductive nephrectomy in patients with metastatic renal cancer: a combined analysis. *J Urol.* 2004;171(3):1071–1076.

95. Kovacs G, Akhtar M, Beckwith BJ, et al. The Heidelberg classification of renal cell tumours. *J Pathol.* 1997;183(2):131–133.

96. Cohen HT, McGovern FJ. Renal-cell carcinoma. *N Engl J Med.* 2005;353(23):2477–2490.

97. Linehan WM, Grubb RL, Coleman JA, et al. The genetic basis of cancer of kidney cancer: implications for gene-specific clinical management. *BJU Int.* 2005;95(Suppl 2):2–7.

98. Kim WY, Kaelin WG. Role of VHL gene mutation in human cancer. *J Clin Oncol.* 2004;22(24):4991–5004.

99. Hudson CC, Liu M, Chiang GG, et al. Regulation of hypoxia-inducible factor 1 alpha expression and function by the mammalian target of rapamycin. *Mol Cell Biol.* 2002;22(20):7004–7014.

100. Schmidt L, Duh FM, Chen F, et al. Germline and somatic mutations in the tyrosine kinase domain of the MET proto-oncogene in papillary renal carcinomas. *Nat Genet.* 1997;16(1):68–73.

101. Wei MH, Toure O, Glenn GM, et al. Novel mutations in FH and expansion of the spectrum of phenotypes expressed in families with hereditary leiomyomatosis and renal cell cancer. *J Med Genet.* 2006;43(1):18–27.

102. Nickerson ML, Warren MB, Toro JR, et al. Mutations in a novel gene lead to kidney tumors, lung wall defects, and benign tumors of the hair follicle in patients with the Birt-Hogg-Dube syndrome. *Cancer Cell.* 2002;2(2):157–164.

103. Cindolo L, de la Taille A, Schips L, et al. Chromophobe renal cell carcinoma: comprehensive analysis of 104 cases from multicenter European database. *Urology.* 2005;65(4):681–686.

104. Kim HL, Seligson D, Liu X, et al. Using tumor markers to predict the survival of patients with metastatic renal cell carcinoma. *J Urol.* 2005;173(5):1496–1501.

105. Jones J, Otu H, Spentzos D, et al. Gene signatures of progression and metastasis in renal cell cancer. *Clin Cancer Res.* 2005;11(16):5730–5739.

106. Beck SD, Patel MI, Snyder ME, et al. Effect of papillary and chromophobe cell type on disease-free survival after nephrectomy for renal cell carcinoma. *Ann Surg Oncol.* 2004;11(1):71–77.

107. Yang XJ, Tan MH, Kim HL, et al. A molecular classification of papillary renal cell carcinoma. *Cancer Res.* 2005;65(13):5628–5637.

108. Motzer RJ, Bacik J, Mariani T, et al. Treatment outcome and survival associated with metastatic renal cell carcinoma of non-clear-cell histology. *J Clin Oncol.* 2002;20(9):2376–2381.

109. Motzer RJ, Mazumdar M, Bacik J, et al. Survival and prognostic stratification of 670 patients with advanced renal cell carcinoma. 1999; 17(8):2530.

110. Nanus DM, Garino A, Milowsky MI, et al. Active chemotherapy for sarcomatoid and rapidly progressing renal cell carcinoma. *Cancer.* 2004;101(7):1545–1551.

111. Stadler WM, Halabi S, Rini B, et al. A phase II study of gemcitabine and capecitabine in metastatic renal cancer: a report of Cancer and Leukemia Group B protocol 90008. *Cancer.* 2006;107(6):1273–1279.

112. Pyrhonen S, Salminen E, Ruutu M, et al. Prospective randomized trial of interferon alfa-2a plus vinblastine versus vinblastine alone in patients with advanced renal cell cancer. *J Clin Oncol.* 1999; 17(9):2859.

113. Interferon-alpha and survival in metastatic renal carcinoma: early results of a randomised controlled trial. Medical Research Council Renal Cancer Collaborators. *Lancet.* 1999;353(9146):14–17.

114. Gitlitz BJ, Figlin RA. Cytokine-based therapy for metastatic renal cell cancer. *Urol Clin North Am.* 2003;30(3):589–600.

115. McDermott DF, Regan MM, Clark JI, et al. Randomized phase III trial of high-dose interleukin-2 versus subcutaneous interleukin-2 and interferon in patients with metastatic renal cell carcinoma. *J Clin Oncol.* 2005;23(1):133–141.

116. Atkins M, Regan M, McDermott D, et al. Carbonic anhydrase IX expression predicts outcome of interleukin 2 therapy for renal cancer. *Clin Cancer Res.* 2005;11(10):3714–3721.

117. Atkins MB, Dutcher J, Weiss G, et al. Kidney cancer: the Cytokine Working Group experience (1986–2001): part I. IL-2-based clinical trials. *Med Oncol.* 2001;18(3):197–207.

118. Yang JC, Haworth L, Sherry RM, et al. A randomized trial of bevacizumab, an anti-vascular endothelial growth factor antibody, for metastatic renal cancer. *N Engl J Med.* 2003;349(5):427–434.

119. Hainsworth JD, Sosman JA, Spigel DR, et al. Treatment of metastatic renal cell carcinoma with a combination of bevacizumab and erlotinib. *J Clin Oncol.* 2005;23(31):7889–7896.

120. Journal of Clinical Oncology, 2006 *ASCO Annual Meeting Proceedings.* Vol 24, No. 18S (June 20 Supplement), 2006:4523.

121. Journal of Clinical Oncology, 2007 *ASCO Annual Meeting Proceedings.* Vol 25, No. 18S (June 20 Supplement), 2007:2.

122. Motzer RJ, Michaelson MD, Redman BG, et al. Activity of SU11248, a multitargeted inhibitor of vascular endothelial growth factor receptor and platelet-derived growth factor receptor, in patients with metastatic renal cell carcinoma. *J Clin Oncol.* 2006;24(1):16–24.

123. Motzer RJ, Rini BI, Bukowski RM, et al. Sunitinib in patients with metastatic renal cell carcinoma. *JAMA.* 2006;295(21):2516–2524.

124. Motzer RJ, Hutson TE, Tomczak P, et al. Sunitinib versus interferon alfa in metastatic renal cell carcinoma. *N Engl J Med.* 2007;356 (2):115–124.

125. Ratain MJ, Eisen T, Stadler WM, et al. Phase II placebo-controlled randomized discontinuation trial of sorafenib in patients with metastatic renal cell carcinoma. *J Clin Oncol.* 2006;24(16): 2505–2512.

126. Journal of Clinical Oncology, 2006 *ASCO Annual Meeting Proceedings.* Vol 24, No. 18S (June 20 Supplement), 2006:4510.

127. Atkins MB, Hidalgo M, Stadler WM, et al. Randomized phase II study of multiple dose levels of CCI-779, a novel mammalian target of rapamycin kinase inhibitor, in patients with advanced refractory renal cell carcinoma. *J Clin Oncol.* 2004;22(5):909–918.

128. Hudes G, Carducci M, Tomczak P, et al. Temsirolimus, interferon alfa, or both for advanced renal-cell carcinoma. *N Engl J Med.* 2007; 356(22):2271–2281.

129. Lipton A, Zheng M, Seaman J. Zoledronic acid delays the onset of skeletal-related events and progression of skeletal disease in patients with advanced renal cell carcinoma. *Cancer.* 2003;98(5):962–969.

130. Chan JM, Gann PH, Giovannucci EL. Role of diet in prostate cancer development and progression. *J Clin Oncol.* 2005;23(32):8152–8160.

131. DeMarzo AM, Nelson WG, Isaacs WB, et al. Pathological and molecular aspects of prostate cancer. *Lancet.* 2003;361(9361):955–964.

132. Bastian PJ, Yegnasubramanian S, Palapattu GS, et al. Molecular biomarker in prostate cancer: the role of CpG island hypermethylation. *Eur Urol.* 2004;46(6):698–708.

133. Huppi K, Chandramouli GV. Molecular profiling of prostate cancer. *Curr Urol Rep.* 2004;5(1):45–51.

134. Stephenson AJ, Smith A, Kattan MW, et al. Integration of gene expression profiling and clinical variables to predict prostate carcinoma recurrence after radical prostatectomy. *Cancer.* 2005;104(2):290–298.

135. Tomlins SA, Rhodes DR, Perner S, et al. Recurrent fusion of TMPRSS2 and ETS transcription factor genes in prostate cancer. *Science.* 2005;310(5748):644–648.

136. Feldman BJ, Feldman D. The development of androgen-independent prostate cancer. *Nat Rev Cancer.* 2001;1(1):34–45.

137. Scher HI, Sawyers CL. Biology of progressive, castration-resistant prostate cancer: directed therapies targeting the androgen-receptor signaling axis. *J Clin Oncol.* 2005;23(32):8253–8261.

138. Scher HI. Prostate carcinoma: defining therapeutic objectives and improving overall outcomes. *Cancer.* 2003;97(3 Suppl):758–771.

139. McDonnell TJ, Troncoso P, Brisbay SM, et al. Expression of the protooncogene bcl-2 in the prostate and its association with emergence of androgen-independent prostate cancer. *Cancer Res.* 1992; 52(24):6940–6944.

140. Morris MJ, Reuter VE, Kelly WK, et al. HER-2 profiling and targeting in prostate carcinoma. *Cancer.* 2002;94(4):980–986.

141. Ross JS, Gray KE, Webb IJ, et al. Antibody-based therapeutics: focus on prostate cancer. *Cancer Metastasis Rev.* 2005;24(4):521–537.

142. Iyer RV, Hanlon AL, Pinover WH, et al. Outcome evaluation of the 1997 American Joint Committee on Cancer staging system for prostate carcinoma treated by radiation therapy. *Cancer.* 1999;85(8): 1816–1821.

143. Chan EC, Sulmasy DP. What should men know about prostate-specific antigen screening before giving informed consent? *Am J Med.* 1998;105(4):266–274.

144. Bahnson RR, Hanks GE, Huben RP, et al. NCCN Practice Guidelines for Prostate Cancer. *Oncology* (Williston Park). 2004;14(11A):111–119.

145. Eastham JA, Riedel E, Scardino PT, et al. Variation of serum prostate-specific antigen levels: an evaluation of year-to-year fluctuations. *JAMA.* 2003;289(20):2695–2700.

146. Thompson IM, Goodman PJ, Tangen CM, et al. The influence of finasteride on the development of prostate cancer. *N Engl J Med.* 2003;349(3):215–224.

147. Singh H, Canto EI, Shariat SF, et al. Improved detection of clinically significant, curable prostate cancer with systematic 12-core biopsy. *J Urol.* 2004;171(3):1089–1092.

148. Cupp MR, Oesterling JE. Prostate-specific antigen, digital rectal examination, and transrectal ultrasonography: their roles in diagnosing early prostate cancer. *Mayo Clin Proc.* 1993;68(3):297–306.

149. Ohori M, Scardino PT. Localized prostate cancer. *Curr Probl Surg.* 2002;39(9):833–957.

150. Miller DC, Hafez KS, Stewart A, et al. Prostate carcinoma presentation, diagnosis, and staging: an update form the National Cancer Data Base. *Cancer.* 2003;98(6):1169 1178.

151. Schroder FH. Detection of prostate cancer: the impact of the European Randomized Study of Screening for Prostate Cancer (ERSPC). *Can J Urol.* 2005;Suppl 1:2-6; discussion 92–93.

152. Seaman E, Whang M, Olsson CA, Katz A, Cooner WH, Benson MC. PSA density (PSAD). Role in patient evaluation and management. *Urol Clin North Am.* 1993;20:653–663.

153. Oesterling JE, Jacobsen SJ, Chute CG et al. Serum prostate-specific antigen in a community-based population of healthy men. Establishment of age-specific reference ranges. *JAMA.* 1993;270:860–864.

154. Carter HB, Morrell CH, Pearson JD, et al. Estimation of prostatic growth using serial prostate-specific antigen measurements in men with and without prostate disease. *Cancer Res.* 1992;52(12): 3323–3328.

155. Catalona WJ, Partin AW, Slawin KM, et al. Use of the percentage of free prostate-specific antigen to enhance differentiation of prostate cancer from benign prostatic disease: a prospective multicenter clinical trial. *JAMA.* 1998;279(19):1542–1547.

156. Andriole G, Bostwick D, Brawley O, et al. Chemoprevention of prostate cancer in men at high risk: rationale and design of the reduction by dutasteride of prostate cancer events (REDUCE) trial. *J Urol.* 2004;172(4 Pt 1):1314–1317.

157. Lippman SM, Goodman PJ, Klein EA, et al. Designing the Selenium and Vitamin E Cancer Prevention Trial (SELECT). *J Natl Cancer Inst.* 2005;97(2):94–102.

158. Stephenson AJ, Kattan MW. Nomograms for prostate cancer. *BJU Int.* 2006;98(1):39–46.

159. Harisinghani MG, Barentsz J, Hahn PF, et al. Noninvasive detection of clinically occult lymph-node metastases in prostate cancer. *N Engl J Med.* 2003;348(25):2491–2499.

160. Ross R, Harisinghani M. New clinical imaging modalities in prostate cancer. *Hematol Oncol Clin North Am.* 2006;20(4):811–830.

161. Freeman LM, Krynyckyi BR, Li Y, et al. The role of (111) In Capromab Pendetide (Prosta-ScintR) immunoscintigraphy in the management of prostate cancer. *Q J Nucl Med.* 2002;46(2):131–137.

162. Keane TE, Rosner IL, Wingo MS, et al. The emergence of radioimmunoscintigraphy for prostate cancer. *Rev Urol.* 2006;8 Suppl 1: S20–S28.

163. Oesterling JE. Using PSA to eliminate the staging radionuclide bone scan. Significant economic implications. *Urol Clin North Am.* 1993; 20(4):705–711.

164. Middleton RG, Thompson IM, Austenfeld MS, et al. Prostate Cancer Clinical Guidelines Panel Summary report on the management of clinically localized prostate cancer. The American Urological Association. *J Urol.* 1995;154(6):2144–2148.

165. Sim HG, Kliot M, Lange PH, et al. Two-year outcome of unilateral sural nerve interposition graft after radical prostatectomy. *Urology.* 2006;68(6):1290–1294.

166. Menon M, Shrivastava A, Tewari A. Laparoscopic radical prostatectomy: conventional and robotic. *Urology.* 2005;66(5 Suppl):101–104.

167. Speight JL, Roach M 3rd. Radiotherapy in the management of clinically localized prostate cancer: evolving standards, consensus, controversies and new directions. *J Clin Oncol.* 2005;23(32):8176–8185.

168. D'Amico AV, Loffredo M, Renshaw AA, et al. Six-month androgen suppression plus radiation therapy compared with radiation therapy alone for men with prostate cancer and a rapidly increasing pretreatment prostate-specific antigen level. *J Clin Oncol.* 2006;24(25): 4190–4195.

169. Lawton CA, Winter K, Grignon D, et al. Androgen suppression plus radiation versus radiation alone for patients with stage D1/pathologic node-positive adenocarcinoma of the prostate: updated results based on national prospective randomized trial Radiation Therapy Oncology Group 85–31. *J Clin Oncol.* 2005;23(34):800–807.

170. Messing EM, Manola J, Yao J, et al. Immediate versus deferred androgen deprivation treatment in patients with node-positive prostate cancer after radical prostatectomy and pelvic lymphadenectomy. *Lancet Oncol.* 2006;7(6):472–479.

171. Chodak GW, Thisted RA, Gerber GS, et al. Results of conservative management of clinically localized prostate cancer. *N Engl J Med.* 1994;330(4):242–248.

172. Albertsen PC, Hanley JA, Fine J. 20-year outcomes following conservative management of clinically localized prostate cancer. *JAMA.* 2005;293(17):2095–2101.

173. Klotz L. Active surveillance for prostate cancer: for whom? *J Clin Oncol.* 2005;23(32):8165–8169.

174. Wong YN, Mitra N, Hudes G, et al. Survival associated with treatment vs observation of localized prostate cancer in elderly men. *JAMA.* 2006;296(22):2683–2693.

175. Bill-Axelson A, Holmberg L, Ruutu M, et al. Radical prostatectomy versus watchful waiting in early prostate cancer. *N Engl J Med.* 2005;352(19):1977–1984.

176. Pound CR, Partin AW, Eisenberger MA, et al. Natural history of progression after PSA elevation following radical prostatectomy. *JAMA.* 1999;281(17):1591–1597.

177. Stephenson AJ, Shariat SF, Zelefsky MJ, et al. Salvage radiotherapy for recurrent prostate cancer after radical prostatectomy. *JAMA.* 2004;291(11):1325–1332.

178. Lee AK, D'Amico AV. Utility of prostate-specific antigen kinetics in addition to clinical factors in the selection of patients for salvage local therapy. *J Clin Oncol.* 2005;23(32):8192–8197.

179. Loblaw DA, Virgo KS, Nam R, et al. Initial hormonal management of androgen-sensitive metastatic, recurrent, or progressive prostate cancer: 2006 update of an American Society of Clinical Oncology practice guideline. *J Clin Oncol.* 2007;25(12):1596–1605.

180. Smith MR. Treatment-related osteoporosis in men with prostate cancer. *Clin Cancer Res.* 2006;12(20 Pt 2):6315s–6319s.

181. Michaelson MD, Kaufman DS, Lee H, et al. Randomized controlled trial of annual zoledronic acid to prevent gonadotropin-releasing hormone agonist-induced bone loss in men with prostate cancer. *J Clin Oncol.* 2007;25(9):1038–1042.

182. Tyrrell CJ, Kaisary AV, Iversen P, et al. A randomised comparison of 'Casodex' (bicalutamide) 150 mg monotherapy versus castration in the treatment of metastatic and locally advanced prostate cancer. *Eur Urol.* 1998;33(5):447–456.

183. Ryan CJ, Small EJ. Early versus delayed androgen deprivation for prostate cancer: new fuel for an old debate. *J Clin Oncol.* 2005;23(32): 8225–8231.

184. Immediate versus deferred treatment for advanced prostatic cancer: initial results of the Medical Research Council Trial. The Medical Research Council Prostate Cancer Working Party Investigators Group. *Br J Urol.* 1997;79(2):235–246.

185. Bolla M, Collette L, Blank L, et al. Long-term results with immediate androgen suppression and external irradiation in patients with locally advanced prostate cancer (an EORTC study): a phase III randomised trial. *Lancet.* 2002;360(9327):103–106.

186. Lawton CA, Winter K, Grignon D, Pilepich MV. Androgen suppression plus radiation versus radiation alone for patients with stage D1/pathologic node-positive adenocarcinoma of the prostate: updated results based on national prospective randomized trial Radiation Therapy Oncology Group 85–31. *J Clin Oncol.* 2005; 23(4): 800–807.

187. See WA, Wirth MP, McLeod DG, et al. Bicalutamide as immediate therapy either alone or as adjuvant to standard care of patients with localized or locally advanced prostate cancer: first analysis of the early prostate cancer program. *J Urol.* 2002;168(2):429–435.

188. Iversen P, Wirth MP, See WA, et al. Is the efficacy of hormonal therapy affected by lymph node status? data from the bicalutamide (Casodex) Early Prostate Cancer program. *Urology.* 2004;63(5):928–933.

189. McLeod DG, See WA, Klimberg I, et al. The bicalutamide 150 mg early prostate cancer program: findings of the North American trial at 7.7-year median followup. *J Urol.* 2006;176(1):75–80.

190. Kelly WK, Curley T, Slovin S, et al. Paclitaxel, estramustine phosphate, and carboplatin in patients with advanced prostate cancer. *J Clin Oncol.* 2001;19(1):44–53.

191. Tannock IF, Osoba D, Stockler MR, et al. Chemotherapy with mitoxantrone plus prednisone or prednisone alone for symptomatic hormone-resistant prostate cancer: a Canadian randomized trial with palliative end points. *J Clin Oncol.* 1996;14(16):1756–1764.

192. Petrylak DP, Tangen CM, Hussain MH, et al. Docetaxel and estramustine compared with mitoxantrone and prednisone for advanced refractory prostate cancer. *N Engl J Med.* 2004;351(15):1513–1520.

193. Tannock IF, de Wit R, Berry WR, et al. Docetaxel plus prednisone or mitoxantrone plus prednisone for advanced prostate cancer. *N Engl J Med.* 2004;351(15):1502–1512.

194. Berry DL, Moinpour CM, Jiang CS, et al. Quality of life and pain in advanced stage prostate cancer: results of a Southwest Oncology Group randomized trial comparing docetaxel and estramustine to mitoxantrone and prednisone. *J Clin Oncol.* 2006;24(18):2828–2835.

195. Berthold DR, Sternberg CN, Tannock IF. Management of advanced prostate cancer after first-line chemotherapy. *J Clin Oncol.* 2005;23(32):8247–8252.

196. Nakabayashi M, Ling J, Xie W, et al. Response to vinorelbine with or without estramustine as second-line chemotherapy in patients with hormone-refractory prostate cancer. *Cancer J.* 2007;13(2):125–129.

197. Oh WK, Tay MH, Huang J. Is there a role for platinum chemotherapy in the treatment of patients with hormone-refractory prostate cancer? *Cancer.* 2007;109(3):477–486.

198. Papandreou CN, Daliani DD, Thall PF, et al. Results of a phase II study with doxorubicin, etoposide, and cisplatin in patients with fully characterized small-cell carcinoma of the prostate. *J Clin Oncol.* 2002;20(14):3072–3080.

199. Steineck G, Reuter V, Kelly WK, et al. Cytotoxic treatment of aggressive prostate tumors with or without neuroendocrine elements. *Acta Oncol.* 2002;41(7–8):668–674.

200. Tannock IF, Osoba D, Stockler MR, et al. Chemotherapy with mitoxantrone plus prednisone or prednisone alone for symptomatic hormone-resistant prostate cancer: a Canadian randomized trial with palliative end points. *J Clin Oncol.* 1996;14(6):1756–1764.

201. Saad F, Gleason DM, Murray R, et al. Long-term efficacy of zoledronic acid for the prevention of skeletal complications in patients with metastatic hormone-refractory prostate cancer. *J Natl Cancer Inst.* 2004;96(11):879–882.

202. Bamias A, Kastritis E, Bamia C, et al. Osteonecrosis of the jaw in cancer after treatment with bisphosphonates: incidence and risk factors. *J Clin Oncol.* 2005;23(34):8580–8587.

203. Basaria S, Lieb J, Tang AM, et al. Long-term effects of androgen deprivation therapy in prostate cancer patients. *Clin Endocrinol (Oxf).* 2002;56(6):779–786.

204. Braga-Basaria M, Dobs AS, Muller DC, et al. Metabolic syndrome in men with prostate cancer undergoing long-term androgen-deprivation therapy. *J Clin Oncol.* 2006;24(24):3979–3983.

10

GYNECOLOGIC CANCERS

Maurie Markman, MD

LEARNING OBJECTIVES

After reviewing this chapter, the reader should be able to

- Recommend appropriate screening for cervical cancer
- Explain the importance of human papillomavirus (HPV) vaccine strategies for the prevention of cervical cancer
- Select the most appropriate management options for cervical cancer based on stage and patient prognosis
- Advise patients regarding the risk factors for endometrial cancer
- Develop and implement appropriate management strategies for endometrial cancer
- Review the epidemiology of ovarian cancer
- Summarize the role of surgical staging and cytoreduction for the management of ovarian cancer
- Determine when both primary and second-line chemotherapy are appropriate options for the treatment of ovarian cancer

Cervical cancer is the most common cause of death from gynecologic cancers worldwide. It is estimated that more than 450,000 new cases of invasive cervical cancer are diagnosed throughout the world each year.[1] Unfortunately, because many developing countries lack satisfactory screening strategies and reporting mechanisms, the total incidence of this disease probably is underestimated. With the routine use of Pap smears, the incidence of cervical cancer in the United States has steadily declined over the past several decades. There were approximately 11,200 new cases and 3,700 deaths in 2007.[2] The mean age at the time of diagnosis of cervical cancer is approximately 50 years. Older women tend to present with higher-stage disease, which suggests a lack of screening in that patient population.

CERVICAL CANCER

EPIDEMIOLOGY AND RISK FACTORS

The risk factors for cervical cancer are the same as those for human papillomavirus (HPV) infection, which is essentially a sexually transmitted disease. These include early coitarche, multiple sexual partners, having partners who have had multiple sexual partners, and immunosuppression including human immunodeficiency virus (HIV) infection. Additionally, smoking causes dysplastic changes to persist and progress and is, therefore, also associated with cervical cancer.

SCREENING AND PREINVASIVE DISEASE

Pap smears are effective for detecting preinvasive cervical changes. Cytologists generally report Pap smear results via the Bethesda system, which accounts for specimen adequacy as well as for cytologic read (Table 10-1). The advent of liquid-based cytology has resulted in fewer inadequate samples. Furthermore, the incorporation of HPV testing into the screening process has helped guide management. Following an abnormal Pap smear, a patient is referred to colposcopy for directed biopsies. If a colposcopy shows low-grade changes or cervical intraepithelial neoplasia (CIN) I, the patient usually is observed because two-thirds of these changes will resolve spontaneously. CIN is characterized by dysplastic changes in the epithelium. The more severe the morphologic changes, which are labeled CIN I, CIN II, and CIN III, the greater the risk for ultimate transformation into invasive cervical cancer. A diagnosis of CIN II or III requires an excisional procedure, usually a loop electrosurgical excision procedure or a cone biopsy. It should be noted that CIN is a histologic diagnosis obtained from a colposcopic-guided biopsy. Treatment is not determined by the cytologic diagnosis.

KEY POINTS

- Optimal use of established screening guidelines will substantially reduce the risk of invasive cervical cancer.
- Vaccination against specific human papillomavirus serotypes has been shown to be an effective strategy to prevent the development of premalignant cervical abnormalities in adolescent girls and young women not previously infected with the virus.

TABLE 10–1 Bethesda System for Reporting Cervical Cytologic Diagnosis

Statement of Specimen Adequacy

General categorization
- Within normal limits
- Benign cellular changes
- Epithelial cell abnormality

Descriptive diagnosis
- Benign cellular changes
- Infection
- Reactive changes

Epithelial Cell Abnormalities

Squamous cell
- Atypical squamous cells of undetermined significance (ASCUS)
- Low-grade squamous intraepithelial lesion
- High-grade squamous intraepithelial lesion
- Squamous cell carcinoma

Glandular cell
- Benign endometrial cells
- Atypical glandular cells of undetermined significance (AGUS)
- Adenocarcinoma

Other malignant neoplasms

HUMAN PAPILLOMAVIRUS (HPV)

An association between cervical cancer and infection with many HPV types (i.e., 16, 18, 45, 31, 33, 52, 58, 35) is well established.[3] Existing evidence suggests that high-risk HPV types that produce viral proteins (E6, E7), as well as those types that are capable of binding to and inactivating tumor suppressor proteins (RB1, TP53), may be essential for the initiation of carcinogenesis. In specific clinical settings, checking for the presence of HPV infection is considered an important component of screening for cervical cancer.

The positive results from randomized phase III trials of HPV vaccination have revealed the importance of this strategy for prevention of premalignant lesions in the cervix, vagina, and vulva.[4–7] Several national and international health organizations have strongly endorsed the concept of routine immunization of all girls and young women as an effective approach to reduce the worldwide burden associated with cervical cancer.

INVASIVE DISEASE

The most common presenting symptom of invasive cervical cancer is abnormal vaginal bleeding (i.e., postmenopausal, intermenstrual, or postcoital). Bleeding accompanied by other symptoms, such as pelvic pain and vaginal discharge, usually represents more advanced disease. Because the rate of false-negative findings of Pap smears may be as high as 50% for women with invasive cancer, negative findings should not preclude further diagnostic evaluation of a woman with signs and symptoms consistent with cervical cancer.

Clinical staging of cervical cancer does not require high-tech equipment because the disease is most common in the developing world where such modalities are not available. Surgical staging (i.e., sampling of paraaortic lymph nodes) is practiced in some centers, but evidence does not support this more invasive approach.

Patients with very early-stage disease (IA1 without lymphvascular space invasion) can be treated with a simple hysterectomy because the risk of lymph node involvement is low. If a patient with early-stage disease wishes to maintain fertility, observation following conization may be considered. The rate of long-term survival for patients with early-stage disease is greater than 95%.

Patients with stages IA1 (with lymphvascular space invasion), IA2, and IB1 disease are candidates for radical hysterectomy, as well as for pelvic and paraaortic lymphadenectomy. The ideal treatment of patients with IB2 disease is controversial; in some centers, primary chemoradiation is practiced but, in others, primary surgery with adjuvant radiation or chemoradiation is used. The long-term survival rate ranges from 80% to 90%. With extensive local disease (stages IIB and beyond) there is no role for primary surgery, and standard treatment includes the simultaneous delivery of external beam radiation plus weekly chemotherapy to be followed by brachytherapy. Several phase III randomized trials have demonstrated that the addition of cisplatin-based chemotherapy, which is used as a radiosensitizer, improves both progression-free and overall survival rates for patients with invasive disease.[8–12]

METASTATIC AND RECURRENT CERVICAL CANCER

The prognosis is poor for patients with metastatic cervical cancer or for those who have recurrence following primary treatment of localized disease. For carefully selected patients who have an isolated recurrence within a previously radiated field, aggressive resection (i.e., pelvic exenteration) can be considered because it offers the potential to provide long-term disease-free survival. Additionally, patients who have not undergone radiation therapy may undergo salvage radiation.

A number of cytotoxic agents have been evaluated for activity against cervical cancer. Cisplatin, which is associated with a 20% objective response rate, is the most widely used. Other drugs with demonstrated activity include carboplatin, paclitaxel, topotecan, vinorelbine, gemcitabine, and ifosfamide. Although palliation of symptoms can be achieved with these drugs, the duration of response generally is less than 3 to 4 months. The toxicity of therapy must be considered for patients who have metastatic disease because they frequently have a marginal performance status.

An objective response is more likely to be noted in a nonirradiated area and in patients who have never received chemotherapy. Because cisplatin is now routinely used as a component of primary therapy for locally advanced cervical cancer,[8–12] the activity of any chemotherapy agent used to treat recurrent disease following radiation plus cisplatin remains an unresolved question.

For patients with metastatic and recurrent cervical cancer, cisplatin plus topotecan has produced a significantly higher objective response rate, as well as superior progression-free and overall survival rates compared with single-agent cisplatin ($p = 0.017$).[13] The combination of cisplatin plus paclitaxel also is associated with a higher response rate and better progression-free survival, compared with single-agent cisplatin, but this regimen was not shown to improve overall survival.[14]

ENDOMETRIAL CANCER

In 2007, there were approximately 39,100 new cases of endometrial cancer and 7,400 deaths in the United States.[1] The pathogenesis of endometrial cancer appears to be related to the effects of unopposed estrogen on the glandular cells of the organ, which accounts for the fact that 95% of cancers are adenocarcinomas. Estrogen stimulation leads to endometrial hyperplasia and atypical adenomatosis hyperplasia, which may be regarded as in situ carcinoma of the endometrium.

RISK FACTORS

The risk factors for endometrial cancer include obesity (which is associated with higher levels of endogenous estrogen), low parity, early menarche, and late menopause. Prolonged administration of exogenous estrogen, without progesterone, increases the risk of endometrial cancer by 4-fold to 8-fold. Combined oral contraceptives appear to protect against endometrial cancer.

Although the disease is increasingly common in a younger patient population, 75% of patients with endometrial cancer are postmenopausal. The risk of endometrial cancer is 40% lower for black women than for white women, but the death rate is 50% higher for black women; this increased mortality is attributed to the fact that black women usually have a more advanced stage of disease at the time of diagnosis. The incidence of endometrial cancer in developing countries, such as India and Southeast Asia, is 4 to 5 times lower than the incidence in the United States.[1]

The most common symptom associated with endometrial cancer is postmenopausal bleeding, which requires careful evaluation. Most endometrial cancers are localized at the time of diagnosis, have a well-differentiated histologic appearance with a lower propensity to spread, and are curable

KEY POINTS

- Sustained exposure to endogenous and exogenous estrogen is the major risk factor for endometrial cancer.
- Most women (80%) with endometrial cancer present with stage I disease.
- Chemotherapy for recurrent/metastatic endometrial cancer has an important role in the management of the disease.

with currently available therapy. High-grade cancers, including the papillary serous subtype, are more likely to demonstrate deep myometrial invasion, lymph node involvement, and metastatic spread at the time of diagnosis.

TAMOXIFEN AND ENDOMETRIAL CANCER

A number of studies have demonstrated that the risk of endometrial cancer is 3-fold to 7-fold higher for women receiving tamoxifen than for women who do not take the drug. Although this finding causes some concern, these cancers are usually well-differentiated neoplasms that present in an early stage at the time of diagnosis and are highly treatable. However, not all studies have supported the generally favorable outcome of treatment for tamoxifen-associated endometrial cancer.[15] It is important for oncologists who care for women who receive tamoxifen to ask these patients about abnormal vaginal bleeding, which should result in immediate evaluation. No clinical data are available to justify routine screening for uterine cancer of women taking tamoxifen.[16] In the Study of Tamoxifen and Raloxifene, there was no statistically significant difference in the incidence of endometrial cancer between individuals receiving tamoxifen or raloxifene.[17]

TREATMENT

Surgical staging and treatment is indicated for most patients with endometrial cancer when they are first seen by an oncologist. The standard surgical staging procedure includes hysterectomy, bilateral salpingo-oophorectomy, washings, pelvic and paraaortic lymph node dissection, and examination of the entire abdominal cavity (Table 10-2). Patients whose performance statuses do not permit surgery can be treated with radiation primarily.

Adjuvant treatment is based on the tumor stage and grade. Options can include no further treatment, cuff and/or pelvic radiation, or chemotherapy. A phase III trial conducted by the Gynecologic Oncology Group (GOG) revealed the superiority of chemotherapy (cisplatin plus doxorubicin) compared with whole-abdominal radiation therapy following surgical resection of stage III endometrial cancer (with small volume residual disease remaining within the peritoneal cavity).[18]

TABLE 10-2 Surgical Staging for Endometrial Cancer

Stage	Description
IA	Tumor limited to the endometrium
IB	Invasion of < 50% of the myometrium
IC	Invasion of ≥ 50% of the myometrium
IIA	Endocervical glandular involvement only
IIB	Cervical stromal invasion
IIIA	Tumor invading serous or adnexa or positive findings on cytologic analysis
IIIB	Vaginal metastasis
IIIC	Positive pelvic or paraaortic nodes
IVA	Invasion of bladder or bowel mucosa
IVB	Distant metastasis

Approximately 80% of patients with endometrial cancer have stage I disease at the time of initial diagnosis. Stages II, III, and IV are found in 11%, 6%, and 2% of patients, respectively.

Survival is substantially influenced by stage. Five-year survival is 83% for patients with stage I disease, 73% for those with stage II disease, 52% for those with stage III disease, and 27% for those with stage IV disease. Age, tumor grade, vascular invasion, hormone receptor status, and specific histologic subtypes (e.g., papillary serous and clear cell) also have been demonstrated to have an independent effect on prognosis.

Surgery alone is generally considered adequate treatment for grade 1 or 2 endometrial cancers that have less than 50% muscle invasion. Postoperative radiation of the pelvis alone or of the pelvis plus intracavitary radiation frequently is added when unfavorable prognostic features are present, such as more than 50% muscle invasion, grade 3 cancer, and papillary serous or clear cell histology. However, the previously noted data that demonstrated the superiority of combination chemotherapy compared with whole-abdominal radiotherapy suggest a more prominent role for chemotherapy in the presence of unfavorable features. Unfortunately, randomized trial data defining the optimal chemotherapy regimen and the effect of such therapy in patients with high-risk stages I and/or II disease are unavailable.

METASTATIC OR RECURRENT DISEASE

Endometrial cancer is a hormonally sensitive malignant disease. Overall, 10% to 30% of patients will have a response to treatment with a progestational agent, but the likelihood of response is strongly influenced by tumor grade. Grade 3 or undifferentiated cancers rarely respond to hormone therapy, and chemotherapy should be the primary treatment for most patients with metastatic disease. Clinical features that are predictors of response to a progestational agent include a long disease-free interval from the date of the original diagnosis to evidence of metastatic disease, as well as the presence of estrogen or progesterone receptors on the tumor cells.

A number of chemotherapy agents have demonstrated biologic activity in endometrial cancer, including the platinum drugs (i.e., cisplatin and carboplatin), paclitaxel, and doxorubicin. The overall activity of these single agents is 25% to 35%. In metastatic or recurrent endometrial cancer, the combination of cisplatin plus doxorubicin produced a higher objective response rate and a limited improvement in progression free-survival but no difference in overall survival when compared with doxorubicin alone. A recently reported study has revealed that combination cisplatin and doxorubicin improves both progression-free and overall survival rates when compared with whole-abdominal radiation therapy for women with stages III to IV endometrial cancer (maximum 2 cm residual tumor following surgical cytoreduction).[18] In a report of a randomized trial conducted by the GOG, researchers noted that the combination of cisplatin, doxorubicin, and paclitaxel (delivered as a 3-hour infusion) resulted in a small but significant improvement in overall survival compared with combination cisplatin plus doxorubicin ($p = 0.037$).[19] However, this triple-agent regimen was associated with a particularly unfavorable side effect profile, including a high incidence of clinically relevant neurotoxicity.

OVARIAN CANCER

Ovarian cancer is the sixth most common cancer overall for women in the United States, comprising 4% of all cancers in women and 25% of cancers of the female genital organs.[2] There are more deaths from ovarian cancer in the United States each year than from endometrial and cervical cancers combined. Epithelial ovarian cancer accounts for 90% of all cases of malignant tumors of the ovaries.

The peak age for the development of ovarian cancer is 55 to 60 years. The age-specific risk of the disease steadily increases from ages 20 to 80 and then declines. More than 80% of ovarian cancers occur after age 40, with 30% to 40% of them developing in women older than 65. Conversely, less than 1% of ovarian cancers occur in women younger than age 20. For reasons that are not clear, patients older than 65 with ovarian cancer present with higher-grade tumors that are more aggressive than the tumors seen in younger patients. This difference is independent of other known unfavorable risk factors.

SYMPTOMS AND PHYSICAL FINDINGS

Patients with early-stage ovarian cancer often have nonspecific discomfort, including irregular menses (in a premenopausal woman), or urinary frequency and constipation, which are caused by an enlarging pelvic mass. With advanced disease, patients may note abdominal pain, bloating, dyspnea, emesis, early satiety, anorexia, and constipation. In early-stage disease, the major physical finding is a pelvic mass; there may be considerable ascites in patients with advanced disease. Because symptoms referable to the upper abdomen often are predominant at the time of presentation in patients with advanced ovarian cancer, this clinical feature may delay the time before a definitive diagnosis is established.

KEY POINTS

- Surgery plays a unique role in the management of ovarian cancer.
- Standard primary chemotherapy for advanced ovarian cancer includes a platinum agent (carboplatin or cisplatin) and a taxane (paclitaxel or docetaxel). Intravenous and, in certain situations, intraperitoneal administration may be used.
- Optimal second-line chemotherapy for ovarian cancer must be individualized.

DIAGNOSIS

In women who are premenopausal, the majority of ovarian masses are functional cysts that usually decrease in size after several menstrual cycles. Performing a transvaginal ultrasound can assist in the differential diagnosis of cysts that do not spontaneously regress. For those women who are postmenopausal, a palpable pelvic mass is of greater concern for the presence of malignant disease. Based on the signs and symptoms of the disease process, other diagnostic procedures may be indicated, including a computerized tomography (CT) scan of the abdomen and pelvis, radiographic or endoscopic studies of either the upper or lower gastrointestinal tract, or both. In a patient with ascites, a paracentesis may be performed to enable cytologic analysis of the fluid and to provide short-term symptomatic relief.

The serum cancer antigen 125 (CA-125) level is likely to be elevated in more than 80% of patients with advanced ovarian cancer, but it also is abnormal in other cancers and benign conditions. Also, 50% of patients with early-stage ovarian cancer will have a normal serum level of CA-125. Therefore, the absence of an elevated CA-125 level should not interfere with a decision to evaluate a suspicious pelvic mass.

SCREENING

A variety of screening approaches for the early detection of ovarian cancer have been advocated, including the routine performance of a transvaginal ultrasound or measurement of the serum CA-125 level, but there is no clinical evidence to suggest that screening for the presence of ovarian cancer decreases mortality. However, because of concern for the development of ovarian cancer in women with a strong family history of the disease or a documented genetic abnormality that predicts for a greater risk (i.e., *BRCA1* mutation), some investigators have recommended regular transvaginal ultrasounds and serum CA-125 evaluation in an effort to detect the disease at an earlier stage. This approach may be reasonable, but existing data do not support the clinical value of screening, even for this high-risk population. False-positive results on screening tests have the potential to lead to further diagnostic evaluation, including unnecessary invasive procedures, such as laparoscopy or laparotomy.

FAMILY HISTORY AND GENETIC TESTING

A family history of ovarian cancer is the single most important risk factor for the disease. Although 90% to 95% of ovarian cancers are sporadic and not hereditary, the lifetime risk for the disease increases 3-fold to 4-fold for women who have one first-degree relative with ovarian cancer compared with women who do not have such a history. The lifetime risk is approximately 40% for women who have two first-degree relatives with ovarian cancer.

There is solid evidence that the presence of either a *BRCA1* or *BRCA2* mutation is a strong predictor of a heightened susceptibility to ovarian cancer.[20] For example, studies have shown that the lifetime risk of ovarian cancer may be as high as 50% for women with a *BRCA1* mutation. The presence of a *BRCA2* mutation appears to be a predictor of a lower cumulative lifetime risk of the disease.

For a woman with more than one family member with either ovarian cancer or early-onset breast cancer, it may be reasonable to consider genetic testing to determine the presence or absence of a *BRCA1* or *BRCA2* mutation. Unless a specific genetic abnormality has been identified in a particular family, testing for one of the numerous defects identified in these genes can be difficult. One exception to this rule is the relatively common genetic defects in *BRCA1* identified in Ashkenzi Jewish women who have a family history of ovarian cancer.[21]

The value of discovering the presence of a *BRCA1* or *BRCA2* abnormality is increasingly recognized as providing useful information for subsequent management. Although the value of intensive screening programs (e.g., routine vaginal ultrasounds) in such individuals is unclear, several studies have provided the first indication that performing a bilateral prophylactic oophorectomy in women with these genetic abnormalities may substantially reduce their risk of ovarian cancer (approximately 80% lower risk with follow-up of less than 10 years from surgical procedure).[22–24] Because of concern for the later development of primary peritoneal cancer, long-term follow-up of a large population of women who have elected to have this prophylactic procedure will be required to determine the extent of risk reduction associated with this surgery.[24] In addition, the consequences of estrogen deprivation, which can include bone loss and cardiac effects, must not be ignored, especially because hormone-replacement therapy may not be considered an appropriate option because of the heightened risk of breast cancer in this patient population.[25,26]

PROGNOSTIC FACTORS

A number of important prognostic factors have been identified in patients with ovarian cancer, including:

- stage at the time of diagnosis,
- extent of disease at the completion of primary surgical cytoreduction,
- patient age,
- performance status, and
- tumor grade.

Certain morphologic variants, including clear cell and mucinous subtypes, appear to have a particularly poor prognosis when ovarian cancer is diagnosed at an advanced stage. Several studies have shown that the prognosis is more favorable for women with a *BRCA1* abnormality, which is independent of other known prognostic factors.[27,28] However, the findings of other studies challenge these conclusions, and their relevance in defining prognosis and treatment must be further clarified.[29,30]

PRIMARY SURGERY

The importance of appropriate surgical staging in ovarian cancer, particularly in cases of apparent early-stage disease, cannot be overemphasized. The prognosis is relatively good for patients who have had an appropriate staging procedure and in whom disease is confined to the ovary, especially if the tumor is low grade. Failure to perform complete surgical staging may result in the need for chemotherapy when it may be unnecessary or may lead to an inappropriate decision to withhold adjuvant chemotherapy when disease in the abdominal cavity or regional lymph nodes has gone undetected. In the United States, national surveys indicate that an appropriate and complete staging procedure is carried out in less than 15% of women with suspected early-stage ovarian cancer.[31]

In a patient with known or suspected ovarian cancer, a vertical midline incision is required for inspection of the entire contents of the abdominal cavity. A thorough staging procedure includes the following steps:

- careful inspection of the upper abdomen and undersurface of the diaphragm;
- cytologic analysis of fluid and peritoneal washings;
- removal of the ovaries, uterus, fallopian tubes, omentum, and any mass lesions;
- fertility – sparing surgery (in select cases);
- sampling of pelvic and paraaortic lymph nodes; and
- peritoneal biopsies.

For patients with advanced disease that is documented prior to or during the initial surgical procedure, the importance of attempting aggressive surgical cytoreduction before initiating cytotoxic chemotherapy remains controversial.[32] Considerable retrospective data have documented that survival is better for women who begin receiving chemotherapy after surgery in the presence of low-volume intraperitoneal disease than it is for women who do not have surgery or for whom surgery was unsuccessful. These data strongly support the conclusion that a reasonable attempt at maximal cytoreduction is a critically important component in treating patients with ovarian cancer.

However, for patients in whom it is possible to carry out optimal cytoreduction and achieve small-volume residual cancer, it remains uncertain whether the survival is better because of the surgery itself or because biologic factors that permit a successful surgery (such as the local growth pattern of the tumor) also are responsible for its overall chemosensitivity, risk of inherent or acquired resistance to chemotherapy, and the rate of disease progression.

For example, cytoreduction would most likely be unsuccessful for a patient with ovarian cancer in whom the disease at presentation is characterized by massive intra-abdominal carcinomatosis, large and widespread pelvic and retroperitoneal adenopathy, and extensive hepatic involvement. The duration of response to chemotherapy also would be relatively short for such a patient, even if the cytotoxic drugs yielded limited symptomatic benefits. The question to be asked in the setting of advanced disease is whether the ultimate outcome is the result of the failure to perform an optimal cytoreduction before administering chemotherapy, or the result of the negative biologic features of the cancer.

In the absence of definitive randomized trials that might directly address this highly relevant issue, some investigators have questioned the choice of aggressive surgery for patients with advanced ovarian cancer for whom optimal surgical cytoreduction probably cannot be achieved, and they have suggested an alternative treatment approach for such women.[33,34] Following a presumptive diagnosis of ovarian cancer or primary peritoneal cancer (based on physical examination, radiographic findings, and histologic confirmation of adenocarcinoma through cytologic analysis of peritoneal fluid), the patient should be treated with cytotoxic chemotherapy, such as a platinum agent plus a taxane. For patients who have a partial response to neoadjuvant chemotherapy, it may be appropriate to attempt surgical removal of residual macroscopic cancer that is evident on physical examination or radiographic evaluation. In the absence of data from randomized trials, the decision about whether to attempt initial surgical cytoreduction or to use primary chemotherapy to treat advanced ovarian cancer must be individualized on the basis of specific clinical characteristics, such as the extent of intra-abdominal disease and pre-existing comorbid medical conditions.

In summary, on the basis of extensive retrospective experience and in the absence of contraindications to this approach, the standard of care for ovarian cancer must be surgical cytoreduction followed by chemotherapy. However, available data support the concept of modification of this strategy for appropriately selected patients.

SECONDARY SURGICAL PROCEDURES

In addition to its importance in staging and primary cytoreduction for ovarian cancer, surgery has additional roles in the management of ovarian cancer. As noted previously, when there has been a response to neoadjuvant chemotherapy, the patient may be a candidate for surgical resection of residual macroscopic disease. In such patients, a residual mass may not be an area of resistant disease; rather, it may be a necrotic or poorly vascularized region where potentially chemosensitive cancer cells have not been exposed to cytotoxic drugs. Thus, removal of bulky residual tumors may improve the clinical outcome for inherently chemosensitive cancers. A European randomized trial has provided limited confirmation of this theory by demonstrating a survival advantage with interval surgical cytoreduction — performed after three cycles of cytotoxic drugs — for women with advanced ovarian cancer who have evidence of an initial response to chemotherapy.[35]

Although it is reasonable to suggest that a secondary surgery might be clinically useful for treating recurrence of ovarian cancer after a prolonged progression-free interval, randomized phase III trial data are not available to either support or refute such approaches.

In the past, women in whom a clinically defined complete response was achieved following primary chemotherapy underwent second-look laparotomy. It was hoped that this procedure would clearly define the ultimate prognosis and provide critical data to assist in future management. However, it is known that relapse will occur in 50% to 60% of women with grade 3 cancers who have no evidence of disease at the time of a second-look procedure (no visible cancer and negative findings on analysis of tissue obtained at biopsy). Therefore, the prognostic value of negative findings on second-look surgery is limited. In addition, no reports of phase III trials have indicated that survival rates are better for patients who have a second-look procedure than for patients who do not undergo this procedure.[36]

CHEMOTHERAPY FOR ADVANCED DISEASE

Based on the results of several randomized phase III trials, standard treatment of advanced ovarian cancer includes the administration of a platinum agent (cisplatin or carboplatin) and a taxane.[37–42] Although they have comparable efficacy with respect to progression-free and overall survival, carboplatin-based regimens are generally preferred to cisplatin regimens because their toxicity profile is better (less emesis, neurotoxicity, and nephrotoxicity), and they are easier to administer. In addition, when paclitaxel is given with cisplatin to treat ovarian cancer, a long (24-hour) infusion is required. With shorter programs (3 hours), the incidence of severe (grade 3) peripheral neuropathy is unacceptably high (more than 20%).[41]

An objective response to this therapy will be achieved and disease-related symptoms will be improved for approximately 60% to 80% of patients with advanced ovarian cancer. No data from randomized trials have supported the benefit of any systemic dose-intense or high-dose chemotherapy strategy to treat the disease, nor are there data to demonstrate that adding a third drug to a standard regimen of a platinum agent and a taxane results in a superior outcome.

The median progression-free survival is 26 months, and the overall survival is approximately 60 months for women with advanced ovarian cancer when the amount of residual tumor is optimum (the remaining tumor mass in the peritoneal cavity before the start of chemotherapy is less than 1 cm in diameter). The corresponding values are 18 months and 38 months when the amount of residual tumor is suboptimal (the remaining tumor mass is more than 1 cm in diameter) or for stage IV disease.

It is important to note the results of one phase III trial that has raised a question regarding the requirement of the addition of paclitaxel to carboplatin in the front-line management of ovarian cancer.[43] This large randomized study, which included more than 2,000 patients, failed to demonstrate a survival advantage for the two-drug combination compared with single-agent carboplatin (control arm). However, several concerns with this trial have been noted, including the issue of appropriate quality control and the fact that paclitaxel was ultimately given to one-third of the patients in the control arm. Thus, one possible interpretation of this study is that it provides support for a previously proposed concept that sequential chemotherapy in ovarian cancer (i.e., administering a platinum agent followed by paclitaxel) results in an equivalent outcome when compared with combination therapy (i.e., a platinum agent given together with paclitaxel).[44]

CHEMOTHERAPY FOR HIGH-RISK, EARLY-STAGE DISEASE

Although a number of randomized trials have demonstrated that adjuvant chemotherapy can prolong the time to progression for women with high-risk, early–stage ovarian cancer (stage I [grade 3] or stage II disease), no single study has definitively established the effect of this treatment strategy on overall survival. However, an analysis of data from more than 900 patients with high-risk, early-stage disease showed that adjuvant platinum-based chemotherapy administered postoperatively led to an 11% improvement in 5-year progression-free survival and an 8% improvement in 5-year overall survival, compared with a strategy of observation until evidence of disease recurrence.[45–47] These data strongly support the argument that the administration of adjuvant platinum-based chemotherapy after initial surgery is the standard of care for high-risk, early-stage ovarian cancer.

INTRAPERITONEAL CHEMOTHERAPY

Managing ovarian cancer by delivering drugs directly into the peritoneal cavity has particular appeal for treating a disease that is largely confined to that region. Phases I and II clinical trials have demonstrated the biologic activity and safety — as well as the important limitations — of using this approach. The limitations include catheter malfunction, development of bacterial and chemical peritonitis, and the fact that antineoplastic effects are limited to patients with relatively small–volume residual disease when the regional treatment program is initiated.

In several randomized phase III clinical trials, intraperitoneally and systemically delivered cisplatin-based chemotherapy have been compared as primary therapy for small-volume residual advanced ovarian cancer.[48–50] These studies have demonstrated that the regional treatment approach results in superior progression-free and overall survival rates (approximate 20% reduction in risk of death) compared with intravenous treatment. Although concern has been raised about excessive local toxicity, the requirement for catheter placement, and the use of cisplatin rather than carboplatin for the standard management of ovarian cancer, available data demonstrate intraperitoneal therapy can be safely administered outside the setting of a clinical trial, and the use of this strategy improves survival when employed as primary treatment of small-volume residual cancer.

CONSOLIDATION CHEMOTHERAPY

Disease will subsequently recur in 70% of women with advanced ovarian cancer who have a clinically defined complete response to standard chemotherapy with a platinum agent and a taxane. Therefore, it is reasonable to question whether using some form of consolidation therapy to treat this highly chemosensitive disease may improve both time to symptomatic disease progression and overall survival.

To critically examine this issue, the Southwest Oncology Group (SWOG) and the GOG conducted a phase III randomized trial to compare three and 12 cycles of single-agent paclitaxel (175 mg/m^2 infused over a 3-hour period) given every 28 days for patients who had a clinically defined complete response to standard chemotherapy with a platinum agent and paclitaxel.[51] The study was closed early by the SWOG Data Safety and Monitoring Committee when it was found that there was a 50% reduction in the risk of disease recurrence for patients who received the 12 months of consolidation chemotherapy. The median progression-free survival (from the time of study entry) was 21 months for the patients who were treated for 3 months compared with 28 months for the patients who were treated for 12 months ($p = 0.0023$; hazard ratio, 2.31). At the time of study closure, there was no difference in overall survival between the trial arms, but there were less than 20 deaths in the entire study population.

The somewhat controversial decision to close this study early has substantially reduced any possibility that longer follow-up will demonstrate a survival benefit for the prolonged maintenance strategy, because women randomly assigned to the 3-month regimen will almost certainly elect to receive additional treatment when informed of the trial results. In assessing the effect of the study on standard treatment, it is reasonable to suggest that oncologists should discuss the results of the trial with appropriately selected patients and allow them to decide for themselves whether the potential for improved progression-free survival associated with the consolidation approach justifies the negative effects of continued treatment, which include peripheral neuropathy and alopecia.

TREATMENT OF RECURRENT OR RESISTANT DISEASE

Approximately 20% to 40% of women with advanced ovarian cancer do not have a response to initial chemotherapy; for the patients who do have a response, relapse subsequently occurs. As a result, second-line treatment of ovarian cancer is common. A variety of management strategies may be associated with improved survival, but there is no evidence that any of these approaches have curative potential.

Although recurrent or resistant ovarian cancer is not curable, there are several reasonable goals for treatment.

- To reduce or eliminate cancer-related symptoms
- To prolong the time to disease progression and ultimate survival
- To optimize overall quality of life, including minimizing treatment-related side effects

The treatment of patients with recurrent or resistant ovarian cancer must be individualized.[52] For women who have had a long treatment-free interval (more than 6 to 12 months) after the completion of primary chemotherapy, the response rate is reasonably high (more than 20%) for retreatment (using the same or similar drugs that were used in the initial chemotherapy regimen). Phase III trial data reveal that the delivery of a carboplatin-based combination regimen (with paclitaxel or gemcitabine) improves outcome (either progression-free or overall survival) compared with carboplatin alone.[53,54]

Conversely, the projected response rate to any antineoplastic drug regimen will be low (less than 20%) for patients whose disease progresses during primary therapy or for those who have new signs or symptoms of disease following a short treatment-free interval (less than 4 months to 6 months). Many chemotherapy agents have demonstrated a reasonable level of biologic activity in platinum-resistant ovarian cancer and may be considered rational treatment options (Table 10-3).[52] There are no data to support the administration of a combination chemotherapy regimen for women with platinum-resistant ovarian cancer outside the setting of a clinical trial.

TABLE 10-3 Antineoplastic Agents with Demonstrated Activity (More than 10% Objective Response Rate) in Platinum-resistant Ovarian Cancer

- Altretamine
- Bevacizumab
- Docetaxel
- Epirubicin
- Etoposide (oral, 21 days)
- Gemcitabine
- Ifosfamide
- Irinotecan
- Liposomal doxorubicin
- Paclitaxel (every 3 weeks or weekly)
- Tamoxifen
- Topotecan
- Vinorelbine

It is likely that patients will receive several second-line chemotherapy regimens when disease recurrence or primary resistance is documented. The selection of optimal therapy and the sequencing of available drugs must be individualized on the basis of several considerations.

- Side effects that previously occurred in the patient
- Known toxicity of the active agents
- Convenience for the patient and her family
- Cost
- Patient choice

External beam radiation may be the optimal treatment for women in whom a painful local tumor develops, particularly in the presence of resistant disease, for which the anticipated response rate to additional cytotoxic therapy is low. When a progressive tumor has caused bowel obstruction, judicious use of surgery, such as colostomy, ileostomy, or gastrostomy, also can be an effective palliative maneuver.

LOW MALIGNANT POTENTIAL TUMORS OF THE OVARY

Standard treatment of low malignant potential (LMP) tumors of the ovary includes surgical resection of all macroscopic disease. Fortunately, most women with LMP tumors have early-stage disease when first seen; the 5-year survival rate associated with early-stage disease exceeds 90%. There is no evidence that any adjuvant treatment (chemotherapy or radiotherapy) is beneficial with respect to either time to progression or overall survival for patients with LMP tumors of the ovary. For a young woman who wishes to preserve child-bearing potential, it is reasonable to manage an LMP tumor of the ovary with a unilateral oophorectomy.

For women who have more advanced LMP tumors, maximal surgical cytoreduction should be attempted. Even for patients presenting with stage III and IV disease, the approximate 5-year survival rate is 75%. The benefit of delivering chemotherapy following optimal surgery of stage III disease has not been demonstrated because this type of tumor progresses slowly in most patients, despite documented residual disease. With subsequent disease progression, cytotoxic chemotherapy may improve disease-related symptoms, but it remains uncertain if it prolongs survival.

GERM CELL TUMORS OF THE OVARY

Germ cell tumors are relatively uncommon malignant lesions that affect adolescent girls and young women. Serum levels of human chorionic gonadotropin (HCG) and alpha-fetoprotein (AFP) can be helpful in diagnosing and following the course of the disease. Unilateral cancers, the most common form at the time of presentation, usually can be managed with a unilateral salpingo-oophorectomy, which preserves fertility.

As with their male counterpart, ovarian germ cell tumors are highly chemosensitive. The standard regimens used to treat men also are used to treat women who have germ cell tumors. Although data to define optimal management for ovarian germ cell tumors are limited, most experts agree that an attempt at maximal surgical cytoreduction should be carried out before administering chemotherapy in patients who have advanced disease confined to the peritoneal cavity. For patients with documented stage IV disease, such as lung metastases, chemotherapy may be administered immediately after a histologic diagnosis is confirmed and before surgery is done to remove tumor bulk. *(For a discussion of germ cell tumors in men, please see Chapter 9: Genitourinary Cancers.)*

Nondysgerminomatous germ cell tumors rarely remain localized to the ovary, despite findings at the time of initial surgical staging. Because the recurrence rate for stage I disease is 80%, chemotherapy is necessary for all patients who are found to have a nondysgerminomatous germ cell tumor of any stage or grade, with the exception of stage I, grade 1 immature teratomas. Depending on the presence or absence of gross residual disease when treatment is initiated, standard chemotherapy includes three or four cycles of a bleomycin, etoposide, and cisplatin regimen.

Dysgerminomas also are highly chemosensitive. Because the recurrence rate for apparently localized disease is 15% to 25%, surgery alone is appropriate for patients who have stage I disease at the time of presentation. Chemotherapy may be initiated when recurrence is documented.

STROMAL TUMORS OF THE OVARY

Ovarian stromal tumors (granulosa cell and Sertoli-Leidig) are uncommon and are managed principally with surgery, even for advanced-stage disease. The prognosis is excellent, as most ovarian stromal tumors are localized at the time of diagnosis. As with borderline ovarian tumors and although the disease may respond to chemotherapy, with important palliation of cancer-related symptoms, it remains unknown if survival is influenced by this treatment because these cancers often progress slowly, even in the presence of residual macroscopic disease following surgery. Although there is no standard chemotherapy for ovarian stromal tumors, the response rate to a regimen of bleomycin, etoposide, and cisplatin has been high.[55]

REFERENCES

1. World Health Organization Web site: http://www.who.int. Accessed: October 4, 2007.
2. American Cancer Society. *Cancer Facts & Figures 2007*. Atlanta:American Cancer Society;2007.
3. Munoz N, Bosch FX, de Sanjose S, et al. Epidemiologic classification of human papillomavirus types associated with cervical cancer. *N Engl J Med.* 2003;348(6):518–527.
4. Koutsky LA, Ault KA, Wheeler CM, et al. A controlled trial of a human papillomavirus type 16 vaccine. *N Engl J Med.* 2002;347(21): 1645–1651.
5. Villa LL, Costa RL, Petta CA, et al. Prophylactic quadrivalent human papillomavirus (types 6, 11, 16, and 18) L1 virus-like particle vaccine in young women: a randomised double-blind placebo-controlled multicentre phase II efficacy trial. *Lancet Oncol.* 2005;6(5):271–278.
6. Harper DM, Franco EL, Wheeler CM, et al. Efficacy of a bivalent L1 virus-like particle vaccine in prevention of infection with human papillomavirus types 16 and 18 in young women: a randomised controlled trial. *Lancet.* 2004;364(9447):1757–1765.
7. Harper DM, Franco EL, Wheeler CM, et al. Sustained efficacy up to 4.5 years of a bivalent L1 virus-like particle vaccine against human papillomavirus types 16 and 18: follow-up from a randomised control trial. *Lancet.* 2006;367(9518):1247–1255.
8. Keys HM, Bundy BN, Stehman FB, et al. Cisplatin, radiation, and adjuvant hysterectomy compared with radiation and adjuvant hysterectomy for bulky stage IB cervical carcinoma. *N Engl J Med.* 1999;340(15):1154–1161.
9. Morris M, Eifel PJ, Lu J, et al. Pelvic radiation with concurrent chemotherapy compared with pelvic and para-aortic radiation for high-risk cervical cancer. *N Engl J Med.* 1999;340(15):1137–1143.
10. Rose PG, Bundy BN, Watkins EB, et al. Concurrent cisplatin-based radiotherapy and chemotherapy for locally advanced cervical cancer. *N Engl J Med.* 1999;340(15):1144–1153.
11. Peters WA III, Liu PY, Barrett RJ II, et al. Concurrent chemotherapy and pelvic radiation therapy compared with pelvic radiation therapy alone as adjuvant therapy after radical surgery in high-risk early-stage cancer of the cervix. *J Clin Oncol.* 2000;18(8):1606–1613.
12. Green JA, Kirwan JM, Tierney JF, et al. Survival and recurrence after concomitant chemotherapy and radiotherapy for cancer of the uterine cervix: a systematic review and meta-analysis. *Lancet.* 2001;358(9284): 781–786.
13. Long HJ 3rd, Bundy BN, Grendys EC Jr, et al. Randomized phase III trial of cisplatin with or without topotecan in carcinoma of the uterine cervix: a Gynecologic Oncology Group study. *J Clin Oncol.* 2005;23(21):4626–4633.
14. Moore DH, Blessing JA, McQuellon RP, et al. Phase III study of cisplatin with or without paclitaxel in stage IVB, recurrent, or persistent squamous cell carcinoma of the cervix: a gynecologic group study. *J Clin Oncol.* 2004;22(15):3113–3119.
15. Bergman L, Beelen ML, Gallee MP, et al. Risk and prognosis of endometrial cancer after tamoxifen for breast cancer. Comprehensive Cancer Centres' ALERT Group. Assessment of Liver and Endometrial cancer Risk following Tamoxifen. *Lancet.* 2000;356(9233):881–887.
16. Suh-Burgmann EJ, Goodman A. Surveillance for endometrial cancer in women receiving tamoxifen. *Ann Intern Med.* 1999;131(2):127–135.
17. Vogel VG, Costantino JP, Wickerham DL, et al. Effect of tamoxifen vs raloxifene on the risk of developing invasive breast cancer and other disease outcomes: the NSABP Study of Tamoxifen and Raloxifene (STAR) P-2 trial. *JAMA* 2006;295(23):2727–2741.
18. Randall ME, Filiaci VL, Muss H, et al. Randomized phase III trial of whole-abdominal irradiation versus doxorubicin and cisplatin chemotherapy in advanced endometrial carcinoma: a Gynecologic Oncology Group Study. *J Clin Oncol.* 2006; 24(1)36–44.
19. Fleming GF, Brunetto VL, Cella D, et al. Phase III trial of doxorubicin plus cisplatin with or without paclitaxel plus filgrastim in advanced endometrial carcinoma: a Gynecologic Oncology Group Study. *J Clin Oncol.* 2004;22(11):2159–2166.
20. Reedy M, Gallion H, Fowler JM, et al. Contribution of BRCA1 and BRCA2 to familial ovarian cancer: a gynecologic oncology group study. *Gynecol Oncol.* 2002;85(2):255–259.

21. Satagopan JM, Boyd J, Kauff ND, et al. Ovarian cancer risk in Ashkenazi Jewish carriers of BRCA1 and BRCA2 mutations. *Clin Cancer Res.* 2002;8(12):3776–3781.

22. Rebbeck TR, Lynch HT, Neuhausen SL, et al. Prophylactic oophorectomy in carriers of BRCA1 or BRCA2 mutations. *N Engl J Med.* 2002;346(21):1616–1622.

23. Kauff ND, Satagopan JM, Robson ME, et al. Risk-reducing salpingo-oophorectomy in women with a BRCA1 or BRCA2 mutation. *N Engl J Med.* 2002;346(21):1609–1615.

24. Finch A, Beiner M, Lubinski J, et al. Salpingo-oophorectomy and the risk of ovarian, fallopian tube, and peritoneal cancers in women with a BRCA1 or BRCA2 mutation. *JAMA.* 2006;296(2):185–192.

25. Eisen A, Rebbeck TR, Wood WC, Weber BL. Prophylactic surgery in women with a hereditary predisposition to breast and ovarian cancer. *J Clin Oncol.* 2000;18(9):1980–1995.

26. Rocca WA, Grossardt BR, de Andrade M, et al. Survival patterns after oophorectomy in premenopausal women: a population-based cohort study. *Lancet Oncol.* 2006;7(10):821–828.

27. Boyd J, Sonoda Y, Federici MG, et al. Clinicopathologic features of BRCA-linked and sporadic ovarian cancer. *JAMA.* 2000;283(17): 2260–2265.

28. Cass I, Baldwin RL, Varkey T, et al. Improved survival in women with BRCA-associated ovarian carcinoma. *Cancer.* 2003;97(9):2187–2195.

29. Johannsson OT, Ranstam J, Borg A, Olsson H. Survival of BRCA1 breast and ovarian cancer patients: a population-based study from southern Sweden. *J Clin Oncol.* 1998;16(2):397–404.

30. Buller RE, Shahin MS, Geisler JP, et al. Failure of BRCA1 dysfunction to alter ovarian cancer survival. *Clin Cancer Res.* 2002;8(5):1196–1202.

31. Munoz KA, Harlan LC, Trimble EL. Patterns of care for women with ovarian cancer in the United States. *J Clin Oncol.* 1997;15(11): 3408–3415.

32. Covens AL. A critique of surgical cytoreduction in advanced ovarian cancer. *Gynecol Oncol.* 2000;78(3 Pt 1):269–274.

33. Ansquer Y, Leblanc E, Clough K, et al. Neoadjuvant chemotherapy for unresectable ovarian carcinoma: a French multicenter study. *Cancer.* 2001;91(12):2329–2334.

34. Chan YM, Ng TY, Ngan HY, et al. Quality of life in women treated with neoadjuvant chemotherapy for advanced ovarian cancer: A prospective longitudinal study. *Gynecol Oncol.* 2003;88(1):9–16.

35. van der Burg ME, van Lent M, Buyse M, et al. The effect of debulking surgery after induction chemotherapy on the prognosis in advanced epithelial ovarian cancer. Gynecological Cancer Cooperative Group of the European Organization for Research and Treatment of Cancer. *N Engl J Med.* 1995;332(10):629–634.

36. Rubin SC, Hoskins WJ, Hakes TB, et al. Recurrence after negative second-look laparotomy for overian cancer: analysis of risk factors. *Am J Obstet Gynecol.* 1998;159(5):1094–1098.

37. Covens A, Carey M, Bryson P, et al. Systematic review of first-line chemotherapy for newly diagnosed postoperative patients with stage II, III, or IV epithelial ovarian cancer. *Gynecol Oncol.* 2002;85(1):71–80.

38. McGuire WP, Hoskins WJ, Brady MF, et al. Cyclophosphamide and cisplatin compared with paclitaxel and cisplatin in patients with stage III and stage IV ovarian cancer. *N Engl J Med.* 1996;334(1):1–6.

39. du Bois A, Luck H-J, Meier W, et al. A randomized clinical trial of cisplatin/paclitaxel versus carboplatin/ paclitaxel as first-line treatment of ovarian cancer. *J Natl Cancer Inst.* 2003;95(17):1320–1330.

40. Ozols RF, Bundy BN, Greer BE, et al. Phase III trial of carboplatin and paclitaxel compared with cisplatin and paclitaxel in patients with optimally resected stage III ovarian cancer: a Gynecologic Oncology Group study. *J Clin Oncol.* 2003;21(17):3194–3200.

41. Piccart MJ, Bertelsen K, James K, et al. Randomized intergroup trial of cisplatin-paclitaxel versus cisplatin-cyclophosphamide in women with advanced epithelial ovarian cancer: three-year results. *J Natl Cancer Inst.* 2000;92(9):699–708.

42. Vasey PA, Jayson GC, Gordon A, et al. Phase III randomized trial of docetaxel-carboplatin versus paclitaxel-carboplatin as first-line chemotherapy for ovarian carcinoma. *J Natl Cancer Inst.* 2004;96(22):1682–1691.

43. The International Collaborative Ovarian Neoplasm (ICON) Group. Paclitaxel plus carboplatin versus standard chemotherapy with single-agent carboplatin or cyclophosphamide, doxorubicin, and cisplatin in women with ovarian cancer: the ICON3 randomised trial. *Lancet.* 2002;360:505–515.

44. Muggia FM, Braly PS, Brady MF, et al. Phase III randomized study of cisplatin versus paclitaxel versus cisplatin and paclitaxel in patients with suboptimal stage III or IV ovarian cancer: a Gynecologic Oncology Group study. *J Clin Oncol.* 2000;18(1):106–115.

45. International Collaborative Ovarian Neoplasm 1 (ICON1) and European Organization for Research and Treatment of Cancer Collaborators-adjuvant Chemotherapy in Ovarian Neoplasm (EORTC-ACTION). International collaborative ovarian neoplasm trial 1 and adjuvant chemotherapy in ovarian neoplasm trial: two parallel randomized phase III trials of adjuvant chemotherapy in patients with early-stage ovarian carcinoma. *J Natl Cancer Inst.* 2003;95:105–112.

46. Trimbos JB, Vergote I, Bolis G, et al. Impact of adjuvant chemotherapy and surgical staging in early-stage ovarian carcinoma: European Organisation for Research and Treatment of Cancer-Adjuvant Chemotherapy in Ovarian Neoplasm Trial. *J Natl Cancer Inst.* 2003;95(2):113–125.

47. International Collaborative Ovarian Neoplasm (ICON1) Collaborators. International collaborative ovarian neoplasm trial 1: a randomized trial of adjuvant chemotherapy in women with early-stage ovarian cancer. *J Natl Cancer Inst.* 2003;95:125–132.

48. Alberts DS, Liu PY, Hannigan EV, et al. Intraperitoneal cisplatin plus intravenous cyclophosphamide versus intravenous cisplatin plus intravenous cyclophosphamide for stage III ovarian cancer. *N Engl J Med.* 1996;335(26):1950–1955.

49. Markman M, Bundy BN, Alberts DS, et al. Phase III trial of standard-dose intravenous cisplatin plus paclitaxel versus moderately high dose carboplatin followed by intravenous paclitaxel and intraperitoneal cisplatin in small-volume stage III ovarian carcinoma: an intergroup study of the Gynecologic Oncology Group, Southwestern Oncology Group, and Eastern Cooperative Oncology Group. *J Clin Oncol.* 2001;19(4): 1001–1007.

50. Armstrong DK, Bundy B, Wenzel L, et al. Intraperitoneal cisplatin and paclitaxel in ovarian cancer. *N Engl J Med.* 2006;354(1):34–43.

51. Markman M, Liu PY, Wilczynski S, et al. Phase III randomized trial of 12 versus 3 months of maintenance paclitaxel in patients with advanced overian cancer after complete response to platinum and paclitaxel-based chemotherapy: a Southwest Oncology Group and Gynecologic Oncology Group trial. *J Clin Oncol.* 2003;2(13): 2460–2465.

52. Markman M, Bookman MA. Second-line treatment of ovarian cancer. *Oncologist.* 2000;5(1):26–35.

53. Parmar MK, Ledermann JA, Colombo N, et al. Paclitaxel plus platinum-based chemotherapy versus conventional platinum-based chemotherapy in women with relapsed ovarian cancer. the OCON4/AGO-OVAR-2.2 trial. *Lancet.* 2003;361(9375):2099–2106.

54. Pfisterer J, Plante M, Vergote I, et al. Gemcitabine plus carboplatin compared with carboplatin in patients with platinum-sensitive recurrent ovarian cancer: an Intergroup trial of the AGO-OVAR, the NCIC CTG, and the EORTC GCG. *J Clin Oncol.* 2006;24(29):4699–4707.

55. Homesley HD, Bundy BN, Hurteau JA, et al. Bleomycin, etoposide, and cisplatin combination therapy of ovarian granulosa cell tumors and other stromal malignancies: A Gynecologic Oncology Group study. *Gynecol Oncol.* 1999;72(2):131–137.

11

MALIGNANT MELANOMA

Lynn M. Schuchter, MD

LEARNING OBJECTIVES

After reviewing this chapter, the reader should be able to

- Advise patients regarding the epidemiology and risk factors for melanoma
- Evaluate biologic pathways in melanoma that may become important targets for future treatment
- Select the appropriate diagnostic evaluation for patients with melanoma to include appropriate staging
- Summarize the role of surgery in the management of melanoma
- Recommend appropriate treatment options to patients with high-risk and metastatic melanoma

Current estimates are that one out of 58 men and one out of every 82 women will be diagnosed with melanoma in their lifetimes. Approximately 59,940 new cases of invasive melanoma will be diagnosed in 2007, and 8,110 patients will die from melanoma in the United States.[1] The incidence of melanoma continues to rise dramatically. Melanoma is the leading cause of death from cutaneous malignancies and accounts for 1% to 2% of all cancer deaths in the United States. Melanoma affects all age groups; the median age at diagnosis is 50 years.

EPIDEMIOLOGY, RISK FACTORS, AND GENETICS OF MELANOMA

Exposure to sunlight (ultraviolet radiation [UV]) has been strongly implicated as a causative factor in the development of melanoma. Ultraviolet B radiation (UVB; defined as radiation with wavelengths of 290 to 320 nanometers) appears to more closely associated with the development of melanoma than ultraviolet A radiation (UVA; defined as radiation with wavelengths of 320 to 400 nanometers).[2] This is supported by the higher incidence of melanoma in equatorial regions than in latitudes farther from the equator; UVB radiation is

KEY POINT

- Risk factors for melanoma include dysplastic (atypical) nevi, an increased number of benign nevi, family history of melanoma, and fair skin that burns.

most intense at the equator, whereas UVA radiation intensity varies less across latitudes.

Although UVB appears to be more important than UVA as a risk factor, a causal link to UVA exposure also is supported by data from patients who used tanning beds and/or who were treated with a combination of psoralene, which is applied or taken orally to sensitize the skin, and UVA (PUVA) for psoriasis. Worldwide, the incidence of melanoma in white individuals generally correlates inversely with geographic latitude: rates are generally higher in areas closer to the equator and become progressively lower in areas near the poles. The rates of melanoma are higher for individuals with a tendency to burn rather than tan when exposed to sunlight, including those people with fair complexion, blond or red hair, blue eyes, and freckles. The pattern of sun exposure also may be important. Intermittent intense exposure and sunburns in areas exposed to the sun only sporadically (e.g., the back for men and the legs for women) rather than chronic exposure may carry more risk of melanoma. Blistering sunburns, particularly in childhood, are associated with an increased risk of melanoma. However, melanoma can occur in any ethnic group and without significant sun exposure.

Pigmented lesions are another factor linked to melanoma risk. This risk is increased for individuals with increased number of benign moles (melanocytic nevi). The proportion of melanomas that arise from melanocytic nevi ranges from 18% to 85%. Atypical moles or dysplastic nevi are important precursor lesions of melanoma and also serve as markers for increasing risk. The presence of dysplastic nevi are associated with a 6% lifetime chance of melanoma.[3] This risk is as high as 80% for individuals who have dysplastic nevi and a family history of melanoma. Other risk factors for melanoma include a personal history of the disease, nonmelanoma skin cancers, immunosuppression, and xeroderma pigmentosa.

HEREDITARY BASIS OF MELANOMA: GENES INVOLVED IN MELANOMA SUSCEPTIBILITY

Approximately 10% of patients with melanoma have a family history of the disease. Some cases occur in the setting of the familial atypical mole and melanoma syndrome or the dysplastic nevus syndrome. Several genetic loci determine susceptibility to melanoma, the most important of these being *p16/CDKN2A*, a gene located on chromosome 9p21. *CDKN2A* gene encodes two proteins, p16 and p14ARF, which are cell-cycle inhibitors. Of the members of melanoma-prone families, 25% to 40% have mutations in this gene.[4] A few rare kindreds have mutations in *CDK4*. Both of these genes are considered tumor suppressor genes. Pancreatic cancer also is seen in melanoma-prone families with *CDKN2A* germ-line mutations. Testing for mutations in the *p16/CDKN2A* locus is available on a commercial basis. However, the clinical utility of genetic testing for melanoma susceptibility is limited at this time and, therefore, is not recommended.[5] In addition, *BRAC2* gene carriers have an increased risk of cutaneous melanoma.

GENES INVOLVED IN SPORADIC MELANOMA

A number of genetic changes recently have been described in primary melanomas.[7,8] The *BRAF* oncogene is the most common somatic mutation in melanoma, present in approximately 60% of cases. This serine-threonine kinase mediates signaling through the mitogen-activated protein kinases (MAPK) pathway. Immediately upstream of *BRAF* is *NRAS*, which is mutated and activated in 15% of melanomas. Mutations of both *NRAS* and *BRAF* virtually never occur together. Recent work has linked molecular alterations in melanoma with subtypes of melanoma, anatomic location, and sun exposure. For example, activating mutations in *BRAF* are more common in melanomas arising in skin that has little chronic sun-induced damage and are less frequent in melanomas associated with severe chronic solar damage. Recently identified is that melanomas on mucosal membranes, acral skin (soles, palms, and nail bed), and skin with chronic sun-induced damage (i.e., lentigo maligna melanoma) have frequent mutations in KIT,[9] and these types of melanoma lack mutation in *BRAF* or *NRAS*. Microphthalmia-associated transcription factor (*MITF*) is an oncogene in melanoma, and loss of PTEN expression also has been described in primary melanomas. Presently, there is no correlation between oncogene expression, overall prognosis, or selection of therapy. Figure. 11-1 summarizes the signaling pathways and examples of targeted therapies in melanoma.

Prevention and Screening

The most important preventive measures are to reduce excessive sun exposure and avoid sunburns. Strategies to reduce exposure include avoiding the midday sun, using sunscreen products with a sun-protection factor (SPF) of more than 15 on a regular basis, and wearing protective clothing. It has been difficult to prove that regular use of sunscreen protects against melanoma, although data suggest that sunscreens may prevent nonmelanoma skin cancer.[6]

Screening for skin cancer, whether by self-examination or by a health care provider, is a controversial area. Individuals with clinically atypical nevi, particularly if they have a family history of melanoma, require a regular surveillance program. Regular skin examinations should be performed every 6 to

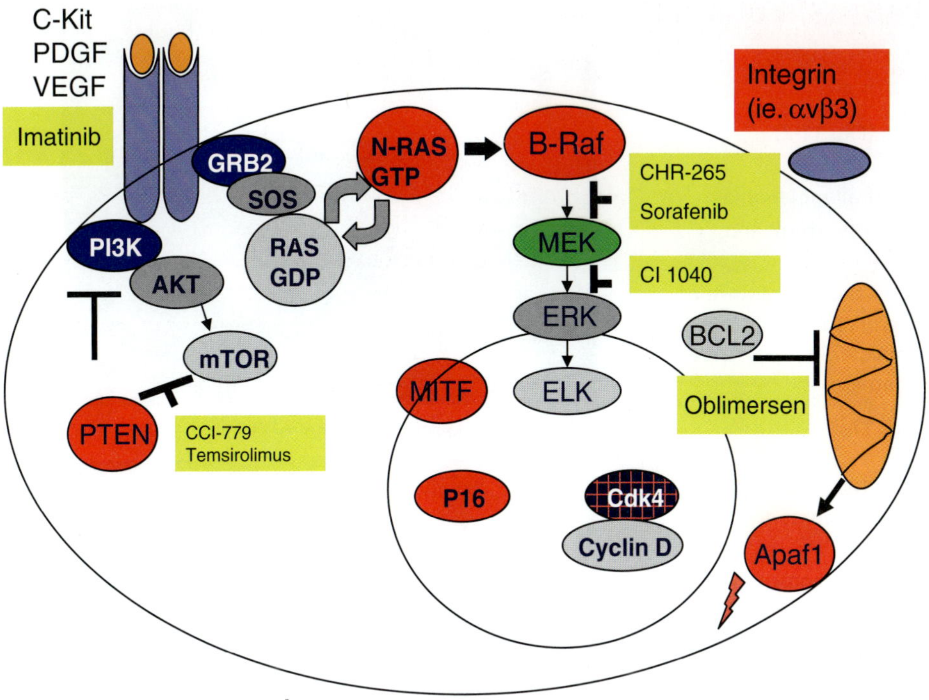

FIG. 11-1 Signaling pathways and examples of targeted therapies in melanoma.

12 months and can be supplemented with photographs of the atypical nevi.

CLINICAL PRESENTATION AND DIAGNOSIS

Early detection and recognition of melanoma is the key to improving overall survival of patients with malignant disease. The signs of early melanoma are based on the clinical appearance of the pigmented lesion in addition to a history of change in an existing mole, including change in shape, color, or surface. More than 70% of melanomas are associated with an increase in size and a change in color. Most patients report having a pre-existing mole at the site of the melanoma. Itching, burning, or pain in a pigmented lesion should increase suspicion, although melanomas often are not associated with local discomfort. Bleeding and ulceration are signs of a more advanced melanoma. Most melanomas are varying shades of brown, but they also may be black, blue, or pink. The "ABCDE's" for the recognition of melanoma are asymetry, border, color, diameter, and evolution.

A biopsy should be performed on any skin lesion suspicious for melanoma. The proper biopsy is essential not only to establish a diagnosis but also to allow precise histologic interpretation that will determine the prognosis and plan of therapy. For most clinically suspicious skin lesions, complete excision with a 1-mm to 2-mm margin of normal skin is best. Shallow shave biopsy or curettage is contraindicated for lesions suspicious for melanoma.

Cutaneous melanoma has been divided into four subtypes based on distinct clinical and histologic features. In descending order of frequency, these are superficial spreading melanoma, nodular melanoma, lentigo maligna melanoma, and acral lentiginous melanoma (Table 11-1 and Figs. 11-2 to 11-6). Histologic subtype does not directly correlate with clinical behavior; however, new data suggest that histologic subtype may correlate with specific genetic abnormalities. Primary melanomas also can arise from mucosal epithelial cells lining the respiratory, alimentary, and genitourinary tracts, although such melanomas are rare. Ocular melanomas arise from the pigmented layer of the eye that includes the iris, ciliary body, and choroid; these lesions are referred to as uveal melanomas. Uveal melanoma is the most common primary intraocular malignancy of adults.

KEY POINT

- A history of recent change in a pigmented lesion or a new pigmented lesion should alert the clinician that a biopsy is needed. Changes in size, color, and border are important clues to the diagnosis of melanoma.

KEY POINT

- Staging is based primarily on tumor depth, tumor ulceration, and on whether the melanoma involves regional lymph nodes or has metastasized to distant sites.

Table 11-1 Four Histologic Subtypes of Cutaneous Melanoma

Superficial Spreading Melanoma (Fig. 11-2)

- Incidence: Accounts for 70% of all melanomas
- Anatomic site: Any, predominantly trunk and extremities
- Clinical appearance: Change in the appearance of a large mole, asymmetry, irregular border, variegated color (brown, black, pink,white, gray, blue), often arising in a precursor mole

Lentigo Maligna Melanoma (Fig. 11-3)

- Incidence: Accounts for 4% to 10% of all melanoma; tends to occur more commonly in older patients
- Anatomic site: Areas with chronic exposure to the sun, head and neck regions and distal extremities
- Clinical appearance: Macular (flat) lesion, arising in a lentigo maligna, which often appears as a flat, light brown skin lesion

Nodular Melanoma (Fig. 11-4)

- Incidence: Accounts for 15% of melanomas
- Anatomic site: Any
- Clinical appearance: Rapidly enlarging, elevated, or polypoid lesion, often arising in normal skin, often blue or black (The A-B-C-D-E rule does not apply*)

Acral Lentiginous Melanoma (Figs. 11-5 and 11-6)

- Incidence: 5% to 10%
- Anatomic site: Most commonly on the palms, soles, or subungual under the nail bed) or mucous membranes
- Clinical appearance: Darkly pigmented, flat to nodular lesion, highly irregular borders

* The A-B-C-D-E rule is defined as the following: A, asymmetry; B, border (irregular); C, color (heterogenous,variegated); D, diameter greater than 5 mm; and E, evolution.

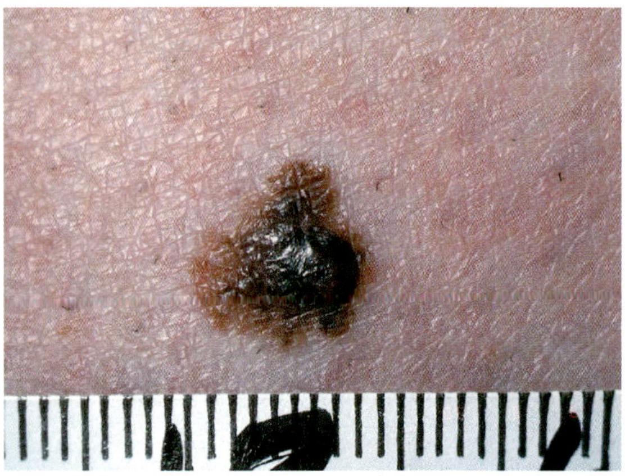

FIG. 11-2 Superficial spreading melanoma

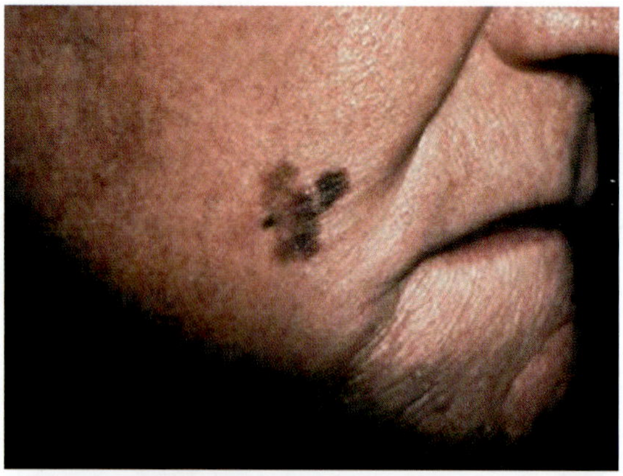

FIG. 11-3 Lentigo maligna melanoma

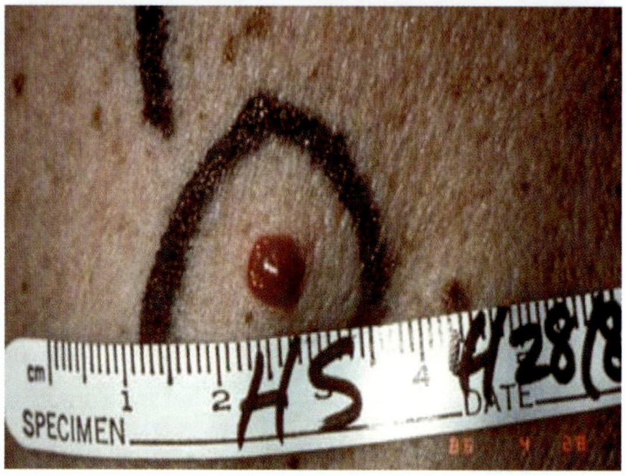

FIG. 11-4 Nodular melanoma

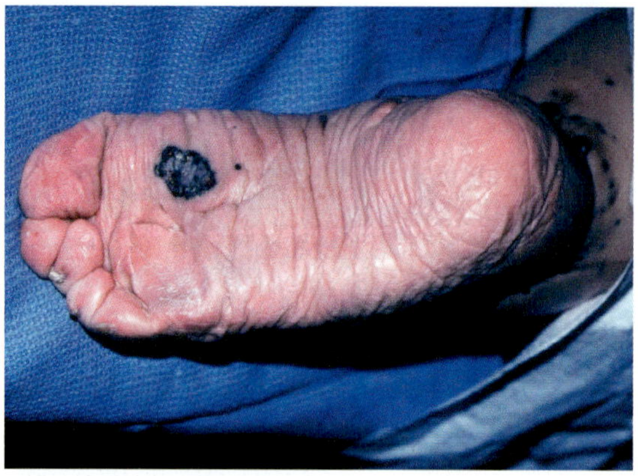

FIG. 11-5 Acral lentiginous melanoma

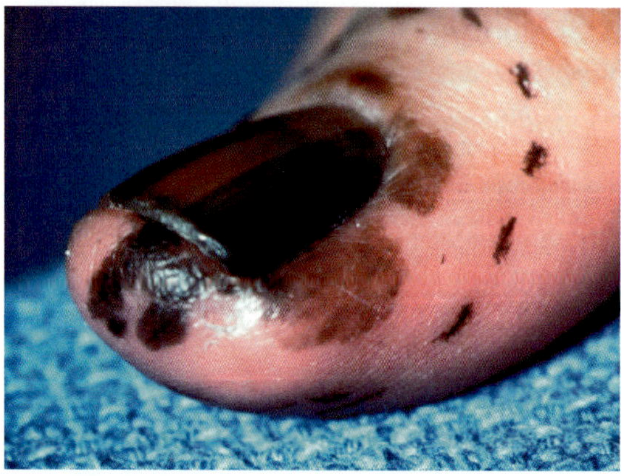

FIG. 11-6 Acral lentiginous melanoma

PROGNOSTIC FACTORS

A number of clinical and histologic factors have been associated with the probability of survival of a patient with melanoma. The single most predictive factor is the depth of invasion (Breslow thickness) of the original lesion, measured in millimeters from the uppermost layer of the epidermis to the deepest melanoma cell in the underlying dermis. Increasing thickness is associated with a higher risk of recurrence of melanoma and, therefore, death (Table 11-2). In addition, the thicker the primary melanoma, the more likely there is microscopic involvement of the lymph nodes. Ulcerated melanomas are associated with a poorer prognosis. This feature of the primary melanoma is now incorporated into the staging system for melanoma. Other poor prognostic factors include increasing level of invasion (Clark level), high mitotic rate, lack of tumor infiltrating lymphocytes, and presence of microscopic satellites. Primary tumor location, patient age, and gender are clinical variables associated with prognosis. In general, patients with primary melanoma of the extremities have a significantly better clinical prognosis than those with primary lesions of the trunk and head. Increased patient age and male sex is associated with a worse outcome. The involvement of regional lymph nodes is a poor prognostic sign, regardless of the thickness or the level of the primary melanoma. In addition, the number of involved lymph nodes correlates with the risk of distant metastatic disease and, therefore, survival. Patients with one regional lymph node have an approximate 50% risk of systemic recurrence. Patients with multiple lymph nodes have a 75% risk of systemic recurrence.

STAGING SYSTEM

The staging system for melanoma, which was developed by the American Joint Committee on Cancer (AJCC) and updated in 2002, now more accurately classifies patients into groups with similar survival (Table 11-2).[10] Stages I and II indicate clinically localized primary melanoma to the skin, and stage III melanoma indicates regional involvement (lymph nodes or in-transit metastases). Stage IV is metastatic disease beyond regional lymph nodes (i.e., lung, liver, and brain). The 5-year survival rates associated with each of the four stages also are noted in the staging system in Table 11-2. It is estimated that 82% to 85% of patients with melanoma present with localized disease (stage I or II), 10% to 13% present with regional lymph nodes disease (stage III), and 2% to 5 % present with distant metastatic disease.

PATIENT EVALUATION

The initial evaluation of a patient with melanoma includes personal and family histories and an appropriate physical

Table 11-2 American Joint Committee on Cancer Staging System for Cutaneous Melanoma

Stage	TNM Classification	Definition	Five-Year Survival Rate, % ± SE
IA	T1a N0 M0	< 1mm; no ulceration (Clark level II/III)	95.3 ± 0.4
IB	T1b N0 M0	≤ 1mm with ulceration or Clark level IV/V	90.9 ± 1.0
	T2a N0 M0	1.01 to 2 mm; no ulceration	89.0 ± 0.7
IIA	T2b N0 M0	1.01 to 2 mm with ulceration	77.4 ± 1.7
	T3a N0 M0	2.01 to 4 mm; no ulceration	78.7 ± 1.2
IIB	T3b N0 M0	2.01 to 4 mm with ulceration	63.0 ± 1.5
	T4a N0 M0	> 4 mm; no ulceration	67.4 ± 2.4
IIC	T4b N0 M0	> 4 mm with ulceration	45.1 ± 1.9
IIIA	T1-4a N1a M0	Single micronode; no ulceration	69.5 ± 3.7
	T1-4a N2a M0	2 to 3 micronodes; no ulceration	63.3 ± 5.6
IIIB	T1-4a N1b–2c M0	1 to 3 macronodes or in-transit mets; no ulcer	40 – 60
	T1-4b N1a–2a M0	1 to 3 micronodes; ulceration	40 – 55
IIIC	T1-4b N1b–2b M0	1 to 3 macronodes; ulceration	20 – 35
	Any T N3 M0	≥ 4 nodes, matted, or nodes plus in-transit metastasis	26.7 ± 2.5
IV	Any T Any N M1a–1b	Distant skin, SC, nodal, or lung metastasis	5 – 20
	Any T Any N M1c	All visceral mets or elevated LDH with metastasis	9.5 ± 1.1

Abbreviations: TNM, tumor, node, metastases; SE, standard error; SC, subcutaneous; LDH, lactate acid dehydrogenase.
Adapted with permission from Balch CM, Buzaid AC, Soong S-J, et al. Final version of the American Joint Committee on Cancer staging system for cutaneous melanoma. J Clin Oncol. 2001;19:3635–3648.

examination including a total skin examination and palpation of regional (draining) lymph nodes. The focus of this evaluation is to identify risk factors, signs or symptoms of metastases, dysplastic nevi, and additional primary melanomas. The extent of the work-up for patients with the initial diagnosis of melanoma is based on the risk of recurrence associated with the primary melanoma. In general, for low-risk melanomas, (i.e., less than 1.0 mm and no ulceration) no further search for occult metastatic disease is indicated. In patients with higher-risk primary melanomas, a chest x-ray, liver function tests, and measurement of lactate dehydrogenase often are performed; however there are no data to support this common practice. A more extensive staging evaluation with computerized tomography (CT) alone or in combination with positron emission tomography (PET) scans of the chest, abdomen, or pelvis can be considered for patients with thick primary melanoma (more than 4 mm, high-risk stage II melanoma) or node-positive disease (stage III melanoma), for whom the risk of distant metastatic disease is higher. Again, there are no data to support this approach, and there is considerable variation in clinical practice. CT or PET imaging is not indicated for patients with stage I melanoma and most patients with stage II melanoma. Currently, no tumor markers are sensitive and specific for melanoma. Assays to detect molecular markers of melanoma cells in the blood and sentinel lymph nodes are being investigated. PET is useful in evaluating metastatic disease, but its role in screening has not yet been defined.

TREATMENT

Once melanoma has been diagnosed, the standard treatment is surgical excision of the primary lesion. The extent of surgery depends on the thickness of the primary melanoma. Large surgical excisions are no longer necessary, and most wide excisions can be performed with primary closure. Findings from randomized clinical studies of optimal surgical margins have demonstrated that less radical surgery results in excellent local control with no adverse effect on survival.[11,12] Current recommendations for the optimal width of surgical margins are summarized in Table 11-3.

The wide excision should include underlying subcutaneous tissue down to fascia. In cosmetically sensitive areas, such as the face, or anatomically difficult areas, such as the ears and hands, it may be difficult to achieve the desired margin. In those situations, at least a 1-cm margin should be obtained.

TABLE 11-3 Recommended Surgical Margins for Primary Melanoma

Tumor Thickness	Surgical Margin
In situ	0.5 to 1.0 cm
≤ 1.0 mm	1.0 cm
1.01 to 2.0 mm	1.0 to 2.0 cm
2.01 to 4.0 mm	2.0 cm
> 4.0 mm	At least 2.0 cm

KEY POINT

- Surgery is the mainstay of treatment of early melanoma. The extent of surgical margins depends on the depth of the primary lesion, but the overall trend is for narrower surgical margins.

MANAGEMENT OF REGIONAL LYMPH NODES

CLINICALLY NORMAL (NEGATIVE) REGIONAL LYMPH NODES

For decades, the management of clinically normal lymph nodes in patients with melanoma has been debated. For approximately 15% to 20% of patients with melanoma who do not have clinically apparent lymph node involvement, the regional lymph nodes will contain occult micrometastases. The risk of occult lymph node involvement increases with greater tumor thickness. The results of randomized clinical trials have not shown a survival benefit from elective, or prophylactic, lymph node dissection for patients with melanoma.[13] These results provide evidence against the routine use of elective lymph node dissection for patients with clinically negative lymph nodes.

Sentinel lymph node mapping has largely replaced elective lymph node dissection for patients with early-stage melanoma and is a useful staging procedure. Sentinel lymph node mapping is generally considered for patients with melanomas that are more than 1 mm thick. For melanomas that are less than 1 mm thick, the likelihood of regional lymph node involvement is low (less than 5%), and, thus, sentinel node mapping is generally not indicated unless there are worrisome histologic features, such as ulceration of the primary melanoma or a Clark level of IV or V. The false-negative rate for sentinel lymph node mapping is approximately 4%. A recently reported study evaluated the role of sentinel lymph node mapping compared with observation in patients with intermediate-thickness melanoma. Patients were randomly assigned to wide excision followed by observation of regional lymph nodes with lymphadenectomy if nodal relapse occurred, or to wide excision and sentinel node biopsy with immediate lymphadenectomy if nodal micrometastases were detected on biopsy. Overall, the 5-year melanoma-specific survival rates were similar for the two groups. However, among patients with nodal metastases, the 5-year survival rate was higher among those who underwent immediate lymphadenectomy than among those in whom lymphadenectomy was delayed.[14]

The sentinel lymph node procedure should be performed before the wide excision because the surgery can

> **KEY POINTS**
>
> - Sentinel lymph node mapping is a useful staging procedure for melanomas and provides important prognostic information.
> - There is no role for prophylactic lymph node dissection in patients with melanoma because of the associated morbidity and lack of survival benefit of this procedure.

alter the lymphatic drainage pattern, which affects the reliability of the procedure. If the sentinel lymph node is negative for melanoma, no further lymph node surgery is required. If melanoma is detected in the sentinel lymph node, a completion lymph node dissection of the involved nodal basin is recommended.

CLINICALLY ENLARGED (POSITIVE) REGIONAL LYMPH NODES

For patients who present with palpable regional lymph nodes metastases, a therapeutic lymph node dissection should be performed. The goal of nodal dissection is to provide long-term, disease-free survival and possibly to cure or provide optimum local-regional control of disease. Satellite metastases and in-transit metastases are usually surgically resected. Negative margins are generally sufficient without large, wide excisions.

ADJUVANT THERAPY FOLLOWING SURGERY

The primary treatment for most patients with stages I and II melanoma is surgical resection. Postoperative adjuvant therapy can be considered for patients at high risk for recurrent melanoma. High risk is generally defined as melanomas that are more than 4 mm thick or node-positive (stage III) disease. Adjuvant therapy options include high-dose interferon-alfa-2b, a clinical trial, or observation. Similar treatment options are considered for patients with resected in-transit melanoma or for those patients with stage IV disease who are free of disease following surgical resection of metastases.

ADJUVANT INTERFERON THERAPY

On the basis of the potent immunologic effects of interferon and its documented activity against metastatic melanoma, numerous studies with this drug have been conducted in the postoperative adjuvant setting. The U.S. Food and Drug Administration (FDA) recommended approval for interferon-alfa2b in 1995 based on study E1684 conducted by the Eastern Cooperative Oncology Group (ECOG).[15] In that study, 280 patients with thick primary melanoma (more than 4 mm) and node-negative disease (T4, stage IIB) or with node-positive disease (stage III) were randomly assigned to receive either dose-intensive interferon-alpha2b for 1 year or to be observed only. All patients had wide excision of the primary melanoma and regional lymphadenectomy. An intensive regimen was deliberately chosen in order to deliver interferon at the maximally tolerated dose to achieve peak drug levels. The patients were treated with an intravenous induction phase of 20 million U/m^2, 5 days a week, for 1 month, followed by an 11-month course of 10 million U/m^2 given subcutaneously 3 days a week. For patients who were treated with interferon, the median survival was significantly longer (3 years compared with 4 years; $p = 0.02$) and the relapse-free survival was better (1 year compared with 2 years; $p = 0.002$). Treatment with interferon was associated with an increase in the 5-year survival rate from 36% to 47%. This trial was the first study of adjuvant therapy for melanoma in which an improvement in overall survival was demonstrated. However with longer follow-up, this survival advantage is no longer statistically significant. In a subsequent Intergroup adjuvant trial, E1690, high-dose interferon therapy was compared with a lower-dose regimen (three million IU/m^2 three times a week for 2 years) and compared with observation after complete resection of all known disease. The results of that trial confirmed the disease-free survival advantage of high-dose interferon seen in study E1684 but not the overall survival advantage.[16] This discrepancy may be the result of differences in eligibility criteria for the two studies and the subsequent availability of cross-over treatment with interferon after relapse in the E1690 trial. There was no benefit from low-dose interferon.

A third trial, E1694, evaluated a 1-year course of high-dose interferon compared with a 2-year course of treatment with a ganglioside GM2 vaccine.[17] After 2 years of median follow-up, high-dose interferon was associated with a highly significant improvement in both relapse-free survival and overall survival, and the study was terminated early. Thus, the results from a series of randomized clinical trials in which the role of high-dose interferon has been evaluated indicate improvement in relapse-free survival and possibly overall survival. However, these results do not come without substantial cost regarding toxicity, which has limited the acceptance of high-dose interferon therapy by patients and physicians. Patients may have flu-like symptoms such as fatigue, fever, chills, myalgia, anorexia, nausea, vomiting, and headache. In addition, high-dose interferon therapy may cause or exacerbate depression. Suicidal ideation and suicide also have been associated with the treatment. Significant laboratory abnormalities include elevated levels of hepatic transaminases,

> **KEY POINT**
>
> - Interferon therapy may be considered as adjuvant therapy following surgery for patients with primary melanomas that are thick (more than 4 mm) or for patients with stage III, node-positive disease.

neutropenia, elevated triglyceride levels, and anemia. It is critical that patients who are treated with high-dose interferon be monitored closely and that the dose of interferon be modified appropriately for toxicity. It has recently been reported that the development of auto antibodies (i.e., antinuclear antibodies, antithyroglobin, and anticardiolipin antibodies) and/or the clinical manifestations of autoimmunity (e.g., vitiligo, autoimmune thrombocytopenia, and retinopathy) during treatment with high-dose interferon was associated with improvement in both recurrence-free and overall survival rates when compared with patients who did not develop autoimmune manifestations. The median time to detection of findings of autoantibody after initiation of interferon was 3 months, and the development of clinical manifestations of autoimmunity was 9 months.[18]

A randomized controlled trial evaluated low-dose interferon-alfa2a compared with observation, and there was no improvement in recurrence-free or overall survivals.[19] Ongoing studies are exploring alternative schedules and doses of interferon.

Thus, the decision regarding the use of high-dose adjuvant interferon should be made carefully and involves a thorough conversation between the patient and physician that includes review of risks and benefits, as well as potential contraindications to treatment with interferon.

ADJUVANT VACCINE THERAPY

Vaccine therapy, particularly in the adjuvant setting, continues to be explored as a treatment option for patients with melanoma. In general, two approaches are under clinical investigation, whole-cell vaccines (autologous or allogeneic) and peptide-based, or defined, antigens.[20] Vaccine approaches should be considered experimental because no benefit in overall survival has been established.

SURVEILLANCE AFTER PRIMARY THERAPY

Patients with a history of melanoma should be followed regularly for evidence of local-regional recurrence, distant metastatic disease, and a second primary melanoma. The most important components of surveillance are the history and physical examination. The physical examination should include a thorough skin examination because the risk of second primary melanoma is increased for individuals who have a history of melanoma. An annual skin exam is recommended for life or, more often, based on individual patient risk factors. Regional lymph nodes should be thoroughly examined, especially in patients who have not had surgical resection of nodes. The remainder of the examination should be comprehensive, with awareness of frequent metastases to the lung, liver, and brain. Patient education is an integral part of the treatment of patients with melanoma, and they should receive instruction on how to perform monthly self-examinations of the skin for detection of new primary melanomas and recurrent disease. They also should be taught about the clinical characteristics of melanoma and the importance of safe-sun strategies. Educating family members about melanoma risk factors and changes in sun behavior also is important.

The optimal follow-up and surveillance program for patients with melanoma has not been defined. To date, there are no data to show that regular screening with radiologic studies affects overall survival for patients with melanoma. The follow-up schedule and the extent of the evaluation (i.e., blood test or radiographic evaluation) is influenced by the risk of recurrence. For patients with thin melanomas, no specific radiologic or laboratory investigations to detect occult disease are recommended. For patients with melanomas more than 1 mm in size, follow-up studies generally include a complete blood count, serum chemistry analyses with liver function tests, and a serum lactate dehydrogenase level. An elevated level of lactate dehydrogenase is suggestive of metastatic melanoma. Because the lungs are the most frequent sites of distant disease, periodic chest x-rays can be considered. The routine use of screening CT, magnetic resonance imaging, PET (with or without CT), or bone scanning is not viewed as necessary but certainly can be performed as clinically indicated. The National Comprehensive Cancer Network has proposed surveillance guidelines (Fig. 11-7). In general, for patients with stage I or stage II melanoma, regular physical examination and annual skin exam are recommended. Chest x-ray and blood tests for lactate dehydrogenase levels are optional. In addition to these tests, CT or PET (or a combination of both) scanning can be considered for patients with stage III melanoma. There is significant variability in clinical practice so these guidelines allow for flexibility in follow-up. The clinician should choose follow-up schedule and selection of tests based on patient's risk of recurrence, symptoms, and the physician's experience.

KEY POINTS

- The median survival for patients with metastatic melanoma (stage IV disease) is influenced by many factors but is approximately 9 months.
- Treatment options for metastatic melanoma include: observation; resection of solitary metastasis; dacarbazine-based or temozolomide-based therapy; immunologic treatments, such as interleukin-2; and participation in clinical trials.
- There is no evidence that combination chemotherapy is superior to single-agent dacarbazine or temozolomide for patients with metastatic melanoma.
- There is no survival benefit of biochemotherapy compared with chemotherapy or immunotherapy in patients with metastatic melanoma.

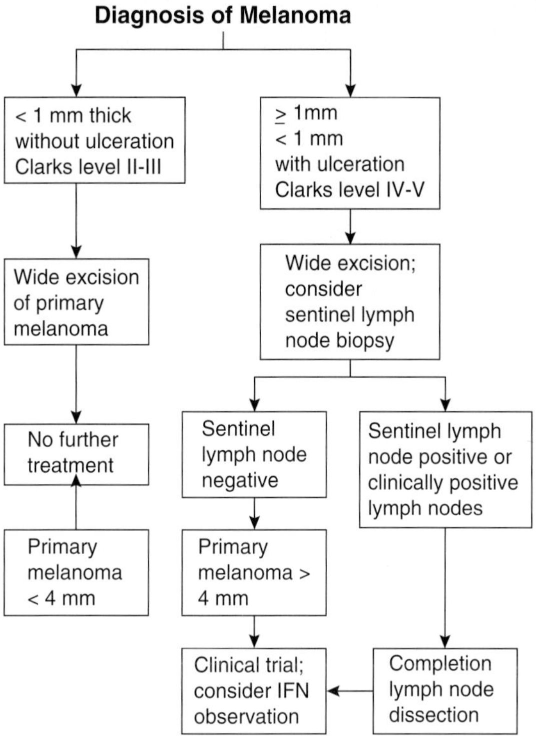

FIG. 11-7 Treatment algorithm for patients with newly diagnosed melanoma.

TREATMENT OF METASTATIC MELANOMA

The treatment of patients with metastatic melanoma depends on multiple factors, including the overall condition and age of the patient, the sites and number of metastases, the pace of the disease, and the patient's wishes for treatment. The goals of treatment are directed toward palliation of symptoms because there is no evidence that treatment of metastatic melanoma has an effect on prolonging survival.[21] Metastatic melanoma can affect virtually any organ of the body, with the most common site being the lung; the skin, liver, and brain also are common sites of metastases. The overall survival for patients with metastatic melanoma ranges from 5 to 11 months, with a median survival of 9 months. The estimated 5-year survival rate for patients with stage IV disease is 5% to 15%. Long-term survival has been reported for highly selected patients. Treatment options include chemotherapy, immunotherapy, biochemotherapy, radiation therapy, surgical resection of isolated metastases, isolated limb perfusion, and participation in a clinical trial. Patients with metastatic melanoma have a particularly high incidence of brain metastases. Surgery or radiation therapy (whole brain or sterotactic radiosurgery) may be considered based on symptoms, number of lesions present, and location of lesions.

CHEMOTHERAPY

Numerous chemotherapy agents have demonstrated modest activity in the treatment of metastatic melanoma. However, no single agent has consistently yielded response rates of greater than 20%. Dacarbazine remains the only chemotherapy agent approved by the FDA for the treatment of metastatic melanoma. The results from clinical trials have demonstrated overall response rates of approximately 10% to 20%. Responses are not durable, lasting a median of 3 to 4 months, and long-term complete responses are seen in only 1% to 2% of patients.[22] Dose and schedules of dacarbazine vary widely, with no data to suggest that response rates are influenced by these variables. The most commonly used regimen is 800 to 1,000 mg/m^2 intravenously repeated every 3 to 4 weeks, or 200 mg/m^2 intravenously for 5 days every 3 to 4 weeks. Dacarbazine is generally well tolerated. The most frequent side effects are nausea and vomiting, which can be severe. Mild to moderate myelosuppression is a common dose-related side effect.

Temozolomide is an oral analogue of dacarbazine, which crosses the blood–brain barrier. Temozolomide was approved by the FDA in 1999 for the treatment of primary brain tumors. The results from several phase II studies suggest that temozolomide is at least as effective as dacarbazine in metastatic disease, with an overall response rate of 21%, including a 5% complete response rate. Temozolomide is easy to administer because it is given orally, and the standard daily dose is 150 to 200 mg/m^2 on days 1 to 5. Courses are repeated every 3 to 4 weeks. The major side effect is mild to moderate myelosuppression. Mild nausea and vomiting also are common but can be readily controlled with standard antiemetic therapy. Temozolomide was compared with dacarbazine in a phase III clinical trial of 305 patients with stage IV melanoma. Temozolomide was associated with a nonsignificant improvement in median survival (7.7 months compared with 6.4 months with dacarbazine). Response rates were 13.5% and 12.1 %, respectively.[23] Additional schedules of temozolomide also have been investigated, lower dose for prolonged periods (75 mg/m^2 daily for 6 weeks on, 2 weeks off). This dosage is associated with lymphopenia, and opportunistic infections have been reported. Temozolomide has not been approved by the FDA for the management of melanoma. Newer approaches combine temozolomide and other agents, including sorafenib, thalidomide, and immunotherapeutic agents. In a recent phase III trial, 771 patients with stage IV melanoma were randomly assigned to treatment with dacarbazine combined with oblimersen — an antisense oligonucleotide directed against BCL-2 mRNA — or with dacarbazine alone. The findings showed that the combination arm had an increase in response rate (13.5% vs. 7.5%, $p = 0.007$) and in progression-free survival (median, 2.6 months vs. 1.6 months; $p = 0.001$) but only a trend for overall survival (median, 9.0 vs. 7.8 months; $p = 0.077$).[24] Other chemotherapy drugs with single-agent activity include cisplatin, the taxanes, carmustine (BCNU), fotemustine, lomustine (CCNU), and vinblastine.

Several combination chemotherapy regimens have been evaluated in patients with metastatic melanoma. Examples include the "Dartmouth regimen," which includes cisplatin, dacarbazine, carmustine, and tamoxifen, or combination cisplatin, vinblastine, and dacarbazine. Initial phase II studies of these regimens were associated with response rates in the range of 30% to 50% range. However, over the past several years as data from larger, multicenter clinical studies have accumulated, the high response rates reported in these initial studies have not been reproduced. A phase III study conducted by Intergroup/ECOG compared the Dartmouth regimen with dacarbazine alone for patients with metastatic melanoma.[25] There was no difference in survival between the two groups and only a small, nonsignificant increase in tumor response in patients treated with the Dartmouth regimen. Based on these data, at the present time, there is no evidence that any combination chemotherapy regimen is superior to single-agent dacarbazine or temozolomide.

IMMUNOTHERAPY

Interferon has been evaluated extensively for patients with metastatic melanoma. In a series of phase II studies involving a variety of doses and schedules, the response rates have ranged from 10% to 25%. Most of the responses have been partial, with a complete response rate of less than 5%. Although interferon has been approved by the FDA for the adjuvant treatment of patients with high-risk melanoma, it is designated as an orphan drug by the FDA for use in combination with aldesleukin, or interleukin-2, for patients with metastatic disease.

Aldesleukin, a potent T-cell activator, is approved by the FDA for the treatment of metastatic melanoma. Long-term follow-up data for 270 patients with metastatic melanoma treated with high-dose aldesleukin show an overall response rate of 16%, with a 6% complete response rate.[26] Durable complete responses have been observed in a small percentage of patients receiving this treatment. The median response duration was 9 months (range, 2 months to more than 106 months).

The current FDA-approved regimen consists of two 5-day courses of aldesleukin separated by a rest period of 7 to 10 days. Two high-dose regimens have been used: 600,000 IU/kg or 720,000 IU/kg, administered every 8 hours for 14 or 15 doses per cycle. Repeat courses can be given at 8 to 12 weeks if the disease responds to treatment. Typically, two or three courses are given when there is a good response, with a maximum of five courses. The toxicity of aldesleukin is clearly dose related. The most common side effects include hypotension, diarrhea, renal dysfunction with oliguria, respiratory failure, fever, chills, and vomiting. Many of the adverse effects of this treatment result from a capillary-leak syndrome caused by the drug. Aldesleukin also is associated with an increased risk of infection, most commonly *Staphylococcus aureus*, because of catheter-related to infection. Most of the side effects are self-limiting and resolve after discontinuation. Because of low response rates and the substantial toxicity of high-dose aldesleukin, its use should be restricted to carefully selected patients and should be administered by experienced clinicians at established cancer treatment centers. Careful assessment of cardiac and pulmonary function is mandatory prior to initiation of high-dose aldesleukin therapy.

Other dosing regimens include continuous intravenous infusion or subcutaneous administration with lower doses of aldesleukin. Less serious side effects with these alternative doses and methods of delivery have been reported in some studies, but it remains unclear whether the efficacy is comparable. Ongoing clinical trials are investigating the role of adoptive immunotherapy — activated T cells, autologous tumor infiltrating lymphocytes (TILS), treatment with anti-CTLA-4 monoclonal antibody with or without peptide vaccine, and lymphodepleting chemotherapy followed by the transfer of autologous tumor reactive lymphocytes.[27]

BIOCHEMOTHERAPY

Biochemotherapy, the combination of immunotherapy and cytotoxic chemotherapy, has been studied in patients with metastatic melanoma. Initial results from multiple phase II studies were encouraging regarding tumor response rates. However, the results of randomized phase III clinical trials in which biochemotherapy was compared with either aldesleukin and interferon or with chemotherapy have been disappointing, with no evidence that this approach improves overall survival of patients with metastatic disease.[28] Biochemotherapy is associated with considerable toxicity including myelosuppression, nausea, vomiting, rash, hypotension, and fluid retention. Thus, given the lack of survival benefit along with the toxicity, biochemotherapy is not the standard of care for patients with stage IV melanoma. However, biochemotherapy continues to be evaluated in the adjuvant and neoadjuvant settings in clinical trials.

NEW DIRECTION: MOLECULARLY TARGETED THERAPY

A number of new approaches for the treatment of stage IV melanoma are undergoing evaluation in clinical trials. An important focus is on drugs that target specific molecular signaling pathways, which are perturbed in melanoma, such as the activating mutation of *BRAF* in the majority of melanomas. The MAPK (i.e., Ras-Raf-Erk) pathway is an attractive target for the treatment of melanoma based on extensive preclinical studies and emerging clinical data. Ongoing studies in patients with melanoma are exploring the role of sorafenib, an oral multikinase inhibitor that targets vascular endothelial growth factor (VEGF) and was the first BRAF inhibitor. Sorafenib is approved by the FDA for the treatment of advanced renal cancer based on its effects on VEGF. As a single agent, sorafenib has little activity against melanoma. Sorafenib has been combined with chemotherapy based on preclinical studies conducted in vitro and in animal models that demonstrate that sorafenib can enhance the activity of chemotherapy. Several clinical trials are completed or are ongoing. The most extensively evaluated combinations are sorafenib with carboplatin and paclitaxel and sorafenib combined with dacarbazine or temozolomide. Encouraging results from these studies have been reported.[29] Other agents that are more potent and specific inhibitors of BRAF also are undergoing clinical testing in patients with advanced melanoma. In some studies, selection of patients is based on the mutation status of *BRAF*. An alternative strategy to targeting BRAF is inhibition of MEK (MAPK/extracellular signal-regulated kinase), the immediate downstream signaling component in the MAPK pathway. Ongoing studies are exploring MEK inhibitor in patients with metastatic melanoma.

RADIATION THERAPY

The main indication for radiation therapy for patients with metastatic disease is the treatment of symptomatic lesions, including painful bone, skin, or subcutaneous metastases. Whole-brain radiation therapy or gamma knife radiation is very helpful in palliating the symptoms of brain metastases in most patients. Overall, 60% to 70% of patients have measurable improvement in their performance status. However, durable local control of brain metastases is rarely achieved. Radiation therapy also is indicated for spinal cord compression.

SURGICAL RESECTION

Surgical resection is a very effective palliative treatment for isolated metastases, offering quick palliation and, in some patients, long-lasting survival. Surgical excision of solitary metastases in visceral organs can lead to survival of more than 5 years in 5% to 20% of patients.

ISOLATED LIMB PERFUSION

Isolated limb perfusion chemotherapy is used to treat patients with melanoma that is confined to a limb, such as local recurrence and in-transit metastases. The most commonly used chemotherapy agent is melphalan, which is used in conjunction with hyperthermia. Response rates have ranged from 40% to 80%. In a recently completed randomized clinical trial that compared melphalan-based hyperthermic isolated limb perfusion with or without tumor necrosis factor (TNF)-alpha in 124 patients with locally advanced extremity melanoma, there was no difference in the overall response rate. The response rate was 65% in the melphalan-alone arm and 69% in the combination arm ($p = 0.435$). Thus, there is no benefit to the addition of TNF–alpha, which was associated with a higher complication rate.[30]

REFERENCES

1. American Cancer Society. *Cancer Facts and Figures, 2007.* Atlanta, GA: American Cancer Society; 2007.
2. Gilchrest BA, Eller MS, Geller AC, et al. The pathogenesis of melanoma induced by ultraviolet radiation. *N Engl J Med.* 1999; 340(17):1341–1348.
3. Naeyaert JM, Brochez L. Clinical practice. Dysplastic nevi. *N Engl J Med.* 2003;349(23):2233–2240.
4. Haluska FG, Hodi FS. Molecular genetics of familial cutaneous melanoma. *J Clin Oncol.* 1998;16(2):670–682.
5. Statement of the American Society of Clinical Oncology: genetic testing for cancer susceptibility. *J Clin Oncol.* 1996;14(5):1730.
6. Meves A, Repacholi MH, Rehfuess EA. Promoting safe and effective sun protection strategies. *J Am Acad Dermatol.* 2003;49(6):1203–1204.
7. Haluska FG, Tsao H, Wu H, et al. Genetic alterations in signaling pathways in melanoma. *Clin Cancer Res.* 2006;12(7 Pt 2):2301s–2307s.
8. Curtin JA, Fridlyand J, Kageshita T, et al. Distinct sets of genetic alterations in melanoma. *N Engl J Med.* 2005;353(20):2135–2147.
9. Curtin JA, Busam K, Pinkel D, et al. Somatic activation of KIT in distinct subtypes of melanoma. *J Clin Oncol.* 2006;24(26):4340–4346.
10. Balch CM, Buzaid AC, Soong SJ, et al. Final version of the American Joint Committee on Cancer staging system for cutaneous melanoma. *J Clin Oncol.* 2001;19(16):3635–3648.
11. Balch CM, Soong SJ, Smith T, et al. Long-term results of a prospective surgical trial comparing 2 cm vs. 4 cm excision margins for 740 patients with 1-4 mm melanomas. *Ann Surg Oncol.* 2001;8(2):101–108.
12. Thomas JM, Newton-Bishop J, A'Hern R, et al. Excision margins in high-risk malignant melanoma. *N Engl J Med.* 2004;350(8):757–766.
13. Balch CM, Soong SJ, Bartolucci AA, et al. Efficacy of an elective regional lymph node dissection of 1 to 4 mm thick melanomas for patients 60 years of age and younger. *Ann Surg.* 1996;224(3):255–263.
14. Morton DL, Thompson JF, Cochran AJ, et al. Sentinel-node biopsy or nodal observation in melanoma. *N Engl J Med.* 2006;355(13): 1307–1317.
15. Kirkwood JM, Strawderman MH, Ernstoff MS, et al. Interferon alfa-2b adjuvant therapy of high-risk resected cutaneous melanoma: the Eastern Cooperative Oncology Group Trial EST 1684. *J Clin Oncol.* 1996; 14(1):7–17.
16. Kirkwood JM, Ibrahim J, Sondak V, et al. High- and low-dose interferon alfa-2b in high-risk melanoma: first analysis of Intergroup Trial E1690/S9111/C9190. *J Clin Oncol.* 2000;18(12):2444–2458.
17. Kirkwood JM, Ibrahim JG, Sosman JA, et al. High-dose interferon alfa-2b significantly prolongs relapse-free and overall survival compared with the GM2-KLH/QS21 vaccine in patients with resected stage IIB/III melanoma: results of intergroup trial E1694/S9512/C509801. *J Clin Oncol.* 2001;19(9):2370–2380.
18. Gogas H, Ioannovich J, Dafni U, et. al. Prognostic significance of autoimmunity during treatment of melanoma with interferon. *N Engl J Med.* 2006;354(7):709–718.
19. Hancock BW, Wheatley K, Harris S, et al. Adjuvant interferon in high-risk melanoma: the AIM HIGH study—United Kingdom Coordinating Committee on Cancer Research randomized study of adjuvant low-dose extended-duration interferon alfa-2a in high-risk resected malignant melanoma. *J Clin Oncol.* 2004;22(1):53–61.
20. Terando A, Sabel MS, Sondak VK. Melanoma: adjuvant therapy and other treatment options. *Curr Treat Options Oncol.* 2003;4(3):187–199.
21. Eigentler TK, Caroli UM, Radny P, et al. Palliative therapy of disseminated malignant melanoma: a systematic review of 41 randomised clinical trials. *Lancet Oncol.* 2003;4(12):748–759.

22. Sun W, Schuchter LM. Metastatic melanoma. *Curr Treat Options Oncol.* 2001;2(3):193–202.

23. Middleton MR, Grob JJ, Aaronson N, et al. Randomized phase III study of temozolomide versus dacarbazine in the treatment of patients with advanced metastatic malignant melanoma. *J Clin Oncol.* 2000; 18(1):158–166.

24. Bedikian AY, Millward M, Pehamberger H, et al. Bcl-2 antisense (oblimersen sodium) plus dacarbazine in patients with advanced melanoma: the Oblimersen melanoma study group. *J Clin Oncol.* 2006; 24(29):4738–4745.

25. Chapman PB, Einhorn LH, Meyers ML, et al. Phase III multicenter randomized trial of the Dartmouth regimen versus dacarbazine in patients with metastatic melanoma. *J Clin Oncol.* 1999;17(9):2745–2751.

26. Atkins MB, Lotze M, Dutcher JP, et al. High-dose recombinant interleukin-2 therapy for patients with metastatic melanoma: analysis of 270 patients treated from 1985–1993. *J Clin Oncol.* 1999;17(7):2105–2116.

27. Morgan RA, Dudley ME, Wunderlich JR, et al. Cancer regression in patients after transfer of genetically engineered lymphocytes. *Science.* 2006;314(5796):126–129.

28. Atkins MB. Cytokine based therapy and biochemotherapy for advanced melanoma. *Clin Cancer Res.* 2006;12(7 Pt 2):2353s–2358s.

29. Panka DJ, Atkins MB, Mier JW. Targeting the mitogen-activated protein kinase pathway in the treatment of malignant melanoma. *Clin Cancer Res.* 2006;12(7 Pt 2):2371s–2375s.

30. Cornett WR, McCall LM, Petersen RP, et al. Randomized multicenter trial of hyperthermic isolated limb perfusion with melphalan alone compared with melphalan plus tumor necrosis factor: American College of Surgeons Oncology Group Trial Z0020. *J Clin Oncol.* 2006;24(25):4196–201.

12

SARCOMA

Robert G. Maki, MD, PhD

LEARNING OBJECTIVES

After reviewing this section, the reader should be able to

- Specify etiologic factors associated with sarcomas
- Understand the significance of different sarcoma diagnostic (histologic and/or genetic) subtypes
- Recognize the controversy regarding use of adjuvant chemotherapy for extremity soft tissue sarcomas
- Identify the most active agents for treatment of specific metastatic soft tissue sarcomas
- Exploit the unique relationship between *c-kit* mutation status and response to tyrosine kinase inhibitors in gastrointestinal stromal tumor
- Compare and contrast the diagnosis and treatment of osteogenic sarcoma and Ewing's sarcoma

Sarcoma is the term used for cancers arising from connective tissue. Sarcomas of soft tissue and bone are uncommon, constituting less than 1% of all cancers. They are remarkably heterogeneous, with more than 50 recognized subtypes, and are named for the normal tissue counterpart they most resemble. In adults, soft tissue sarcomas are more than 3 times more common than sarcomas of bone (9,220 compared with 2,370 cases in 2007).[1] The most common subtypes of soft tissue sarcoma include gastrointestinal stromal tumors (GIST), leiomyosarcoma, liposarcoma, and high-grade undifferentiated pleomorphic sarcoma (previously called malignant fibrous histiocytoma [MFH]), each representing 15% to 20% of soft tissue sarcomas. Approximately 10% to 15% of soft tissue sarcomas cannot be characterized beyond noting that they are sarcomas (soft tissue sarcoma, not otherwise specified). Other relatively common subtypes of soft tissue sarcoma include synovial sarcoma, fibrosarcoma, malignant peripheral nerve sheath tumor, and angiosarcoma. Osteogenic sarcomas (osteosarcomas) and chondrosarcomas are the two most common

KEY POINT

- Therapeutic radiation confers a small but measurable risk for the development of sarcomas.

sarcomas arising from osseous elements in adults. Ewing's sarcoma can arise in either bone or soft tissue. Figure 12-1 indicates the relative frequency of some of these sarcoma subtypes.

Most sarcomas arise spontaneously. The incidence of soft tissue sarcomas increases with age, although specific subtypes, such as Ewing's sarcoma, rhabdomyosarcoma, and osteosarcoma, occur almost exclusively in children and young adults. Adults younger than 35 are at a greater risk of synovial sarcoma and desmoplastic small round cell tumors; individuals older than 60 are at a greater risk of myxofibrosarcoma, undifferentiated pleomorphic sarcoma, and sarcoma not otherwise specified. Genetic syndromes associated with soft tissue sarcoma include Li-Fraumeni syndrome (*p53* mutation), and neurofibromatosis type I (*NF1* mutation), as well as mutations in a series of helicases.[2] Despite the presence of an *NF1* mutation, probands have only a 5% to 10% risk of developing a soft tissue sarcoma in their lifetimes.

According to the National Comprehensive Cancer Network (NCCN) guidelines for evidence strength, study results can be labeled as belonging to one of four categories: Category 1, which means that there is uniform consensus based on high-level evidence; Category 2A, which indicates uniform consensus based on lower-level data; Category 2B, meaning nonuniform consensus but no major disagreement; and Category 3, which indicates major disagreement. With this in mind, there is epidemiologic evidence that associates vinyl chloride with hepatic angiosarcoma (Category 2A), but few other environmental exposures are associated with the development of sarcomas. Some studies have linked dioxins or phenoxyacetic acid herbicides, such as Agent Orange, to the development of sarcomas, but others have not; meta-analyses of such data remain inconclusive (Category 3).

There is a small but measurable long-term risk of soft tissue or bone sarcoma after radiation therapy (Category 2A). The mean latency time is 16 years (range: 4 to 30 or more years), and the mean radiation exposure is 40 Gy (range: 12 to 60 Gy). Although one-half of such sarcomas are high grade, their prognosis does not appear to be worse than that of sporadic soft tissue sarcomas of the same stage, although the local control issues can be considerable. Other risk factors for the development of soft tissue sarcoma include lymphedema (e.g., Stewart-Treves syndrome), and, in the case of Kaposi's sarcoma, human herpes virus-8 (HHV-8). Trauma does not appear to cause sarcomas; rather it may signal presence of a sarcoma.

EPIDEMIOLOGY AND ETIOLOGY

GENETIC CHARACTERISTICS

GIST usually contain a *c-kit* or platelet-derived growth factor receptor mutation, and approximately 30% of other soft tissue sarcomas are associated with specific genetic alterations. This is perhaps more than any other type of solid tumor save prostate cancer because of its recently recognized *ETS* family translocations (Table 12-1). Given the broad differential diagnosis for many sarcomas, molecular analysis has proven extremely useful in the definitive diagnosis of specific sarcoma subtypes. Most analyses of chromosomal translocations require fresh-frozen tissue, although fluorescent in situ hybridization (FISH) can sometimes provide information from fixed tissue. cDNA, oligonucleotide, and protein arrays may add to diagnosis and prognostication for sarcomas in the near future as genes characteristic of each subtype of sarcoma are recognized and validated.

CLINICAL PRESENTATION AND DIAGNOSIS

Soft tissue sarcomas generally present as painless, growing masses. They are generally differentiated from benign tumors, such as lipomas, by either their texture (generally firmer) or their location (typically deeper than subcutaneous fat).

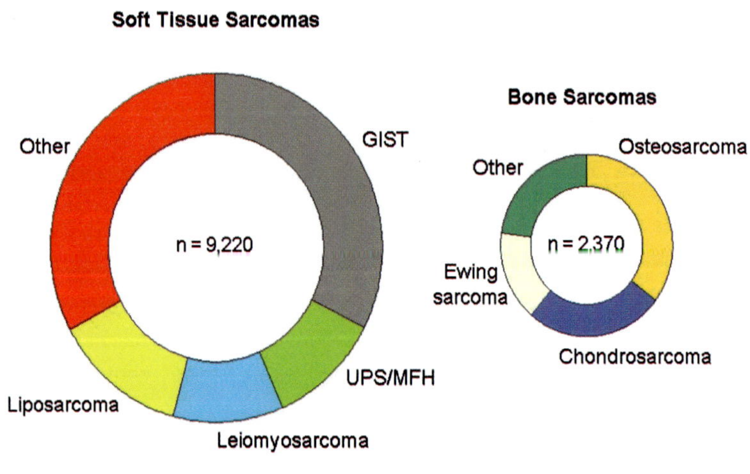

FIG. 12-1 Soft tissue and bone sarcomas: relative frequency.
The number of estimated cases and breakdown of subtypes for soft tissue and bone sarcomas is indicated. The area of each circle is proportional to the frequency of such tumors. Abbreviations: GIST, gastrointestinal stromal tumor; UPS, undifferentiated pleomorphic sarcoma; MFH, malignant fibrous histiocytoma.

TABLE 12-1 Representative Genetic Alterations in Sarcomas[2]		
Sarcoma Subtype	**Genetic alteration**	**Frequency**
Gastrointestinal stromal tumor (GIST)	*CD117* (*c-kit*) mutation, exon 11 or 9	> 80%
Well differentiated/dedifferentiated liposarcoma	Giant or ring chromosomes (*CDK4, MDM2* amplification)	> 70%
Synovial sarcoma	t(X;18) *SYT-SSX1* or *SYT-SSX2*	> 90%
Myxoid/round cell liposarcoma	t(12;16) *TLS-CHOP*	> 75%
Ewing sarcoma	t(11;22) *EWS-FLI1*	> 85%
Alveolar rhabdomyosarcoma	t(2;13)(q35;q14) *PAX3-FOXO1A* or	Approximately 60%
	t(1;13)(p36;q14) *PAX7-FOXO1A*	Approximately 20%

Lipomas remain at least 100 times more common than their neoplastic counterpart. For many masses, a diagnosis of sarcoma can be rendered with a core needle biopsy, although this procedure may not yield specific information about subtype. When diagnostic material cannot be obtained by core needle biopsy, incisional or excisional biopsy is performed, with the understanding that the procedure may have to encompass the prior biopsy site. Fine-needle aspiration is generally inadequate to confirm the diagnosis of sarcoma, and its use is generally limited to confirming recurrence of sarcomas. Similarly, attention must be paid to the biopsy technique when attempting to diagnose a sarcoma of the bone because it has implications for the extent of definitive surgery to follow.

PATHOLOGIC FEATURES AND PROGNOSTIC FACTORS

Because of the diversity of sarcoma subtypes and their differential diagnosis, such as sarcomatoid carcinoma (which is treated like other carcinomas), carcinosarcoma, melanoma, or lymphoma, the pathologist is a critical contributor to patient care. Important considerations for sarcoma staging include an evaluation of sarcoma grade and histologic subtype. It is important to recognize that pathologists may use different grading systems, with two grades (low and high), three grades (low, intermediate, and high), or four grades (grades 1 to 4). The specific grading system used by individual pathologists is unlikely to change, but all such differences of grading are captured by the staging system noted further in the chapter (and in Table 12-2).

Immunohistochemical staining will demonstrate features of sarcomas that are not obvious with routine staining, and this technique is an important component in the determination of sarcoma subtype. Cytogenetic or similar molecular analyses are the gold standard for diagnosing several specific sarcoma subtypes.

Of primary importance in determining overall survival is the grade of the primary tumor. The American Joint Committee on Cancer (AJCC) staging system for soft tissue sarcoma includes the tumor grade, size, and location of the tumor (superficial or deep to any overlying investing fascia),

TABLE 12-2 American Joint Committee on Cancer Staging System for Soft Tissue Sarcoma[3]						
Stage:	**Four-grade System**	**Three-grade System**	**Two-grade System**	**T***	**N†**	**M‡**
I	Grades 1 and 2	Grade 1	Low	T1a, T1b, T2a, T2b	N0	M0
II	Grades 3 and 4	Grades 2 and 3	High	T1a, T1b, T2a	N0	M0
III	Grades 3 and 4	Grades 2 and 3	High	T2b	N0	M0
IV	Any grade	Any grade	Any	Any	N1	Any
	Any grade	Any grade	Any	Any	Any	M1

*T1 = tumor of no more than 5 cm in greatest dimension, T2 = tumor of more than 5 cm in greatest dimension, a = superficial to investing fascia, b = deep to investing fascia.
†N0 = no lymph node metastasis, N1 = lymph node metastasis.
‡M0 = no distant metastasis, M1 = distant metastasis.

TABLE 12-3 Five-year Disease-free Survival Rates According to Size of High-grade Soft Tissue Sarcoma[4,5]

Size of Tumor (cm)	Five-year Disease-free Survival Rate (%)
2.6 to 4.9	77
5.0 to 9.9	62
10.0 to 14.9	51
15.0 to 20.0	42

Tumors 5 cm or less were generally treated with surgery; tumors larger than 5 cm were typically treated with surgery and radiation.

as well as presence of nodal disease or overt metastatic disease (Table 12-2).[3] Nodal metastatic disease is a nearly equal unfavorable prognostic feature compared with bloodborne metastases, but nodal metastatic disease is observed in less than 10% of patients with soft tissue sarcomas. Some subtypes of sarcoma with a propensity for growing in lymph nodes include epithelioid sarcoma, rhabdomyosarcoma, and angiosarcoma.

Histology and grade are the most important factors in determining risk of relapse. Overall survival after diagnosis of soft tissue sarcoma also is dependent on the initial size and location of the tumor. For example, as the size of the primary tumor increases, the risk of relapse increases, even within a given stage (Table 12-3).[4-5] It is important to recognize that sarcomas of different primary sites (and typically different histologic subtypes) are associated with different patterns of distant and local failure (Table 12-4).

Several staging systems have been employed for sarcomas of the bone (Table 12-5). As with soft tissue sarcomas, metastases of osteosarcomas to lymph nodes are extremely unusual and constitute stage IV disease. Lung metastases are treated differently from other metastases because surgical resection of these metastases can be curative for selected patients.

Other prognostic factors for soft tissue sarcomas include specific histologic subtype, age of the patient, and site of the tumor, but these variables are heterogeneous with respect to different subtypes and are difficult to incorporate into a staging system. Molecular markers may prove to be prognostic for survival or for response to chemotherapy but remain an area of investigation.

TREATMENT OF NON-GIST SOFT TISSUE SARCOMAS

GENERAL PRINCIPLES

The primary treatment for most sarcomas of bone or soft tissue is surgery. With advances in surgical technique during the past 20 to 30 years, limb-sparing procedures have replaced amputation for more than 90% of patients with sarcomas of the extremities.[6]

TABLE 12-4 Site of Recurrence According to Primary Site of Soft Tissue Sarcoma

Primary Site	Local	Lung	Other	Multiple Sites
Extremity (%)	10	70	15	5
Trunk (%)	41	29	12	18
Retroperitoneum (%)	30	17	6	47

Radiation generally is not used to treat bone sarcomas. However, radiation to the site of the primary tumor is a standard of care for all sarcomas of the extremities or trunk that are larger than 5 cm, independent of the grade (Category 1). Radiation therapy has been effective as an adjuvant to surgery for soft tissue sarcomas of the extremity in randomized studies involving external beam radiation[7] and brachytherapy.[8] The issue of whether to employ radiation before or after surgery was clarified by a study from Canada, which determined that long-term success with either approach appeared similar. The risk of wound complications is increased with preoperative radiation, but the treated field is smaller, and the dose is lower than in the postoperative setting.[9] Therefore, it is not surprising that the risk of late complications, such as fibrosis, appears greater with the larger fields treated using postoperative radiation.[10]

In contrast to the benefit of radiation for soft tissue sarcomas of the extremities, there is no clear role for radiation for abdominal or visceral sarcomas; the doses that can be used for

TABLE 12-5 American Joint Commission on Cancer Staging System for Bone[3]

Stage	Grade (Four Tiers)	T*	N†	M‡
IA	1 to 2 (low)	T1	N0	M0
IB	1 to 2	T2	N0	M0
IIA	3 to 4 (high)	T1	N0	M0
IIB	3 to 4	T2	N0	M0
III	Any	T3	N0	M0
IVA	Any	Any	N0	M1a
IVB	Any	Any	N1	Any
	Any	Any	Any	M1b

*T1 = tumor of no more than 8 cm in dimension, T2 = tumor of more than 8 cm in greatest dimension, T3 = discontinuous tumor in primary bone site.
†N0 = no lymph node metastasis, N1 = lymph node metastasis.
‡M0 = no distant metastasis, M1a = lung metastasis, M1b = other distant metastasis.

KEY POINTS

- Surgery remains the standard of care for most sarcomas. Adjuvant or neoadjuvant external beam radiation is used for larger tumors (more than 5 cm in greatest dimension, regardless of grade) in areas where tumoricidal doses can be delivered.
- Adjuvant chemotherapy is mandatory for most pediatric sarcomas (i.e., osteosarcoma, Ewing sarcoma, and rhabdomyosarcoma). Its use for adult soft tissue sarcomas remains controversial.
- Doxorubicin and ifosfamide are the most effective drugs for metastatic non-GIST soft tissue sarcomas. The benefit of such drugs appears additive, not synergistic.

abdominal disease are generally not tumoricidal and are toxic to the abdominal viscera. However, for very large abdominal or retroperitoneal sarcomas, preoperative radiation may be considered because the tumor serves as its own tissue expander, pushing normal abdominal components, such as bowel, out of the radiation field. This anatomic finding increases the likelihood that a tumoricidal dose of radiation can be delivered to the abdomen. Intraoperative radiation and new techniques, such as neoadjuvant intensity-modulated radiation therapy, remain investigational.

ADJUVANT CHEMOTHERAPY

The role of chemotherapy in the adjuvant setting for standard adult soft tissue sarcoma remains controversial (Category 3). Although a meta-analysis showed no statistically significant benefit in overall survival outcomes for doxorubicin-based adjuvant chemotherapy for sarcomas overall, most patients had not received ifosfamide.[11] In a subset analysis of extremity sarcomas from the same meta-analysis, a 7% absolute survival benefit was found. The subset analysis was unplanned, and no central pathology review was undertaken in this meta-analysis, which could mitigate the reported benefit. A more recent study demonstrated a survival benefit for patients with large (median diameter, 10 cm) soft tissue sarcomas of the extremities or the pelvic girdle who were receiving adjuvant epirubicin and ifosfamide.[12] With longer follow-up, the survival advantage is no longer significant, indicating that for most patients adjuvant chemotherapy may shrink, but not eliminate, microscopic metastatic disease. However, the 5-year overall survival remains statistically superior for the study arm employing adjuvant chemotherapy (66% vs. 46%; $p = 0.04$).[13] Two other smaller randomized studies following the meta-analysis did not show a benefit for overall survival after chemotherapy but were underpowered to detect a small difference in survival.[14,15] In addition, a large study from Europe recently indicated that there was no benefit in overall survival when comparing combination doxorubicin and ifosfamide with observation alone.[16]

Given the lack of definitive benefit from chemotherapy in the adjuvant setting, the use of surgery and radiation alone remains a good standard of care for most patients. Any small potential benefit from adjuvant chemotherapy should be discussed with the patient on an individual basis with respect to the significant toxicity associated with adjuvant therapy. There are situations in which adjuvant therapy clearly is not indicated. For example, there appears to be no benefit of adjuvant chemotherapy for soft tissue sarcomas that arise from visceral or abdominal sites, and surgery alone remains the standard of care (Category 2B). Retrospective data indicate that people with specific subtypes of adult soft tissue sarcomas may benefit from adjuvant chemotherapy,[17] specifically synovial sarcoma and high-grade myxoid/round cell liposarcoma, but randomized data are lacking. When used, the author employs 25 mg/m^2 doxorubicin intravenously as an intravenous push or 24-hour continuous infusion, daily every 3 days and 3,000 mg/m^2 of infosfamide over 3 hours daily for 3 days, with support of mesna and growth factors.

In contrast to adjuvant therapy for adult soft tissue sarcoma, adjuvant or neoadjuvant chemotherapy has dramatically improved overall survival for patients with sarcomas typically seen in the pediatric population, (e.g., rhabdomyosarcoma, Ewing's sarcoma, and osteosarcoma) regardless of the age of the patient at the time of diagnosis (Category 1). Although found less frequently in adults than in children, treatment of adults with these diagnoses follows the schedules of therapy administered to pediatric patients, when feasible. Neoadjuvant/adjuvant chemotherapy should be administered to all patients with this diagnosis who have good clinical performance status and sufficient bone marrow reserve to tolerate such therapy. Based on phase III data (Category 1), combination vincristine, dactinomycin, and cyclophosphamide form the backbone of therapy for most patients with primary rhabdomyosarcomas.[18] The five-drug combination of alternating vincristine, doxorubicin, and cyclophosphamide with ifosfamide and etoposide is the standard of care for primary Ewing sarcoma (Category 1).[19]

METASTATIC DISEASE

As single drugs or in combination, anthracyclines, such as doxorubicin and the alkylating agent ifosfamide, yield the best response rates for metastatic sarcoma (rates of 10% to 25% for each drug in various studies).[6] Single-agent therapy may be as useful as combination therapy because doxorubicin and ifosfamide are not synergistic, although combinations are generally used when patients are symptomatic. Standard doses of doxorubicin are 75 mg/m^2 per cycle, usually administered in split daily doses or by continuous intravenous infusion to minimize cardiac toxicity. Ifosfamide is administered in a variety of schedules, from 5 g/m^2 over 24 hours once every 3 weeks to 2 to 4 g/m^2 per day to a total dose per cycle of 6 to 16 g/m^2, with support of mesna, and usually with growth factor support.

Certain chemotherapy agents have greater or lesser activity against specific sarcoma subtypes. Ifosfamide is particularly active for synovial sarcoma and myxoid/round cell liposarcoma and appears to be less active for leiomyosarcomas.[20,21] At least three studies have confirmed the activity of the combination of gemcitabine and docetaxel in leiomyosarcoma (Category 1); the combination also has activity against undifferentiated pleomorphic sarcoma. Dacarbazine has modest activity against leiomyosarcoma. Taxanes and vinorelbine are active against angiosarcomas and generally inactive against other sarcomas. Because sarcomas are proving to be a very heterogeneous group of diseases as they pertain to systemic chemotherapy, it is not surprising that specific sarcoma subtypes have distinct sensitivity patterns to chemotherapy.

GASTROINTESTINAL STROMAL TUMORS (GIST)

During the past several years, it has become clear that a group of sarcomas of the gastrointestinal tract is very distinct from leiomyosarcomas of the gastrointestinal tract. Now called gastrointestinal stromal tumors (GIST), these sarcomas are characterized by the presence of the CD117 (*c-kit*) immunohistochemical marker, most of which are positive for stem cell marker CD34. With their increasing recognition, they appear to be the most common form of sarcoma (as many as 3,000 to 3,500 cases per year in the United States). These tumors appear to arise from the interstitial cells of Cajal, the pacemaker cells of the gastrointestinal tract. Approximately 65% of GIST arise from the stomach, 25% arise from the small bowel, and the remainder arise from other sites along the gastrointestinal tract or in the abdomen. The primary treatment for these tumors is surgery, but the majority will recur in the peritoneum, liver, or both.

Cytotoxic chemotherapy (even intraperitoneal chemotherapy) is ineffective for the vast majority of GIST, but imatinib, which was found to be effective for chronic myelogenous leukemia, has remarkable activity against GIST. In early-phase studies of imatinib therapy for metastatic GIST, the response rates were approximately 60%, which is at least 5-fold to 10-fold greater than rates associated with previously available therapy.[22] In randomized phase II and phase III studies, a once-daily dose of 400 mg was as effective as 600 or 800 mg of imatinib daily.[23,24] As a result, 400 mg daily of oral imatinib is the standard of care for metastatic GIST (Category 1). Dose-limiting side effects of imatinib include nausea and vomiting, diarrhea, rash, mucositis, and/or diuretic-resistant peripheral edema. Of note, the *c-kit* phenotype of a GIST predicts for the responsiveness of the tumor to imatinib. Patients with exon 11 mutations in *c-kit* have a greater chance of response to imatinib than patients with exon 9 *c-kit* mutations or wild-type *c-kit*.[25] The response rate to imatinib for patients with platelet-derived growth factor receptor mutations appears to be lower than that for patients with exon 11 *c-kit* mutations as well.

For GIST resistant to imatinib at an oral dose of 400 mg daily, a conventional approach is to increase the dose to a total daily dose of 800 mg (or 600 mg if the higher dose is not tolerated) (Category 2A).[22] For patients with imatinib refractory or intolerant disease, sunitinib is a good standard of care (Category 1) because sunitinib was shown to be superior to placebo in a phase III study in this setting.[26] Patients with exon 9 mutations in *c-kit* and wild-type *c-kit* had the best response to sunitinib.[27] However, in this setting, patients entering the phase III sunitinib study with mutations in exon 11 often had more than one mutation in *c-kit*, making it difficult to speculate on the potential efficacy of sunitinib when compared with imatinib as first-line therapy.

The role of imatinib in the adjuvant or neoadjuvant setting is a subject of ongoing phase III studies involving imatinib compared with placebo (in the United States and in Europe). Imatinib has been tested in the adjuvant setting for patients with primary resected GIST at moderate to high risk of recurrence. This large, randomized, prospective, placebo-controlled trial was stopped early because of a positive effect of imatinib on delaying disease recurrence. Three percent of patients who received imatinib progressed at 1 year (the end of the mandated treatment) compared with 17% of those patients who received observation alone. Importantly, there was no demonstrable survival benefit. As a result, it is difficult to recommend imatinib for 1 year in the adjuvant setting without further follow-up data from this study or from other clinical trials. Further details from this large clinical trial include whether specific subsets of patients following primary resection of GIST might benefit more than others.[28] Two ongoing studies in Europe are examining observation compared with 2 years of imatinib, as well as 1 year compared with 3 years of treatment with imatinib in the adjuvant setting.

KEY POINTS

- Imatinib is the standard of care for patients with newly diagnosed metastatic GIST; for progressive disease the dose of imatinib is generally increased before switching to sunitinib.
- Surgery is the treatment of choice for primary disease. It also can play a role for patients with progressive metastatic disease.
- Sunitinib is approved for second-line therapy for patients with imatinib-refractory GIST or with imatinib intolerance.

Surgery can play a role in the treatment of metastatic disease. Some patients progress with limited disease (e.g., one or two deposits of progression in the background of responding disease). Patients with this pattern of progression may have a long period before further progression (Category 2A). For those patients with multiple sites of disease progression, a change in systemic therapy appears to be warranted because patients with resection of disease have evidence of further progression within a few months (Category 2A).[29]

BONE SARCOMAS

OSTEOSARCOMA

Osteosarcomas are the most common tumors of bone, with two peaks of incidence, one between the ages of 10 and 20 and a smaller one between the ages of 60 and 80. Disease in the latter age-group often is associated with Paget's disease of bone. Osteosarcomas generally arise in the metaphysis of the bone (between the end of the bone [epiphysis] and the shaft [diaphysis]). They are characterized by lytic and blastic features in admixed bone. If the tumors extend to soft tissue, they can cause both a periosteal reaction (Codman triangle) and ossification in a pattern perpendicular to the surface of the bone (sunburst pattern) (Fig. 12-2).

Adjuvant or neoadjuvant chemotherapy is a standard of care for most patients with osteosarcomas (Category 1). The exception is superficial low-grade osteosarcomas, for which adjuvant chemotherapy is not indicated.[30] For conventional osteosarcomas, the combination of neoadjuvant and adjuvant cisplatin and doxorubicin was found to be as effective as a more complex methotrexate-containing regimen in one randomized multicenter study.[31] The data regarding the use of methotrexate are somewhat controversial; functionally, methotrexate most frequently is used for younger patients, owing to possible nephrotoxicity and acute lung toxicity in adults. Ifosfamide is effective for osteosarcomas, but its role in standard neoadjuvant and adjuvant therapy remains under investigation.[32]

> **KEY POINTS**
>
> - Common sarcomas of bone include osteosarcoma, chondrosarcoma, and Ewing sarcoma. (Ewing sarcoma frequently arises in soft tissue in adults as well.) Osteosarcoma affects the metaphysis (between the bone endplate and the shaft) and causes lytic and blastic changes, whereas Ewing sarcoma affects the diaphysis (mid-shaft) and causes an infiltrative pattern.
> - Chemotherapy always is used in the adjuvant or neoadjuvant setting to manage Ewing sarcoma and osteosarcoma; typically, surgery alone is used to manage chondrosarcoma.

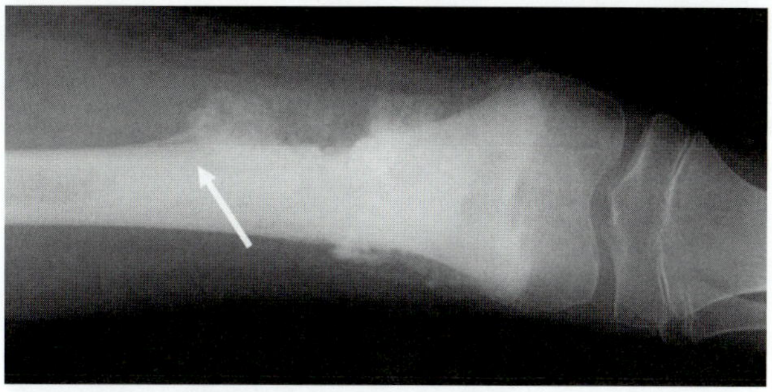

FIG. 12-2 Plain radiograph of osteogenic sarcoma of the distal part of the femur.

Note the Codman triangle (arrow) and the blastic changes in the bone and soft tissue.

The response of osteosarcomas to neoadjuvant chemotherapy can be assessed by pathologic examination at the time of operation, with decisions regarding continuing or changing postoperative therapy based on the amount of necrosis found. However, there is no evidence that changing therapy can help improve overall survival after disease has been resistant to neoadjuvant chemotherapy. Osteosarcomas typically metastasize to the lung. Resection of pulmonary metastases (stage IVA disease) is one of the few examples in oncology of possible cure if the number of metastases is limited.[33]

CHONDROSARCOMA

Chondrosarcomas are the second most common tumor of the bone and usually affect patients older than age 60. There is no role for chemotherapy in the management of most chondrosarcomas, which are typically low-grade to intermediate grade tumors that resemble cartilage both macro-scopically and microscopically. On radiographs, chondrosarcomas generally appear as a radiolucent area with obvious bony destruction and a moderate number of discrete calcified areas, and they often involve the medullary cavity. They often have scalloped edges consistent with a multinodular growth pattern. Patients with dedifferentiated chondrosarcoma occasionally respond to chemotherapy used for osteogenic sarcomas, as can patients with mesenchymal chondrosarcoma (another high-grade variant). With routine staining, mesenchymal chondrosarcoma resembles Ewing's sarcoma. They occasionally respond to chemotherapy typically used for Ewing's sarcoma, although, after surgery (when feasible) a completely viable low-grade component typically is found.

EWING'S SARCOMA

Ewing's sarcoma and extracranial primitive neuroectodermal tumors typically arise in the bones of children, but occur more commonly in soft tissues in adults. These tumors are part of a spectrum of diseases characterized by a varying degree of differentiation and always are considered high grade. They usually affect the shaft of the bone in an

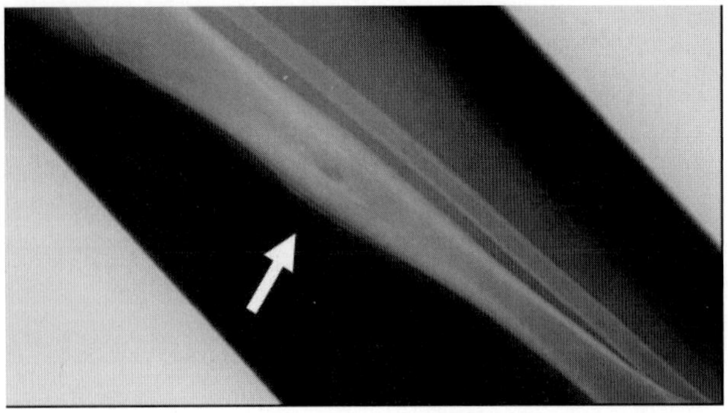

FIG. 12-3 Plain radiograph of Ewing's sarcoma of the tibia.
Note the diffuse infiltrative changes in the middle part of the shaft, or "onion-skinning" characteristic of Ewing sarcoma (arrow).

infiltrative pattern called "onion-skinning," which is easily visible on computerized tomography scans (less so on plain x-rays; Fig. 12-3). Multimodality therapy with surgery, chemotherapy, and radiation is the best standard of care for this disease (Category 1). The addition of ifosfamide and etoposide to the regimen of vincristine, doxorubicin, and cyclophosphamide yields better results than the regimen alone as the form of neoadjuvant and adjuvant chemotherapy for patients with primary localized Ewing sarcoma and is a good standard of care.[34] For metastatic Ewing's sarcomas, combination vincristine, doxorubicin, and cyclophosphamide was shown to be as efficacious as the five-drug combination used for primary disease, probably because patients progressing on the triple-drug regimen could cross over to ifosfamide and etoposide at time of progression.[34] Assuming patients have received the standard multidrug regimens for osteogenic sarcoma and Ewing's sarcoma, options for therapy are very limited, and these patients are good candidates for clinical trials. Assuming the standard agents have already been given as (neo)adjuvant therapy, patients with either histology may occasionally respond to gemcitabine and docetaxel, and patients with Ewing's sarcoma may respond to topoisomerase I inhibitors, either as single agents or in combination.[35]

REFERENCES

1. Jemal A, Siegel R, Ward E, et al. Cancer satistics, 2007. *CA Cancer J Clin.* 2007;57(1):43–66.
2. Bennicelli JL, Barr FG. Chromosomal translocations and sarcomas. *Curr Opin Oncol.* 2002;14(4):412–419.
3. Greene FL, Page DL, Fleming ID, et al, eds. *AJCC Cancer Staging Handbook*, 6th edition. New York, NY: Springer; 2002.
4. Brennan MF. Staging of soft tissue sarcomas. *Ann of Surg Oncol.* 1999;6(1):8–9.
5. Pisters P, Leung D, Woodruff J, et al. Analysis of prognostic factors in 1,041 patients with localized soft tissue sarcomas of the extremities. *J Clin Oncol.* 1996;14(5):1679–1689.
6. Brennan MF, Alektiar K, Maki RG, O'Sullivan B. Soft tissue sarcoma. In: DeVita VT Jr., Hellman S, Rosenberg SA, eds. *Cancer: Principles and Practice of Oncology*, 7th edition. Philadelphia, PA: Lippincott, Williams, & Wilkins; 2005:1581–1637.
7. Yang J, Chang AE, Baker AR, et al. Randomized prospective study of the benefit of adjuvant radiation therapy in the treatment of soft tissue sarcomas of the extremity. *J Clin Oncol.* 1998;16(1):197–203.
8. Pisters PW, Harrison LB, Leung DH, et al. Long-term results of a prospective randomized trial of adjuvant brachytherapy in soft tissue sarcoma. *J Clin Oncol.* 1996;14(3):859–868.
9. O'Sullivan B, Davis AM, Turcotte R, et al. Preoperative versus postoperative radiotherapy in soft-tissue sarcoma of the limbs: a randomised trial. *Lancet.* 2002;359(9325):2235–2241.
10. Davis AM, O'Sullivan B, Turcotte R, et al. Late radiation morbidity following randomization to preoperative versus postoperative radiotherapy in extremity soft tissue sarcoma. *Radiother Oncol.* 2005;75(1):48–53.
11. Adjuvant chemotherapy for localised resectable soft-tissue sarcoma of adults: meta-analysis of individual data. Sarcoma Meta-analysis Collaboration. *Lancet.* 1997;350(9092):1647–1654.
12. Frustaci S, Gherlinzoni F, De Paoli A, et al. Adjuvant chemotherapy for adult soft tissue sarcomas of the extremities and girdles: results of the Italian randomized cooperative trial. *J Clin Oncol.* 2001;19(5): 1238–1247.
13. Frustaci S, De Paoli A, Bidoli E, et al. Ifosfamide in the adjuvant therapy of soft tissue sarcomas. *Oncology.* 2003;65(Suppl 2):80–84.
14. Gortzak E, Azzarelli A, Buesa J, et al. A randomised phase II study on neo-adjuvant chemotherapy for 'high-risk' adult soft-tissue sarcoma. *Eur J Cancer.* 2001; 37(9):1096–1103.
15. Brodowicz T, Schwameis E, Joachim W, et al. Intensified adjuvant IFADIC chemotherapy for adult soft tissue sarcoma: a prospective randomized feasibility trial. *Sarcoma.* 2000;4:151–160.
16. Woll PJ, van Glabbeke M, Hohenberger P, et al. Adjuvant chemotherapy with doxorubicin and ifosfamide in resected soft tissue sarcoma: Interim analysis of a randomised phase III trial. *J Clin Oncol.* 2007;25(18S):10008.
17. Eilber FC, Eilber FR, Eckardt J, et al. The impact of chemotherapy on the survival of patients with high-grade primary extremity liposarcoma. *Ann Surg.* 2004;240(4):695–697.
18. Crist WM, Anderson JR, Meza JL, et al. Intergroup rhabdomyosarcoma study-IV: results for patients with nonmetastatic disease. *J Clin Oncol.* 2001;19(12):3091–3102.
19. Grier HE, Krailo MD, Tarbell NJ, et al. Addition of ifosfamide and etoposide to standard chemotherapy for Ewing's sarcoma and primitive neuroectodermal tumor of bone. *N Engl J Med.* 2003;348(8): 694–701.
20. Patel SR, Vadhan-Raj S, Papadopolous N, et al. High-dose ifosfamide in bone and soft tissue sarcomas: results of phase II and pilot studies — dose-response and schedule dependence. *J Clin Oncol.* 1997;15(6): 2378–2384.
21. Edmonson JH, Ryan LM, Blum RH, et al. Randomized comparison of doxorubicin alone versus ifosfamide plus doxorubicin or mitomycin, doxorubicin, and cisplatin against advanced soft tissue sarcomas. *J Clin Oncol.* 1993;11(7): 1269–1275.
22. Verweij J, Casali PG, Zalcberg J, et al. Progression-free survival in gastrointestinal stromal tumours with high-dose imatinib: randomised trial. *Lancet.* 2004;364(9440):1127–1134.
23. Blay JY, Le Cesne A, Verweij J, et al. A phase II study of ET-743/-trabectedin ('Yondelis') for patients with advanced gastrointestinal stromal tumours. *Eur J Cancer.* 2004;40(9):1327–1331.

24. Demetri GD, von Mehren M, Blanke CD, et al. Efficacy and safety of imatinib mesylate in advanced gastrointestinal stromal tumors. *N Engl J Med.* 2002;347(7):472–480.

25. Heinrich MC, Corless CL, Demetri GD, et al. Kinase mutations and imatinib response in patients with metastatic gastrointestinal stromal tumor. *J Clin Oncol.* 2003;21(23):4342–4349.

26. Demetri GD, van Oosterom AT, Garrett CR, et al. Efficacy and safety of sunitinib in patients with advanced gastrointestinal stromal tumour after failure of imatinib: a randomised controlled trial. *Lancet.* 2006;368(9544):1329–1338.

27. Heinrich MC, Maki RG, Corless CL, et al. Sunitinib (SU) response in imatinib-resistant (IM-R) GIST correlates with *KIT* and *PDGFRA* mutation status. *J Clin. Oncol.* 2006;24(18S):9502.

28. DeMatteo R, Owzar K, Maki R, et al. Adjuvant imatinib mesylate increases recurrence free survival in patients with completely resected localized primary gastrointestinal stromal tumor: North American Intergroup Phase III trial ACOSOG Z9001. *J Clin. Oncol.* 2007;25(185):10079.

29. DeMatteo RP, Maki RG, Singer S, et al. Results of tyrosine kinase inhibitor therapy followed by surgical resection for metastatic gastrointestinal stromal tumor. *Ann Surg.* 2007;245(3):347–352.

30. Okada K, Frassica FJ, Sim FH, et al. Parosteal osteosarcoma: a clinicopathological study. *J Bone Joint Surg Am.* 1994;76(3):366–378.

31. Souhami RL, Craft AW, Van der Eijken JW, et al. Randomised trial of two regimens of chemotherapy in operable osteosarcoma: a study of the European Osteosarcoma Intergroup. *Lancet.* 1997;350(9082):911–917.

32. Meyers PA, Schwartz CL, Krailo M, et al. Osteosarcoma: a randomized, prospective trial of the addition of ifosfamide and/or muramyl tripeptide to cisplatin, doxorubicin, and high-dose methotrexate. *J Clin Oncol.* 2005;23(9):2004–2011.

33. Pastorino U, Gasparini M, Tavecchio L, et al. The contribution of salvage surgery to the management of childhood osteosarcoma. *J Clin Oncol.* 1991;9(8):1357–1362.

34. Grier HE, Krailo MD, Tarbell NJ, et al. Addition of ifosfamide and etoposide to standard chemotherapy for Ewing's sarcoma and primitive neuroectodermal tumor of bone. *N Engl J Med.* 2003;348(8):694–701.

35. Bisogno G, Riccardi R, Ruggiero A, et al. Phase II study of a protracted irinotecan schedule in children with refractory or recurrent soft tissue sarcoma. *Cancer.* 2006;106(3):703–707.

13

AIDS-RELATED MALIGNANCIES: NON-HODGKIN'S LYMPHOMA AND KAPOSI'S SARCOMA

David Aboulafia, MD

LEARNING OBJECTIVES

After reviewing this chapter, the reader should be able to

- Identify and accurately diagnose the clinical spectrum of AIDS-related Kaposi's sarcoma and non-Hodgkin's lymphoma
- Examine and interpret data regarding the changing incidence of AIDS-related Kaposi's sarcoma and non-Hodgkin's lymphoma in the era of highly active antiretroviral therapy (HAART)
- Make appropriate changes in treatment plans for patients with AIDS-related Kaposi's sarcoma and non-Hodgkin's lymphoma for patients who have received HAART

Patients infected with human immunodeficiency virus (HIV) are at significantly increased risk of developing neoplasms compared with the general population. In 1982, the U.S. Centers for Disease Control and Prevention (CDC) proposed initial case definition for acquired immune deficiency syndrome (AIDS), including AIDS-defining malignancies such as Kaposi's sarcoma (KS) and primary central nervous system lymphoma (PCNSL).[1] Subsequent revisions of the CDC case definition of AIDS resulted in the additions of peripheral intermediate and high-grade B-cell non-Hodgkin's lymphoma (NHL)[2, 3] and cervical cancer.[3]

The introduction of two new classes of antiretroviral agents (non-nucleoside reverse transcriptase inhibitors and HIV protease inhibitors) in the mid-1990s led to the use of combination highly active antiretroviral therapy (HAART). In economically advanced countries, HAART has had a profound effect on the treatment of HIV regarding overall survival, incidence of opportunistic infections, and quality of life. However, only a small subset of the estimated 42 million people infected with HIV worldwide are receiving HAART. In addition to changing the natural history of HIV infection, HAART has influenced the epidemiology of AIDS-associated malignancies and affected outcomes of these tumors. For those

The American Society of Clinical Oncology and Dr. Aboulafia would like to gratefully acknowledge Parkash Gill, MD, for his contributions to the original content of this chapter.

TABLE 13-1 Clinical Effects of Highly Active Antiretroviral Therapy on AIDS-associated Kaposi's Sarcoma and Non-Hodgkin's Lymphoma

	Kaposi's Sarcoma	Non-Hodgkin's Lymphoma
Tumor incidence	Significantly decreased	Decreased
Incidence of concomitant opportunistic infections	Significantly decreased	Significantly decreased
Patient tolerance to cytotoxic chemotherapy	Improved	Improved
Tumor response to treatment	Improved	Improved
Overall patient survival	Improved	Improved

countries with access to HAART, there has been a significant decrease in incidence of KS and PCNSL, and a lesser decline in AIDS-related lymphomas (ARL).[4,5] Despite recent declines in incidence of KS and AIDS-related lymphomas, these two tumors remain the most common malignancies associated with AIDS. Uniformly, KS is associated with human herpes virus type-8 (HHV-8) and with a lesser subset of ARL, which is, in turn, associated with Epstein-Barr virus (EBV). Concomitant advances in chemotherapy, antiretroviral drugs, and supportive care allow for more aggressive management of AIDS-related cancers compared with management in the pre-HAART era (Table 13-1). Ironically, as patients live longer with chronic HIV infection and sustain fewer opportunistic infections in the HAART era, AIDS-defining and non-AIDS-defining malignancies in this population are becoming an increasingly important cause of mortality.[6]

KEY POINTS

- Kaposi's sarcoma is uniformly associated with human herpes virus type-8.
- AIDS-related non-Hodgkin's lymphoma is frequently but not invariably associated with Epstein-Barr virus.
- Despite declines in Kaposi's sarcoma and in AIDS-related lymphoma incidence in the era of highly active antiretroviral therapy, these two tumors remain the most common malignancies associated with HIV infection.

AIDS-RELATED LYMPHOMAS

EPIDEMIOLOGY AND ETIOLOGY

NHL is associated with both congenital and iatrogenic immunosuppression; therefore, it was perhaps not surprising that an increased incidence was demonstrated early in the AIDS epidemic (Table 13-2). Registry linkage studies in the pre-HAART era found that the incidence of AIDS-related lymphoma varied by histologic subtype, ranging from a 14-fold increased risk for low-grade NHL, to a 145-fold increased risk for diffuse large B-cell lymphoma (DLBCL), to a 627-fold increased risk for immunoblastic NHL.[7]

A subsequent meta-analysis of 23 cohort studies, which included 47,936 patients with HIV, found a decline in AIDS-related lymphoma between the periods of 1992 and 1996 and 1997 and 1999.[8] In this analysis, the decline since the widespread introduction of HAART was most marked for PCNSL (from 0.17% to 0.07%) and other immunoblastic NHL (from 0.3% to 0.17%) but not as marked for Burkitt's lymphoma. The change in NHL incidence, most notable for only some subsets, underscores a possible differential involvement of immune function and tumor development.

In a recent cohort analysis of 9,621 patients with HIV followed since 1996, in which 102 developed ARL,[9] three factors were significantly associated with NHL development: age, nadir CD4-positive cell count, and no prior HAART. Moreover, non-nucleoside reverse transcriptase inhibitor-based HAART was as protective as protease inhibitor-based HAART, and these were significantly more protective than nucleoside analogs alone or no antiretrovirals ($p = 0.001$). This may explain the declining incidence of NHL since the introduction of HAART because it is thought that the immune restoration that accompanies HAART protects against the development of AIDS-related lymphoma.[10] However, these data should be interpreted

KEY POINTS

- AIDS-related lymphoma is characterized by intermediate or high-grade B-cell histology and extranodal involvement; patients most often present with fevers, night sweats, and weight loss.
- Treatment of AIDS-related lymphoma has improved in the HAART era, and complete response rates now approach those of individuals with non-Hodgkin's lymphoma without HIV infection.

TABLE 13-2 AIDS-related Lymphomas

Burkitt's Lymphoma
Classic Burkitt's lymphoma
Burkitt's lymphoma with plasmacytoid differentiation
Atypical Burkitt's lymphoma
Diffuse Large B-cell Lymphoma
Centroblastic
Immunoblastic (includes most cases of primary central nervous system lymphoma)
Primary effusion lymphoma/body cavity lymphoma
Plasmablastic lymphoma of the oral cavity
Polymorphic B-cell lymphoma

with caution, because only with longer follow-up analyses will the true effect of HAART on the incidence of AIDS-related lymphoma be known, particularly as patients with HIV survive longer with milder degrees of immuno deficiency. Clearly, such patients retain a substantial risk of AIDS-related lymphoma development.[11,12] Despite the salutary effect of HAART on the survival of patients with HIV, AIDS-related lymphoma continues to be a major source of morbidity and mortality, accounting for as many as 23% of AIDS-related deaths. [13] In medically underserved continents, such as Africa, the risk of AIDS-related lymphoma appears to be much lower than in economically developed countries, but earlier deaths from other AIDS manifestations may partly explain this disparity in incidence.[11]

The true rate of HIV-associated PCNSL is uncertain; many cases were previously not diagnosed antemortem, and autopsies of patients with central nervous system lesions were not frequently performed. This may be a lesser issue in the HAART era because of the considerable decline in the incidence of PCNSL. In an analysis of 4,026 patients with HIV, the incidence of PCNSL declined from 5.6 cases per 1,000 person-years in the pre-HAART era to 2.1 cases per 1,000 person-years in the post-HAART era (Fig. 13-1).[14]

Although Hodgkin's lymphoma is not recognized by the CDC as an AIDS-defining cancer, its incidence is elevated 5- to 15-fold in people with AIDS compared with the general population. The relative risk of Hodgkin's lymphoma increases with time following HIV infection.[15] Ironically, in the era of HAART, incidence of Hodgkin's lymphoma is increasing. It appears that the cytokine and chemokine milieu of a reconstituting immune system may provide the impetus for growth and proliferation of the malignant Reed-Sternberg cell.[16]

ETIOLOGY

Several pathogenesis models for ARL have been proposed. The heterogeneity of ARL likely reflects the various important pathologic mechanisms that promote lymphomagenesis, including HIV-induced immunosuppression, chronic antigenic stimulation, genetic abnormalities, cytokine release and dysregulation, dendritic cell impairment, and the role of herpes viruses, including EBV- and KS-associated HHV-8.

According to the classic antigen-driven model of AIDS-related lymphoma, chronic antigenic stimulation of B lymphocytes and macrophages induced by EBV, HIV, and other infectious agents elicits the continuous release of various growth factors and cytokines promoting B-cell proliferation.[17-19] The multicenter AIDS cohort study evaluated the cytokine profile of men who have sex with men and in whom ARL developed within a 6-month period.[20] Markers

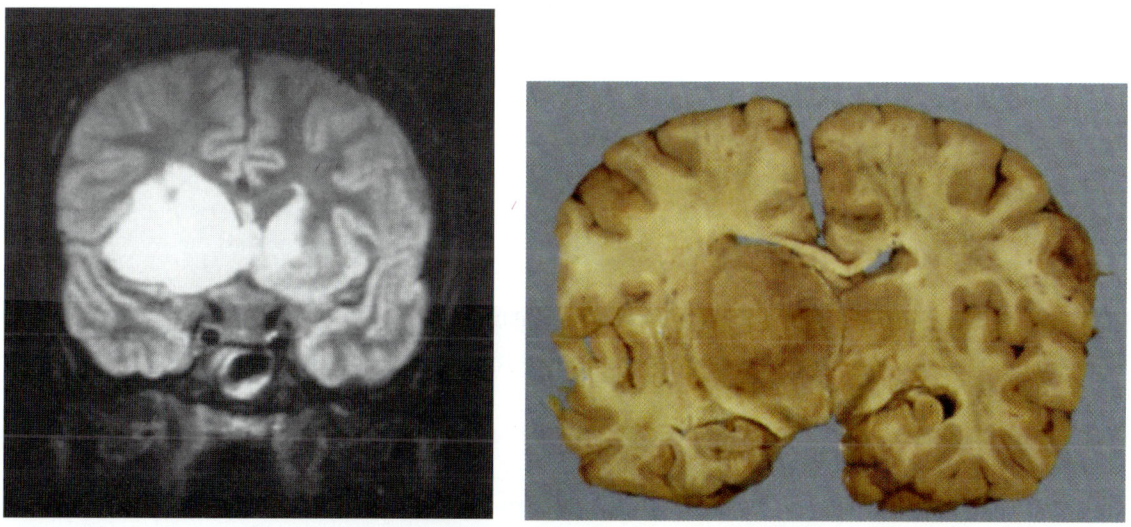

FIG. 13-1 Radiologic and pathologic findings of AIDS-associated primary central nervous system lymphoma. *(Left) Nuclear magnetic resonance imaging scan of brain shows a large tumor mass in the basal ganglia. (Right) Autopsy shows extent of basal ganglia mass lesion. Adapted with permission from the AIDS Images Library, www.aids-images.ch.*

of B-cell activation including interleukin (IL)-6 and IL-10 and soluble CD30 were increased compared with HIV-positive controls in whom NHL did not develop. In addition to contributing to chronic B-cell hyperactivation in HIV infection, the overproduction of B-cell stimulatory cytokines has the potential to enhance the growth and viability of nascent lymphoma cells. IL-6 and IL-10 are both antiapoptotic factors for B-cells and are potent growth factors for AIDS-related lymphoma cells in vitro.[21, 22] Soluble CD30 could be an important biomarker for an immune system environment conducive to B-cell hyperactivation and for the development of this type of lymphoma.

Host factors in cytokine genes also may influence lymphomagenesis. People with HIV who are heterozygous for a deletion in the chemokine receptor CCR5 have a 3-fold lesser risk of NHL compared with people without this mutation.[23] In contrast, those with stromal cell-derived factor-1 mutations have a 2- to 4-fold greater likelihood of developing NHL.[24] HAART may modify lymphomagenic stimuli and may improve the responsiveness of EBV-specific cytotoxic T-cell lymphocytes. In addition, HAART may increase EBV-specific antibodies and can improve immune perturbations that may contribute to B-cell proliferation.[25]

The association between various subtypes of AIDS-related lymphoma and particular viruses supports the notion that antigenic stimulation may underlie the propensity for NHL in people with HIV. HIV viral proteins may induce B-cell proliferation through gene alterations in T-cells, which in turn augment activation of B-cell growth factors. In addition, certain DNA viruses are more commonly associated with various lymphoma histologies and anatomic sites. Specifically, EBV is invariably associated with PCNSL and HHV-8 is highly associated with primary effusion lymphoma (Table 13-3). However, 50% of patients with ARL are negative for EBV or HHV-8. Therefore, other factors must be important in lymphomagenesis including HIV-induced polyclonal B-cell expansion and impaired T-cell immunosurveillance. Although the molecular steps responsible for B-cell transformation associated with AIDS-related lymphoma have not been completely elucidated, this process often is associated with various molecular lesions, including *c-myc* immunoglobulin gene chromosomal translocations, *Bcl-6* mutations and translocations, and inactivation of the *p53* tumor-suppressor gene.[22, 26]

CLINICAL PRESENTATION

In contrast to KS, which is most common in men who have sex with men, NHL distributes homogenously throughout the spectrum of HIV-risk groups. The absolute risk of AIDS-related lymphoma is highest in men and increases with age, duration of HIV infection, and decline in immune competence.[27] Although most often a late manifestation of HIV infection, AIDS-related lymphoma can occur at any CD4-positive cell count. Burkitt and Burkitt-like NHL tend to occur at relatively higher CD4-positive cell counts (greater than 200/µL), whereas immunoblastic NHL, including PCNSL, more often is associated with a lesser CD4-positive cell count (less than 50/µL).

TABLE 13-3 Features Associated with AIDS-related Lymphoma (ARL)

Lymphoma Type	Frequency of ARL	Virus (%)	Comment
Classic Burkitt's lymphoma	30%	EBV (30%)	Neoplastic cells may be found circulating in peripheral blood. Frequently associated with leptomeningeal and bone marrow involvement. Seen most frequently in earlier stages of HIV infection.
Burkitt's with plasmacytoid differentiation	20%	EBV (50%-70%)	
Burkitt-like (atypical)	< 10%	EBV (30%-50%)	
Diffuse Large B-cell			
Centroblastic	25%	EBV (30%)	Most often associated with primary central nervous system lymphoma.
Immunoblastic	10%	EBV (> 90%)	
CD30-positive anaplastic large cell	< 5%	EBV (30%)	
Primary effusion lymphoma/body cavity lymphoma	< 5%	HHV-8 (90%)	May be associated with Castleman's disease and KS. Malignant effusions contain large pleomorphic cells which stain for CD45 and plasma cell markers, but usually negative for B-cell markers. Occurs in late stages of HIV infection.
Plasmablastic lymphoma of the oral cavity	< 5%	HHV-8 (10%)	Rare tumor of oral cavity with aggressive phenotype and plasmacytoid features.

Abbreviations: EBV, Epstein-Barr virus; HIV, human immunodeficiency virus; HHV-8, human herpes virus type 8; KS, Kaposi's sarcoma.

The clinical presentation of patients with AIDS-related lymphoma overlaps with that of the general population with intermediate and high-grade NHL.[28] The majority of patients present with advanced-stage disease, fevers, night sweats, and greater than 10% weight loss over a 3-month period. The presenting symptoms of AIDS-related lymphoma are not appreciably affected by HAART. Patients in the HAART era, however,are less likely to have a prior AIDS diagnosis, are older, and have a higher CD4-positive cell counts at lymphoma presentation than their pre-HAART counterparts.[29] AIDS-related lymphoma may be divided into several clinical categories by site of disease, including systemic DLBCL, which represents at least 80% of cases, PCNSL, plasmablastic lymphoma of the oral cavity, and primary effusion lymphoma/body-cavity lymphoma (Fig. 13-2). The latter lymphoma is a rare subset of AIDS-related lymphoma that predominately grows in the pleural, pericardial, and peritoneal cavities, usually without a contiguous tumor mass.

The most common site of extranodal systemic AIDS-related lymphoma is the gastrointestinal tract, particularly the stomach, anorectum, Waldeyers' ring, and liver.[30,31] Twenty percent to 30% of patients will have bone marrow involvement. Leptomeningeal involvement is seen in 10% of patients; those who are at highest risk for leptomeningeal involvement are patients whose primary tumors are EBV positive and patients whose tumors are located adjacent to paranasal, epidural, or testicular sites.[32]

Histologic subtypes of AIDS-related lymphoma have discriminating patterns of involvement. For example, large cell lymphomas often involve the gastrointestinal tract and central nervous system; small non-cleaved cell lymphomas tend to gravitate to bone marrow and meninges (Fig. 13-3).[19,25]

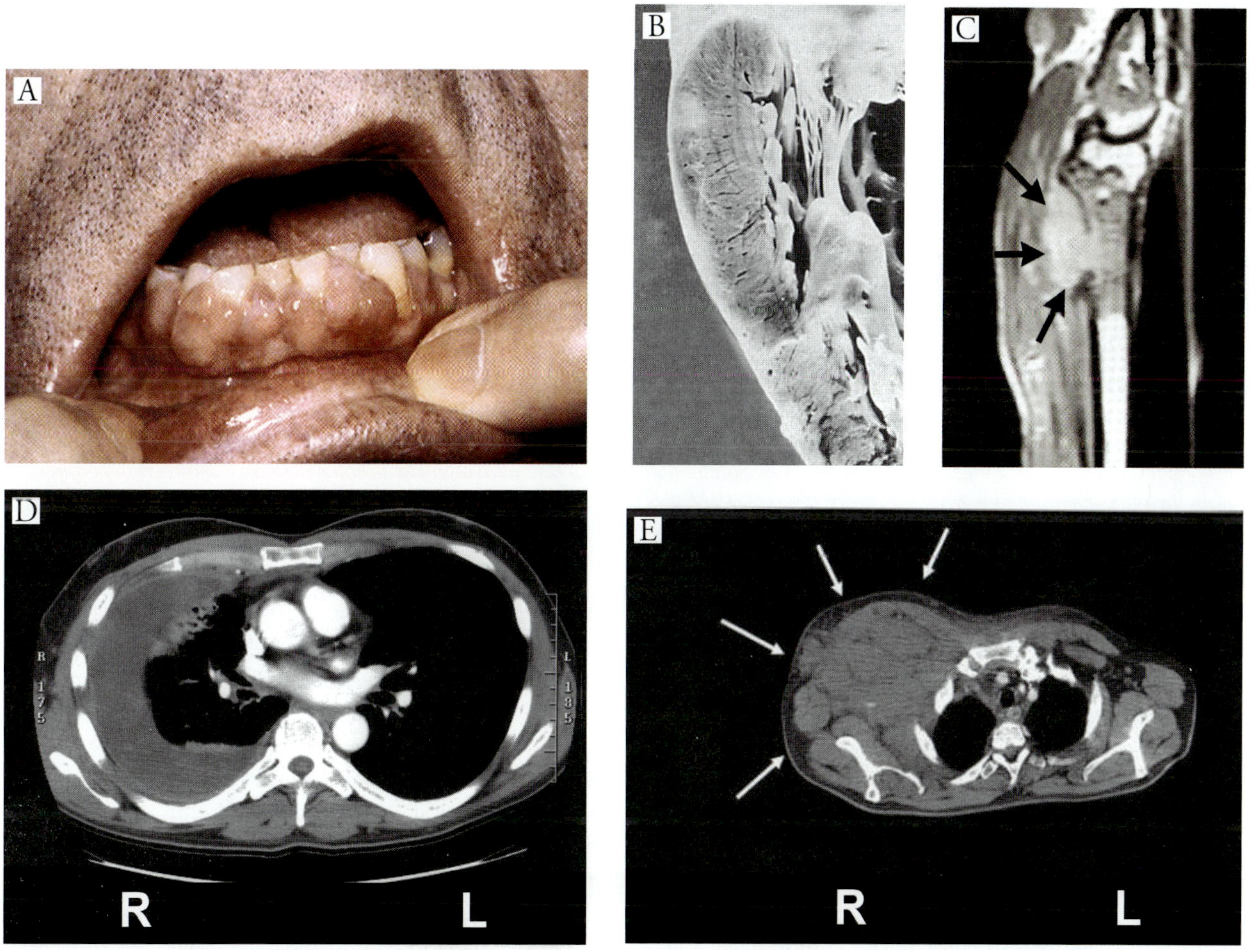

FIG. 13-2 Varied manifestations of AIDS-related lymphomas. *Adapted with permission from the AIDS Images Library, www.aids-images.ch.*

A. Plasmablastic lymphoma of the oral cavity.

B. Diffuse large B-cell lymphoma involving the myocardium (see arrows) in a patient who succumbed after developing electro-mechanical dissociation.

C. Primary lymphoma of fibula in an HIV-seropositive drug user.

D. Computerized tomography scan of a loculated pleural effusion. Cytology was indicative of HHV-8 associated primary effusion lymphoma.

E. Large B-cell lymphoma involving right axilla and thoracic wall.

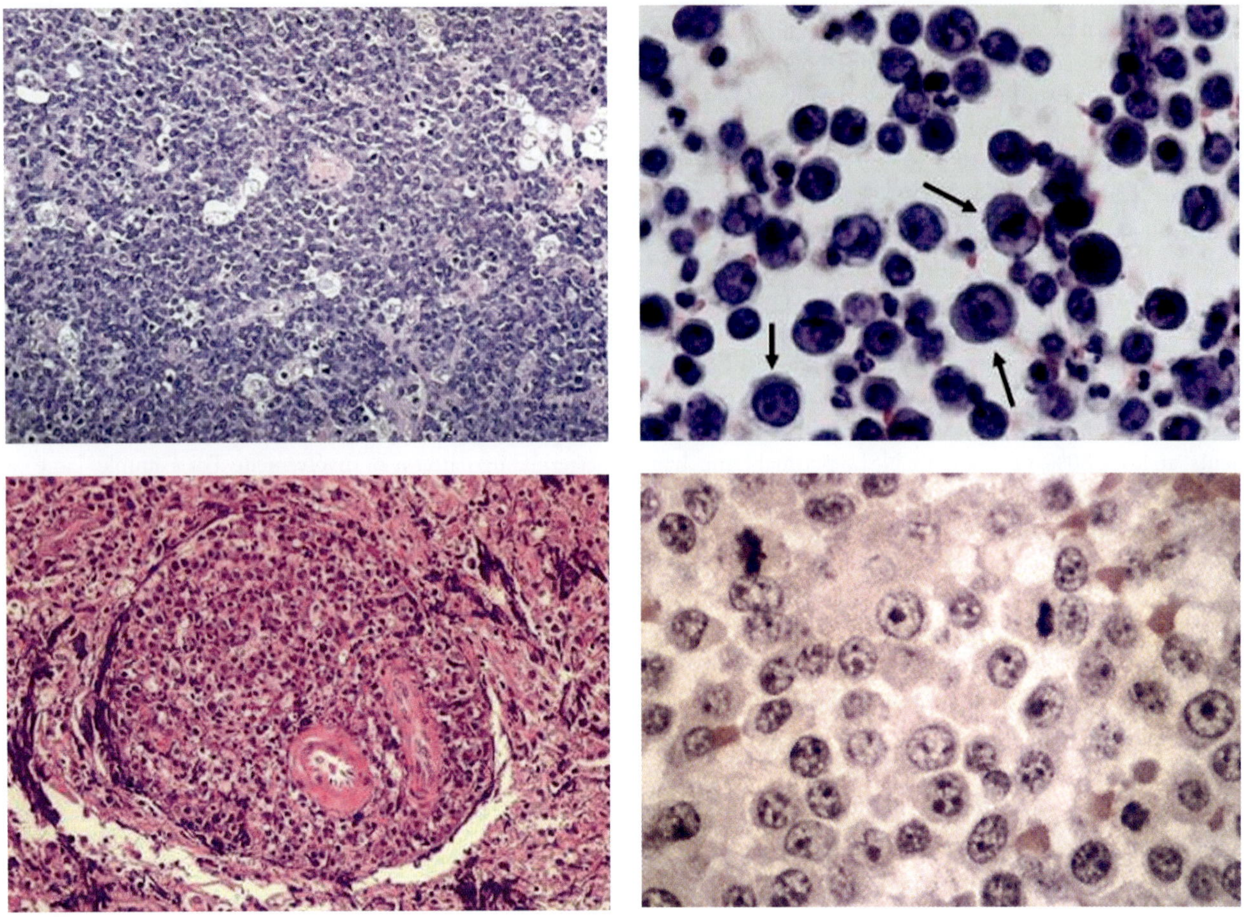

FIG. 13-3 Pathology of AIDS-related lymphomas.

Burkitt-like lymphoma (top left): the predominant malignant lymphocytes have little cytoplasm and appear blue, interspersed with macrophages with more cytoplasm. This aspect has been compared to a "starry sky." (bottom left) Perivascular lymphoma infiltration in primary central nervous system lymphoma (top right). Cytology of pericardial effusion etc, containing large cells with basophilic cytoplasm and prominent nucleoli (bottom left). These cells stained negative for CD20, but positive for CD38. This is suggestive of primary effusions lymphoma. Plasmablastic lymphoma of the oral cavity (bottom right). Tumor cells have prominent central nucleoli. Adapted with permission from the AIDS Images Library, www.aids-images.ch.

PROGNOSTIC FACTORS

Early in the HAART era, adverse prognostic factors for AIDS-related lymphoma included a CD4-positive count of less than 100 cells/μL, age older than 35, a history of injection drug use, poor performance status, elevated levels of lactate dehydrogenase (LDH), advanced lymphoma stage at diagnosis, and prior AIDS diagnosis.[33] When zero or one of these factors was present, overall survival was 46 weeks; when three or four factors were present, patient survival was 18 weeks. The international prognostic index (which incorporates age, performance status, tumor stage, LDH level, and the number of sites of extranodal disease) is a useful means of stratifying risk in aggressive lymphoma in the non-HIV and in the HIV settings.[34]

More recently, control of HIV viral replication through HAART has emerged as a major positive prognostic factor for patients with AIDS-related lymphoma.[35,36] In a retrospective analysis of 235 patients diagnosed between 1988 and 1999, multivariate Cox proportional hazards model showed dramatic improvements in overall survival among those who received HAART.[37] The improvement in survival was most marked for those patients with DLBCL and may not extend to the same degree for patients with AIDS-related Burkitt's lymphoma.[38] HAART also favorably affects the survival of patients with PCNSL. In a retrospective analysis and after a median follow-up of 667 days, six out of seven patients with PCNSL who were treated with HAART were alive, compared with none of 18 patients who did not receive HAART.[39]

TREATMENT

Initial attempts to treat patients with AIDS-related lymphoma using aggressive chemotherapy led to unacceptable toxicity and early death. Subsequent efforts with low-dose chemotherapy regimens yielded modest benefit — only 10% of patients survived 2 years.[40] With the advent of

HAART and anticipated restored immunity, more recent regimens have reported the use of standard-dose chemotherapies without excessive toxicity.

In 2001, the AIDS Malignancy Consortium reported the feasibility of combining cyclophosphamide, doxorubicin, vincristine, and prednisone (CHOP) chemotherapy (dose-reduced or full-dose CHOP) with concomitant HAART in 65 patients.[41] Complete response rates were 30% and 48% in the reduced-dose and full-dose groups, respectively. Only one opportunistic infection occurred during chemotherapy administration. Cyclophosphamide clearance was reduced compared with historical controls, without clinical significance. Importantly, this study demonstrated that combining chemotherapy with HAART was feasible and that a change in cyclophosphamide metabolism was not associated with increased toxicity. No long-term outcomes have been reported in this study. Other studies of CHOP-based chemotherapy and HAART have yielded median survival periods of approximately 2 years.[35,42] Infusional regimens of combination cyclophosphamide, doxorubicin, and etoposide (CDE) also have confirmed the feasibility of combining chemotherapy and HAART.[43] For patients who continue HAART while they receive chemotherapy, CD4-positive cell counts decline by 50% during chemotherapy, but these values gradually improve within several months of completing treatment.[44] For patients who continue to receive effective HAART during chemotherapy, HIV viral replication tends to remain suppressed below the limits of detection using commercial-based polymerase chain reaction assays.[44,45]

Chemotherapy without concomitant HAART also has been studied. Reasons for HAART omission include concerns of drug interactions with chemotherapy and poor patient compliance regarding antiretrovirals, potentially leading to heightened toxicity and the emergence of multidrug-resistant HIV quasispecies. The National Cancer Institute (NCI) described a dose-adjusted regimen consisting of a 4-day infusion of etoposide, vincristine, and doxorubicin in addition to daily oral prednisone for 5 days; the infusion was followed by an adjusted dose of cyclophosphamide (EPOCH) according to initial CD4-positive cell count.[46] Twenty-nine out of 38 patients (74%) achieved a complete remission. Even more impressive, among the 29 patients who achieved a complete response, there was a 60% probability of survival without disease and a 92% probability of durable remission at 53 months. As anticipated, the HIV viral load increased and CD4-positive cell counts decreased while patients were receiving chemotherapy, but both parameters improved rapidly following the reintroduction of HAART at the completion of chemotherapy. In the hands of NCI investigators, the temporary discontinuation of HAART for 4 to 6 months while patients received chemotherapy did not lead to obvious deleterious effects.

Whether it is preferable for HAART to be administered concomitantly with chemotherapy or immediately restarted after chemotherapy is completed remains unclear. As experience has mounted, most community oncologists are increasingly combining chemotherapy with HAART. However, outcomes data between these two approaches have not been studied prospectively to know if one approach is superior to another.

Recent studies also have sought to combine the CD20 chimeric monoclonal antibody rituximab with chemotherapy. In the AIDS Associated Malignancies Clinical Trials Consortium Study 010, investigators evaluated the role of rituximab therapy for patients with AIDS-related lymphoma. Patients were randomly assigned to CHOP or to CHOP and 375 mg/m^2 of rituximab administered with each chemotherapy cycle (for a total of six to eight cycles, with an additional three monthly doses after complete response was obtained).[47] Results are provocative because, although there was a trend toward a higher complete response rate for the rituximab arm (58% vs. 47%, respectively), there also was substantially more treatment-related infectious deaths in the rituximab arm (14% vs. 2%; $p = 0.027$). The majority of these deaths were in patients with CD4-positive counts of less than 50 cells/µL at entry. There was no significant difference in the rate of grade 4 neutropenia, febrile neutropenia, or infections between the arms.

A French study of rituximab in conjunction with CHOP yielded a complete remission in 40 out of 52 (77%) accessible patients with AIDS-related lymphoma, and the addition of rituximab to CHOP also demonstrated an excellent 2-year survival rate of 75%.[48] Eighteen patients died — 16 as a result of NHL, one as a result of encephalitis and, unlike Study 010, only one patient died as a result of infection.

Also, in contrast to Study 010, investigators at the National Institutes of Health have reported preliminary results with rituximab plus EPOCH that demonstrated a benefit for rituximab for patients with CD4-positive counts of greater than 100 cells/µL.[49] Compared with historical controls, rituximab improved survival at 19 months median follow-up from 16% to 57%. No additional benefit was seen for patients with CD4-positive counts of greater than 100 cells/µL, but these patients had cure rates already approaching 90%. Increased neutropenia during and after chemotherapy was observed with rituximab plus EPOCH but without patient deaths.

Rituximab has been shown to improve response rates and overall survival for patients with aggressive NHL who were HIV negative and treated with CHOP, without an increased risk of infectious complications. Rituximab, when given sequentially with chemotherapy, may contribute to improved control of AIDS-related lymphoma but possibly accounts for a higher risk of severe infection than has been seen for patients with NHL who were HIV negative. Most oncologists favor administration of rituximab concurrently with chemotherapy for these patients, although caution should be demonstrated regarding patients with CD4-positive cell counts of less than 50 cells/μL. Table 13-4 lists common chemotherapy regimens used for AIDS-related lymphoma.

Prospective studies of AIDS-related lymphoma generally have combined the high-grade DLBCL and Burkitt's lymphoma/Burkitt-like lymphoma histologies, with little difference in outcome between the subtypes. In contrast,

TABLE 13-4 Common Chemotherapy Regimens for AIDS-related Non-Hodgkin's Lymphoma

	R-CHOP[48]	Dose-adjusted R-EPOCH[49]	R-CDE[43]
Regimen	— Rituximab, 375 mg/m^2 intravenously on day 1 — Cyclophosphamide, 750 mg/m^2 intravenously on day 1 — Adriamycin, 50 mg/m^2 intravenously on day 1 — Vincristine, 1.4 mg/m^2 (maximum, 2 mg) intravenously on day 1 — Prednisone, 40 mg/m^2 orally four times daily on days 1 through 5 — IT, central nervous system prophylaxis not routine — TMP-SMZ, orally, administration recommended but not required — G-CSF, 5 mcg/kg subcutaneously four times daily on days 6 through 12 Administer every 3 weeks for six cycles	— Rituximab, 375 mg/m^2 intravenously on day 1 — Etoposide, 50 mg/m^2 per day continuous infusion for days 1 through 4 — Prednisone, 60 mg/m^2 per day orally on days 1 through 5 — Vincristine, 0.4 mg/m^2 per day continuous infusion for days 1 through 4 — Doxorubicin, 10 mg/m^2 per day continuous infusion for days 1 through 4 — Cyclophosphamide, 750 mg/m^2 intravenously for 15 minutes on day 5 — IT MTX, 12 mg on days 1 and 5 of cycles 3 to 6 — TMP-SMZ, 1 tablet orally twice daily, three times weekly — G-CSF 5 mcg/kg subcutaneously every day beginning on day 6 until ANC $>$ 5,000/L Administer every 3 weeks for four to eight cycles Dose-adjustment paradigm based on twice weekly CBC (dose adjustment above starting doses apply to etoposide, doxorubicin, and cyclophosphamide. Dose adjustment below starting doses apply to cyclophosphamide. If nadir ANC $>$ 500/L, 20% increase in etoposide, doxorubicin, and cyclophosphamide. If nadir ANC $<$ 500/L on one or two measurements, same doses as last cycle. If nadir ANC $<$ 500/L on at least three measurements, or nadir platelet $<$ 25,000/L on day 1 measurement, 20% decrease in cyclophosphamide dose below last cycle.	— Rituximab, 375 mg/m^2 intravenously on day 1 — Cyclophosphamide, 187.5 mg/m^2 continuous infusion on days 1 through 4 — Doxorubicin, 12.5 mg/m^2 continuous infusion on days 1 through 4 — Etoposide, 60 mg/m^2 continuous infusion on days 1 through 4 — IT MTX, 12 mg every cycle or — IT AraC, 50 mg on days 1 and 4 on cycles 1 and 2 for patients with Burkitt's lymphoma or bone marrow involvement — TMP-SMZ, 1 tab by mouth 3 times per week — Fluconazole, 100 mg orally per day Administer every 4 weeks for six cycles

Abbreviations: R-CHOP, rituximab plus combination cyclophosphamide, doxorubicin, vincristine, and prednisone; R-EPOCH, rituximab plus combination etoposide, vincristine, doxorubicin, prednisone, and cyclophosphamide; R-CDE, rituximab plus combination cyclophosphamide, doxorubicin, and etoposide; IT, intrathecal; MTX, methotrexate; TMP-SMZ, trimethoprim-sulfamethoxazole (160/180 mg); AraC, cytarabine; G-CSF, granulocyte-colony stimulating factor; ANC, absolute neutrophil count; CBC, complete blood count.

two retrospective reviews demonstrated substantially inferior outcomes for HIV-associated Burkitt lymphoma in the HAART era in comparison with HIV-associated DLBCL if CHOP-like treatments were used.[38,50] Median survival was 5.7 months and 8 months for those with Burkitt lymphoma compared with 43.2 months and 22 months for those with DLBCL. Small retrospective and phase II studies reported the feasibility of using dose-intensive protocols with or without HAART, with response rates of approximately 70%.[51–53] There are no prospective studies demonstrating superior response with high-dose compared with standard-dose regimens, but these pilot study results are compelling. For patients with an adequate Karnofsky performance status, intensive chemotherapy akin to what is offered to patients with Burkitt's lymphoma who are HIV negative is recommended.

Attention to supportive care measures is essential in this patient population. The judicious use of hematopoietic stimulants including the newer formulations of pegylated granulocyte-colony stimulating factor (G-CSF) and erythropoietin may help ameliorate chemotherapy-induced cytopenias. To minimize cardiac toxicity, pegylated anthracyclines may be safely and effectively substituted for doxorubicin.[54,55] It is possible that infectious complications may be minimized with antibiotic prophylaxis during periods of severe neutropenia. Recently published data suggest a clinical benefit from the use of this approach in non-immunocompromised patients with solid tumors and lymphomas.[56,57] Table 13-5 lists measures that may lead to improved outcomes or less treatment-associated toxicity.

TABLE 13-5 AIDS-related Lymphoma: Minimizing Treatment-related Side Effects

- Avoid drugs that aggravate cytopenias if possible (e.g., zidovudine and trimethoprim-sulfamethoxazol); granulocyte-colony stimulating factor and erythropoietin may ameliorate cytopenias.
- Avoid drugs with overlapping toxicities with chemotherapy (e.g., didanosine and stavudine may exacerbate neuropathy; zidovudine can aggravate anemia).
- Use leuko-reduced blood products for the rare patient who is cytomegalovirus seronegative.
- All patients should receive *Pneumocystis jiroveci* prophylaxis regardless of initial CD4-positive cell count (e.g., dapsone, inhaled pentamidine, and atovaquone).
- Consider the use of prophylactic fluoroquinolone antibiotics and azoles during periods of neutropenia.

Patients with relapsed or refractory AIDS-related lymphoma can be considered for high-dose therapy with stem cell support if they have chemosensitive disease and have not exhausted HAART options. HAART therapy is feasible throughout the transplant process. In one report, 16 out of 19 patients remained in remission after 2 years of follow-up.[59] Infectious complications were comparable with those reported in the HIV-negative NHL populations, and no long-term deterioration in immune function was found. Larger studies with longer follow-up in a focused intent-to-treat analysis are needed to better define the optimal AIDS-related lymphoma conditioning regimen and to better delineate patient selection criteria.

Prior to the HAART era, whole-brain radiation therapy was a standard of care for PCNSL, but patient median survival was typically limited to 2 to 4 months, owing to progressive lymphoma or uncontrolled opportunistic infections. As noted previously, epidemiologic studies have shown a significant decline in the incidence of AIDS-associated PCNSL in the HAART era. Retrospective studies also have demonstrated improved survival for such patients who receive HAART. In a multicenter study of 29 patients with histologically confirmed AIDS-related PCNSL, six received HAART and had a greater median survival time (1,093 days) compared with those patients who received whole-brain radiation therapy alone (132 days) or supportive care (33 days).[60] A single-institution study also reported that six out of seven patients with PCNSL who were treated with HAART were alive compared with zero out of 18 untreated patients at a median follow-up of 667 days.[61] A survival benefit was seen for patients who had a decrease in HIV viral load of 0.5 $\log_{10}$ copies/mL or greater after diagnosis and for patients with a CD4 positive count rebound of 50 cells/μL or greater.

In the HAART era, radiotherapy remains the treatment of choice for patients with PCNSL, but it is now preferred in conjunction with HAART. There also is renewed interest in offering chemotherapy to the rare patient who has a well preserved CD4-positive count of greater than 100 cells/μL and effective HAART options. Rare reports also describe spontaneous regression of PCNSL with HAART alone.[62]

KAPOSI'S SARCOMA

EPIDEMIOLOGY

Although the prevalence of KS in North American men with AIDS has dramatically decreased in the past decade, it remains the most common AIDS-associated cancer. It also is a persistent cause of morbidity and mortality, particularly in sub-Saharan Africa. Prior to the widespread use of HAART in 1996, KS was 100,000-fold greater among individuals with HIV compared with the general population. This risk appeared most strongly concentrated in men who have sex with men. Specifically, KS was noted to be 20 times more prevalent in these men than among heterosexual patients with hemophilia who were HIV negative, and 20 times

KEY POINTS

- Kaposi's sarcoma most commonly involves the skin.
- First-line treatment for AIDS-related Kaposi's sarcoma is highly active antiretroviral therapy.
- Chemotherapy is most commonly reserved for patients with advancing Kaposi's sarcoma despite the use of highly active antiretroviral therapy, patients with problematic lymphedema, and patients with symptomatic Kaposi's sarcoma involving visceral organs.

more prevalent in HIV-seropositive men than HIV-seropositive women.[63,64] A recent analysis of 13,894 serum samples from the United States general population who participated in the National Health and Nutrition Examination Survey III confirmed that HHV-8 transmission may occur through sexual activity, particularly through sex with other men. No evidence was observed for heterosexual transmission to women.[65]

In the United States, up to 40% of men who have sex with men who received an AIDS diagnosis in the early 1980s presented with KS at the time of their initial AIDS diagnosis. Ten years later, the percentage of people with HIV infection with KS as their initial AIDS-defining illness had decreased to less than 20%. Factors that may have contributed to this phenomenon that antedated the HAART era include expansion of the AIDS case definition to encompass conditions that may be diagnosed earlier than KS, a decrease in identification or reporting of relatively minor KS lesions, and the decline in exposure to environmental factors associated with KS. In particular, the adoption of "safer" sex practices, which may have reduced the rate of HHV-8 transmission is considered to be an important modifier of incidence.[63]

The declining incidence of KS, in part, preceded the introduction of HAART, but this well documented decline has persisted HAART era. The annual reduction of KS incidence between 1994 and 2003 in the pan-European multicenter EuroSIDA group of 9,803 people with HIV was 39%.[66] Moreover, most patients who developed KS while receiving HAART began with low CD4-positive cell counts and developed KS within 6 months of starting HAART. This is similar to previous studies demonstrating that HAART reduced the risk of KS and that most patients who received HAART and who developed KS have evidence of HIV virologic failure.[67] In the Swiss HIV group, the standardized incidence ratio for KS was 239 for patients with HIV who did not receive HAART and 25 for those who did.[68]

ETIOLOGY

An increased risk of KS in a subpopulation of individuals at risk for HIV suggested the presence of a second infectious agent as the cause.[64] These findings were confirmed by the identification of HHV-8 in the tumor tissue of KS but not in adjacent normal tissue.[69] In contrast to other viruses previously linked to KS pathogenesis (including EBV, cytomegalovirus and human papillomavirus), HHV-8 consistently has been detected in all forms of KS. In addition, HHV-8 DNA is present in the lymphoid system, peripheral blood mononuclear cells, saliva, and semen of patients with KS.[70] In HIV-infected individuals who do not receive HAART, the presence of antibodies to this virus is predictive of KS development.[71]

Important advances in our understanding of the factors that contribute to KS initiation occurred when investigators perfected laboratory techniques to sustain the growth of large numbers of KS cells in culture.[72] Subsequent studies demonstrated that cultured spindle cells from KS lesions were abnormally responsive to a variety of growth factors and that transformed culture medium promoted normal endothelial cells to acquire the features of the KS genotype.[73] These factors, which include Oncostatin M, gamma interferon, IL-1, IL-6 and IL-8, tumor necrosis factor, granulocyte-macrophage-CSF, platelet derived growth factor (PDGF), basic fibroblast growth factor (bFGF), and vascular endothelial growth factor (VEGF) also are found in the inflammatory cell infiltrates of KS lesions. The ability of this inflammatory infiltrate to promote KS growth was illustrated in experiments in which nude mice were inoculated with KS cells and with the media used to support growth of the cells; the mice subsequently developed cutaneous KS-like lesions.[74]

In the early stages, KS behaves more like a hyperplastic proliferative disease than a true cancer. PDGF and VEGF mediate spindle-cell growth, angiogenesis, and KS-associated angiodema. The abnormal cytokine milieu of HIV infection and the mitogenic effects of HIV TAT protein may further act synergistically to stimulate KS spindle cell growth through autocrine and paracrine loops, leading to an increased frequency and aggressiveness of KS.[75,76] In one model of KS pathogenesis, circulating KS progenitor cells latently infected with HHV-8 migrate to inflammatory sites.[77] Exposure to various inflammatory cytokines results in dedifferentiation of these latently infected cells into KS-like spindle cells and induces HHV-8 reactivation. Reactivation of HHV-8 leads to the expression of pathogenic early genes, including viral IL-6, which can further activate VEGF and induce angiogenesis. Viral lytic replication in the same cells increases proinflammatory conditions, which further serves to stimulate angiogenesis. The HIV TAT protein enhances this inflammatory-angiogenic state by increasing the angiogenic activities of VEGF, bFGF and gamma interferon and by increasing the expression of matrix metalloproteinases.[78]

The precise role that HHV-8 plays in stimulating KS growth is becoming increasingly clear. The genetic sequence of HHV-8 largely has been determined, and portions of its genome are analogous to DNA sequences believed to have oncogenic potential. The open reading frame 74 of HHV-8 encodes for the G-protein coupled receptor (GPCR) that stimulates the production of angiogenic factors, including VEGF.[79] When mouse kidney cells are transfected with the GPCR HHV-8 gene and bathed with VEGF, they transform and induce angiogenesis. However, the recognition that KS lesions are clonagenic and KS-like cells can be detected in the peripheral blood of patients with AIDS-associated KS provides further evidence for the malignant potential of KS spindle cell proliferation.[80]

CLINICAL FEATURES

KS most often involves the skin and, in the setting of AIDS, tends to be multicentric (Figure 13-4). Patients may have small and innocuous looking skin blemishes that are easily overlooked. Alternatively, they may possess large and complex cutaneous lesions that scatter over the body and manifest as red, purple, or brown patches, plaques, or nodules. These unsightly lesions are rarely painful, but their resulting disfigurement can have profound psychologic effects. In some patients, only a few skin lesions are apparent, and the lesions may remain unchanged for several years; in others, lesions appear rapidly, particularly during periods of heightened illness and immunosuppression. In most patients, new lesions appear gradually over several weeks to months.[81]

KS often involves the head and neck, including the tip of the nose and the retroauricular and periorbital areas. KS involving the eyelid or conjunctiva can interfere with vision. Examination of the oropharynx may uncover clinically silent hard- and soft-palate lesions; if allowed to grow, these lesions can interfere with eating but rarely cause airway obstruction. Lymphatic involvement may produce debilitating and cosmetically unacceptable edema, particularly in the periorbital and genital areas, as well as the lower extremities. Edema may be complicated by skin breakdown and cellulitis. Foot lesions are common. Approximately 30% of patients with cutaneous KS also will have gastrointestinal involvement. These tumors may be a source of dysphagia, blood loss, or obstipation.

Involvement of the tracheobronchial tree, pulmonary parenchyma, and pleura are late and serious KS complications.

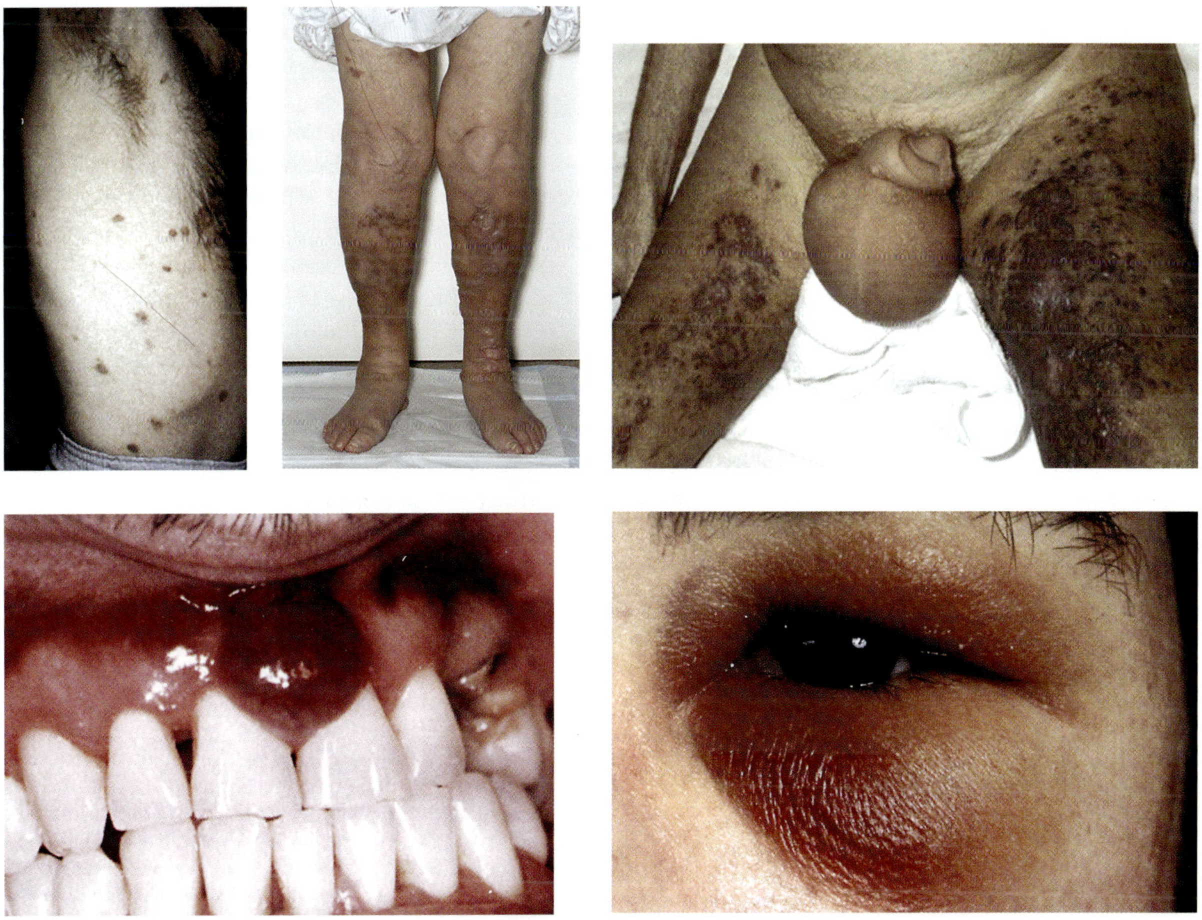

FIG. 13-4 Varied manifestations of Kaposi's sarcoma.

Kaposi's sarcoma lesions scattered across trunk (top left). Kaposi's sarcoma-associated lymphedema involving lower extremities (top middle). Kaposi's sarcoma involving thighs and causing scrotal edema (top right). Asymptomatic Kaposi's sarcoma of the gingiva (bottom left). Kaposi's sarcoma involving the head and neck and contributing to periorbital erythema and lymphedema (bottom right). Adapted with permission from the AIDS Images Library, www.aids-images.ch.

Fortunately, in the era of HAART, such events are uncommon. Patients may have dyspnea, hemorrhagic pleural effusions, and fever. Even in the absence of symptoms, the presence of hilar adenopathy, diffuse interstitial infiltrates, or prominent parenchymal nodularity on chest radiograph should heighten clinical suspicion, particularly for patients with a CD4-positive cell count of less than 50 cells/µL and with uncontrolled HIV infection.[82]

There has been little change in the initial clinical features of KS since the introduction of HAART, especially because most patients are not yet receiving HAART when diagnosed with KS. Patients diagnosed with KS in the HAART era do not have significantly different CD4-positive cell counts or HIV viral loads compared with the pre-HAART era, but their risk of dying is significantly reduced.[83]

PATHOLOGIC FEATURES

KS is an angioproliferative tumor that is characterized by slit-like neovascular processes and the presence of proliferating endothelial cells, fibroblasts, infiltrating leukocytes, and a population of spindle-shaped tumor cells. In the early stages, cutaneous KS is characterized by inflammatory cell infiltration, extravasation of red blood cells, endothelial cell activation, and angiogenesis. This is followed by the appearance of the typical spindle-shaped cells that represent a heterogeneous population dominated by activated endothelial cells mixed with macrophages and dendritic cells.[84] In advancing lesions, spindle cells tend to become the predominant cell type, although angiogenesis always remains a prominent feature. The ability to reliably diagnose KS has improved with the use of immunostains directed at HHV-8 and tumor endothelium (Fig. 13-5).

PROGNOSTIC FACTORS

Prior to the introduction of HAART, a diagnosis of AIDS-related KS was associated with median survival of 12 to 18 months. Patients most often died from opportunistic infections rather than KS. The prognosis has improved dramatically with 3-year overall survival of more than 80% in one series.[85] In another group from Seattle, the 1-year overall survival was 79% in the post-HAART era, and this compared favorably with 59% in the pre-HAART era controls.[83] A staging system that classifies risk according to such factors as extent of the tumor, the immune status, and systemic illness has long been used.[86] More recently, the prognosis of KS diagnosed in the HAART era has been evaluated, and only poor tumor stage (T1) and systemic symptoms (S1) were associated with unfavorable outcomes. CD4-positive cell counts appear not to be a prognostic factor as long as the patient continues to receive effective HAART.[85]

TREATMENT

Even for the patient with severe immunodeficiency, both the abundance of lesions and the rate of KS progression are highly variable. The role of HAART alone in the management of early-stage KS is well established with durable clinical response rates of more than 60%.[87] HAART-induced KS regression is generally durable and gradually increases with time. Occasionally, and sometimes dramatically, patients with KS who subsequently receive HAART experience a sudden flare or burst in KS lesion growth. This phenomenon may occur in patients with KS, typically within weeks to a few months after initiation of HAART, despite control of virologic and immunologic parameters.

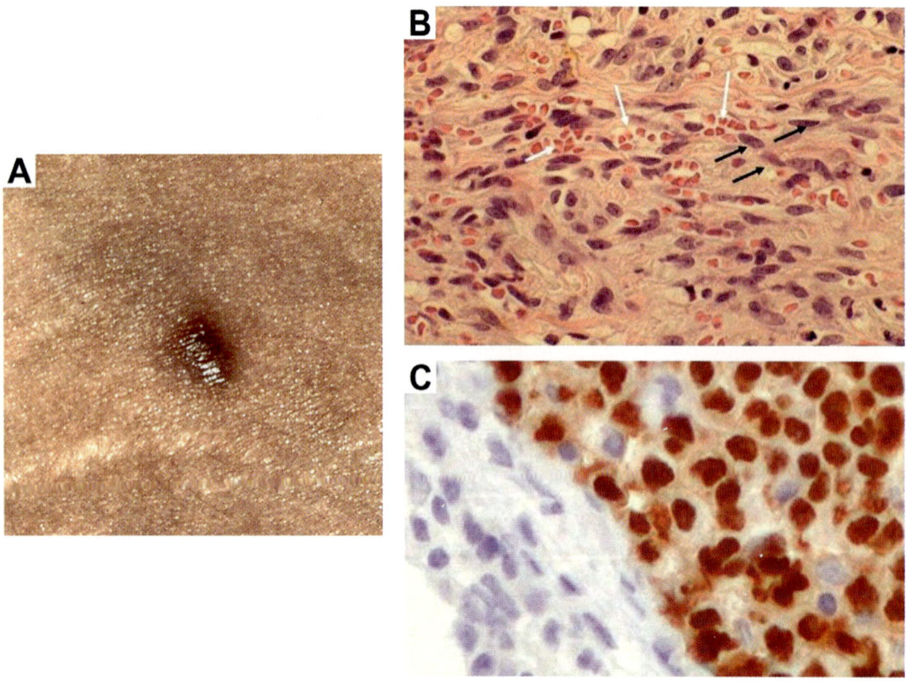

FIG. 13-5 A. A single Kaposi's sarcoma lesion involving the dorsum of hand. B. Punch biopsy of the lesion. Note fusiform cells (black arrows) and vascular spaces filled with erythrocytes (white arrows) contributing to the typical reddish-brown color of Kaposi's sarcoma. C. Kaposi's sarcoma. Staining with an antibody directed against a protein of HHV-8 (ORF 73, LANA). Images 5B and 5C. Adapted with permission from the AIDS Images Library, www.aids-images.ch.

This clinical response, known as the immune reconstitution inflammatory syndrome (IRIS), occurs secondary to an immune response against previously diagnosed pathogens. In a cohort study of 150 patients with HIV-associated KS who began HAART as the sole treatment for KS, 10 patients (6.6%) developed progressive IRIS-associated KS.[88] In such instances, HAART usually can be successfully continued, although for a time, chemotherapy also may be required to control KS growth.[89]

Although HAART plays an important role as a primary therapy for AIDS-associated KS, it often is insufficient for patients with aggressive disease that requires tumor-specific therapy. The decision to provide local or systemic treatment should be based on several factors, including assessment of disease abundance, site of the disease, rate of disease progression, patient-specific psychologic factors, and presence of organ dysfunction.[90]

Local treatment may be possible for individuals who have limited, nonbulky, and accessible lesions. Alitretinoin gel (0.1%) is the only topical patient-administered therapy approved by the U.S. Food and Drug Administration for the treatment of KS. Alitretinoin is a retinoid-receptor panagonist. It is presumably this unique receptor-binding profile that gives alitretinoin its efficacy for the topical treatment of KS. It has been shown to be beneficial for several patient populations, including treatment-naïve populations, patients who received one or more prior anti-KS therapies, and patients who were treatment refractory.[91] Most patients require 4 to 8 weeks of treatment before responses are noted. Dermal irritation is common at the site of application of the gel and, because minimal drug is absorbed systemically, the gel does not affect the growth of new lesions in untreated areas. It also is exceptionally expensive. At the time this publication was released, a 30-g tube cost approximately $2,000 (U.S.)

Other local treatments include intralesional chemotherapy, radiation therapy, laser therapy, and cryotherapy, all of which can be quite effective at controlling local tumor growth. Vinblastine probably is the most widely used intralesional agent and, in the pre-HAART era, was associated with a response rate of 70%.[92] Treated lesions will usually fade and regress, although they typically will not resolve completely. In the HAART era, this approach is rarely employed because small KS lesions will often regress with effective HAART. Radiation therapy can effectively palliate symptomatic disease that is too extensive to be treated with intralesional chemotherapy but not extensive enough to warrant systemic therapy.[93] In a series of 36 patients with KS of the feet, a fractionation schedule of three fractions a week at 3.5 Gy/fraction up to a total dose of 21.0 Gy yielded an overall response rate of 91% (complete response rate, 80%). Although discomfort from radiation therapy was frequent, it usually resolved without intervention within 2 weeks of completion of the therapy.[94] Poor wound healing and woody induration are most problematic for patients with large KS lesions, particularly for patients who already suffer from KS-associated lymphedema.

Patients with KS-associated edema, extensive mucocutaneous disease, or symptomatic pulmonary or gastrointestinal involvement need a rapid response that is achieved best with systemic chemotherapy. A number of cytotoxic chemotherapy agents have moderate activity in AIDS-related KS, including bleomycin, vinca alkaloids, etoposide, taxanes, and anthracyclines.[95] For patients with extensive or advanced disease or for patients who require rapid tumor shrinkage, liposomal formulations of doxorubicin and daunorubicin are the gold standard of clinical treatment. Paclitaxel is an established second-line therapy for KS treatment (Table 13-6). In randomized multicenter trials, each of the two available liposomal anthracyclines proved superior to conventional chemotherapy (bleomycin and vincristine, with or without nonliposomal doxorubicin) regarding response rates and toxicity profiles.[96-98] Recommended dosage of liposomal doxorubicin is 20 mg/m^2 every 3 weeks and that of liposomal daunorubicin is 40 mg/m^2 every 2 weeks.

When administered in conjunction with HAART, liposomal anthracyclines reliably shrink KS tumors, and, more importantly, each improves lymphedema, gastrointestinal involvement, and lesion-associated pain. However, longstanding lymphedema may not improve as dramatically as disfiguring lesions. Side effects are, in general, quite mild. Alopecia and neuropathies, in particular, are unusual with these preparations compared with conventional chemotherapies. Further, at higher cumulative doses, these agents typically

TABLE 13-6 Therapies for the Treatment of Patients with Widespread or Advanced Kaposi's Sarcoma (KS)

Therapy	Comment
HAART	Should be incorporated into treatment schemes whenever possible for all patients with AIDS and KS
Liposomal anthracyclines: Doxorubicin Daunorubicin	Often used as first-line therapy patients requiring cytotoxic chemotherapy
Paclitaxel	Responses seen in patients who have failed anthracycline therapy; associated with greater toxicity (i.e., neutropenia and alopecia) than liposomal anthracyclines
Gemcitabine	A treatment option for which further clinical trials are being considered

Abbreviation: HAART, highly active antiretroviral therapy.

have not been associated with the cardiomyopathies that have frequently limited the use of nonliposomal anthracyclines.

Paclitaxel has shown striking efficacy even for patients with anthracycline-resistant disease. The response rate in two trials were 59% and 71%, respectively, for patients in whom one previous systemic chemotherapeutic regimen had failed.[99,100] Paclitaxel is well tolerated. However, at the recommended dose of 100 mg/m^2 every 2 weeks or 135 mg/m^2 every 3 weeks, the increased incidence of alopecia, myalgia, and arthralgia make this a less favored option than liposomal anthracyclines as initial therapy for disseminated KS.

Improved understanding of factors that promote KS growth have led to a variety of novel pathogenesis-based treatments. Small clinical trials using drugs with anti-angiogenic potential (e.g., thalidomide and Col-3) and drugs (imatinib mesylate) which downregulate oncogenes (c-kit) or block growth receptors (PDGF and VEGF) recently have been studied.[101-103] Also intriguing is a recent publication that showed that patients with transplant-associated KS who did not have HIV can respond to replacement of cyclosporine immunosuppression with sirolimus, an inhibitor of mammalian target of rapamycin (mTOR) with both immunosuppressive and antineoplastic activity.[104] Finally, another treatment area being explored involves antiviral therapy to target HHV-8. This approach is buttressed by the observation that the use of genciclovir and foscarnet for the treatment of cytomegalovirus disease in patients with AIDS reduced their risk of KS.[105]

REFERENCES

1. CDC. Update on acquired immune deficiency syndrome (AIDS) – United States. Morbidity and Mortality Weekly Report 1982;31: 507–514.
2. CDC. Revision of the CDC surveillance case definition for acquired immune deficiency syndrome. Morbidity and Mortality Weekly Report 1987;36:1s–15s.
3. CDC. 1993 revised classification system for HIV infection and expanded surveillance case definitions for AIDS among adolescents and adults. Morbidity and Mortality Weekly Report 1992;41:961–962.
4. Jaffe ES, Harris NL, Stein H, et al. World Health Organization Classification of Tumours. Pathology and Genetics of Tumours of Haematopoietic and Lymphoid Tissues. Lyon, France: International Agency for Research on Cancer; 2001.
5. Ledergerber B, Telonti A, Egger M. Risk of HIV-related Kaposi's sarcoma and non-Hodgkin's lymphoma with potent antiretroviral therapy: prospective cohort study. Swiss HIV Cohort Study. *BMJ*. 1999;319(7201):23–24.
6. Lewden C, Salmon D, Morlat P, et al. Causes of death among human immunodeficiency virus (HIV) –infected adults in the era of potent antiretroviral therapy: emerging role of hepatitis and cancers, persistent role of AIDS. *Int J Epidemiol.* 2005;34(1):121–130.
7. Cote TR, Biggar RJ, Rosenberg PS, et al. Non-Hodgkins lymphoma among people with AIDS: incidence, presentation and public health burden. AIDS/Cancer Study Group. *Int J Cancer.* 1997;73(5):645–650.
8. International Collaboration of HIV and Cancer. Highly active antiretroviral therapy and incidence of cancer in human immunodeficiency virus-infected adults. *J Natl Cancer Inst.* 2000;92(22):1823–1830.
9. Stebbing J, Gazzard B, Mandalia S, et al. Antiretroviral treatment regimens and immune parameters in the prevention of systemic AIDS-related non-Hodgkin's lymphoma. *J Clin Oncol.* 2004;22(11): 2177–2183.
10. Bower M, Palmieri C, Dhillon T. AIDS-related malignancies: changing epidemiology and the impact of highly active antiretroviral therapy. *Curr Opin Infect Dis.* 2006;19(1):14–19.
11. Mbulaiteye SM, Parkin DM, Rabkin CS. Epidemiology of AIDS-related malignancies: an international perspective. *Hematol Oncol Clin North Am.* 2003;17(3):673–696.
12. Laurence J. Impact of HAART on HIV-linked malignancies. *AIDS Read.* 2003;13(5):202–205.
13. Sackoff JE, Hanna DB, Pfeiffer MR, Torian LV. Causes of death among persons with AIDS in the era of highly active antiretroviral therapy: New York City. *Ann Intern Med.* 2006;145(6):397–406.
14. Kirk O, Pedersen C, Cozzi-Lepri A, et al. EuroSIDA Study Group. Non-Hodgkin lymphoma in HIV-infected patients in the era of highly active antiretroviral therapy. *Blood.* 2001;98(12):3406–3412.
15. Glaser SL, Clarke CA, Gulley ML, et al. Population based patterns of human immunodeficiency virus-related Hodgkin lymphoma in the Greater San Francisco Bay Area, 1988–1998. *Cancer.* 2003;98(2):300–309.
16. Biggar RJ, Jaffe ES, Goedert JJ, et al. Hodgkin lymphoma and immunodeficiency in persons with HIV/AIDS. *Blood.* 2006;108(12):3786–3791.
17. Carbone A. AIDS-related non-Hodgkin's lymphomas. from pathology and molecular pathogenesis to treatment. *Human Pathol.* 2002;33(4): 392–404.
18. Gates AE, Kaplan LD. Biology and management of AIDS-associated non-Hodgkin's lymphoma. *Hematol Oncol Clin North Am.* 2003;17(3): 821–841.
19. Knowles DM. Etiology and pathogenesis of AIDS-related non-Hodgkin's lymphoma. *Hematol Oncol Clin North Am.* 2003;17(3): 785–820.
20. Breen EC, Fatahi S, Epeldegui M, et al. Elevated serum soluble CD30 precedes the development of AIDS-associated non-Hodgkin's B cell lymphoma. *Tumor Biol.* 2006;27(4):187–194.
21. Martinez-Maza O, Breen EC. B-cell activation and lymphoma in patients with HIV. *Curr Opin Oncol.* 2002;14(5):528–532.
22. Epeldegui M, Widney DP, Martinez-Maza O. Pathogenesis of AIDS lymphoma: role of oncogenic viruses and B cell activation-associated molecular lesions. *Curr Opin Oncol.* 2006;18(5):444–448.
23. Dean M, Jacobson LP, McFarlane G, et al. Reduced risk of AIDS lymphoma in individuals heterozygous for the CCR5-delta32 mutation. *Cancer Res.* 1999;59(15):3561–3564.
24. Rabkin CS, Yang Q, Goedert JJ, et al. Chemokine and chemokine receptor gene variants and risk of non-Hodgkin's lymphoma in human immunodeficiency virus-1-infected individuals. *Blood.* 1999;93(6): 1838–1842.
25. Tirelli U, Bernardi D, Spina M, et al. AIDS-related tumors: integrating antiviral and anticancer therapy. *Crit Rev Oncol Hematol.* 2002;41(3): 299–315.
26. Carbone A, Cloghini A. AIDS-related lymphoma: from pathogenesis to pathology. *Br J Haematol.* 2005;130(5):662–670.
27. Biggar RJ. AIDS-related cancers in the era of highly active antiretroviral therapy. *Oncology (Williston Park).* 2001;15(4):439–449.
28. Aboulafia DM, Pantanowitz L, Dezube B. AIDS-related non-Hodgkin lymphoma: still a problem in the era of HAART. *AIDS Read.* 2004;14(11):605–617.
29. Barclay LR, Buskin SE, Kahle EM, et al. Clinical and immunologic profile of AIDS-related lymphoma in the era of highly active antiretroviral therapy. *Clin Lymphoma Myeloma.* 2007;7(4):1–8.

30. Knowles DM, Chamulak GA, Subar M, et al. Lymphoid neoplasia associated with the acquired immunodeficiency syndrome (AIDS). The New York University Medical Center experience with 105 patients (1981–1986). *Ann Intern Med.* 1988;108(5):744–753.

31. Levine AM, Wernz JC, Kaplan L, et al. Low-dose chemotherapy with central nervous system prophylaxis and zidovudine maintenance in AIDS-related lymphoma. A prospective multi-institutional trial. *JAMA.* 1991;266(1):84–88.

32. Scadden DT. Epstein-Barr virus, the CNS, and AIDS-related lymphomas: as close as flame to smoke. *J Clin Oncol.* 2000;18(19): 3323–3324.

33. Straus DJ, Huang J, Testa MA. Prognostic factors in the treatment of human immunodeficiency virus-associated non-Hodgkin's lymphoma: analysis of AIDS Clinical Trials Group protocol 142–low-dose versus standard-dose m-BACOD plus granulocyte-macrophage colony-stimulating factor. National Institute of Allergy and Infectious Diseases. *J Clin Oncol.* 1998;16(11):3601–3606.

34. Rossi G, Donisi A, Casari S, et al. The International Prognostic Index can be used as a guide to treatment decisions regarding patients with human immunodeficiency virus-related systemic non-Hodgkin lymphoma. *Cancer.* 1999;86(11):2391–2397.

35. Besson C, Goubar A, Gabarre J, et al. Changes in AIDS-related lymphoma since the era of highly active antiretroviral therapy. *Blood.* 2001;98(8):2339–2344.

36. Hoffmann C, Wolf E, Faetkenheuer G, et al. Response to highly active antiretroviral therapy strongly predicts outcome in patients with AIDS-related lymphoma. *AIDS.* 2003;17(10):1521–1529.

37. Vaccher E, Spina M, Talamini R, et al. Improvement of systemic human immunodeficiency virus-related non-Hodgkin lymphoma outcome in the era of highly active antiretroviral therapy. *Clin Infect Dis.* 2003;37(11):1556–1564.

38. Lim ST, Karim R, Nathwani BN, et al. AIDS-related Burkitt's lymphoma versus diffuse large-cell lymphoma in the pre-highly active antiretroviral therapy (HAART) and HAART eras: significant differences in survival with standard chemotherapy. *J Cln Oncol.* 2005;23(19): 4430–4438.

39. Skiest DJ, Crosby C. Survival is prolonged by highly active antiretroviral therapy in AIDS patients with primary central nervous system lymphoma. *AIDS.* 2003;17(12):1787–1793.

40. Kaplan LD, Straus DJ, Testa MA, et al. Low-dose compared with standard-dose m-BACOD chemotherapy for non-Hodgkin's lymphoma associated with human immunodeficiency virus infection. National Institute of Allergy and Infectious Diseases. AIDS Clinical Trials Group. *N Engl J Med.* 1997;336(23):1641–1648.

41. Ratner L, Lee J, Tang S, et al. Chemotherapy for human immunodeficiency virus-associated non-Hodgkin's lymphoma in combination with highly active antiretroviral therapy. *J Clin Oncol.* 2001;19(8):2171–2178.

42. Vaccher E, Spina M, di Gennaro G. Concomitant cyclophosphamide, doxorubicin, vincristine, and prednisone chemotherapy plus highly active antiretroviral therapy in patients with human immunodeficiency virus-related non-Hodgkin lymphoma. *Cancer.* 2001;91(1):155–163.

43. Spina M, Jaeger U, Sparano JA, et al. Rituximab plus infusional cyclophosphamide, doxorubicin, and etoposide in HIV-associated non-Hodgkin's lymphoma: pooled results from 3 phase 2 trials. *Blood.* 2005;105(5):1891–1897.

44. Cheung MC, Pantanowitz L, Dezube BJ. AIDS-related malignancies: emerging challenges in the era of highly active antiretroviral therapy. *Oncologist.* 2005;10(6):412–426.

45. Powles T, Imami N, Nelson M, et al. Effects of combination chemotherapy and highly active antiretroviral therapy on immune parameters in HIV-1 associated lymphoma. *AIDS.* 2002;16(4):531–536.

46. Little RF, Pittaluga S, Grant N, et al. Highly effective treatment of acquired immunodeficiency syndrome-related lymphoma with dose-adjusted EPOCH: impact of antiretroviral therapy suspension and tumor biology. *Blood.* 2003;101(12):4653–4659.

47. Kaplan LD, Lee JY, Ambinder RF, et al. Rituximab does not improve clinical outcome in a randomized phase 3 trial of CHOP with or without rituximab in patients with HIV-associated non Hodgkin lymphoma: AIDS-Malignancies Consortium Trial 010. *Blood.* 2005; 106(5):1538–1543.

48. Boue F, Gabarre J, Gisselbrecht C, et al. Phase II trial of CHOP plus rituximab in patients with HIV-associated non-Hodgkins lymphoma. *J Clin Oncol.* 2006;24(25):4123–4128.

49. Dunleavy K, Wilson WH, Kaplan LD. The case for rituximab in AIDS-related lymphoma. *Blood.* 2006;107(7):3014–3015.

50. Spina M, Simonelli C, Talamini R, Tirelli U. Patients with HIV with Burkitt's lymphoma have a worse outcome than those with diffuse large-cell lymphoma also in the highly active antiretroviral therapy era. *J Clin Oncol.* 2005;23(31):8132–8133; Author reply 8133–8134.

51. Bower M, Gazzard B, Mandalia S, et al. A prognostic index for systemic AIDS-related non-Hodgkin lymphoma treated in the era of highly active antiretroviral therapy. *Ann Intern Med.* 2005;143(4):265–273.

52. Cortes J, Thomas D, Rios A, et al. Hyperfractionated cyclophosphamide, vincristine, doxorubicin, and dexamethasone and highly active antiretroviral therapy for patients with acquired immunodeficiency syndrome-related Burkitt lymphoma/leukemia. *Cancer.* 2002;94 (5):1492–1499.

53. Wang ES, Straus DJ, Teruya-Feldstein J, et al. Intensive chemotherapy with cyclophosphamide, doxorubicin, high-dose methotrexate/ifosfamide, etoposide, and high-dose cytarabine (CODOX-M/IVAC) for human immunodeficiency virus-associated Burkitt lymphoma. *Cancer.* 2003;98:1196–1205.

54. Levine AM, Tulpule A, Espina B, et al. Liposome-encapsulated doxorubicin in combination with standard agents (cyclophosphamide, vincristine, prednisone) in patients with newly diagnosed AIDS-related non-Hodgkin's lymphoma: results of therapy and correlates of response. *J Clin Oncol.* 2004;22(13):2662–2670.

55. Combs S, Neil N, Aboulafia DM. Liposomal doxorubicin, cyclophosphamide, and etoposide and antiretroviral therapy for patients with AIDS-related lymphoma: a pilot study. *Oncologist.* 2006;11(6):666–673.

56. Cullen M, Steven N, Billingham L, et al. Antibacterial prophylaxis after chemotherapy for solid tumors and lymphomas. *N Engl J Med.* 2005;353(10):988–998.

57. Bucaneve G, Micozzi A, Menichetti F, et al. Levofloxacin to prevent bacterial infection in patients with cancer and neutropenia. *N Engl J Med.* 2005;353(10):977–987.

58. Krishnan A, Zaia J, Forman SJ. Should HIV-positive patients with lymphoma be offered stem cell transplants? *Bone Marrow Transplant.* 2003;32(8):741–748.

59. Krishnan A, Molina A, Forman SJ. Organ transplantation in HIV-infected patients. *N Engl J Med.* 2002;347(22):1801–1803.

60. Hoffmann C, Tabrizian S, Wolf E, et al. Survival of AIDS patients with primary central nervous system lymphoma is dramatically improved by HAART-induced immune recovery. *AIDS.* 2001;15(16): 2119–2127.

61. Skiest DJ, Crosby C. Survival is prolonged by highly active antiretroviral therapy in AIDS patients with primary central nervous system lymphoma. *AIDS.* 2003;17(12):1787–1793.

62. Aboulafia DM, Puswella AL. Highly active antiretroviral therapy (HAART) as the sole treatment for AIDS-related primary central nervous system lymphoma: a case report with implication for treatment. AIDS Patient Care and STDs 2007: In press.

63. Beral V, Bull D, Darby S, et al. Risk of Kaposi's sarcoma and sexual practices associated with fecal contact in homosexual or bisexual men with AIDS. *Lancet.* 1992;339(8794):632–635.

64. Beral V, Peterman TA, Berkelman RL, Jaffe HW. Kaposi's sarcoma among persons with AIDS: a sexually transmitted infection? *Lancet.* 1990;335(8682):123–128.

65. Engels EA, Atkinson JO, Graubard BI, et al. Risk factors for human herpesvirus 8 infection among adults in the United States and evidence for sexual transmission. *J Infect Dis.* 2007;196(2):199–207.

66. Mocroft A, Kirk O, Clumeck N, et al. The changing pattern of Kaposi sarcoma in patients with HIV, 1994-2003: the EuroSIDA Study. *Cancer.* 2004;100(12):2644–2654.

67. Portsmouth S, Stebbing J, Gill J, et al. A comparison of regimens based on non-nucleoside reverse transcriptase inhibitors or protease inhibitors in preventing Kaposi's sarcoma. *AIDS.* 2003;17(11):F17–22.

68. Clifford GM, Polesel J, Rickenbach M, et al. Cancer risk in the Swiss HIV cohort study: associations with immunodeficiency, smoking, and highly active antiretroviral therapy. *J Natl Cancer Inst.* 2005;97(6):425–432.

69. Moore PS, Chang Y. Detection of herpesvirus-like sequences in Kaposi's sarcoma in patients with and without HIV infection. *N Engl J Med.* 1995;332(18):1181–1185.

70. Huang YQ, Li JJ, Poiesz BJ, et al. Detection of the herpesvirus-like DNA sequences in matched specimens of semen and blood from patients with AIDS-related Kaposi's sarcoma by polymerase chain reaction in situ hybridization. *Am J Pathol.* 1997;150(1):147–53.

71. Sitas F, Carrara H, Beral V, et al. Antibodies against human herpesvirus 8 in black South African patients with cancer. *N Engl J Med.* 1999;340(24):1863–1871.

72. Nakamura S, Salahuddin SZ, Biberfeld P, et al. Kaposi's sarcoma cells: long-term culture with growth factor from retrovirus-infected CD4+ T cells. *Science.* 1988;242(4877):426–430.

73. Gallo RC. The enigmas of Kaposi's Sarcoma. *Science.* 1998;282(5395): 1837–1839.

74. Salahuddin SZ, Nakamura S, Biberfeld P, et al. Angiogenic properties of Kaposi's sarcoma-derived cells after long-term culture in vitro. *Science.* 1988;242(4877):430–433.

75. Ensoli B, Nakamura S, Salahuddin SZ, et al. AIDS-Kaposi's sarcoma-derived cells express cytokines with autocrine and paracrine growth effects. *Science.* 1989;243(4888):223–226.

76. Cornali E, Zeitz C, Benelli R, et al. Vascular endothelial growth factor regulates angiogenesis and vascular permeability in Kaposi's sarcoma. *Am J Pathol.* 1996:149(6);1851–1869.

77. Mesri EA. Inflammatory reactivation and angiogenicity of Kaposi's sarcoma-associated herpesvirus/HHV8: a missing link in the pathogenesis of acquired immune deficiency syndrome-associated Kaposi's sarcoma. *Blood.* 1999;93(12):4031–4033.

78. Dezube BJ. The role of human immunodeficiency virus-I in the pathogenesis of acquired immunodeficiency syndrome-related Kaposi's sarcoma: the importance of an inflammatory and angiogenic milieu. *Semin Oncol.* 2000;27(4):420–423.

79. Bais C, Santomasso B, Coso O, et al. G-protein-coupled receptors of Kaposi's sarcoma-associated herpesvirus is a viral oncogene and angiogenesis activator. *Nature.* 1998;391(6662):86–89.

80. Rabkin CS, Janz S, Lash A, et al. Monoclonal origin of multicentric Kaposi's sarcoma lesions. *N Engl J Med.* 1997;336(14):988-993.

81. Aboulafia DM. Kaposi's sarcoma. Clinics in Dermatology 2001;19: 269–283.

82. Aboulafia DM. The epidemiologic, pathologic, and clinical features of AIDS-associated pulmonary Kaposi's sarcoma. *Chest.* 2000;117(4): 1128–1145.

83. Gallafent JH, Buskin SE, De Turk PB, Aboulafia DM. Profile of patients with Kaposi's sarcoma in the era of highly active antiretroviral therapy. *J Clin Oncol.* 2005;23(6):1253–1260.

84. Kaaya EE, Parravicini C, Ordonez C, et al. Heterogeneity of spindle cells in Kaposi's sarcoma: comparison of cells in lesions and in culture. *J Acquir Immune Defic Syndr Hum Retrovirol.* 1995:10(3); 295–305.

85. Nasti G, Talamini R, Antinori A, et al. AIDS-related Kaposi's sarcoma: evaluation of potential new prognostic factors and assessment of the AIDS Clinical Trial Group Staging System in the Haart Era – the Italian Cooperative Group on AIDS and Tumors and the Italian Cohort of Patients Naïve From Antiretrovirals. *J Clin Oncol.* 2003;21(15): 2876–2882.

86. Krown SE, Testa MA, Huang J. AIDS-related Kaposi's sarcoma: prospective validation of the AIDS Clinical Trials Group staging classification. AIDS Clinical Trials Group Oncology Committee. *J Clin Oncol.* 1997;15(9):3085–3092.

87. Aversa SM, Cattelan AM, Salvagno L, et al. Treatments of AIDS-related Kaposi's sarcoma. *Crit Rev Oncol Hematol.* 2005;53(3): 253–265.

88. Bower M, Nelson M, Young AM, et al. Immune reconstitution inflammatory syndrome associated with Kaposi's sarcoma. *J Clin Oncol.* 2005;23(22):5224–5228.

89. Leidner R, Aboulafia DM. Recrudescent Kaposi's sarcoma after initiation of HAART: a manifestation of immune reconstitution syndrome. *AIDS Patient Care and STDs.* 2005;19(10):635–644.

90. Dezube BJ, Pantanowitz L, Aboulafia DM. Management of AIDS-related Kaposi's sarcoma: advances in target discovery and treatment. *AIDS Read.* 2004;14(5):236–253.

91. Walmsley S, Northfelt DW, Melosky B, et al. Treatment of AIDS-related cutaneous Kaposi's sarcoma with topical alitretinoin (9-cis-retinoic acid) gel. Panretin Gel North American Study Group. *J Acquir Immune Defic Syndr.* 1999;22(3):235–246.

92. Boudreaux AA, Smith LL, Cosby CD, et al. Intralesional vinblastine for cutaneous Kaposi's sarcoma associated with acquired immunodeficiency syndrome. A clinical trial to evaluate efficacy and discomfort associated with infection. *J Am Acad Dermatol.* 1993;28(1):61–65.

93. Swift PS. The role of radiation therapy in the management of HIV-related Kaposi's sarcoma. *Hematol Oncol Clin North Am.* 1996;10(5): 1069–1080.

94. Gressen EL, Rosenstock JG, Xie Y, et al. Palliative treatment of epidemic Kaposi sarcoma of the feet. *Am J Clin Oncol.* 1999;22(3): 286–290.

95. Lee FC, Mitsuyasu RT. Chemotherapy of AIDS-related Kaposi's sarcoma. *Hematol Oncol Clin North Am.* 1996;10(5):1051–1068.

96. Gill PS, Wernz J, Scadden DT, et al. Randomized phase III trial of liposomal daunorubicin versus doxorubicin, bleomycin, and vincristine in AIDS-related Kaposi's sarcoma. *J Clin Oncol.* 1996;14(8): 2353–2364.

97. Northfelt DW, Dezube BJ, Thommes JA, et al. Pegylated-liposomal doxorubicin versus doxorubicin, bleomycin, and vincristine in the treatment of AIDS-related Kaposi's sarcoma: results of a randomized phase III clinical trial. *J Clin Oncol.* 1998;16(7):2445–2451.

98. Stewart S, Jablonowski H, Goebel FD, et al. Randomized comparative trial of pegylated liposomal doxorubicin versus bleomycin and vincristine in the treatment of AIDS-related Kaposi's sarcoma. International Pegylated Liposomal Doxorubicin Study Group. *J Clin Oncol.* 1998;16(2):683–691.

99. Gill PS, Tulpule A, Espina BM, et al. Paclitaxel is safe and effective in the treatment of advanced AIDS-related Kaposi's sarcoma. *J Clin Oncol.* 1999;17(6):1876–1883.

100. Welles L, Saville MW, Lietzau J, et al. Phase II trial with dose titration of paclitaxel for the therapy of human immunodeficiency virus-associated Kaposi's sarcoma. *J Clin Oncol.* 1998;16(3):1112–1121.

101. Little RF, Wyvill KM, Pluda JM, et al. Activity of Thalidomide in AIDS-related Kaposi's sarcoma. *J Clin Oncol.* 2000;18(13):2593–2602.

102. Dezube B, Krown SE, Lee JY, et al. Randomized phase II trial of matrix metalloproteinase inhibitor COL-3 in AIDS-related Kaposi's Sarcoma: an AIDS Malignancy Consortium Study. *J Clin Oncol.* 2006;24(9):1389–1394.

103. Koon HB, Bubley GJ, Pantanowitz L, et al. Imatinib-induced regression of AIDS-related Kaposi's sarcoma. *J Clin Oncol.* 2005;23(5): 982–989.

104. Stallone G, Schena A, Infante B, et al. Sirolimus for Kaposi's sarcoma in renal-transplant recipients. *N Engl J Med.* 2005;352(13): 1317–1323.

105. Glesby MJ, Hoover DR, Weng S, et al. Use of antiherpes drugs and the risk of Kaposi's sarcoma: data from the Multicenter AIDS Cohort Study. *J Infect Dis.* 1996;173(6):1477–1480.

14

CENTRAL NERVOUS SYSTEM TUMORS

Jan C. Buckner, MD

> **LEARNING OBJECTIVES**
>
> After reviewing this chapter, the reader should be able to
>
> - Compare and contrast the types and frequency of primary brain tumors
> - Select the appropriate diagnostic evaluation for patients with primary and metastatic brain tumors
> - Discuss prognosis with patients who have various histologic subtypes of primary brain tumors and central nervous system (CNS) metastases
> - Recommend the most appropriate therapeutic options for patients with primary and metastatic brain tumors
> - Understand appropriate diagnostic and therapeutic tools for patients with leptomeningeal malignant tumors

Primary malignant central nervous system (CNS) tumors represent approximately 2% of all cancers but account for a disproportionate share of morbidity and mortality. They may occur in any age group, from infants to individuals older than 65. They are the most common solid tumor in children and are the second leading cause of death in children, with leukemia being the first. CNS tumors are the third leading cause of cancer-related death for adolescents and adults who are age 15 to 34 and occur more frequently in men than in women. The median age-adjusted incidence for primary brain tumors is four or five cases per 100,000 individuals per year. Diffuse astrocytomas represent approximately 80% of primary brain tumors in adults (Fig 14-1).[1]

Genetic predisposition to these tumors appears relatively uncommon, although gliomas may be inherited as a part of several familial diseases. Specifically, type 1 neurofibromatosis, Turcot's syndrome, and Li-Fraumeni syndrome are associated with the greatest risk of brain tumors. It has been difficult to identify environmental factors associated with primary brain tumors. One factor, exposure to vinyl chloride, has been associated with an

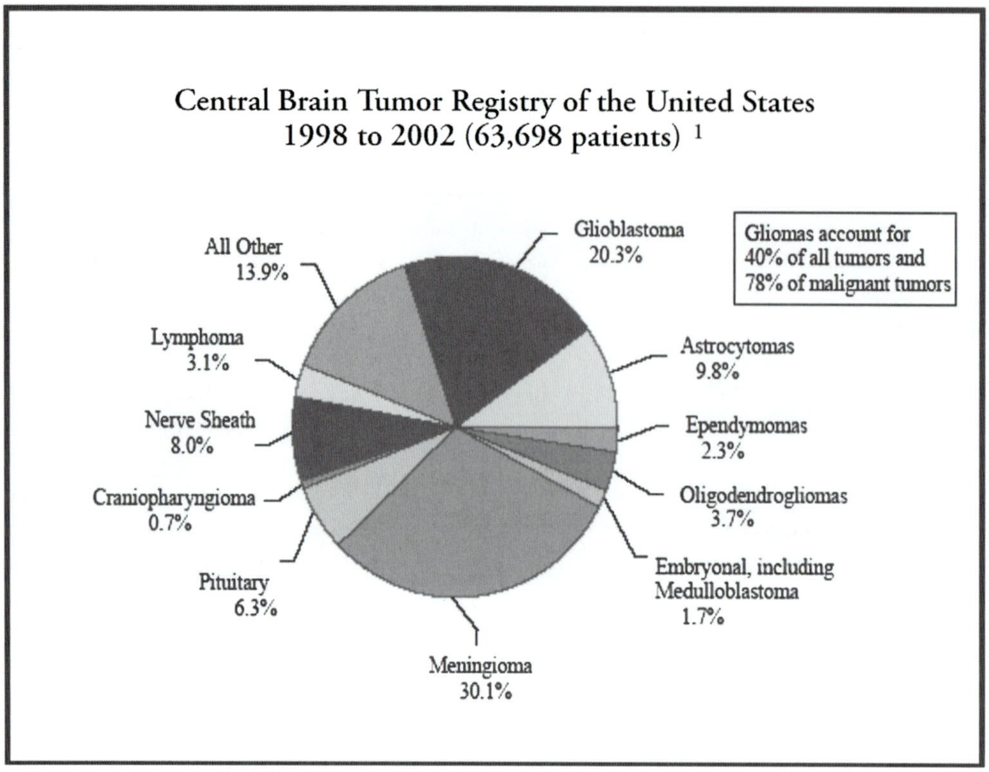

FIG. 14-1 Distribution of all brain and central nervous system tumors by histology. Reprinted with permission from the Central Brain Tumor Registry of the United States.

increased incidence of high-grade gliomas. Also, ionizing radiation has been identified as a rare cause of primary brain tumors. For example, radiation treatment for children with tinea capitis, acute lymphocytic leukemia, craniopharyngioma, or non-Hodgkin's lymphoma has been associated with an increased risk of subsequent brain tumors, especially gliomas. The risk of primary CNS lymphoma, but not other types of primary brain tumors, is increased for patients infected with the human immunodeficiency virus (HIV).[2]

It appears that most malignant CNS tumors arise as a consequence of acquired somatic mutations in genes responsible for control of cell growth proliferation. Mutations in the *NF1* gene are very uncommon in most sporadic brain tumors. However, mutations in *TP53* are frequently detected in many gliomas.

KEY POINTS

- The etiology of most primary CNS tumors remains unknown with the exception of the associations between astrocytomas and neurofibromatosis and between CNS lymphoma and HIV infections.
- Experienced neuropathology review of tumor tissue is essential to appropriate diagnosis and treatment of patients with brain tumors.

Primary CNS tumors consist of a diverse range of pathologic entities, each with a distinct natural history. For simplicity, primary CNS tumors may be classified as gliomas or nongliomas. The most common gliomas are astrocytoma, oligodendroglioma (or mixtures of oligodendroglioma and astrocytoma elements), and ependymoma. Uncommon astrocytoma variants, including pilocytic astrocytoma, pleomorphic xanthoastrocytoma, and subependymal giant cell astrocytoma, tend to be well circumscribed and may be excised with curative intent. Unfortunately, most gliomas are characterized by diffuse infiltration of white matter tracts, making surgical extirpation impossible. Nongliomas consist of typically benign tumors, such as meningioma and pituitary adenoma, as well as malignant tumors, such as primitive neuroectodermal tumors (medulloblastoma), primary CNS lymphoma, and the seldom-occurring CNS germ cell tumors.

Accurate pathologic diagnosis requires the review of an experienced tumor neuropathologist, as the rate of discordance between general pathologists and neuropathologists is very high. The diagnosis may change substantially for at least one-third of patients when pathologic review is performed by an experienced neuropathologist.

DIAGNOSIS AND STAGING

The presenting symptoms of a brain tumor are related to mass effect, parenchymal infiltration, hydrocephalus, and tissue destruction. The most common presenting symptom is related to mass effect and includes headache, which occurs in approximately 35% of patients. The sudden onset of headaches in a patient who has not previously had headaches is most characteristic, especially if the headaches are more severe in the morning and are associated with nausea, vomiting, or focal neurologic deficits. Seizures occur in approximately one-third of patients with gliomas, especially in patients with low-grade tumors. However, seizures may be associated with any CNS tumor. Focal neurologic deficits are related to the location of the tumor. Altered mental status may develop in 15% to 20% of patients with gliomas. Posterior fossa masses, and occasionally supratentorial masses, may obstruct the third or fourth ventricle and may result in hydrocephalus, with headache, nausea, vomiting, and somnolence, lethargy, or coma.

Computerized tomography (CT) of the brain typically shows a mass that may or may not enhance with use of contrast medium. Low-grade gliomas may be isodense with normal brain parenchyma and may not enhance with contrast medium. Consequently, the findings on CT may not indicate the diagnosis. Also, lesions in the posterior fossa may not be identifiable on CT scans. Magnetic resonance imaging (MRI) is more sensitive than CT for confirming the presence of a brain tumor. On T1-weighted MRI scans, a brain tumor appears as a mass lesion that may or may not enhance with contrast; there also may be signal abnormality on T2-weighted scans. As a rule, the amount of contrast enhancement increases with higher grades of malignant disease; however, low-grade (benign) tumors, such as pilocytic astrocytoma, also may demonstrate contrast enhancement. Ring enhancement is characteristic of glioblastoma multiforme.

MRI perfusion scans may demonstrate increased blood flow in high-grade tumors, whereas MRI diffusion shows reduced water movement, presumably secondary to increased cellularity and increased interstitial pressure. Both MRI spectroscopy and positron emission tomography (PET) scans provide physiologic information about the tumor. To date, the sensitivity and specificity of these techniques for particular tumor histology or radiation necrosis are too low to recommend their routine use in the clinic. Definitive diagnosis still requires a surgical biopsy or resection with histologic examination of the tissue in nearly all patients. Patients with brainstem gliomas may not be candidates for biopsy, both because of the associated risk to the patient and because of the characteristic imaging findings. Also, patients with CNS germ cell tumors may have elevated serum or cerebrospinal fluid alpha-fetoprotein or human chorionic gonadotropin levels, which confirms the diagnosis.

Because most primary brain tumors remain localized, extensive staging procedures are not necessary. Primitive neuroectodermal tumors, such as medulloblastoma, CNS germ cell tumors, ependymoma, and primary CNS lymphoma, frequently spread by way of the subarachnoid space to the leptomeninges. Consequently, MRI of the spine and cytologic examination of cerebrospinal fluid should be performed for all patients with these diagnoses.

KEY POINT

- The best imaging tool for CNS tumors is magnetic resonance imaging (MRI), and contrast enhancement on MRI scans is the primary imaging hallmark of high-grade tumors. Physiologic imaging methods, such as position emission tomography (PET) and MRI spectroscopy, remain under investigation.

TREATMENT

SURGERY

The goals of surgery are to obtain tissue for histologic diagnosis, to reduce mass effect while preserving neurologic function, to cytoreduce the tumor, and to treat hydrocephalus, if present. Surgery remains the initial therapy for nearly all patients with brain tumors and can be curative for most benign tumors including meningiomas. Because of the infiltrative nature of most primary brain tumors, relief of mass effect and debulking results in symptomatic improvement and permits time for safe administration of subsequent treatment. Current stereotactic technique allows for biopsy specimens to be obtained from nearly any part of the brain, including the brainstem. Biopsy alone is generally reserved for patients with tumors in critical functional portions of the brain, where resection would result in unacceptable

KEY POINTS

- The primary roles of surgery are to obtain tissue for diagnosis, reduce mass effect, and reduce the tumor cell burden.
- Radiation therapy plays a key role in treatment of most patients with brain tumors. It results in increased survival for most patients, as well as in cure for some patients.
- Chemotherapy, especially temozolomide, produces clinical improvement and prolonged survival in many patients with gliomas.

neurologic deficit. In addition, patients with primary CNS lymphoma or CNS germ cell tumors may need biopsy alone because primary treatment usually involves radiation therapy, chemotherapy, or both.

RADIATION THERAPY

External beam radiation therapy is an essential component of treatment for many patients with brain tumors. It can be curative for some patients, and it prolongs survival for most. Radiation often is the primary treatment modality for patients with metastatic brain tumors, epidural spinal cord compression, and leptomeningeal metastases. Whereas whole-brain radiation may be administered for certain tumors, such as medulloblastoma or primary CNS lymphoma, involved-field radiation using multiple field techniques has become the standard of treatment for most patients with glioma. Involved-field radiation has been as effective as whole-brain radiation and reduces the dose of radiation to normal brain tissue, potentially reducing late neurotoxic effects. Radionecrosis presents as a focal mass lesion with contrast enhancement and mass effect. The clinical scenario is difficult to distinguish from recurrent tumor and may require surgical resection to relieve mass effect, as well as to establish a histologic diagnosis. Radiation-induced leukoencephalopathy often occurs months to years after treatment, and usually appears as more diffuse increased T2 signal abnormality on MRI with associated atrophy. Patients with characteristic MRI changes may be asymptomatic or may be severely compromised with dementia, gait instability, and urinary incontinence. The frequency of radiation injury is related to total radiation dose, fraction size, volume of brain irradiated, treatment technique, and age. In general, morbidity is reduced by using smaller fraction size, lower total dose, and smaller treatment volumes. No information regarding frequency, although relevant, is included here because of the limited scope of the chapter. Stereotactic radiotherapy techniques have demonstrated efficacy for well circumscribed lesions, such as meningioma or limited brain metastases. However, for the infiltrative malignant tumors, the role of stereotactic radiotherapy remains under investigation. In a phase III trial, investigators found no survival advantage for patients receiving radiation with stereotactic boost compared with patients receiving standard radiation.[3] Similarly, the clinical benefits of other focal radiation therapy techniques, such as the use of radioactive isotopes, are being investigated and are not recommended for routine clinical use. Of note, brachytherapy using the Gliasite balloon method remains under investigation, but is beyond the scope of this chapter.

CHEMOTHERAPY

Although chemotherapy provides only modest benefit for many patients with brain tumors, it has an increasing role in palliation and in the adjuvant setting, as well as in combination with surgery and radiation therapy. The most commonly used agent is temozolomide. Temozolomide penetrates the intact blood–brain barrier and produces benefit in many patients with gliomas. Nitrosoureas, such as carmustine and lomustine, also have modest antitumor activity, especially in patients with oligodendroglioma. Platinum drugs have antitumor efficacy for medulloblastoma and germ cell tumors. High-dose methotrexate regimens result in clear clinical benefit for patients with primary CNS lymphomas. Nevertheless, chemotherapy results in durable benefit for only a small portion of patients with glioma. Multiple agents that target aberrant signaling pathways, such as epidermal growth factor receptor inhibitors and angiogenesis inhibitors, are under investigation and demonstrate promise in early-phase clinical trials. In addition, there have been many efforts to improve efficacy by using methods to improve the delivery of antineoplastic agents through the variably disrupted blood–tumor barrier. These techniques have included intra–arterial chemotherapy with or without blood–brain barrier disruption, intratumoral administration of agents by convection-enhanced delivery, and placement of intratumoral biodegradable polymers. The efficacy of local administration of various agents directly into brain tumors has generally been modest. However, the U.S. Food Drug Administration (FDA) has approved the use of carmustine-impregnated degradable polymers for the treatment of newly diagnosed gliomas and recurrent glioblastoma multiforme. Even so, the median survival associated with that treatment is only slightly better than that associated with placebo, and the benefits do not last long.

OTHER THERAPEUTIC AGENTS

Corticosteroids, anticonvulsant drugs, and anticoagulant drugs are important ancillary agents for the treatment of patients with brain tumors. Corticosteroids are indispensable for controlling increased intracranial pressure and mass effect. Unfortunately, the long-term use of these agents can result in substantial toxic effects. Anticonvulsant drugs are administered prophylactically following surgical procedures and for the treatment of seizure disorders. The use of routine prophylactic anticonvulsant therapy for patients in whom seizures have not occurred remains variable, although clinical trials have demonstrated no discernible benefit. Clinical trials have demonstrated that some anticonvulsant agents, including phenytoin, phenobarbital, and carbamazepine, induce common hepatic enzyme systems, such as cytochrome P-450 (especially cyp3A4/5) and glucuronidation enzymes. Induction of these enzymes results in decreased exposure to chemotherapy agents and other drugs metabolized by the same enzyme systems, such as warfarin and small molecule inhibitors. The use of anticonvulsant drugs clearly reduces the blood concentration of camptothecins (topotecan and irinotecan), as well as taxanes (paclitaxel). At this point, it is not known if the reduced drug concentration affects efficacy. Other anticonvulsant drugs, such as levetiracetam, do not result in drug interactions and may simplify other pharmaceutical interventions.

Clinically apparent deep-vein thrombosis or pulmonary emboli that requires treatment with anticoagulation drugs may occur in 20% to 30% of patients with primary brain tumors. Presumably, injury to brain parenchyma results in the release of tissue thromboplastins and increases the risk for clotting. Conventional therapy with heparin and warfarin is usually effective and well tolerated. For patients who have serum levels of anticoagulant agents that are within the therapeutic range, the risk of intracranial bleeding does not appear to be higher than that for patients who do not need anticoagulant drugs.[4]

ASTROCYTOMAS

The use of different grading systems for astrocytomas has resulted in considerable confusion in the past. Since 1993, the World Health Organization (WHO) classification system has been the most widely accepted, although variably used, four-tiered grading system. Four key histologic features are documented.

- Increased cellularity
- Mitoses
- Endothelial proliferation
- Necrosis

The WHO classification system defines grades as the following: grade 1 astrocytomas, such as pilocytic astrocytoma, are typically benign; grade 2 astrocytomas are diffuse infiltrating low-grade tumors with only increased cellularity; grade 3 (anaplastic) astrocytomas have mitoses; and grade 4 astrocytomas (glioblastoma multiforme) have evidence of endothelial proliferation, tumor necrosis, or both.

LOW-GRADE ASTROCYTOMAS

Most patients with diffuse infiltrating low-grade astrocytomas (grade 2) are young adults (in their 20s and 30s) and typically present with seizures. Favorable prognostic features include younger age at diagnosis, tumor size of less than 5 cm, and, possibly, greater extent of tumor resection. The median survival is approximately 5 years. Late recurrences are relatively common, and patients should be followed for at least 15 years. Circumscribed astrocytomas, such as pilocytic astrocytoma, are more common in children.

> **KEY POINT**
>
> - Treatment of low-grade glioma remains controversial, and reasonable options include biopsy or surgical removal alone, immediate or delayed radiotherapy, or chemotherapy.

Low-grade astrocytomas may be either well circumscribed or diffusely infiltrating. The circumscribed tumors include pilocytic astrocytoma, pleomorphic xanthoastrocytoma, subependymal giant cell astrocytoma, and subependymoma. These tumors are uncommon, and it is important to note that resection often leads to cure. Even if resection is incomplete, the tumor may remain indolent or may be successfully treated with radiation. In the rare instances in which local treatment fails, the value of chemotherapy is unclear, although the combination of carboplatin and vincristine has been reported to be of benefit for children.[5]

On CT scans, diffuse infiltrating low-grade astrocytomas typically appear as lesions with low attenuation or with isodensity. On MRI (the preferred diagnostic procedure) these tumors may not be contrast enhanced, or the contrast enhancement may be wispy and faint. Focal intense enhancement may indicate areas of increased anaplasia. When feasible, biopsy should be done to obtain a sample of the contrast-enhanced portion, because the prognosis is typically related to the most anaplastic part of the tumor.

Therapy for patients with low-grade astrocytoma is controversial. Despite their relatively indolent course, most astrocytomas eventually evolve into more anaplastic lesions and are incurable despite surgery and radiation therapy. The role of complete surgical resection has been debated. The findings of some studies suggest that maximum tumor debulking is optimal.[6] However, complete resection may be limited to a select group of patients with small unilateral tumors or tumors that do not involve critical brain structures. A practical approach is to resect as much of the abnormal tissue as possible without causing substantial neurologic deficit. Radiation therapy that begins immediately after diagnosis has been shown to extend the time to recurrence compared with radiation that is delayed until the time of tumor progression. However, there is no convincing evidence that early radiation therapy improves overall survival (Fig. 14-2).[7] For patients with minimal or no symptoms or with seizures that are controlled with anticonvulsant drugs, deferring radiation until there is evidence of symptomatic tumor growth is acceptable. The rationale for delaying radiation is to reduce the risk of radiation-induced neurologic damage. Emerging evidence suggests that the risk of neurologic injury for patients treated with carefully planned involved-field radiation therapy is low; therefore, that rationale becomes questionable.[8] Two prospective randomized trials failed to demonstrate a benefit for higher-dose radiotherapy compared with intermediate-dose radiotherapy (Fig. 14-3).[9,10] Typically, doses of 45 to 54 Gy, delivered in 1.8 to 2.0 Gy fractions, are considered acceptable. The role of adjuvant chemotherapy for patients with low-grade astrocytomas remains under investigation. A phase III trial in which radiation alone was compared with radiation followed by chemotherapy with procarbazine, lomustine, and vincristine (PCV) has completed accrual.

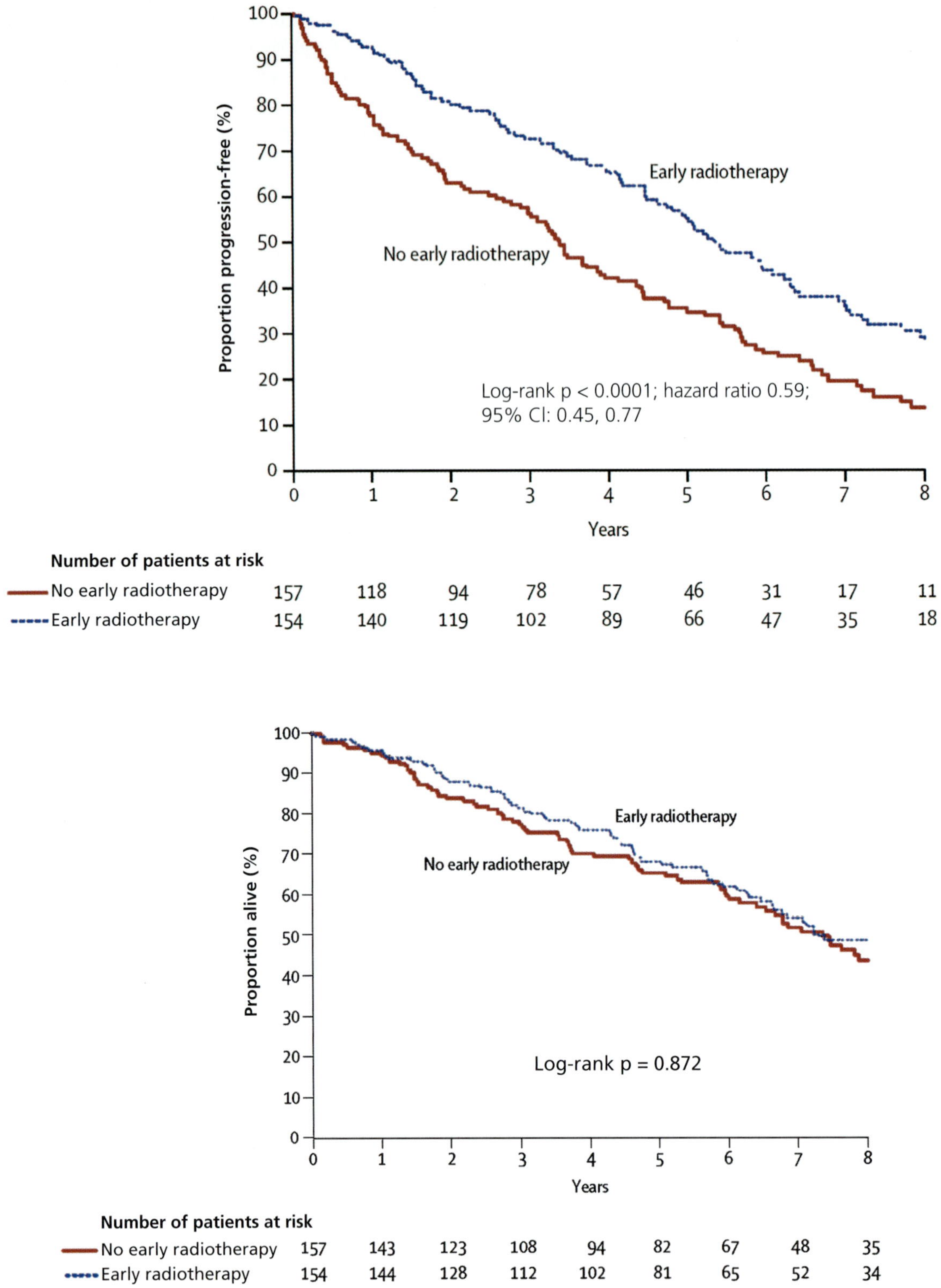

FIG. 14-2 Progression-free survival by intention-to-treat analysis (top). Number of events: 80 for control group, 76 for early radiotherapy group. Overall survival by intention-to-treat analysis (bottom). Number of events: 121 for control group, 96 for early radiotherapy group.[7]
Reprinted with permission from Elsevier.

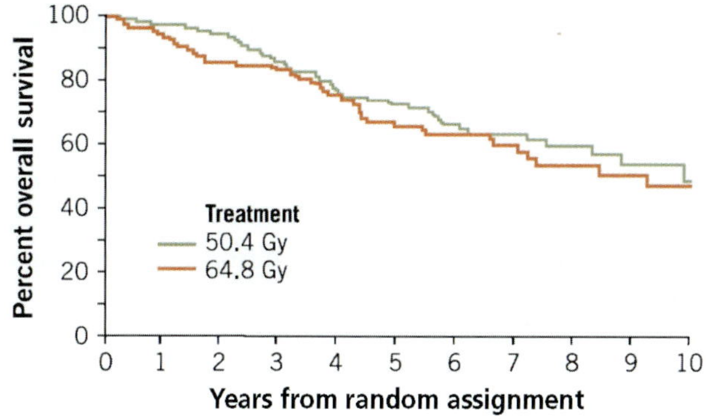

50.4 Gy	N(t)	101	94	60
	S(t)		94%	72%
	CI		90% to 99%	63% to 81%
64.8 Gy	N(t)	102	83	54
	S(t)		85%	65%
	CI		78% to 92%	56% to 75%

FIG. 14-3 Kaplan-Meier estimates of overall survival for two arms of a trial in which patients with supratentorial low-grade gliomas were randomly assigned to an intermediate dose (50.4 Gy in 28 fractions) or a high dose (64.8 Gy in 36 fractions) of localized radiation therapy ($p = 0.48$, two-sided log-rank test). [9]

Abbreviations: N(t), number of patients; S(t), Kaplan-Meier survival; CI, 95% confidence interval. Modified with permission from Shaw E, Arusell R, Scheithauer B, et al. Prospective randomized trial of low- versus high-dose radiation therapy in adults with supratentorial low-grade glioma: initial report of a North Central Cancer Treatment Group/Radiation Therapy Oncology Group/Eastern Cooperative Oncology Group study. J Clin Oncol. 2002;20:2271.

Preliminary results suggest that PCV resulted in superior progression-free survival, but not overall survival.[11] Because of the toxicity associated with PCV, many practitioners recommend the use of temozolomide either as initial therapy or at recurrence.

ANAPLASTIC ASTROCYTOMA

Patients with anaplastic astrocytomas may present with seizures, focal neurologic deficit, headaches, or changes in mental status. The median age at the time of diagnosis is approximately 45 years. MRI usually indicates a contrast-enhanced mass lesion, although some lesions may not be contrast enhanced. Biopsy or surgical resection is necessary to establish the diagnosis. The presence of mitoses in anaplastic astrocytomas distinguishes them from low-grade astrocytomas (Fig. 14-4). Because of the high propensity of these lesions to undergo further anaplastic transformation, removal of sufficient tissue for thorough pathologic evaluation is necessary to distinguish anaplastic astrocytoma from glioblastoma multiforme. In particular, histologic diagnosis of anaplastic astrocytoma in patients with ring-enhancing mass lesions on MRI suggests glioblastoma and suggests that tissue representative of the true diagnosis has not been obtained.

Poor prognostic variables include older age, poor performance score, and severe neurologic impairment. In general, the outcome is better for more complete surgical

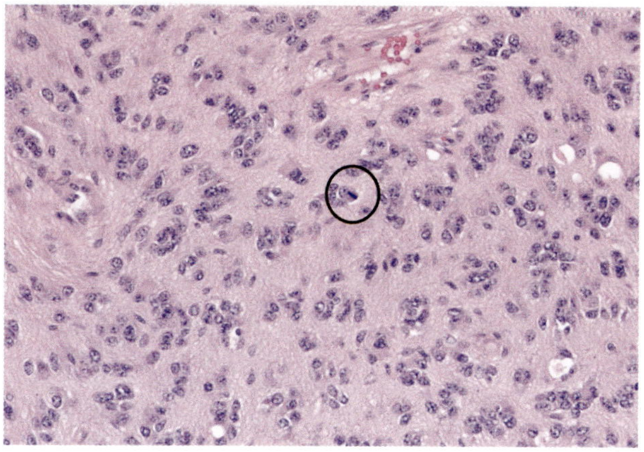

FIG. 14-4 Photomicrograph of an anaplastic astrocytoma specimen, mitotic figure in center.

resection, but it remains uncertain whether the better outcome is associated with the surgery itself or is a result of the clinical scenario that permitted more complete resection.

The standard initial treatment remains maximum surgical debulking without increasing neurologic deficit. In this setting, radiation therapy has been demonstrated to prolong survival and is a standard component of treatment. The role of adjuvant chemotherapy remains controversial. Some phase III trials have demonstrated no benefit of adjuvant chemotherapy compared with radiation alone, whereas others have demonstrated benefit. Both single-agent carmustine and the combination regimen of PCV are associated with prolonged survival in some series and meta-analyses. The results for the two options have been similar (Fig. 14-5).[12] Most recently, a meta-analysis by the Glioma Meta-Analysis Trialists' Group[13] demonstrated an approximate 6% absolute increase in 1-year and 2-year survival

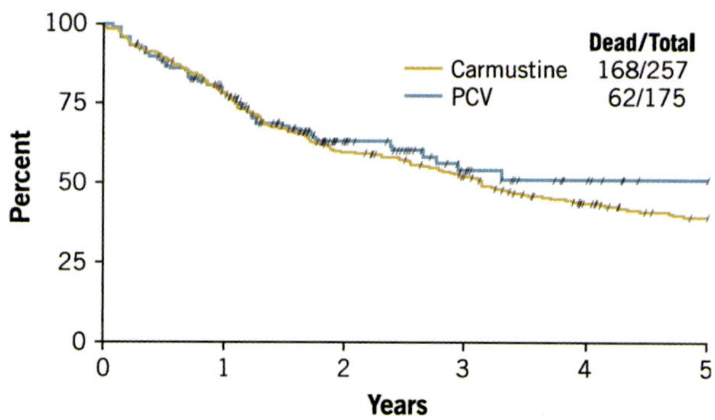

FIG. 14-5 Overall survival for patients with anaplastic astrocytoma who were treated with adjuvant carmustine (BCNU) or a regimen of procarbazine, lomustine, and vincristine (PCV). *The difference in survival was not significant ($p = 0.5460$).[12] Modified with permission from Prados MD, Scott C, Curran WJ Jr, et al. Procarbazine, lomustine, and vincristine (PCV) chemotherapy for anaplastic astrocytoma: a retrospective review of Radiation Therapy Oncology Group protocols comparing survival with carmustine or PCV adjuvant chemotherapy. J Clin Oncol. 1999;17:3394.*

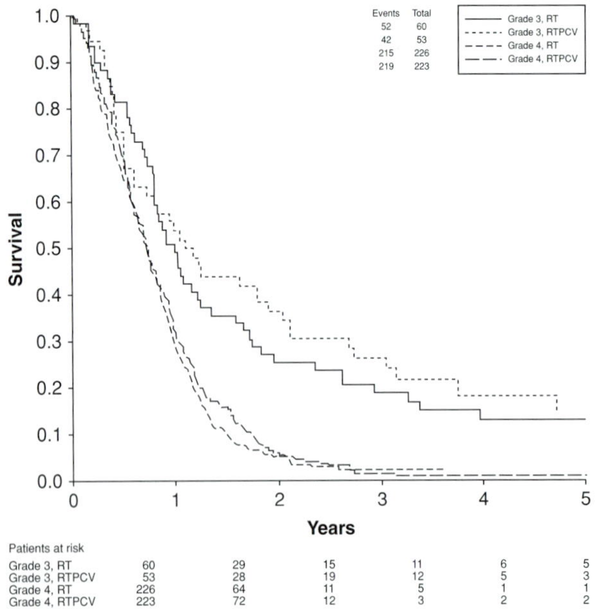

FIG. 14-6 Survival in patients with anaplastic astrocytoma or glioblastoma multiforme treated with radiation alone (RT) or radiation plus procarbazine, CCNU (lomustine), and vincristine (RT-PCV).[14]

Medical Research Council Brain Tumor Working Party. Randomized trial of procarbazine, lomustine, and vincristine in the adjuvant treatment of high-grade astrocytoma: a Medical Research Council trial. J Clin Oncol. 2001;19:509-518.

rates for patients with anaplastic astrocytoma who received chemotherapy. Two-year survival was better for those patients who received radiation plus chemotherapy than for those who received radiation alone (37% compared with 31%). However, a large randomized trial by the Medical Research Council found no benefit of adjuvant PCV compared with radiation therapy alone (Fig. 14-6).[14] In general, the median survival has ranged from 24 months to more than 36 months. The breadth of the range in survival likely reflects patient selection criteria, which are influenced by the interpretation of pathologic analyses, patient age, performance score, and referral bias. At the present time, clinical trials do not confirm a therapeutic benefit for adjuvant chemotherapy. Although temozolomide is effective for the treatment of recurrent anaplastic astrocytoma, its role as an adjuvant to radiation therapy has not been rigorously assessed. One major clinical trial (R9813) is underway to compare radiation plus carmustine with radiation plus temozolomide.

As with low-grade astrocytoma, chemotherapy for anaplastic astrocytoma that recurs following radiation is of benefit, and both nitrosourea-based regimens and temozolomide have demonstrated efficacy. In fact, the FDA granted accelerated approval for temozolomide on the basis of its activity in recurrent anaplastic astrocytoma; the response rate was 35% for patients who had not received chemotherapy and 20% for patients who had received nitrosurea-based therapy (Table 14-1).[15] Other agents have not shown consistent antitumor activity for recurrent anaplastic astrocytoma.

GLIOBLASTOMA MULTIFORME

Glioblastoma multiforme is the most common and most malignant of the primary brain tumors. The average age at the time of diagnosis is approximately 55 years, but the tumor occurs in all age groups. The onset of symptoms often is abrupt and is most commonly related to mass effect and focal neurologic symptoms. Seizures also are relatively common. Intracranial bleeding may be the presenting symptom for less than 3% of patients. The duration of symptoms before diagnosis is usually short, ranging from a few days to a few weeks.

TABLE 14-1 Response to Temozolomide in Patients with Malignant Astrocytoma at First Relapse[15]

		Patients with Eligible Histology*		
Central Reviewer's Assessment	Patients in Intent-to-treat Population with Response (162 patients)	Patients with Anaplastic Astrocytoma with Response (97 patients)	Patients with Mixed Anaplastic Oligoastrocytoma with Response (14 patients)	Total Number of Patients with Response
Complete response	13 (8%)	6 (6%)	2 (14%)	8 (7%)
Partial response	44 (27%)	27 (28%)	4 (29%)	31 (28%)
Stable disease	44 (27%)	31 (32%)	1 (7%)	32 (29%)
Total	101 (62%)	64 (66%)	7 (50%)	71 (64%)

*Disease was confirmed on central histologic review.

Modified with permission from Yung WK, Prados MD, Yaya-Tur R, et al. Multicenter phase II trial of temozolomide in patients with anaplastic astrocytoma or anaplastic oligoastrocytoma at first relapse. Temodal Brain Tumor Group. J Clin Oncol. 1999;17:2766

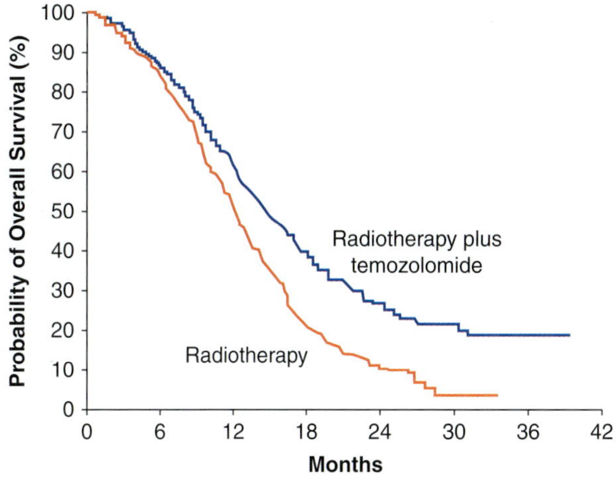

No. at risk

Radiotherapy	286	240	144	59	23	2	0
Radiotherapy plus temozolomide	287	246	174	109	57	27	4

FIG. 14-7 Overall survival in patients with glioblastoma multiforme treated with radiation therapy (RT) alone compared with radiation therapy plus temozolomide.[16]

Stupp R, Mason WP, van den Bent MJ, et al. Radiotherapy plus concomitant and adjuvant temozolomide for glioblastoma. N Engl J Med. 2005;352:987–996. Copyright © 2005. Massachusetts Medical Society. All rights reserved.

Pathologic features include increased cellularity with marked nuclear pleomorphism, frequent mitoses, endothelial proliferation, and areas of palisading necrosis. Characteristic genetic alterations include epidermal growth factor receptor amplification and mutation or loss of the phosphatase and tensin homolog (*PTEN*) tumor suppressor gene. Both of these abnormalities are characteristic of glioblastoma multiforme. Anaplastic astrocytoma with these genetic alterations may behave more like glioblastoma multiforme than anaplastic astrocytoma. Poor prognostic variables include increasing age, poor performance status, increased severity of neurologic deficits at the time of diagnosis, and the inability to achieve substantial tumor resection.

T1-weighted MRI scans with use of gadolinium typically show a ring-enhanced mass lesion with low signal intensity in the center and surrounding the ring-enhanced component. In specimens obtained by biopsy, the central portion of the lesion often contains tumor necrosis, the ring-enhanced portion is associated with increased vascular permability, and the surrounding low-signal component corresponds to intact brain parenchyma diffusely infiltrated by tumor cells. Studies involving the use of serial stereotactic biopsies have demonstrated isolated tumor cells well beyond any signal abnormality visible on T2-weighted scans.

The mainstay of treatment remains surgical removal without creating an unacceptable neurologic deficit. The extremely infiltrative nature of this tumor, as well as that of other infiltrating astrocytomas, make complete surgical removal impossible. Radiation therapy has been the standard treatment since the early-phase III clinical trials in which the Brain Tumor Study Group[17] compared treatment with postoperative supportive care only, carmustine alone, radiation therapy alone, and radiation therapy plus carmustine. The 1-year survival for each of these treatment arms was 3%, 12%, 24%, and 25%, respectively. Currently, radiation consisting of 60 Gy delivered as 2 Gy fractions over 30 treatment days is commonly administered. Multiple attempts to improve the therapeutic efficacy of radiation by using higher doses, altered fraction schemes, and use of radiation sensitizers have failed to produce better results. A phase III randomized trial of patients with glioblastoma multiforme showed no benefit to adding stereotactic radiosurgery to radiation plus carmustine.[3] Moreover, such radiosurgical boost can result in tumor and brain necrosis which contribute to increased focal deficit and increased intracranial pressure, sometimes requiring surgical debulking.

The benefit of adjuvant temozolomide for patients with glioblastoma multiforme has been demonstrated convincingly in the recent past. In a landmark trial, patients were randomly assigned after surgery to receive radiotherapy alone or radiotherapy plus concurrent temozolomide followed by six cycles of adjuvant temozolomide. Median and 2-year survival rates were increased by 2.5 months and 16.1%, respectively, in patients receiving temozolomide (Fig. 14-7).[16] These results changed the standard of care for treatment of these patients. Moreover, a companion correlative laboratory study demonstrated that methylation of the promoter region of the methyl guanine methyl transferase (*MGMT*) gene in the tumor specimen is associated with superior survival, regardless of treatment received (Fig. 14-8).[18] *MGMT* removes the methyl group from the O6 position of guanine, reversing the effects of methylating agents, such as temozolomide. Methylation prevents transcription of the *MGMT* gene and prevents its

KEY POINTS

- The primary treatment of anaplastic astrocytoma is surgical debulking when possible, followed by radiation therapy with or without adjuvant chemotherapy.
- The current standard of treatment for glioblastoma is radiation with concurrent and adjuvant temozolomide.

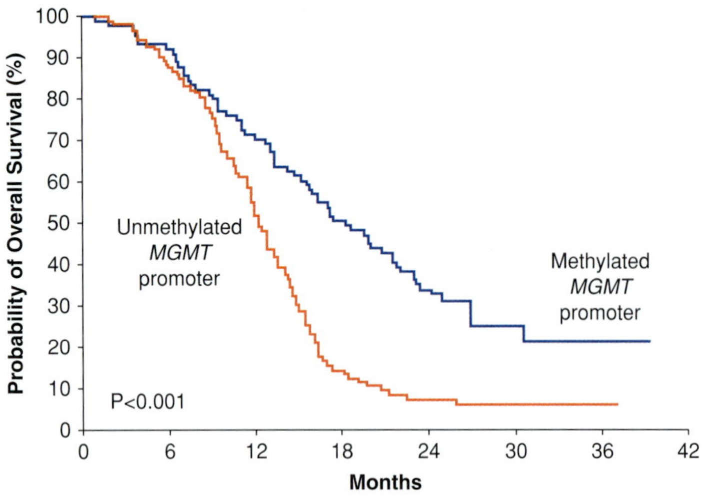

No. at risk							
Unmethylated	114	100	59	16	7	4	1
Methylated	92	84	64	46	24	7	1

FIG. 14-8 Survival in patients with glioblastoma multiforme with and without methylation of the MGMT as determined by methylation-specific PCR.[18]

Abbreviation: MGMT, methyl guanine methyl transferase. Hegi ME, Diserens AC, Gorlia T, et al. MGMT gene silencing and benefit from temozolomide in glioblastoma. N Engl J Med. 2005;352:997–1003.

expression. Consequently, we would expect patients whose tumors express *MGMT* to have less benefit from temozolomide than those whose tumors do not express *MGMT*. In this trial, however, survival also was better in patients receiving temozolomide in addition to radiation with or without methylation of *MGMT* (Fig 14-9). The underlying biology of MGMT methylation and the associated clinical outcomes remain under investigation.

The findings of individual phase III trials have shown no or modest benefit with the use of nitrosourea-based regimens. When compared with radiation therapy alone, adjuvant chemotherapy in addition to radiation was associated with a better 1-year survival rate (35% vs. 41%, respectively) and a better 2-year survival rate (9% vs. 13%, respectively) compared with radiation therapy alone in the Glioma Meta-Analysis Trialists' Group study (Fig. 14-10).[13] At best, the benefit of adjuvant nitrosourea-based chemotherapy is small, whether given systemically or as an implantable carmustine-impregnated polymer (Gliadel) wafer.[19] The benefits and risks of the combination of carmustine-impregnated wafers in combination with temozolomide are under investigation.

Treatment options for glioblastoma recurrent after radiation and temozolomide must be tailored to the individual. Because all therapies have limited benefits, symptom control with end-of-life care may be appropriate. For patients with resectable disease, good neurologic status, and good performance score, a second resection, with or without placement of carmustine-impregnated wafers, can be done. The value of additional radiation therapy or chemotherapy remains under investigation. Participation in a well-designed clinical trial should be considered.

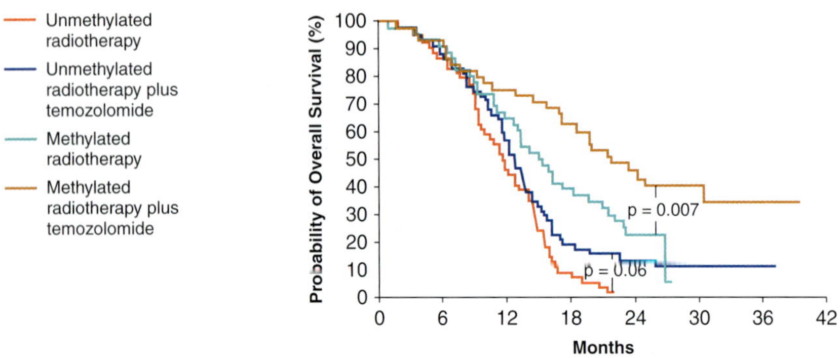

No. at risk							
Unmethylated radiotherapy	54	47	25	5	0	0	0
Unmethylated radiotherapy plus temozolomide	60	53	34	11	7	4	1
Methylated radiotherapy	46	42	30	18	8	0	0
Methylated radiotherapy plus temozolomide	46	42	34	28	16	7	1

FIG. 14-9 Survival in patients with glioblastoma multiforme by MGMT methylation status and treatment (radiation alone or radiation plus temozolomide).[18]

Abbreviation: MGMT, methyl guanine methyl transferase. Hegi ME, Diserens AC, Gorlia T, et al. MGMT gene silencing and benefit from temozolomide in glioblastoma. N Engl J Med. 2005;352:997–1003.

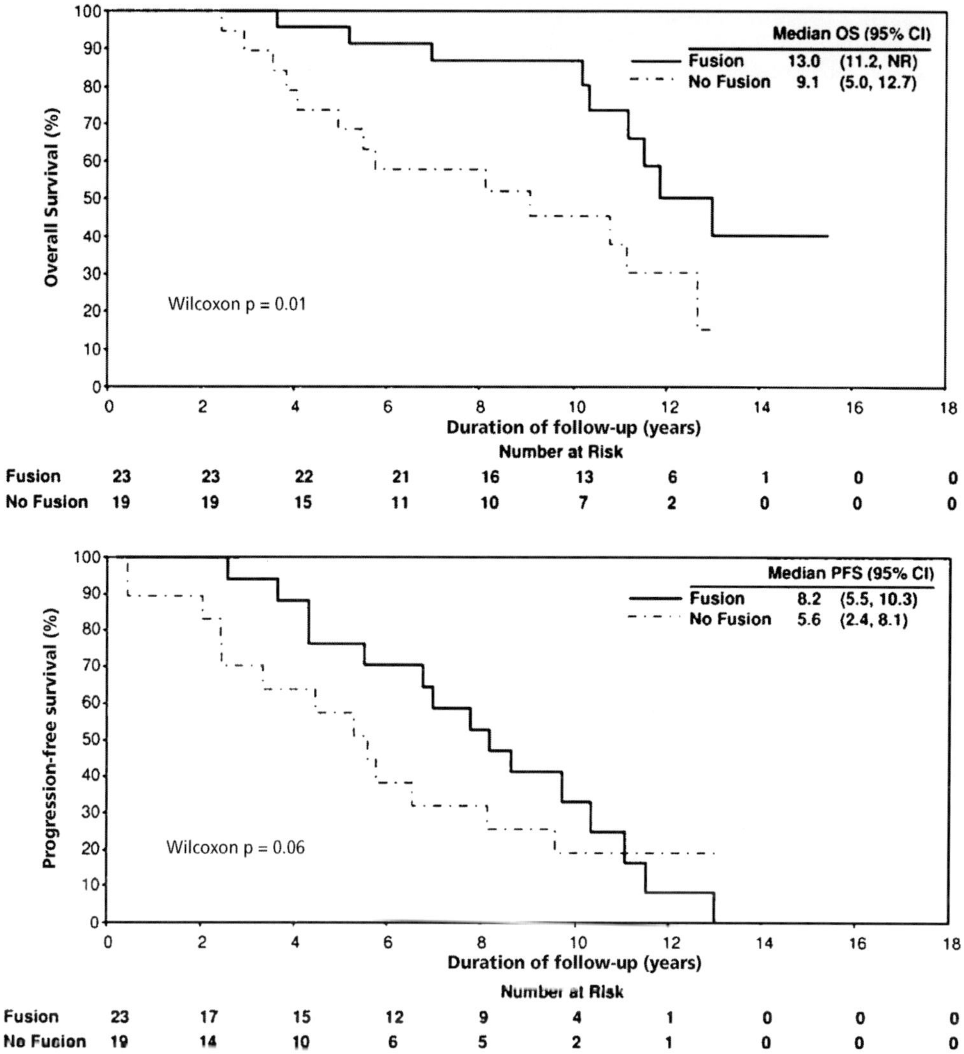

FIG. 14-10 Survival distribution in low-grade oligodendroglioma/oligoastrocytoma by 1p/19q status.[20] Abbreviations: NR, not reported; PFS, progression-free survival.

Reprinted with permission from the American Association for Cancer Research. Jenkins RB, Blair H, Ballman KV, et al. A t(1;19)(q10;p10) mediates the combined deletions of 1p and 19q and predicts a better prognosis of patients with oligodendroglioma. Cancer Res. 2006;66(20):9852–9861.

OLIGODENDROGLIOMAS AND OLIGOASTROCYTOMAS

Tumors containing oligodendroglial elements are relatively uncommon, probably accounting for no more than 10% of primary brain tumors. Nevertheless, they are important to note because of their unique natural history and sensitivity to chemotherapy. They are classified as either low grade or anaplastic. Anaplastic oligodendrogliomas demonstrate high cellularity, nuclear pleomorphism, frequent mitoses, abundant endothelial proliferation, and tumor necrosis. Approximately one-half of oligodendrogliomas are characterized by loss of heterozygosity of chromosomes 1p and 19q, a pathognomonic diagnostic feature. Recently, the loss of heterozygosity was demonstrated to be secondary to an unbalanced pericentromeric translocation.[20]

Most oligodendrogliomas originate as low-grade tumors. Mixed oligoastrocytomas contain both oligodendroglial and astrocytic elements; the percentage of each component needed to classify a tumor as mixed has not been clearly defined.

LOW-GRADE OLIGODENDROGLIOMAS AND OLIGOASTROCYTOMAS

The average age at the time of diagnosis of low-grade oligodendroglioma is approximately 35 years. Patients typically present with seizures, although focal neurologic deficits, changes in mental status or personality, or symptoms of increased intracranial pressure can occur. The median survival for patients with pure low-grade oligodendrogliomas is approximately 10 years; median survival for patients with mixed oligoastrocytoma is approximately 8 years, which is intermediate between pure oligodendroglioma and pure astrocytoma. Deletion or translocation of 1p and 19q in the tumor is associated with superior survival compared with absence of deletion or translocation (Fig. 14-10).[20] MRI is

KEY POINTS

- Increasing histologic grade is a potent predictor of survival for patients with astrocytoma and those with oligodendroglioma.
- Oligodendrogliomas are more sensitive to current chemotherapy regimens than astrocytomas.
- Deletion or translocation of 1p and 19q occurs in one-half of oligodendrogliomas and portends a better prognosis.

the preferred imaging modality because these tumors may not be visible on CT scans. The tumor is most visible as increased signal intensity on T2-weighted scans. There may be a decreased signal on T1-weighted scans and occasional scant contrast enhancement. Signal void from calcification may or may not be present.

As with low-grade astrocytoma, controversy exists regarding optimum management. Because these tumors are even more indolent than astrocytoma, symptom control with anticonvulsant drugs without additional antitumor therapy has been common. More complete surgical resection has been suggested as beneficial, although removal of smaller tumors from regions of the brain that are less likely to cause neurologic deficits may result in selection bias. The early results of a European trial of immediate radiation compared with delayed radiation failed to demonstrate a survival benefit for early radiation, although immediate radiation was associated with a longer time to tumor progression.[7] No benefit for higher-dose radiation when compared with intermediate-dose radiation was found in two other trials.[9,10] Data from several studies indicate that initial therapy with temozolomide or PCV may shrink these tumors in 31% to 61% of patients with either oligodendroglioma or oligoastrocytoma.[21-25]

Whether such tumor response improves time to progression or overall survival remains to be determined. A clinical trial designed to compare radiation only with radiation followed by PCV has been reported.[11] Although progression-free survival was superior in the PCV treatment arm, survival was not different between the two groups. Presumably, treatment at recurrence is effective, resulting in similar outcomes regardless of the timing of chemotherapy. In addition, because temozolomide produces tumor responses and is less toxic, many practitioners advocate its use rather than that of PCV. Thus, current options for initial treatment include symptom control only with anticonvulsant agents, radiation therapy alone, chemotherapy alone, or the combination of chemotherapy and radiation.

Surgery, radiation, and chemotherapy may each play an important role for recurrent oligodendroglial tumors. Primary or secondary debulking may reduce symptoms. If radiation therapy was not administered as initial therapy, it is likely to be effective for recurrent disease. Response to PCV has occurred in 50% to 90% of patients with low-grade oligodendrgliomas recurrent after radiation. A response rate of approximately 50% has been reported for temozolomide given after radiation therapy has failed.[26]

ANAPLASTIC OLIGODENDROGLIOMA/ OLIGOASTROCYTOMA

Mass effect or seizures are typically seen at presentation with anaplastic oligodendroglial tumors. Average age at diagnosis is approximately 45 years. Despite the chemosensitivity of these tumors, the median survival is only 3 to 5 years. MRI reveals a variably contrast-enhancing mass lesion in most patients. Current treatment includes optimal surgical debulking followed by radiation therapy. In two recent phase III trials, one conducted in North America and the other in Europe, radiation alone was compared with radiation plus PCV. In the North America trial, patients received PCV for four cycles prior to radiation. Although progression-free survival rates were better in the PCV arm, survival rates in the two groups were the same (Fig. 14-11).[27] Notably, patients with 1p and 19q deletions had significantly better outcomes, regardless of treatment. The improvement in progression-free survival was most notable in patients with 1p and 19q deletions. There also was better progression-free survival with PCV in patients without 1p and 19q deletion (Fig. 14-12).[27]

In the European trial, patients received PCV after radiation. Results were nearly identical to the North American results. Progression-free survival was better in the PCV group, but overall survival was not different between the two groups. Patients with 1p and 19q deletion had superior survival, regardless of treatment arm. The difference in progression-free survival for the treatment arm did not differ according to presence or absence of 1p and 19q deletions.[28] Taken together, these studies demonstrate that chemotherapy improves progression-free survival, but that salvage treatment at recurrence results in equivalent survival. Importantly, both trials confirm the prognostic value of 1p and 19q, but do not clearly demonstrate that only patients with 1p and 19q deletions benefit from chemotherapy.

Prospective trials have demonstrated that approximately 50% to 70% of patients with anaplastic oligodendrogliomas that recur after radiotherapy respond to chemotherapy with either temozolomide or PCV.[26,29] Although there is no evidence that the sequence of temozolomide and PCV is important in terms of efficacy, the absence of cumulative myelosuppression with temozolomide argues for its use initially in the setting of recurrent disease.

EPENDYMOMA

Ependymomas may occur anywhere in the spinal axis. In children, this tumor is more commonly found in the posterior fossa and spinal cord; in adults, the tumor is somewhat more common in the supratentorial brain. The tumors can be classified as either low-grade or anaplastic. For low-grade lesions,

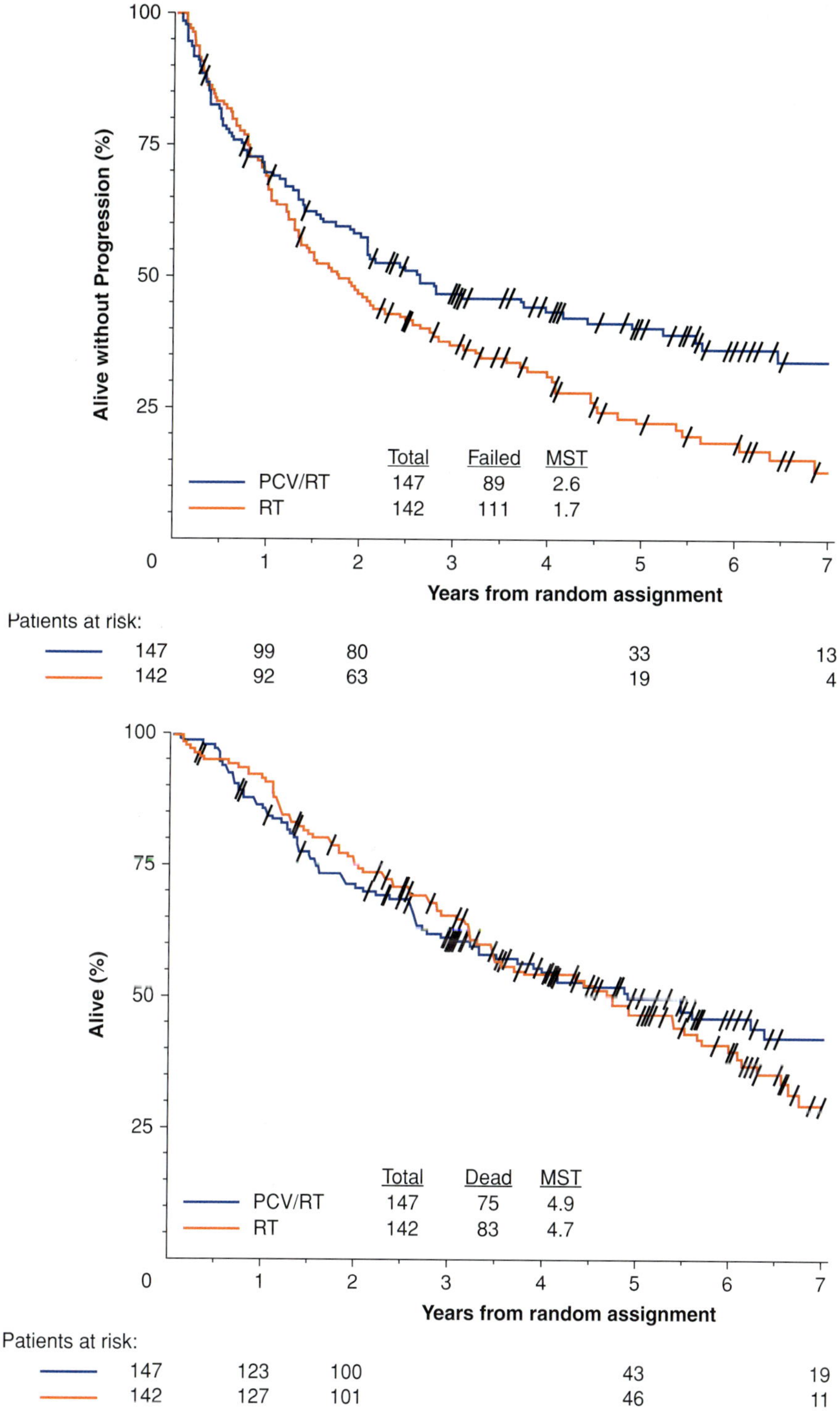

FIG. 14-11 Progression-free survival (top) and overall survival (bottom) in patients receiving radiation therapy compared with four cycles of procarbazine, CCNU, and vincristine followed by radiation therapy as initial treatment for anaplastic oligodendroglioma/ anaplastic oligoastrocytoma.[27]

Abbreviations: MST, median survival time; PCV, procarbazine, CCNU (lomustine) and vincristine; RT, radiation therapy. Cairncross G, Berkey B, Shaw E, et al. A randomized clinical trial of chemotherapy plus radiotherapy (RT) versus RT alone for pure and mixed anaplastic oligodendroglioma: an Intergroup trial by the RTOG, NCCTG, SWOG, NCIC CTG and ECOG. J Clin Oncol. 2006;24(18):2707–2714.

surgical resection alone may provide cure. Both the low-grade and anaplastic lesions may disseminate along the leptomeningeal surfaces. Low-grade completely resected ependymomas are usually treated with surgery alone. Incompletely resected, anaplastic, or disseminated disease is usually treated with radiation therapy. Studies have shown that ependymomas may respond to platinum-based chemotherapy regimens, but the clinical benefit of chemotherapy remains speculative.[30] Overall, the response to chemotherapy is less than 20%.

MENINGIOMA

Meningiomas are usually benign and originate in the dura covering the brain and spinal cord. The incidence of the tumor is approximately two cases per 100,000 individuals. They are most common for women in the sixth and seventh decades of life. Loss of chromosome 22 is characteristic of meningiomas, although the prognostic significance of this finding is not clear. Also, the frequency of meningioma is increased for patients with type 2

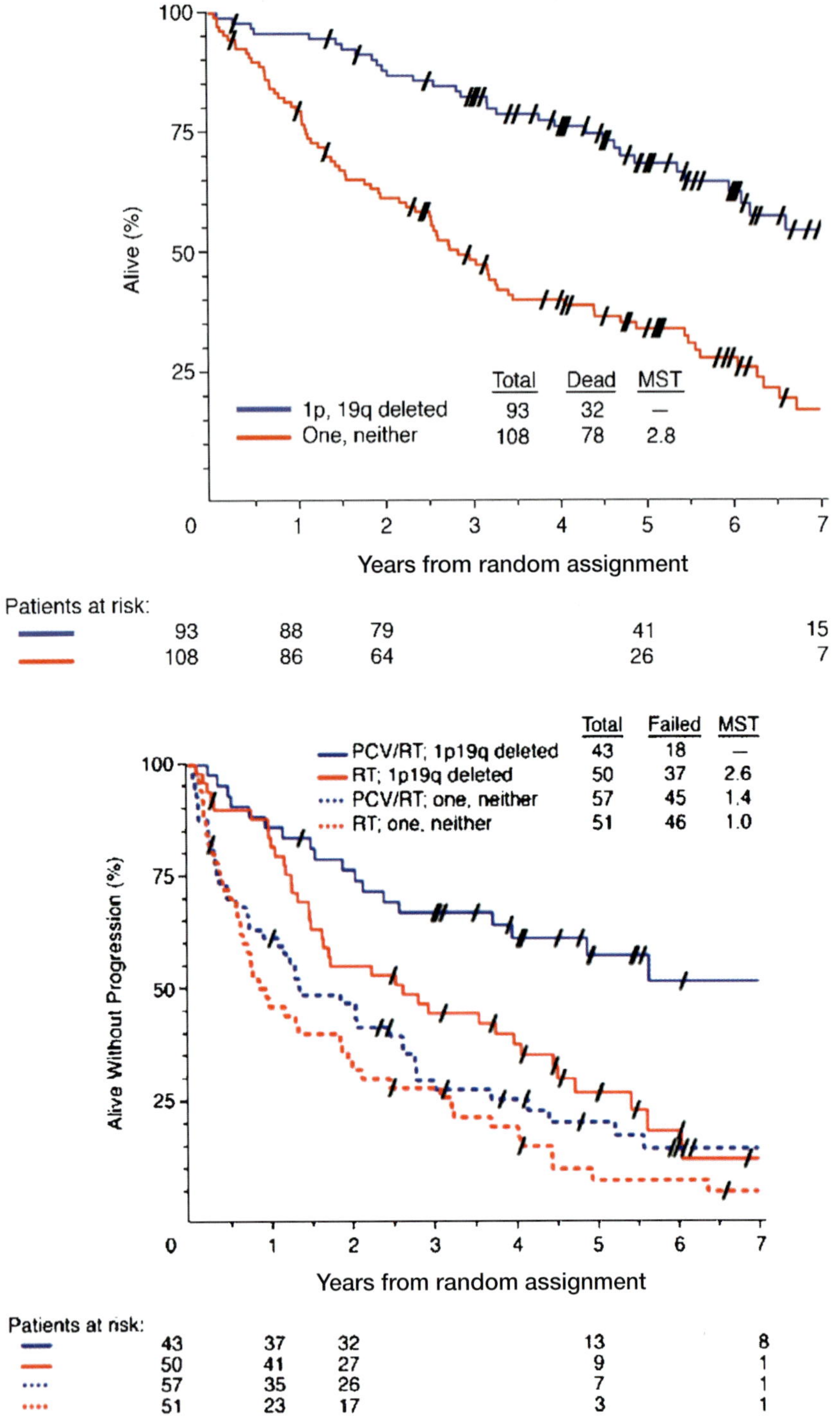

FIG. 14-12 Survival distributions by 1p/19q status in all patients with oligodendroglioma/oligoastrocytoma (top) and by treatment arm (bottom).[27]

Abbreviations: MST, median survival time; RT, radiation therapy; RT-PCV, radiation plus procarbazine, CCNU (lomustine) and vincristine. Cairncross G, Berkey B, Shaw E, et al. A randomized clinical trial of chemotherapy plus radiotherapy (RT) versus RT alone for pure and mixed anaplastic oligodendroglioma: an Intergroup trial by the RTOG, NCCTG, SWOG, NCIC CTG and ECOG. J Clin Oncol. 2006;24(18):2707–2714.

neurofibromatosis. Although meningiomas can express receptors for androgen, estrogen, progesterone, and somatostatin, hormone therapies directed at these receptors have not yet demonstrated therapeutic efficacy.

Patients with meningiomas may present with typical features of mass lesions in the brain, including seizures or focal neurologic deficits. Meningiomas also may be asymptomatic and are detected incidentally on CT or MRI scans that are obtained for other reasons. The tumors have a characteristic MRI appearance usually consisting of uniform contrast enhancement along the dura, with distinct separation from brain parenchyma. Contrast enhancement extending from the mass lesion, known as the dural tail, is characteristic but not present in all cases. There may be marked parenchymal edema as a result of the mass effect.

Many meningiomas that are noted incidentally do not require treatment. For patients with asymptomatic meningioma, observation may be appropriate. Epidemiologic

KEY POINTS

- Meningiomas are typically benign dura-based tumors, usually occurring in older women.
- In most patients with meningioma, observation only is appropriate. For patients who are symptomatic, surgical removal is most commonly the treatment of choice.

evidence suggests that as many as two-thirds of these patients will not have symptoms over time.[31] When there is substantial mass effect with or without symptoms, the treatment of choice is usually complete resection. Surgery often is feasible if the meningioma is located over the cortical convexity, olfactory groove, anterior sagittal sinus, or posterior fossa. However, resection may be more difficult for tumors in other sites, such as sphenoid, parasagittal, orbital, tentorial, or clivus locations. Under those circumstances, external beam radiation therapy or focal stereotactic radiotherapy may be extremely useful for tumor control. No pharmaceutical interventions have reproducibly demonstrated antitumor efficacy for meningiomas.

Rarely, meningiomas may have atypical histologic features or may be frankly malignant. Meningiomas can be highly aggressive, and the approach to such tumors is identical to that for benign meningiomas, although early radiation often is used.

PITUITARY TUMORS

Pituitary tumors are typically either functional or nonfunctional adenomas. Endocrine abnormalities may be found at presentation if the tumors are producing peptides, such as prolactin, growth hormone, or adrenocorticotropic hormone. Also present may be ocular manifestations—classically bitemporal hemianopsia—because of compression of the medial and posterior aspects of the optic chiasm. A diagnosis may be confirmed by an assay of pituitary hormones, CT scans, or MRI scans of the sella. Neuroimaging studies usually demonstrate a mass lesion arising in or just above the sella turcica with either displacement or obliteration of the normal pituitary gland. Also, these tumors may be noted incidentally on scans obtained for other reasons.

Therapy should be tailored to the individual. For patients with asymptomatic pituitary tumors, observation only may be appropriate. Patients with prolactinoma may benefit from bromocriptine. Surgery should be considered for either functional or nonfunctional lesions that threaten the visual pathways.

PRIMARY CNS LYMPHOMA

CNS lymphomas constitute approximately 2% to 3% of all brain tumors in patients who have an adequate immune system. The tumor is more common for men who are age 55 to 60, and nearly one-half of all CNS lymphomas occur in patients older than 60. The incidence appears to be increasing. Patients with a compromised immune system are at risk for CNS lymphoma, including patients who have had solid organ transplant, who have congenital immunodeficiency or an autoimmune disorder, or who are infected with HIV. HIV-associated CNS lymphomas are related to the Epstein Barr virus, particularly if the CD4 count is less than 500 cells/μL.[5] Most CNS lymphomas are of the large B-cell variety.

Patients present with a variety of symptoms characteristic of either focal or multifocal mass lesions. The MRI scan usually shows homogeneous contrast-enhanced tumors within the periventricular deep white matter. Multifocality is common. Inhomogeneous contrast enhancement is not uncommon, especially in patients with a compromised immune system. It is extremely important to consider CNS lymphoma in the differential diagnosis of brain tumors. Administration of corticosteroids may result in complete disappearance of the contrast-enhanced lesion, making the diagnosis difficult. Consequently, when CNS lymphoma is considered in the differential diagnosis, corticosteroids should be avoided, unless a mass effect is causing serious and immediate injury to the patient. Obtaining specimens of suspected lesions by biopsy is critically important because many malignant and nonmalignant CNS conditions can mimic a CNS lymphoma. Unlike systemic large B-cell lymphomas, for which both chemotherapy and radiation therapy are effective and treatment for localized disease is curative, CNS lymphoma will usually respond to initial therapy but then typically relapses. As with systemic lymphoma, the role of surgery is restricted primarily to obtaining appropriate tissue for diagnosis. The mainstay of treatment has been whole-brain radiation therapy. Unfortunately, even with localized lesions, the median survival with radiation alone is approximately 1 year. Relapse at sites other than the primary lesion is common. The regimen of

KEY POINTS

- Primary CNS lymphoma is increasing in frequency among patients who have an adequate immune system.
- Primary CNS lymphomas are usually B-cell type.
- High-dose methotrexate-based chemotherapy regimens appear to improve survival for patients with CNS lymphoma who have an adequate immune systems.
- Epstein-Barr virus (EBV)-associated B-cell lymphoma is a hallmark feature of patients with chronic immunosuppression, including patients who have AIDS or who have had organ transplantation.

TABLE 14-2 Survival for 98 Patients with Primary Central Nervous System Lymphoma Who Were Treated with Chemotherapy and Whole-brain Radiation Therapy[23]

	Progression-free Survival		Overall Survival	
No. of Years after Treatment	*Rate (%)*	*No. of Patients at Risk*	*Rate (%)*	*No. of Patients at Risk*
0	100	98	100	98
1	64	63	79	77
2	50	49	64	62
3	41	40	52	50
4	33	27	39	32
5	25	11	32	13

Modified with permission from DeAngelis LM, Seiferheld W, Schold SC, et al. Combination chemotherapy and radiotherapy for primary central nervous system lymphoma: Radiation Therapy Oncology Group Study 93–10. *J Clin Oncol.* 2002;20:4645.

rituximab plus cyclophosphamide, doxorubicin, vincristine, and prednisone (R-CHOP) often is effective for systemic lymphoma, however, similar approaches for patients with primary CNS lymphoma have been unsuccessful in producing durable disease control

Studies have examined the incorporation of high-dose methotrexate into the following treatment regimens: single-agent methotrexate;[33] methotrexate plus high-dose cytarabine; procarbazine, with or without intrathecal methotrexate;[32] or intra-arterial chemotherapy following blood–brain barrier modification with mannitol.[34] Results have demonstrated superior overall survival compared with historical results for radiation therapy alone. With methotrexate-containing regimens, the median survival (range, 24 to 40 months) exceeded that associated with radiation therapy alone (Table 14-2).[33] In some cases, radiation therapy was used only at recurrence if complete regression had been achieved with chemotherapy; long-term survival was reported for some patients without the use of radiation therapy.[32–34] Because the diffuse nature of CNS lymphoma requires whole-brain radiation therapy, the risk of later neurologic toxicity with dementia secondary to leukoencephalopathy is relatively common, occurring in one-third of patients or more.[35] Consequently, strategies that avoid the use of whole-brain radiation and still result in tumor control could improve the overall result. Initial therapy for patients with compromised immune systems is reduction of the cause of immunosuppression. The prognosis for such patients is usually worse that that for patients who have an adequate immune systems. Because of comorbid infections and generally poor performance status, the use of chemotherapy for patients with a compromised immune system often is not feasible.

MEDULLOBLASTOMA (PRIMITIVE NEUROECTODERMAL TUMOR)

Medulloblastoma and other CNS primitive neuroectodermal tumors, such as pineoblastoma and cerebral neuroblastoma, are very uncommon primary CNS malignant tumors. Medulloblastoma is more common in children, but young adults also are at risk. This tumor occurs in the posterior fossa. It may be located in either the cerebellar hemisphere or the vermis and may involve the fourth ventricle. Because of the proximity of the fourth ventricle, obstructive hydrocephalus is relatively common. Symptoms at presentation include loss of balance, incoordination, diplopia, dysarthria, and signs of hydrocephalus, including headache, nausea, vomiting, and gait instability.

MRI usually shows a contrast-enhanced mass lesion involving the cerebellum, although some medulloblastomas do not enhance. Other locations of primitive neuroectodermal tumors include the pineal region and supratentorial sites. These tumors have a high propensity to seed the leptomeninges focally as well as to spread through the subarachnoid space to involve the ventricle, cerebral convexity, and spinal leptomeningeal surfaces. MRI of the entire craniospinal axis is necessary.

KEY POINTS

- Medulloblastoma typically occurs in the cerebellum of children.
- Treatment for medulloblastoma includes complete surgical debulking when feasible, followed by radiation of the craniospinal axis and chemotherapy.

Surgical removal of as much of the mass lesion as possible is important, because residual tumor after surgery confers a worse prognosis. Also associated with a worse prognosis are positive findings on cytologic analysis of cerebrospinal fluid or the presence of leptomeningeal metastases on an MRI scan. Surgery alone is rarely curative; however, surgical resection followed by radiation to the craniospinal axis with a boost to the site of the primary tumor can be curative. In addition, adjuvant chemotherapy (following radiation therapy) with a platinum drug (cisplatin or carboplatin), etoposide, and an alkylating agent (either cyclophosphamide or lomustine) plus vincristine has increased the cure rate compared with the use of radiation therapy alone. With appropriate initial therapy, long-term survival is achieved in 60% to 80% of patients with medulloblastoma.[36]

METASTATIC DISEASE TO THE NERVOUS SYSTEM

BRAIN METASTASES

Metastases to the brain are the most common intracranial tumors in adults and are 10 times more common than primary tumors. There have been substantial advances in the diagnosis and treatment of these lesions. As a result, duration of life and symptom control for patients with brain metastases can be substantially improved. Brain metastases occur in 20% to 40% of adults with cancer and are most commonly associated with cancers of the lung, breast, or unknown primary site, and melanoma. These lesions result from hematogenous spread and are most common at the junction of the gray and white matter where the caliber of blood vessels change, thereby trapping tumor emboli.

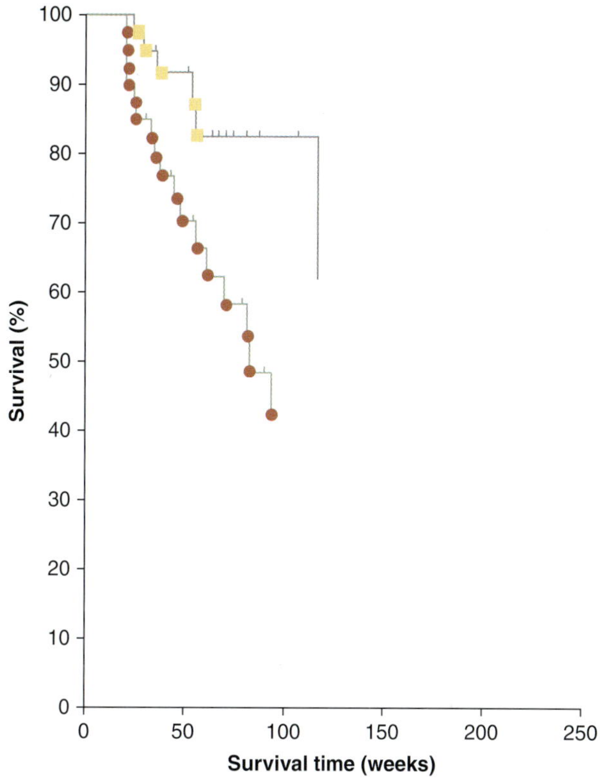

FIG. 14-13 Survival for patients with single brain metastasis who were randomly assigned to postoperative radiation treatment (squares) or observation (circles). When only those deaths attributed to neurologic causes were used as endpoints and data on patients who died from nonneurologic causes were censored, the difference in survival was significant (p = 0.03).[37] *The median survival was more than 115 weeks for patients who were treated with radiation and 81 weeks for patients observed only following surgery (relative risk of death from neurologic causes, 2.62; 95% CI: 1.03, 6.64). The length of survival was measured from the beginning of treatment for the original brain metastasis. Tick marks indicate patients who did not die of neurologic causes or the last follow-up evaluation for living patients. Reprinted with permission form the Journal of the American Medical Association.*

KEY POINTS

- Brain metastases are 10 times more common than primary brain tumors. The most common primary tumors are lung and breast cancers, melanoma, and cancer of unknown primary site.
- Surgical resection or stereotactic radiosurgery are of benefit to patients with a single brain metastasis who have a good Karnofsky performance score and controlled or absent primary tumor.
- Leptomeningeal metastases are manifested by symptoms and signs of injury to brain parenchyma, cranial nerves, or spinal nerves.
- Treatment of leptomeningeal metastases frequently is limited to symptom control because it is minimally effective and because leptomeningeal metastases frequently occur in the context of widespread systemic metastases.

Eighty percent of the brain lesions occur in the cerebral hemispheres, 15% in the cerebellum, and 5% in the brainstem. Approximately 80% of patients have a history of a systemic cancer, and 70% have multiple brain metastases that are evident on MRI scans.

The presenting signs and symptoms of these lesions are similar to those of other mass lesions in the brain. The best diagnostic test is MRI with use of a contrast medium; however, not all brain lesions in patients with cancer are metastases. In one prospective study of patients with systemic cancer who were thought to have single brain metastasis, 11% of biopsy specimens of brain tissue showed primary brain tumors or infections.[37] Two randomized prospective studies have shown that surgery plus whole-brain radiation is the treatment of choice for patients with surgically accessible single brain metastasis, because survival was substantially better than that associated with radiation alone.[37, 38]

However, nearly 50% of patients with one or two brain metastases are not candidates for surgery because the tumor is inaccessible, there is extensive systemic disease, or other complicating factors exist. Moreover, patients with tumors that disseminate widely in almost all cases, such as small cell lung cancer and lymphoma, are not candidates for surgical resection. These patients and others with multiple brain metastases should receive whole-brain radiation as standard therapy. There is considerable controversy regarding the role of whole-brain radiation to prevent the growth of micrometastases after complete resection of a single metastatic lesion.[38] Although radiation does reduce the recurrence of brain metastases, survival is not improved. Other techniques for delivering focal radiation therapy (i.e., radiosurgery and brachytherapy) may be effective in treating unresectable lesions. Stereotactic radiosurgery also appears to improve outcomes compared with whole-brain radiation therapy alone.[39] Chemotherapy rarely is used as primary therapy for brain metastases. Many tumors that metastasize to the brain (e.g., non-small cell lung cancer, a tumor of an unknown primary site, and melanoma) are not sensitive to chemotherapy or have been heavily pretreated with potentially effective agents.

LEPTOMENINGEAL METASTASES

Involvement of the leptomeninges occurs in approximately 5% of patients with cancer and is being recognized more commonly as patients with cancer live longer and as diagnostic studies improve. The leptomeninges are most commonly involved by cancer of the breast and lung and by melanoma. Tumor reaches the leptomeninges by hematogenous spread or by direct extension from pre-existing tumor deposits. Tumor cells are disseminated throughout the neuroaxis by the flow of the cerebrospinal fluid. Patients present with signs and symptoms referable to one or more of the following:

- local injury to nerves traveling through the spinal fluid (cranial nerve palsies, weakness, paresthesias, or pain),
- direct invasion into the brain or spinal tissues or interruption of blood supply to those tissues (focal findings or seizures),
- obstruction of normal cerebrospinal fluid flow pathways (headache and increased intracranial pressure), and
- interference of normal brain function (encephalopathy).

The diagnosis is made by examination of the cerebrospinal fluid or MRI of the brain and spinal cord. Initial analysis of cerebrospinal fluid demonstrates malignant cells in 50% of affected patients; however, in nearly 10% of patients with leptomeningeal involvement, the cytologic examination remains persistently negative. Increasing the number of lumbar punctures (up to six) and the volume of cerebrospinal fluid removed (10 cc per lumbar puncture) increases the yield of positive diagnosis. The protein concentration in the cerebrospinal fluid usually is elevated, there is a pleocytosis, and the glucose concentration may be low. Radiographic studies may demonstrate hydrocephalus without a mass lesion or diffuse contrast enhancement of the leptomeninges.

Without therapy, the median survival is 4 to 6 weeks, with death the result of progressive neurologic dysfunction. Often, leptomeningeal metastases are a manifestation of end-stage disease. Symptom management may be the most appropriate care. Corticosteroids and analgesics may offer limited temporary palliation. For patients who have minimal systemic disease and an acceptable performance status, treatment may improve symptoms and prolong survival. Radiation therapy to areas of bulky disease identified on neuroimaging studies and symptomatic sites, and intrathecal therapy with methotrexate, cytarabine, or thiotepa increases the median survival to 3 to 6 months. However, many patients die of advanced systemic disease. Drugs can be administered intrathecally through an Ommaya reservoir or by repeated lumbar punctures. Blockage of cerebrospinal fluid flow by tumor deposits in the subarachnoid space reduce drug delivery and increase the risk of toxicity. The major complication of intrathecal methotrexate is a necrotizing leukoencephalopathy that may develop after months of therapy in those few patients who do have prolonged survival. This devastating toxic effect is most common for patients who receive radiation therapy before or concurrently with intrathecal methotrexate.

REFERENCES

1. Central Brain Tumor Registry of the United States. Statistical Report: Primary Brain Tumors in the United States, 1998-2002. http://www.cbtrus.org/reports//2005-2006/2006 report.pdf. Accessed October 3, 2007.
2. Wrensch M, Minn Y, Chew T, et al. Epidemiology of primary brain tumors: current concepts and review of the literature. *Neuro Oncol.* 2002;4(4):278–299.
3. Souhami L, Seiferheld W, Brachman D, et al. Randomized comparison of stereotactic radiosurgery followed by conventional radiotherapy with carmustine to conventional radiotheraphy with carmustine for patients with glioblastoma multiforme: Report of Radiation Therapy Oncology Group 93–05 protocol. *Int J Radiat Oncol Biol Phys.* 2004; 60(3): 158-860.
4. Wen PY, Schiff D, Kesari S, et al. Medical management of patients with brain tumors. *J Neurooncol.* 2006;80(3):313–332.
5. Packer RJ, Ater J, Allen J et al. Carboplatin and vincristine chemotherapy for children with newly diagnosed progressive low-grade gliomas. *J Neurosurg.* 1997;86(5):747–754.
6. Keles GE, Lamborn KR, Berger MS. Low-grade hemispheric gliomas in adults: a critical review of extent of resection as a factor influencing outcome. *J Neurosurg.* 2001;95(5):735–745.
7. Van den Bent MJ, Afra D, de Witte O, et al. Long-term efficacy of early versus delayed radiotherapy for low-grade astrocytoma and oligodendroglioma in adults: the EORTC 22845 randomised trial. *Lancet.* 2005;366(9490):985–990.
8. Klein M, Heimans JJ, Aaronson NK, et al. Effect of radiotherapy and other treatment-related factors on mid-term to long-term cognitive

sequelae in low-grade gliomas: a comparative study. *Lancet.* 2002; 360(9343):1361–1368.

9. Shaw E, Arusell R, Scheithauer B, et al. Prospective randomized trial of low- versus high-dose radiation therapy in adults with supratentorial low-grade glioma: initial report of a North Central Cancer Treatment Group/Radiation Therapy Oncology Group Study. *J Clin Oncol.* 2002;20(9):2267–2276.

10. Karim AB, Maat B, Hatlevoll R, et al. A randomized trial on dose-response in radiation therapy of low-grade cerebral glioma: European Organization for Research and Treatment of Cancer (EORTC) Study 22844. *Int J Radiat Oncol Biol Phys.* 1996;36(3):549–556.

11. Shaw EG, Berkey BA, Coons SW, et al. Initial report of Radiation Therapy Oncology Group (RTOG) 9802: Prospective studies in adult low-grade glioma. *J Clin Oncol.* 2006;24(18s, pt I):63s (abstract 1500).

12. Prados MD, Scott C, Curran WJ Jr, et al. Procarbazine, lomustine, and vincristine (PCV) chemotherapy for anaplastic astrocytoma: A retrospective review of Radiation Therapy Oncology Group protocols comparing survival with carmustine or PCV adjuvant chemotherapy. *J Clin Oncol.* 1999;17(11):3389–3395.

13. Stewart LA. Chemotherapy in adult high-grade glioma: a systemic review and meta-analysis of individual patient data from 12 randomised trials. *Lancet.* 2002;359(9311):1011–1018.

14. Medical Research Council Brain Tumor Working Party. Randomized trial of procarbazine, lomustine, and vincristine in the adjuvant treatment of high-grade astrocytoma: a Medical Research Council trial. *J Clin Oncol.* 2001;19(2):509–518.

15. Yung WK, Prados MD, Yaya-Tur R, et al. Multicenter phase II trial of temozolomide in patients with anaplastic astrocytoma or anaplastic oligoastrocytoma at first relapse. Temodal Brain Tumor Group. *J Clin Oncol.* 1999;17(9):2762–2771.

16. Stupp R, Mason WP, van den Bent MJ, et al. Radiotherapy plus concomitant and adjuvant temozolomide for glioblastoma. *N Engl J Med.* 2005;352(10):987–996.

17. Walker MD, Alexander E Jr, Hunt WE, et al. Evaluation of BCNU and/or radiotherapy in the treatment of anaplastic gliomas. A cooperative clinical trial. *J Neurosurg.* 1978;49(3):333–343.

18. Hegi ME, Diserens AC, Gorlia T, et al. MGMT gene silencing and benefit from temozolomide in glioblastoma. *N Engl J Med.* 2005;352(10): 997–1003.

19. Westphal M, Hilt DC, Bortey E, et al. A phase 3 trial of local chemotherapy with biodegradable carmustine (BCNU) wafers (Gliadel wafers) in patients with primary malignant glioma. *Neuro Oncol.* 2003; 5(2):79–88.

20. Jenkins RB, Blair H, Ballman KV, et al. A t(1;19)(q10;p10) mediates the combined deletions of 1p and 19q and predicts a better prognosis of patients with oligodendroglioma. *Cancer Res.* 2006;66(20):9852–9861.

21. Hoang-Xuan K, Capelle L, Kujas M, et al. Temozolomide as initial treatment for adults with low-grade oligodendrogliomas or oligoastrocytomas and correlation with chromosome 1p deletions. *J Clin Oncol.* 2004; 22(15):3133–3138.

22. Quinn JA, Reardon DA, Friedman AH, et al. Phase II trial of temozolomide in patients with progressive low-grade glioma. *J Clin Oncol.* 2003;21(4):646–651.

23. Pace A, Vidiri A, Galiè E, et al. Temozolomide chemotherapy for progressive low-grade glioma: clinical benefits and radiological response. *Ann Oncol.* 2003;14(12):1722–1726.

24. Brada M, Viviers L, Abson C, et al. Phase II study of primary temozolomide chemotherapy in patients with WHO grade II glioma. *Ann Oncol.* 2003;14(12):1715–1721.

25. Buckner JC, Gesme D Jr, O'Fallon JR, et al. Phase II trial of procarbazine, lomustine, and vincristine as initial therapy for patients with low-grade oligodendroglioma or oligoastrocytoma: efficacy and associations with chromosomal abnormalities. *J Clin Oncol.* 2003;21(2):251–255.

26. van den Bent MJ, Taphoorn MJ, Brandes AA, et al. Phase II study of first-line chemotherapy with temozolomide in recurrent oligodendroglial tumors: the European Organization for Research and Treatment of Cancer Brain Tumor Group Study 26971. *J Clin Oncol.* 2003;21(13):2525–2528.

27. Cairncross G, Berkey B, Shaw E, et al. Phase III trial of chemotherapy plus radiotherapy compared with radiotherapy alone for pure and mixed anaplastic oligodendroglioma: Intergroup Radiation Therapy Oncology Group Trial 9402. *J Clin Oncol.* 2006;24(18):2707–2714.

28. van den Bent MJ, Carpentier AF, Brandes AA, et al. Adjuvant procarbazine, lomustine, and vincristine improves progression-free survival but not overall survival in newly diagnosed anaplastic oligodendrogliomas and oligoastrocytomas: a randomized European Organisation for Research and Treatment of Cancer phase III trial. *J Clin Oncol.* 2006;24(18):2715–2722.

29. Cairncross G, Macdonald D, Ludwin S, et al. Chemotherapy for anaplastic oligodendroglioma. National Cancer Institute of Canada Clinical Trials Group. *J Clin Oncol.* 1994; 12(10):2013–2021.

30. Gornet MK, Buckner JC, Marks RS, et al. Chemotherapy for advanced CNS ependymoma. *J Neurooncol.* 1999;45(1):61–67.

31. Go RS, Taylor BV, Kimmel DW. The natural history of asymptomatic meningiomas in Olmsted County, Minnesota. *Neurology.* 1998;51(6): 1718–1720.

32. DeAngelis LM, Seiferheld W, Schold SC, et al. Combination chemotherapy and radiotherapy for primary central nervous system lymphoma: Radiation Therapy Oncology Group Study 93–10. *J Clin Oncol.* 2002;20(24):4643–4648.

33. Batchelor T, Carson K, O'Neill A, et al. Treatment of primary CNS lymphoma with methotrexate and deferred radiotherapy: a report of NABTT 96–07. *J Clin Oncol.* 2003;21(6):1044–1049.

34. Doolittle ND, Miner ME, Siegal T, et al. Safety and efficacy of a multicenter study using intraarterial chemotherapy in conjunction with osmotic opening of the blood-brain barrier for the treatment of patients with malignant brain tumors. *Cancer.* 2000;88(3):637–647.

35. Abrey LE, DeAngelis LM, Yahalom J. Long-term survival in primary CNS lymphoma. *J Clin Oncol.* 1998;16(3):855–863.

36. Packer RJ, Cogen P, Vezina G, et al. Medulloblastoma: clinical and biological aspects. *Neuro Oncol.* 1999;1(3):232–250.

37. Patchell RA, Tibbs PA, Walsh JW, et al. A randomized trial of surgery in the treatment of single metastases to the brain. *N Engl J Med.* 1990;322(8):494–500.

38. Patchell RA, Tibbs PA, Regine WF, et al. Postoperative radiotherapy in the treatment of single metastases to the brain: a randomized trial. *JAMA.* 1998;280(17):1485–1489.

39. Andrews DW, Scott CB, Sperduto PW, et al. Whole brain radiation therapy with or without stereotactic radiosurgery boost for patients with one to three brain metastases: phase III results of the RTOG 9508 randomised trial. *Lancet.* 2004;363(9422):1665–1672.

15

LEUKEMIAS

Frederick R. Appelbaum, MD

LEARNING OBJECTIVES

After reviewing this chapter, the reader should be able to:

- Compare and contrast the molecular abnormalities associated with the various subtypes of leukemia
- Select the appropriate therapy for each subtype of leukemia
- Identify the features of leukemia that are the most accurate predictors of therapeutic outcome
- Monitor patients for minimal residual disease based on current clinical evidence

The cause of leukemia is usually unknown, but some individuals have a genetic predisposition for its development. For example, if the disease develops before age 10 in a patient with an identical twin, there is a one in five chance that the disease will develop in the unaffected twin.[1] Several single-gene leukemia syndromes have been described, including an autosomal-recessive syndrome of myelodysplasia with monosomy 7 and a familial syndrome of erythroleukemia. An autosomal-dominant syndrome of an aspirin-like platelet disorder with thrombocytopenia and a propensity for the development of acute myeloid leukemia (AML) are the results of germline mutations in the *Runx-1* (formerly *AML-1*) gene.[2] Inherent chromosome instability exists in several autosomal-recessive disorders, including Fanconi anemia, ataxia telangiectasia, and Bloom syndrome; in these cases, an increased incidence of acute leukemia has been identified.[3] An increased incidence of acute leukemia also has been identified in congenital immunodeficiency disorders, such as infantile X-linked agammaglobulinemia and Down's syndrome.

ETIOLOGY

ONCOGENIC VIRUSES

Human T-cell lymphotropic virus type I (HTLV I) is a causative agent of adult T-cell leukemia. This enveloped, single-strand RNA virus is associated with a distinct form of leukemia found in geographic clusters in southwestern Japan, the Caribbean basin, and Africa. The virus can be spread horizontally by sexual contact or through blood products

KEY POINT

- Although the cause of leukemia is unknown in most cases, the incidence of myelodysplasia and acute myeloid leukemia secondary to prior therapy is increasing as chemotherapy is used more widely to manage other diseases.

as well as vertically from mother to fetus. Although the virus is endemic in the geographic clusters mentioned, adult T-cell leukemia will develop in only 2% to 4% of patients infected with the virus. The latency period is very long, estimated at 30 years or more.[4]

RADIATION

Ionizing radiation is leukemogenic.[5] The incidences of AML, chronic myeloid leukemia (CML), and acute lymphoid leukemia (ALL) were all higher for patients who received radiation therapy for ankylosing spondylitis and for survivors of the atomic bomb blasts of Hiroshima and Nagasaki. Increased incidences of leukemia were associated with higher doses of radiation, particularly if the radiation was absorbed over a shorter period of time. Younger individuals appear more susceptible to the leukemogenic effects of radiation. Following radiation exposure, leukemia may develop within several years, and the incidence appears to peak between 5 and 10 years after exposure, regardless of patient age. The incidence of chromosome aberrations has been reported to be higher than expected for individuals living in areas of high natural background radiation, often because of radon, but a higher incidence of acute leukemia has not been found consistently.

Another concern has been the possible leukemogenic effects of extremely low-frequency, nonionizing electromagnetic fields emitted by high-energy wires and step-down transformers. Several studies have been conducted, and if there is any leukemogenic effect of such radiation, the magnitude of the effect appears to be small.

CHEMICALS

Extensive occupational exposure to benzene and benzene-containing compounds may lead to marrow damage that can eventually manifest as aplastic anemia, myelodysplasia, or AML. Benzene is widely used in industry — particularly for organic synthesis and as a solvent — and constitutes 1% of unleaded gasoline. Other associations between occupational exposure to chemicals and subsequent leukemia are not as persuasive. Most studies have found a small but consistent increase in AML among cigarette smokers.

DRUG AND THERAPY-RELATED LEUKEMIAS

Therapy with antineoplastic agents is a major identifiable cause of acute leukemia. In general, alkylating agents are the class of drugs most commonly associated with secondary leukemia.[6] Among the various alkylating agents, melphalan and the nitrosoureas appear to be particularly associated with increased risk; however, all alkylating agents are likely leukemogenic, with an increased incidence of leukemia observed after prolonged exposure and the use of dose-intense regimens. The secondary leukemias associated with alkylating agents often present initially as a myelodysplastic syndrome (MDS) before progressing to AML; they have no other distinct morphologic features and frequently exhibit cytogenetic abnormalities of chromosomes 5, 7, and, to a lesser extent, 8. These leukemias typically develop 4 to 6 years after chemotherapy and tend to have lower therapeutic response rates than de novo disease.

Patients treated with topoisomerase II inhibitors also are at risk of therapy-related leukemia. In contrast to leukemias associated with alkylating agents, disease caused by topoisomerase II inhibitors tends to have a shorter latency period (1 to 2 years), lacks a myelodysplastic phase, carries a monocytic morphology, and involves abnormalities of the long arm of chromosome 11 (band q23), or, less commonly, translocations of 21q22.[7] Patients with lymphoma who receive autologous hematopoietic cell transplant are at increased risk of leukemia, with a cumulative incidence as high as 15%. Leukemias typically associated with exposure to alkylating agents and topoisomerase II inhibitors have both been reported. Registry data demonstrate that the type and extent of therapy administered before autologous hematopoietic cell transplant is the greatest risk factor. An association between acute promyelocytic leukemia (APL) and previous treatment of psoriasis with bimolane (a dioxopiperazine derivative) has been reported.

ACUTE LEUKEMIA

BIOLOGY, CYTOGENETICS, AND MOLECULAR GENETICS

Acute leukemia is the result of a malignant process that occurs in an early hematopoietic precursor. The affected cell gives rise to progeny that fail to differentiate and continue to proliferate in an uncontrolled fashion. This results in replacement of normal bone marrow with a clonal population of immature myeloid or lymphoid cells. The subsequent loss of normal marrow function results in the common clinical signs of acute disease: anemia, infection, and bleeding. If untreated, acute leukemia results in death within several months; however, with appropriate therapy, many patients can be cured.

Acute leukemias can be categorized according to morphology, histochemistry, cell-surface markers, cytogenetics, and oncogene expression.

Morphology

The difference between AML and ALL is the most important morphologic distinction. AML cells are typically 12 to 20 μm

KEY POINT

- In most cases of acute leukemia, a clonal abnormality in chromosome number or structure can be found. These cytogenetic abnormalities have emerged as the single most important prognostic factor in acute leukemia and are indispensable in making therapeutic decisions.

in diameter with discrete nuclear chromatin, multiple nucleoli, and azurophilic granules in the cytoplasm. The French-American-British (FAB) group recognizes eight morphologic subtypes of AML (Table 15-1, Fig. 15-1). The leukemia cells in ALL are typically smaller than AML blasts and are devoid of granules. Three forms of ALL are recognized by the FAB (Table 15-1, Fig. 15-2).[8]

Histochemistry

Specific patterns of reactivity with histochemical stains are also noted for the acute leukemias. Myeloperoxidase reacts specifically with FAB types M1, M2, M3, and M4, and fails to react with lymphoid leukemias. Nonspecific esterase predominantly stains cells of monocytic lineage, specifically FAB subtypes M4 and M5. Periodic acid-Schiff staining is more variable, with the greatest reactivity seen in FAB subtype L1 disease.

Cell-surface Markers

Acute leukemias can be further categorized using monoclonal antibodies that are reactive with cell-surface antigens. In general, these antigens are identical to antigens found on normal immature hematopoietic cells and reflect the level of differentiation of the acute leukemia cells. Most cases of AML express antigens found on normal immature myeloid cells, including CD13, CD33, and CD34.[9] AML with monocytic characteristics expresses CD14. Erythroid leukemias frequently express CD36, CD71, and the blood group H antigen, whereas megakaryocytic leukemias express CD41a and CD61. Although the antigens detected on leukemic blasts generally represent antigens found on normal immature hematopoietic cells, abnormal combinations frequently are identified on leukemic blasts. Of the cases of AML, 10% to 20% also express antigens usually restricted to B- or T-cell lineages. Expression of lymphoid antigens by AML cells does not appear to influence either the natural history or therapeutic response of these leukemias.

Approximately 60% of ALLs express common ALL antigen (CALLA or CD10), a glycoprotein normally found on early B lymphocytes and on other nonhematopoietic tissue.[10] Most cases of CALLA-positive ALL are thought to represent an early pre–B-cell (or pro-B) differentiation state. Approximately 20% of CALLA-positive ALL cases have intracytoplasmic immunoglobulin; therefore, they are called

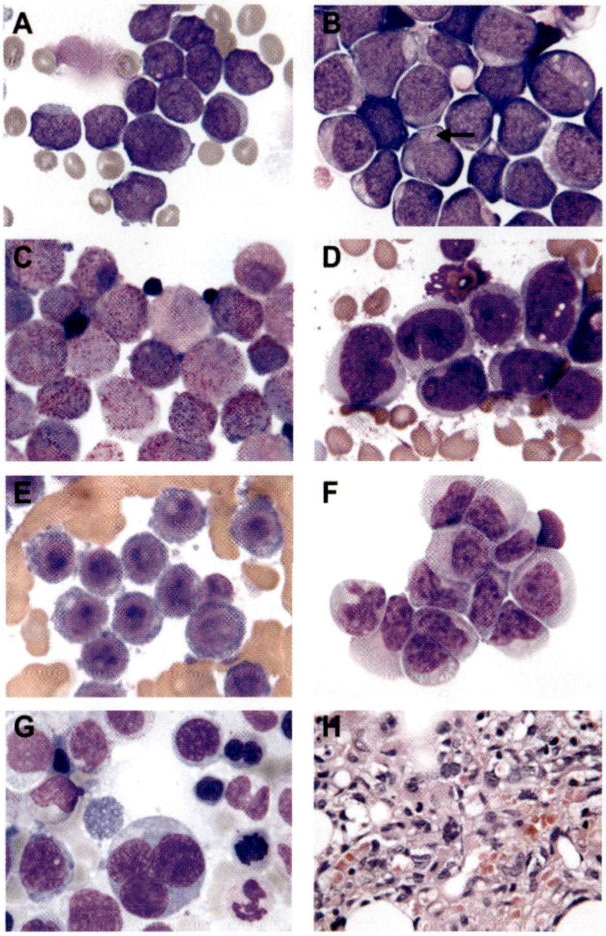

FIG. 15-1 The morphologic spectrum of the acute myeloid leukemias (AML) in bone marrow aspirates (A-G) and a marrow biopsy (H).

(A) Acute myeloblastic leukemia with minimal (French-American-British [FAB] AML-MI) or no (FAB AML-MO) maturation. The cells are myeloblasts with dispersed chromatin and variable amounts of agranular cytoplasm. Some display medium-sized, poorly defined nucleoli. (B) Acute myeloblastic leukemia with maturation (FAB AML-M2). Some of the blasts contain azurophilic granules, and there are promyelocytes. More mature neutrophils were present in other fields. Note the Auer rod (arrow). (C) Acute promyelocytic leukemia (FAB AML-M3). All of these cells are promyelocytes containing coarse cytoplasmic granules which sometimes obscure the nuclei. (D) Acute myelomonocytic leukemia (FAB AML-M4). Promonocytes with indented nuclei are present with myeloblasts. The dense nuclear staining is unusual. (E) Acute monoblastic leukemia (FAB AML-M5a). These characteristic monoblasts have round nuclei with delicate chromatin and prominent nucleoli. Cytoplasm is abundant. Nonspecific esterase staining was intense (not shown). (F) Acute monocytic leukemia (FAB AML-M5b). Most of the cells in this field are promonocytes. Monoblasts and an abnormal monocyte also are present. (G) Acute erythroid leukemia (FAB AML-M6). Dysplastic multinucleated erythroid precursors with megaloblastoid nuclei are present. (H) Acute megakaryoblastic leukemia (FAB AML-M7). In this marrow biopsy, there are large and small blasts as well as atypical megakaryocytes.

TABLE 15-1 French-American-British (FAB) Classification of Acute Leukemias

Subtype	Morphology	Histochemistry: Myeloperoxidase	Histochemistry: Nonspecific Esterase	Histochemistry: PAS	Monoclonal Reactivity	Cytogenetic Abnormalities
M0, acute undifferentiated leukemia	Uniform, very undifferentiated	–	–	–	For subtypes M0-M5b, approximately 90% of cases will react with at least one of the following monoclonal antibodies: Anti-CD13, Anti-CD14, Anti-CD33, Anti-CD34	Various
M1, acute myeloid leukemia with minimal differentiation	Very undifferentiated, few various azurophilic granules	+/–	+/–	–		Various
M2, acute myeloid leukemia with differentiation	Granulated blasts predominate; auer rods may be seen	+++	+/–	+		Various
M3, acute promyelocytic leukemia	Hypergranular promyelocytes predominate	+++	+	+		t(15;17)
M4, acute myelomonocytic leukemia	Both monoblasts and myeloblasts present	++	+++	++		various inv/del(16)
M4E	Like M4 but with eosinophils					
M5, acute monocytic leukemia	Monoblasts predominate	+/–	+++	++		t(9;11), t(11q23)
M5a	> 80% monoblasts					
M5b	> 20% promonocytes					
M6, acute erythroleukemia	Erythroblasts and megaloblastic red cell precursors seen	–	–	++	Antiglycophorin, antispectrin	5/del(5q), 7/del(7q)
M7, acute megakaryocytic leukemia	Undifferentiated blasts	–	+/–	+	Antiplatelet GpIIb/IIIa	Various, t(1;22)
L1, acute lymphoid leukemia, childhood variant	Small, uniform blasts, nucleoli indistinct	–	–	+++	60% react with anti-CD10 (anti-CALLA)	Various
L2, acute lymphoid leukemia, adult variant	Larger, more irregular nucleoli present	–	–	++	20% react with anti-CD5, anti-CD3, or anti-CD2 (anti-T cell)	Various
L3, Burkitt-like acute lymphoid leukemia	Large with strongly basophilic cytoplasm and vacuoles	–	–	–	Antisurface immunoglobulin, anti-CD19, anti-CD20	t(8;14)

Abbreviations: PAS, periodic acid-Schiff; CALLA, common ALL antigen.
Reprinted with permission from Cheson BC, ed. Oncology MKSAP, 2nd ed. Philadelphia, Pa: American College of Physicians; 1999:239.

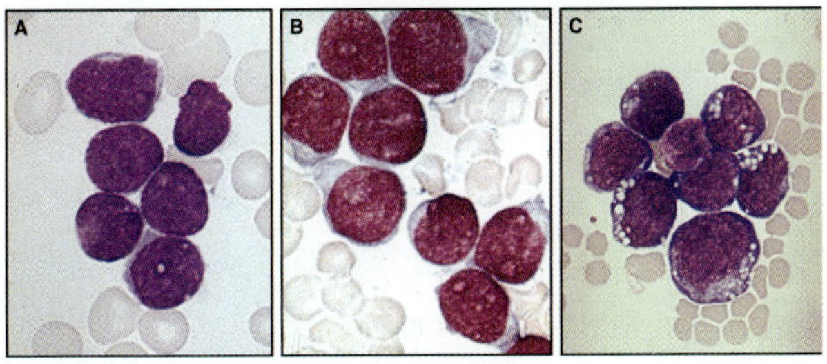

FIG. 15-2 Morphology of acute lymphoblastic leukemia (ALL) in adults.

A. ALL childhood variant. The cells are small, homogeneous, with inconspicuous nucleoli (FAB-L1). B. ALL adult variant. The cells are pleomorphic with some cytoplasm and prominent nucleoli (FAB-L2). C. Burkitt-like leukemia. The cells are homogeneous with multiple nucleoli, deep blue cytoplasm and sharply defined vacuoles (FAB-L3).

pre–B-cell ALL (as opposed to pro-B-cell). Another 5% express surface immunoglobulin and are termed B-cell ALL. T-cell antigens are found on 20% of ALL cases, whereas the remaining 20% express neither CALLA nor T-cell antigens, but they do express the B-cell marker CD19. In 25% of ALL cases, myeloid antigens can be detected. Although some studies suggest that myeloid antigens are a negative prognostic factor, the bulk of evidence suggests no independent significance for their presence. Discordant combinations of antigens on leukemic blasts allow detection of small numbers of blasts in a morphologically normal marrow using multidimensional flow cytometry. Studies suggest that presence of residual disease detected by flow cytometry following induction chemotherapy can predict shorter remission durations for both AML and ALL.

Cytogenetics and Molecular Biology

In most cases of acute leukemia, an acquired abnormality in chromosome number or structure is found. These abnormalities are clonal, involving essentially all of the malignant cells, and are not found in normal cells. Certain abnormalities are seen repeatedly and are associated with distinct morphologic or clinical subtypes of leukemia. They may be simply the result of the gain or loss of a whole chromosome, but more often include translocations, deletions, or inversions (*See Chapter 2, "Molecular Genetics" for more information*).

Certain chromosome abnormalities are associated with specific syndromes in AML. APL (FAB subtype M3) accounts for approximately 8% of AML cases and virtually always has a translocation involving the promyelocytic leukemia (*PML*) gene on chromosome 15 and the retinoic acid receptor alpha gene (*RAR-alpha*) on chromosome 17, t(15;17)(q22;q11-12). The resultant abnormal fusion protein acts as a dominant negative inhibitor of normal *PML* and *RAR-alpha* function.[11] The fusion protein of *PML* and *RAR-alpha* appears to recruit nuclear corepressors and histone deacetylase, inhibiting the transcription of genes needed for myeloid differentiation. All-trans retinoic acid binds to the fusion protein, changing its configuration and thereby allowing release of the nuclear corepressor and histone deacetylase complexes, thus permitting resumption of transcription. Acute myelomonocytic leukemia with abnormal eosinophilia is associated with an inversion in chromosome 16 (inv[16][q13q22]), and some patients with M2 AML have a translocation between chromosomes 8 and 21, t(8;21)(q22;q22). These two translocations result in abnormalities in a transcription factor made up of core-binding factors (CBF) alpha or beta. t(8;21) results in fusion of the CBF-alpha subunit on chromosome 21 with the *MTG8* (formerly *ETO*) gene on chromosome 8, whereas inv(16) results in fusion of CBF-beta on the q arm of chromosome 16 with MYH11 on the p arm. t(8;21) and inv(16) each account for 5% to 8% of AML cases, are more prominent among younger patients, and have a relatively favorable prognosis.[12] Some cases of t(8;21) or inv(16) AML also have mutations in the receptor tyrosine kinase gene *KIT*; such cases do not have as favorable an outcome.[13] Translocations involving the *MLL* gene located at 11q23 and several partners constitute approximately 7% of adult AML cases.[14] Trisomy 8 is seen in approximately 9% of AML cases and carries an intermediate prognosis. Partial or full deletions of chromosomes 5 and 7 each account for 6% to 8% of AML cases. These abnormalities are more common in older patients with AML and in cases associated with prior exposure to alkylating agents, and they typically indicate poor prognosis.

Nonrandom mutations undetectable by routine cytogenetics also have been identified in AML cases. FLT3 is a receptor tyrosine kinase, and activating mutations in *FLT3* have been found in 20% to 40% of cases. These mutations may be internal tandem repeats (15% to 30%) or point mutations (5% to 10%), are somewhat more common in older patients, and are associated with a higher blast count at diagnosis as well as a less favorable response to treatment.[15] Mutations in H-ras, K-ras, or N-ras — cellular proteins involved with signal transduction — are seen in 10% to 15% of AML cases, whereas *CEBPA* — a gene encoding a leucine zipper transcription factor — is mutated in 4% to 15% of AML cases and may be associated with a favorable prognosis. Mutations in the nucleophosmin gene (*NPM1*) have been identified in 20% to 30% of AML cases, usually those with a normal karyotype, and appear to be associated with a favorable clinical outcome.[16]

Between 20% and 30% of adults with ALL have the Philadelphia (Ph) chromosome. The Ph chromosome now is understood to result from a specific translocation, t(9;22)(q34;q11), which involves the movement of most of the *ABL* proto-oncogene from chromosome 9 adjacent to the 5' portion of the *BCR* gene on chromosome 22. The breakpoint on chromosome 9 is highly variable and occurs anywhere over a region of 200 kilobase or more, usually

Table 15-2 World Health Organization (WHO) Classification of Acute Leukemia with Corresponding FAB Classification Subtypes

WHO Classification	Usual FAB Subtypes
Precursor lymphoblastic leukemia/lymphoblastic lymphoma	
Precursor B-cell acute lymphoblastic leukemia/lymphoblastic lymphoma	L1, L2
Precursor T-cell lymphoblastic leukemia/lymphoblastic lymphoma	L1, L2
Burkitt's lymphoma/leukemia	
Endemic Burkitt's lymphoma/leukemia	L3
Sporadic Burkitt's lymphoma/leukemia	L3
Immunodeficiency-associated Burkitt's lymphoma/leukemia	L3
AML with recurrent genetic abnormalities	
AML with t(8;21)(q22;q22); AML1-ETO	M2, M1
AML with abnormal marrow eosinophilia and inv(16)(p13q22) or t(16;16)(p13q22): CBFβ-MYH11	M4Eo, M4
Acute promyelocytic leukemia with t(15;17)(q22;q12); PML-RARα	M3
AML with 11q23 abnormalities; MLL rearrangements	M5, M4
AML with multilineage dysplasia	
Following a myelodysplastic syndrome of myeloproliferative disorder or without antecedent myelodysplastic syndrome	M2, M4
AML and myelodysplastic syndrome, therapy related	
Alkylating agent-related	M2, M4
Topoisomerase type II inhibitor-related	M5, M4, M2
Other types	
AML not otherwise categorized	
Acute myeloid leukemia without maturation	M0
Acute myeloid leukemia minimally differentiated	M1
Acute myeloid leukemia with maturation	M2
Acute promyelocytic leukemia	M3
Acute myelomonocytic leukemia	M4
Acute monoblastic leukemia	M5
Acute erythroid leukemia	M6
Acute megakaryoblastic leukemia	M7
Acute basophilic leukemia	—
Acute panmyelosis with myelofibrosis	M7
Myeloid sarcoma	—

Abbreviations: RARα, retinoic acid-receptor alpha; CBFB, core-binding factor beta FAB, French-American-British; AML, acute myeloid leukemia.

within the intron 5' of exon 2. In contrast, the breakpoints in the *BCR* gene on chromosome 22 occur within two regions, one termed the major breakpoint cluster region (M-bcr), and the other the minor breakpoint cluster region (m-bcr). Rearrangements within the M-bcr are transcribed into a chimeric messenger RNA, which produces a hybrid 210-kilodalton protein ($p210^{Bcr\text{-}Abl}$), whereas breaks within the m-bcr express a chimeric messenger RNA that gives rise to a smaller 190-kilodalton protein ($p190^{Bcr\text{-}Abl}$). In chronic myelogenous leukemia (CML), virtually all breakpoints are mapped to the M-bcr, which has been termed the CML-type Ph chromosome. Conversely, in ALL, breakpoints are found within both the M-bcr and m-bcr, and those within the m-bcr are termed the ALL-type Ph chromosome.[17] The relative frequency of the two breakpoints in adult ALL has varied among studies, but overall, the two seem to be represented with equal frequency. Ph-positive ALL with the CML-type of *BCR-ABL* translocation is not simply the lymphoid blast crisis phase of CML. Patients with this disease rarely have a long prediagnostic prodrome and do not routinely have marked splenomegaly; most importantly, when treated with conventional chemotherapy, disease does not enter a Ph-positive chronic phase but instead goes into Ph-negative complete remission. In some studies, the duration of disease-free survival has been found to be shorter for patients with the ALL-type breakpoint than for patients with the CML-type breakpoint, but this has not been found in all studies.[18]

The other most common change observed in patients with ALL is t(12;21), evident in 25% of children with pre–B-cell ALL, which identifies a subgroup of patients with a favorable outcome.[19] t(12;21) involves the genes *TEL* and

Runx1 and, as with AML-associated t(8;21), is thought to result in an abnormal CBF transcription factor. Other abnormalities seen in B-cell ALL include t(8;14) and t(8;22), which result in translocation of the *MYC* gene on chromosome 8, with the immunoglobin enhance response genes on chromosomes 14 or 22, and translocations involving 11q23. T-cell ALLs often have translocations involving chromosomes 7 or 14 at T-cell receptor enhancer gene sites. In approximately 20% of ALL cases, the leukemic cells gain chromosomes in a distinct pattern, often reaching an average of 50 to 60 chromosomes per cell. These hyperdiploid leukemias generally have a favorable prognosis.

In an effort to incorporate etiologic, immunophenotypic, and cytogenetic characteristics, as well as the more traditional morphologic features, into the categorization of acute leukemia, the World Heath Organization (WHO) has adopted the classification schema shown in Table 15-2.[20]

CLINICAL FEATURES

The signs and symptoms of acute leukemia are a result of decreased normal hematopoiesis and infiltration of normal organs by leukemic blasts. Thus, most patients present with anemia and thrombocytopenia. The white blood cell count may be elevated, normal, or low, but most patients will have granulocytopenia, and one-third will present with signs of substantial or life-threatening infection.

In addition to suppressing normal marrow function, leukemic cells may infiltrate normal organs. This process occurs more frequently in ALL than in AML. In ALL, approximately 50% of patients may have enlarged lymph nodes, hepatomegaly, or splenomegaly. Bone pain is commonly reported by patients who have acute disease, particularly younger patients with ALL. Leukemic cells may infiltrate the skin, resulting in a raised, nonpruritic rash (leukemia cutis). Approximately 5% of patients with ALL and a smaller percentage of patients with AML will have involvement of the central nervous system (CNS) at the time of diagnosis; this confers a worse prognosis.

TREATMENT FOR AML

INDUCTION

For almost 3 decades, standard remission induction therapy for AML has been a combination of 7 days of cytarabine at 100 to 200 mg/m^2 daily with 3 days of daunorubicin at 45 to 60 mg/m^2 daily. With this combination, complete remission is achieved for approximately 60% to 75% of patients. Studies designed to improve on these results have involved changes in the dose of cytarabine, alternatives to the use of daunorubicin, the addition of other chemotherapy drugs to the combination, and the use of hematopoietic growth factors.

Investigators in two large randomized trials have asked whether high-dose cytarabine offers an advantage compared with conventional-dose cytarabine when used in combination with daunorubicin for remission induction.[21,22] In both studies, the complete remission rates were not improved with the use of the high-dose regimen. In addition, the higher doses of cytarabine were consistently associated with more toxicity, usually neurotoxicity. Risk factors for neurotoxicity include patient age and the presence of renal insufficiency. In both of these randomized studies, despite the lack of improvement in complete response rate, disease-free survival was longer in the high-dose arms. Neither study attempted to equalize the total dose of cytarabine given throughout therapy; therefore, although some patients may benefit from exposure to higher total doses of cytarabine, there is no evidence that this exposure must occur during induction.

KEY POINTS

- Optimal induction therapy in AML involves the use of an anthracycline and cytarabine.
- The outcome is favorable for patients with leukemias characterized by inv(16) or t(8;21); once remission is achieved, they should be treated with repetitive cycles of consolidation therapy that involves moderate-dose or high-dose cytarabine.
- Younger patients with AML characterized by poor-risk cytogenetic features, such as abnormalities of chromosomes 5 or 7, are best treated with allogeneic transplantation if an appropriate donor can be found.
- The prognosis is poor for patients with recurrent AML, and the likelihood of achieving a second remission is predicted by the length of the first remission. Because of this poor outcome, efforts should be made to perform transplantation for all patients with recurrent AML who are appropriate candidates.

Idarubicin and mitoxantrone have been studied as possible alternatives to daunorubicin. In several studies, idarubicin at a daily dose of 10 to 13 mg/m^2 for 3 days was compared with daunorubicin at 45 mg/m^2 for 3 days, both in combination with standard-dose cytarabine. The results of these studies tended to favor idarubicin. For example, the findings of one large randomized study demonstrated a complete response rate of 67% for patients treated with idarubicin compared with 58% for patients treated with daunorubicin.[23] An important shortcoming of these studies was that the two anthracyclines were not administered at equally toxic — and therefore, perhaps, equally potent — doses. Evidence for this fact comes from the finding that the period of myelosuppression, particularly during consolidation chemotherapy, was much longer in the idarubicin arm. At present, idarubicin can be considered at least equivalent to daunorubicin.

Mitoxantrone is an anthraquinone rather than an anthracycline. In several studies, standard-dose cytarabine plus mitoxantrone at a daily dose of 12 mg/m^2 for 3 days has been compared with cytarabine plus daunorubicin at 45 mg/m^2 daily for 3 days. Overall, the complete response rates for the two regimens were similar; additionally, there were no significant differences in either the incidence or the severity of toxicities between the regimens. The findings of a three-arm study in which daunorubicin, idarubicin, and mitoxantrone were compared as part of the induction regimen for older patients demonstrated no advantage for any arm.[24] Thus, there is little evidence to strongly favor the use of idarubicin, daunorubicin, or mitoxantrone in combination with cytarabine during remission induction of AML.

Etoposide is active in AML and has a different mechanism of action than either cytarabine or the anthracyclines. Therefore, the Australian Leukemia Study Group conducted a randomized trial to determine whether the addition of etoposide at 75 mg/m^2 daily for 7 days to a standard combination of cytarabine plus daunorubicin improved results. In that study, the addition of etoposide did not improve the overall complete remission rate, nor did it affect overall survival. The patients randomly assigned to receive etoposide did have a small but significant improvement in the duration of remission.[25]

For patients older than age 60, clinical trials have been designed to discover induction regimens that would result in less toxicity and maintenance of antileukemic effects. The results of earlier studies suggested that lowering the dose of daunorubicin from 60 mg/m^2 to either 45 or 30 mg/m^2 diminished the incidence of severe toxicities and toxicity-related deaths. This decrease in toxicity more than overcame any decrease in the antileukemic effects from the attenuated dose of the anthracycline. More recently, investigators have explored alternatives to standard-dose cytarabine. In one study, low-dose cytarabine (20 mg daily) was compared with a standard dose of the drug (200 mg/m^2) and was found to result in less toxicity; however, there was a trend toward fewer complete responses, and so there was no improvement in overall survival.[26]

At least 10 large randomized trials have evaluated the effect of the addition of granulocyte colony-stimulating factor (G-CSF) or granulocyte macrophage colony-stimulating factor (GM-CSF) on remission induction in AML. Most of these studies included older patients to whom growth factor was given after induction chemotherapy in an effort to shorten the period of myelosuppression. In virtually all of the studies, the administration of growth factor was associated with a shorter period of granulocytopenia (usually by 4 or 5 days), as well as with fewer days of fever and less antibiotic use. However, the use of myeloid growth factors did not improve the complete response rate or prolong overall survival in most of the studies.[27,28]

CHEMOTHERAPY AFTER REMISSION

The findings of large randomized studies have demonstrated that chemotherapy administered after remission improves both disease-free survival and overall survival.[29] These results are less definitive in terms of which agents are most effective and which dose and schedule are most appropriate. For this discussion, consolidation chemotherapy, late intensification, and maintenance chemotherapy have the following definitions.

- Consolidation chemotherapy: treatment given shortly after induction, in doses sufficient to produce severe myelosuppression, usually requiring hospitalization
- Late intensification: chemotherapy at doses similar to the doses used for consolidation but given after a delay of 6 to 12 months
- Maintenance chemotherapy: chemotherapy administered after remission and given at doses that do not require hospitalization

If no therapy is administered after induction, the median duration of remission is short, and the disease will likely relapse. In a randomized study, the median duration of remission was 4 months for patients who received no therapy after remission, and disease relapsed for all patients.[29] Thus, some form of therapy is clearly indicated after remission. Various studies have explored the use of two to four courses of consolidation therapy using daunomycin and cytarabine with or without additional agents at doses similar to induction doses. Results of these studies have consistently shown a median disease-free survival of approximately 1 year and a median overall survival of 18 months to 2 years. This approach is curative for approximately 15% to 20% of patients in whom complete remission is achieved.[30]

In several studies, consolidation chemotherapy involving high-dose cytarabine alone or in combination with daunomycin was compared with consolidation therapy using conventional-dose cytarabine with or without daunomycin. In one large randomized trial, a single cycle of high-dose cytarabine given at 2 g/m^2 every 12 hours for 6 days with daunomycin offered no apparent advantage compared with conventional-dose cytarabine with daunorubicin. However, patients who received two cycles of high-dose cytarabine appeared to have a marginal benefit.[21] The findings of a second large randomized study suggested that four cycles of high-dose cytarabine administered at 3 g/m^2 every 12 hours on days 1, 3, and 5 yielded a superior outcome compared with less intensive cytarabine therapy given at either 200 or 400 mg/m^2 by continuous infusion for 5 days.[31] This is an intense treatment, and as many as 50% of patients cannot continue therapy on a regular schedule. Nonetheless, for younger patients with AML who are not candidates for transplantation, treatment with multiple cycles of some form of high-dose cytarabine probably represents the most effective form of consolidation therapy available.[32]

Other studies have evaluated consolidation regimens that involve alternative chemotherapy agents that work through different mechanisms. The results of most of these studies have been published only as limited pilot trials, precluding any real conclusions. However, findings from studies that have been conducted as in one large randomized trial have been negative. For example, substituting m-AMSA and 5-azacitidine for daunorubicin and cytarabine during one consolidation cycle offered no advantage.[33]

The findings of prospective randomized trials have shown that low-dose maintenance chemotherapy (given as cytarabine and thioguanine alone or in combination with vincristine and prednisone) prolongs the duration of remission and overall survival for adults with AML. However, these studies enrolled patients who received less intense consolidation chemotherapy than is standard today; thus, the role of low-dose maintenance chemotherapy for patients receiving intensive consolidation chemotherapy is unknown. A similar situation exists concerning the role of late-intensification chemotherapy. In one large randomized study, late intensification with a combination of 6-mercaptopurine, methotrexate, prednisone, and vincristine (POMP) clearly prolonged both disease-free and overall survival for adults with AML.[34] However, as with low-dose maintenance therapy, patients enrolled in this trial were treated with only moderate-dose consolidation chemotherapy. The role of late intensification with POMP remains in question.

Leukemic recurrence occurs in the CNS in less than 10% of adults with AML. The results of randomized trials have not found evidence that CNS prophylaxis improves either disease-free or overall survival for adults with AML, nor is there a role for CNS surveillance for asymptomatic patients.

RISK FACTORS

Several factors — including age, white blood cell count at diagnosis, and prior hematologic abnormalities — correlate with the probability of an initial complete remission and with the duration of that remission (Table 15-3). Clonal cytogenetic abnormalities can be detected in more than 60% of AML cases and are the strongest single predictive factors. Abnormalities involving 16q22, t(8;21), and t(15;17) (the translocation associated with APL) are associated with high remission rates and generally with long survival duration. Loss or partial deletion of chromosomes 5 or 7 and complex abnormalities are associated with low remission rates and with short remission durations (Table 15-4, Fig. 15-3).[35,36] Mutations in *FLT3* appear to predict poor outcome; mutations in *NPM1* appear to indicate the opposite. The importance of immunophenotype on outcome is uncertain. The results of some studies suggest that expression of T-cell markers, particularly CD2, may indicate a favorable outcome and that expression of the stem cell marker CD34 may be unfavorable. However, these associations have not been consistently confirmed in other studies. Several studies report that increased expression of the multidrug resistance gene (*MDR-1*) is associated with a lower rate of complete remission, as well as with shortened duration of remission. Many of these risk factors are linked; for example, increased expression of *MDR-1* tends to occur in older individuals with background dysplasia. Thus, not all of these factors have independent prognostic importance.

CHEMOTHERAPY FOR RECURRENT DISEASE

Patients with recurrent AML can be categorized in a number of ways. Most studies describe patients as experiencing the following:

- primary induction failure if initial induction therapy failed,
- early relapse if the disease recurs within 6 months after diagnosis,
- late relapse if the first complete remission lasts longer than 18 months, and
- refractory disease if the last attempt at reinduction failed.

In general, the prognosis is worse for patients with refractory disease and for patients who have early relapse — regardless of therapy administered — than it is for patients who experience a late relapse. Most chemotherapy studies involving recurrent AML are nonrandomized reports, and many of the suggested differences in outcome are likely influenced as much by patient selection as by differences in therapy.

In the past, standard chemotherapy for recurrent disease was retreatment with daunorubicin and cytarabine. Overall, this approach yields a second complete remission for

Table 15-3 Prognosis for Acute Myeloid Leukemia

	Unfavorable	Favorable
Age	Older	Younger
White blood cell count at diagnosis	High	Low
Multidrug resistance gene (*MDR-1*)	Present	Absent
Previous hematologic disorder	Myelodysplasia	None
Chromosome abnormalities	Chromosome 5, chromosome 7, t(11q23)	t(8;21)(q22;q22), 16q22, t(15;17)(q22;q11–q12)

Modified with permission from Cheson BC, ed. Oncology MKSAP, 2nd ed. Philadelphia, Pa: American College of Physicians; 1999:243.

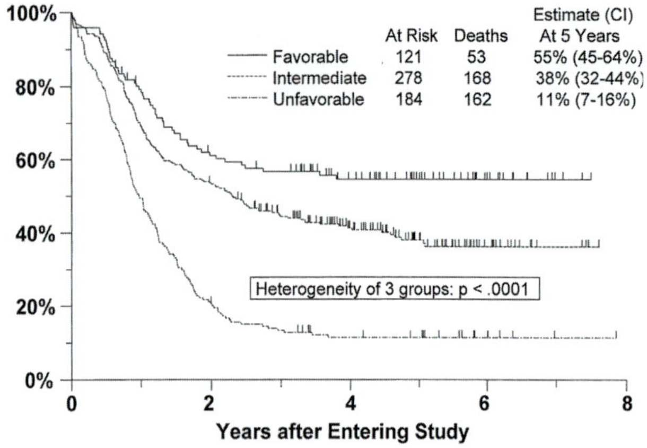

FIG. 15-3 Survival in adult AML according to cytogenetic risk group[36]

approximately 30% to 50% of patients, with an average remission duration of 6 months. If the initial remission was longer (more than 18 months), the rate of complete remission with retreatment is much higher — 64% in one study — and the average duration of second remission tends to be longer (approximately 8 months).[37] Occasionally, patients retreated with daunorubicin and cytarabine may experience complete remission for periods beyond 3 years; rarely, a patient may be cured. If the first complete remission is shorter than 18 months, the chance of successful repeat induction is lower, (averaging 25%) and the average duration of the second remission is only 3 months.

High-dose cytarabine has been studied for management of recurrent AML. Although findings from single-institution pilot studies showed complete response rates as high as 65%, in large cooperative group studies, the complete response rate has been only 40% to 45% and is not appreciably different from what one might expect from conventional-dose cytarabine plus daunomycin. In randomized trials, the addition of either an anthracycline or an anthraquinone to high-dose cytarabine has led to marginally higher complete response rates but has yielded no improvement in overall survival. High-dose cytarabine is unique in that it can, on occasion, result in a complete response for patients with disease refractory to conventional-dose cytarabine.

Mitoxantrone, etoposide, topotecan, and gemtuzumab ozogamicin are all active for recurrent disease. The best approach depends on the patient's clinical characteristics and previous therapy. Patients with a long initial remission should be retreated with intensive induction with either an anthracycline and cytarabine or cytarabine in high doses. Patients with a short first remission are candidates for alternative regimens, such as mitoxantrone plus etoposide. Gemtuzumab ozogamicin is a conjugate composed of a humanized anti-CD33 antibody linked to the antitumor antibiotic calicheamicin. The agent results in complete response for 30% of patients treated for an initial recurrence of AML.[38] Severe myelosuppression is found in all patients treated with gemtuzumab, and the results of liver function tests are elevated for approximately 15%. However, because of the targeted nature of therapy, less mucositis and sepsis are seen, making the drug a reasonable option for patients who are not candidates for intensive therapy. Patients with slowly evolving disease, particularly if they are older or infirm, can sometimes have a reasonable quality of life if treated with supportive care alone; rapid, intensive induction is not always warranted for this population.

Although some patients with recurrent AML may derive long-term benefit from chemotherapy, most do not, and hematopoietic cell transplantation appears to offer such patients a better chance for long-term survival.

HEMATOPOIETIC CELL TRANSPLANTATION

High-dose chemotherapy with or without radiation followed by hematopoietic cell transplantation has become increasingly popular as a therapy for AML. Generic issues of transplantation are discussed in Chapter 17. Specific issues concerning transplantation for AML are discussed here, and

Table 15-4 Cytogenetics and Treatment Outcome in Acute Myeloid Leukemia

Risk Group	Incidence (%)	Complete Response Rate (%)	5-year Survival (%)
Favorable Inv(16) T(8;21), t(15;17)	20	85	60
Intermediate Normal, +8	45	76	30
Unfavorable Del 5q, -5 Del 7q, -7 Complex, 11q23	30	55	12

focus on the timing of transplantation, the source of stem cells, the choice of preparative regimen, and the form of prophylaxis used for graft-versus-host disease.

Timing

Unless otherwise noted, the following discussion of timing concerns transplants between human leukocyte antigen (HLA)-identical siblings. The outcome of allogeneic marrow transplantation depends on the stage of AML at the time of transplant. The best results with transplantation can be expected when it is done during the first complete remission, both because the probability of leukemic relapse is lowest in this group and also because patients are better able to tolerate the transplant procedure. Although results vary slightly, most centers report a disease-free survival rate of 50% to 65% at 5 years. Patients who receive transplants while disease is in an untreated first relapse or in a second remission do not fare as well, with approximately 30% alive and disease-free at 5 years; the outcome is poorest for patients who receive transplants for primary induction failure or for refractory relapse, with 10% to 20% remaining leukemia-free at 5 years.[39]

For almost every patient category, leukemia recurrence is the most common cause of treatment failure, with recurrence rates of 25% for transplantation during first remission, 40% for transplantation during the first relapse or second remission, and more than 50% for transplantation during a refractory relapse. Other frequent causes of death include idiopathic interstitial pneumonia, with an overall mortality rate of approximately 5%; graft-versus-host disease and infection, each with a mortality rate of 5% to 10%; and veno-occlusive disease of the liver, with a mortality rate of approximately 3%.

If complete remission is not achieved with initial induction chemotherapy and the patient has an HLA-identical sibling, marrow transplantation should be strongly considered, because 10% to 15% of such patients can become long-term survivors, whereas second-line chemotherapy offers almost no chance of cure. For those patients in whom a first remission is achieved, the choice of continuing with chemotherapy or having allogeneic transplantation is more difficult. Several prospective comparisons have been published in which allogeneic transplantation for patients with HLA-matched siblings was compared with chemotherapy or autologous transplantation for patients without such a sibling. A meta-analysis of studies conducted since 1995 shows that overall survival is improved with allogeneic hematopoietic cell transplantation in first remission compared with chemotherapy or autologous transplantation, with a hazard ratio of 1.15. This benefit was particularly noted for patients with poor-risk cytogenetics and was not seen for those with favorable-risk cytogenetics.[40]

The results of marrow transplantation in untreated first relapse and second remission are similar, particularly if transplantation is performed during early first relapse. Because a second remission is achieved in approximately 50% of patients with AML who receive chemotherapy and complications precluding subsequent transplantation occur in some of those patients, there appears to be little advantage to administering additional chemotherapy or attempting to achieve a second remission before marrow transplantation if relapse is detected early and a transplant can be performed promptly.

Source of Stem Cells

The source of hematopoietic stem cells for transplantation can be defined in two ways: by their anatomic source and by the relationship of the donor and recipient. In normal circumstances, the highest concentration of hematopoietic stem cells is found in the marrow; therefore, marrow traditionally has been the source of stem cells for transplantation. Hematopoietic stem cells also circulate in the peripheral blood, albeit at low concentrations. However, following administration of hematopoietic growth factors, such as G–CSF or GM-CSF, and during recovery from myelosuppressive chemotherapy, the concentration of stem cells in the peripheral blood increases considerably. The use of such mobilized stem cells from the peripheral blood has largely replaced marrow as the source of stem cells for autologous transplantation because of the ease of collection as well as the fact that their use is associated with quicker engraftment. However, because collections of stem cells in the peripheral blood contain more T cells than marrow, and, in animal models, increasing numbers of T cells in the stem cell inoculum correlate with more graft-versus-host disease, clinicians were initially reluctant to use mobilized peripheral blood stem cells for allogeneic transplantation. Nonetheless, the results of pilot studies suggested that allogeneic peripheral blood stem cell transplantation was possible, and now the findings of three large randomized trials have shown that, compared with marrow, G–CSF-mobilized peripheral blood leads to more rapid engraftment, no increase in acute graft-versus-host disease, and a tendency toward improved overall survival.[41–43]

Approximately 1% of patients will have an identical twin. Except for these rare cases, the preferred source of stem cells for transplantation in AML is from an HLA-identical sibling, which can be found in approximately 35% of cases. Among matched-sibling donors, a less favorable outcome has been associated with parous female donors, largely because of an increased incidence of graft-versus-host disease. This finding is consistent with the view that such donors become sensitized during pregnancy to minor histocompatibility antigens. If patients are seronegative for cytomegalovirus, like donors should be selected, if possible.

For the majority of patients, an HLA-matched donor sibling cannot be found. In approximately 1% of cases, a family member, such as a parent or a child who is an HLA phenotypic but not genotypic match, can be identified. Results of transplants from such donors are virtually identical to the results from genotypically matched donors. In perhaps 2% to 3% of cases, a family member can be identified who is matched with the patient for one complete haplotype but mismatched on the second haplotype for a single antigen. With such donors, there is a slight increase in the incidence of graft rejection and a definite increase in the incidence of graft-versus-host disease. However, the incidence of leukemic relapse is lower, and overall survival with single-antigen mismatched donors is similar to the survival associated with HLA-matched donors. Thus, the indications for transplantation using a donor who is a family member with one mismatched antigen are the same as when using a matched-sibling donor. Use of a family member donor mismatched for two or three loci is associated with a poor overall outcome, principally because of a much higher incidence of graft-versus-host disease, as well as a higher incidence of graft failure or rejection. Thus, the use of donors with two or three mismatched antigens is restricted to younger patients who have no other options for cure.

The use of unrelated, HLA-matched donors has rapidly increased, particularly since the formation of the National Marrow Donor Program. The use of matched, unrelated donors is associated with an increased incidence of graft-versus-host disease and infectious complications, but a lower incidence of disease recurrence. In most studies, the result has been a slightly poorer outcome than the outcome associated with completely matched family-member donors; however, using matched, unrelated donors yields a better outcome than that associated with the use of a family member with two or three mismatched antigens. In the experience of most transplant centers, a period of 2 to 4 months is necessary to identify a matched, unrelated donor and to carry out such transplants. Because of the increased risks associated with unrelated donor transplants, most experts would restrict their use in the setting of AML first remission to patients with higher risk disease. However, once patients have relapsed, matched unrelated transplants should be considered if a completely matched or single-antigen mismatched family member is not available.

Autologous transplantation for AML is now a commonly used approach. This procedure is more widely applicable because donors do not have to be identified, and the incidence of transplant-related complications is lower, with no graft-versus-host disease problems and associated infections. However, autologous transplantation is associated with a higher incidence of relapse after the transplant, likely a result of a lack of a graft-versus-leukemia effect as well as the reinfusion of autologous tumor cells even with carefully manipulated marrow or stem cells from the peripheral blood.

The clearest indication for autologous transplantation for AML is disease in second remission. In this setting, the results of several studies have demonstrated that 30% to 35% of patients will become long-term, disease-free survivors. These studies involved considerable patient selection, and no prospective study has definitively shown an advantage of autologous transplantation in second remission compared with continued chemotherapy; however, most investigators accept the premise that autologous transplantation is more likely to lead to a cure.[44] No prospective trials comparing autologous transplantation in second remission with allogeneic transplantation have been reported. Randomized trials of autologous transplantation in first remission have not shown a clear survival advantage compared with chemotherapy, and appear to result in outcomes somewhat less favorable than those seen with matched related allogeneic transplants.

Considerable effort has gone into developing methods of purging autologous marrow of leukemic progenitors. The two most commonly used methods involve in vitro chemotherapy with an alkylating agent such as 4-hydroperoxycyclophosphamide or the use of antimyeloid antibodies combined with complement. Although both methods are based on solid preclinical models and have a demonstrated ability (according to in vitro assays) to remove tumor cells, they both result in delayed recovery of hematopoiesis, and no randomized study has been published to address whether these approaches result in any benefit.

Preparative Regimen

The preparative regimen given before transplantation for AML ideally should eradicate all disease, suppress the immune system adequately to permit sustained engraftment (in the allogeneic setting), and accomplish these goals with minimal toxicity. A regimen commonly used for the past 3 decades has included cyclophosphamide administered at 60 mg/kg for 2 days, followed by total body radiation at a dose of 10 to 14 Gy given over 3 to 6 days. A number of investigators have substituted single chemotherapy agents for cyclophosphamide, including melphalan (110 mg/m^2), etoposide (60 mg/m^2), or high-dose cytarabine (3 g/m^2 every 12 hours for 12 doses). Although some pilot data have been presented, the only published randomized study compared melphalan plus total body radiation with cyclophosphamide and total body radiation for AML in first remission. Both approaches were found to be equivalent with regard to disease-free survival.[45]

It is possible to avoid total body radiation altogether by combining busulfan at 16 mg/kg with cyclophosphamide at 200 mg/kg. Results with this regimen appear approximately equivalent to the results obtained with cyclophosphamide and total body radiation. A modification of this approach using a lower dose of cyclophosphamide (120 mg/kg) also is widely used. Whereas the results of a prospective, randomized study of cyclophosphamide plus 12 Gy of total body radiation compared with busulfan plus 120 mg/kg of cyclophosphamide showed an advantage to the regimen that included radiotherapy, subsequent registry data including large numbers of patients are not consistent with this finding.[46]

Graft-versus-Host Disease

Graft-versus-host disease considerably affects the outcome of allogeneic hematopoietic cell transplantation for AML, resulting in both increased nonleukemic deaths caused by graft-versus-host disease and its complications and fewer relapses. Therefore, the overall effect depends on the particular clinical situation; if the risk of recurrent leukemia is low, graft-versus-host disease is likely to have a deleterious effect, but if the risk is high, mild disease may even be of some benefit. The overwhelming predictive factor for the development of this complication is the degree of patient and donor matching, with a higher incidence of graft-versus-host disease found for increased degrees of mismatching. Among recipients of HLA-identical marrow, the frequency of graft-versus-host disease rises with increasing patient age and for recipients of marrow from previously pregnant women. Substantial progress has been made in preventing the acute form of graft-versus-host disease. If no immunosuppressive therapy is given after the transplant, acute graft-versus-host disease will develop in essentially all recipients of HLA-identical marrow unless the T cells are removed. A short course of methotrexate can reduce the incidence of this complication; a longer course of methotrexate is more effective. Cyclosporine is equivalent to methotrexate in the prevention of graft-versus-host disease, and in prospective randomized studies, the combination of methotrexate and cyclosporine is superior to either agent alone.[47] Tacrolimus is at least as effective as cyclosporine, and mycophenolate mofetil has been substituted for methotrexate in some regimens. The depletion of T cells in allogeneic bone marrow also is successful for decreasing the incidence of acute graft-versus-host disease. In some settings, this approach has been associated with an increased incidence of both graft failure and leukemic recurrence; there is no proof that depletion of T cells can improve overall survival.

SPECIAL TYPES OF AML

ACUTE PROMYELOCYTIC LEUKEMIA (APL)

APL is a distinct subtype of AML, accounting for 5% to 15% of cases (average, approximately 10%), with unique clinical, morphologic, and cytogenetic features. Compared with most patients with AML, patients with APL tend to be somewhat younger (median age, 30 to 40 years), rarely have a myelodysplastic prodrome, and usually have a lower white blood cell count at the time of diagnosis. Among the different subtypes of AML, APL appears to be over-represented among Hispanics. Whereas many of the other clinical and laboratory features are similar to other forms of AML, APL virtually always presents with some of the following elements of a hemorrhagic syndrome.

- Hypofibrinogenemia
- Decreased normal coagulation factors
- Elevated fibrin degradation products
- Increased platelet consumption

These findings are the result of both disseminated intravascular coagulation as well as primary fibrinolysis. As noted earlier, leukemic blasts virtually always have the characteristic translocation t(15;17)(q22;q11-12). A unique feature of APL is its sensitivity to treatment with all-trans retinoic acid. In previous studies, all-trans retinoic acid as a single agent led to complete response rates of 80% or more for both relapsed disease and previously untreated disease. In these initial studies, correction of coagulation disorders was the earliest sign of the efficacy of this agent, with coagulation parameters improving within several days. An increase in both normal and abnormal granulocytes occurred during the first several weeks and morphologic analysis of bone marrow during the first 3 months demonstrated progressive differentiation of malignant cells. Generally, 2 to 3 months were needed to achieve complete remission using all-trans retinoic acid alone. In these studies, when the agent was used alone, even if continued for maintenance, the median duration of complete remission was only approximately 7 months.[48]

The striking activity of all-trans retinoic acid for patients with recurrent disease led to trials exploring its use in initial therapy. Combining the agent with conventional induction therapy leads to complete responses for approximately 90% of patients and decreases the incidence of substantial bleeding complications. Clinical trials conducted before the availability of all-trans retinoic acid demonstrated that APL is particularly sensitive to anthracycline therapy.[49] Thus, substantial doses of anthracyclines generally are included during the consolidation treatment phase for APL. In addition, there is a clear role for all-trans retinoic acid as maintenance therapy. With current therapies that include all-trans retinoic acid for induction, anthracyclines during consolidation, and all-trans retinoic acid maintenance therapy, 5-year survival rates of 70% or more can be expected.[50] Better outcomes are seen for patients presenting with a white count of less than 10,000 and those younger than age 56.

Arsenic trioxide has been shown to have considerable activity for patients with recurrent disease, leading to complete response for 85% of patients.[51] Treatment with this agent has been complicated by a prolongation of the QT interval and, rarely, by sudden death. Thus, before initiating treatment with arsenic, any electrolyte imbalances should be

KEY POINT

- Patients with APL should receive all-trans retinoic acid as part of both induction and maintenance therapy.

corrected, especially hypomagnesemia and hypocalcemia; other drugs that can prolong the QT interval also should be discontinued.

During induction therapy with either all-trans retinoic acid or arsenic, some patients will experience fever, weight gain, respiratory distress, pulmonary infiltrates, episodic hypotension, and renal failure.[52] This condition is thought to be related to the sudden maturation of promyeloblasts and usually responds to dexamethasone.

TREATMENT-RELATED AML AND AML ARISING FROM MDS

The term "secondary AML" has been used to describe two distinct subtypes of AML: those cases that arise secondary to chemotherapy or radiotherapy (also termed treatment-related AML) and those that develop after an antecedent hematologic disorder, usually myelodysplasia. As noted earlier, there are several categories of treatment-related AML, including those cases that develop after treatment with an alkylating agent and that typically have abnormalities of chromosomes 5 and 7, as well as those cases resulting from exposure to topoisomerase II inhibitors and characterized by abnormalities involving 11q23. Exposure to bimolane, a drug previously used to treat psoriasis but no longer sold in the United States, has been associated with the development of APL with t(15;17) (Table 15-5). Other less common, but recurring, cytogenetic abnormalities are seen as well.

In general, the overall response rate of treatment-related AML and AML arising from MDS is lower than that seen in denovo leukemia, averaging 35% to 40% in several large series. Furthermore, the median disease-free and overall survival with secondary AML is considerably shorter than with de novo AML, and less than 10% of patients can expect to survive disease-free more than 3 years after initiation of chemotherapy. Important exceptions are patients who have secondary leukemias with favorable cytogenetic abnormalities such as t(8;21) or inv(16). These patients have a complete response rate indistinguishable from that seen for patients with de novo leukemia with similar karyotypes. Unfortunately, few patients with secondary disease fall into this category. Although the number of published studies is limited, allogeneic transplantation leads to long-term, disease-free survival for some patients with secondary AML.[53] Thus, allogeneic transplantation from either a matched sibling or a matched unrelated donor should be considered for most cases of secondary AML.

THERAPY FOR ALL

INDUCTION

Standard induction therapy for adult ALL most commonly involves combination chemotherapy including vincristine, prednisone, an anthracycline, and asparaginase. With such regimens, 80% to 90% of patients achieve a first complete remission. Several variations have been reported in which, for example, cyclophosphamide has been added and asparaginase removed (as in the M. D. Anderson Hyper-CVAD approach) or high-dose mitoxantrone and high-dose cytarabine combined (as in a study from Memorial Sloan-Kettering Cancer Center).[54,55] No prospective randomized trial has identified any superior regimen. A number of investigators have explored the use of hematopoietic growth factors

KEY POINTS

- Induction therapy in adult ALL should generally include vincristine, prednisone, an anthracycline and asparaginase. With such regimens, complete remission can be achieved in 80% to 90% of patients.
- Adults with high-risk ALL, including those with Ph-positive ALL or t(4;11), should receive allogeneic transplantation during first remission, if possible.
- In adult ALL, complete response rates average 90%, and 5-year disease-free survival rates are 30% to 35%.

TABLE 15-5 Features of Therapy-related Leukemias

	Causative Agents		
	Alkylating Agents	Topoisomerase II Inhibitors	Bimolane
Chromosome abnormality	del(5q),-5 del(7q),-7	11q23 21q22	t(15;17)
Preleukemia phase	Myelodysplastic syndromes	None	None
FAB morphology	Not classifiable	Usually M4, M5	M3
Latency	5 - 7 years	6 months to 3 years	2 to 3 years
Response to induction therapy	Poor	Good	Good
Long-term survival	Poor	Poor	Good

Abbreviation: FAB, French-American-British

Reprinted with permission from Cheson BC, ed. Oncology MKSAP, 2nd ed. Philadelphia, Pa: American College of Physicians; 1999:248.

immediately following induction chemotherapy. Similar to the findings for AML, the results of such studies demonstrate accelerated myeloid recovery and a decrease in the incidence of febrile neutropenia. In some trials, the complete response rate was improved, but no findings have indicated an improvement in disease-free or overall survival.[56]

THERAPY AFTER REMISSION

After achievement of remission, the following principles apply:

- Some form of therapy is needed after remission. If induction alone is used, the duration of remission is invariably short.
- Therapy after remission should include prophylaxis for the CNS, because although such a complication is less common for adults with ALL than children, without prophylaxis, CNS disease will develop in at least 35% of adults. At highest risk are patients with a high tumor burden at diagnosis as reflected by an elevated level of lactate dehydrogenase. With prophylaxis, relapse in the CNS as an isolated event is uncommon in adults, seen in less than 10% of patients.
- Intensive consolidation therapy seems warranted. The best form of intensive consolidation has not been demonstrated, but many studies use combinations of cytarabine, cyclophosphamide, and an anthracycline.
- Although maintenance therapy may be important, neither the duration nor intensity of such therapy has been precisely defined. With current treatment regimens, approximately 35% of adult patients will have ALL in complete remission for longer than 5 years.[57]

RISK FACTORS

Various risk factors have been shown to affect the probability of achieving and maintaining a complete remission (Table 15-6).[56] Age has consistently been found to be an important prognostic factor for adults with ALL. Older individuals have both a lower likelihood of experiencing a complete remission and, if they do experience a complete remission, of remaining in it. The influence of peripheral white count at diagnosis is more variable. In most studies, an elevated white count has no effect or a weak effect on the chance of achieving a complete remission, whereas an elevated white count at diagnosis has consistently been associated with a shorter duration of remission.[56]

The immunophenotype of leukemic blasts also is of prognostic value. In the past, the prognosis was thought to be worse for patients with T-cell leukemia, but with current, more intensive regimens — perhaps because of the addition of cytarabine and cyclophosphamide to consolidation — the prognosis for patients with T-cell disease is similar to that for patients with B-cell disease. The presence of myeloid antigens on leukemic blasts can be seen in approximately 20% of cases. Myeloid antigens, particularly CD13 and CD33, can be found in both T-cell and B-cell ALLs. Myeloid antigens are more commonly associated with FAB subtype L2 morphology, as well as with leukemic blasts that are Ph-positive or *BCR-ABL*–positive. In most, but not all studies, the likelihood of complete remission is lower for patients in whom blasts bear myeloid antigens, as is the probability of remaining in complete remission.[56]

Cytogenetic characteristics also have important prognostic significance (Fig. 15-4)[58]: 10% to 20% of ALL cases are Ph-positive (5% of childhood cases, 25% of adult cases), and the incidence of Ph positivity increases with age, which may explain the importance of age as a prognostic variable. In studies conducted prior to the availability of imatinib, the likelihood of complete remission was somewhat lower for patients with Ph-positive ALL, and the probability of remaining in complete remission was much lower. Studies designed to find molecular evidence of the *BCR-ABL* rearrangement have shown that at least 25% to 30% of adults with ALL

Table 15-6 Prognosis in Acute Lymphocytic Leukemia

	Unfavorable	Favorable
Age	Older	Younger
White blood cell count at time of diagnosis	High	Low
Myeloid antigens	Present	Absent
Achievement of complete response	Late	Early
Chromosome abnormalities	t(9;22)(q34;q11) t(4;11)(q21;q23) t(8;14)(q24;q32) t(1;19)(q23;p13)	Hyperdiploidy (50 to 60 chromosomes) t(12;21)

Modified with permission from Cheson BC, ed. Oncology MKSAP, 2nd ed. Philadelphia, Pa: American College of Physicians; 1999:249.

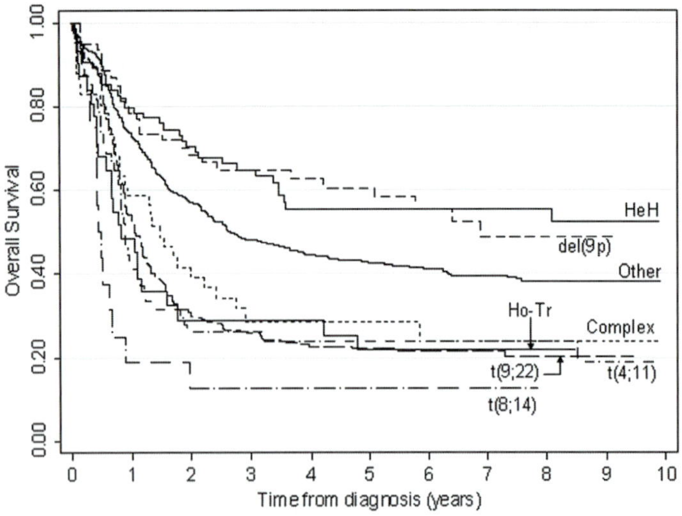

FIG. 15-4 Survival in adult ALL according to cytogenetic abnormality. HeH = high hyperdiploidy; Ho-Tr = hypodiploidy/near triploidy.[58]

will be *BCR-ABL*–positive. Therefore, up to 10% of cases that are Ph-negative, normal, or inadequate by cytogenetic analysis will, nonetheless, have the *BCR-ABL* rearrangement.

The prognosis is as poor for patients who are Ph-negative by conventional cytogenetics and *BCR ABL*–positive according to molecular studies as it is for patients who are Ph-positive. Although Ph-positive ALL has a very poor prognosis when treated with conventional ALL therapy, results of recent trials that combine imatinib with standard induction are sufficiently encouraging to warrant inclusion of imatinib in the initial treatment of Ph-positive ALL.[59] Other cytogenetic abnormalities of adult ALL that carry a poor prognosis, both in terms of achieving a complete remission and of staying in complete remission, include t(4;11), t(8;14) and having complex cytogentics with 5 or more abnormalities.

Adults with high hyperdiploidy or del(9p) seem to have a more favorable prognosis.[60] A fusion of the *ETV6* gene on chromosome 12, band p13, and the *CBFA* gene on chromosome 21, band q22, has been identified in 25% of precursor B-cell ALL in children (formerly referred to as *TEL-AML1* fusion). This rearrangement is the result of a cryptic translocation, t(12;21)(p13;q22), that is not easily detectable by cytogenetic analysis but can be detected by polymerase chain reaction (PCR) assay. The *ETV6-CBFA* fusion frequently is associated with age (2 to 9 years) and immunophenotype (CD10 positive, CD19 positive, HLA-DR positive, CD2 negative, and CD33 negative). Half of these patients fall into standard-risk groups, whereas the other half fall into a high-risk group by standard criteria. Nevertheless, the *ETV6-CBFA* fusion identifies a subset of patients with a highly favorable outcome.

STEM CELL TRANSPLANTATION

As with AML, the results of stem cell transplantation for ALL depend largely on the remission status of the patient, the source of stem cells, and, perhaps, the choice of preparative regimen. The most experience has been with the use of HLA-identical sibling donors. If such transplants are carried out for patients with disease that is resistant to conventional chemotherapy, long-term disease-free survival can be obtained for 10% to 20% of patients. These results are clearly superior to the results obtained with chemotherapy, but only a small fraction of patients ultimately benefit. The major cause of treatment failure is recurrent leukemia, with an actuarial relapse rate in excess of 60%. If transplants are carried out while patients are in a second remission, the 5-year disease-free survival is approximately 35%.

In the pediatric setting, chemotherapy can be curative for patients in second remission who have had a long first remission (in excess of 18 months); whether such patients should have transplantation during second remission is controversial. However, among adult patients, the likelihood of cure with conventional chemotherapy during second remission is substantially less, and most investigators agree that such patients should receive a transplant if a suitable donor is available, regardless of the length of the initial remission.

The best results with allogeneic transplantation have been obtained for patients in first remission, with reports ranging from 35% to 65% for long-term disease-free survival. The largest collection of cases has been reported by the International Bone Marrow Transplant Registry (IBMTR), in which approximately 50% of patients who received a transplant remain in complete remission 4 years later and the actuarial relapse rate is 25%.[61] However, considerable patient selection, both positive and negative, probably influenced the results of the registry data.

The first prospective trial to address the role of transplantation during first remission was the French LALA87 trial. In that trial, patients between the ages of 15 and 40 were assigned to allogeneic transplantation if they had a matched sibling and were randomly assigned to further chemotherapy or autologous transplantation if they did not. When patients were analyzed according to protocol intent, allogeneic transplantation was marginally better than chemotherapy or autologous transplantation (10-year survival, 46% compared with 31%). High-risk patients particularly benefited from allogeneic transplantation (10-year survival, 44% compared with 11%), whereas no form of therapy was particularly advantageous for patients with standard-risk disease.[62] More recently, an Eastern Cooperative Oncology Group, UK ALL trial has demonstrated improved survival among patients with matched siblings who undergo transplantation in first remission compared with those treated with chemotherapy, including both high-risk and standard-risk patients.

The best preparative regimen for transplantation for patients with ALL is uncertain. Most experience has been gained with use of the standard regimen of cyclophosphamide and total body radiation. There are suggestions that substituting etoposide for cyclophosphamide may offer some advantage. However, no controlled trials have been conducted to provide evidence supporting this theory.

The role of autologous transplantation in ALL is difficult to evaluate. The results for patients with multiple relapses are poor, largely owing to a high incidence of leukemic relapse. In second remission, long-term disease-free survival has been reported for 20% to 30% of patients, and probably represents an advantage compared with conventional chemotherapy. The disease-free survival rate for patients in first remission in the only prospective studies published to date has averaged approximately 30% and shows no obvious advantage compared with conventional chemotherapy.[63] In some studies, autologous marrow is purged using either antibodies plus complement, antibodies linked to magnetic beads or toxins, or in vitro chemotherapy. The clinical value of ex vivo treatment of autologous bone marrow to prevent relapse after transplantation has not been tested in prospective randomized trials.

MYELODYSPLASTIC SYNDROMES

BIOLOGY, CYTOGENETICS, AND MOLECULAR BIOLOGY

The myelodysplastic syndromes (MDS) are a group of clonal, acquired hematopoietic disorders. Clonality has been demonstrated by the presence of clonal cytogenetic abnormalities, as well as by studies of G6PD heterozygosity in black women and other X-linked polymorphisms. There are likely multiple steps in the development of clinically evident MDS, with an early step in its development leading to the expansion of a genetically unstable clone beginning close to, if not at, the level of the stem cell, followed by acquisition of chromosome abnormalities that may confer selective growth advantages to these clones.

G6PD studies of MDS have shown clonality not only of the myeloid lineage, but also, in some cases, of B cells and even T cells. Clonal chromosome abnormalities are detected in 40% to 70% of patients with MDS at the time of diagnosis. The frequency of clonal abnormalities varies among the subtypes of MDS and is lowest (approximately 10%) for patients with refractory anemia with ringed sideroblasts and highest (approximately 60%) for patients with refractory anemia with excess blasts. Trisomy 8, loss or deletion of chromosomes 5 and 7, as well as deletions in chromosomes 13 and 20 are particularly frequent.

> **KEY POINT**
>
> - The three most important factors that predict outcome for patients with myelodysplasia are percentage of marrow blasts, karyotype, and number of peripheral cytopenias.

Although many of these abnormalities also are seen among patients with AML, other specific structural rearrangements that are closely associated with distinct morphologic subtypes of AML, such as t(8;21), are almost never seen in MDS. Some of the chromosome abnormalities in MDS are of prognostic importance. Abnormalities of chromosomes 5 or 7 are associated with the shortest survival; the outcome is intermediate for patients with other abnormalities, and the longest survival is found for patients with a normal karyotype, -y, del (5q), or del (20q) as a sole abnormality. Chromosome abnormalities also are associated with an increased risk of progression to acute leukemia.

Links between cytogenetic abnormalities and the MDS phenotype are beginning to emerge. In many MDS cases, deletions involving 5q31 have been noted. Although the genes encoding for GM-CSF, interleukin (IL)-3, IL-4, IL-5, and IL-9 all are located within this region, these genes are not included in the smallest commonly depleted segment of 5q; thus, they are unlikely to be involved in the pathogenesis of these disorders. Mutations affecting *N-RAS* are found in 30% to 40% of patients with MDS. Mutant *RAS* alleles are detected in all subtypes of MDS. The frequency of leukemic conversion appears to be somewhat higher for patients who have mutant *RAS* alleles. Normal *RAS* gene products are guanine nucleotide-binding proteins that couple membrane receptors to phospholipase C and to MAP kinase signal-transduction pathways. The growth-promoting effect of these oncoproteins may derive from their ability to augment protein kinase C activation. Another proto-oncogene mutated in many cases of MDS is *C-FMS*, which encodes a receptor that has ligand-dependent tyrosine kinase activity. The *FMS* gene is located on the long arm of chromosome 5. Mutations of *FMS* are found in 10% to 15% of patients with MDS.

CLASSIFICATION AND PROGNOSIS

Traditionally, MDS was classified according to recommendations of the FAB Morphology Group[64], was based solely on morphology, and recognized five categories of MDS.

- Refractory anemia
- Refractory anemia with ringed sideroblasts
- Refractory anemia with excess blasts
- Refractory anemia with excess blasts in transition
- Chronic myelomonocytic leukemia

This system has been revised by the WHO (Table 15-7), but remains morphologically based.[65] In an effort to provide greater prognostic accuracy, an International Prognostic Scoring System has been developed on the basis of outcomes of 816 patients with primary MDS. In this analysis, the three major factors affecting outcome were percentage of bone marrow blasts, karyotype, and number of cytopenias (Table 15-8). On the basis of these features, patients can be categorized into four risk groups with the median survivals as listed here.[66]

- Low risk: 5.7 years
- Intermediate risk 1: 3.5 years
- Intermediate risk 2: 1.2 years
- High risk: 0.4 years

Findings from additional studies suggest that, stage for stage, the prognosis is somewhat worse for patients with therapy-related MDS than for patients with primary MDS.

THERAPY

An array of therapies have been tested for the treatment of MDS. For patients with early-stage disease (low risk or intermediate risk 1) or patients who are frail or elderly, supportive care with red blood cell and platelet transfusions as necessary generally is recommended. Recently, three drugs have been approved for treatment of MDS. Lenalidomide, a 4-aminoglutarimide analog of thalidomide, has been approved for treatment of transfusion-dependent low-risk or intermediate-risk 1 MDS associated with chromosome 5q31.1 deletion. In a pivotal study of 148 such patients treated with lenalidomide, 64% became transfusion independent, and 75% experienced a cytogenetic response, half of which were complete.[67] The mechanism of action is uncertain, but side effects include myelosuppression, pruritus, diarrhea, and urticaria. 5-azacytidine and decitabine both are thought to have utility in MDS via their DNA demethylating activity, which leads to re-expression of key genes otherwise inactivated in MDS by hypermethylation.[68,69] The effects of azacytidine were documented in a phase III trial that found improved partial responses and a larger time to AML progression than seen with supportive care alone for patients with intermediate risk 2 or high-risk disease. Similar results have been presented with decitabine.

The median duration of response seen with 5-azcytabine and decitabine is measured in months, not years, and none of the approved agents are curative. Other therapies that have been studied include hematopoietic growth factors, immunosuppressive therapy, various biologic response modifiers, and chemotherapies other than those already mentioned.

Erythropoietin can improve the anemia associated with MDS in 20% to 30% of cases.[70] For patients who do not have a response after 4 to 6 weeks, the addition of a myeloid growth factor may result in responses for 20% to 30%. Myeloid growth factors, including G-CSF and GM-CSF, have been used in an effort to treat the neutropenia that sometimes accompanies MDS. The results of a randomized trial of the prophylactic use of G-CSF showed no advantage to its use and a possible shortening of survival for patients with advanced disease.[71] Thus, myeloid growth factors

TABLE 15-7 Myelodysplastic Syndrome World Health Organization Classification 2000

Category	Peripheral Blood	Bone Marrow
1a. Refractory anemia without dysplasia	Blasts < 1%; monocytes < 1,000/mm³	Blasts < 5%; ringed sideroblasts < 15%
1b. Refractory anemia with dysplasia	Same + dysgranulocytes and/or giant platelets	Same + dysgranulocytes and/or dysmegakaryocyte
2a. Refractory anemia with ringed sideroblasts wiithout dysplasia	Blasts < 1%; monocytes < 1,000/mm³	Blasts < 5%; > 15% ringed sideroblasts
2b. Refractory anemia with ringed sideroblasts with dysplasia	Same + dysgranulocytes and/or giant platelets	Same + dysgranulocytes and/or dysmegakaryocytes
3a. Refractory anemia with excess blasts in transition	Blasts 1%–5%; monocytes < 1,000/mm³	Blasts 5%–10%
3b. Refractory anemia with excess blasts	Blasts 6%–20%; monocyte < 1,000/mm³	Blasts 11%–20%
4. Chronic myelomonocytic leukemia	Blasts < 1%–20%; monocytes > 1,000/mm³	Blasts 0%–20%

TABLE 15-8 International Prognostic Scoring System for Myelodysplastic Syndromes

	Score Value				
Variable	0	0.5	1.0	1.5	2.0
Percentage of blasts in the bone marrow	< 5	5–10	—	11–20	21–30
Karyotype*	Good	Intermediate	Poor	—	—
Cytopenia	0/1	2/3	—	—	—

*Good = -y, del(5q), del(20q); intermediate = neither good nor poor; poor = chromosome 7 abnormalities or complex abnormalities.
Scores by group: low = 0; intermediate 1 = 0.5–1.0; intermediate 2 = 1.5–2.0; high = ≥ 2.5.

should probably be restricted to patients with recurrent infections. Platelets have responded to low-dose IL-11.

Based on the hypothesis that the pancytopenia seen in MDS (in a manner analogous to aplastic anemia) may be the result of T cells inhibiting hematopoiesis, trials of immunosuppressive therapy using antithymocyte globulin, cyclosporine, or the two agents in combination have been conducted. Responses, sometimes enduring, have been documented for approximately one-third of patients, particularly those who express HLA-DR15.[72,73]

A variety of biologic-response modifiers have been studied in MDS, including agents developed to reduce levels of tumor necrosis factor (TNF), as well as antiangiogenesis agents, retinoic acid, amifostine, and interferon. Although occasional responses have been seen with each of these, none have resulted in sustained responses for substantial proportions of patients nor have they been shown in randomized trials to alter the course of the disease.

Low-dose cytarabine has been studied as a treatment option for MDS, with responses seen in 10% to 20% of cases. Patients with refractory anemia with excess blasts type I or II have, in some cases, been treated with AML-like induction chemotherapy. Although response rates are lower than the rates seen with de novo AML, complete responses in 40% to 50% of patients have been reported for some studies.[74] Whether this results in an overall improvement in survival has not been prospectively tested.

Hematopoietic Cell Transplantation

Allogeneic hematopoietic cell transplantation was initially attempted for the treatment of MDS because the disease is incurable with conventional measures and transplantation can cure other forms of otherwise incurable hematologic cancer. A considerable number of studies have now shown the results of allogeneic transplantation for patients with MDS, and investigators report long-term disease-free survival for 20% to 65% of patients, with many patients alive without evidence of disease for more than 5 years after transplantation, and some for as long as 25 years.[75,76] This positive survival outcome offers strong evidence that MDS is curable with hematopoietic cell transplantation. The factor that appears to have the greatest effect on outcome is disease stage, with the best chance for long-term disease-free survival being associated with transplantation earlier in the course of disease. However, low-risk patients also can survive for long periods without transplant. In general, transplantation should be strongly considered for all patients with intermediate risk 2 or high-risk disease and for younger patients with intermediate risk 1 disease. The overall utility of marrow transplantation for myelodysplasia is limited by the age of the patient (many with MDS are older than age 65) and by the need to find an appropriately matched allogeneic donor. Autologous transplantation in MDS has no demonstrative role.

CHRONIC MYELOID LEUKEMIA (CML)

BIOLOGY, CYTOGENETICS, AND MOLECULAR GENETICS

CML was the first malignant disease found to be consistently associated with a specific cytogenetic abnormality, the Ph chromosome. The abnormal chromosome is the product of a translocation between chromosomes 9 and 22 (t[9;22][q34;q11]), which places the *ABL* proto-oncogene from chromosome 9 contiguous with the 5' portion of the

KEY POINTS

- Imatinib mesylate is a small-molecule inhibitor of the ABL protein tyrosine kinase and is remarkably effective in newly diagnosed CML, leading to complete hematologic and cytogenetic responses for most patients. However, continued therapy and careful follow-up are necessary.
- Although allogeneic transplantation remains the only curative approach to CML, because of the high response rate and favorable toxicity profile of imatinib, this agent has become the initial treatment of choice of most patients with newly diagnosed CML.

BCR gene on chromosome 22. The breakpoint on chromosome 9 is highly variable and occurs anywhere over a region of 200 kilobase or more, usually located in a large intron 5′ of exon 2. In contrast, the breakpoint in the *BCR* gene occurs within one of two relatively short sequences. One is a 5.8-kilobase sequence, the major breakpoint cluster region (M-bcr). This breakpoint is associated with Ph-positive CML, approximately half of the cases of Ph-positive ALL, and occasionally, cases of Ph-positive AML. The other breakpoint within the *BCR* gene, the minor breakpoint cluster region (m-bcr), is virtually never associated with CML, but is seen in approximately half of the cases of Ph-positive ALL.

Studies have shown that, in most cases of Ph-negative CML, a molecular rearrangement can still be found, even though the translocation is masked at the karyotypic level. Whether a true *BCR-ABL*–negative CML exists must be investigated further. The transcription of the chimeric *BCR-ABL* gene results in a hybrid messenger RNA that is translated into a hybrid p210 protein. Both the messenger RNA and the protein, which is an activated form of the ABL protein tyrosine kinase, are unique to cells of the leukemic clone. There is now definitive evidence that these changes are more than just a marker of the disease and are part of its pathogenesis. Transgenic expression of the 190-kilodalton BCR-ABL protein in mice causes acute leukemia at birth. Retroviral transfer of BCR-ABL into hematopoietic stem cells of normal mice leads to the development of a variety of acute and chronic leukemias. The BCR-ABL protein transforms hematopoietic cells so that their growth in vitro becomes cytokine independent, protects cells from apoptotic responses to DNA damage, and increases adhesion of cells to the extracellular matrix. The persistent and increased activity of the ABL protein tyrosine kinase appears to result in the continuous activation of a number of cytoplasmic and nuclear signal-transduction pathways involved in cell growth and survival, including STAT, RAS, JUN kinase, and MYC.

CLINICAL FEATURES

The natural history of untreated CML is a relatively benign chronic phase lasting approximately 3 years, followed by an accelerated phase lasting several months and finally, a rapidly fatal blast crisis. At the time of diagnosis, more than 90% of patients are in the chronic phase, and as many as 50% are diagnosed incidentally during routine screening. Symptoms, when present, include fatigue, weight loss, bone aches, and abdominal discomfort from splenomegaly. Patients typically have leukocytosis, thrombocytosis, and anemia at the time of presentation. The marrow is virtually always hypercellular and the Ph chromosome is found in 90% of cases. In the remaining 10%, cryptic or complex translocations can be detected by fluorescence in situ hybridization (FISH) or PCR assays.

The accelerated phase is characterized by fever, night sweats, weight loss, bone pain, difficulty controlling blood counts, increased numbers of blasts and early myeloid cells in the marrow and peripheral blood, as well as evidence of karyotypic evolution. The most common cytogenetic changes associated with disease evolution are an additional Ph chromosome, trisomy 8, i(17q), and trisomy 19. Blast crisis is defined as having more than 30% blasts and promyelocytes in the bone marrow or peripheral blood or the development of extramedullary blastic infiltrates. In most cases (more than 60%), the blasts are of myeloid lineage as determined by morphology and cell surface markers. In 25% to 30% of cases, the blasts are of lymphoid lineage, and in the remaining cases, blasts may be biphenotypic or undifferentiated. Determination of the blast lineage is important for selecting appropriate therapy.

TREATMENT

Conventional Chemotherapy

Before the introduction of interferon alpha in the late 1980s, palliative therapy for CML involved the use of either busulfan, starting at a daily dose of 2 to 4 mg/m^2, or hydroxyurea, starting at a daily dose of 1 to 2 g/m^2. With these therapies, the duration of the chronic phase was approximately 4 years, and, once blast crisis supervened, survival averaged approximately 6 months. Sokal et al. conducted a study of 625 patients between the ages of 5 and 50, which includes the ages of most recipients of marrow transplants, and identified five variables useful for predicting survival of patients with CML treated with busulfan or hydroxyurea (i.e., before the availability of interferon or imatinib).[77]

- Sex of the patient
- Size of the spleen
- Platelet count
- Hematocrit
- Percentage of circulating blasts

Approximately two-thirds of patients were categorized as poor risk — with a 5-year survival rate of less than 40% — and few survived beyond 7 years. One-third of patients were identified as being in a better-risk group, with a 5-year survival rate of 60%. These figures are important for evaluating the results of newer therapies.

Interferon

Interferon was first shown to have activity for CML in the late 1980s. Interferon induces a complete hematologic response in 50% to 80% of patients — a lower percentage of response than seen with conventional chemotherapy. However, with interferon therapy, 10% to 25% of patients become cytogenetically negative for the Ph chromosome, a result almost never seen with busulfan or hydroxyurea. The effectiveness of interferon alpha is dose dependent, and the best responses are usually seen at daily doses of 5,000,000 U/m^2.

A meta-analysis of seven randomized studies in which interferon was compared with hydroxyurea or busulfan showed an improvement in 5-year survival with the use of interferon (57% compared with 42%).[78] However, interferon is associated with several complications, including fever, chills, malaise, headache, anorexia, joint pain, myalgias, and, rarely, autoimmune disorders such as hypothyroidism, hemolytic anemia, and depression. These side effects can be diminished by slow dose increments and with the addition of acetaminophen. Usually, the symptoms resolve over 6 to 8 weeks, but as many as 20% of patients find the side effects of interferon intolerable.

Imatinib Mesylate

Imatinib mesylate is a small molecule inhibitor of several protein tyrosine kinases, including the ABL protein tyrosine kinase.[79] In a phase I trial initiated in 1998 for patients with CML for whom interferon therapy had failed, a complete hematologic response was achieved in 53 of 54 patients receiving a daily oral dose of imatinib of 300 mg or more. Furthermore, cytogenetic responses were seen in 54% of patients.[80] A large randomized trial in which imatinib was compared with interferon plus low-dose cytarabine demonstrated disease progression at 6 months for 1% of patients who received imatinib compared with 10% of patients who received interferon. The crossover to the alternative therapy because of intolerance was 1% for patients who received imatinib compared with 19% for patients who received interferon, and cytogenetic responses were seen in 63% of imatinib-treated patients compared with 10% of interferon-treated patients. Based primarily on the differences in disease progression, the study was closed with the conclusion that imatinib at a daily dose of 400 mg is the nontransplant treatment of choice for patients with newly diagnosed CML.[81] After 54 months of follow-up, the progression-free survival was 84% and overall survival was 90% among patients in early chronic phase treated with imatinib at a dose of 400 mg daily. For patients first exposed to imatinib in accelerated phase, the results are less encouraging, with a 37% complete hematologic response rate and a progression-free survival rate of 40% at 3 years.[79] For patients in blast crisis, complete hematologic responses to imatinib are seen in 25%, but the duration of response is short, averaging only 7 to 10 months.[82]

Among patients in early chronic phase treated with imatinib, complete cytogenetic response will occur for roughly 75% after 1 year of therapy. In approximately 50% of complete cytogenetic responders, a "major molecular response" (defined as 3-log reduction in *BCR-ABL* transcripts in peripheral blood) will be seen. The actual frequency of true molecular remissions in which no residual *BCR-ABL* transcripts can be detected using the most sensitive available methods is uncertain but seems to be uncommon, occurring in perhaps 10% of patients.[83] In those few cases in which imatinib therapy has been stopped after achievement of complete cytogenetic response, rapid disease recurrence has been seen.

In an effort to achieve higher rates of complete cytogenetic and major molecular responses, higher doses of imatinib (600 mg or 800 mg) have been explored. Although some patients seem to respond after dose escalation, it is unknown whether higher doses of imatinib will result in an increased incidence of complete cytogenetic or major molecular responses. Prospective randomized trials are in progress addressing this point. Imatinib-related toxcities include nausea, diarrhea, muscle cramps, and peripheral edema and are more common and more severe at higher doses.

Imatinib resistance can be the result of *BCR-ABL* mutations in the kinase domain interfering with imatinib binding, *BCR-ABL* amplification or overexpression, decreased drug bioavailability, or drug efflux. In as many as 50% of cases, the reasons for resistance are unclear. Mutations in *BCR-ABL* appear to be the most common identifiable reason for resistance and can be detected in samples collected before treatment, suggesting that the delayed imatinib failure may reflect the considerable amount of time required for outgrowth of these selected clones.[84,85] Not all mutations in *BCR-ABL* have the same significance; mutations at *T315I* and those affecting the P-loop appear to confer the greatest degree of imatinib resistance, whereas others can be overcome by a dose increase or are functionally irrelevant.

Some patients with CML will have additional chromosome abnormalities (ACA) in Ph-positive cells. The presence of ACA is predictive of a lower response rate to imatinib and a shorter response duration.[86] Patients treated with imatinib can develop other chromosome abnormalities (OCA) in Ph-negative cells in about 5% of cases. Approximately 50% of OCAs are trisomy 8 alone. About 10% will include trisomy 8 plus another abnormality, and an additional 15% will involve deletion of chromosome 7 alone or with other abnormalities. The implications of OCA are unclear. In some cases, particularly those involving chromosome 7, OCA has been predictive of myelodysplastic syndrome development, but in other cases, patients have remained stable or the OCA clone has disappeared.[87]

Recently, two BCR-ABL tyrosine kinase inhibitors with greater potency than imatinib have been shown to have activity in imatinib-resistant CML.[88] Therapy with dasatinib or nilotinib results in hematologic responses for the majority of patients with CML in chronic phase who are resistant to imatinib, and as many as one-third will achieve a cytogenetic response. Response rates in accelerated phase or blast crisis CML do not occur as frequently. In vitro studies show that dasatinib or nilotinib have activity against most *BCR-ABL* mutations except *T315I*.

Patients in lymphoid blast crisis resistant to all tyrosine kinase inhibitors sometimes respond to ALL-type therapy, whereas AML-type induction results in temporary complete remission for 15% to 20% of patients in myeloid blast crisis. Allogeneic hematopoietic cell transplantation, as noted below, is the only known curative therapy for patients in advanced phase.

Hematopoietic Cell Transplantation

Allogeneic transplantation is the only known cure for CML. Most published studies have been limited to patients age 65 or younger. When patients undergo transplantation during blast crisis and the donor is a matched sibling, approximately 10% to 15% become long-term survivors. Transplantation for accelerated-phase CML yields somewhat better results, with cure rates of 30% to 45%.[89] Transplantation performed during chronic phase yields considerably better results. Data involving more than 1,000 patients from the IBMTR suggest that long-term disease-free survival is possible for approximately 65% to 70% of patients who undergo transplantation during the chronic phase when the donor is a matched sibling.[61] In single-institution trials, a long-term survival rate of 80% has been documented. The probability of relapse for such patients is approximately 10%, and the probability of death from transplant-related complications is approximately 15%.[90]

Both the IBMTR[61] and the Seattle series[89] have been analyzed with regard to factors predictive of long-term survival. In both series, age is a significant factor, but the overall effect of age up to 65 is relatively small. In most series, there is a relationship between the interval from diagnosis to transplantation and outcome. Patients who receive transplants within the first 2 years after diagnosis consistently do better than patients who receive them after longer intervals in chronic phase. Delay not only jeopardizes the results of transplantation in chronic phase, but also carries the risk of disease entering the accelerated phase or blast crisis before transplantation is carried out.

Neither the best regimen nor the best way to protect against graft-versus-host disease in CML has been defined. The results of studies in which cyclophosphamide and total body radiation were compared with busulfan and cyclophosphamide have shown a small advantage for the latter combination.[91] The combination of methotrexate and cyclosporine is a commonly used and effective means of preventing graft-versus-host disease. There is no evidence that any other combination results in better survival, although a combination of methotrexate with tacrolimus provides similar control for this complication. The use of donor marrow that has had ex vivo depletion of T cells decreases the incidence of acute graft-versus-host disease but has consistently been associated with an increased risk of graft rejection and, more importantly, an increase in tumor recurrence. Therefore, most centers do not deplete T cells if an HLA-identical sibling donor is available.

As with transplantation for other disorders, a phenotypically matched family member or one with a single mismatched antigen can be used with essentially the same results as a genotypically matched family member. Results with family member donors mismatched for two or three antigens are markedly worse, and such donors cannot be recommended for transplantation during the chronic phase of the disease. Many patients have received transplants from an HLA-matched unrelated donor. As typing and supportive measures have improved, the differences in outcomes between recipients of transplants from matched-related and matched-unrelated donors have decreased and, at some centers, there is no appreciable difference in cure rates with the two approaches.[92]

Various studies have demonstrated that BCR-ABL fusion messenger RNAs can be detected by PCR assays in some patients after allogeneic marrow transplantation. Of interest, in many cases, BCR-ABL could be detected only transiently and, with time, no BCR-ABL transcripts are detected in some patients. In other cases, there was sustained evidence of BCR-ABL transcripts detected by PCR assays over several years without disease progressing to clinical relapse. Most of the current evidence suggests that detection of BCR-ABL transcripts during the first 3 months after transplant is not prognostically significant. In contrast, at 6 and 12 months after transplant, detection of BCR-ABL transcripts is associated with a 40% chance of subsequent relapse compared with a 5% chance for patients who are BCR-ABL–negative by the same assay.[93]

Reports suggest that several options are available for patients with chronic-phase CML who have disease recurrence after marrow transplantation. Occasionally, patients have received second transplants with success. Several reports suggest that for patients who experience relapse after allogeneic transplantation, disease is particularly sensitive to interferon therapy. If such patients are treated for hematologic relapse, most have a response, and 35% become Ph-negative.[94] If interferon is used to treat patients for cytogenetic relapse before the development of clinical relapse, complete cytogenetic responses for 70% of patients have been documented.

Another approach to the treatment of relapse after transplantation in CML is the infusion of viable donor leukocytes. Such infusions lead to complete cytogenetic remission for approximately 75% of cases. These responses appear to be enduring, lasting more than 3 years for most patients. Donor leukocyte infusions can be complicated by marrow failure or severe graft-versus-host disease. These risks can be reduced by limiting the number of leukocytes or administering them on a fractionated basis. Imatinib mesylate is another very effective alternative for patients who have relapse following allogeneic hematopoietic cell transplantation, at least for patients who previously have not been exposed to the drug.

Although allogeneic transplantation remains the only curative approach to CML, because of the high response rate and favorable toxicity profile of imatinib, imatinib mesylate has become the initial treatment of choice for most patients with newly diagnosed CML. However, allogeneic transplantation should be strongly considered for patients who fail to respond at 400 mg/day, and an increased dose of imatinib or transplantation should be considered for those who have a suboptimal response as defined in Table 15-9.[95]

CHRONIC LYMPHOCYTIC LEUKEMIA (CLL)

> **KEY POINTS**
>
> - Distinguishing CLL from other diseases, notably hairy cell leukemia or the leukemic phases of marginal zone lymphoma or mantle cell lymphoma, is based on the morphologic appearance of the cells and the distinct immunophenotype of the malignant cells.
> - Although the outcome for patients with CLL has improved modestly during the past few years, the disease is not curable with currently available therapies.

Chronic lymphocytic leukemia (CLL) is the most common adult leukemia in Western countries, with an estimated 8,190 new cases in the United States in 2004 and 4,800 deaths each year.[96] CLL is more common in men than in women (ratio of 1.7 to 1), with a steep age-specific incidence. There is a higher incidence in Jewish people of Russian or Eastern European ancestry, but it is rare in Asian countries, where T-cell chronic leukemias are more common.

There are no known risk factors for CLL. Indeed, CLL is one of the few leukemias that does not appear to be associated with exposure to ionizing radiation, chemicals, or drugs, although data suggest a possible relationship with Agent Orange. Although there are no clear genetic factors, an increased familial incidence has been reported.[97]

DIAGNOSIS

The diagnosis of CLL requires a sustained increase in mature-appearing lymphocytes in the peripheral blood to more than 5000/mm^3. It is not unusual that a small percentage of larger atypical cells, cleaved cells or prolymphocytes also may be present. The majority of CLL cases are B-CLL. The predominant cell population expresses B-cell markers (CD19, CD20, and CD23) and the CD5 antigen but not other pan T-cell markers. The B cells are monoclonal as evidenced by expressing either kappa or lambda light chains and characteristically express surface immunoglobulin (sIg), CD79b, CD20, and CD22 with low density. The bone marrow usually is infiltrated by at least 30% lymphocytes. Whereas a bone marrow aspirate and biopsy are not needed to make the diagnosis, they are strongly recommended if cytopenias in other cell lines are present prior to starting therapy. Neither lymph node biopsy nor CT scanning is needed in the initial evaluation and should only be performed if clinically indicated.

CYTOGENETIC AND MOLECULAR ABNORMALITIES IN CLL

Conventional banding techniques detect cytogenetic abnormalities in more than 50% of CLL cases. More recently, FISH allows for identification of cytogenetic abnormalities in more than 80% of cases.[98] The most common abnormality is deletions of 13q, which is present in 55% of cases, either alone or in combination with other abnormalities. The disease course is more benign for patients with 13q14 abnormalities, and such patients often have a normal life span. Next in frequency of abnormalities are deletions of 11q, which are identified in 15% to 20% of cases. Deletions of 11q23 are associated with massive lymphadenopathy, often out of proportion to the increase in the

TABLE 15-9 Operational Definition of Failure or Suboptimal Response to Imatinib in Previously Untreated Patients with Chronic Phase CML[1]

Time	Failure	Suboptimal Response
3 months	No HR	less than CHR
6 months	less than CHR, no CgR	less than PCgR
12 months	less than PCgR	less than CCgR
18 months	less than CCgR	less than MMolR
Anytime	loss of CHR, loss of CCgR	ACA in Ph+ cells, loss of MMolR

Abbreviations: HR, hematologic response; CHR, complete hematologic response; CgR, any cytogenetic response; PCgR, partial (> 65% Ph-) cytogenetic response; CCgR, complete (100% Ph-) cytogenetic response; ACA, additional chromosome abnormality Ph, Philadelphia chromosome; MMolR, major molecular response.

peripheral blood lymphocyte count. Trisomy 12 can be detected in 15% to 20% of cases. Structural abnormalities of chromosome 17 occur in at least 15% of patients when FISH testing is performed. 17p13 deletions lead to disruption of the *TP53* gene and are found more frequently in cases of atypical CLL, which is associated with a higher likelihood of Richter's transformation, more prolymphocytes, advanced stage, resistance to chemotherapy, and a poor prognosis. More than one-third of patients have complex abnormalities.

Translocations associated with *BCL-2* (t[14;18][q32;q21]) and *BCL-3* (t[14;19][q32;q13.1]) have been detected in only 5% to 10% of cases. However, overexpression of the *BCL-2* gene is present in more than 70% of cases, even in the absence of the chromosome rearrangement. The ratio of the antiapoptotic gene *BCL-2* to the proapoptotic gene *BAX* is increased in CLL cells, which favors cell survival. These findings support the concept that CLL is more a disorder of prolonged cell survival than a hyperproliferative disease, although both factors probably contribute.

Lymphocytes from about half of patients with CLL are naïve and have unmutated V_H genes; the other half contain V_H genes that are mutated, postgerminal center B cells. These two populations are characterized by markedly different clinical outcomes, with the survival significantly shorter for the group with unmutated V_H genes. DNA microarray analyses have shown that ZAP-70 accurately distinguishes the mutated from the unmutated populations of patients with CLL.[99] ZAP-70 is associated with enhanced signal transduction through the BCR complex, which may contribute to an aggressive course.[100] The overall incidence of genomic aberrations is similar in the mutated and unmutated groups; however, the unfavorable cytogenetic abnormalities (e.g., 17p- and 11q-) occur in the unmutated group, whereas the more favorable mutations (e.g., 13q-) occur in the mutated group.[101] Lymphocytes with trisomy 12 tend to have unmutated V_H genes, whereas those with 13q14 have evidence of somatic mutations. CD38 is expressed more commonly in CLL cells that are ZAP70-positive and have unmutated V_H genes.

STAGING AND PROGNOSIS

Several characteristics have been used to stratify patients with CLL into groups according to different clinical outcomes that may require different therapeutic approaches. The five-stage Rai classification[102] is most commonly used in the United States (Table 15-10), and the Binet system[103] is most often applied in Europe (Table 15-11). A major difference between the two systems is that the latter does not include a category for patients with Rai stage 0 disease. Patients classified under Binet stage A include all patients in Rai stage 0, two-thirds of patients in Rai stage I, and one-third of patients in Rai stage II. Nevertheless, the two systems have similar prognostic value.

About 10% to 15% of patients with CLL are younger than age 50, and 20% are younger than age 55. Younger patients are more likely to die from CLL-related events, whereas older patients more often die from secondary malignant diseases and non-CLL causes.

As noted in the previous section, several prognostic factors separate patients into clinically meaningful risk groups even within a clinical stage. The outcome is poor for patients with CLL with unmutated heavy chain genes and expression of CD38, regardless of clinical stage; the clinical course is more indolent for patients with mutated genes and no CD38 expression.[104] CD38 and gene mutational status are independent factors.[105] Favorable cytogenetic abnormalities tend to occur in patients with mutated immunoglobulin genes and patients who do not have expression of CD38, whereas unfavorable abnormalities occur with unmutated genes and expression of CD38.[68,70] Other potential prognostic factors include sex, race, performance status, cellular morphology, pattern of bone marrow infiltration, lymphocyte doubling time, serum beta$_2$-microglobulin, and soluble CD23.

CLINICAL FEATURES

Clinical Presentation

Most patients with CLL are generally asymptomatic at the time of presentation, and the diagnosis is often made incidentally when lymphocytosis is noted during a routine evaluation. The findings on physical examination are normal for

TABLE 15-10 Rai Classification for Staging CLL

Stage	Clinical Features	Median Survival (Years)
0	Lymphocytosis only	> 12.5
I	Lymphadenopathy	8.5
II	Splenomegaly with or without hepatomegaly	6
III*	Anemia	1.5
IV*	Thrombocytopenia	1.5

* The anemia or thrombocytopenia cannot be immune-mediated. Abbreviation: CLL, chronic lymphocytic leukemia.

TABLE 15-11 Binet Classification for Staging Chronic Lymphocytic Leukemia

Stage	Symptoms	Median Survival (Years)
A	< 3 node-bearing areas	> 10
B	≥ 3 node-bearing areas	5
C	Anemia and/or thrombocytopenia	2

20% to 30% of patients, with lymphadenopathy and/or hepatosplenomegaly observed in an additional 40% to 50% of patients. However, as disease progresses, generalized lymphadenopathy and splenomegaly become common features. Involvement of other organs is unusual and should suggest the possibility of transformation to Richter's syndrome.

Infections

Increased susceptibility to infections reflects the hypogammaglobulinemia that worsens with disease progression and abnormal activation of complement. Historically, the most common pathogens have been those that require opsonization for bacterial killing, such as *Staphylococcus pneumoniae, S. aureus,* and *Haemophilus influenzae.* The increased use of immunosuppressive agents such as fludarabine, 2-chlorodeoxyadenosine (2-CdA; cladribine), 2′-deoxycoformycin (DCF; pentostatin), and alemtuzumab has markedly increased the number of infections with opportunistic organisms such as *Candida, Listeria, Pneumocystis carinii,* cytomegalovirus, *Aspergillus,* herpes viruses, and others.

The prophylactic use of intravenous immunoglobulins or antimicrobial agents should be reserved for select patients with documented, repeated bacterial infections.

Aggressive Transformation

In 3% to 15% of patients with CLL, disease will evolve into a more aggressive lymphoid malignant process, most often Richter's syndrome, which characteristically presents with increasing lymphadenopathy, hepatosplenomegaly, fever, abdominal pain, weight loss, progressive anemia and thrombocytopenia with a rapid rise in the peripheral blood lymphocyte count, and an increased serum LDH level. Evaluation of lymph node tissue obtained by biopsy indicates a large cell lymphoma. This transformation is not clearly related to either the nature or extent of previous therapy. The large cell lymphoma shares immunologic, cytogenetic, and molecular features with the original CLL clone in half of the cases. For patients with Richter's syndrome, response to systemic therapy is poor, with a median survival of 4 to 5 months when treatment involves alkylating agents; survival may be longer after use of nucleoside analog-based regimens.

CLL also may evolve into prolymphocytic leukemia (PLL), which is associated with progressive anemia and thrombocytopenia, with at least 55% prolymphocytes in the peripheral blood. Clinical features include lymphadenopathy, hepatosplenomegaly, a wasting syndrome, and an increasing resistance to therapy. Transformation to acute lymphoblastic leukemia, plasma cell leukemia, multiple myeloma, or Hodgkin's disease has been noted in anecdotal reports.

Autoimmunity

A positive Coombs' antiglobulin test is present in 20% to 30% of CLL cases, with clinical hemolysis in 10% to 25% of patients. The frequency of immune thrombocytopenia appears to be about 2%. In most cases, these antibodies are polyclonal; therefore, they are not produced by the malignant B cells.

Autoimmune anemia or thrombocytopenia generally responds to corticosteroids such as prednisone at a dose of 60 mg to 100 mg/day, which may be tapered after 1 or 2 weeks following evidence of response. Patients who do not experience a response to corticosteroids may experience a response to high-dose intravenous immunoglobulins. Reports suggest impressive results following therapy with rituximab. Splenectomy may be considered when systemic approaches fail. Radiation therapy to the spleen induces only transient responses.

Pure Red Cell Aplasia

Pure red cell aplasia is an uncommon occurrence in CLL. It is characterized by severe anemia without a reticulocyte response or bone marrow normoblasts and without neutropenia or thrombocytopenia. Corticosteroids as well as cyclosporine and rituximab may be effective.

Secondary Malignant Diseases

Secondary malignant diseases occur with increased frequency in patients with CLL, related both to the immune defects of the disease as well as to the consequences of therapy. The most frequent tumors are skin cancer (including melanomas), colon cancers, and lung cancers.

THERAPY

CLL is not curable with currently available therapies, with the exception of allogeneic hematopoietic cell transplantation, nor is there evidence that treatment of patients with early-stage disease (Rai 0-2 or Binet A) extends life expectancy. Therefore, asymptomatic patients with early-stage disease should be monitored but not treated unless enrolled on a clinical trial. Early-stage patients with disease-related symptoms including B-symptoms; weight loss; pronounced fatigue; symptoms or complications from hepatomegaly, splenomegaly or lymphadenopathy; autoimmune anemia or thrombocytopenia; or recurrent infections may be candidates for treatment. A rapid lymphocyte doubling time (less than 6 months) also may support the decision to treat.

INITIAL THERAPY

Fludarabine and Other Purine Analogues

Fludarabine is the most active chemotherapy agent for the treatment of CLL and is generally administered as an intravenous bolus of 25 mg/m^2 daily for 5 consecutive days once a month. When used as a single agent, the response rate to fludarabine as initial treatment is about 70%, including a 5% to 30% rate of complete response.[106,107] The major toxicities associated with fludarabine are moderate myelosuppression and severe immunosuppression, with occasional neurotoxicity, particularly when used at doses that are higher than recommended. The number of lymphocyte cells, notably CD4, decreases within weeks, and the count does not return to normal for 1 year or more after treatment has been discontinued. Fludarabine has not been found to be more myelotoxic than alkylating agent-based regimens, but it has been associated with increased opportunistic infections.[107,108] Nevertheless, prophylactic antimicrobial therapy should be reserved for patients who have had extensive prior therapy, are taking concurrent corticosteroids, or have a history of infection.

Tumor lysis syndrome occurs in less than 0.4% of patients with CLL who are treated with fludarabine. This syndrome may be fatal and is not consistently preventable with the use of prophylactic allopurinol and/or hydration. Fludarabine may be associated with autoimmune hemolytic anemia and thrombocytopenia. Whether patients with these conditions can continue to receive the drug is controversial.

Despite the profound immunosuppression associated with single-agent fludarabine, the risk of secondary malignant disease does not appear to be increased.[109]

Both cladribine and pentostatin are active in CLL, although to a lesser extent than fludarabine. There is limited activity but considerable toxicity from these agents when used to treat patients for whom fludarabine has failed.

Alkylating Agents

Administration of oral chlorambucil, either at a dose of 4 to 8 mg/m^2 daily for 4 to 8 weeks or as pulses of 15 to 30 mg/m^2 every 2 to 4 weeks, achieves response in approximately 20% to 70% of previously untreated patients, although few of these responses are complete. In a large prospective trial, chlorambucil was found to be inferior to fludarabine in terms of response rates and time to disease progression.[107]

Fludarabine-alkylating Agent Combinations

Various combinations of fludarabine and alkylating agents have been studied and compared with single-agent fludarabine. The most thoroughly studied combination is fludarabine plus cyclophosphamide, which in two prospective randomized trials has been found to result in higher complete response rates and overall response rates, as well as longer response durations than fludarabine alone.[110] To date, no differences in overall survival have emerged.

Rituximab-containing Combinations

Unless very high doses are used, rituximab has only modest single-agent modest activity in CLL.[111] However, the combination of rituximab plus fludarabine appears very active in CLL. A recent retrospective comparison of 104 patients treated on two phase II trials of fludarabine plus rituximab with 178 patients treated with fludarabine alone on a previous trial using exactly the same study criteria showed improved 2-year progression-free and overall survival with the combination.[112] Although this survival advantage has not yet been confirmed in prospective randomized trials, the combination of fludarabine plus rituximab has become a popular first-line therapy for CLL.

Other Combinations

Other combinations under study include the three-drug combination of fludarabine/rituximab/cyclophosphamide or combinations that include the anti-CD52 antibody alemtuzumab (see below). High levels of activity been have reported in phase II trials, but increased toxicities also have been reported. Whether these combinations represent a therapeutic advantage is unclear.

TREATMENT FOR RELAPSED OR REFRACTORY DISEASE

Treatment is not necessarily needed for relapsed or refractory disease after initial therapy; treatment in this setting is based on the same indications as for initial treatment. The most appropriate treatment for such patients is a clinical research study. For patients who are not eligible for a trial or who are unwilling to participate in clinical research, salvage therapy is determined on the type of primary therapy received and the duration of the initial response. In general, patients who have long first remissions can be retreated with the same agents as used initially with a reasonable chance of response. Patients who relapse within 6 months of previous therapy should be switched to an alternative regimen. Patients initially treated with only alkylating agents should receive a fludarabine-containing regimen. Patients refractory to therapy with fludarabine sometimes respond to the rituximab/cyclophosphamide/fludarabine combination or should be switched to alemtuzumab.[113]

Alemtuzumab is a humanized anti-CD52 monoclonal antibody that has been approved by the U.S. Food and Drug

Administration for the treatment of fludarabine-refractory CLL. CD52 is an antigen of unknown function that is expressed on virtually all lymphocytes at various stages of differentiation, as well as monocytes, macrophages, and eosinophils, but not hematopoietic stem cells, erythrocytes, or platelets.

Alemtuzumab is generally administered at doses of 3 mg on the first day, 10 mg on the second day, and 30 mg three times a week as soon as the infusion-related reactions are tolerable. Patients are premedicated with acetaminophen and diphenhydramine. The use of hydrocortisone also has been recommended. Antimicrobial prophylaxis should include trimethoprim sulfamethoxazole and acyclovir. Alemtuzumab is administered for 4 to 12 weeks, although studies suggest that there is additional benefit when therapy is extended to 18 weeks.[114]

The pivotal trial of alemtuzumab included 93 patients for whom prior therapy with fludarabine had failed and who also had received alkylating agents.[115] The response rate was 33%, including a 2% rate of complete response. An additional six patients had clearing of CLL from all sites but had persistent anemia or thrombocytopenia that improved during long-term follow-up. The median duration of response was 9 months; the median survival was 16 months for all patients and 32 months for patients who had a response. Toxicities can be either acute and related to the infusions or delayed and associated with myelosuppression and immunosuppression. The most frequent adverse events include rigors (90% of patients), fever (85%), nausea (53%), vomiting (38%), and rash (33%). These events decrease over the duration of treatment. Infections also are common — often with opportunistic organisms — notably reactivation of cytomegalovirus (CMV) that may occur in as many as 25% of patients. Routine monitoring for CMV should be performed weekly by PCR as well as intervention with gancyclovir in the setting of a positive test or after the onset of clinical symptoms.

Alemtuzumab appears to be as active when administered subcutaneously as when given intravenously, but with fewer infusional complications. However, mild to moderate cutaneous reactions may occur, lasting up to 2 weeks.[114]

Other agents under investigation for CLL include lenalidomide, flavopiridol, and depsipeptide.

HEMATOPOIETIC CELL TRANSPLANTATION

Initial trials of ablative allogeneic hematopoietic cell transplantation for refractory CLL showed substantial non-relapse mortality but prolonged disease-free survival for a significant proportion of patients. A study from Seattle, for example, demonstrated 32% 5-year disease-free survival for patients with refractory CLL.[116] Studies from M. D. Anderson Cancer Center, Dana-Farber Cancer Institute, and the IBMTR provide further evidence that prolonged disease-free survival can be achieved in CLL with allogeneic transplantation.[117,118]

Given that the median age at diagnosis of CLL is older than 60, ablative transplantation for this disease has been limited to a minority of patients. The more recent advent of reduced-intensity transplantation has widened the possible application of transplantation. In a study from Seattle, 64 patients with advanced CLL were treated with a reduced intensity regimen, with a 52% disease-free survival rate at 2 years post-transplant.[119] Thus, reduced-intensity allogeneic transplantation appears to be a reasonable option for patients with fludarabine-refractory disease who are otherwise in reasonably good health.

SUPPORTIVE MEASURES

Splenectomy

Splenectomy may provide important palliation for patients with CLL for whom systemic treatment has failed and who have persistent splenomegaly or cytopenia that precludes chemotherapy. The procedure also should be considered for patients with autoimmune thrombocytopenia or hemolytic anemia who do not experience a response to more conservative measures, such as corticosteroids, intravenous immunoglobulins, or rituximab.

Leukapheresis

Leukapheresis results in only transient reductions in circulating lymphocytes and is not recommended for general practice. As patients with CLL rarely experience tumor cell aggregates, regardless of the number of circulating cells, systemic treatment is usually adequate to reduce the number of circulating lymphocytes, when indicated.

Erythropoietin

Erythropoietin may reduce transfusion requirements for approximately two-thirds of patients with CLL, and a trial involving this agent can be considered for patients who have CLL with anemia and no other obvious correctable cause.[120]

ASSESSMENT OF RESPONSE TO THERAPY IN CLL

The National Cancer Institute Working Group eligibility, response, and toxicity criteria are used worldwide for dose modifications for drug-related myelosuppression and as a grading system for infectious complications. As more information is gathered on the effect of attaining minimal residual disease and molecular remission, these criteria may need to be modified.[121]

PROLYMPHOCYTIC LEUKEMIA (PLL)

Patients with prolymphocytic leukemia (PLL) tend to be older than patients with CLL (median age, 70 years). At the time of presentation, the primary symptoms include abdominal discomfort, fever, and weight loss. Disease pres-

KEY POINTS

- Prolymphocytic leukemia can occur as a transformation from CLL but is more commonly de novo.
- Therapeutic activity with alemtuzumab and purine analogs has been noted but tends to be transient.

ents at an advanced stage for virtually all patients. PLL is associated with a larger spleen and a higher white blood cell count than CLL; however, there is less lymphadenopathy. PLL cells are large, with a round nucleus and a prominent nucleolus. In de novo PLL, most of the peripheral blood mononuclear cells tend to be prolymphocytes; in the setting of an aggressive transformation from CLL, there is a dimorphic population in the peripheral blood. The immunophenotype is different from CLL; the cells are positive for CD19, CD20, and CD24, and they strongly express CD22, surface immunoglobulins, and FMC7. CD5 or CD23 is expressed in less than one-third of cases.

Patients with PLL are generally treated with the same regimens used to treat CLL, but response rates tend to be lower and response durations usually are shorter. Therapeutic activity with alemtuzumab and purine analogs has been noted but tends to be transient.

HAIRY CELL LEUKEMIA

Hairy cell leukemia occurs in about 500 new patients each year in the United States, generally in older persons, with a strong predominance in men. Patients generally present with symptoms referable to cytopenias, including infections (29%) and weakness or fatigue (27%); less common presentations include pain in the left upper quadrant related to splenomegaly (5%) or bleeding related to thrombocytopenia (4%). The incidence of secondary malignant disease is increased. The most common signs include palpable splenomegaly (72% to 86%); hepatomegaly (13% to 20%); hairy cells in the peripheral blood (85% to 89%); thrombocytopenia, defined as less than 100,000/mm^3 (53%); anemia, defined as hemoglobin of less than 12 g/dL (71% to 77%); and neutropenia, defined as an absolute neutrophil count of less than 500/mm^3 (32% to 39%).

KEY POINTS

- Hairy cell leukemia is highly responsive to cladribine (2-CdA) or pentostatin (DCF).
- Patients with refractory disease who require treatment may have a response to rituximab or to an anti-CD22 immunotoxin.

The cells in the peripheral blood generally have an eccentric, spongiform kidney-shaped nucleus, with characteristic filamentous cytoplasmic projections. A bone marrow biopsy usually is needed to make the diagnosis, because an aspirate often cannot be obtained. The malignant cells are of B-cell origin, expressing CD19 and CD20, as well as the monocyte antigen CD11c. The most specific marker is CD103. It is most difficult to distinguish hairy cell leukemia from hairy cell variant; the latter often is associated with a high circulating white blood cell count, cells containing bilobed nuclei with prominent nucleoli, a bone marrow with interstitial infiltration of clumped cells, and resistance to treatment with interferon-alpha, cladribine, and pentostatin.

Treatment is indicated in the setting of massive or progressive splenomegaly, worsening blood counts, recurrent infection, more than 20,000 hairy cells/mm^3 of peripheral blood, or bulky lymphadenopathy. Until the early 1980s, splenectomy was the standard treatment for hairy cell leukemia. This procedure improves symptoms related to splenomegaly and peripheral blood counts — often for prolonged periods of time — but it does not affect the disease itself. Splenectomy is now reserved for the rare occasion when a patient has disease that is refractory to treatment and has splenomegaly that is either symptomatic or is resulting in cytopenias.

Interferon was the first systemic therapy to demonstrate activity in hairy cell leukemia. At doses of 2×10^6 U/m^2/d or 3×10^6 U three times a week, interferon induces response in 80% of patients; however, only 10% are complete remissions. Although response generally occurs within 3 to 4 months, therapy may be needed for more than 1 year before a maximal effect is achieved. Hairy cell leukemia invariably recurs after interferon therapy has been discontinued, and maintenance therapy is associated with excessive toxicity and expense without any apparent survival benefit.

Purine analogs revolutionized the treatment of patients with hairy cell leukemia. Pentostatin at doses of 4 mg/m^2 intravenously every other week for 4 to 6 months achieves complete remission in 60% to 89% of previously treated or untreated patients, including those for whom interferon has failed, with an overall response rate of 80% to 90%. Approximately 25% of patients experience relapse during more than 5 years of follow-up. In an Intergroup trial, 350 previously untreated patients with hairy cell leukemia were randomly assigned to treatment with interferon or with pentostatin. The complete remission rate was approximately 11% for interferon compared with 76% for pentostatin, with a significant advantage to the latter therapy in terms of the durability of response.[122] The lack of a survival advantage reflects the high number of patients treated with interferon who receive salvage therapy with pentostatin.

Cladribine also is highly effective for hairy cell leukemia. Using a 7-day infusion or a 2-hour infusion for 5 to 7 days achieves response for approximately 80% to 90% of patients, with a complete remission rate of 65% to 80%. The responses tend to be durable, with relapse occurring in 20% to 30% of patients during prolonged follow-up. In many cases, relapse is characterized only by an increase in hairy cells in the bone marrow, with no indication for treatment. A second durable response is achieved for most patients who need repeat treatment. The results with pentostatin are equivalent to those with cladribine. The shorter duration of treatment makes the latter drug somewhat more attractive, although it may be associated with greater toxicity.

An anti-CD22 pseudomonas exotoxin immunoconjugate induces response for most patients for whom purine analog therapy has failed.[123] Rituximab also has shown promise for such patients or for patients with hairy cell variant.

CHRONIC T-CELL LEUKEMIAS

The chronic T-cell leukemias consist of mycosis fungoides, T-PLL, adult T-cell leukemia/lymphoma (ATLL), various subtypes of large granular lymphocytosis, and natural killer (NK) cell leukemia. T-PLL tends to occur in older persons (median age, 63 years). The presenting features include widespread lymphadenopathy (50% of cases) and splenomegaly (approximately 80%); the lymphocyte count is often more than 100,000/mm^3. Anemia and thrombocytopenia also are common. T-PLL is associated with recurrent chromosome abnormalities, notably inversion of chromosome 14 with breakpoints at the long arm at q11 and q32, in 80% of patients. In more than half of cases, abnormalities of chromosome 8 can be identified (i(8q)), trisomy 8, t(8;8)(p11;q32), or add(8)(p11). Treatment is, in general, unsatisfactory. Alemtuzumab has demonstrated impressive activity in T-PLL, with response rates of 50% to 70%.[124]

Large granular lymphocytosis can be divided into two major subsets: those that are CD3-positive representing in vivo activated cytotoxic T cells (T-large granular lymphocytosis) and NK-large granular lymphocytosis that are CD3-negative. T-large granular lymphocytosis tends to occur in older persons, and most patients (60%) are symptomatic at diagnosis. There is an association with recurrent infections, related in part to chronic neutropenia, as well as to anemia and rheumatoid arthritis with Felty's syndrome. The phenotype includes CD3-positive, CD8-positive, CD57-positive, with clonal rearrangement of T-cell receptor genes. NK-large granular lymphocytosis accounts for approximately 15% of the disease and includes aggressive NK-cell leukemia and a more indolent NK lymphocytosis. The cells are CD3-negative, CD8-positive, CD16-positive, CD56-positive, and CD57-positive/-negative. Rearrangements of *TCR* genes are absent. In the aggressive form of the disease, patients tend to be younger and do not have rheumatoid arthritis. Infiltration of the gastrointestinal tract and bone marrow are common. Neutropenia is modest in comparison with the severity of anemia and thrombocytopenia. Patients often die from multiorgan failure with a coagulopathy, generally within a few months of diagnosis, despite aggressive chemotherapy. Approximately 5% of large granular lymphocytosis is a nonclonal expansion of CD3-positive large granular lymphocytosis that is generally unaccompanied by lymphadenopathy or hepatosplenomegaly. The features of the cells are CD3-negative, CD4-negative, CD8-negative, CD16++, and CD56-positive. The disease is indolent, rarely requiring intervention unless accompanied by neutropenia. Prednisone and immunosuppressive agents have been used. It is not clear if this disorder is actually neoplastic.

ATLL is endemic in Japan, the Caribbean, parts of central Africa, and the southeastern United States. It is linked to the prevalence of HTLV-1. There are a number of clinical variants that range from a chronic, smoldering disorder, to an aggressive, leukemic disease. The levels of serum calcium and LDH are prognostic for outcome. The major causes of death are related to infection. Combination chemotherapy and pentostatin have had limited success.

KEY POINT

- Chronic T-cell leukemias consist of mycosis fungoides, T-PLL, adult T-cell leukemia/lymphoma, various subtypes of large granular lymphocytosis, and natural killer cell leukemia.

REFERENCES

1. Buckley JD, Buckley CM, Breslow NE, et al. Concordance for childhood cancer in twins. *Med Pediatr Oncol.* 1996;26(4):223–229.
2. Song WJ, Sullivan MG, Legare RD, et al. Haploinsufficiency of CBFA2 causes familial thrombocytopenia with propensity to develop acute myelogenous leukaemia. *Nat.Genet.* 1999;23(2):166–175.
3. Taylor AM, Metcalfe JA, Thick J, et al. Leukemia and lymphoma in ataxia telangiectasia (Review). *Blood.* 1996;87(2):423–438.
4. Mortreux F, Gabet AS, Wattel E. Molecular and cellular aspects of HTLV-1 associated leukemogenesis in vivo (Review). *Leukemia.* 2003;17(1):26–38.
5. Cronkite EP, Moloney W, Bond VP. Radiation leukemogenesis: an analysis of the problem. *Am J Med.* 1960;28:673–682.
6. Leone G, Mele L, Pulsoni A, et al. The incidence of secondary leukemias (Review). *Haematologica.* 1999;84(10):937–945.
7. Larson RA, Le Beau MM, Ratain MJ, Rowley JD. Balanced translocations involving chromosome bands 11q23 and 21q22 in therapy-related leukemia. *Blood.* 1992;79(7):1892–1893.
8. Bennett JM, Catovsky D, Daniel MT, et al. Proposals for the classification of the acute leukaemias. French-American-British (FAB) cooperative group. *Br J Haematol.*1976;33(4):451–458.
9. Campos L, Guyotat D, Archimbaud E, et al. Surface marker expression in adult acute myeloid leukaemia: correlations with initial characteristics, morphology and response to therapy. *Br J Haematol.* 1989;72(2):161–166.

10. Boucheix C, David B, Sebban C, et al. Immunophenotype of adult acute lymphoblastic leukemia, clinical parameters, and outcome: an analysis of a prospective trial incuding 562 tested patients (LALA87). French Group on Therapy for Adult Acute Lymphoblastic Leukemia. *Blood.* 1994;84(5):1603–1612.

11. de The H, Lavau C, Marchio A, et al. The PML-RAR alpha fusion mRNA generated by the t(15;17) translocation in acute promyelocytic leukemia encodes a functionally altered RAR. *Cell.* 1991;66(4): 675–684.

12. Appelbaum FR, Kopecky KJ, Tallman MS, et al. The clinical spectrum of adult acute myeloid leukaemia associated with core binding factor translocations. *Br J Haematol.* 2006;135(2):165–173.

13. Paschka P, Marcucci G, Ruppert A, et al. Adverse prognostic significance of KIT mutations in adult acute myeloid leukemia with inv(16) and t(8;21): a Cancer and Leukemia Group B Study. *J Clin Oncol.* 2006;24(24):3904–3911.

14. Ernst P, Wang J, Korsmeyer SJ. The role of MLL in hematopoiesis and leukemia (Review). *Curr Opin Hematol.* 2002;9(4):282–287.

15. Kottaridis PD, Gale RE, Frew ME, et al. The presence of a FLT3 internal tandem duplication in patients with acute myeloid leukemia (AML) adds important prognostic information to cytogenetic risk group and response to the first cycle of chemotherapy: analysis of 854 patients from the United Kingdom Medical Research Council AML 10 and 12 trials. *Blood.* 2001;98(6):1752–1759.

16. Thiede C, Koch S, Creutzig E, et al. Prevalence and prognostic impact of NPM1 mutations in 1485 adult patients with acute myeloid leukemia (AML). *Blood.* 2006;107(10):4011–4020.

17. Chan LC, Karhi KK, Rayter SI, et al. A novel abl protein expressed in Philadelphia chromosome positive acute lymphoblastic leukaemia. *Nature.* 1987;325(6105):635–637.

18. Radich JP, Kopecky KJ, Boldt DH, et al. Detection of BCR-ABL fusion genes in adult acute lymphoblastic leukemia by the polymerase chain reaction. *Leukemia.* 1994;8(10):1688–1695.

19. Pui CH, Relling MV, Downing JR, et al. Acute lymphoblastic leukemia. *N Engl J Med.* 2004;350(15):1535–1548.

20. Vardiman JW, Harris NL, Brunning RD. The World Health Organization (WHO) classification of the myeloid neoplasms *Blood.* 2002; 100(7):2292–2302.

21. Weick JK, Kopecky KJ, Appelbaum FR, et al. A randomized investigation of high-dose versus standard-dose cytosine arabinoside with daunorubicin in patients with previously untreated acute myeloid leukemia: A Southwest Oncology Group Study. *Blood.*1996;88(8): 2841–2851.

22. Bishop JF, Matthews JP, Young GA, et al. A randomized study of high-dose cytarabine in induction in acute myeloid leukemia. *Blood.* 1996;87(5):1710–1717.

23. Wiernik PH, Banks PL, Case DC, Jr, et al. Cytarabine plus idarubicin or daunorubicin as induction and consolidation therapy for previously untreated adult patients with acute myeloid leukemia. Blood. 1992; 79(2):313–319.

24. Rowe JM, Neuberg D, Friedenberg W, et al. A phase 3 study of three induction regimens and of priming with GM-CSF in older adults with acute myeloid leukemia: a trial by the Eastern Cooperative Oncology Group. Blood. 2004;103(2):479-485.

25. Bishop JF, Lowenthal RM, Joshua D, et al. Etoposide in acute nonlymphocytic leukemia. Australian Leukemia Study Group. *Blood.* 1990; 75(1):27–32.

26. Tilly H, Castaigne S, Bordessoule D, et al. Low-dose cytarabine versus intensive chemotherapy in the treatment of acute nonlymphocytic leukemia in the elderly. *J Clin Oncol.* 1990;8(2):272–279.

27. Godwin JE, Kopecky KJ, Head DR, et al. A double-blind placebo-controlled trial of granulocyte colony-stimulating factor in elderly patients with previously untreated acute myeloid leukemia: a Southwest Oncology Group Study (9031). *Blood.* 1998;91(10): 3607–3615.

28. Heil G, Hoelzer D, Sanz MA, et al. A randomized, double-blind, placebo-controlled, phase III study of filgrastim in remission induction and consolidation therapy for adults with de novo acute myeloid leukemia. The International Acute Myeloid Leukemia Study Group. *Blood.* 1997;90(12):4710–4718.

29. Cassileth PA, Hines JD, Oken MM, et al. Maintenance chemotherapy prolongs remission duration in adult acute nonlymphocytic leukemia. *J Clin Oncol.* 1998;6(4):583–587.

30. Appelbaum FR. Acute myeloid leukemia in adults, in Abeloff MD, Armitage JO, Niederhuber JE, et al (eds). *Clinical Oncology.* (edThird). Philadelphia, PA, Elsevier Churchill Livingstone. 2004;2825–2848.

31. Mayer RJ, Davis RB, Schiffer CA, et al. Intensive post-remission chemotherapy in adults with acute myeloid leukemia. Cancer and Leukemia Group B. *N Engl J Med.* 1994;331(14):896–903.

32. O'Donnell MR, Appelbaum FR, Baer MR, et al. NCCN practice guidelines for acute myelogenous leukemia. Oncology, NCCN Proceedings. 2000;14:53–61.

33. Rees JK, Gray RG, Wheatley K. Dose intensification in acute myeloid leukemia: greater effectiveness at lower cost. Principal report of the Medical Research Council's AML9 study. MRC Leukemia in Adults Working Party. *Br J Haematol.* 1996;94(1):89–98.

34. Morrison FS, Kopecky KJ, Head DR, et al. Late intensification with POMP chemotherapy prolongs survival in acute myelogenous leukemia - results of a Southwest Oncology Group study of rubidazone versus adriamycin for remission induction, prophylactic intrathecal therapy, late intensification, and levamisole maintenance. *Leukemia.* 1992;6(7): 708–714.

35. Grimwade D, Walker H, Oliver F, et al. The importance of diagnostic cytogenetics on outcome in AML: analysis of 1,612 patients entered into the MRC AML 10 trial. The Medical Research Council Adult and Children's Leukaemia Working Parties. *Blood.* 1998;92(7): 2322–2333.

36. Slovak ML, Kopecky KJ, Cassileth PA, et al. Karyotypic analysis predicts outcome of preremission and postremission therapy in adult acute myeloid leukemia: a Southwest Oncology Group/Eastern Cooperative Oncology Group Study. *Blood.* 2000;96(13):4075–4083.

37. Estey EH. Treatment of relapsed and refractory acute myelogenous leukemia (Review). *Leukemia.* 2000;14(3):476–479.

38. Larson RA, Sievers EL, Stadtmauer EA, et al. Final report of the efficacy and safety of gemtuzumab ozogamicin (Mylotarg) in patients with CD33-positive acute myeloid leukemia in first recurrence. *Cancer.* 2005;104(7):1442–1452.

39. Appelbaum FR. The current status of hematopoietic cell transplantation. *Annu Rev Med.* 2003;54:491–512.

40. Yanada M, Matsuo K, Emi N, et al. Efficacy of allogeneic hematopoietic stem cell transplantation depends on cytogenetic risk for acute myeloid leukemia in first disease remission: a metaanalysis. *Cancer.* 2005;103(8): 1652–1658.

41. Bensinger WI, Martin PJ, Storer B, et al. Transplantation of bone marrow as compared with peripheral blood cells from HLA-identical relatives in patients with hematologic cancers. *N Engl J Med.* 2001; 344(3): 175–181.

42. Schmitz N, Beksac M, Hasenclever D, et al. Transplantation of mobilized peripheral blood cells to HLA-identical siblings with standard-risk leukemia. *Blood.* 2002;100(3):761–767.

43. Couban S, Simpson DR, Barnett MJ, et al. A randomized multicenter comparison of bone marrow and peripheral blood in recipients of matched sibling allogeneic transplants for myeloid malignancies. *Blood.* 2002;100(5):1525–1531.

44. Gorin NC. Autologous stem cell transplantation in acute myelocytic leukemia (Review). *Blood.* 1998;92(4):1073–1090.

45. Helenglass G, Powles RL, McElwain TJ, et al. Melphalan and total body irradiation (TBI) versus cyclophosphamide and TBI as conditioning for allogeneic matched sibling bone marrow transplants for acute myeloblastic leukaemia in first remission. *Bone Marrow Transplant.* 1988;3(1):21–29.

46. Ringden O, Labopin M, Tura S, et al. A comparison of busulphan versus total body irradiation combined with cyclophosphamide as conditioning for autograft or allograft bone marrow transplantation in patients with acute leukaemia. Acute Leukaemia Working Party of the European Group for Blood and Marrow Transplantation (EBMT). *Br J Haematol.* 1996;93(3):637–645.

47. Storb R, Deeg HJ, Whitehead J, et al. Methotrexate and cyclosporine compared with cyclosporine alone for prophylaxis of acute graft versus host disease after marrow transplantation for leukemia. *N Engl J Med.* 1986;314(12):729–735.

48. Warrell RP Jr, Frankel SR, Miller WH Jr, et al. Differentiation therapy of acute promyelocytic leukemia with tretinoin (all-trans-retinoic acid). *N Engl J Med.* 1991;324(20):1385–1393.

49. Head D, Kopecky KJ, Weick J, et al. Effect of aggressive daunomycin therapy on survival in acute promyelocytic leukemia. *Blood.* 1995;86(5): 1717–1728.

50. Tallman MS, Nabhan C, Feusner JH, et al. Acute promyelocytic leukemia: evolving therapeutic strategies. *Blood.* 2002;99(3):759–767.

51. Soignet SL, Frankel SR, Douer D, et al. United States multicenter study of arsenic trioxide in relapsed acute promyelocytic leukemia. *J Clin Oncol.* 2001;19(18):3852–3860.

52. Tallman MS, Andersen JW, Schiffer CA, et al. Clinical description of 44 patients with acute promyelocytic leukemia who developed the retinoic acid syndrome. *Blood.* 2000;95(1):90–95.

53. Witherspoon RP, Deeg HJ, Storer B, et al. Hematopoietic stem-cell transplantation for treatment-related leukemia or myelodysplasia. *J Clin Oncol.* 2001;19(8):2134–2141.

54. Kantarjian HM, O'Brien S, Smith TL, et al. Results of treatment with hyper-CVAD, a dose-intensive regimen, in adult acute lymphocytic leukemia. *J Clin Oncol.* 2000;18(3):547–561.

55. Weiss M, Maslak P, Feldman E, et al. Cytarabine with high-dose mitoxantrone induces rapid complete remissions in adult acute lymphoblastic leukemia without the use of vincristine or prednisone. *J Clin Oncol.* 1996;14(9):2480–2485.

56. Larson RA, Dodge RK, Linker CA, et al. A randomized controlled trial of filgrastim during remission induction and consolidation chemotherapy for adults with acute lymphoblastic leukemia: CALGB study 9111. *Blood.* 1998;92(5):1556–1564.

57. Hoelzer D, Gökbuget N. Treatment of adult acute lymphoblastic leukemia: perspective 2, in Pui C-H. (ed): Treatment of Acute Leukemias: New Directions for Clinical Research. Totowa, NJ, Humana Press Inc., 2003:pp 143–157.

58. Moorman AV, Harrison CJ, Buck GA, et al. Karyotype is an independent prognostic factor in adult lymphoblastic leukemia (ALL): analysis of cytogenetic data from patients treated on the Medical Research Council (MRC) UKALLXII/Eastern Cooperative Oncology Group (ECOG) 2993 trial. *Blood.* 2007;109(8):3189-3197.

59. Yanada M, Takeuchi J, Sugiura I, et al. High complete remission rate and promising outcome by combination of imatinib and chemotherapy for newly diagnosed BCR-ABL-positive acute lymphoblastic leukemia: a phase II study by the Japan Adult Leukemia Study Group. *J Clin Oncol.* 2006;24(3):460–466.

60. Mancini M, Scappaticci D, Cimino G, et al. A comprehensive genetic classification of adult acute lymphoblastic leukemia (ALL): analysis of the GIMEMA 0496 protocol. *Blood.* 2005;105(9):3434–3441.

61. International Bone Marrow Transplantation Registry/Autologous Blood and Marrow Registry. Available at http://www.ibmtr.org. Accessed November 7, 2006.

62. Thiebaut A, Vernant JP, Degos L, et al. Adult acute lymphocytic leukemia study testing chemotherapy and autologous and allogeneic transplantation. A follow-up report of the French protocol LALA 87 (Review). *Hematol Oncol Clin North Am.* 2000;14(6):1353–1366.

63. Livesey EA, Brook CG. Thyroid dysfunction after radiotherapy and chemotherapy of brain tumours. *Arch Dis Child.* 1989;64(4): 593–595.

64. Bennett JM, Catovsky D, Daniel MT, et al. Proposals for the classification of the myelodysplastic syndromes. *Br J Haematol.* 1982;51(2): 189–199.

65. Bennett JM. World Health Organization classification of the acute leukemias and myelodysplastic syndrome. *Int J Hematol.* 2000;72(2): 131–133.

66. Greenberg P, Cox C, LeBeau MM, et al. International scoring system for evaluating prognosis in myelodysplastic syndromes (erratum appears in *Blood.* 1998;91(3):1100). *Blood.* 1997;89(6):2079–2088.

67. List A, Kurtin S, Roe DJ, et al. Efficacy of lenalidomide in myelodysplastic syndromes. *N Engl J Med.* 2005;352(6):549–557.

68. Silverman LR, Demakos EP, Peterson BL, et al. Randomized controlled trial of azacitidine in patients with the myelodysplastic syndrome: a study of the cancer and leukemia group B. *J Clin Oncol.* 2002;20(10): 2429–2440.

69. Saba H, Rosenfeld C, Issa J-P, et al. First report of the phase III North American trial of decitabine in advanced myelodysplastic syndrome (MDS). *Blood.* 2004;104(Part 1):23a, #67 (abstr).

70. Hellstrom-Lindberg E, Gulbrandsen N, Lindberg G, et al. A validated decision model for treating the anaemia of myelodysplastic syndromes with erythropoietin + granulocyte colony-stimulating factor: significant effects on quality of life. *Br J Haematol.* 2003;120(6): 1037–1046.

71. Greenberg P, Taylor K, Larson R, et al. Phase III randomized multicenter trial of G-CSF vs. observation for MDS. *Blood.* 1993;82:196a.

72. Molldrem JJ, Leifer E, Bahceci E, et al. Antithymocyte globulin for treatment of the bone marrow failure associated with myelodysplastic syndrome [summary for patients in Ann Intern Med. 2002;137(3): I-27]. *Ann Intern Med.* 2002;137(3):156–163.

73. Saunthararajah Y, Nakamura R, Nam JM, et al. HLA-DR15 (DR2) is overrepresented in myelodysplastic syndrome and aplastic anemia and predicts a response to immunosuppression in myelodysplastic syndrome. *Blood.* 2002;100(5):1570–1574.

74. Estey EH, Thall PF, Cortes JE, et al. Comparison of idarubicin + ara-C-, fludarabine + ara-C-, and topotecan + ara-C-based regimens in treatment of newly diagnosed acute myeloid leukemia, refractory anemia with excess blasts in transformation, or refractory anemia with excess blasts. *Blood.* 2001;98(13):3575–3583.

75. Appelbaum FR, Anderson J. Allogeneic bone marrow transplantation for myelodysplastic syndrome: outcomes analysis according to IPSS score. *Leukemia.* 1998;12(Suppl 1):S25–S29.

76. Deeg HJ, Storer B, Slattery JT, et al. Conditioning with targeted busulfan and cyclophosphamide for hemopoietic stem cell transplantation from related and unrelated donors in patients with myelodysplastic syndrome. *Blood.* 2002;100(4):1201–1207.

77. Sokal JE, Cox EB, Baccarani M, et al. Prognostic discrimination in "good-risk" chronic granulocytic leukemia. *Blood.* 1984;63(4)789-799.

78. Interferon alfa versus chemotherapy for chronic myeloid leukemia: a meta-analysis of seven randomized trials: Chonic Myeloid Leukemia Trialists' Collaborative Group. *J Natl Cancer Inst.* 1997;89(21):1616–1620.

79. Savage DG, Antman KH. Imatinib mesylate—a new oral targeted therapy (Review). *N Engl J Med.* 2002;346(9):683–693.

80. Druker BJ, Talpaz M, Resta DJ, et al. Efficacy and safety of a specific inhibitor of the BCR-ABL tyrosine kinase in chronic myeloid leukemia. *N Engl J Med.* 2001;344(14):1031–1037.

81. O'Brien SG, Guilhot F, Larson RA, et al. Imatinib compared with interferon and low-dose cytarabine for newly diagnosed chronic-phase chronic myeloid leukemia. *N Engl J Med.* 2003;348(11):994–1004.

82. Druker BJ, Sawyers CL, Kantarjian H, et al. Activity of a specific inhibitor of the BCR-ABL tyrosine kinase in the blast crisis of chronic myeloid leukemia and acute lymphoblastic leukemia with the Philadelphia chromosome. *N Engl J Med.* 2001;344(14):1038–1042.

83. Hughes TP, Kaeda J, Branford S, et al. Frequency of major molecular responses to imatinib or interferon alfa plus cytarabine in newly diagnosed chronic myeloid leukemia. *N Engl J Med.* 2003;349: 1423–1432.

84. Gorre ME, Mohammed M, Ellwood K, et al. Clinical resistance to STI-571 cancer therapy caused by BCR-ABL gene mutation or amplification. *Science.* 2001;293(5531):876–880.

85. Branford S, Rudzki Z, Walsh S, et al. Detection of BCR-ABL mutations in patients with CML treated with imatinib is virtually always accompanied by clinical resistance, and mutations in the ATP phosphate-binding loop (P-loop) are associated with a poor prognosis. *Blood.* 2003;102(1): 276–283.

86. O'Dwyer ME, Mauro MJ, Blasdel C, et al. Clonal evolution and lack of cytogenetic response are adverse prognostic factors for hematologic relapse of chronic phase CML patients treated with imatinib mesylate. *Blood.* 2004;103(2):451–455.

87. Bacher U, Hochhaus A, Berger U, et al. Clonal aberrations in Philadelphia chromosome negative hematopoiesis in patients with chronic myeloid leukemia treated with imatinib or interferon alpha. *Leukemia.* 2005;19(3):460–463.

88. O'Hare T, Walters DK, Stoffregen EP, et al. In vitro activity of Bcr-Abl inhibitors AMN107 and BMS-354825 against clinically relevant imatinib-resistant Abl kinase domain mutants. *Cancer Res.* 2005; 65(11): 4500–4505.

89. Clift RA, Buckner CD, Thomas ED, et al. Marrow transplantation for patients in accelerated phase of chronic myeloid leukemia. *Blood.* 1994;84(12):4368–4373.

90. Radich JP, Gooley T, Bensinger W, et al. HLA-matched related hematopoietic cell transplantation for chronic-phase CML using a targeted busulfan and cyclophosphamide preparative regimen. *Blood.* 2003;102(1):31–35.

91. Clift RA, Buckner CD, Thomas ED, et al. Marrow transplantation for chronic myeloid leukemia: a randomized study comparing cyclophosphamide and total body irradiation with busulfan and cyclophosphamide. *Blood.* 1994;84(6):2036–2043.

92. Hansen JA, Gooley TA, Martin PJ, et al. Bone marrow transplants from unrelated donors for patients with chronic myeloid leukemia. *N Engl J Med.* 1998;338(14):962–968.

93. Radich JP, Gehly G, Gooley T, et al. Polymerase chain reaction detection of the BCR-ABL fusion transcript after allogeneic marrow transplantation for chronic myeloid leukemia: results and implications in 346 patients. *Blood.* 1995;85(9):2632–2638.

94. Higano CS, Chielens D, Raskind W, et al. Use of alpha-2a-interferon to treat cytogenetic relapse of chronic myeloid leukemia after marrow transplantation. *Blood.* 1997;90(7):2549–2554.

95. Baccarani M, Saglio G, Goldman J, et al. Evolving concepts in the management of chronic myeloid leukemia: recommendations from an expert panel on behalf of the European LeukemiaNet. *Blood.* 2006; 108(6):1809–1820.

96. Jemal A, Thomas A, Murray T, Thun M. Cancer statistics, 2002. *CA Cancer J Clin.* 2002;52(1):23–47.

97. Yuille MR, Matutes E, Marossy A, et al. Familial chronic lymphocytic leukaemia: a survey and review of published studies. *Br J Haematol.* 2000;109(4):794–799.

98. Dohner H, Stilgenbauer S, Benner A, et al. Genomic aberrations and survival in chronic lymphocytic leukemia. *N Engl J Med.* 2000;343(26): 1910–1916.

99. Rosenwald A, Alizadeh AA, Widhopf G, et al. Relation of gene expression phenotype to immunoglobulin mutation genotype in B cell chronic lymphocytic leukemia. *J Exp Med.* 2001;194(11): 1639–1647.

100. Chen L, Widhopf G, Huynh L, et al. Expression of ZAP-70 is associated with increased B-cell receptor signaling in chronic lymphocytic leukemia. *Blood.* 2002;100(13): 4609–4614.

101. Kröber A, Seiler T, Benner A, et al. V(H) mutation status, CD38 expression level, genomic aberrations, and survival in chronic lymphocytic leukemia. *Blood.* 2002;100(4):1410–1416.

102. Rai KR, Sawitsky A, Cronkite EP, et al. Clinical staging of chronic lymphocytic leukemia. *Blood.* 1975;46(2):219–234.

103. Binet JL, Auquier A, Dighiero G, et al. A new prognostic classification of chronic lymphocytic leukemia derived from a multivariate survival analysis. *Cancer.* 1981;48(1):198–206.

104. Ibrahim S, Keating M, Do KA, et al. CD38 expression as an important prognostic factor in B-cell chronic lymphocytic leukemia. *Blood.* 2001;98(1):181–186.

105. Oscier DG, Gardiner AC, Mould SJ, et al. Multivariate analysis of prognostic factors in CLL: clinical stage, IGVH gene mutational status, and loss or mutation of the p53 gene are independent prognostic factors. *Blood.* 2002;100(4):1177–1184.

106. Leporrier M, Chevret S, Cazin B, et al. Randomized comparison of fludarabine, CAP, and ChOP in 938 previously untreated stage B and C chronic lymphocytic leukemia patients. *Blood.* 2001;98(8): 2319–2325.

107. Rai KR, Peterson BL, Appelbaum FR, et al. Fludarabine compared with chlorambucil as primary therapy for chronic lymphocytic leukemia. *N Engl J Med.* 2000;343(24):1750–1757.

108. Morrison VA, Rai KR, Peterson BL, et al. Impact of therapy with chlorambucil, fludarabine, or fludarabine plus chlorambucil on infections in patients with chronic lymphocytic leukemia: Intergroup Study Cancer and Leukemia Group B 9011. *J Clin Oncol.* 2001; 19(16):3611–3621.

109. Morrison VA, Rai KR, Peterson BL, et al. Therapy-related myeloid leukemias are observed in patients with chronic lymphocytic leukemia after treatement with fludarabine and chlorambucil: results of an Intergroup Study, Cancer and Leukemia Group B 9011. *J Clin Oncol.* 20(18):3878–3884.

110. Eichhorst F, Busch R, Hopfinger G, et al. Fludarabine plus cyclophosphamide versus fludarabine alone in first line therapy of younger patients with chronic lymphocytic leukemia. *Blood.* 2006;107: 885–889.

111. O'Brien S, Kantarjian H, Thomas DA, et al. Rituximab dose-escalation trial in chronic lymphocytic leukaemia. *J Clin Oncol.* 2001;19(8): 2165–2170.

112. Byrd JC, Rai K, Peterson BL, et al. Addition of rituximab to fludarabine may prolong progression-free survival and overall survival in patients with previously untreated chronic lymphocytic leukemia: an updated retrospective comparative analysis of CALBG 9712 and CALBG 9011. *Blood.* 2005;105(1):49–53.

113. O'Brien SM, Kantarjian HM, Cortes J, et al. Results of the fludarabine and cyclophosphamide combination regimen in chronic lymphocytic leukemia. *J Clin Oncol.* 2001;19(5):1414–1420.

114. Lundin J, Kimby E, Björkholm M, et al. Phase II trial of subcutaneous anti-CD52 monoclonal antibody alemtuzumab (CAMPATH-1H) as first-line treatment for patients with B-cell chronic lymphocytic leukemia (B-CLL). *Blood.* 2002;100(3):768–773.

115. Keating MJ, Flinn I, Jain V, et al. Therapeutic role of alemtuzumab (Campath-1H) in patients who have failed fludarabine: results of a large international study. *Blood.* 2002;99(10):3554–3561.

116. Doney KC, Chauncey T, Appelbaum FR. Allogeneic related donor hematopoietic stem cell transplantation for treatment of chronic lymphocytic leukemia. *Bone Marrow Transplant.* 2002;29(10): 817–823.

117. Michallet M, Archimbaud E, Bandini G, et al. HLA-identical sibling bone marrow transplantation in younger patients with chronic lymphocytic leukemia. European Group for Blood and Marrow Transplantation and the International Bone Marrow Transplant Registry. *Ann Intern Med.* 1996;124(3):311–315.

118. Khouri IF, Przepiorka D, van Besien K, et al. Allogeneic blood or marrow transplantation for chronic lymphocytic leukaemia: timing of transplantation and potential effect of fludarabine on acute graft-versus-host disease. *Br J Haematol.* 1997;97(2):466–473.

119. Sorror ML, Maris MB, Sandmaier BM, et al. Hematopoietic cell transplantation after nonmyeloablative conditioning for advanced chronic lymphocytic leukemia. *J Clin Oncol.* 2005;23(16): 3819–3829.

120. Österborg A, Brandberg Y, Molostova V, et al. Randomized, double-blind, placebo-controlled trial of recombinant human erythropoietin, epoietin Beta, in hematologic malignancies. *J Clin Oncol.* 2002; 20(10):2486–2494.

121. Cheson BD, Bennett JM, Grever M, et al. National Cancer Institute-sponsored Working Group guidelines for chronic lymphocytic leukemia: revised guidelines for diagnosis and treatment. *Blood.* 1996;87(12):4990–4997.

122. Flinn IW, Kopecky KJ, Foucar K, et al. Long-term follow-up of remission, duration, mortality and second malignancies in hairy cell leukemia patients treated with pentostatin. Blood. 2000;96: 2981–2986.

123. Kreitman RJ, Wilson WH, Bergeron K, et al. Efficacy of the anti-CD22 recombinant immunotoxin BL22 in chemotherapy-resistant hairy-cell leukemia. *New Engl J Med.* 2001;345(4):241–247.

124. Keating MJ, Cazin B, Coutré S, et al. Campath-1H treatment of T cell prolymphocytic leukemia in patients for whom at least one prior chemotherapy regimen has failed. *J Clin Oncol.* 2002;20(1): 205–213.

16

LYMPHOMAS AND MYELOMA

Bruce D. Cheson, MD

LEARNING OBJECTIVES

After reviewing this chapter, the reader should be able to

- Describe the natural history and biology of Hodgkin's lymphoma, non-Hodgkin's lymphoma, and multiple myeloma
- Accurately classify and stage Hodgkin's lymphoma, non-Hodgkin's lymphoma, and multiple myeloma
- Implement the standard therapeutic approaches to Hodgkin's lymphoma, non-Hodgkin's lymphoma, and multiple myeloma

Hodgkin's lymphoma accounts for 14% of lymphomas with an estimated 8,190 new cases in 2007 and an estimated 1,070 deaths.[1] The etiology of Hodgkin's lymphoma is not known. There is an association with the Epstein Barr virus (EBV), and the likelihood of developing Hodgkin's lymphoma is increased 3-fold for people with a history of infectious mononucleosis. Half of all Hodgkin's lymphoma nodes show evidence of EBV DNA in the genome of the Reed-Sternberg (R-S) cell. However, because many cases of Hodgkin's lymphoma are EBV negative, controversy remains as to whether there is a causative relationship. There also appears to be an increased frequency of the disease in patients with acquired immunodeficiency syndrome (AIDS) and patients who have had bone marrow transplantation. In patients infected with the human immunodeficiency virus (HIV) or AIDS, Hodgkin's lymphoma tends to involve extranodal sites and to exhibit an aggressive clinical course with a poor outcome. There are no clear relationships with environmental exposures, although an increase in the incidence of Hodgkin's lymphoma has been reported in wood workers/carpenters, farmers, and meat processors.

HODGKIN'S LYMPHOMA

DIAGNOSIS AND CLASSIFICATION

Hodgkin's lymphoma should be considered in the differential diagnosis of persistent, unexplained lymphadenopathy. Although enlarged lymph nodes may be noted by the patient, they are commonly an incidental finding during a physical evaluation or an examination for an unrelated condition. The size of a normal node varies somewhat according to location, but, in general, is approximately 1 cm in the longest axis. The presence of fevers, night sweats, unexplained

KEY POINTS

- Hodgkin's lymphoma is composed of classical Hodgkin's lymphoma and nodular lymphocyte-predominant Hodgkin's lymphoma, each of which has different clinical presentations, treatment approaches, and prognosis.
- Hodgkin's lymphoma of any stage is curable in most patients.
- Combination doxorubicin, bleomycin, vinblastine, and dacarbazine ABVD is the standard chemotherapy.
- The number of courses of treatment varies with the stage of the disease.
- Evaluation of the role of radiation therapy in the management of Hodgkin's lymphoma is ongoing.

weight loss (defined as more than 10% of body weight) — generally referred to as B symptoms — also should increase the level of suspicion for this diagnosis. Other disease-associated symptoms not categorized within in the B-designation include chills, pruritus, or pain in a lymph node-bearing area that is associated with alcohol consumption. Laboratory findings may indicate a mild lymphocytosis, eosinophilia, and an elevated erythrocyte sedimentation rate.

After other causes, such as infection or inflammation, are ruled out, a biopsy is needed to exclude the possibility of malignant disease. To make the pathologic diagnosis of lymphoma, an excisional biopsy is required because it provides a more representative sample for assessment of lymph node architecture and supplies adequate tissue for other studies, including immunophenotyping.[2] A core biopsy may be useful to document recurrent disease.

The distinctive pathologic finding in Hodgkin's lymphoma is the classic R-S cell, a multinucleate giant cell characterized by abundant eosinophilic cytoplasm and large blue nucleoli, giving the appearance of an owl eye. Studies of immunoglobulin (Ig) heavy-chain gene rearrangements demonstrate that the R-S cells are derived from a precursor B cell.

From 1965 to 1994, Hodgkin's lymphoma was distinguished by subtype according to the Rye Classification. In 1994, the International Lymphoma Study Group introduced the Revised European American Lymphoma (REAL) Classification. This classification schema retained the four distinct histologic subtypes of the Rye Classification system and added a provisional category of lymphocyte-rich classical Hodgkin's lymphoma and another category for unclassifiable cases. The World Health Organization (WHO) classification of 1999 recommended a name change, from Hodgkin's disease to Hodgkin lymphoma (although Hodgkin's lymphoma is still widely used) and proposed two categories: classical Hodgkin's lymphoma and nodular lymphocyte-predominant Hodgkin's lymphoma, with the first category comprising four subcategories (Table 16-1).[3]

TABLE 16-1 World Health Organization (WHO) Classification of Hodgkin's Lymphoma

Classical Hodgkin's lymphoma
- Nodular-sclerosis Hodgkin's lymphoma
- Mixed-cellularity Hodgkin's lymphoma
- Lymphocyte depletion Hodgkin's lymphoma
- Lymphocyte-rich Hodgkin's lymphoma

Nodular lymphocyte-predominant Hodgkin's lymphoma

Classical Hodgkin's Lymphoma

Classical Hodgkin's lymphoma represents approximately 95% of all cases. More than 60% of patients with classical Hodgkin's lymphoma present with the nodular-sclerosis subtype, which is most common in women, adolescents, and young adults. At the time of presentation, patients characteristically have an anterior mediastinal mass that may be symptomatic. The histologic pattern of nodular-sclerosis Hodgkin's lymphoma is at least partially nodular with fibrous bands. Diffuse areas and necrosis also may be present. The characteristic R-S cell is the lacunar variant, which are giant cells with a multilobulated nucleus. The nucleus is surrounded by a clear area that is an artifact of formalin fixation. Nucleoli are less prominent than in the so-called classical R-S cell. The tumor cells are CD30+, CD15±, and CD45–. Epithelial membrane antigen (EMA) expression is rare.

Mixed-cellularity Hodgkin's lymphoma represents approximately 20% of cases and is more common in men. The histologic appearance is of a diffuse, or vaguely nodular, infiltrate. R-S cells are primarily of the classic variety. The cells are CD30+, CD15±, and CD45–. In contrast to the other histologic subtypes, EBV genomic DNA is detectable in 60% to 70% of mixed-cellularity Hodgkin's lymphoma. Patients tend to present with disseminated disease, and the clinical course may be aggressive; however, this subtype is still curable.

The growth pattern in lymphocyte-rich classic Hodgkin's lymphoma commonly is nodular, but may be diffuse, with a phenotype of CD30+, CD15±, and CD20±. The small lymphocytes exhibit the features of mantle cells (IgM+D+) as the nodules represent the extended mantle zone of the node. This subtype is more common in older males and presents at an early stage of disease. Other findings are similar to nodular lymphocyte-predominant Hodgkin's lymphoma, except that patients are slightly older (40 years) at the time of diagnosis, and the presenting mass is more frequently located in the mediastinum. Late relapses are less common but more often fatal.

Lymphocyte-depleted Hodgkin's lymphoma accounts for less than 5% of cases of Hodgkin's lymphoma. It occurs more often in older men, and in people who are infected with HIV. It also is more common in nonindustrialized countries. At the time of presentation, patients have abdominal adenopathy but with less peripheral adenopathy than is found with other types of Hodgkin's lymphoma. Hepatosplenomegaly may be prominent, and the bone marrow is often infiltrated with disease. The histologic appearance of the lymph nodes is characterized by a diffuse infiltrate, which may appear hypocellular. R-S cells, CD30+, CD15±, and CD45– are plentiful and may have a malignant appearance.

Nodular Lymphocyte-predominant Hodgkin's Lymphoma

Nodular lymphocyte-predominant Hodgkin's lymphoma is a unique form of Hodgkin's lymphoma that accounts for approximately 5% of cases. The histology is characterized by a nodular growth pattern, with or without diffuse areas, and rare R-S cells. The atypical lymphocytic and histiocytic cells — called popcorn cells — express B-cell antigens such as CD20 but rarely CD15 or CD30, and are negative for serum Ig and CD45. EMA is positive in half of the cases. This type of lymphoma is more common in adults than in children and occurs more often in men than in women. Median patient age is 34 years. The disease more often is localized than disseminated at the time of diagnosis (more than 70% of cases are stage I or II). The course of disease is slowly progressive, and the outcome is extremely favorable. Mediastinal masses are noted in fewer than 20% of cases. Although survival tends to be long, late relapses are more common than for other histologic subtypes, and progression to large B-cell non-Hodgkin's lymphoma occurs in 35% of cases. Rituximab is active in relapsed nodular lymphocyte-predominant Hodgkin's lymphoma.[4] Response rates were as high as 86%, half of which were complete and durable.

STAGING AND PROGNOSIS

Although the Ann Arbor staging system, which denotes four clinical and pathologic stages of Hodgkin's lymphoma, has been used for more than 30 years, the stages of Hodgkin's lymphoma actually fall into the following three prognostic groups that correlate better to treatment planning and survival.

- Favorable: stages IA and IIA
- Intermediate risk: stages III and IV and any stage with B symptoms
- Less favorable: any stage with bulky disease, defined as a mass larger than 10 cm in diameter or greater than one-third the transverse diameter of the chest at the fifth and sixth thoracic vertebral levels

The Cotswolds staging system, developed in 1989, emphasizes the unfavorable prognostic effect of tumor bulk by incorporating an X designation to each stage.

To determine the extent of involvement, staging should include computerized tomography (CT) scans of the chest, abdomen, and pelvis, as well as 18-fluorodeoxyglucose (FDG) positron emission tomography (PET) scan assessment following therapy to predict outcome. Bone marrow biopsy can be reserved for patients with clinical stages III and IV disease or stage II disease with B symptoms. Because of the availability of CT and PET scans, as well as because of the more frequent use of systemic therapy, a staging laparotomy with splenectomy (previously used in this patient population) is no longer needed.

An International Prognostic Scoring System identified seven risk factors predictive of outcome for patients with advanced Hodgkin's lymphoma.

- Albumin less than 4 g/dL
- Hemoglobin less than 10.5 g/dL
- Male sex
- Age of 45 or older
- Stage IV disease
- White blood cell count higher than 15,000/μL
- Lymphocyte count of less than 600/mm^3 or less than 8% of the white blood cell count

The expected 5-year survival correlates with the number of factors present (Table 16-2).

TREATMENT

Early-stage Disease (Nonbulky IA and IIA)

Radiation therapy has been the standard approach for patients with early-stage Hodgkin's lymphoma. This approach yields complete response in more than 95% of patients with limited disease. The failure-free survival and overall survival rates are 75% and greater than 90%, respectively, beyond 20 years. For patients with lower risk disease, the efficacy of involved-field radiation is comparable with that of extended-field radiation, and it also is associated with a lower incidence of toxicity.

Several randomized trials involving patients with early-stage disease have been conducted. In one study, patients were randomly assigned to treatment with either four cycles of combination doxorubicin, bleomycin, vinblastine, and dacarbazine (ABVD) or with two cycles of ABVD plus extended-field radiation. The combination treatment was associated with longer progression-free survival (93% compared with 87%)

TABLE 16-2 Survival Correlated to Risk Factors Predictive of Outcome for Hodgkin's Lymphoma

Number of Risk Factors	Five-Year Survival Rate (%)
0	84
1	77
2	67
3	60
4	51
5, 6, or 7	42

See text for list of risk factors.

but with no apparent difference in overall survival.[5] Thus, with this approach, 90% of patients can be spared the toxicities associated with radiation therapy.

For patients with early-stage disease but less favorable features (age older than 50, bulky disease, absence of B symptoms, and an erythrocyte sedimentation rate of more than 50 mm per hour or presence of B symptoms and an erythrocyte sedimentation rate of more than 30 mm per hour), treatment with four cycles of ABVD and involved-field radiation results in a failure-free survival rate of more than 90% and an overall survival rate of 95%. The Stanford V regimen followed by radiation to sites of bulky disease appears to produce results comparable to ABVD but with a shorter duration of therapy; however, if the radiation is not applied as originally described, the outcome is inferior, demonstrating the importance of radiation in this strategy.

The presence of tumor bulk is predictive of poor outcome following single-modality therapy, even for patients with early-stage disease. For patients with stage IIX Hodgkin's lymphoma, there is a 50% to 75% chance of relapse after radiation therapy alone and a 40% chance following chemotherapy alone. The findings from uncontrolled trials suggest that chemotherapy is effective as salvage treatment after failure of radiation in 50% to 80% of cases. Studies have shown that the combination of radiation therapy and chemotherapy with mechlorethamine, vincristine, procarbazine, and prednisone (MOPP) yields a longer disease-free survival rate than is expected with either therapy alone. Anthracycline-based regimens have replaced MOPP, and the risks of secondary malignant disease from the combined-modality approach are minimal. However, the risk of cardiotoxicity is greater for patients treated with radiation to the mediastinum. Although combined-modality therapy is the standard approach for patients with bulky disease, the role of radiation is being re-evaluated given the increased efficacy of more recent chemotherapy regimens.

Advanced-stage Disease

Advanced-stage disease refers to stage III or IV disease, as well as disease accompanied by B symptoms and/or bulky disease. ABVD has become the standard chemotherapy for advanced-stage disease as a result of the following advantages:

- intravenous administration (better compliance);
- less cumulative myelotoxicity;
- low risk of secondary malignant diseases, such as acute myeloid leukemia or solid tumors; and
- low rate of infertility compared with regimens, such as MOPP.

ABVD can induce complete response in 80% to 85% of patients, with a 5-year progression-free survival rate of 61% and an overall 5-year survival rate of 73%.[6]

The escalated regimen of bleomycin, etoposide, doxorubicin, cyclophosphamide, vincristine, procarbazine, and prednisone (BEACOPP), with involved field irradiation to prior sites of bulky disease, leads to a better failure-free survival rate than cyclophosphamide, vincristine, procarbazine, and prednisone (COPP)/ABVD but is associated with an increased risk of secondary acute myeloid leukemia (AML) or myelodysplastic syndrome (MDS) and solid tumors.[7] The rate of progression during treatment is 2%. In addition, the relapse rate is 5% following completion of therapy, the time-to-treatment failure is 88% at 3 years, and the overall survival is almost 95% at 5 years. A randomized trial is comparing ABVD and BEACOPP. For most patients who have had a partial response, radiation therapy to sites of residual disease can lead to a complete response. Radiation as part of consolidation therapy to prior bulky disease may prolong disease-free survival in those sites, but it does not have an effect on the overall survival rate of patients with stage IV disease.

In summary, the approach for patients with stage IA or IIA Hodgkin's lymphoma involves four cycles of ABVD. For patients with B symptoms or those with stage III or IV disease, treatment involves ABVD for six cycles. Treatment for patients with stage I or II and bulky disease involves chemotherapy with six cycles of ABVD and involved-field radiation therapy. Whether radiation therapy is required for such patients is the subject of ongoing study.

Residual Mass

In approximately 80% of patients with bulky mediastinal or retroperitoneal disease who have an initial response to therapy, a radiographic abnormality persists. In more than half of those cases, there may be no evidence of disease progression for more than 1 year. The residual mass generally represents fibrotic tumor, and such patients tend to do as well as patients who have a clinical complete response. A PET scan can be useful to discriminate between fibrosis and active disease in patients with a tumor that had been positive on PET scan prior to therapy.[8]

In such cases, additional therapy should not be given unless there are positive findings on biopsy or until there is clear evidence of active disease. For some patients, notably those younger than 25, a mediastinal radiographic density may actually increase within 6 months following therapy. This finding may represent regenerating thymus and can be confused with disease progression, creating a diagnostic dilemma, as the thymus may be positive on PET scan (Fig. 16-1). Careful follow-up with repeat PET or CT scans is necessary to confirm this possibility, and treatment intervention is generally not needed. Therapy may be indicated if the mass continues to enlarge or if disease becomes apparent outside of the radiated field. A CT-guided biopsy may provide useful information.

Relapsed or Refractory Disease

Although Hodgkin's lymphoma is a relatively curable disease, a complete or partial response is never achieved in 20% to 30% of patients, and another 20% to 30% have relapse following an initial complete response. The type of initial

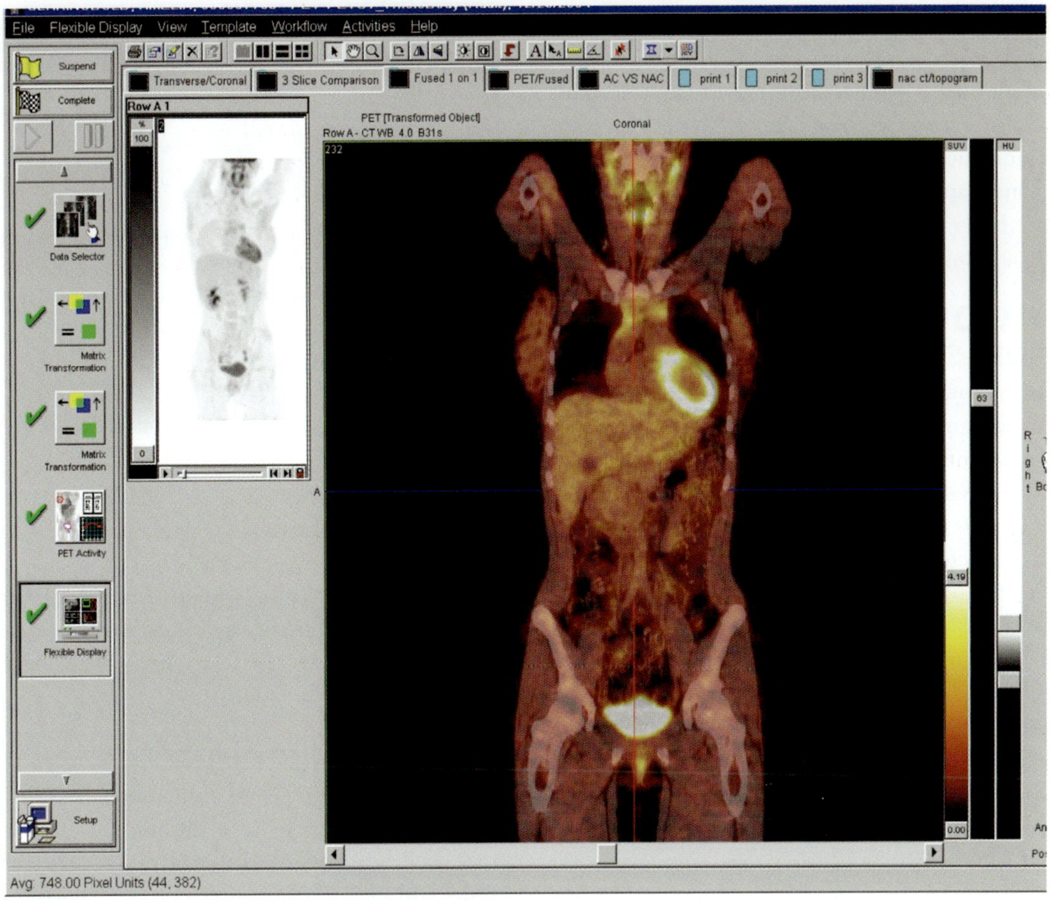

FIG. 16-1 18-fluorodeoxyglucose (FDG) positron emission tomography (PET) scan in a woman with nodular sclerosing Hodgkin's lymphoma 6 weeks following therapy demonstrating the persistent FDG-avidity of thymic hyperplasia. *The patient remains in continuous complete remission for more than 3 years.*[8]

therapy given and the duration of the initial response play major roles in determining the appropriate second-line program. The likelihood of long-term disease-free survival after treatment with ABVD is 50% to 80% for patients who have relapse after radiation therapy alone.

Late relapses (more than 12 months) after complete response or a durable partial response following initial chemotherapy may be treated successfully with a different combination chemotherapy. Disease will remain in remission at 5 years for approximately 15% of patients who have a response to treatment for late relapse.

High-dose therapy with autologous stem cell support should be considered for patients in whom disease relapses but who remain sensitive to chemotherapy. This approach has been associated with a 5-year relapse-free survival rate of 20% to 40%, which can vary based on prognostic factors such as performance status, tumor bulk, and number and type of prior chemotherapy regimens. The likelihood of successful transplantation is higher for patients who first received ABVD than for those who received escalated BEACOPP. However, high-dose chemotherapy with autologous stem cell support does not appear to have an effective role in the initial treatment of high-risk patients. Allogeneic bone marrow transplant for patients who have refractory disease is associated with a poor outcome because of excessive treatment-related morbidity and mortality.

Gemcitabine induces response in approximately half of patients with relapsed or refractory disease, and the drug is being incorporated into multiagent regimens. Newer approaches also involve anti-CD30 monoclonal antibodies and bispecific monoclonal antibodies.

Radiation therapy alone is generally not associated with treatment-related secondary leukemia, and AML does not appear to complicate treatment with ABVD or similar regimens. However, secondary diffuse aggressive non-Hodgkin's lymphomas occur with a cumulative risk rate of 4% to 5% at 10 years. The frequency of solid tumors following first-line treatment increases from 2% at 10 years to 13% at 19 years. Radiation therapy, with or without chemotherapy, is the major contributor to cancers (e.g., lung and breast cancers, soft tissue sarcomas, and melanomas) that develop in the irradiated field. Unlike women with primary breast cancer, these breast cancers are more often bilateral. Regular breast examination and mammography, even at an early age, are recommended as part of routine follow-up care for patients with Hodgkin's lymphoma.

More than two-thirds of patients who receive mantle radiation will be diagnosed with thyroid disease, including hypothyroidism, Graves' disease, silent thyrotoxicosis, and nodules, with a 2% risk rate of secondary cancer. Myelosuppression caused by radiation therapy correlates with the amount of irradiated bone marrow. Long-term toxicities associated with radiation are likely to be reduced with current equipment, lower doses, and smaller treatment fields.

NON-HODGKIN'S LYMPHOMAS

EPIDEMIOLOGY

Non-Hodgkin's lymphoma is the fifth most common tumor type diagnosed annually in men in the United States, and the sixth most common type in women. Approximately 63,190 new cases were diagnosed in the United States in 2007, with 18,660 deaths reported.[1] Despite the continued increase in frequency, non-Hodgkin's lymphoma has decreased from the fifth and sixth to the eighth and seventh leading cause of cancer deaths in men and women, respectively. The reasons for the increase in frequency of diagnosis of non-Hodgkin's lymphoma are unknown, but this increase is primarily in cases of diffuse large B-cell lymphoma and notably in older individuals. The median age of patients who are diagnosed with lymphoma varies according to the histologic subtype.

ETIOLOGY

For most patients with non-Hodgkin's lymphoma, the etiology is unknown. Pesticides and agricultural chemicals, exercise, smoking, hair dyes, and other toxins have not been conclusively associated with the disease — the pattern of use of these agents has not paralleled the pattern of diagnoses. However, there is a marked increase in the frequency of diagnosed aggressive non-Hodgkin's lymphoma in patients who receive continual immunosuppressive agents, who have had autologous stem cell transplant or solid organ transplantation, and who have inherited immune defects, rheumatoid arthritis, or HIV/AIDS. In a small fraction of patients, there also is an association between a variety of infectious agents and the occurrence of lymphomas (Table 16-3).

KEY POINTS

- Non-Hodgkin's lymphomas comprise a group of heterogeneous diseases that vary widely with respect to clinical presentation, therapy, and prognosis.
- Advances in the diagnosis and classification of these diseases are facilitated by immunophenotyping and by newer molecular genetic approaches.
- Marked advances have been made in the treatment of these diseases over the past few years, largely because of the availability of monoclonal antibodies and related agents.

DIAGNOSIS AND CLASSIFICATION

Most patients who will be diagnosed with non-Hodgkin's lymphoma are initially seen because of signs or symptoms associated with lymphadenopathy, although the enlarged nodes are often painless. Because numerous infections, benign inflammatory conditions, and nonlymphomatous tumors also can cause enlarged nodes, precise diagnosis and classification of non-Hodgkin's lymphoma requires evaluation of lymph node tissue obtained at biopsy. An excisional biopsy is necessary because fine-needle aspirations have a high false-negative rate. Fine-needle aspirations also fail to distinguish between nodular and diffuse histologic subtypes in lesions with substantial fibrosis or sclerosis, in cases of T-cell non-Hodgkin's lymphoma, or T-cell rich B-cell non-Hodgkin's lymphoma, as well as in cases in which

TABLE 16-3 Infectious Agents Associated with Specific Types of Non-Hodgkin's Lymphoma

Infectious Agent	Type of Non-Hodgkin's Lymphoma
Epstein-Barr virus	Hodgkin's lymphoma and post-transplant lymphoproliferative disorders
Human herpesvirus-8	Body cavity lymphoma, Castleman disease
Hepatitis C	Immunocytoma, splenic marginal zone lymphoma
Human T-cell lymphoma virus-I (HTLV-I)	Adult T-cell leukemia/lymphoma
Helicobacter pylori	Gastric mucosa-associated lymphoid tissue (MALT) lymphoma
Chlamydia psitacci	Orbital adnexal lymphoma
Campylobacter jejuni	Immunoproliferative small bowel disease
Borrelia burgdorferi	Cutaneous MALT lymphoma

the lymph nodes are only partially involved with disease. Although an excisional biopsy is preferred, evaluation of tissue obtained by a core-needle biopsy may be sufficient to confirm a suspected recurrence in patients with previously diagnosed lymphoma. The increased use of flow cytometry and molecular genetic studies has made it possible to diagnose a lymphoma in the mediastinal, retroperitoneal, or other deep locations through analysis of tissue obtained by core-needle biopsy.

In 1982, the National Cancer Institute (NCI) Working Formulation was adopted to facilitate communication among investigators, although the Kiel classification was still widely used in Europe. The Revised European-American Lymphoma (REAL) Classification (1994) was used to distinguish the non-Hodgkin's lymphomas using morphology, immunophenotype, genetic characteristics, and clinical features. The REAL Classification was modified by the WHO Classification (1999), and the latter is the universally adopted system (Table 16-4).[3]

TABLE 16-4 WHO Classification of Non-Hodgkin's Lymphoma[3]*

B-Cell Neoplasms

- Precursor B-cell neoplasm
- Precursor B-lymphoblastic leukemia/lymphoma (precursor B-cell acute lymphoblastic leukemia)
- Mature (peripheral) B-cell neoplasms†
- B-cell chronic lymphocytic leukemia/small lymphocytic lymphoma
- B-cell prolymphocytic leukemia
- Lymphoplasmacytic lymphoma
- Splenic marginal zone B-cell lymphoma (with or without villous lymphocytes)
- Hairy cell leukemia
- Plasma cell myeloma/plasmacytoma
- Extranodal marginal zone B-cell lymphoma of mucosa-associated lymphoid tissue (MALT) type
- Nodal marginal zone B-cell lymphoma (with or without monocytoid B cells)
- Follicular lymphoma
- Mantle cell lymphoma
- Diffuse large B-cell lymphoma
- Mediastinal large B-cell lymphoma
- Primary effusion lymphoma
- Burkitt's lymphoma/Burkitt cell leukemia

T-Cell and Natural Killer (NK) Cell Neoplasms

- Precursor T-cell neoplasm
- Precursor T-lymphoblastic lymphoma/leukemia (precursor T-cell acute lymphoblastic leukemia)
- Mature (peripheral) T-cell neoplasms†
- T-cell prolymphocytic leukemia
- T-cell granular lymphocytic leukemia
- Aggressive NK cell leukemia
- Adult T-cell lymphoma/leukemia (HTLV1+)
- Extranodal NK/T-cell lymphoma, nasal type
- Enteropathy-type T-cell lymphoma
- Hepatosplenic gamma-delta T-cell lymphoma
- Subcutaneous panniculitis-like T-cell lymphoma
- Mycosis fungoides/Sézary syndrome
- Anaplastic large-cell lymphoma, T/null cell, primary cutaneous type
- Peripheral T-cell lymphoma, not otherwise characterized
- Angioimmunoblastic T-cell lymphoma
- Anaplastic large-cell lymphoma, T/null cell, primary systemic type

*Only major categories are included.
†B-cell and T-cell/NK cell neoplasms are grouped according to major clinical presentations (predominantly disseminated/leukemic, primary extranodal, and predominantly nodal).

STAGING AND PROGNOSIS

The Ann Arbor staging system is used for non-Hodgkin's lymphoma, but it is less relevant than in Hodgkin's lymphoma because non-Hodgkin's lymphoma is more often at an advanced stage at the time of presentation. Staging for non-Hodgkin's lymphoma requires CT scans of the neck, chest, abdomen, and pelvis and an adequate amount (more than 2 cm) of unilateral bone marrow biopsy. Flow cytometric analysis of a biopsy specimen may be useful when immunohistochemistry is equivocal. PET scanning has replaced gallium scanning because it is more sensitive and practical.[9] The usefulness of PET scanning varies with the histologic subtype of non-Hodgkin's lymphoma[10]; it consistently identifies more sites of disease than CT scan in FDG-avid lymphomas when used for staging. However, stage is altered in fewer than one-fourth of patients, and treatment is changed on the basis of this information in only a small fraction of cases with no clear effect on outcome. PET may be valuable in confirming if the patient has stage I disease and if the patient may be a candidate for radiation therapy. PET is more useful in assessing response in diffuse large B-cell lymphoma and in Hodgkin's lymphoma where a complete remission may translate into cure. However, PET scans will demonstrate evidence of disease in less than one-half of marginal zone non-Hodgkin's lymphoma, small lymphocytic lymphoma, and peripheral T-cell non-Hodgkin's lymphoma. Whereas PET scan results following one or more cycles of multiagent chemotherapy may be predictive of outcome, there are no data to suggest that altering therapy on the basis of this information has an effect on patient survival.

INDOLENT NON-HODGKIN'S LYMPHOMA

The International Prognostic Index, although initially developed for aggressive non-Hodgkin's lymphoma, also is used for classifying indolent subtypes of non-Hodgkin's lymphomas into risk groups with markedly different outcomes. However, most patients have low-risk disease at the time of presentation, and there is no evidence that the associated International Prognostic Index risk group can be used to effectively direct therapy. Somewhat better separation of prognostic groups has been reported with the Follicular Lymphoma International Prognostic Index.[11] This index is based on age (60 or older), stage (III and IV), serum lactate dehydrogenase (LDH) level, hemoglobin, and the number of extranodal sites (Fig. 16-2). However, this index is not useful in directing optimal treatment approaches for the various risk groups.

The indolent histologic subtypes of non-Hodgkin's lymphoma are considered to include follicular grade I (formerly follicular small cleaved cell), grade II (formerly follicular mixed), and grade IIIa. However, the approach to these patients is the same as outcome following therapy. On the other hand, those patients with follicular grade IIIb disease have a clinical course that is more consistent with diffuse

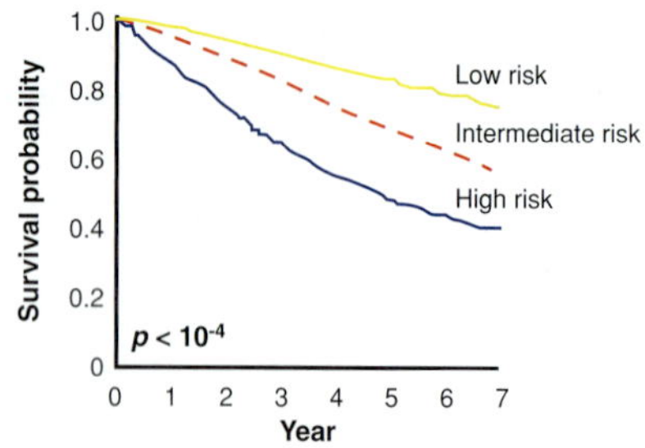

Risk Group	Number of Factors	Patients (%)	5-year Overall Survival (%)	10-year Overall Survivl (%)
Low	0 to 1	36	90.6	70.7
Intermediate	2	37	77.8	50.9
High	3 to 5	27	52.5	35.5

Reprinted with permission from the American Society of Hematology.

FIG. 16-2 Overall Survival According to FLIPI: Clinical Prognosis Factors[12] Reprinted with permission from the American Society of Hematology.

large B-cell non-Hodgkin's lymphoma. Also included are marginal zone lymphoma, lymphoplasmacytic lymphomas (including immunocytoma and Waldenström's macroglobulinemia), and small lymphocytic lymphoma.

Follicular Non-Hodgkin's Lymphoma

The follicular non-Hodgkin's lymphomas are the second most common subset of this disease and the most common of the indolent types. They are characterized by a follicular growth pattern on lymph node biopsy, although diffuse areas also may be present and should be reported by the pathologist. The characteristic immunophenotype is CD20+, CD5–, CD23–, CD10+, and commonly *Bcl-6* positive. *Bcl-2* is overexpressed in more than 85% of patients. This gene is the result of the t(14;18)(q32;q21), which can be detected by fluorescent in situ hybridization of polymerase chain reaction technology.

Approximately 10% to 15% of patients with follicular lymphoma have stage I or nonbulky stage II disease at the time of initial presentation. Involved-field or extended-field radiation therapy produces a 10-year failure-free survival rate of 50% to 60% and an overall survival rate of 60% to 80%. Nevertheless, because it is not clear whether radiation is required in all of these patients, they can be observed without treatment and treated at the time of disease progression. The remaining 85% to 90% of patients with follicular grade I or II non-Hodgkin's lymphoma have advanced-stage disease (bulky stage II and stages III and IV) at the time of presentation. The median time to progression of non-Hodgkin's lymphoma in these patients was 4 to 6 years, with an overall survival of 6 to 10 years prior to the availability of antibody-containing regimens. Despite this relatively long natural history, these lymphomas are incurable.

Early intervention with therapy using an alkylating agent does not appear to prolong survival for asymptomatic patients. Therefore, the conventional approach has been to wait and watch until therapy is indicated by the presence of increasing adenopathy, disease-related symptoms, organ compromise, or bone marrow failure. The Groupe d'Etudes

des Lymphomes Folliculaires (GELF) criteria have been suggested to be effective in the identification of patients who may benefit from earlier intervention. Treatment may be deferred for patients with all of the following: maximum diameter of any site of disease less than 7 cm, fewer than three nodal sites greater than 3 cm in diameter, absence of systemic symptoms, spleen smaller than 16 cm, no pleural effusions, no risk of local compressive symptoms, and no circulating lymphoma cells or cytopenias related to the disease.[12]

The availability of an increasing number of active biologic agents, particularly monoclonal antibodies and radioimmunoconjugates, has markedly altered the therapeutic approach for patients with non-Hodgkin's lymphoma (Table 16-5). Although antibodies in clinical use may be derived from mice (murine), they are more often chimeric, which reduces the likelihood of forming neutralizing antibodies, such as human anti-mouse antibody (HAMA). The newest antibodies are either humanized or human in order to reduce immunogenicity. The most commonly targeted antigen associated with lymphoma is CD20, which is first expressed during the pre-B-cell stage of development and is no longer detectable on plasma cells.

Rituximab is a chimeric anti-CD20 monoclonal antibody that has been used most extensively in the treatment of B-cell malignant diseases. When used as monotherapy for the initial treatment for patients with follicular and low-grade non-Hodgkin's lymphoma, the response rate ranges from 50% to 70%, with a median duration of response of 1.0 to 2.5 years, depending on patient selection criteria and on whether additional cycles of antibody are delivered as maintenance following the initial four infusions. Thus, this approach is inadequate therapy for many patients. The use of rituximab as maintenance treatment — as a single infusion every 2 months for 8 months, as four weekly infusions every 6 months for 2 years, or as a single infusion every 3 months for 2 years — may prolong the time to progression and event-free survival following either single-agent rituximab or cyclophosphamide, vincristine, and prednisone (CVP) chemotherapy for initial therapy, but additional follow-up is needed to determine the effect on overall survival.[13,14] The Rituximab Extended Schedule or Retreatment (RESORT) trial is randomly assigning patients with low-risk follicular non-Hodgkin's lymphoma to four weekly infusions followed by maintenance with one infusion every 3 months until disease progression, with retreatment on progression.

TABLE 16-5 Monoclonal Antibodies and Radioimmunoconjugates for the Treatment of Non-Hodgkin's Lymphoma

Monoclonal Antibody	Antigen
Rituximab	CD20
Other humanized anti-CD20s	CD20
Alemtuzumab	CD52
Epratuzumab	CD22
Lumiliximab	CD23
Apolizumab	HLA-DR
Galiximab	CD80
SGN-40	CD40
Bevacizumab	VEGF
Monoclonal Antibody with Radioimmunoconjugate	
Iodine-131 (^{131}I)- tositumomab	CD20
Yttrium-90 (^{90}Y)-ibritumomab tiuxetan	CD20

Abbreviations: HLA-DR, human leukocyte antigen-DR; VEGF, vascular endothelial growth factor.

Rituximab is generally well tolerated; the major side effects are fevers and chills during infusion. Some patients may have a cytokine-release syndrome that can be life-threatening, but this side effect is rare and does not generally recur with subsequent doses of the drug. Patients with a high number of circulating malignant cells have been reported to have a rapid tumor clearance syndrome, with abnormal renal function, electrolyte abnormalities, and coagulopathy.

Several randomized studies have clearly demonstrated an advantage in progression-free, event-free survival, with a suggestion of an overall survival benefit from combinations of rituximab and chemotherapy regimens, such as CVP and combination cyclophosphamide, doxorubicin, vincristine, and prednisone (CHOP).[15-17] However, the use of an anthracycline during initial treatment is controversial because these agents may subsequently be needed for treatment in the event of histologic transformation. The risk of histologic transformation is constant at approximately 3% per year. The optimal regimen for the initial treatment of patients with follicular lymphoma is unknown. However, R-CHOP is probably preferable in the setting of bulky disease and disease-related symptoms.

Relapsed and Refractory Follicular and Low-grade Lymphoma

Patients with follicular and low-grade non-Hodgkin's lymphoma invariably relapse because these diseases are not curable. The choice of salvage therapy is dependent on a number of factors, including the initial treatment regimen and the quality of response to that regimen, as well as patient factors including performance status, organ function, and extent of bone marrow involvement. Although most patients have recurrence with a similar histologic subtype as that at the time of initial diagnosis, there is a constant risk that a high-grade non-Hodgkin's lymphoma may develop, which is generally an ominous event. If disease is diagnosed and treated early, however, a small percentage of patients with transformed non-Hodgkin's lymphoma may have prolonged disease-free survival.

A variety of aggressive combination regimens have been used to treat relapsed or refractory disease, but there is no evidence that indicates a major advantage among them. New agents with promising activity include bendamustine bortezomib and lenalidomide.

Other approaches to relapsed or refractory disease include monoclonal antibodies, radioimmunotherapy, interferon, biologic therapies, and stem cell transplantation.

Monoclonal Antibodies. Rituximab has been approved by the U.S. Food and Drug Administration (FDA) for the treatment of relapsed and refractory follicular and low-grade non-Hodgkin's lymphoma. This approval was based on the results of a pivotal trial that evaluated 166 patients for whom previous treatment had failed. Four weekly infusions of rituximab were administered at a dose of 375 mg/m^2. The response rate was 46%, including an 8% rate of complete response and a median time to progression of approximately 1 year.

The best response to rituximab in patients with relapsed or refractory disease has occurred in patients with a follicular subtype. Only 12% of patients with small lymphocytic lymphoma have a response to the drug. There was no clear advantage to eight weekly infusions compared with the standard four infusions. For 40% of patients who have a relapse after an initial response to the antibody lasting at least 6 months, a second response may be achieved, lasting at least as long as the initial one. However, because most patients now receive rituximab as part of their initial treatment regimen and because many also have been treated with maintenance, the role of single-agent rituximab in relapsed patients may be reduced. Rituximab maintenance appears to prolong the survival of patients who receive either CHOP or rituximab plus CHOP (R-CHOP) for disease that has recurred following a non-anthracyline based regimen.[18]

Other monoclonal antibodies are being evaluated for relapsed and refractory follicular and low-grade non-Hodgkin's lymphoma include epratuzumab, galiximab, anti-CD40, and several humanized anti-CD20 monoclonal antibodies.

Radioimmunotherapy. Treatment with monoclonal antibodies labeled with isotopes, such as iodine-131 (^{131}I) and yttrium-90 (^{90}Y), has provided promising results. The FDA has approved ^{90}Y-ibritumomab tiuxetan for the treatment of relapsed and refractory follicular and low-grade non-Hodgkin's lymphoma, transformed non-Hodgkin's lymphoma, and disease that has not responded to rituximab. Response rates of more than 80%, with a 26% rate of complete response, were achieved for patients with relapsed and refractory indolent non-Hodgkin's lymphoma.[19] In a randomized study, the rates of complete and overall response were higher with ^{90}Y-ibritumomab than with rituximab, but there was no difference in time to progression.

^{131}I-tositumomab also has been approved by the FDA, and response rates for patients with relapsed or refractory follicular or low-grade non-Hodgkin's lymphoma have been greater than 70%, with an approximate 30% rate of complete response, lasting a median of 9 months.[20] In a series of 76 patients who received ^{131}I-tositumomab as initial therapy, 95% responded, with a complete remission rate of 75%, and almost 60% of patients were free from progression at 5 years.[21] An ongoing study to compare R-CHOP with CHOP followed by ^{131}I-tositumomab may define the initial treatment for follicular lymphoma. When administered at doses appropriate for myeloablation with stem cell support, ^{131}I-tositumomab antibody also has yielded promising results.

Because these agents are myelosuppressive, patients who may be considered for treatment with them must have less than 25% lymphoma involvement in the bone marrow, cellularity of more than 15%, more than 100,000 platelets/mm^3 (more than 1,500 neutrophils/mm^3), and no history of stem cell support or a failed stem cell harvest. Toxicities associated with ^{90}Y-ibritumomab tiuxetan are primarily of a myelosuppressive nature, with nadirs occurring 7 to 9 weeks after therapy. Secondary AML and MDS are partially related to previous therapy. Treatment with ^{131}I-tositumomab also may result in hypothyroidism. The lack of severe nausea, vomiting, or mucositis with these agents is likely responsible for the low incidence of severe infections. The relative role of radioimmunoconjugates and unconjugated antibodies is under investigation.

Interferon. Despite extensive study, the role for interferon as a treatment for indolent non-Hodgkin's lymphoma remains unclear, and it is not commonly used.

Other Biologic Therapies. New promising biologic approaches in development include anti-idiotype vaccines and several agents that target the apoptotic pathways.

Stem Cell Transplantation. Few data related to the use of allogeneic bone marrow transplantation for the treatment of indolent non-Hodgkin's lymphomas are available because of several factors: the low likelihood of finding a donor, greater rates of morbidity and mortality associated with allogeneic bone marrow transplantation compared with autologous stem cell transplantation, and a relatively long natural history of the disease. Although disease-free survival may be prolonged for approximately 40% of patients in whom disease failed to respond to previous chemotherapy, the mortality rate ranges from 20% to 40%. Therefore, careful patient selection and informed consent are essential.

The use of autologous stem cell transplantation for the treatment of relapsed or refractory low-grade non-Hodgkin's lymphoma is supported primarily by nonrandomized studies with long term follow-up. In a collaborative study of 126 adult patients conducted by St. Bartholomew's Hospital and the Dana-Farber Cancer Institute, there was an apparent plateau on the remission duration curve of 48% at a median follow-up of 13.5 years.[22] Survival appeared to be longer among patients transplanted in second compared with subsequent remissions. This approach also has been tested in a single trial of 89 patients, in which many but not all participants were randomly assigned, that demonstrated survival advantage for autologous transplantation compared with three cycles of chemotherapy. When used as part of initial therapy for high-risk patients, randomized studies demonstrate a prolongation of progression-free survival, but without a prolongation of survival.[23,24] Short-term and long-term complications of autologous stem cell transplantation include treatment-related mortality, prolonged anemia or thrombocytopenia, and a substantial increase in the incidence of secondary myelodysplasia and AML, which ranges from 7% to 19%.

When bone marrow transplantation and autologous stem cell transplantation are compared, the long-term survival rates are comparable. Autologous stem cell transplantation is associated with a greater likelihood of dying from recurrent disease, and allogeneic bone marrow transplantation results in a high frequency of death from graft-versus-host disease, infection, and venoocclusive disease. The potential benefit from a moderate amount of graft-versus-host disease in the form of graft-versus-lymphoma effect has been exploited in the use of submyeloablative transplantation.

Marginal Zone Lymphomas

The marginal zone lymphomas consist of extranodal marginal zone lymphomas (mucosa-associated lymphoid tissue [MALT]), nodal marginal zone non-Hodgkin's lymphomas, and primary splenic lymphoma. These tumors are CD5–, CD10–, CD23–, and CD11c±. Trisomy 3 and t(11;18) have been reported in 60% of extranodal cases. Other cytogenetic abnormalities have included translocations and abnormalities of 1p or 7. The t(11;18)(q21;q21), the most common of the structural abnormalities, produces a fusion between API2 on 11q21 and MLT (MALT lymphoma-associated translocation) on chromosome 18q21, also known as MALT1. IAPI2 belongs to the family of inhibitors of apoptosis (IAPs), and MALT1 is a pro-caspase–like protease. Bcl-10 also can bind to MALT1, resulting in an increase in translocation of nuclear factor (NF)-kappa B to the nucleus, impairing apoptosis and leading to the elaboration of a number of cytokines that favor the proliferation and longevity of the malignant cells.

Extranodal marginal zone (MALT) lymphomas affect the gastrointestinal and respiratory tracts, salivary glands, kidney, prostate, and other organs. Many patients have an associated autoimmune disease, such as Sjögren's syndrome or Hashimoto's thyroiditis. Unlike with most indolent non-Hodgkin's lymphoma, nearly all patients with marginal zone lymphoma have stage I or II disease at the time of presentation, although dissemination, often to other extranodal sites, can be detected at diagnosis or can subsequently occur in more than one-third of patients. MALT lymphomas account for approximately 80% of cases of indolent non-Hodgkin's lymphoma of the stomach, most of which occur in association with *Helicobacter pylori* infection. MALT lymphomas of the stomach are highly responsive to double or triple antibiotic therapy (e.g., omeprazole plus amoxicillin, or omeprazole, metronidazole, and clarithromycin), and the response is prolonged in more than 60% of patients. For patients in whom antibiotic therapy is not successful, alternative treatment approaches include single-agent rituximab, combination chemotherapy with rituximab, or local radiation therapy. However, MALT lymphomas arising from or involving other sites appear to require systemic chemotherapy. Histologic follow-up of gastric MALT lymphomas appears to be superior to follow-up with polymerase chain reaction analysis in the identification of persistent or recurrent disease. Two chromosomal translocations that are predictive of treatment failure also may be predictive of response to antibiotic therapy for *H. pylori*: bcl-10 t(1;14) (p22;q14) and t(11;18)(q21;q21).

Nodal marginal zone non-Hodgkin's lymphomas are the nodal counterpart of MALT lymphomas. Dissemination may occur in extranodal sites and may represent the nodal spread of MALT lymphomas. There is no standard chemotherapy, and patients with this disease tend to be treated with regimens used for follicular non-Hodgkin's lymphoma. The outcome following therapy is inferior to the extranodal marginal zone lymphoma.

Splenic lymphoma may be diagnosed in the presence of circulating villous lymphocytes that share phenotypic features with other marginal zone non-Hodgkin's lymphomas, but which have a distinct histologic appearance with cytoplasmic projections and can be confused with hairy cell leukemia cells. Patients typically have peripheral blood and bone marrow involvement, as well as a massively enlarged spleen. Splenectomy may result in a prolonged clinical remission, but systemic chemotherapy is eventually required in most patients. Small reports suggest response from treatment with fludarabine or rituximab.

Lymphoplasmacytic Lymphomas

Lymphoplasmacytic lymphomas include immunocytomas and Waldenström's macroglobulinemia. These lymphomas tend to occur in older people (median age, 63 years) and account for 1.5% of non-Hodgkin's lymphoma. Most patients present with a monoclonal immunoglobulin M (IgM) spike, with hyperviscosity syndrome in approximately 30% of patients. The disease also may be complicated by neuropathy, amyloidosis, cryoglobulinemia, and cold agglutinin disease. In most cases, the etiology of lymphoplasmacytic lymphomas is unknown, but an association with hepatitis C has been documented, especially for patients with cryoglobulinemia. Lymphoplasmacytic lymphomas are associated with a specific cytogenetic abnormality in 50% of cases, with t(9;14) (p13;q32) and rearrangement of the *PAX* gene. The *PAX-5* gene encodes the B-cell–specific activator protein.

When signs and symptoms reflect the concentration of IgM in the blood, generally over 3 CP, treatment is directed against the paraprotein, using plasmapheresis, although usually with systemic therapy. Treatment is indicated with enlarging organomegaly or lymphadenopathy, a rising IgM, symptomatic hyperviscosity, or other disease-related symptoms. Plasmapheresis may provide acute, symptomatic relief for the symptoms of hyperviscosity. Therapeutic options include nucleoside analog-based therapy, often in combination with rituximab, rituximab as a single agent, thalidomide or lenalidomide, bortezomib, or alkylating-agent based therapy.[25]

The prognosis for lymphoplasmacytic lymphomas is similar regardless of the presence of an associated paraprotein. Although disease is initially responsive to therapy, relapse is inevitable, and most patients die from the disease. The prognosis is worse for patients in whom disease transforms to large-cell non-Hodgkin's lymphoma (approximately 24% of cases).

Small Lymphocytic Lymphoma

Small lymphocytic lymphoma, the tissue counterpart of chronic lymphocytic leukemia (CLL), is characterized by an accumulation of small, mature-appearing lymphocytes in the blood, bone marrow, and lymph nodes. The immunophenotypic feature of small lymphocytic lymphoma and CLL is expression of CD19, CD20, CD5, and CD23. The distinctions between the two entities is the number of circulating clonal B-cells with a threshold of more than 5,000/mm^3 for the diagnosis of CLL. (See Chapter 15, Leukemias.) Thus, the diagnosis of small lymphocytic lymphoma can be made in the absence of blood or bone marrow involvement. Although small lymphocytic lymphoma often is included in clinical trials with the follicular and other low-grade non-Hodgkin's lymphomas, its biology and response to various therapies differ enough from those of the other indolent non-Hodgkin's lymphomas that it is better treated as CLL.

DIFFUSE LARGE B-CELL LYMPHOMA

Diffuse large B-cell non-Hodgkin's lymphoma is the most common form of non-Hodgkin's lymphoma in adults, accounting for 35% to 40% of cases. In up to 40% of patients, the disease may initially present in an extranodal site, most commonly in the gastrointestinal tract, but also in the central nervous system, genitourinary or reproductive tracts, lung, or other sties.

Morphologically, this tumor typically effaces the normal architecture of the lymph node. The characteristic immunophenotype is positive for CD19 and CD20, and negative for CD5 and CD23, with *Bcl-2* and *Bcl-6* both positive in the majority of cases. Those that are positive for CD10+ are of germinal center origin.

The International Prognostic Index (IPI) is widely used to classify patients with aggressive B-cell non-Hodgkin's lymphoma into four groups according to risk: low, low-intermediate, high-intermediate, and high (Table 16-6).[26] The identified parameters include:

- age (younger than 60 or older than 60),
- serum LDH level (normal or increased),
- performance status (0 to 1 or 2 to 4),
- number of extranodal sites (none or one compared with more than one), and
- tumor stage (I or II compared with III or IV).

It should be noted that these figures were derived from patients treated in the pre-rituximab era. A schema for patients treated with rituximab has recently been proposed.[27]

Although the IPI separates diffuse large B-cell lymphoma into clinically meaningful risk groups, there is considerable heterogeneity within those groups.

Studies using DNA microarray analyses suggest that there are at least two and perhaps three distinct subgroups within diffuse large B-cell lymphoma — namely a germinal center like B cell, an intermediate group, and an activated B-cell type — with a pattern in patients with primary mediastinal B-cell non-Hodgkin's lymphoma that more closely resembles that seen in Hodgkin's lymphoma. The activated B-cell type is associated with a worse prognosis even within

TABLE 16-6 Outcome According to Risk Group Defined by the International Prognostic Index[26]*

			Complete Response			Survival	
			Rate (%)	Relapse-free Survival			
Risk Group	Risk Factors	Distribution of Patients (%)		2-year Rate (%)	5-year Rate (%)	2-year Rate (%)	5-year Rate (%)
Low	0 or 1	35	87	79	70	84	73
Low-intermediate	2	27	67	66	50	66	51
High-intermediate	3	22	55	59	49	54	43
High	4 or 5	16	44	58	40	34	26

* The total of patients includes 1,385 in a training sample and 646 in a validation sample. *Reprinted with permission from the New England Journal of Medicine.*

subgroups of the IPI.[28] However, most of the data with molecular profiling are retrospective and prior to the widespread use of rituximab-based therapies. Whether the prognostic effect persists with more effective treatments remains to be determined.

Limited Disease

Approximately 20% of patients with diffuse large B-cell lymphoma have limited disease (stage I or nonbulky stage II) at the time of presentation. The likelihood of cure is more than 80% for patients with clinical stage I disease when treated with either involved-field or extended-field radiation therapy. However, one-third to one-half of patients with stage II disease treated with radiation therapy alone subsequently have relapse. A study conducted by the Southwest Oncology Group suggested a survival advantage for three cyles of CHOP followed by involved-field radiation compared with eight cycles of CHOP alone; however, although the benefit of combined modality therapy persists from 1 to 7 years, the curves merge at year 10.[29] More recently, a Groupe d'Etudes des Lymphomes de l'Adulte (GELA) study compared four cycles of CHOP chemotherapy with or without involved-field radiation in older patients with stages I to II aggressive non-Hodgkin's lymphoma and failed to demonstrate benefit from the addition of radiation, but with associated excess toxicity, even in patients with bulky tumors.[30]

Advanced-stage Disease

The first major progress in the treatment of advanced-stage, aggressive B-cell non-Hodgkin's lymphoma came in the 1970s when doxorubicin was combined with other drugs to form regimens such as CHOP. Complete response was achieved in 50% to 70% of patients, with a plateau on the disease-free survival curve at approximately 30%. Other combination regimens — including various doses and schedules of other standard agents — failed to demonstrate benefit compared with CHOP and were more toxic and expensive. Thus, CHOP remained the standard treatment for more than a decade. Single-agent activity with rituximab as well as promising phase II data for R-CHOP led to randomized studies in which this combination was compared with CHOP. The GELA randomly assigned 399 patients (age 60 to 80) to receive either CHOP alone or R-CHOP.[31] The rates of complete response, time to progression, and overall survival were better for patients treated with the combination chemotherapy-rituximab strategy, although this effect was most pronounced for patients in the low-risk category. Several trials have now confirmed the benefit of rituximab in the treatment of diffuse large B-cell lymphoma. A revised prognostic system may be more relevant for patients treated with R-CHOP, aggregating patients with no negative factors, one or two negative factors, or three or more negative factors.[27]

Promising data with a 14-day schedule are being validated in a randomized trial by comparing the previously mentioned regimen with the standard 21-day cycle. It is not clear whether using autologous stem cell transplantation for advanced stage, aggressive B-cell non-Hodgkin's lymphoma to consolidate initial complete response prolongs survival; therefore, this approach should not be part of routine management.

Relapsed or Refractory Disease

R-CHOP cures approximately 65% of patients with diffuse large B-cell non-Hodgkin's lymphoma. Because 10% to 25% of patients who have late recurrence have a low-grade histologic subtype, a repeat biopsy is necessary to plan appropriate treatment.

Therapy for patients with relapsed or refractory disease remains unsatisfactory. Several combination salvage regimens have been studied, and all have comparable results, considering the differences in patient selection. For approximately 40% of patients with chemosensitive disease, high-dose chemotherapy with autologous stem cell support results in long-term disease-free survival, but this treatment is not effective for patients with primary refractory disease. The outlook is poor for patients who have relapse after autologous transplantation. Single-agent rituximab induces response in 30% of patients, but the response is of brief duration.

MANTLE CELL LYMPHOMA

Mantle cell lymphoma comprises approximately 4% to 6% of non-Hodgkin's lymphoma. The characteristic phenotype is CD20+ and CD5+, a feature shared with CLL. However, mantle cell lymphoma does not express CD23, which is a feature of CLL, or CD10, found on cells of follicular lymphoma. Mantle cell lymphoma is usually associated with t(11;14)(q13,q32) and with overexpression of cyclin D1. Patients with mantle cell lymphoma may present with diffuse bowel involvement (lymphomatous polyposis), and central nervous system (CNS) involvement has been noted in almost 20% of cases but generally is initially asymptomatic. Mantle cell lymphoma is an incurable lymphoma with a clinical course that is usually aggressive. With the use of aggressive combination chemotherapy, response can be achieved in as many as 80% to 90% of patients, with complete response occurring in more than one-half of patients. However, responses are not available, with a median survival of 3.5 to 4.0 years. The addition of rituximab to CHOP for initial therapy does not clearly prolong survival. Data with aggressive acute leukemia-like regimens such as HyperCVAD, with transplant or rituximab, have produced promising results. In relapsed patients, a regimen of fludarabine, cyclophosphamide, and mitoxantrone with rituximab and rituximab maintenance improves response rate and duration of response, with an apparent prolongation of survival.[32] Bortezomib has been approved for relapsed and refractory mantle cell lymphoma, with several published studies showing response rates of 30% to almost 50%.[33] Other promising therapies include temsirolimus, lenalidomide, and radioimmunotherapy.

LYMPHOBLASTIC LYMPHOMAS

Patients who have lymphoblastic lymphoma generally have symptoms referable to a mediastinal mass. The distinction between lymphoblastic lymphomas and acute lymphoblastic leukemia is based on an arbitrary number of bone marrow lymphoblasts (generally with a 25% to 30% threshold). The presence of an elevated serum LDH level and bone marrow or CNS involvement confers a poorer prognosis. Complete response can be achieved in more than 90% of patients with low-risk disease with use of an aggressive, multiagent chemotherapy regimen. Disease is cured in more than 80% of patients. Relapse rarely occurs after 1 year. In contrast, although complete response can be achieved in most patients with high-risk disease, the 5-year survival rate is only 20%. Patients with high-risk disease are suitable candidates for investigational therapy. The results of autologous stem cell transplantation during second complete response are better than those associated with other salvage approaches; however, the long-term survival rate is only 15% for patients with resistant disease, compared with 63% for patients who have transplantation during first complete response and 31% for patients who have transplantation during second complete response. A role for high-dose therapy during first complete response has not been demonstrated but is under investigation.

BURKITT'S LYMPHOMA

Burkitt's lymphoma is a highly aggressive tumor. Those tumors with a high expression of Ki-67 and classical morphology — including a diffuse infiltration with a "starry-sky" appearance in the endemic setting, sporadic cases, and in patients with HIV — are considered "classical" Burkitt's. Other cases with an atypical morphology but a high expression of Ki-67 have been considered Burkitt-like tumors, although this diagnosis is not highly reproducible. The distinction may be made using DNA-microarray analysis.[34] All cases of classical Burkitt's have a translocation of *MYC* at band q24 t(8;14), and less commonly at t(2;8) or t(8;22). Epstein-Barr virus is routinely demonstrated in endemic cases but in only 25% to 40% of immunodeficiency-associated cases and in less than 30% of sporadic cases. Thus, the role of Epstein-Barr virus in the pathogenesis of this disorder remains unclear.

Treatment usually involves intensive therapy similar to that used to manage acute lymphoblastic leukemia, including CNS prophylaxis. (See Chapter 15, Leukemias.) The rate of complete response is 85% to 95%, with 47% failure-free survival at 5 years. Involvement of the CNS and/or bone marrow largely is responsible for the poor outlook for this patient group. The survival rate is 74% for adults treated with aggressive chemotherapy, consolidation, and maintenance, as well as with CNS prophylaxis. The 3-year survival rate is 100% for patients with stage I or II disease, 80% for patients with stage III disease, and 57% for patients with stage IV disease or ALL. Addition of rituximab to aggressive chemotherapy regimens appears to increase the response rate and duration.

Burkitt's lymphomas are characterized by a rapid growth rate, and treatment may be associated with potentially fatal tumor lysis syndrome, renal failure, hyperuricemia, and hyperkalemia. Biochemical abnormalities should be corrected rapidly before treatment, and patients should receive prophylactic xanthine oxidase and hydration. For patients who have relapse after initial therapy, high-dose chemotherapy with stem cell support should be considered.

PRIMARY CNS LYMPHOMA

Primary CNS lymphoma may occur de novo or in the setting of immunodeficiency, such as in HIV-positive patients, in those patients who received immunosuppressive therapy following organ transplantation, or for those patients with immunologic or rheumatologic disorders. The factors most consistently predictive of outcome include age younger than 50 and performance status.[35] Historically, the standard approach has been radiation therapy, with no additional benefit from regimens such as CHOP. The concurrent administration of high-dose methotrexate and radiation also is associated with unacceptable toxicity. However, in patients younger than 65, high-dose methotrexate followed by whole-brain irradiation has been associated with favorable results (median, 51 months).[36] In older patients, radiation should be deferred until recurrence. A number of radiation-sparing regimens are in development. Drugs being tested in the salvage setting include rituximab and temozolomide.

PERIPHERAL T-CELL NON-HODGKIN'S LYMPHOMA

The term peripheral T-cell lymphoma is used to refer to a diverse group of post-thymic T-cell tumors that have a mature T-cell phenotype in common. Patients with these lymphomas generally present with advanced-stage disease and B symptoms. The prognosis for patients with peripheral T-cell lymphoma is less promising than it is for patients with B-cell lymphoma. Patients tend to have higher scores on the IPI, B symptoms, advanced-stage disease, and high serum beta2-microglobulin. In general, patients with peripheral T cell lymphoma are treated with an aggressive multiagent chemotherapy, such as CHOP, similar to what is used to treat aggressive B-cell malignant diseases. However, patients with this disease have poor treatment response and a high rate of relapse, with few sustained remissions. Newer agents with activity include gemcitabine, nelarabine, alemtuzumab, and pralatrexate. The largest subgroup is peripheral T-cell lymphoma, not otherwise specified (NOS). The second most common is angioimmunoblastic T-cell lymphoma. Patients tend to present with generalized lyhmphadenopathy, fevers, weight loss, and rash, with autoimmune features including hypergammaglobulinemia and a positive Coombs' test. The course is typically complicated by serious and often fatal infections. Extranodal NK/T-cell lymphomas are characteristically positive for Epstein-Barr virus. These patients most often present with nasal symptoms, including obstruction and bleeding. Treatment includes both radiation therapy and combination chemotherapy; nevertheless, the outlook is poor. Hepatosplenic T-cell lymphoma is a rare entity that typically occurs in young men with splenomegaly, half of whom have systemic symptoms. Cytopenias, especially thrombocytopenia, are typical. A hemophagocytic syndrome has been reported in several cases. Because this disorder is relatively rare, there is no standard treatment approach, and virtually all patients diagnosed with it die within approximately 1 year. However, there are several less aggressive histologic subtypes, including subcutaneous panniculitis T-cell lymphoma of the alpha/beta type.

Anaplastic Large-cell Lymphoma

Anaplastic large-cell lymphoma (Ki-1, CD30+) can either be limited to the skin or can present as an aggressive lymphoma. The usual phenotype includes expression of T-cell antigens and CD30. The characteristic cytogenetic abnormality, t(2;5)(p23;q35), is associated with expression of a nucleoplasmin-anaplastic lymphoma kinase (NPM-ALK) protein, which is associated with a favorable outcome. ALK-positive anaplastic large cell lymphoma is one of the more favorable histologic subtypes of aggressive non-Hodgkin's lymphoma. Combination chemotherapy regimens, such as CHOP, induce complete response in more than 70% of patients, with more than half alive and disease-free at 5 years. Patients with ALK-negative disease have a worse prognosis.

CUTANEOUS T-CELL NON-HODGKIN'S LYMPHOMA

The cutaneous T-cell lymphomas are a heterogeneous group of lymphomas characterized by infiltration of the skin and other organs by mature T cells. In the WHO classification, these disorders are considered indolent T-cell malignant diseases and include mycosis fungoides and Sézary syndrome. In most cases, the diagnosis is made after a prolonged period of ill-defined skin disorders. Subsequently, patches or plaques characteristic of mycosis fungoides develop. At the time of diagnosis, fewer than one-half of patients have limited plaques, one-third have extensive plaques, and 10% to 15% have generalized erythroderma. The spleen, liver, and lymph nodes also may be involved, especially in patients with advanced skin disease and circulating malignant cells. When the peripheral blood becomes extensively involved with the malignant T cells, Sézary syndrome can be diagnosed. These patients often have erythroderma.

Most patients with cutaneous T-cell lymphoma are initially treated with topical measures, including steroids, photochemotherapy with oral methoxypsoralen therapy followed by ultraviolet light, mechlorethamine, bexarotene creme, or electron-beam radiation. Systemic therapy is needed when these approaches fail or when patients have major organ involvement, diffuse lymphadenopathy, or transformation to a large-cell non-Hodgkin's lymphoma. Treatment options include extracorporeal irradiation, interferon, nucleoside analogs, alemtuzumab, bexarotene, denileukin diftitox, or combination chemotherapy. The oral histone deacetylate inhibitor vorinostat has recently been approved by the FDA for treatment of this condition.[37] These patients often die from infections that can be minimized earlier, to some extent, by good skin care.

MULTIPLE MYELOMA

Multiple myeloma is an uncommon B-cell malignant disease of unknown etiology that accounts for 1% of all cancers and 14% of hematologic malignancies. Approximately 19,900 cases were diagnosed in the United States in 2007, with 10,790 deaths.[1] The incidence of multiple myeloma increases with advancing age. The median age of patients at the time of diagnosis is 65, and fewer than 2% of patients are younger than 40 at the time of diagnosis. Multiple myeloma is twice as common in black patients as in white patients.

There are no clear predisposing factors to the development of multiple myeloma, although there may be a genetic susceptibility. Exposure to radiation has been linked to the development of multiple myeloma, although the relationship between multiple myeloma and other environmental factors is controversial.

DIFFERENTIAL DIAGNOSIS

Not all patients with a monoclonal protein in the serum or urine have multiple myeloma. A monoclonal gammopathy of undetermined significance (MGUS) occurs in approximately 2% of the general population older than 50 and in 3% of people older than 70. It is associated with evidence of

KEY POINTS

- Monoclonal gammopathy of undetermined significance (MGUS) occurs in 2% of the population older than 50, with a lymphoid malignancy (including multiple myeloma) occurring in more than 8% of such patients.
- Newer and more effective therapies for multiple myeloma include thalidomide, lenalidomide, and bortezomib.

genomic instability, with 14q32 in half of patients and hyperdiploidy in 40%. Distinguishing between MGUS and asymptomatic multiple myeloma can be determined by comparing several characteristics.[38]

A diagnosis of MGUS requires that the results of all tests consistent with multiple myeloma must be normal, including bone marrow with normal cytogenetics, MRI, bone scan, and a paraprotein level of 3 g/dL or less. However, studies of MGUS involving the use of fluorescent in situ hybridization (FISH) have demonstrated cytogenetic abnormalities similar to those abnormalities seen in patients with multiple myeloma. In a large, retrospective review of 1,384 patients, MGUS progressed to multiple myeloma, CLL, primary amyloidosis, macroglobulinemia, or plasmacytoma in 8% of patients.[39] In 32 additional patients, either the paraprotein increased to more than 3 g/dL or the bone marrow plasma cells increased to more than 10% without evidence of progression. Thus, the risk of progression is approximately 1% per year, although approximately one-third of patients with multiple myeloma have a history of MGUS and the initial paraprotein concentration is predictive of progression.

The diagnosis of multiple myeloma requires a serum paraprotein of at least 3 g/dL, except in true cases of non-secretory disease, at least 10% plasma cells, and evidence of end-organ disease including lytic bone lesions, renal failure, or hypercalcemia (Table 16-7).[39]

EVALUATION AND STAGING

The initial evaluation of patients who have multiple myeloma requires a careful history and physical examination. Laboratory studies include a complete blood count and serum chemistries, with particular attention to serum calcium, albumin, renal function, LDH, and uric acid. The serum calcium concentration must be corrected for the serum albumin because of the possibility of a falsely high value. An ionized calcium result will help confirm the impression of possible hypercalcemia. Renal function studies — including a serum blood urea nitrogen and creatinine test and a 24-hour urine collection to determine protein and creatinine clearance — will help identify patients with renal dysfunction caused by multiple myeloma. A serum beta2-microglobulin provides useful prognostic information for patients with normal renal function, but it is less valuable for monitoring the course of the disease.

Serum protein electrophoresis may identify an M-spike, generally in the gamma region, and quantitative immunoglobulins are needed to determine the concentrations of the various immunoglobulin subtypes. Sixty percent to 80% of patients with multiple myeloma have an IgG M-component, and 20% have an IgA M-component. Light chain excretion in the urine in the absence of a serum paraprotein occurs in 15% of patients; approximately 1% do not secrete a monoclonal immunoglobulin. Serum-free light chain assays may be useful in patients who produce low or otherwise nondetectable levels of M-protein. This assay has been proposed as a replacement for the more cumbersome urine protein estimation.

Cytogenetic analysis is now considered an important part of initial analysis, as results may have an effect on therapy selection. Chromosome 13 deletions by FISH can be identified in one-half of newly diagnosed patients who have an abnormal karyotype. Abnormalities of chromosome 13 are associated with a poor prognosis, even with stem cell transplantation, although this prognostic effect appears to be strongest when detected by karyotype rather than by FISH. These deletions also can be reliably detected by gene-expression profiling. Translocations involving the immunoglobulin heavy chain gene, including t(11;14)(q13;q32), may be more common in patients with light-chain myeloma and in patients with amyloidosis. Another poor prognostic cytogenetic abnormality is t(4;14), which is present in 15% of patients. Gene-expression profiling also may be of future use in identifying patients most likely to respond to therapies such as bortezomib.[40]

Radiographic studies should include a chest x-ray and a bone survey. Radionuclide bone scans are not useful for assessing bone involvement in multiple myeloma. The most common finding on bone radiographs is osteopenia, often with vertebral body compression; however, the most characteristic

TABLE 16-7 Diagnosis Criteria for MGUS, Smoldering Multiple Myeloma , and Multiple Myeloma

	MGUS	SMM	MM
Serum Monoclonal Protein Level	< 3 g/dL	≥ 3 g/dL	
Bone Marrow Plasma Cells	< 10%	≥ 10%	≥ 10%
End Organ Damage	No	No	1 or more of the following
Lytic Bone Lesions	No	No	Yes
Renal Failure	No	No	Yes
Hypercalcemia	No	No	Yes

Abbreviations: MGUS, monoclonal gammopathy of undetermined significance; SMM, smoldering multiple myeloma; MM, multiple myeloma.

abnormalities are lytic lesions. In some patients with multiple myeloma, osteoblastic lesions may be present instead. An MRI may provide valuable prognostic information about bone marrow involvement and prognosis. Patients who have multiple myeloma should not be permitted to become dehydrated. Also, patients who are suspected to have multiple myeloma and patients who have been diagnosed with the disease should not have contrast studies (if possible), such as intravenous pyelography and CT scans, because of the possibility of precipitating or worsening renal failure. MRI and FDG-PET scans also may be useful in determining the extent of disease, especially when there is suspicion of a plasmacytoma.

Traditionally, patients with multiple myeloma have been staged according to the Durie-Salmon system, which is based on the concentration of paraprotein in the blood and/or urine, the number of bone lesions, serum calcium (corrected for albumin), and hemoglobin. The level of serum creatinine also is used to further separate patients into a subclassification category within a stage (A, serum creatinine levels less than 2.0 mg/dL; or B, serum creatinine ≥ 2.0 mg/dL).

More recent staging systems that incorporate serum beta2-microglobulin and cytogenetic characteristics have been proposed.[41] In a study of patients receiving high-dose chemotherapy as part of initial treatment, chromosome 13 abnormalities were the most reliable predictor of survival, followed by beta2-microglobulin.[42] The expected median survival of 111 months was not reached by patients who had either of these adverse factors. The median survival was 47 months for patients with one factor and 25 months for patients with two factors.

Additional studies, including those to evaluate C-reactive protein and plasma cell labeling index, have been used to identify patients in different risk groups. One of the most reliable prognostic factors is cytogenetic features, especially translocations or partial deletions of 13q.

A new international staging system for multiple myeloma has been widely adopted based on the serum beta2-microglobulin and serum albumin (Table 16-8).[41]

TABLE 16-8 International Staging System for Multiple Myeloma[41]

Stage	Criteria	Median Survival (months)
I	Serum β_2-microglobulin < 3.5 mg/L Serum albumin ≥ 3.5 g/dL	62
II	Not stage I or II	44
III	Serum β_2-microglobulin ≥ 5.5 mg/L	29

There are two categories for stage II: serum beta2-microglobulin < 3.5 mg/L but serum albumin < 3.5 g/dL; or serum beta2-microglobulin 3.5-<5.5 mg/L irrespective of the serum albumin level.

This system provides a more equal distribution among stages when compared with the previously used Durie-Salmon system and should be considered the new standard.

COMPLICATIONS OF MULTIPLE MYELOMA

Multiple myeloma can affect many organ systems and functions, and complications include plasmacytomas, renal insufficiency, hypercalcemia, life-threatening infections, anemia, painful bone lesions, and neurologic symptoms.

Plasmacytomas

Plasmacytomas, or solid tumor masses of plasma cells, can occur either in soft tissues (extramedullary plasmacytomas) or in bone. Plasmacytomas of the soft tissue are curable with local radiation therapy. Plasmacytomas may present with symptoms associated with spinal cord compression, which is an oncologic emergency requiring neurosurgical intervention and radiation therapy. The diagnosis of a solitary plasmacytoma can be made only on evaluation of tissue obtained at biopsy; the diagnosis is confirmed by the presence of a plasma cell infiltrate with no evidence of bone lesions on radiographs or myeloma at another site. The level of M-protein in blood or urine should be absent or low, with normal concentrations of residual immunoglobulins.

Local radiation is the treatment of choice. If the presence of M-protein persists after radiation, there is a high likelihood that overt multiple myeloma will subsequently develop. The most common outcome is the subsequent development of multiple bone lesions, with a median time to progression of 2 to 3 years. However, progression may occur as long as 15 years after the initial diagnosis.

Renal Insufficiency

Patients with multiple myeloma may have renal insufficiency attributable to a number of conditions.

- Hypercalcemia
- Hyperuricemia
- Obstruction of the tubules with multiple myeloma protein ("myeloma kidney")
- Amyloidosis
- Nephrotic syndrome
- Infiltration of the kidneys by plasma cells
- Obstruction by a plasmacytoma
- Pyelonephritis
- CT scan with contrast

Hypercalcemia

Hypercalcemia occurs in 10% to 20% of patients with multiple myeloma and often is accompanied by symptoms of confusion, dehydration, and constipation. It is related to the production of cytokines, such as tumor necrosis factor-alpha and interleukin (IL)-1. Treatment requires rapid correction with hydration, diuresis, and bishphosphonate therapy, if the latter is not already prescribed. Treatment of the underlying multiple myeloma is critical for an optimal response, which is related, in part, to the use of high doses of corticosteroids.

Infections

The risk of life-threatening infections, most often with encapsulated bacteria such as *Streptococcus pneumoniae*, is present until therapy has started. While undergoing therapy, patients also are subject to the development of gram-negative organisms and fungal infections. Predisposition to infections in this population is related to an impaired ability to produce specific immunoglobulins, defective activation of the complement system, and therapy-related neutropenia. The use of high-dose intravenous immunoglobulins should be limited to patients with recurrent bacterial infections that are unresponsive to prophylactic antibiotics. Vaccines against pneumococcus or other organisms are generally ineffective because of a poor response to bacterial antigens.

Anemia

Anemia subsequently occurs in most patients with multiple myeloma, and the cause is multifactoral. Anemia can be related to bone marrow infiltration by plasma cells or, less often, to amyloidosis. Anemia of chronic disease, which is a consequence of therapy, and renal failure also can be related. Randomized studies have demonstrated the efficacy of exogenous recombinant erythropoietin in this setting. Doses in these trials were either 10,000 U per day given subcutaneously for 7 days, or 2,000 U per day for 8 weeks. Treatment with erythropoietin resulted in an increase in hemoglobin concentration by at least 2 g/dL in 75% of patients. Alternative dosing may include 40,000 U subcutaneously, administered weekly. The longer-acting darbepoietin alpha (200 mg every other week or 300 mg every 3 weeks) is a more convenient and comparably effective option.

Bone Lesions

The vertebral bodies, ribs, and long bones are the most frequent sites of painful bone lesions. Radiation therapy is effective for palliation; however, unless there is an impending fracture of a weight-bearing bone, radiation should be deferred until systemic chemotherapy has had a chance to be effective because radiation can reduce bone marrow reserves, which limits the amount of chemotherapy that can be administered. Potential fractures to long bones can be treated with radiation therapy alone or with internal fixation.

Neurologic Symptoms

The most severe neurologic symptoms associated with multiple myeloma are spinal cord compression, requiring emergency intervention with surgery and radiation therapy, followed by systemic therapy. Hyperviscosity occurs more often with IgAI than with IgGI multiple myeloma. The clinical manifestations can be reversed with plasmapheresis, generally in conjunction with treatment of the underlying multiple myeloma. Amyloidosis and polyneuropathy, organomegaly, endocrinopathy, monoclonal component, and skin changes (POEMS) syndrome also may lead to neuropathy. Amyloidosis can affect multiple organ sites, including the heart, kidneys, and tongue, and can result in renal failure and cardiac decompensation. Diagnosis is made by performing a Congo Red stain on the bone marrow specimen, a kidney biopsy, a rectal biopsy, or an abdominal fat pad biopsy.

TREATMENT

Although treatment is eventually needed for almost all patients with multiple myeloma, observation alone is sufficient until signs of disease progression for individuals who have asymptomatic, smoldering disease, characterized by the following:

- serum M-protein levels greater than 3 g/dL,
- plasma cells in the bone marrow of less than 10%,
- normal level of serum calcium,
- normal hemoglobin concentration,
- no lytic bone lesions, and
- normal plasma cell labeling index.

Such patients should be monitored at 3-month intervals until therapy is indicated as a result of disease progression.

Treatment is generally initiated for patients with progressive or symptomatic disease, such as disease with any of the symptoms listed.

- Increasing M-protein concentration in the blood or urine
- Worsening anemia
- Bone lesions with fractures
- Bone marrow failure with neutropenia and/or thrombocytopenia
- Bone pain or fracture
- Recurrent infections
- Development of plasmacytomas

Standardized criteria for assessment of response have recently been published.[43] The response criteria rely on measurements of serum and urine M-proteins, plasma cells in bone marrow, and the size of soft tissue plasmacytomes. Measurement of these criteria allow the response to be categorized as one of the following: stringent complete response, complete response, very good partial response, and stable disease. Relapse criteria define progressive disease and clinical relapse using the same criteria noted previously, along with the progression of bone lesions and development of hypercalcemia, anemia, or renal insufficiency.[44]

The administration of bisphosphonate is important for all patients with active multiple myeloma. Studies with pamidronate (a monthly dose of 90 mg, administered as a 4-hour intravenous infusion) demonstrated a significant delay to the first skeletal event and an improvement in quality of life. Zoledronic acid (4 mg every 3 to 4 weeks) may be preferable despite its increased cost because of a shorter infusion time (15 minutes compared with 2 hours). However, it cannot be given to patients with impaired renal function. Bisphosphonate therapy, especially with zoledronic acid, may be complicated by osteonecrosis of the jaw, often following dental procedures or trauma; therefore, this agent should only be used on a long-term basis in patients with active disease.

The optimal initial chemotherapy treatment for multiple myeloma is evolving. Corticosteroids (e.g., dexamethasone at a dose of 40 mg orally, taken every other day, or taken daily for 4 days every 2 weeks) induces responses in up to 40% of patients when used as initial therapy and in 20% to 40% of patients for whom primary therapy has failed.

Melphalan (8 mg/m^2 daily for 4 days) and prednisone (60 mg/m^2 daily for 4 days) repeated every 3 to 4 weeks was the standard treatment for multiple myeloma for decades but was supplanted by combination vincristine, doxorubicin (adriamycin), and dexamethasone (VAD), which includes a 4-day continuous infusion of vincristine (0.4 mg/day) and doxorubicin (9 mg/m^2 daily) — both of which are administered through an indwelling catheter — along with oral dexamethasone (40 mg each morning for 4 days and repeated on days 9 and 17 of each cycle). VAD cycles are repeated every 21 days, for four cycles beyond best response. Dexamethasone accounts for approximately 80% of activity this regimen's activity. The outcome following VAD is not clearly superior to that following melphalan and prednisone, but it is less toxic to the bone marrow stem cells, thus permitting autologous stem cell transplantation in a greater number of patients.

Based on encouraging data about the use of thalidomide to treat relapsed and refractory multiple myeloma, the combination of thalidomide and dexamethasone was compared with dexamethasone alone in a phase III study conducted by the Eastern Cooperative Oncology Group (ECOG) that accrued 207 patients. The response rate with the combination was 63% compared with 41% with dexamethasone alone. However, the incidence of deep venous thrombosis, or any grade 4 to 5 toxicity, was greater with the combination therapy (45% vs. 21%). Other notable toxicities with thalidomide have included constipation, sedation, neurologic complications, rash, and infections.[45] Unfortunately, the study was not designed to compare survival; patients were allowed to discontinue therapy to receive stem cell transplantation. Although the combination was more active, the increase in toxicity must be weighed in the treatment decision.

Recent data suggest promising activity for the second generation immunomodulatory agent lenalidomide, with response rates of about 25% in relapsed and refractory patients and an advantage for lenalidomide plus dexamethasone over dexamethasone alone.[46] When used as initial therapy, response rates as high as 90% have been reported, with 6% of patients achieving complete remissions and 32% achieving a very good partial response or near complete response.[47] Significant peripheral neuropathy or thrombosis were rare occurrences. Thus, the choice of initial treatment may depend on whether the patient is considered a candidate for autologous stem cell transplantation. For those who are deemed suitable, treatment generally consists of thalidomide and dexamethasone or lenalidomide and dexamethasone. Newer data suggest high response rates with bortezomib in combination with dexamethasone and with doxorubicin. For nontransplant candidates, therapy may include melphalan and prednisone alone or in combination with thalidomide or thalidomide plus dexamethasone.

Relapsed and Refractory Disease

The treatment for patients for whom primary therapy has failed is determined to some extent by the initial therapy. Patients treated with melphalan and prednisone have a 40% chance of having a response to VAD. Patients in whom disease failed to respond to VAD are less likely to have a response to melphalan and prednisone, but they can be treated with single-agent dexamethasone. Thalidomide induces response in approximately one-third of patients with relapsed or refractory disease, but the duration of response is only approximately 3 months. The combination of thalidomide and dexamethasone also has been successful. The FDA approved bortezomib for the treatment of relapsed and refractory multiple myeloma based on a series of 202 patients, more than half of whom had autologous stem cell transplantation that had failed.[48] Treatment with thalidomide had failed for almost three-quarters of these patients. The response rate with bortezomib was approximately 30%, including a 13% rate of complete response or near-complete response (complete response with positive immunofixation). The performance status, hemoglobin, and quality of life also were better, and in some patients, bone lesions resolved. In a phase III trial, bortezomib was superior to dexamethasone in relapsed and refractory patients. Combinations of this agent with other drugs are being developed. For example, the FDA recently approved the combination of bortezomib with liposomal doxorubicin based on a randomized trial in which this regimen yielded prolonged survival for patients with relapsed/refractory multiple myeloma compared with bortezomib alone.[49]

Hematopoietic Stem Cell Transplantation

Stem cell transplants for myeloma have included single autologous, tandem autologous, allogeneic, nonmyeloablative allogeneic, and autologous followed by allogeneic. Several randomized trials have supported autologous transplant as part of the initial therapy for patients with multiple myeloma.[50,51]

The relative efficacy of autologous transplant over standard therapy has not been uniformly observed. In a North American Intergroup trial that included more than 500 patients, no benefit was noted for high-dose therapy compared with standard chemotherapy, either as initial treatment or in the salvage setting.[52] Similarly, in a large French study in patients between the ages of 55 and 65, high-dose therapy prolonged event-free survival but did not improve overall survival,[53] and a Dutch-Belgian trial also did not show survival benefit.[54] Differences among these studies may reflect variability in treatment regimens, patient-related features, or other factors.

In patients age 65 and older, the combination of melphalan, prednisone, and thalidomide appears to be superior to both melphalan and prednisone alone and autologous stem cell transplantation.[55]

Despite preliminary results suggesting an advantage for tandem autologous transplants over a single transplant, a survival benefit has been difficult to demonstrate.[56]

Allogeneic stem cell transplants have been evaluated in multiple myeloma, but the associated mortality of 20% to 40% has tempered enthusiasm for using this approach as part of routine therapy. However, promising data have been reported for the use of submyeloablative transplants, either alone or following autologous stem cell transplantation, because of apparent efficacy and reduced toxicity.[57] In one study, an autologous stem cell transplant followed by an allogeneic transplant was superior to tandem autologous transplants with respect to patient survival.[58] Other studies failed to confirm this advantage.[59]

POEMS SYNDROME

POEMS syndrome is an entity of uncertain etiology and includes the association of a plasma cell disorder and peripheral neuropathy with at least one of the following: osteosclerotic multiple myeloma, Castleman's disease, organomegaly, endocrinopathy (excluding diabetes or hypothyroidism), edema, skin changes, or papilledema. It is diagnosed at a median age of 51. In a review of 99 cases of the syndrome, the median survival was 165 months, with no presenting feature — other than response to therapy — accurately predicting survival.[30] Other findings associated with POEMS syndrome include pulmonary hypertension with clubbing, renal failure, thrombotic events, testicular atrophy, gynecomastia, hypertrichosis, thrombocytosis, and congestive heart failure. Approximately 50% of patients with POEMS syndrome have a response to radiation of localized lesions. The associated bone lesions are generally osteosclerotic rather than the more characteristic osteolytic lesions associated with multiple myeloma. A number of cytokines are increased in this disease, including tumor-necrosis factor, interleukin (IL)-6 and IL-1. Vascular endothelial growth factor (VEGF) also has been implicated in the pathogenesis of this disorder, and elevated levels of VEGF are commonly detected. There is no specific treatment for this syndrome, although local radiation to limited areas of disease or to associated plasmacytomas may provide clinical improvement. Drugs that have been used are generally those used to treat myeloma.

SYSTEMIC AMYLOIDOSIS

Amyloidosis results from deposition of a fibrillar amyloid protein in the kidneys, heart, tongue, nerves, and other organs. This protein is detectable with a Congo red stain demonstrating birefringent crystals under polarized light. The specific organ that is involved may result from the type of germline light chain V gene. Amyloidosis occurs at a median age of 65 and coexists in approximately 10% of patients with multiple myeloma. Systemic manifestations include nephrotic syndrome; cardiomyopathy; hepatomegaly; neurologic abnormalities, including carpal tunnel syndrome; and purpura, notably periorbital.

The outcome has been disappointing after therapy using alkylating agents, interferon, or colchicine. Data from studies of dexamethasone and interferon are encouraging. Thalidomide has limited activity but considerable toxicity in this patient group. Stem cell transplantation also has been recommended for the treatment of systemic amyloidosis; however, any benefit appears to be related to patient selection. Preliminary data suggest activity for lenalidomide in this disorder.[60]

REFERENCES

1. Jemal A, Siegel R, Ward E, et al. Cancer statistics, 2007. *CA Cancer J Clin.* 2007:57(1):43–66.
2. Hehn ST, Grogan TM, Miller TP. Utility of fine-needle aspiration as a diagnostic technique in lymphoma. *J Clin Oncol.* 2004;22(15): 3046–3052.
3. Jaffe ES. *Pathology and Genetics: Tumours of Haematopoietic and Lymphoid Tissues (World Health Organization Classification of Tumours).* Lyon, France: IARC Press; 2001.
4. Ekstrand BC, Lucas JB, Horwitz SM, et al. Rituximab in lymphocyte-predominant Hodgkin disease: results of a phase 2 trial. *Blood.* 2003; 101(11):4285–4289.
5. Meyer RM, Gospodarowicz MK, Connors JM, et al. Randomized comparison of ABVD chemotherapy with a strategy that includes radiation therapy in patients with limited-stage Hodgkin's lymphoma: National Cancer Institute of Canada Clinical Trials Group and the Eastern Cooperative Oncology Group. *J Clin Oncol.* 2005;23(21): 4634–4642.
6. Duggan DB, Petroni GR, Johnson JL, et al. Randomized comparison of ABVD and MOPP/ABV hybrid for the treatment of advanced Hodgkin's disease: report of an Intergroup trial. *J Clin Oncol.* 2003; 21(4):607–614.
7. Diehl V, Franklin J, Pfreundschuh M, et al. Standard and increased-dose BEACOPP chemotherapy compared with COPP-ABVD for advanced Hodgkin's disease. *New Engl J Med.* 2003;348(24):2386–2395.

8. Juweid ME, Stroobants S, Hoekstra OS, et al. Use of positron emission tomography for response assessment of lymphoma: consensus recommendations of the Imaging Subcommittee of the International Harmonization Project in Lymphoma. *J Clin Oncol.* 2007;25(5):571–578.

9. Juweid M, Stroobants S, Mottaghy F, et al. Recommendations of the imaging committee of the International Harmonization Project (IHP) for FDG-PET (PET) use in patients with lymphoma. *Proc Eur Soc Nuc Med.* 2006:24.

10. Elstrom R, Guan L, Baker G, et al. Utility of FDG-PET scanning in lymphoma by WHO classification. *Blood.* 2003;101(10):3875–3876.

11. Solal-Céligny P, Roy P, Colombat P, et al. Follicular lymphoma international prognostic index. *Blood.* 2004;104(5):1258–1265.

12. Brice P, Bastion Y, Lepage E, et al. Comparison in low-tumor-burden follicular lymphomas between an initial no-treatment policy, prednimustine, or interferon alfa: a randomized study from the Group D'Etude des Lymphomes Folliculares. *J Clin Oncol.* 1997;15(3):1110–1117.

13. Ghielmini M, Schmitz SF, Cogliatti SB, et al. Prolonged treatment with rituximab in patients with follicular lymphoma significantly increases event-free survival and response duration compared with weekly × 4 schedule. *Blood.* 2004;103(12):4416–4423.

14. Hochster HS, Weller E, Gascoyne RD, et al. Maintenance rituximab after CVP results in superior clinical outcome in advanced follicular lymphoma (FL): results of the E1496 phase III trial from the Eastern Cooperative Oncology Group and the Cancer and Leukemia Group B. *Blood.* 2005;106(146a):abstract 349.

15. Marcus RE, Solal-Celigny P, Imrie K, et al. MabThera (rituximab) plus cyclophosphamide, vincristine and prednisone (CVP) chemotherapy improves survival in previously untreated patients with advanced follicular non-Hodgkin's lymphoma (NHL). *Blood.* 2006;108(146a):abstract 481.

16. Hiddemann W, Kneba M, Dreyling M, et al. Frontline therapy with rituximab added to the combination of cylophosphamide, doxorubicin, vincristine, and prednisone (CHOP) significantly improves the outcome for patients with advanced-stage follicular lymphoma compared with therapy with CHOP alone: results of a prospective randomized study of the German Low-Grade Lymphoma Study Group. *Blood.* 2005;106(12):3725–3732.

17. Herold M, Haas A, Srock S, et al. Rituximab added to first-line mitoxantrone, chlorambucil, and prednisolone chemotherapy followed by interferon maintenance prolongs survival in patients with advanced follicular lymphoma: an East german Study Group Hematology and Oncology study. *J Clin Oncol.* 2007;25(15):1986–1992.

18. van Oers MH, Klasa R, Marcus RE, et al. Rituximab maintenance improves clinical outcome of relapsed/refractory follicular non-Hodgkin's lymphoma in patientes both with and without rituximab during induction: results of a prospective randomized phase 3 intergroup trial. *Blood.* 2006;108(10):3295–3301.

19. Cheson BD. Radioimmunotherapy of non-Hodgkin's lymphomas. *Curr Drug Targets.* 2006;7(10):1293–1300.

20. Fisher RI, Kaminski MS, Wahl RL, et al. Tositumomab and iodine 131 tositumomab produces durable complete remission in heavily pretreated patients with low-grade and transformed low-grade non-Hodgkin's lymphoma. *J Clin Oncol.* 2005;23(30):7565–7573.

21. Kaminski M, Tuck M, Estes J, et al. 131I-tositumomab as initial treatment for follicular lymphoma. *New Engl J Med.* 2005;352(5):441–449.

22. Rohatiner AZ, Nadler LM, Davies AJ, et al. Myeloablative therapy with autologous bone marrow transplantation for follicular lymphoma at the time of second or subsequent remission: long-term follow-up. *J Clin Oncol.* E-pub ahead of print, 2007.

23. Lenz G, Dreyling M, Schiegnitz E, et al. Myeloablative radiochemotherapy followed by autologous stem cell transplantation in first remission prolongs progression-free survival in follicular lymphoma: results of a prospective, randomized trial of the German Low-Grade Lymphoma Study Group. *Blood.* 2004;104(9):2667–2674.

24. Deconinck E, Foussard C, Milpied N, et al. High-dose therapy followed by autologous purged stem-cell transplantation and doxorubicin-based cheemotherapy in patients with advanced follicular lymphoma: a randomized multicenter study by GOELAMS. *Blood.* 2005;105(10): 3817–3823.

25. Treon SP, Gertz MA, Dimopoulos M, et al. Update on treatment recommendations from the Third International Workshop on Waldenstrom's macroglobulinemia. *Blood.* 2006;107(9):3442–3446.

26. A predictive model for aggressive non-Hodgkins lymphoma: The International Non-Hodgkins Lymphoma Prognostic Factors Project. *N. Engl J Med.* 1993;329:987–994.

27. Sehn LH, Berry B, Chhanabhai M, et al. The revised International Prognostic Index (R-IPI) is a better predictor of outcome than the stnadard IPI for patients with diffuse large B-cell lymphoma treated with R-CHOP. *Blood.* 2007;109(5):1857–1861.

28. Rosenwald A, Wright G, Chan WC, et al. The use of molecular profiling to predict survival after chemotherapy for large B-cell lymphoma. *New Engl J Med.* 2002;346(25):1937–1947.

29. Miller TP, Dahlberg S, Cassady JR, et al. Chemotherapy alone compared with chemotherapy plus radiotherapy for localized intermediate- and high-grade non-Hodgkin's lymphoma. *N Engl J Med.* 1998; 339(1):31–26.

30. Bonnet C, Fillet G, Mounier N, et al. CHOP alone compared with CHOP plus radiotherapy for localized aggressive lymphoma in elderly patientse: a study by the Groupe d'Etude des Lymphomes de l'Adulte. *J Clin Oncol.* 2007;25(7):787–792.

31. Feugier P, Van Hoof A, Sebban C, et al. Long-term results of the R-CHOP study in the treatment of elderly patients with diffuse large B-cell lymphoma: a study by the Groupe d'Eetude des Lymphomes de l'Adulte. *J Clin Oncol.* 2005;23(18):4117–4126.

32. Forstpointner R, Unterhalt M, Dreyling M, et al. Maintenance therapy with rituximab leads to a significant prolongation of response duration after saslvage therapy with a combination of rituximabd, fludarabine, cyclophosphamide, and mitoxangtrone (R-FCM) in patients with recurring and refractory follicular and mantle cell lymphomas: Results of a prospective randomized study of the German Low Grade Lymphoma Study Group (GLSG). *Blood.* 2006;108(13): 4003–4008.

33. Fisher RI, Bernstein SH, Kahl BS, et al. Multicenter phase II study of bortezomib in patients with relapsed or refractory mantle cell lymphoma. *J Clin Oncol.* 2006;24(30):4867–4874.

34. Dave SS, Fu K, Wright GW, et al. Molecular diagnosis of Burkitt's lymphoma. *New Engl J Med.* 2006;354(23):2431–2442.

35. Abrey LE, Ben-Porat L, Panageas KS, et al. Primary central nervous system lymphoma: the Memorial Sloan-Kettering Cancer Center prognostic model. *J Clin Oncol.* 2006;24(36):5711–5715.

36. Gavrilovic IT, Hormigo A, Yahalom J, et al. Long-term follow-up of high-dose methotrexate-based therapy with and without whole brain irradiation for newly diagnosed primary CNS lymphoma. *J Clin Oncol.* 2006;24(28):4570–4574.

37. Zhang C, Richon V, Ni X, et al. Phase 2 trial of oral vironostat (suberoylanilide hydroxamic acid, SAHA) for refractory cutaneous T-cell lymphoma (CTCL). *Blood.* 2007;109(1):31–39.

38. Rajkumar SV, Dispenzieri A, Kyle RA. Monoclonal gammopathy of undetermined significance, Waldenstrom macroglobulinemia, AL amyloidosis, and related plasma cell disorders: diagnosis and treatment. *Mayo Clin Proc.* 2006;81(5):693–703.

39. International Myeloma Working Group. Criteria for the classification of monoclonal gammopathies, multiple myeloma and related disorders: a report of the International Myeloma Working Group. *Br J Haematol.* 2003;121(5):749–757.

40. Mulligan G, Mitsiades C, Bryant B, et al. Gene expression profiling and correlation with outcome in clinical trials of the proteasome inhibitor bortezomib. *Blood.* 2007;109(8):3177–3188.

41. Greipp PR, San Miguel J, Durie BG, et al. International staging system for multiple myeloma. *J Clin Oncol.* 2005;23(15):3412–3420.

42. Facon T, A Vet-Loiseau H, Guillerm G, et al. Chromosome 13 abnormalities identified by FISH analysis and serum beta2-microglobulin produce a powerful myeloma staging system for patients receiving high-dose therapy. *Blood.* 2001;97(6):1566–1571.

43. Durie BG, Harousseau JL, Miguel JS, et al. International uniform response criteria for multiple myeloma. *Leukemia.* 2006;20(9):1467–1473.

44. National Comprehensive Cancer Network. NCCN Clinical Practice Guidelines in Oncology: Multiple Myeloma. Version 2008. Available at: www.nccn.org/professionals/physician_gls/PDF/myeloma.pdf. Accessed October 11, 2007.

45. Rajkumar SV, Blood E, Vesole D, et al. Phase III clinical trial of thalidomide plus dexamethasone compared with dexamethasone alone in newly diagnosed multiple myeloma: a clinical trial coordinated by the Eastern Cooperative Oncology Group. *J Clin Oncol.* 2006;24(3): 431–436.

46. Dimopoulos MA, Spencer A, Attal M, et al. Study of Lenalidomide Plus Dexamethasone Versus Dexamethasone Alone in Relapsed or Refractory Multiple Myeloma (MM): Results of a Phase 3 Study (MM-010). *Blood* (*ASH Annual Meeting Abstracts*). 2005;106:Abstract 6.

47. Rajkumar SV, Hayman SR, Lacy MQ, et al. Combination therapy with lenalidomide plus dexamethasone (Rev/Ddex) for newly diagnosed patients. *Blood.* 2005;106(13):4050–4053.

48. Richardson PG, Sonneveld P, Schuster M, et al. Extended follow-up of a phase 3 trial in relapsed multiple myeloma: final time-to-event results of the APEX trial. *Blood*. 2007;[Epub ahead of print].

49. Harousseau JL, Nagler A, Sonneveld P, et al. Effect of the combination of pegylated liposomal doxorubicin and bortezomib on time to progression (TTP) and overall survival of patients with relapsed/refractory multiple myeloma compared with bortezomib alone. *J Clin Oncol.* 2007;24(441s):abstract 8002.

50. Attal M, Harousseau JL, Stoppa AM, et al. A prospective, randomized trial of autologous bone marrow transplantation and chemotherapy in multiple myeloma. *New Engl J Med.* 1996;335(2):91–97.

51. Child JA, Morgan G, Davies F, et al. High-dose chemotherapy with hematopoietc stem-cell rescue for multiple myeloma. *New Engl J Med.* 2003;348(19):1875–1883.

52. Barlogie B, Kyle RA, Anderson KC, et al. Standard chemotherapy compared with high-dose chemoradiotherapy for multiple myeloma: final results of phase III US intergroup trial S9321. *J Clin Oncol.* 2006;24(6):929–936.

53. Fermand JP, Katsahian S, Divine M, et al. High-dose therapy and autologous blood stem-cell transplantation comapred with conventional treatment in myeloma patients aged 55 to 65 years: long-term results of a randomized control trial from the Group Myelome-Autogreffe. *J Clin Oncol.* 2005;23(36):9227–9233.

54. Segeren CM, Sonneveld P, van der Holt B, et al. Overall and event-free survival are not improved by the use of myeloablative therapy following intensified chemotherapy in previously untreated patients with multiple myeloma: a prospective randomized phase 3 study. *Blood.* 2003;101(6): 2144–2151.

55. Facon T, Mary J, Harousseau J, et al. Superiority of melphalan-prednisone (MP) + thalidomide (THAL) over MP and autologous stem cell transplantation in the treatment of newly diagnosed elderly patients with multiple myeloma. *J Clin Oncol.* 2006;24(1s):abstract 1.

56. Cavo M, Tosi P, Zamagni E, et al. Prospective, randomized studey of single compared with double autologous stem-cell transplantation for multiple myeloma: Bologna 96 clinical study. *J Clin Oncol.* 2007; 25(17)2434–2441.

57. Maloney DG, Molina AJ, Sahebi F, et al. Allografting with nonmyeloablative conditioning following cytoreductive autografts for the treatment of patients with multiple myeloma. *Blood.* 2003; 102(9): 3447-3454.

58. Bruno B, Rotta M, Patriarca F, et al. A comparison of allografting with autografting for newly diagnosed myeloma. *New Engl J Med.* 2007; 356(11):1110–1120.

59. Garban F, Attal M, Michallet M, et al. Prospective comparison of autologous stem cell transplantation followed by dose-reduced allograft (IFM99-03 trial) with tandem autologous stem cell transplantation (IFM99–04 trial) in high-risk de novo multiple myeloma. *Blood.* 2006;107(9):3474–3480.

60. Dispenzieri A, Lacy MQ, Zeldenrust SR, et al. The activity of lenalidomide with or without dexamethasone in patients with primary systemic amyloidosis. *Blood.* 2007;109(2):492–496.

17

HEMATOPOIETIC CELL TRANSPLANTATION

Frederick R. Appelbaum, MD

LEARNING OBJECTIVES

After reviewing this chapter, the reader should be able to

- Recommend hematopoietic transplantation to patients who are appropriate candidates
- Secure an appropriate source of hematopoietic stem cells for transplantation
- Explain the general process of transplantation
- Advise patients regarding the major complications of hematopoietic cell transplantation

Until recently, the term "bone marrow transplantation" was used to describe the process of transferring the lymphohematopoietic system from one individual to another. With the demonstration that peripheral blood and umbilical cord blood also can serve as sources of the stem cells necessary to accomplish this transfer, the term "hematopoietic cell transplantation" may be more appropriate. Hematopoietic cell transplantation is used to replace an abnormal but nonmalignant hematopoietic system with a normal one, or to treat a variety of malignancies because it allows administration of higher doses of chemotherapy and radiotherapy than would otherwise be possible and, in the setting of allogeneic transplantation, confers an immunologic graft-versus-tumor effect. Worldwide, approximately 45,000 to 50,000 patients received hematopoietic cell transplants in 2005.[1] The general categories of diseases for which transplantation is routinely used are described in this chapter. The specific role of transplantation in each of these disorders is discussed in greater detail in the chapters focused on the specific diseases.

INDICATIONS

IMMUNODEFICIENCY STATES

Allogeneic transplantation can successfully establish a normal immune system in patients with severe combined immunodeficiency disorders as well as correct the abnormalities associated with Wiskott-Aldrich syndrome and other immunodeficiency states.[2,3]

> **KEY POINT**
>
> - All diseases of hematopoiesis, both nonmalignant and malignant, are potentially curable with hematopoietic cell transplantation.

NONMALIGNANT DISORDERS OF HEMATOPOIESIS

Ninety percent of patients with severe aplastic anemia can be cured with allogeneic transplantation from a matched sibling.[4] Allogeneic hematopoietic cell transplantation cures 70% to 90% of patients with thalassemia major, with the best results achieved for patients who have previously received adequate iron chelation therapy and who received the transplant before the development of hepatomegaly or portal fibrosis.[5] Although data for sickle-cell disease are more limited, a European study of 100 patients showed survival at 2 years as 90%, with 80% of patients disease-free at that time.[6] Cures also have been obtained for other nonmalignant disorders of hematopoiesis, including Fanconi anemia, Blackfan-Diamond syndrome, chronic granulomatous disease, Kostmann's syndrome, and leukocyte adhesion deficiency.[7]

ENZYMATIC DISORDERS

Allogeneic hematopoietic cell transplantation can replace the abnormal enzyme systems and result in cure for patients with mucopolysaccharidosis and Gaucher's disease.

MALIGNANT DISEASES

The most frequent use of hematopoietic cell transplantation has been for the treatment of malignant diseases. Allogeneic transplantation can cure disease in 10% to 30% of patients with acute myeloid leukemia (AML) or acute lymphoblastic leukemia (ALL) in relapse, as well as patients with chronic myeloid leukemia (CML) in blast crisis. If transplantation is carried out early in the course of disease, the results are better. For example, transplantation consistently achieves 5-year disease-free survival rates of 50% to 70% when it is performed for AML and ALL in first remission or CML in chronic phase.[8–10] Cure rates of 40% to 60% have been reported for patients with myelodysplastic syndrome and for patients with non-Hodgkin's lymphoma or Hodgkin's disease that recurred following first-line therapy.[11] In addition, cure has been reported for patients with chronic lymphocytic leukemia (CLL), hairy cell leukemia, myelofibrosis, multiple myeloma, testicular cancer, and neuroblastoma.[12–15]

SOURCE OF STEM CELLS

Hematopoietic stem cells used for transplantation can be categorized according to the relationship between the donor and the recipient or according to anatomic source. In those rare cases where the patient has an identical (syngeneic) twin, hematopoietic cell transplantation can be conducted without the risks of graft rejection or graft-versus-host disease.

When the marrow of a patient is clearly abnormal, as in aplastic anemia and most cases of leukemia, allogeneic transplantation from a human leukocyte antigen (HLA)-identical sibling is usually preferred. The role of HLA molecules enable it to display both exogenous peptides (e.g., from an infecting organism) and endogenous peptides, presenting them to T cells to initiate an immune response. If two persons are HLA nonidentical, T cells from one person will react vigorously to the mismatched molecules on the surface of cells from the second individual. The HLA molecules themselves are termed "major HLA determinants." Even though nontwin siblings may be HLA matched, the endogenous peptides presented by the HLA antigens will differ, resulting in T-cell responses against "minor HLA determinants." The genes encoding HLA class I (*HLA-A, HLA-B,* and *HLA-C*) and class II (*HLA-DP, HLA-DQ,* and *HLA-DR*) are located on chromosome 6, are tightly linked, and tend to be inherited as haplotypes with low recombination frequency (see Fig. 17-1). Thus, for any given patient, the likelihood that any one sibling will be HLA matched with the patient is 25%. The likelihood of finding a matched sibling for a patient can be calculated by the formula $x = 1 - 0.75^n$, where x equals the probability of finding a matched sibling, and n equals the number of siblings. Overall, the chance that a matched sibling can be identified for any patient is approximately 30%. Hematopoietic cell transplantation can be carried out across ABO blood group barriers without difficulty.

> **KEY POINTS**
>
> - Both graft rejection and graft-versus-host disease are more common with use of cells from unrelated donors than with use of cells from matched siblings because of increased disparities in minor histocompatibility antigens.
> - Use of granulocyte-colony stimulating factor (G-CSF)-mobilized peripheral blood for allogeneic transplantation is associated with faster engraftment and less infection. However, such transplantation is perhaps associated with a greater frequency of chronic graft-versus-host disease.

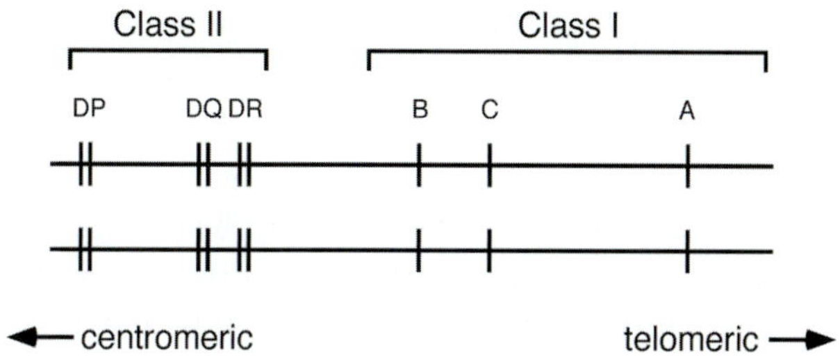

Fig. 17.1 The human major histocompatibility complex on the short arm of chromosome 6.

Family members who are genotypically identical to the patient for one HLA haplotype and are either phenotypically identical or partially matched on the other HLA haplotype have been used as donors. The overall results for transplantation for most hematologic malignancies are essentially the same when the donor is a relative who is phenotypically identical or mismatched for a single antigen, as when the donor is a completely matched HLA-identical sibling. If donors are mismatched for two or three antigens, the incidences of graft-versus-host disease and graft rejection are higher, and the results are considerably worse (Table 17-1).[16,17] Such transplants should be restricted to patients for whom there are no other options.

Donors who are totally unrelated to the patient but are matched for *HLA-A*, *HLA-B*, and *HLA-D* have been used in an increasing number of cases with promising results. Since the formation of the National Marrow Donor Program and other national registries, more than 8 million healthy individuals have volunteered to serve as stem cell donors. With improvements in donor selection and supportive care, the difference in outcome between matched sibling and matched unrelated donor transplants has diminished.[7] It is estimated that a matched unrelated donor can be found for more than 60% of individuals, with somewhat higher rates for white individuals and decreased rates for both Hispanic and black individuals, in part because of underrepresentation of these groups in the registries, but also because of greater HLA diversity in these populations.[18] The rates of graft-versus-host disease and graft rejection are higher after transplantation from matched unrelated donors than for those after transplantation from matched sibling donors. Prior to 1998, *HLA*-typing largely relied on serologic methods incapable of identifying all *HLA* subtypes. More recent studies using automated direct sequencing of *HLA-A*, *HLA-B*, *HLA-C*, *HLA-DRB1*, and *HLA-DQB1* demonstrate that approximately 30% of serologically matched donors are, in fact, mismatched for one or more alleles.[19,20] These results indicate that improvements in donor selection should further improve the outcome of transplants from unrelated donors. On average, the period of time between initiating the search for an unrelated matched donor and performing the transplant is 3 to 4 months.

The use of a patient's own (autologous) stem cells for transplantation also is possible. Autologous transplantation was initially and primarily used for the treatment of lymphoma and other tumors in which marrow was not overtly involved in the disease. The technique also has been explored as a treatment option for patients with AML and ALL using stem cells collected during remission. In the cases of AML and ALL, enough patients have received transplants with either allogeneic or autologous marrow to allow for comparisons of the two therapies. In general, autologous transplantation is associated with fewer complications; graft-versus-host disease does not occur, and the incidence of infectious complications, idiopathic interstitial pneumonia, and veno-occlusive disease of the liver are lower. However, the risk of tumor recurrence is higher with autologous transplantation, likely because of a lack of a graft-versus-tumor effect and tumor contamination of the reinfused stem cell product. Gene marking studies have demonstrated that tumor cells within the transplanted marrow can contribute to relapse.[21] Ex vivo treatment of autologous stem cell collections to remove contaminating cells, although based on sound preclinical models, has never been adequately tested in prospective randomized clinical studies.

TABLE 17-1 Effect of Human Leukocyte Antigen (HLA) Matching on Graft Rejection and Graft-versus-host Disease (GVHD) following Transplantation for Leukemia[17]

HLA Match	Graft Failure (%)	Acute GVHD (Grade III or more)*(%)
Genotypic match	2	7
Phenotypic match	7	7
Mismatch of 1 locus mismatch	9	32
Mismatch of 2 or 3 locus	21	62
Matched, unrelated	3	36
Mismatch of 1 locus, unrelated	5	51

*See Table 17-3 for definition of grades.
Modified with permission from the American College of Physicians.

BONE MARROW

Because bone marrow is rich in hematopoietic stem cells, it has traditionally served as the source of stem cells for transplantation. Marrow for transplantation usually is obtained through multiple aspirations from the posterior and sometimes anterior iliac crests. To obtain as many marrow cells with as little peripheral blood contamination as possible, the collection from each aspiration site is normally limited to 5 to 10 mL, and a total collection usually comprises approximately 1 L of marrow from a healthy adult man. The marrow is heparinized and filtered through screens to remove osseous spicules and fat globules before either being infused to the patient or cryopreserved for later transplantation. In some studies, the marrow has been treated before infusion or cryopreservation to test whether removal of T cells from allogeneic marrow can improve outcome by reducing graft-versus-host disease or whether tumor cells can be removed prior to autologous transplantation.[22] The risks associated with marrow donation are minimal. Of the first 1,220 marrow donations in Seattle, Washington, no donor died and there were only six cases of complications, mostly local hematomas or infection that required hospitalization.

PERIPHERAL BLOOD

Hematopoietic stem cells circulate in the peripheral blood, albeit in small numbers. During recovery from drug-induced cytopenias or after exposure to hematopoietic growth factors, such as granulocyte macrophage-colony stimulating factor (GM-CSF) or granulocyte-colony stimulating factor (G-CSF), the number of hematopoietic progenitor cells in the peripheral blood increases considerably. With the use of these mobilizing techniques, followed by leukapheresis, it is possible to collect sufficient stem cells from the peripheral blood to permit successful transplantation. Because peripheral blood has a higher proportion of T cells than marrow does, the first trials of peripheral blood stem cell transplantation were performed in the autologous setting, in which graft-versus-host disease is not a concern. These studies demonstrated that such transplantation is not only possible but also results in faster engraftment than is seen with marrow.[23] When more than 5.0×10^6 CD34+ cells/kg are infused, recovery to 0.5×10^3 granulocytes/μL and 20×10^3 platelets/μL is generally seen by less than 2 weeks after transplantation. Because of the increased safety and decreased costs associated with peripheral blood stem cell transplantation, it has largely replaced marrow as the source of stem cells for autologous transplantation. However, few randomized studies have been performed to compare autologous marrow and autologous peripheral blood stem cells in terms of the rate of relapse and disease-free survival.

Given the rapid recovery associated with the use of autologous peripheral blood stem cells, pilot studies of allogeneic peripheral blood stem cell transplantation using HLA-identical sibling donors were performed.[24] The results of these studies demonstrated rapid engraftment without an apparent increase in the incidence of acute graft-versus-host disease, and randomized trials have confirmed these findings.[25] In most studies, the incidence of chronic graft-versus-host disease associated with allogeneic peripheral blood stem cell transplantation is higher, but both disease-free and overall survival rates appear to be improved, particularly in patients who received transplants for more advanced-stage diseases.[26]

UMBILICAL CORD BLOOD

Umbilical cord blood also is rich in hematopoietic stem cells, and studies have shown that cord blood can serve as a source of stem cells for transplantation. Cord blood has relatively few mature T cells; as a result, the risk of graft-versus-host disease with cord blood appears to be somewhat less than that associated with marrow, although the risk of graft rejection or failure may be greater. In an analysis of 562 recipients of transplants from unrelated cord blood, the number of cells per kilogram infused was found to have a considerable influence on the outcome, as did patient age and degree of match with donors, with improved survival associated with higher cell dose, younger patient age, and greater degree of matching.[27] The low cell content in most collections of cord blood has limited this approach to children and smaller adults.[28] Recent trials exploring the use of double cord transplants show promise. Although only one cord ultimately engrafts, the use of two cords appears to reduce the risk of graft failure.[29]

PREPARATIVE REGIMEN

The form of treatment administered to patients directly before transplantation depends on the disease being treated and the source of stem cells. Patients with severe combined immunodeficiency diseases often require no therapy before transplantation because there is no abnormal cell population that must be eradicated and because their immune system is so severely compromised that the infused marrow rarely is rejected if the donor is an HLA-matched sibling. In the setting of aplastic anemia, patients are sufficiently immunocompetent to reject allogeneic marrow if no pretransplant immunosuppression is given. Thus, high-dose cyclophosphamide alone or combined with antithymocyte globulin (ATG) often is used as the preparative regimen for allogeneic transplantation. When transplantation is applied to the treatment of leukemia or other malignant diseases, the regimen must be both immunosuppressive

KEY POINT

- The purpose of the preparative regimen used prior to hematopoietic transplantation is to help eliminate the underlying disease and in the case of allogeneic transplantation, to provide sufficient immunosuppression to prevent graft rejection.

(in the setting of allogeneic transplantation) and capable of eradicating the malignant disease. Commonly used regimens involve high doses of cyclophosphamide, etoposide, busulfan, and total-body radiation therapy, in various combinations. The choice of specific regimens is discussed more completely in chapters focused on the particular diseases for which transplantation is used.

Although high-dose myeloablative preparative regimens have traditionally been used in transplantation for malignant diseases, the observation that some of the antitumor effects following allogeneic transplantation are the result of a graft-versus-tumor response has led to investigations of whether reduced intensity regimens might be effective and less toxic. Evidence for the existence of a graft-versus-tumor effect includes the finding that relapse rates following allogeneic transplantation are the lowest when acute and chronic graft-versus-host disease develops, greater if no graft-versus-host disease develops, and greater still if T cell-depleted allogeneic or syngeneic marrow is used.[8,30] Additional evidence of a potent graft-versus-tumor effect comes from the use of viable donor lymphocyte infusions. The simple transfusion of as few as 1×10^7 viable donor lymphocytes/kg as treatment for patients who have relapsed after allogeneic transplantation can result in complete remission in as many as 70% of patients with CML and in a smaller but still substantial portion of patients with AML, myelodysplasia, or multiple myeloma.[31]

A variety of approaches of reduced intensity transplantation are being studied, ranging from regimens of the minimum intensity necessary to achieve engraftment (for example, fludarabine plus low-dose total body radiation therapy) to regimens of intermediate intensity, such as fludarabine plus melphalan. Studies have demonstrated that engraftment can be reliably obtained in most cases with less toxicity than occurs with myeloablative transplantation and that complete remission can be achieved for many patients with a variety of hematologic malignancies, particularly indolent diseases such as CML, CLL, and follicular lymphoma. The exact response rate associated with any particular category of disease, as well as the exact role of this approach, is being defined.[32,33]

ENGRAFTMENT

Following administration of a myeloablative preparative regimen and the infusion of stem cells, a period of profound myelosuppression ensues. Within 1 to 2 weeks after transplantation, the peripheral leukocyte count begins to increase, signifying engraftment. When stem cells are procured from marrow and no hematopoietic growth factors are used after transplantation, the granulocyte count reaches $0.1 \times 10^3/\mu L$ by day 16 and $1.0 \times 10^3/\mu L$ by day 26. Administration of G-CSF or GM-CSF to the recipient can accelerate the recovery of peripheral granulocyte counts by as much as 1 week. The platelet count recovers simultaneously with or shortly after recovery of granulocytes.

> **KEY POINTS**
>
> - In patients beginning transplantation without latent cytomegalovirus (CMV) infection (as evidenced by lack of antibodies to CMV), death from CMV infection can be prevented by using only blood products from donors similarly without latent CMV. In patients beginning transplantation with latent CMV infection, death also can be substantially reduced by administering ganciclovir at the time of CMV reactivation.
> - Graft-versus-host disease results from T cells in the donor graft reacting against allogeneic targets on the genetically different host. It can be prevented in many cases by removing T cells from the donor graft or by administering various combinations of immunosuppressants for several months after transplantation.

When peripheral blood is the source of stem cells, engraftment is more rapid, with a granulocyte count of $0.5 \times 10^3/\mu L$ and a platelet count of $20 \times 10^3/\mu L$ achieved by day 12, on average. Use of growth factors after transplantation have less of an effect when peripheral blood stem cells are used. Engraftment of allogeneic stem cells can be documented using cytogenetic techniques, which are relatively simple to conduct if the donor and the recipient are different sexes. When the donor and the recipient are the same sex, unique chromosome polymorphisms can be identified by banding techniques. With the use of DNA restriction fragment-length polymorphisms or analysis of variable nucleotide tandem repeats, the origin of populations of cells can now be determined in virtually all cases.

COMPLICATIONS OF MARROW TRANSPLANTATION

Both the nature and the degree of complications associated with marrow transplantation depend on the health of the patient, the specific preparative regimen used, and the source of stem cells. The frequency of complications is higher and the rate of survival is lower for patients with a Karnofsky score of less than 80% and in patients with significant comorbidities.[34] Graft-versus-host disease is normally seen only after allogeneic transplantation and is associated with an increased incidence of infection. The extent of other specific organ toxicities is largely dependent on the specific preparative regimen used. Figure 17-2 illustrates the approximate timing of possible toxicities after allogeneic transplantation using a typical intensive preparative regimen. The following sections include a discussion of these issues in more detail.

GRAFT FAILURE

In some instances, the transplanted graft functions briefly, but after a period of days or weeks, marrow function is lost and myeloid elements are absent on evaluation of marrow

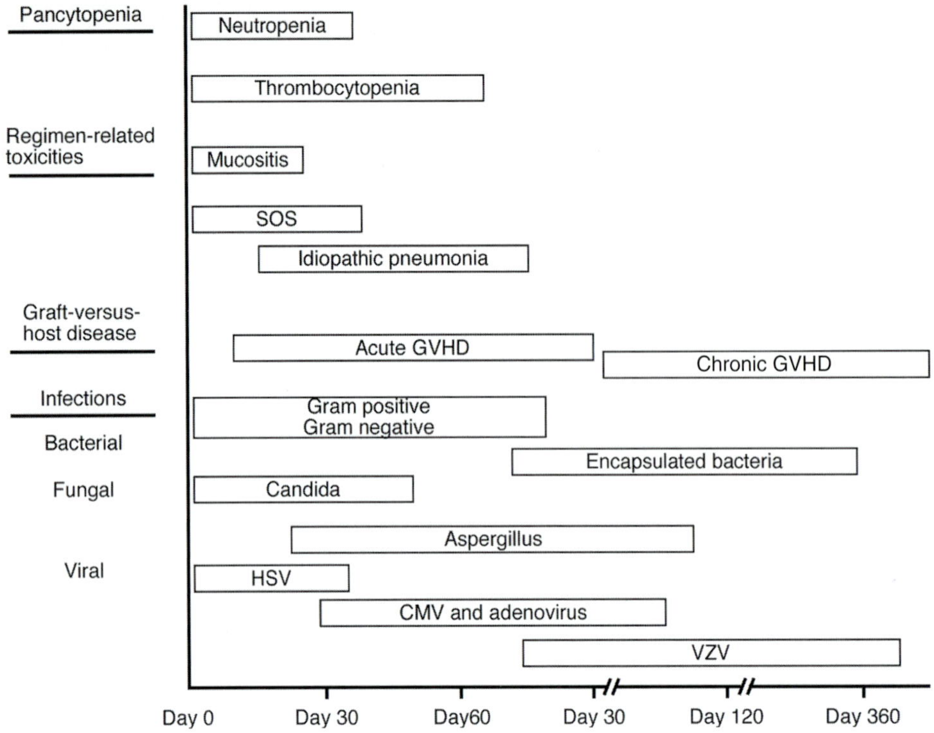

Fig. 17-2 The major syndromes that complicate ablative allogeneic hematopoietic cell transplantation and the approximate periods in which they develop.

Abbreviations: SOS, sinusoidal obstructive syndrome; GVHD, graft versus host disease; HSV, herpes simplex virus; CMV, cytomegalovirus; VZV, varicella zoster virus.

obtained by biopsy. In the setting of allogeneic transplantation, failure of the graft often is the result of residual host immune elements rejecting the marrow, a phenomenon termed graft rejection. Following transplantation involving an HLA-identical donor, graft rejection occurs most commonly when the patient has received multiple transfusions and when the preparative regimen is less immunosuppressive, such as with the use of cyclophosphamide alone before transplantation for aplastic anemia. The greater the disparity in HLA antigens between donor and recipient, the greater the chance of rejection.[16] Also, because donor T cells react with and help eliminate host immune competent cells not eradicated by the preparative regimen, T cell depletion of donor marrow prior to transplantation can lead to persistence of host immunity, resulting in an increased chance of graft rejection.

Graft failure also occurs in some recipients of autologous transplants. A single cause often is difficult to identify, but several have been implicated, including prior exposure to stem cell poisons, marrow damage during in vitro processing and cryopreservation, drug toxicity after transplantation, and viral infections.

Patients with graft failure but not immunologically mediated graft rejection sometimes have a response to treatment with a hematopoietic growth factor, such as GM-CSF, and have had an increase in the granulocyte count that may be sustained even after discontinuation of the growth factor. If persistent host lymphocytes are detected, which documents graft rejection, a second marrow transplant following an immunosuppressive preparative regimen may be successful.

GRAFT-VERSUS-HOST DISEASE

Graft-versus-host disease is a complication usually restricted to allogeneic transplants and is the result of allogeneic T cells that were transfused with the graft reacting against targets on the genetically different host. Acute graft-versus-host disease develops within the first 3 weeks after transplantation using an ablative preparative regimen, but can be more delayed in onset with the use of reduced intensity regimens. The syndrome is associated with characteristic lesions of the skin, gastrointestinal tract, and liver (Table 17-2).

Acute graft-versus-host disease usually is staged and graded using a modification of the original Seattle system (Tables 17-3 and 17-4). The most commonly used regimens to prevent graft-versus-host disease include a combination of an antimetabolite (methotrexate or mycophenolate mofetil) and a calcineurin inhibitor (cyclosporine or tacrolimus).

If no evidence of acute graft-versus-host disease develops, these drugs are usually continued for approximately 3 months and then tapered, until discontinuation at 6 months. With use of these regimens, moderate graft-versus-host disease requiring therapy occurs in approximately 30% of patients who have transplants from a matched-sibling donor. Lethal acute graft-versus-host disease is uncommon in patients who have

TABLE 17-2 Signs of Acute Graft-versus-host Disease

Skin

- Erythematous maculopapular rash (including on palms or soles)

Gastrointestinal Tract

- Anorexia
- Nausea and vomiting
- Diarrhea
- Abdominal pain
- Ileus

Liver

- Increased levels of serum bilirubin, transaminases, and alkaline phosphatase

Pathologic Evaluation

- Lymphocytic and monocytic infiltration into
  1. perivascular spaces in the dermis and dermal-epidermal junction of the skin
  2. base of the intestinal crypts in the small and large bowels
  3. periportal areas of the liver

transplants from an HLA-identical donor, occurring in less than 10% of patients.

Another approach to preventing acute graft versus-host disease is the removal of T cells from the donor marrow. Although effective, this approach has been associated with an increased risk of graft rejection and tumor recurrence following transplantation. Factors associated with an increased risk of moderate or severe acute graft-versus-host disease include the following:

- older age of patient and donor;
- multiparous woman as the donor; and
- exposure to more intensive conditioning regimens.

Responses have been reported after many treatment options for established acute graft-versus-host disease, and none have yet been shown to be superior (Table 17-5).

Chronic graft-versus-host disease affects 20% to 40% of matched sibling transplant recipients and resembles a collagen vascular disease, with symptoms such as:

- skin changes (e.g., malar erythema, sclerodermatous changes, cutaneous ulcers);
- alopecia;
- sicca syndrome;
- polyserositis; and
- liver dysfunction.

Chronic graft-versus-host disease is seen more frequently in older patients and patients who have had prior episodes of acute graft-versus-host disease. If chronic graft-versus-host disease develops while cyclosporine is being tapered, increasing cyclosporine to therapeutic levels often is effective. Prednisone alone or in combination with azathioprine or cyclophosphamide can control chronic graft-versus-host disease in 50% to 70% of cases. Bacterial infection frequently occurs in patients with chronic graft-versus-host disease, and prophylactic treatment with antibiotics should be prescribed.

As noted earlier, the incidence of both acute and chronic graft-versus-host disease is increased in recipients of transplants from mismatched or unrelated donors (Table 17-1). A mild graft-versus-host disease-like syndrome develops in some patients after autologous transplantation. The syndrome nearly always resolves with a short course of prednisone and does not affect overall transplant outcome.

INFECTIOUS COMPLICATIONS

Infection is a major risk for nearly all transplant recipients. Recipients of autologous transplants are at risk for the early bacterial and fungal infections common to all patients with granulocytopenia. Recipients of allogeneic hematopoietic grafts, particularly patients in whom graft-versus-host disease develops, also are at risk for late bacterial, fungal, and viral diseases.

During the early granulocytopenic period following transplantation, patients are likely to become febrile, and one episode of bacteremia will occur in at least 50% of patients. Therefore, at most transplant centers, treatment with antibiotics is begun once patients become granulocytopenic, even if they are afebrile. Prophylaxis with fluconazole reduces the incidence of both superficial and invasive fungal infections.[35] Patients who become or remain febrile

TABLE 17-3 Clinical Staging of Acute Graft-versus-host Disease[17]

Clinical Stage	Skin (Erythmatous Rash)	Liver (Serum Bilirubin)	Gut (Diarrhea)
1	< 25% of body surface	2–3 mg/dL	500–1,000 mL per day
2	25% to 50% of body survace	3–6 mg/dL	1,000–1,500 mL per day
3	Generalized	6–15 mg/dL	> 1,500 mL per day
4	Desquamation and bullae	> 15 mg/dL	(Pain or ileus)

Modified with permission from the American College of Physicians.

despite treatment with broad-spectrum antibiotics and have no obvious source of infection are usually treated with amphotericin or voriconazole or other antifungal agents.

Although laminar airflow isolation and prophylactic granulocyte transfusions can prevent early infection, neither action influences overall survival and thus, in general, neither approach is recommended. With current methods of supportive care, the risk of death as a result of infection during the early granulocytopenic period after transplantation is less than 3% for recipients of either allogeneic or autologous transplants.

Herpes simplex infection, which contributed to the severity of oral mucositis in the past, can be prevented with the use of systemic acyclovir 250 mg/m^2 every 8 hours intravenously, beginning 1 week before transplant and continuing for 1 month after transplantation.[36]

In the past, symptomatic cytomegalovirus (CMV) infection, which typically involves either the gastrointestinal tract or the lungs, occurred in approximately 25% of patients who received allogeneic transplant and led to death (typically from CMV pneumonia) in 10% to 15% of patients. Primary CMV infection in the setting where both donor and recipient are without latent CMV infection (as evidenced by having no detectable antibodies to CMV before transplantation) can be prevented by using only blood products that come from donors without latent CMV, or by using blood products that have been filtered to remove all leukocytes. For patients with evidence of latent CMV before transplantation, the use of prophylactic ganciclovir, starting either at the time of initial engraftment or at the time of CMV reactivation, can substantially reduce the risk of CMV disease. Prophylactic ganciclovir is not without toxicities, however, and granulocytopenia is more common for patients receiving prophylactic ganciclovir than for patients in control groups.[37] Prophylactic ganciclovir is not generally recommended for patients who have an autologous transplant, except for those cases in which T cells are removed from the stem cell inoculum. Foscarnet is effective for some patients in whom CMV infection develops despite the use of ganciclovir, as well as for patients who cannot tolerate ganciclovir.

Pneumonia as a result of *Pneumocystis carinii*, previously seen in 5% to 10% of transplant recipients, can be prevented by treatment with oral trimethoprim-sulfamethoxazole for 1 week before transplantation and resuming treatment once the granulocyte count exceeds $0.5 \times 10^3/\mu L$. Treatment 2 days per week while patients are taking immunosuppressive drugs after transplantation usually is sufficient to prevent pneumocystis disease. Allergic reactions to trimethoprim-sulfamethoxazole are common but can usually be managed with desensitization. Dapsone can serve as a substitute for trimethoprim-sulfamethoxazole.

Late infections, occurring more than 3 months after transplant, usually are restricted to varicella zoster virus or, in patients with chronic graft-versus-host disease, to recurrent bacterial or fungal infections. The use of prophylactic trimethoprim-sulfamethoxazole or penicillin, or both, can reduce the incidence of late bacterial infections for patients with chronic graft-versus-host disease.

CHEMORADIOTHERAPY TOXICITIES

Following most standard preparative regimens, immediate toxicities, such as nausea, vomiting, fever, and mild skin erythema, are common. Unusual toxicities associated with high-dose cyclophosphamide include hemorrhagic cystitis and, rarely, acute hemorrhagic carditis. Parotitis commonly is seen in patients receiving total-body radiation therapy.

Oral mucositis requiring narcotic analgesia typically develops 5 to 7 days following transplantation using myeloablative preparative regimes. Patient-controlled analgesia provides the greatest patient satisfaction and results in lower cumulative doses of narcotics. Keratinocyte growth factor (palifermin) significantly shortens the duration of severe mucositis following ablative transplant regimens.[38]

Sinusoidal obstruction syndrome, previously termed veno-occlusive disease of the liver, can develop within 1 to 4 weeks of treatment with many of the currently used preparative regimens, and its symptoms include ascites, tender hepatomegaly, and jaundice. The overall incidence of sinusoidal obstruction syndrome is approximately 10%, but varies according to the preparative regimen. In general, the incidence is higher for patients with abnormal results of liver function tests before transplant and for patients with an active infection at the time of transplant.[39] No therapy for sinusoidal obstruction syndrome has been demonstrated to be effective, although the results of studies with defibrotide appear to be encouraging.[40]

Idiopathic interstitial pneumonia, which is thought to be a toxicity directly related to chemoradiotherapy, occurs 30 to 90 days after transplant in 5% to 10% of patients. As with other toxicities, the incidence of idiopathic interstitial pneumonia is dependent, in part, on the preparative regimen, occurring more frequently after use of regimens that include high doses of total-body radiation therapy. Pre-existing lung disease, prior radiation therapy to the thorax, and increased age also seem to be associated with an increased risk of idiopathic interstitial pneumonia, whereas fractionated radiation instead of single-dose radiation appears to decrease the risk. The mortality rate associated with idiopathic interstitial pneumonia is approximately 50%, and no available treatments are clearly effective, although early results with tumor necrosis factor blockade show some promise.[41]

Late complications attributable to the preparative regimens include decreased growth velocity in children and delayed development of secondary sexual characteristics. Most postpubescent women will have ovarian failure and few men regain spermatogenesis. Cataracts occur in as many as one-third of patients, although the incidence associated with use of fractionated radiation is lower. Thyroid dysfunction, usually well compensated, also may occur. Patients treated with high-dose chemoradiotherapy and hematopoietic stem cell transplantation are at an increased risk for the development of second cancers. This risk is highest for patients receiving T cell-depleted allogeneic transplants and for patients who receive multiple cycles of highly immunosuppressive drugs to treat graft-versus-host disease. In the latter instance, a high incidence of Epstein-Barr virus-associated lymphoproliferative disease has been reported.[42] A smaller increase in solid tumors has been reported after transplantation, with a 3% 10-year cumulative rate. A high incidence of myelodysplasia (nearly 10%) has been reported following autologous transplantation for lymphoma, but whether myelodysplasia is a complication of transplantation or is the long-term effect of chemotherapy used before transplantation is unknown.[43]

TABLE 17-4 Clinical Grading of Acute Graft-versus-host Disease[17]

	Clinical Stage		
Clinical Grade	**Skin**	**Liver**	**Gut**
I (Mild)	1 or 2	0	0
II (Moderate)	3 or	1 or	1
III (Severe)	1, 2, or 3	2 or 3	2–4
IV (Life-threatening)	4 or	4	

Modified with permission from the American College of Physicians.

LONG-TERM SURVIVORS

Case control studies of patients who survive more than 10 years from transplant show that survivors are, in most respects, indistinguishable from controls reporting similar rates of osteoporosis, hypothyroidism, employment, marital satisfaction, divorce, and psychological problems. Transplant survivors do report an increased incidence of musculoskeletal problems and sexual dysfunction.[44]

RELAPSE AFTER TRANSPLANTATION

There is a substantial risk of recurrent malignant disease after transplantation, particularly when transplantation is performed at the time of relapse rather than earlier in the course of the disease. The appropriate management of relapse after transplantation depends on the disease and type of transplant. Patients in whom disease recurs after autologous transplantation may have a response to subsequent chemotherapy and, occasionally, such responses are surprisingly complete and prolonged, particularly if the duration of remission after transplantation was long.

Patients taking immunosuppressive drugs who have recurrent disease after allogeneic transplantation will, on occasion, have a second complete remission after discontinuation of immunosuppressive therapy. Infusions of viable lymphocytes from the original stem cell donors can result in complete remission in many patients. In a European study involving 135 patients, the rate of complete response was 70% for patients with chronic-phase CML, 12% for patients with advanced-phase CML, 29% for patients with AML or myelodysplasia, and 0% for patients with ALL.[31] Occasionally, patients with myeloma and non-Hodgkin's lymphoma also have a response. Most experts recommend that patients with recurrent acute leukemia undergo reinduction chemotherapy prior to use of donor lymphocyte infusions. Some form of graft-versus-host disease develops in approximately 60% of patients after infusion of donor lymphocytes; of those patients, 50% require therapy for graft-versus-host disease, and 15% have life-threatening graft-versus-host disease. In addition, marrow aplasia occurs in 35% of patients, and the overall mortality associated with infusion of donor lymphocytes is 20%. Administration of fewer lymphocytes or administration on a fractionated schedule can decrease the risk of graft-versus-host disease. For patients with CML who have relapse after transplant, the disease appears to be sensitive to interferon therapy, with complete cytogenetic responses

TABLE 17-5 Treatment Options for Graft-versus-host Disease

Acute Graft-versus-Host Disease

- Prednisone
- Antithymocyte globulin (ATG)
- Cyclosporine
- Mycophenolate mofetil
- Rapamycin
- Monoclonal antibodies against T cells

Chronic Graft-versus-Host Disease

- Cyclosporine
- Prednisone
- Prednisone with either azathioprine or cyclophosphamide
- Thalidomide

reported for 35% of patients treated for hematologic relapse and 70% for patients treated for cytogenetic relapse. Imatinib also is highly effective, at least for patients who have not previously had resistance to the drug before transplantation.[45]

A number of patients have had a second transplant as treatment for relapse after the first transplant. Such transplants, if performed within 1 year of the original transplant, have been associated with an extremely high risk of severe or fatal transplant-related toxicities, including veno-occlusive disease and idiopathic interstitial pneumonia. However, the results are better when the second transplant is performed more than 1 year after the original transplant, with prolonged subsequent remissions reported for as many as 25% of patients.[46] More recently, reduced intensity allogeneic transplants have been found to be tolerable and sometimes effective for patients in whom a prior autologous transplantation has failed.[47]

REFERENCES

1. Appelbaum FR. Hematopoietic-cell transplantation at 50. *N Engl J Med.* 2007;357(15):1472–1475.
2. Buckley RH, Schiff SE, Schiff RI, et al. Hematopoietic stem-cell transplantation for the treatment of severe combined immunodeficiency. *N Engl J Med.* 1999;340:508–516.
3. Grunebaum E, Mazzolari E, Porta F, et al. Bone marrow transplantation for severe combined immune deficiency. *JAMA.* 2006;295:508–518.
4. Storb R, Etzioni R, Anasetti C, et al. Cyclophosphamide combined with antithymocyte globulin in preparation for allogeneic marrow transplants in patients with aplastic anemia. *Blood.* 1994;84:941–949.
5. Lucarelli G, Galimberti M, Polchi P, et al. Marrow transplantation in patients with Thalassemia responsive to iron chelation therapy. *N Engl J Med.* 1993;329:840–844.
6. Walters MC, Patience M, Leisenring W, et al. Bone marrow transplantation for sickle cell disease. *N Engl J Med.* 1996;335:369–376.
7. Guardiola P, Pasquini R, Dokal I, et al. Outcome of 69 allogeneic stem cell transplantations for Fanconi anemia using HLA-matched unrelated donors: a study on behalf of the European Group for Blood and Marrow Transplantation. *Blood.* 2000;95:422–429.
8. Appelbaum FR. Haematopoietic cell transplantation as immunotherapy. *Nature.* 2001;411:385–389.
9. Hansen JA, Gooley TA, Martin PJ, et al. Bone marrow transplants from unrelated donors for patients with chronic myeloid leukemia. *N Engl J Med.* 1998;338:962–968.
10. Yanada M, Matsuo K, Emi N, Naoe T. Efficacy of allogeneic hematopoietic stem cell transplantation depends on cytogenetic risk for acute myeloid leukemia in first disease remission: a metaanalysis. *Cancer.* 2005;103:1652–1658.
11. Philip T, Guglielmi C, Hagenbeek A, et al. Autologous bone marrow transplantation as compared with salvage chemotherapy in relapses of chemotherapy-sensitive non-Hodgkin's lymphoma. *N Engl J Med.* 1995;333:1540–1545.
12. Appelbaum FR. The current status of hematopoietic cell transplantation. *Annu Rev Med.* 2003;54:491–512.
13. Attal M, Harousseau J-L, Stoppa A-M, et al. A prospective, randomized trial of autologous bone marrow transplantation and chemotherapy in multiple myeloma. *N Engl J Med.* 1996;335:91–97.
14. Child JA, Morgan GJ, Davies FE, et al. High-dose chemotherapy with hematopoietic stem-cell rescue for multiple myeloma. *N Engl J Med.* 2003;348:1875–1883.
15. Michallet M, Archimbaud E, Bandini G, et al. HLA-identical sibling bone marrow transplantation in younger patients with chronic lymphocytic leukemia. European Group for Blood and Marrow Transplantation and the International Bone Marrow Transplant Registry. *Ann Intern Med.* 1996;124:311–315.
16. Anasetti C, Amos D, Beatty PG, et al. Effect of HLA compatibility on engraftment of bone marrow transplants in patients with leukemia or lymphoma. *N Engl J Med.* 1989;320:197–204.
17. Cheson BD, ed. *Oncology MKSAP,* 2nd ed. Philadelphia, PA: American College of Physicians; 1999;293–296.
18. Chell JW. Hematopoietic cell donor registries. In: Blume KG, Forman SJ, Appelbaum FR, eds. *Thomas' Hematopoietic Cell Transplantation.* Oxford, UK: Blackwell Publishing Ltd.; 2004:624–631.
19. Petersdorf EW, Hansen JA, Martin PJ, et al. Major-histocompatibility-complex class I alleles and antigens in hematopoietic-cell transplantation. *N Engl J Med.* 2001;345:1794–1800.
20. Petersdorf EW, Anasetti C, Martin PJ, et al. Limits of HLA mismatching in unrelated hematopoietic cell transplantation. *Blood.* 2004;104:2976–2980.
21. Brenner MK, Rill DR, Moen RC, et al. Gene-marking to trace origin of relapse after autologous bone-marrow transplantation. *Lancet.* 1993;341:85–86.
22. Gribben JG, Freedman AS, Neuberg D, et al. Immunologic purging of marrow assessed by PCR before autologous bone marrow transplantation for B-cell lymphoma. *N Engl J Med.* 1991;325:1525–1533.
23. Bensinger WI, Longin K, Appelbaum F, et al. Peripheral blood stem cells (PBSCs) collected after recombinant granulocyte colony stimulating factor (rhG-CSF): an analysis of factors correlating with the tempo of engraftment after transplantation. *Br J Haematol.* 1994;87:825–831.
24. Bensinger WI, Weaver CH, Appelbaum FR, et al. Transplantation of allogeneic peripheral blood stem cells mobilized by recombinant human granulocyte colony-stimulating factor. *Blood.* 1995;85:1655–1658.

25. Bensinger WI, Martin PJ, Storer B, et al. Transplantation of bone marrow as compared with peripheral-blood cells from HLA-identical relatives in patients with hematologic cancers. *N Engl J Med.* 2001;344:175–181.

26. Stem Cell Trialists' Collaborative Group. Allogeneic peripheral blood stem-cell compared with bone marrow transplantation in the management of hematologic malignancies: an individual patient data meta-analysis of nine randomized trials. *J Clin Oncol.* 2005;23:5074–5087.

27. Rubinstein P, Carrier C, Scaradavou A, et al. Outcomes among 562 recipients of placental-blood transplants from unrelated donors. *N Engl J Med.* 1998;339:1565–1577.

28. Rocha V, Labopin M, Sanz G, et al. Transplants of umbilical-cord blood or bone marrow from unrelated donors in adults with acute leukemia. *N Engl J Med.* 2004;351:2276–2285.

29. Barker JN, Weisdorf DJ, Defor TE, et al. Transplantation of 2 partially HLA-matched umbilical cord blood units to enhance engraftment in adults with hematologic malignancy. *Blood.* 2005;105:1343–1347.

30. Horowitz MM, Gale RP, Sondel PM, et al. Graft-versus-leukemia reactions after bone marrow transplantation. *Blood.* 1990;75:555–562.

31. Kolb HJ, Schattenberg A, Goldman JM, et al. Graft-versus-leukemia effect of donor lymphocyte transfusions in marrow grafted patients. European Group for Blood and Marrow Transplantation Working Party Chronic Leukemia. *Blood.* 1995;86:2041–2050.

32. McSweeney PA, Niederwieser D, Shizuru JA, et al. Hematopoietic cell transplantation in older patients with hematologic malignancies: replacing high-dose cytotoxic therapy with graft-versus-tumor effects. *Blood.* 2001;97:3390–3400.

33. Giralt S, Thall PF, Khouri I, et al. Melphalan and purine analog-containing preparative regimens: reduced-intensity conditioning for patients with hematologic malignancies undergoing allogeneic progenitor cell transplantation. *Blood.* 2001;97:631–637.

34. Sorror ML, Sandmaier BM, Storer BE, et al. Comorbidity and disease status-based risk stratification of outcomes among patients with acute myeloid leukemia or myelodysplasia receiving allogeneic hematopoietic cell transplantation. *J Clin Oncol.* In press.

35. Goodman JL, Winston DJ, Greenfield RA, et al. A controlled trial of fluconazole to prevent fungal infections in patients undergoing bone marrow transplantation. *N Engl J Med.* 1992;326:845–851.

36. Wade JC, Newton B, Flournoy N, Meyers JD. Oral acyclovir for prevention of herpes simplex virus reactivation after marrow transplant. *Ann Intern Med.* 1984;100:823–828.

37. Goodrich JM, Bowden RA, Fisher L, Keller C, Schoch G, Meyers JD. Ganciclovir prophylaxis to prevent cytomegalovirus disease after allogeneic marrow transplant. *Ann Intern Med.* 1993;118:173–178.

38. Spielberger R, Stiff P, Bensinger W, et al. Palifermin for oral mucositis after intensive therapy for hematologic cancers. *N Engl J Med.* 2004; 351:2590–2598.

39. Bearman SI. The syndrome of hepatic veno-occlusive disease after marrow transplantation. *Blood.* 1995;85:3005–3020.

40. Richardson PG, Murakami C, Jin Z, et al. Multi-institutional use of defibrotide in 88 patients after stem cell transplantation with severe veno-occlusive disease and multisystem organ failure: response without significant toxicity in a high-risk population and factors predictive of outcome. *Blood.* 2002;100:4337–4343.

41. Crawford SW, Hackman RC. Clinical course of idiopathic pneumonia after bone marrow transplantation. *Am Rev Respir Dis.* 1993;147: 1393–1400.

42. Witherspoon RP, Fisher LD, Schoch G, et al. Secondary cancers after bone marrow transplantation for leukemia or aplastic anemia. *N Engl J Med.* 1989;321:784–789.

43. Metayer C, Curtis RE, Vose J, et al. Myelodysplastic syndrome and acute myeloid leukemia after autotransplantation for lymphoma: a multicenter case-control study. *Blood.* 2003;101:2015–2023.

44. Syrjala KL, Langer SL, Abrams JR, et al. Late effects of hematopoietic cell transplantation among 10-year adult survivors compared with case-matched controls. *J Clin Oncol.* 2005;23:6596–6606.

45. Carpenter PA, Snyder DS, Flowers MED, et al. Prophylactic administration of imatinib after hematopoietic cell transplantation for high-risk Philadelphia chromosome-positive leukemia. *Blood.* 2007; 109:2791–2793.

46. Radich JP, Gooley T, Sanders JE, et al. Second allogeneic transplantation after failure of first autologous transplantation. *Biol Blood Marrow Transplant.* 2000;6:272–279.

47. Baron F, Storb R, Storer BE, et al. Factors associated with outcomes in allogeneic hematopoietic cell transplantation with nonmyeloablative conditioning after failed myeloablative hematopietic cell transplantation. *J Clin Oncol.* 2006;24:4150–4157.

18

SYMPTOM MANAGEMENT

Charles L. Loprinzi, MD

LEARNING OBJECTIVES

After reviewing this chapter, the reader should be able to

- Recognize, evaluate, and develop treatment strategies for symptoms due to cancer and/or cancer-related therapies
- Evaluate and treat patients with cancer-related pain, malignant bowel obstruction, malignant ascites, cancer-associated anemia, dyspnea, cancer fatigue, and cancer-related anorexia and cachexia
- Recommend, when appropriate, nonestrogenic treatment of hormone-deprivation syndromes for women with hormone-sensitive cancers and for men who have received androgen-ablation therapy for prostate cancer
- Develop and implement appropriate treatment modalities for diarrhea related to radiation therapy, chemotherapy, or cancer itself and anti-emetic treatment for patients receiving emetogenic cancer therapy
- Mitigate bone health issues in patients with hormone-dependent cancer using current standards of care

Approximately 30% to 40% of patients have cancer-related pain at the time of diagnosis, and as many as 65% to 85% of patients with advanced disease have cancer-related pain. It is one of the most common and feared symptoms. Cancer-related pain and its treatment contribute to and are, in turn, affected by many other common symptoms associated with cancer, including fatigue, weakness, dyspnea, nausea, constipation, and impaired cognition. Pain can disrupt sleep and hamper movement. The perception of pain is intensified in the presence of such other symptoms.

CANCER-RELATED PAIN

New or recurrent pain may herald a change in the patient's status, necessitating an investigation of the cause and, in many cases, a change in anticancer therapy because of the discovery of metastatic or recurrent disease. Treating the underlying malignant disease, along with the pain, often is appropriate. In addition, not all pain in a patient with cancer is necessarily from the cancer and thus must be properly evaluated so that non-cancer pain, such as an osteoporotic compression fracture, can be appropriately treated.

KEY POINTS

- Cancer-related pain is a prominent clinical problem. Asking the patient about pain is important because pain management cannot readily begin without an understanding of the patient's pain.
- Barriers to cancer pain management include patient reluctance to report pain, patient concerns about pain medications, inadequate assessment of pain, and the lack of knowledge of pain treatment on the part of physicians, nurses, and pharmacists.
- The World Health Organization (WHO) three-step analgesic ladder is an outline for appropriate pain management.
- When strong opioids are used, they should be given on a scheduled, as opposed to on an as-needed basis. Appropriate, fast-acting opioid medications should be available for intermittent pain.
- Other methods of analgesia, such as intrathecal morphine, should be considered for patients with difficult pain problems.

An evaluation of the WHO guidelines for the management of cancer-related pain indicates that an integrated approach of systemic, pharmacologic, and anticancer therapy should manage pain effectively in 85% to 95% of patients. However, when patients were surveyed regarding pain relief, only 40% to 50% thought their pain was adequately relieved. This discrepancy highlights the continued need to aggressively manage treatable cancer-related pain.

BARRIERS TO ADEQUATE PAIN RELIEF

Barriers to relieving pain in patients with cancer include inadequate priority, insufficient education, and inappropriate attitudes. Both health care personnel and patients may contribute at each level because of poor communication, failure to address pain during health care follow-up, and downplaying or underestimating the severity of the pain. Providers should proactively discuss common patient misconceptions about pain management.

The health care system may not have appropriately prioritized the management of cancer-related pain in the past. Frequently, appropriate treatments are not reimbursed or are too expensive for patients to afford. Legislation designed to regulate controlled substances often makes their use complex and burdensome.

Several initiatives to emphasize the importance of pain management have been published by the American Pain Society Quality of Care Committee, the Agency for Healthcare Research and Quality (AHRQ), the National Cancer Care Network (NCCN), and the Wisconsin Cancer Pain Initiative.

A survey conducted in the mid-1990s was designed to evaluate the knowledge of physicians in training with respect to management of cancer-related pain. The results of the survey showed a widespread lack of familiarity with the WHO analgesic ladder and a poor understanding of equianalgesic dosing.[1] In a survey conducted by the Eastern Cooperative Oncology Group (ECOG), as well as in a more recent survey by the Radiation Therapy Oncology Group (RTOG), poor pain assessment was found to be the major barrier to effective pain management.[2,3] Knowledge deficits regarding opioid tolerance and risk of addiction also are common.

Patient education programs have shown benefit by enhancing knowledge about pain, increasing patient compliance, and decreasing pain intensity. Implementing guidelines in algorithmic form for the management of cancer-related pain in the outpatient setting, compared with standard community practice, has been shown to be an effective strategy for reducing pain in patients with cancer.

Patients are frequently reluctant to report discomfort and may fear that unrelieved pain is an indication of disease progression. Often, they are inappropriately concerned about the addictive potential of opioid analgesics, potential side effects, and the development of tolerance.

Physicians often share such concerns and myths. The ECOG[2] and RTOG[3] surveys both found physician reluctance to prescribe opioids as one of the major perceived barriers to adequate pain management. Physicians also may undervalue the contribution of nonpharmacologic treatments of cancer pain. In response to these barriers, the NCCN has developed guidelines for the management of cancer pain.

ASSESSMENT OF PAIN

There are four steps in a clinical strategy for the relief of cancer-related pain. These include: assessment of the pain (believe the patient); the establishment of a plan of care, which includes information for the patient about the use of short- and long-acting medications and about the management of side effects; implementation of the plan of care; and regular reassessment of the patient and modification of the plan of care as necessary. To determine the best way to relieve pain — in addition to carrying out a comprehensive assessment of patients' pain — physicians must determine the extent of cancer, the relationship between the pain and the disease, and the manageability and prognosis of the cancer itself. Concurrent medical problems, such as peptic ulcers, hypertension, renal failure, and cardiac arrhythmias, can affect which coanalgesics and invasive procedures can be used. It is critical to evaluate patients for pre-existing psychologic conditions, spiritual crises, and coping mechanisms.

One of the major problems recognized by clinicians in surveys regarding the management of cancer-related pain is the inability to properly assess the pain. The elements of assessment include the history, physical examination, and psychosocial evaluation (Table 18-1). The intensity of the pain may be evaluated with use of a visual analogue scale that is anchored at one end by "no pain" and at the other end by "worst possible pain," by an 11-point graphic or numeric scale (0 is no pain, 10 is the worst pain), by a simple verbal category scale (none, mild, moderate, severe, or excruciating), or by a pain scale appropriate for the given patient. It should be noted that using numeric scales permits comparisons of pain before and after treatment as well as between results collected by different observers.

TREATMENT

There are three basic approaches to pain control: modifying the source of pain, altering the central perception of pain, and blocking the transmission of pain (Table 18-2). The goals of analgesic therapy are to alleviate persistent pain and to relieve breakthrough discomfort. Pharmacologic treatment of cancer-related pain must be individualized and should be as simple and noninvasive as possible. Equianalgesic tables are a useful guide when changing opioid analgesic drugs and routes of administration. Addiction and tolerance to opioid analgesics are rare. Selection of the appropriate agent depends on the severity of the pain, the etiology of the pain, the current analgesic therapy, the past analgesic therapy, and any comorbid medical conditions (e.g. renal or hepatic dysfunction). In the pharmacologic treatment of cancer-related pain, it is reasonable to follow the WHO three-step analgesic ladder, which designates the type of analgesic based on the severity of pain. The step system reminds clinicians to consider the continued use of nonopioids and adjuvant agents as coanalgesics for more severe levels of pain. If pain persists, other etiologies and treatments are considered. Palliative therapies, adjuvant drugs, psychosocial interventions, and physical modalities may be part of the initial treatment or may be added if pain persists.

WHO Step 1

Nonopioid analgesics have limited value as a treatment of pain for advanced cancer because of their low maximal efficacy. However, they may be useful as adjuncts to opioid therapy. The commonly used nonopioid analgesics include aspirin, acetaminophen, and nonsteroidal anti-inflammatory drugs. Cyclooxygenase (COX)-selective nonsteroidal anti-inflammatory drugs have not, overall, been shown to be superior for cancer-related pain. In addition, they are considerably more expensive than other nonsteroidal anti-inflammatory drugs.

WHO Step 2

Opioids such as codeine are considered to be step 2 therapies and are recommended for moderate pain. They may be useful in combination with step 1 nonopioid analgesics for pain unrelieved by step 1 strategies or as initial therapy for patients who present with moderate discomfort. Propoxyphene and

TABLE 18-1 Assessment of Pain

History (to determine)

- Site, temporal pattern, quality, and severity of pain
- Nature, extent, and prognosis of the malignant disease
- General medical conditions
- Factors that exacerbate or relieve the pain
- Associated symptoms (such as numbness and weakness)
- Prior relief of pain
- What the pain means to the patient and how it may affect his or her lifestyle

Physical examination (to evaluate)

- Neurologic function
- Site of the tumor and of metastases
- Locus of the pain

Psychosocial evaluation (to determine)

- Depression
- Patient perspectives
- Coping mechanisms
- Support systems

TABLE 18-2 Three Approaches to Pain Control

Approach	Methods
Modify the source of pain	Surgery, chemotherapy, radiation, antibiotics, anti-inflammatory agents
Alter the central perception of pain	Analgesics, psychotropic coanalgesics, nonpharmacologic therapies
Block the transmission of pain to the CNS	Anesthetics, neurolytic blockade, surgery

Abbreviation: CNS, central nervous system.

meperidine are not recommended because of the potential buildup of toxic metabolites and/or minimal analgesic effects demonstrated in randomized clinical trials.

One advantage to the use of opioids is that patients usually do not develop tolerance to the analgesic effects of these agents, although patients may become tolerant to many of the side effects. Physical dependence can occur with long-term use, but addiction and psychologic dependence are exceedingly rare in patients with cancer. When opioids or their routes of administration are changed, consulting a table of equianalgesic dosing can provide the necessary information to determine appropriate doses. Because of incomplete cross-tolerance, 50% to 75% of the equianalgesic dose is often used when changing to a new agent.

WHO Step 3

Patients with pain unrelieved by step 2 maneuvers, or who present with moderate to severe discomfort, should be treated with step 3 opioids, which include morphine, oxycodone, hydromorphone, fentanyl, and methadone. Opioids might be best used one at a time because of patient variability in response and overlapping side effects. Some experts believe that rotation of opioids (successive use of different agents) may provide a better balance of efficacy and of side effects for some patients,[4] although this theory is controversial. Meperidine is not recommended because of its short half-life and toxic metabolites.

Morphine has been a commonly used step 3 opioid. The oral dose is approximately three times the parenteral dose because of first-pass metabolism in the liver. Morphine is usually administered every 4 hours when used in an immediate-release formulation because its half-life is approximately 3.5 hours; additional doses are prescribed as needed for breakthrough pain. Both immediate-release and sustained-release forms are available (Table 18-3). A sustained-released formulation of morphine can simplify the regimen for patients and improve adherence. Most sustained-release morphine formulations release medication over 12 hours. Tablets should not be cut, crushed, or chewed because this will negate the sustained-release properties. It should be recognized that sustained-release opioids generally are more expensive than other immediate-release opioids.

When sustained-release formulations are administered, the patient should be provided with an immediate-release opioid for breakthrough doses as needed. The appropriate short-acting opioid dose to be administered for breakthrough pain should be approximately 10% to 20% of the 24-hour morphine-equivalent dose. The appropriate dosing interval should be determined by the time to peak effect of the last dose.[5] This means every hour for oral administration, every 15 minutes for subcutaneous administration, and every 5 to 10 minutes for intravenous administration. To titrate the dose, the sustained-release formulation should be increased if the patient needs more than three or four daily doses of a short-acting opioid. The short-acting dose should then be increased proportionally with the dose of controlled-release morphine.

Oxycodone is considered an overlap opioid, with use appropriate at step 2 and step 3. When it is prepared as a single agent, it can be titrated to maximal effect. It may have fewer side effects than morphine; hallucinations and delirium appear to be less common. It is safer for patients with renal failure because its metabolism is not greatly affected by renal function. In contrast to sustained-release morphine, oral sustained-release oxycodone has a triphasic half-life. In a randomized clinical trial, the oral sustained-release formulations of oxycodone and morphine have proved equally safe and effective for the treatment of cancer-related pain.[6] Oxycodone also is available in an immediate-release formulation. Caution is advised related to the presence of acetaminophen in many of the oxycodone preparations. Hydromorphone has the advantage of requiring less volume for parenteral administration than other opioids because of its potency (four times the potency of morphine) and solubility (six times the solubility of morphine). This is one of the opioids of choice for patients with renal failure. However, a shortcoming of this medication is the lack of a long-acting form.

Fentanyl has the advantage of availability as a transdermal drug-delivery system that provides the equivalent of a subcutaneous infusion without a pump or needle.[7] Because of the long time to peak delivery (12 hours), a patient also should

TABLE 18-3 World Health Organization (WHO) Step 3 Opioids

Drug	Onset of Action	Peak Concentration	Duration of Action	Comments
Morphine (immediate release)				
Oral	30 min.	1 hrs.	3–4 hrs.	Repeat bolus rescue doses every 60 min. as needed
Rectal	20–60 min.	1–1.5 hrs.	3–4 hrs.	Repeat bolus rescue doses every 60 min. as needed
Intravenous	5–10 min.	5–10 min.	3–4 hrs.	Repeat bolus rescue doses every 10 minutes as needed
Subcutaneous	10–15 min.	30–60 min.	3–4 hrs.	Repeat bolus rescue doses every 15 min. as needed
Epidural/intrathecal	15–60 min.		3–7 hrs.	Repeat bolus rescue doses every 8 hrs. as needed
Morphine (controlled release)	1 hrs.	2–3 hrs.	12 hrs.	Add rescue doses of immediate-release morphine every hour as needed
Oxycodone (immediate release)	30 min.	1 hrs.	3–4 hrs.	Add rescue doses of immediate-release opioid every hour as needed
Oxycodone (controlled release)	*1–1.5 hrs.*	*3–4 hrs.*	*12 hrs.*	*Add rescue doses of immediate-release opioid every hour as needed*
Hydromorphone				
Oral	30 min.	1.5–2 hrs.	4 hrs.	In general, 4 times as
Rectal	30 min.	1.5–2 hrs.	4 hrs.	potent as morphine
Intravenous	1–5 min.	10–15 min.	1–2 hrs.	
Fentanyl				
Oral (lozenge on a plastic stick)	5–10 min.	1–2 hrs.	1–2 hrs.	Indicated for relief of breakthrough pain; lower doses available for children
Transdermal	6–12 hrs.	24–48 hrs.	48–72 hrs.	Add rescue doses of immediate-release opioid every hour as needed

initially receive an alternate analgesic. The steady state is reached in 48 to 72 hours. The subcutaneous depot lasts 17 to 24 hours after removal of the transdermal patch. The equianalgesic dose of the fentanyl patch (25 μg per hour) is 45 to 134 mcg of oral morphine daily. However, it appears that, for many patients, the equivalence is on the lower end of the range of 45 to 60 μg. The recommended hourly microgram dose of fentanyl is available in equianalgesic tables. Caution is in order regarding the effects of temperature driving the kinetics of this drug as well as regarding a lack of absorption in patients with severe cachexia because of a lack of subcutaneous fat.

The oral form of fentanyl is absorbed transmucosally, and its bioavailability is 25% by this route. It is an alternative immediate-release opioid that can be used for the relief of breakthrough pain. The optimal dose must be determined by titration. It is provided as a lollipop (a lozenge on a plastic stick), which has some advantage in that patients are not likely to overdose on this agent because they will stop sucking the lollipop if they get somnolent. There also is an oral formulation of fentanyl that is placed between the gums and absorbed transmucosally, rapidly giving serum fentanyl concentrations.

Dosing of Opioids

Lower doses should be used at treatment initiation for patients who have not taken opioids recently, compared with those patients who are tolerant to opioids. Patients who have not recently received opioids will be more sensitive to the pain-relieving effects and will not have developed tolerance to the side effects. The recommended starting oral dose of immediate-release morphine or its equivalent for an opioid-naïve patient is 5 to 10 mg. It can be given hourly until adequate pain relief. For opioid-tolerant patients with new severe pain, the dose should be increased by 50% to 100% of the current opioid dose. If the unrelieved pain is moderate, an appropriate titration amount is to increase the daily dose by 25% to 50% every 24 hours.

The appropriate dose for any patient is based on the current intensity of the pain and on the analgesic therapy. There is no one optimal or maximum dose of any step 3 opioid analgesic. The correct dose at any one time is the dose that provides pain relief throughout its dosing interval without unmanageable side effects.

Routes of Administration for Opioids

The oral route is the most convenient and least expensive. When swallowing is problematic, the transdermal route is both less expensive and less invasive than parenteral routes, although concentrated liquid morphine can provide significant doses in very small volumes as well. Patients who have pain crises or considerable intermittent pain can benefit from subcutaneous or intravenous opioid infusions by a patient-controlled analgesia pump. Many patients with cancer will require more than one route of administration during the course of the disease. An intraspinal route may provide better pain relief and may improve the quality of life for some patients with cancer. This should be considered after aggressive systemic analgesic and coanalgesic therapy have failed.[8]

Maintenance of Analgesia

Once pain relief is obtained, maintenance of analgesia is needed. When pain medication is taken only on an as-needed basis, pain returns before the patient is prompted to take the next dose. The most effective method of preventing pain is by giving around-the-clock dosing once an effective analgesic dose has been determined. Usually, this is most conveniently done with a controlled-release preparation in order to minimize the number of doses needed.

If the response to an opioid is inadequate or if side effects are prominent, a sequential trial of a different opioid should be considered.[4] Physicians should allow for incomplete cross-tolerance when making a change. Patients who have had pain relief but with intolerable side effects from the initial opioid may have pain relief and no side effects from a second opioid at 50% to 75% of its calculated equianalgesic dose. When switching to methadone from high does of another opioid, clinicians should start with a low dose of methadone (5 to 10 μg every 6 hours) and titrate it upwards as indicated. However, use of this drug is not well standardized.[9]

Common indications for dose reductions are adequate pain relief with bothersome side effects, reduction in the source of pain (e.g., by effective chemotherapy or radiation therapy), or interruption of pain transmission by neurolysis or neurosurgery. In order to prevent withdrawal symptoms, when a gradual downward titration is desired after a period of regular use of an opioid, the dose can be decreased by 25% to 50% every 1 to 7 days. This rate of reduction should prevent physical withdrawal symptoms. If more rapid reductions are needed because of the severity of side effects or for other reasons, the dose can be decreased by 50% to 75% every 12 to 24 hours.

True allergy to morphine is rare; however, when it occurs, a structurally unrelated opioid (e.g., fentanyl or methadone) should be considered.

Side Effects of Opioids

The side effects of opioids limit their use and are the primary reason patients do not adhere to treatment. These side effects include constipation, nausea, sedation, confusion, hallucinations, and, less commonly, urinary retention, delirium, myoclonus, seizures, and respiration depression. With appropriate anticipation of these effects, many can be avoided or minimized. Nausea, sedation, and cognitive impairment tend to improve with time as tolerance develops.

Constipation should be managed prophylactically with increased fluid and fiber intake and exercise when possible, as well as a prophylactic regimen to try to maintain normal laxation.[10–13] Typical preventive medications, depending on the opioid dose and on the patient's usual bowel pattern, include senna with or without docusate or casanthranol with or without docusate. Doses of such agents should be titrated upward to try to obtain one soft bowel movement every 1 to 2 days. Two tablets of bisacodyl can be taken orally at bedtime if no bowel movement has occurred for 2 to 3 days, and the dose may be repeated the following morning if there has still been no bowel movement.

If constipation occurs despite a prophylactic regimen, the patient should be assessed for cause and severity. Fecal impaction should be ruled out if no bowel movement has occurred in a 3-day period. Several medications treat constipation.

- Milk of Magnesia (30 to 60 mL orally one or two times daily)
- Lactulose (30 to 60 mL orally two or three times daily)
- Magnesium citrate (8 oz orally once daily)
- Bisacodyl suppositories (one or two administered once or twice daily)
- Phosphosoda enemas (once daily)
- Miralax (polyethylene glycol; one heaping teaspoon dissolved in liquid every few hours until relief)

Nausea and vomiting are frequently associated with opioid use, occurring in up to 40% of patients. Tolerance may develop, typically within a few days. Constipation should be ruled out as an etiology. Dopamine-blocking agents such as prochlorperazine or haloperidol can be prescribed on an as-needed basis. Metoclopramide has been recommended by some as a motility stimulant, although good data demonstrating efficacy in this situation do not exist.

Although delirium may be an opioid-related toxicity, patients should be assessed for other causes of delirium. Rotating opioids may be helpful in this situation. Haloperidol, 0.5 to 2 mg administered orally or intravenously every 4 to 6 hours, can help control symptoms.

There appear to be some cases for which high doses of morphine can actually cause increased pain.[14] Decreasing the narcotic dose or changing to methadone may be helpful in such situations.

Coanalgesic Agents

Coanalgesic agents are commonly used with such cancer-related syndromes as bone metastases, nerve compression, visceral distention, and nerve damage. The most commonly used coanalgesic drugs are nonsteroidal anti-inflammatory drugs, corticosteroids, tricyclic antidepressants, and anticonvulsant agents.

Coanalgesic therapy with nonsteroidal anti-inflammatory drugs may be used for bone metastases, hypertrophic pulmonary osteoarthropathy, soft tissue infiltration, arthritis, serositis, and postoperative pain. Tricyclic antidepressants are useful as adjuvant therapy for neuropathic pain and may be helpful for underlying depression and insomnia. Anticonvulsant agents, such as gabapentin, are used frequently for lancinating or tic-like neuropathic pain and for myoclonic jerks that result from treatment with opioids.

Dexamethasone, given in oral doses of 2 to 8 mg two or three times daily, is commonly used for cancer-pain syndromes such as acute nerve compression, visceral distension, increased intracranial pressure, and soft tissue infiltration. Higher doses given intravenously (10 to 20 mg every 6 hours) are used for acute spinal cord compression and acute, severe, increased intracranial pressure.

Intravenous bisphosphonates have been demonstrated to be effective for patients with multiple myeloma, breast cancer, prostate cancer, and other solid tumors.

Radiation Therapy

External beam radiation therapy can be effective for localized pain. In addition, strontium-89 and samarium-153 may be useful in managing refractory multifocal metastatic bone pain caused by osteoblastic activity. Experience with these agents predominantly has been with prostate and breast cancer.

Neuroablation and Other Invasive Procedures

Neuroablative procedures can be helpful in some patients with localized pain that is not well controlled by medications. Such procedures include: nerve blocks, regional plexus infusions, and neurodestructive procedures. For example, celiac plexus block using an endoscopic approach may be beneficial for pain caused by pancreatic cancer. Verterbroplasty and kyphoplasty can be used to eliminate pain from vertebral collapse due to metastatic cancer or to treatment-induced osteoporosis (assuming the anterior bony cortex is intact to prevent extravasation of the injected material). In addition, radiofrequency ablation of painful bone metastases has been used successfully.

Summary

In summary, most medical oncologists should be able to control pain in most patients. Collaboration with pain and palliative-care experts can help physicians to determine ways to relieve pain in remaining patients. No patient with cancer should live or die with unrelieved pain.

NAUSEA AND VOMITING ASSOCIATED WITH CYTOTOXIC AGENTS

Vomiting is a natural protective mechanism to rid the body of toxic substances. However, in the setting of cancer chemotherapy and radiation therapy, nausea and vomiting become toxicities of major concern. For patients, nausea and vomiting are one of the most feared toxicities related to cancer treatment — an observation described in surveys conducted in the 1980s and confirmed in the 1990s — even after the introduction of antiemetic agents that are considered to be highly effective. Protracted emesis can lead to dehydration, electrolyte imbalance, and other metabolic derangements. Patient withdrawal from chemotherapy also may result. In view of the psychologic and social implications, as well as of the physical detriments associated with nausea and vomiting, appropriate and effective management of this problem continues to be of major importance.

The emetic response can be conceptualized as a brainstem-based reflex arc. The final common pathway begins in the emetic center, a diffuse neural complex located in the brainstem near the nucleus tractus solitarius. Efferent neuronal pathways from the emetic center activate and coordinate the many muscle groups necessary for an effective vomiting response. This reflex arc has multiple afferent pathways that lead to the vomiting center. The chemoreceptor trigger zone, located in the area postrema adjacent to the fourth ventricle, can be activated by humoral mediators that enter the cerebrospinal fluid. Activation signals are then transmitted to the emetic center. The peripheral pathways begin at nerve endings in the upper gastrointestinal tract itself. Vagal pathways, which terminate in the brainstem, allow activation of the emetic center. Other afferent pathways include cerebral cortical-signaling pathways (learned emesis) and vestibular pathways related to motion sickness.

The emetic reflex arc includes synaptic sites through which signals are relayed to receptors by various neurotransmitters. Identification and blockade of these key neurotransmitter receptors have been the major strategies for the development of effective antiemetic agents. Dopaminergic, serotonergic, and neurokinin receptors have been considered to be of major importance in acute vomiting. Other receptors, such as cannabinoid and opiate receptors, also may have a role in emetic pathways.

Emetic potential can be affected by patient characteristics. Of these features, poor control with prior chemotherapy is particularly important. Emesis tends to be more severe in younger patients than in older patients, and in women more than men. A history of motion sickness and/or a history of morning sickness during pregnancy also appears to directly correlate with chemotherapy-induced nausea and vomiting. Findings from several retrospective and prospective studies have suggested that the risk of emesis is lower for patients with a history of excessive alcohol intake than for patients with no such history. However, biochemical and genetic differences that explain these risk factors have not been firmly established.

KEY POINTS

- There are three types of chemotherapy-induced nausea and vomiting — acute, delayed, and anticipatory — with different management for each.
- Serotonin-3 (5-HT3)-receptor antagonists are helpful medications for patients receiving emetogenic chemotherapy. When 5-HT3-receptor antagonists are used, corticosteroids also are recommended.
- Aprepitant is a neurokinin-1 (NK-1) receptor antagonist that is particularly efficacious for preventing delayed nausea and vomiting. It is recommended for patients receiving highly emetogenic chemotherapy, including anthiocycline cyclophosphamide (AC), or for patients with a prior episode of delayed emesis with the same chemotherapy.
- The use of antiemetic guidelines and knowledge of the emetogenic potential of chemotherapy agents is critical to treating patients.

TYPES OF NAUSEA AND VOMITING

There are three different types of nausea and vomiting related to chemotherapy: acute (within 24 hours from chemotherapy), delayed (after 24 hours from chemotherapy), and anticipatory (prior to a subsequent chemotherapy dose).

TREATMENT ACCORDING TO EMETOGENIC POTENTIAL OF CHEMOTHERAPY

In 1999, the American Society of Clinical Oncology (ASCO) convened a multidisciplinary panel to classify the emetogenic potential of chemotherapy agents and to provide recommendations to manage nausea and vomiting.[15] Following an extensive review of the literature and guided by clinical experience, the panel categorized agents based on the incidence with which each chemotherapy regimen caused emesis.[16,17] Regimens containing cisplatin were considered high risk because emesis has been documented to occur in more than 95% of patients receiving such therapy. For non–cisplatin-containing regimens, high-risk agents were defined as those causing emesis in 30% to 90% of patients. In some previous classifications, this level of emetic risk had been considered to include both highly emetogenic and moderately emetogenic chemotherapy. The intermediate-risk category in the present classification includes agents that produced emesis in 10% to 30% of patients; the low-risk category includes agents that produced emesis in fewer than 10% of patients.

The ASCO guidelines were updated in 2006.[18] In this edition, the emetogenic classifications of chemotherapy drug regimens were not modified, but combination doxorubicin/cyclophosphamide chemotherapy, although still considered to be a moderately emetogenic regimen, was singled out to be treated as a highly emetogenic regimen.

Acute Nausea and Vomiting

Acute nausea and vomiting induced by chemotherapy has been defined as that which occurs within the first 24 hours after administration of a chemotherapy agent. This type is generally the most prominent clinical nausea and vomiting problem. Most antiemetic agents, including the dopamine-receptor antagonists and serotonin-receptor antagonists, were developed specifically for the prevention of acute emesis.

Delayed Nausea and Vomiting

Some chemotherapy drugs, such as cisplatin and cyclophosphamide, may cause delayed nausea and vomiting, which is defined as occurring 2 to 5 days after administration of chemotherapy. This delayed emesis is often of lesser intensity and occurs in fewer patients, but it can be of longer duration than acute emesis. In addition, it may appear independent of the acute emetic response. The lack of control of acute emesis, however, is a risk factor for the development of delayed emesis. The relative role of central, as opposed to peripheral, sites of activation for both acute and delayed emesis is controversial. However, the fact that the antiemetic agents that are effective for managing delayed vomiting differ from the agents that are effective for managing acute emesis suggests that different neurotransmitter mechanisms, if not different physical sites, are involved in these two forms of emesis. Delayed emesis remains a challenge to manage. The risk factors are the same as for acute nausea and vomiting and include chemotherapy-related factors and patient characteristics.

Anticipatory Nausea and Vomiting

Anticipatory (learned) emesis is a conditioned reflex that rapidly can be established by poor antiemetic protection during an early course of chemotherapy. It can be triggered by numerous stimuli that come to be associated with chemotherapy and can occur at any time. Anticipatory emesis is similar to conditioned taste aversions that also can be seen among patients with cancer. Although there are treatment strategies for this problem, the best protection against anticipatory emesis is prevention of the conditioning event itself. Thus, appropriately aggressive antiemetic therapy initiated with the first course of chemotherapy is best for an optimal overall antiemetic response.

TREATMENT OF NAUSEA AND VOMITING

The best strategy for managing emesis is prevention. Prevention must begin with the very first course of chemotherapy because, once emesis occurs, it is far more difficult to control. Effective management of emesis reduces not only morbidity but also the medical complications that can result from protracted vomiting. An added benefit is that control of emesis avoids the possibility of a patient prematurely discontinuing chemotherapy.

Most of the antiemetic agents developed in the 1960s and 1970s were antidopaminergic drugs specifically targeted at the dopamine-2 receptor. These agents include the phenothiazines, the butyrophenones, and the substituted benzamides. A dose-response curve for efficacy for phenothiazines and butyrophenones indicates that these two classes of agents have a low therapeutic index. Antidopaminergic toxicity, including extrapyramidal reactions, agitation, and depression, is dose dependent and can be limiting for the use of these agents. Therefore, phenothiazines and butyrophenones generally are used only to control moderately or mildly emetogenic chemotherapy.

The substituted benzamide, metoclopramide, blocks the dopamine-2 receptor and, at high doses, the 5-HT3-receptor as well. Development of the high-dose metoclopramide regimen (2 mg/kg intravenously every 2 hours for five doses) in 1981 was a breakthrough in antiemetic therapy and provided the first effective treatment for control of emesis induced by high-dose cisplatin. However, antidopaminergic toxicity is a major limiting factor with high-dose metoclopramide. In general, metaclopromide has been replaced with the 5-HT3-receptor antagonists (discussed further in this section) because of their improved toxicity profiles.

Antiemetic agents with a high therapeutic index include the 5-HT3-receptor antagonists and corticosteroids (Table 18-4). The 5-HT3-receptor antagonists became available in the 1990s and have become the cornerstone of present-day effective antiemetic therapy for highly emetogenic and moderately emetogenic chemotherapy regimens.

Clinical trials have shown that the efficacy is similar for the three 5-HT3-receptor antagonists that have been available in clinical practice for some time: ondansetron, granisetron, and dolasetron. The classic dose-response curve of 5-HT3-receptor antagonists approximates a logarithmic shape; that is, a steep and linear dose response is present until a threshold (shoulder) value is reached, after which increasing the dose does not further increase efficacy (plateau effect).

Although the modest side-effect profile of the 5-HT3-receptor antagonists allows for dose escalation without a substantial increase in side effects, the most cost-effective dose will be one close to the threshold value; that is, the lowest dose that provides maximum antiemetic protection. However, this value is affected by the emetic potential of the chemotherapy being given and can, therefore, vary for different classes of chemotherapy agents and for high-dose, compared with standard-dose, regimens. As a group, the 5-HT3-receptor antagonists share the same low side-effect profile, including mild headache, transient and asymptomatic elevation of transaminase levels, and constipation.

TABLE 18-4 Antiemetic Agents

Therapeutic Index	Agents
High	5-HT3-receptor antagonists (ondansetron,granisetron, dolasetron, and palonosetron); corticosteroids (dexamethasone and methylprednisolone); neurokinin-1 receptor antagonist (aprepitant)
Limited	Dopamine-2 receptor antagonist (metoclopramide); phenothiazines (chlorpromazine and prochlorperazine); butyrophenones (droperidol)
Adjunctive	Benzodiazepines (anxiolytics); antihistamines

The newest 5-HT3-receptor antagonist, palonosetron, has a longer half-life and a higher receptor-binding affinity than the other three agents. Presently, this drug is only available as an intravenous agent, but an oral formulation may soon be available. Although there are data to demonstrate that this drug is more effective than the other 5-HT3-receptor antagonists, especially when corticosteroids are not given,[19,20] recent ASCO guidelines did not recommend use of this agent over other 5-HT3-receptor antagonists.[18] Corticosteroids can be useful either as a single agent or in combination with a 5-HT3-receptor antagonist or a dopamine-receptor antagonist. With few exceptions, a corticosteroid (e.g., dexamethasone) is recommended to be given whenever a 5-HT3-receptor antagonist is given. Despite this, there may occasionally be significant side effects with corticosteroids, and work is ongoing to try to better delineate the benefits and toxicities of corticosteroids when used as antiemetic agents, especially for patients receiving moderately emetogenic regimens.[21]

The recently available neurokinin-1 receptor antagonist, aprepitant, is a major advance in the prevention of both acute and delayed nausea and vomiting, especially the latter.[22] The newest ASCO guidelines recommend its use for patients receiving highly emetogenic chemotherapy or combination doxorubicin and cyclophosphamide chemotherapy.[18]

Studies show that cannabinoids have a low therapeutic index. In addition, their role is limited by side effects such as dizziness, sedation, hypotension, and dysphoria, especially in older adults.

Occasionally, adjunctive agents, such as benzodiazepines and antihistamines, are a helpful addition to the antiemetic regimen. Of the benzodiazepines, lorazepam is the agent used most widely. Its contribution probably results from its anxiolytic properties. An antihistamine can be used to help prevent dystonic reactions that may occur with use of a dopamine-2 receptor antagonist. However, because those agents are used less frequently, the role of antihistamines is limited.

Regarding the treatment of anticipatory nausea and vomiting, management options include:

- behavioral desensitization,
- relaxation,
- distraction, and
- focusing on enjoyable things.

If the patient is particularly anxious, an anxiolytic agent, such as a benzodiazepine, may be helpful especially within the 1 to 12 hours prior to therapy.

GUIDELINES

Perhaps the best way to ensure the appropriate use of antiemetic agents for patients receiving chemotherapy is to apply guidelines in clinical practice. In addition to ASCO guidelines, several other guidelines are available.[23–26]

Radiation Therapy-induced Nausea and Vomiting

As with chemotherapy, radiation therapy carries an emetogenic risk, the treatment field being one of the major determinants. The dose of radiation therapy administered per fraction and the pattern of fractionation are important risk factors but are less well defined. As with chemotherapy, the risk can be classified as high, intermediate, or low.

The recently revised ASCO guidelines[18] addressed this issue by stating that 5-HT3-receptor antagonists are considered to be the mainstay of therapy for patients receiving radiation with more than a minimal emetogenic risk. Nonetheless, there is a dearth of data regarding this subject and more information is desired. In practice, many radiation oncologists do not treat all patients with prophylactic therapy, but, rather, treat patients if nausea and vomiting become an issue.

For patients receiving radiation with low emetogenic risk, either a 5-HT3-receptor antagonist or a dopamine-receptor antagonist can be used as needed and continued prophylactically for each remaining day of radiation treatment. Because the difference in efficacy between dopamine-receptor antagonists and 5-HT3-receptor antagonists is smaller in this setting, dopamine receptor antagonists are recommended (based on expense), with 5-HT3-receptor antagonists reserved for rescue.

BOWEL OBSTRUCTION

PATHOPHYSIOLOGY

The normal function of the intestine is to move oral intake along the course of the gastrointestinal tract, with secretion of digestive enzymes, fluid, and electrolytes to promote subsequent absorption of nutrients. The purposes of the large intestine are reabsorption of fluid and the elimination of waste and undigested fiber.

Intraluminal fluid is primarily derived from endogenous secretions. The average oral fluid intake is approximately 2 L daily. In comparison, the average daily fluid secretion from gastric and small intestinal epithelium into the lumen is nearly 8 L.

KEY POINTS

- Malignant bowel obstruction can have multiple etiologies related to the tumor itself or adhesions from prior abdominal surgery.
- In general, a nasogastric tube with suction is the initial treatment for patients with bowel obstruction. Medications can be useful for some patients. Scopalamine, glycopyrrolate, or octreotide should be considered.
- There are limitations to the surgical management of malignant bowel obstruction.

In the setting of intestinal obstruction, peristalsis pushes endogenous fluids toward the site of an obstruction. Luminal distention causes pain, nausea, and vomiting, the latter of which is caused primarily through innervation of the vagus nerve and of other nerves in the autonomic nervous system.

It is estimated that 3% of all advanced cancers are complicated by obstruction of the gastrointestinal tract. Of these cancers, ovarian (11% to 42%) and colorectal (5% to 24%) cancers are the ones most often implicated. Symptoms of obstruction also may herald the diagnosis of esophageal cancer. A wide variety of other primary tumor sites may be associated with gastrointestinal tract obstruction, including gastric, endometrial, prostate, and bladder cancers. There is a wide variability in the time of occurrence of obstruction during the overall course of the disease, with primary tumors below the diaphragm often causing obstruction earlier in the disease course than those arising above the diaphragm. If the obstruction is inoperable, it is associated with a poor prognosis and the average survival is approximately 2 months.

Gastrointestinal tract obstruction can be caused by multiple and often coexisting etiologies, such as intraluminal masses, direct infiltration of the bowel wall (colon cancer), external compression of the lumen, carcinomatosis causing dysmotility (ovarian cancer), intra-abdominal adhesion (resulting from postoperative changes), constipation, vascular infarcts, and intussusception. Although the definitive management of obstruction from each cause may differ, the symptom complex is similar.

SYMPTOMS

The symptoms of gastrointestinal tract obstruction result from partial or total occlusion of the bowel lumen, alteration of normal peristaltic motion, and alterations in physiologic intestinal fluid secretion and absorption. The site of obstruction is variable; multiple areas of the tract may be involved.

Most patients (68% to 100%) with intestinal obstruction experience nausea and vomiting. In addition, distention of the bowel wall causes moderate to severe pain for nearly all patients (92%), and many patients (72% to 76%) have periodic flares of increased pain. This discomfort has been termed "colicky" pain, which is the result of peristaltic waves against the obstruction with consequent additional distention of the intestine. The inflammatory response to obstruction in or around the bowel wall may further exacerbate fluid secretion through prostaglandin-mediated increases in membrane permeability with or without additional cellular breakdown. Local inflammation may cause edema and contribute directly to increased tumor bulk, thereby precipitating or exacerbating obstructive physiology.

TREATMENT

Evaluating the patient to differentiate obstruction from ileus caused by treatment (e.g., vinca alkaloids), antiemetics (e.g., 5-HT3 antagonists), opioids, or inactivity and decreased oral fluid intake is the first step in treating patients who present with abdominal pain, distension, vomiting, or decreased bowel movement. If it is determined that obstruction is present, the clinician should first rule out rectal impaction that may respond to a suppository or enema and render a nasogastric tube unnecessary.

Medical management with intravenous fluids and intermittent nasogastric tube suction may need to follow if the patient has repeated episodes of emesis. Decompression of the gas and fluid accumulation in the stomach and intestine is the primary goal of nasogastric tube placement, and the surgeon or oncologist can initiate this treatment while an assessment for operability is being made.[27] If a nasogastric tube is in place, it can be clamped when the nasogastric volume decreases to 100 cc. The tube may be removed if there is no subsequent nausea or vomiting, or at the patient's request.

Many patients (5% to 50%) are either ineligible for surgery or endoscopic procedures because of advanced disease with multiple areas or obstruction, or they decline to have such a procedure. In addition, patients with gastrointestinal tract obstruction are often malnourished and debilitated, and the operative mortality risk is high for such individuals (12% to 33%).[28] Select patients who are not candidates for an operation may be evaluated for placement of a stent across the site of obstruction. This treatment can relieve symptoms in patients with esophageal, gastric, and pancreatic cancers causing upper tract obstruction, or rectal cancers causing distal blockage. In general, candidates for stent placement have an isolated site of partial obstruction that is approachable by endoscopic means. Although the treatment is generally safe, perforation, bleeding, pain, or migration of the stent develops in 18% of patients. Venting gastrostomies, placed percutaneously or surgically, have been advocated for more permanent decompression of the obstruction and prevention of emesis if the patient is not deemed to be a candidate for an operation.

Although these procedures have been recommended to relieve symptoms in patients who are not candidates for an operation, relief is often inadequate. In many cases, emptying the gastric contents alone is not effective in alleviating the obstructive symptoms. Furthermore, not only is a nasogastric tube uncomfortable, its ongoing presence increases the risk of iatrogenic complications and may be unpleasant for the patient and family. Whereas the data supporting venting gastrostomy are more favorable, many patients with advanced disease choose not to have this (or any other) surgical procedure to control their symptoms.[29]

A growing clinical experience suggests that pharmacologic agents can relieve the symptoms associated with gastrointestinal obstruction (Table 18-5). Antiemetics can be used to relieve nausea. Prochlorperazine, however, is not very effective, controlling nausea for only a minority of patients. Agents with prokinetic effects, such as metoclopramide, may be beneficial for nausea related to partial obstruction but have the potential to increase cramping or pain by increasing motility against a fixed obstruction. Corticosteroids, which can relieve nausea through both central and peripheral antiemetic effects, have been recommended to decrease the inflammatory response and resultant edema. Their effectiveness may be the result of reducing the volume of intestinal fluid caused by either a disruption of cellular integrity by the tumor or the inflammatory response. Anecdotal evidence suggests that these agents are relatively well tolerated, but no controlled clinical trials have supported the use of these agents in this setting.

Opioid analgesics control constant pain in many patients but may not be effective for intermittent colicky pain. The mechanism of such pain is thought to be spasms of smooth muscle, as well as bowel-wall distension in response to peristaltic waves converging on the site of obstruction. Thus, antimuscarinic anticholinergic agents can be used in addition to opioids to help manage this symptom complex.

Antimuscarinic anticholinergic agents act by competitively inhibiting the effects of acetylcholine at muscarinic receptors. These parasympatholytic agents functionally block the parasympathetic division of the autonomic nervous system. These agents can be divided into tertiary amines or quaternary ammonium compounds. Tertiary amines readily cross the blood–brain barrier and can have considerable adverse clinical effects, whereas quaternary ammonium compounds do not readily penetrate the central nervous system (CNS). All antimuscarinic agents have variable effects on the parasympathetic nervous system. They inhibit secretions in the salivary, bronchial, and sweat glands, as well as in the gastrointestinal tract. In addition, they affect heart rate and movement of the ocular muscles and restrict the activity of smooth muscle in the bladder and gastrointestinal tract.

Atropine, a racemic mixture of dextrohyoscyamine and levohyoscyamine, is considered to be the prototype gastrointestinal antimuscarinic agent. It can be administered intravenously, subcutaneously, or orally every 4 hours. Its usefulness is limited by its adverse effects, which include the following: xerostomia, blurred vision, cycloplegia, mydriasis,

TABLE 18-5 Treatment of Gastrointestinal Tract Obstruction

Class of Drug	Effect	Specific Agents	Comments
Antiemetics	Relieve nausea	Prochlorperazine metoclopramide, cisapride, and corticosteroids	Limited benefit; should not be used for patients with total obstruction
Corticosteroids	Decrease inflammatory response and resultant edema	Dexamethosone and others	Limited evidence proving benefit
Opioid analgesics	Relieve constant pain	Morphine, hydromorphone, and fentanyl	May not relieve intermittent, so-called colicky pain
Antimuscarinic/ anticholinergic agents			
Tertiary amines	Inhibit secretions and decrease peristalsis	Atropine and hyoscyamine sulfate	Can have considerable adverse side effects
Quaternary ammonium compounds	Inhibit secretions and decrease peristalsis	Scopolamine, Belladonna leaf extract, glycopyrrolate, and ipratopium	Fewer side effects than tertiary amines
Somatostatin analogs	Inhibit secretion of hormones, slow the release of enzymes, decrease peristalsis	Octreotide	May cause mild hyperglycemia

photophobia, anhidrosis, urinary retention, tachycardia, palpitations, constipation, mental confusion, and delirium. Another antimuscarinic anticholinergic drug is scopolamine, which is available in both parenteral and transdermal preparations in the United States. Intravenous or subcutaneous doses in the range of 5 to 100 μg every hour have been reported to be effective. However, this agent is available only as the hydrobromide salt that penetrates the CNS, with the attendant potential for considerable side effects. Glycopyrrolate, a quaternary ammonium compound, has clinical effects similar to those of scopolamine but lacks the side effects related to the CNS. It is commonly used in anesthesia to control secretions perioperatively, and emerging data suggest a potential benefit in bowel obstruction.

Another potential approach to treating symptoms related to gastrointestinal obstruction uses somatostatin analog. Somatostatin functions as a neurotransmitter and a neurohormone, with regulatory effects in the gastrointestinal tract, including both endocrine and exocrine outcomes on the pancreas. It inhibits the glandular secretion of growth hormone, thyrotropin, corticotropin, and prolactin and slows the release of gastrin, cholecystokinin, insulin, glucagon, gastric acid, and pancreatic enzymes. It also may prevent neurotransmission in the peripheral nerves of the gastrointestinal tract, leading to diminished peristalsis and a decrease in splanchnic blood flow. There also is some indication that somatostatin inhibits the function of activated immune cells and may have a central opioid-like function. Somatostatin is the naturally occurring precursor hormone of octreotide.

The dosing regimen of octreotide for gastrointestinal obstruction in patients with cancer is not well established. Nonetheless, therapy can be initiated at 10 μg per hour, either intravenously or subcutaneously, and titrated every 24 hours to control nausea and vomiting. Alternatively, octreotide can be instituted as an intermittent subcutaneous injection at 50 μg every 8 hours and titrated every 24 hours.

Octreotide is generally well tolerated. Most patients report no side effects; the most common side effect is dry mouth, which can be relieved by ice chips and moist troches. Although the drug has been reported to cause nausea, abdominal pain, and diarrhea in 4% to 7% of patients, its use for the treatment of bowel obstruction has improved these symptoms. Long-term therapy has been shown to lead to biliary sludging with formation of gallstones in 15% to 20% of patients. Because of its effects on insulin and glucagon secretion, octreotide may cause mild hyperglycemia. These possible side effects have not been reported to be of clinical importance in the management of gastrointestinal obstruction, even with the use of high doses (up to 150 μg per hour or 3,600 μg daily). The use of octreotide has led to cessation of nausea and vomiting, removal of nasogastric tubes, and, in some cases, the ability of the patient to resume modest oral intake.[30–32] The route of drug delivery is an important consideration when treating nausea and vomiting caused by gastrointestinal obstruction. If intravenous access is established, most treatments can be given by that route. However, for patients without such access, subcutaneous infusion is the preferred route of administration according to much of the Canadian and European literature because octreotide is equally effective when given by that route, issues of venous access are avoided, and the drug can be administered safely at home.

SUMMARY

In summary, gastrointestinal obstruction in patients with cancer presents a considerable challenge with regard to symptom control. Surgery is appropriate for select patients. Skillful use of pharmacologic modalities can relieve symptoms for many patients who are not candidates for an operation. Antisecretory agents, particularly octreotide, are reasonable to use for the medical management of the symptoms from an irreversible underlying pathologic process.

MANAGEMENT OF ESTROGEN-DEPRIVATION SYMPTOMS

HOT FLASHES

Menopausal symptoms are highly prevalent among patients with breast cancer. Couzi et al. surveyed 190 postmenopausal women with local-regional (85%) or in situ (15%) breast cancer, who had been disease free for at least 1 year, to determine the prevalence and severity of menopausal symptoms.[33] Approximately 40% of the women believed that they had a

KEY POINTS

- Hot flashes are a problem for many women with breast cancer and for men who have had androgen-ablation therapy.
- Newer antidepressants, such as venlafaxine and paroxetine, decrease hot flashes by approximately 60% to 70%. Paroxetine should not be given with tamoxifen because it may interfere with the metabolism of tamoxifen to its active compound, endoxifen. Fluoxetine and sertraline, other newer antidepressants, do not appear to decrease hot flashes as well as do venlafaxine and paroxetine.
- Gabapentin, at a dose of 900 mg per day, decreases hot flashes by approximately 50% from baseline.
- Progestational agents decrease hot flashes as does estrogen treatment, but there is some theoretical concern about giving this therapy to breast cancer survivors.
- Vaginal dryness is a substantial problem for some women, who can be treated with local estrogen, but there is concern regarding the use of vaginal estrogen therapy in breast cancer survivors.

physical or emotional problem related to menopause since their diagnosis of breast cancer. Of those women, half wanted treatment for these symptoms. Hot flashes were the most prevalent symptom in the 4 weeks preceding the survey, occurring in 65% of patients. The use of tamoxifen was significantly associated with hot flashes, with 78% of women taking tamoxifen reporting hot flashes compared with 59% of women not taking tamoxifen ($p = 0.009$). Hot flashes also are a problem for men with prostate cancer who have had androgen-deprivation therapy. Approximately 75% of men so treated will have substantial discomfort because of hot flashes. Many times, these hot flashes are severe and may last for a considerable time.[34]

TREATMENT

Estrogens and androgens can alleviate hot flashes for women and men, respectively. Clearly, there is concern about giving estrogen to women who have had breast cancer.[35] Similarly, the administration of androgens to men with prostate cancer defeats the purpose of androgen-deprivation therapy. The consensus among experts is that estrogen-replacement therapy should not generally be recommended for women with a history of breast cancer. In contrast to this recommendation, some data suggest that estrogen therapy is not associated with adverse events for most survivors.[35,36] This means that estrogen can be used by select women, provided that they understand the potential theoretical risks associated with treatment. Nonetheless, additional agents are needed to control hot flashes in these patients (Table 18-6).

Progestational agents appear to alleviate hot flashes about as well as estrogen does.[37] Low doses of megestrol acetate decrease hot flashes by approximately 80%. Despite this efficacy, there is theoretical concern regarding the use of any hormone for patients with breast or prostate cancer. Although megestrol acetate is used at times as a management for metastatic disease, some believe that low doses of this drug may stimulate tumor growth. Further substantiating this concern, men who receive low doses of megestrol acetate may have a marked and prolonged decrease in the prostate-specific antigen (PSA) level when low doses of the drug are withdrawn. This effect is somewhat akin to withdrawal of flutamide causing a reduction of prostate cancer activity.

An alternative way to give progestational agents is to use intramuscular medroxyprogesterone acetate (MPA). The results of randomized studies show that intramuscular MPA injections of 400 to 500 mg control hot flashes for a prolonged period in breast cancer survivors.[38,39] Because this modality can control hot flashes for a prolonged period, relatively short-term progestational therapy is possible, alleviating the concern about long-term, continuous hormone therapy.

Given that there has been a desire to find nonhormonal agents to treat hot flashes, a number of clinical studies have been conducted to explore this possibility. Newer antidepressant medications have been found to be effective for the treatment of hot flashes (Table 18-6). Pilot studies demonstrated that low doses of venlafaxine decreased hot flash intensity and frequency both in breast cancer survivors and in men receiving androgen-deprivation therapy. The results of a randomized, placebo-controlled trial subsequently confirmed these findings, demonstrating a dose-response effect up to 75 mg daily of venlafaxine. This drug resulted in a 60% reduction in the frequency of hot flashes compared with a 27% reduction for the placebo.[40] Paroxetine (10 to 20 mg daily) was associated with a similar reduction in the number of hot flashes in a randomized, placebo-controlled trial.[41] Fluoxetine (20 mg daily) and sertraline (50 mg daily) appear to reduce hot flashes slightly more than does a placebo, but the efficacy of these agents appears to be less than that for venlafaxine or paroxetine.[42,43] Paroxetine, fluoxetine, and sertraline decrease the metabolism of tamoxifen to its active metabolite, endoxifen. Therefore, these agents should be avoided for patients receiving tamoxifen. Venlafaxine, however, does not appear to substantially alter tamoxifen metabolism.[44]

Data from pilot and randomized clinical trials demonstrate that relatively low doses of gabapentin also decrease the frequency of hot flashes, to a degree similar to that with the newer

TABLE 18-6 Pharmacologic Treatment of Hot Flashes (Agents Other Than Estrogen)

- Progestational Agents
  - Megestrol acetate: 20 to 40 mg orally per day
  - Medroxyprogesterone acetate: 400 to 500 mg intramuscular injection (once)
- Antidepressants
  - Venlafaxine: 37.5 mg orally per day for 1 week, then 75 mg orally per day
  - Paroxetine: 10 mg orally per day
- Gabapentin: titrate oral doses up to 900 to 2,400 mg per day
- Clonidine: 0.1 mg orally per day orally

antidepressant agents.[45–48] Gabapentin should be started at 100 to 300 mg daily. After 3 days, the dosing frequency can be increased to twice daily and then, a few days later, to three times daily. Doses of 900 mg daily decrease hot flashes by approximately 50%. New data suggest that doses of 2,400 mg daily decrease hot flashes by an amount comparable to that of estrogen.[49] The study that demonstrated this appeared to be well conducted but had a relatively small number of patients. Therefore, ideally this finding should be confirmed in a subsequent clinical trial.

The results from well-powered, randomized, placebo-controlled trials indicate that clonidine statistically inhibits hot flashes more when compared with placebo ($p = 0.0006$).[50] The magnitude of benefit from clonidine, however, is quite small. In addition, clonidine causes substantially more toxicity (e.g., hypotension, drowsiness, dry mouth, and constipation) than placebo. Because patients were just as likely to choose placebo over clonidine in a double-blind, randomized, crossover clinical trial, enthusiasm for this agent is tempered.

Although the findings from a number of pilot studies suggested that soy products could alleviate hot flashes, the majority of results from large, placebo-controlled clinical trials do not demonstrate any benefit from a phytoestrogen product for breast cancer survivors.[51–52]

Several nonpharmacologic options to prevent hot flashes have been studied for otherwise healthy postmenopausal women but, to date, there is not sufficient evidence to recommend any of them.

VAGINAL DRYNESS

Vaginal dryness from urogenital atrophy is another major symptom of estrogen depletion for some women. It can contribute to pain with intercourse, as well as itching and irritation. Vaginal lubricants are helpful for alleviating symptoms.[53] Nonetheless, these products seem to be less efficacious than estrogen therapy.[54]

New data demonstrating benefit for aromatase inhibitors, which lower postmenopausal estrogen levels, have heightened the concern for giving vaginal estrogen. Whereas patients must be told hypothetical risks of vaginal estrogen therapy, they should be allowed to balance the desire for controlled symptoms against presumably small, potential risks.

New data suggest that pilocarpine may decrease vaginal dryness.[55,56] This subject is being studied with a randomized, double-blind, placebo-controlled trial design.

ORAL MUCOSITIS AND ESOPHAGITIS ASSOCIATED WITH TREATMENT

BACKGROUND

Oral mucositis and esophagitis are common complications of chemotherapy and radiation therapy. The overall incidence of oral mucositis is approximately 40% for patients who receive standard-dose chemotherapy. The incidence varies with the chemotherapy agents used and increases substantially for patients who receive dose-intensified regimens. Mucositis and esophagitis are common in patients receiving irradiation to susceptible areas, and both can be exacerbated by concomitant chemotherapy. Dental evaluation prior to therapy should be encouraged if poor oral hygiene is seen on exam. Mucositis may occur as a result of any of the following:

- direct injury from cytotoxic chemotherapy or radiation therapy,
- secondary infection from treatment-induced myelosuppression, or
- graft-versus-host disease.

The severity of mucositis is dose and treatment specific. Mucositis typically starts 5 to 7 days after the initiation of chemotherapy. It often presents first as erythema on the soft palate, the buccal mucosa, the ventral surface of the tongue, and the floor of the mouth. These symptoms may progress to a generalized desquamation, commonly reaching a maximum on days 11 to 14. More than 90% of ulcerations are localized on nonkeratinized mucosa. Mucositis as the result of chemotherapy can resolve within a few days or last up to 2 to 3 weeks; oral mucositis caused by radiation therapy typically lasts an average of 6 weeks.

Chemotherapy agents frequently associated with mucositis include the antimetabolites fluorouracil and methotrexate and high-dose or prolonged infusions of chemotherapy.

Radiation therapy to the oral cavity frequently causes a host of oral complications, including mucositis, xerostomia, dental caries, tissue necrosis, and taste alterations.

> **KEY POINTS**
>
> - There are multiple causes of mucositis related to cytotoxic therapy.
> - Oral cryotherapy is useful for patients receiving bolus-dose fluorouracil therapy. Several other drugs have been suggested as being helpful for standard chemotherapy-induced mucositis, but the results of randomized trials generally have shown these agents to be ineffective and/or associated with some toxicity.
> - Palifermin decreased oral mucositis in patients receiving a bone marrow-ablative chemotherapy regimen associated with a high incidence of mucositis.
> - Treatment of established mucositis can include analgesics, a saline and baking soda solution mouthwash, and modification of food consistency.

The Multinational Association for Supportive Care of Cancer (MASCC) has developed clinical practice guidelines for the prevention and treatment of cancer therapy-induced oral and gastrointestinal mucositis.[57]

PREVENTION OF CHEMOTHERAPY-ASSOCIATED MUCOSITIS

The prevention of oral mucositis is an important goal because, once present, it can make ingestion of fluids, nutrition, and medications difficult. Three general approaches have been taken to prevent this condition (Table 18-7). Numerous agents have been proposed to prevent chemotherapy-induced mucositis, but most have not been shown to be effective when compared with placebo. Such agents include sucralfate, allopurinol, chamomile tea, glutamine, and vitamin E. One treatment that has been shown in clinical trials to effectively prevent mucositis is oral cryotherapy — sucking on ice chips during administration of chemotherapy. This treatment produces temporary vasoconstriction and thus appears to reduce the delivery of bolus-dose fluorouracil chemotherapy to the oral mucosa. Results from two controlled clinical trials indicated that oral cryotherapy reduced oral mucositis resulting from such treatment by approximately 50%.[58–59] Phase II evidence suggests that oral cryotherapy also decreases edatrexate-associated mucositis.[60–62]

Palifermin, which is a keratinocyte growth factor, is an agent that has been studied in prospective placebo-controlled, double-blinded clinical trials. It is evaluated for patients receiving high-dose chemotherapy as a preparation for bone marrow transplant. This trial demonstrated that palifermin decreased mucositis significantly more than placebo ($p < 0.001$).[63,64] It should be noted that not all high-dose chemotherapy programs induce quite as much mucositis as the one used in this particular trial.

Palifermin also has been studied in a placebo-controlled trial for patients receiving 5-flurouracil. Results from the trial suggest that it decreased mucositis more than placebo. The results, however, were not very impressive. The patients on this trial had not been given oral cryotherapy for alleviating mucositis. This, and the expense of the drug, precludes its generalized use for preventing fluorouracil-induced mucositis, pending data from subsequent trials.[65,66]

PREVENTION OF RADIATION-ASSOCIATED ORAL MUCOSITIS

A dental evaluation before the initiation of radiation therapy to the oral cavity is recommended. Fluoride carriers can provide fluoride for maintaining teeth integrity and, if worn during treatments, may help prevent radiation scatter from metal dental work, thus decreasing the inappropriately high radiation dose to buccal mucosa in the near vicinity of metal dental work.

Effective management of established oral mucositis includes general measures, such as oral hygiene and dietary modification, topical local anesthetics, and systemic analgesics.

PREVENTION OF RADIATION-ASSOCIATED ESOPHAGITIS

The results of a placebo-controlled trial showed no benefit for the use of sucralfate for the prevention of radiation-associated esophagitis.[67] Some evidence suggests that amifostine can mildly decrease radiation-induced esophagitis but at the cost of moderate toxicity, inconvenience, and expense.[68,69]

TREATMENT OF ESTABLISHED MUCOSITIS

General measures to treat oral mucositis include good oral hygiene and dietary modification. Patients should brush gently with a soft-bristled toothbrush and fluoride toothpaste two to three times daily. Gentle flossing daily is encouraged to remove food and bacteria build-up. The mouth can be rinsed every 4 hours with a diluted saline and baking soda solution (one-half teaspoon of salt plus

TABLE 18-7 Steps to Prevent Oral Mucositis

Step	Rationale
Alter the mucosal delivery and excretion of individual chemotherapy agents	The mucous membranes have less exposure to the cytotoxic agent.
Modify the epithelial proliferative capabilities of the mucosa	The rate of basal epithelial cell proliferation correlates with the susceptibility of mucosal tissues to the toxic effects of chemotherapy.
Reduce infectious or inflammatory complications	The presence of microorganisms may contribute indirectly to the inflammatory process.

one-half teaspoon of baking soda in a cup of warm water). This treatment is often soothing (and thought to be cleansing) but has not been formally evaluated. Also, dentures should be removed, particularly at night. It is noteworthy that these recommendations have not been validated by controlled clinical trials but intuitively appear reasonable for recommendation.

The maintenance of adequate caloric intake in the presence of mucositis can be a challenge. The length of time food is allowed to come in contact with the oral mucosa should be limited. The diet should consist of food that requires little or no chewing. Foods that irritate the mucosa chemically or mechanically should be avoided, including foods that are acidic, spicy, salty, coarse, or dry.

Adequate relief of pain associated with mucositis should be sought with pharmacologic agents. Local anesthetic agents, such as cocaine and viscous lidocaine, provide some pain relief, but the effects last for a few hours at best. In addition, cocaine has high abuse potential. Systemic analgesics, including opioids, may be useful when local anesthetics are ineffective. Chlorhexidine is not effective and causes substantial morbidity. The use of hydroxypropyl cellulose films as a mechanical barrier has shown some success, but its effectiveness lasts only a few hours. Sucralfate is not recommended because of lack of evidence of benefit. It is probably best to avoid alcohol-based mouth rinses.

MALIGNANT ASCITES

ETIOLOGY AND DIAGNOSIS

Ascites, the accumulation of fluid in the abdominal cavity, is a common cause of distress for patients with advanced cancer. More than 80% of patients in whom malignant ascites develops have epithelial cancers, particularly of the ovaries, endometrium, breast, colon, gastrointestinal tract, and pancreas.

> **KEY POINTS**
>
> - Diuretics can be useful therapeutic modalities for selected patients with ascites. Spironolactone is the initial diuretic to consider, with furosemide added after treatment with spironolactone is started.
> - For patients with far-advanced cancer, the use of diuretics for malignant ascites may be associated with more disadvantages than benefit.
> - Repeat paracentesis can be a helpful therapeutic modality for patients with symptomatic ascites. Rarely are ascitic shunting procedures useful.
> - New information suggests that octreotide might be helpful for patients with ascites; this deserves further study.

Under physiologic conditions, intravascular and extravascular hydrostatic and colloid osmotic pressures are in balance, preventing accumulation of extravascular fluid. Ascites develops when the influx of abdominal fluid increases or the outflow decreases, causing an accumulation of fluid in the peritoneal space. Ascites may indicate conditions that elevate hydrostatic pressure (e.g., congestive heart failure or cirrhosis), conditions that decrease osmotic pressure (e.g., nephrotic syndrome or malnutrition), or conditions in which fluid production exceeds resorptive capacity (e.g., infections and malignant diseases).

Because of the different pathophysiologic features and treatments, physicians must first distinguish between malignant and nonmalignant ascites. It should not be assumed that cancer is the cause until other common etiologies, such as cirrhosis, heart failure, or peritonitis, have been ruled out.

Clinical determination of the presence or absence of ascites has the advantages of speed, convenience, and cost savings. A focused history and physical examination are required to identify the signs and symptoms of ascites. The clinical history can distinguish patients with high and low probabilities for ascites. For example, ascites is unlikely for patients who report no increase in abdominal girth and for male patients who report no history of ankle swelling.

During physical examination, the clinician should determine if the flanks are bulging, if there is dullness over the flanks on percussion, if there is shifting dullness (dullness on percussion when the patient is rolled to the side), and if a fluid wave can be elicited. Diagnostic imaging may help diagnose ascites, particularly if the physical examination is equivocal, when there is a relatively small amount of fluid, or when loculation is present. A plain radiograph of the abdomen may show a hazy pattern or a pattern with a so-called ground glass appearance. Ultrasound or computerized tomography (CT) of the abdomen may identify even small amounts of free fluid.[70]

When diagnostic confirmation of ascites is needed, analysis of fluid obtained by paracentesis can confirm the presence of ascites and help determine its cause. Ultrasound guidance is helpful if the fluid is difficult to obtain or loculation is suspected. The most specific test to determine whether the ascites is the result of a malignant process is cytologic analysis; however, the absence of malignant cells does not exclude cancer. The fluid should be evaluated for color and for the cell count and total protein concentration; a serum ascites-albumin gradient also should be determined (Table 18-8).

Ascitic fluid indicates a likely malignant etiology when the following are present:

- blood,
- positive findings on cytologic analysis,
- low (negligible) absolute neutrophil count, and/or
- total protein concentration of at least 2.5 g/dL.

TABLE 18-8 Analysis of Fluid Obtained by Paracentesis

Characteristics	Interpretation	Comment
Color		
White, milky	Chylous ascites	Blood also may be caused by
Reddish (bloody)	Malignant disease	abdominal tuberculosis.
Cytologic analysis	Malignant cells indicate cancer	Absence of malignant cells does not exclude cancer.
Absolute neutrophil count of greater than 250 /μL	Bacterial peritonitis	Nonapplicable (NA)
Total protein concentration of 2.5 g/dL or less	Transudative ascites (less likely to have malignant cells)	Less likely to have malignant cells than exudative
Serum-ascites albumin gradient of 11 g/L or greater	Portal hypertension	NA

TREATMENT

Once a diagnosis of malignant ascites is established, treatment is largely directed at relieving symptoms such as dyspnea, abdominal pain, fatigue, anorexia or early satiety, and reduced exercise tolerance. Although treatment is not required for patients with a small amount of ascitic fluid, intervention may be needed to relieve symptoms when a larger amount is present. Because each treatment has adverse effects that must be taken into account for the individual patient, the physician should discuss the prognosis, expected response to treatment, and treatment preferences with the patient and family before making a treatment plan.

Therapeutic interventions for malignant ascites should be carefully selected (Table 18-9), and the use of chemotherapy should be considered in patients with potentially sensitive diseases. Diuretics should be used only for selected patients. The goal of diuretic therapy is to reduce the fluid accumulation; diuretics should not be administered to render the patient totally free of edema and ascites but rather to remove only enough fluid to ensure the patient's comfort. Diuresis should be slow and gradual, not to exceed the patient's capacity to mobilize ascitic fluid. Overly aggressive management of ascites for a patient with liver disease may lead to the hepatorenal syndrome and death.

It is usually best to start with a diuretic that acts at the distal nephron to block the effect of increased aldosterone activity. Spironolactone is often used as a first-line drug, starting with a daily dose of 25 to 50 mg in the morning. Spironolactone is sometimes associated with painful gynecomastia so amiloride at 5 mg daily is an alternative. If the response is suboptimal despite maximal use of distal diuretics, a low dose of a loop diuretic may be added, such as 20 mg of furosemide daily.

TABLE 18-9 Treatment Options for Ascites

Therapeutic Approach	Comment
Sodium Restriction	Potential benefits and burdens of sodium restriction, as well as other treatment options, should first be discussed with the patient.
Chemotherapy	For patients with cancers that are responsive to chemotherapy, such as lymphoma and breast or ovarian cancer.
Diuretics	Well tolerated and particularly useful for patients with cancer in whom ascites arises at least partially from nonmalignant causes; must be used carefully (see text).
Paracentesis	For ascites that is associated with respiratory distress or for symptomatic ascites that is resistant to diuretics.
Surgical Procedure (placement of LeVeen or Denver shunts to drain ascitic fluid from the peritoneal space into the internal jugular vein)	Rarely required; high protein content of malignant ascites may impair the flow of fluid through the shunt and lead to frequent blockage.

The initial dose of the diuretic may be gradually increased over days to weeks until the desired symptomatic relief is achieved. It may take several weeks for a given dose of diuretic to achieve its ultimate effect. Sometimes, very large doses of diuretics are needed to produce an adequate diuresis.

As with any drug therapy in the supportive-care setting, the patient's symptoms and lifestyle should be evaluated to consider the benefits and burdens of the treatment before deciding on medical management of ascites. Diuretic therapy is likely to be burdensome for patients who have limited mobility or urinary tract outflow symptoms, such as hesitancy or frequency, poor appetite or poor oral intake, or difficulties related to polypharmacy (the use of many medications for comorbid conditions).

Diuretic therapy is frequently associated with more disadvantages than benefits for patients with far-advanced cancer and a poor performance status. In these situations, therapy can result in incontinence, lead to sleep deprivation, and cause problems related to self-esteem, skin care, safety, fatigue, hyponatremia, hypokalemia, or symptomatic postural hypotension.

Therapeutic paracentesis may provide symptomatic relief with minimal morbidity and mortality. It may be the only therapeutic modality that is effective for patients with malignant ascites, and it provides symptomatic relief more rapidly than can be achieved with diuretics. As much as 5 L of fluid may safely be removed during a single session. Paracentesis can be performed either in the outpatient clinic setting or in the individual's home. Ascitic fluid, however, may reaccumulate within 1 to 4 days. The frequency of the subsequent drainage depends on the patient's subjective reports of shortness of breath, activity intolerance, or dyspnea on exertion.

Tenckhoff catheters may be beneficial for selected patients for whom repeated large-volume paracentesis is needed for comfort and for whom the prognosis warrants a surgical procedure. The Tenckhoff catheter is a soft, silicone rubber catheter that has two Dacron felt cuffs bonded to the catheter. The catheter is placed by a surgeon or, in some centers, by an interventional radiologist, with an external drain that can be accessed at home by a nurse or the family. Other catheters, such as Port-a-Caths, can be placed at the time of an initial operation if the prognosis is poor and repeated paracentesis is expected.[71] Surgical treatment of malignant ascites is associated with risks and, therefore, is rarely recommended (Table 18-9).

Anecdotal information suggests that octreotide may be helpful in patients with malignant ascites.[72] A randomized, placebo-controlled clinical trial of this subject sponsored by the North Central Cancer Treatment Group (NCCTG) of the National Cancer Institute is ongoing.

Having reviewed all of the treatment options for malignant ascites, it should be noted that ascites can often be a marker of disease progression. It may be appropriate to have a discussion with patients with ascites that focuses on realistic goals and options, such as supportive care and hospice.

ANOREXIA AND CACHEXIA

Involuntary weight loss has long been recognized as an adverse prognostic factor for patients with cancer. It has been reported to occur in 15% to 40% of patients at the time of presentation and in as many as 80% of patients with advanced cancer. Anorexia contributes to the wasting seen in cancer-related cachexia, but it is not the complete cause. In fact, the etiology of involuntary weight loss for patients with cancer is believed to be multifactorial.

In 1980, DeWys et al. reported that decreased survival was a consequence of cancer-associated cachexia. A retrospective analysis of 3,047 patients with 11 different tumor types demonstrated a relationship between tumor type and incidence, as well as between tumor type and degree of weight loss. For each tumor type, survival times were shorter for patients who lost weight compared with patients who had not.[73] In addition to survival, there are several other consequences of involuntary weight loss including the following: decreased response to and tolerance of radiation therapy and chemotherapy, increased frequency of surgical complications, weakness, fatigue, loss of energy, and inability to perform everyday tasks.

There are no strict criteria for the diagnosis of cachexia, but its common clinical manifestations are anorexia, early satiety, chronic nausea, asthenia, changes in body image, involuntary

KEY POINTS

- Anorexia is a prominent clinical problem for many patients with advanced cancer. For patients with far-advanced cancer who are not undergoing therapy, anorexia need only be treated if the patient considers it to be a substantially bothersome symptom.
- The two classes of medications that have been demonstrated to be helpful for cancer-related anorexia and cachexia are corticosteroids and progestational agents. Progestational agents are generally better tolerated than corticosteroids when given for substantial periods of time.
- Deep-vein thrombosis and adrenal suppression are two notable side effects of megestrol acetate.
- Total parenteral nutrition should be used for highly selected patients only.
- Anorexia may cause emotional problems for family members because of a perception of a lost nurturing opportunity. Teaching the family to substitue other nurturing activities (e.g., help with bathing, massage) may allow a good substitute.

weight loss, impaired immune function, poor performance status, and fatigue. Cancer-related cachexia differs from simple starvation because there is a disproportionate loss of lean body mass among patients with cancer-induced cachexia. A host of metabolic alterations are thought to play an important role including: tumor products, including lipolytic and proteolytic factors; humoral factors, such as serotonin and bombesin; and cytokines, such as tumor necrosis factor (TNF), interleukin (IL)-1, IL-6, and interferon-alpha. The end result is a reduction in the synthesis of lipids and proteins and an increase in lipolysis.[74]

Anorexia is a multidimensional symptom that usually results from multiple contributing factors, some of which are directly related to the presence of the tumor and some of which are related to reversible comorbid factors. The potential causes of anorexia/cachexia include constipation, emesis, mucositis, depression, decreased gastric emptying, dysphagia, food aversions, and fat malabsorption. One of the challenges in the clinical assessment of patients with anorexia is to characterize all of the different contributors so that a targeted treatment approach can be implemented.

The intensity of symptoms varies among patients. Although anorexia may be a major problem for many patients, it is not a major concern for all of them, even if cachexia is prominent. The lack of eating is often a bigger problem for the family than for the patient because the patient may not be bothered by a lack of appetite. When patients abstain from eating, the family loses a chance to provide nurturing for their loved one. Teaching the family to substitute other nurturing activities (e.g., help with bathing, massage) may allow a good substitute. In some patients it may be best not to offer medications; it may be one of many symptoms that will transition discussions to supportive care or hospice.

Numerous prospective randomized clinical trials have been conducted to ascertain whether nutritional support would improve the outcome for patients with cancer. In general, the results of these studies have shown that if there is such an effect, it is likely a small one or it is confined to a small subset of patients. Nutritional counseling alone is capable of improving daily caloric intake by approximately 450 calories. However, this advantage is generally short lived and does not appear to translate into improved patient weight, quality of life, or survival.

The use of parenteral nutrition does not have a major role in the care of the vast majority of patients with advanced cancer care.[75] However, it may provide some benefit for selected patients with cancer, such as patients who are unable to maintain adequate nutrition because of bowel obstruction but who do not have other life-threatening metastatic disease. Parenteral nutrition also may have benefit for cachectic patients who have a potentially curable tumor and require short-term nutritional support. In addition, parenteral nutrition is useful preoperatively for patients who will have tumor resection. In this latter indication, parenteral nutrition has been shown, in some situations, to decrease surgical complications and to possibly increase survival.

Enteral nutrition, usually through a gastronomy tube which has been placed endoscopically or by an interventional radiologist, may be considered when food intake is inadequate but the gastrointestinal tract is functionally intact. This often is used in patients with upper aero-digestive tract cancer who may have temporary disruption of eating and swallowing while undergoing radiation therapy. For such patients, there is no evidence that enteral nutrition is less effective than parenteral nutrition, but few prospective studies have been conducted to evaluate the benefits of this form of nutritional support. Enteral nutrition offers several advantages compared with parenteral nutrition (Table 18-10). The major serious complication associated with enteral nutrition is aspiration, with the risk of this complication increasing for patients with delayed gastric emptying. The risk can be reduced by frequent aspiration of the gastric contents during the first days of starting the infusion in order to exclude stasis. If stasis is found, metoclopramide or domperidone can be given to increase gastric emptying. Alternatively, a duodenal tube can be inserted as an alternate route of nutritional support; however, there is no good evidence that placing a tube in the duodenum or jejunum, rather than in the stomach, helps to prevent aspiration. All are associated with increased risk for aspiration pneumonia (as evidenced in dementia studies). Other side effects associated with enteral nutrition include diarrhea or constipation, nausea and vomiting, and abdominal cramping, bloating, or distension.

Because parenteral and enteral nutrition generally do not provide substantial benefit in reversing or stabilizing weight loss in the absence of tumor control, the main goals of the management of cachexia are to increase the general comfort of the patient, alleviate symptoms (particularly those symptoms contributing to anorexia), and provide improved function. In order to achieve these objectives, adaptive and pharmacologic approaches should be considered. However, there are no data that suggest that enteral or parenteral nutrition decrease anorexia in patients with cancer.

Fat malabsorption may occur in patients with pancreatic disease, in patients who have had gastric resection, in patients who have short-bowel syndrome or chronic radiation enteritis, or in patients who have had bone marrow transplantation.

TABLE 18-10 Advantages of Enteral Nutrition Compared with Parenteral Nutrition

- Fewer risks and complications
- Less expensive
- More easily carried out at home by most patients
- Delivers nutrients in a more physiologic manner

If there is increased stool odor, an empiric trial of exogenous pancreatic enzyme should be considered. Eight thousand units of lipase should be administered for every 5 to 7 g of fat in a meal.

TREATMENT OF CANCER-RELATED ANOREXIA

Drugs that have been demonstrated to be helpful for the treatment of cancer anorexia/cachexia are listed in Table 18-11. Megestrol acetate is the drug most widely studied in cancer-related anorexia and cachexia, with at least 12 completed controlled clinical trials. In these studies, megestrol acetate was administered daily over periods ranging from 1 to more than 12 weeks. Increases in appetite and/or body weight were documented in most of the studies.[76] Megestrol acetate provides benefits for appetite, caloric intake, and weight gain over the range of 160 to 1,600 mg daily. In clinical trials, the effect appeared to plateau at approximately 800 mg, suggesting that this amount should be the maximum dose.

Megestrol acetate is commercially available in the United States as 20-mg and 40-mg tablets and as a 40-mg/mL oral suspension. A 160-mg tablet is available in Canada. Several factors should be considered in dose selection.

- Side effects may be dose related.
- High doses are expensive. The suspension is the preferred delivery mode, as it is less expensive and more bioavailable than the tablets.
- Lower doses are effective in stimulating appetite; therefore, it is reasonable to start with a daily dose of 400 mg, with the dose titrated to clinical response.
- There is a newer micronized megestrol acetate formulation (Megace ES) that allows for better drug absorption in the fasting state, but it is more expensive than other forms of this drug.

Megestrol acetate is generally well tolerated, with side effects occurring infrequently and probably in relation to the dose. In clinical trials, patients receiving megestrol acetate generally are no more likely to discontinue treatment because of side effects than are patients receiving placebos. The side effect of most clinical concern is thromboembolic complications. Because of this possibility, megestrol acetate is relatively contraindicated for patients with a history of thromboembolic disease. Also, because the drug can cause adrenal-axis suppression, adrenal insufficiency may occur either while a patient is using the medication or shortly after discontinuing treatment. Thus, in the event of infection, surgery, or trauma, stress doses of corticosteroids should be given. Furthermore, anecdotal experience suggests that megestrol acetate may alter glucose control in patients with diabetes mellitus who require insulin. Of note, this agent has antiemetic efficacy; the findings from randomized, placebo-controlled clinical trials have demonstrated less nausea and vomiting for patients receiving the drug compared with patients receiving placebo preparations.[77,78]

Medroxyprogesterone acetate is another progestational agent that stimulates appetite, but it has been less widely studied than megestrol acetate. It is generally well tolerated with a side-effect profile similar to that of megestrol acetate.

At least five randomized clinical trials have been conducted with various corticosteroids, and the results have indicated that these drugs increase appetite and food intake and enhance the patient's sense of well-being and performance status.[79,80]

In order to compare the activity and tolerability of megestrol acetate and a corticosteroid, a randomized controlled study was conducted in which patients with cancer-related anorexia and cachexia were randomly assigned to

TABLE 18-11 Treatment of Cancer-related Anorexia

Drug	Function	Dosing
Megestrol acetate	Improves appetite, increases caloric intake, decreases nausea and vomiting	Activity seen with range of 160 to 1,600 mg/d; recommended maximum dose, 800 mg/d
Medroxyprotesterone acetate	Stimulates appetite	Activity seen with range of 300 to 1,000 mg; generally well tolerated with a side-effect profile similar to that of megestrol acetate
Corticosteroids	Increase appetite and food intake and improve the sense of well-being and performance status, generally only for a short period of time	
Dexamethasone (oral)		Dexamethasone doses of 2 to 4 mg per day
Prednisolone (oral)		Not supplied (NS)
Methylprednisolone (oral and intravenous)		NS

receive 800 mg of megestrol acetate daily or 0.75 mg of dexamethasone four times daily. Patients were followed at monthly intervals. Both drugs produced similar appetite enhancement and changes in nonfluid weight, with a trend favoring megestrol acetate. Drug discontinuation because of toxicity or patient refusal was significantly higher with dexamethasone than with megestrol acetate (36% compared with 25%; $p = 0.03$). However, deep vein thrombosis was more common with megestrol acetate (5% compared with 1%; $p = 0.06$).[81]

Several factors should be considered when deciding whether to use megestrol acetate or corticosteroids for the treatment of cancer-related cachexia. Megestrol acetate is favored when cachexia is the main symptom, whereas corticosteroids may be useful when other symptoms, such as pain, also are present. Megestrol acetate is preferable for long-term use or when weight gain is desired. Corticosteroids are particularly useful for patients with short expected survival in whom weight gain is not an expected outcome. Corticosteroids should not be used longer than several weeks because longer-term use is associated with unacceptable side effects, such as edema, muscle weakness, dysphoria, hypokalemia, hyperglycemia, and immune suppression. There does not appear to be any advantage to using corticosteroids and megestrol acetate concomitantly.

Cyproheptadine is a serotonin antagonist that has been available for more than 20 years. It has been used in Latin America and Europe as an appetite stimulant for patients with cancer. In a large, randomized controlled study, oral cyproheptadine at a dose of 8 mg three times daily produced a mild increase in appetite and food intake but had no effect on progressive weight loss.[82] As a result of its side effects, notably sedation, and lack of much efficacy, cyproheptadine is not very useful for patients with cancer-related cachexia.

A number of other agents have been proposed to be helpful for cancer-related anorexia and cachexia, but none have been beneficial when tested in controlled clinical trials.[83–86] These drugs include hydrazine sulfate, eicosapentaenoic acid, pentoxifylline, and dronabinol. New reports of trials involving antibodies against tumor necrosis factor (TNF, otherwise known as cachectin), such as etanercept and infliximab, suggest that these drugs also are not helpful.[87] A double-blind, randomized trial of the anabolic agent oxandrolone completed accrual several years ago but has, apparently, never been reported. As this trial was conducted by a pharmaceutical company, the lack of a manuscript being published suggests that this trial was not positive.

DIARRHEA ASSOCIATED WITH CANCER OR CANCER THERAPY

Nonpharmacologic and pharmacologic steps are often required for the management of acute treatment-related diarrhea, and several nonpharmacologic measures can be carried out in clinical practice to manage subacute diarrhea (Table 18-12).[88] Rehydration is important for patients with severe diarrhea that has caused dehydration. Usually, an increased intake of clear liquids is all that is required, but parenteral administration of fluids and electrolytes may be necessary for some patients.

> **KEY POINTS**
>
> - Fluorouracil, irinotecan, and topotecan commonly cause diarrhea. Irinotecan causes two types of diarrhea: an early-onset cholinergic mechanism diarrhea and a more severe diarrhea that generally begins a few days after irinotecan administration.
> - Radiation to the pelvis causes diarrhea for a substantial number of patients.
> - Graft-versus-host disease also can cause diarrhea that can be treated with steroids and octreotide.
> - Multiple clinical trials have demonstrated that many purported antidiarrheal agents are not efficacious and carry some toxicity.
> - Loperamide should be prescribed for patients with chemotherapy-induced diarrhea. Octreotide can be helpful for patients in whom loperamide does not control chemotherapy-induced diarrhea. Octreotide also can be helpful for treating radiation-induced diarrhea.
> - For diarrhea associated with pancreatic insufficiency, 8,000 units of lipase should be administered for every 5 to 7 g of fat in a meal.

CHEMOTHERAPY-INDUCED DIARRHEA

Etiology and Incidence

Chemotherapy can cause diarrhea by irritating or damaging the crypt and villi cells of the intestinal mucosa. The incidence and severity of chemotherapy-induced diarrhea depends on a number of factors, including the drug dose and treatment regimen. In general, diarrhea is most common with regimens that include antimetabolites. Of these agents, fluorouracil is the agent that has been studied the most in terms of this side effect. The risk of diarrhea from fluorouracil increases when leucovorin is given as a modulating agent.

Diarrhea also is common with newer antimetabolites, such as irinotecan and topotecan. With irinotecan, diarrhea may occur immediately after administration through a cholinergic mechanism (early-onset diarrhea), or a more severe, potentially life-threatening form of diarrhea may develop days after administration (late-onset diarrhea). The severity of late-onset diarrhea correlates with peak plasma levels of the irinotecan metabolite, SN38. The incidence of diarrhea associated with these two drugs for patients with metastatic cancer of the colon or rectum ranges from 5% to

TABLE 18-12 Steps in the Treatment of Patients with Diarrhea

- Conduct a comprehensive evaluation of the patient at the first report of diarrhea
- Obtain information about the onset and duration of diarrhea and the number and characteristics of the stool
- Ask the patient about other symptoms, such as fever, abdominal pain, dizziness, and weakness, which could indicate the cause of diarrhea and the risk of dehydration, bowel obstruction, and infection
- Review the patient's diet and medication usage to identify any foods or medicines that may be causing or contributing to the diarrhea
- Advise the patient to eat frequent small meals and to avoid foods that irritate the intestines or stimulate its motility
- Encourage the patient to drink 8 to 10 large glasses of clear liquid per day in order to maintain adequate hydration and to prevent potential dehydration
- Taper or eliminate medications that may cause or exacerbate diarrhea, if medically possible

90% (Table 18-13).[88] In is important to note that patients who have received antibiotics or cisplatin-based therapy may have a Clostridium difficile infection and that patients with neutropenia must be followed closely because of the possibility of developing typhlitis.

Treatment

The choice of effective pharmacologic measures is limited despite the availability of many types of antidiarrheal agents. Opioid-like medications often are useful. Of these agents, loperamide and diphenoxylate are most commonly used for treating acute diarrhea caused by a wide variety of conditions. In addition, side effects, especially with loperamide, are generally minimal. Octreotide also is effective and is generally well tolerated. Loperamide has been compared with octreotide for the treatment of fluorouracil-induced diarrhea. In one clinical trial, 41 patients with grade 2 or greater diarrhea (according to the National Cancer Institute [NCI] Common Toxicity Criteria) resulting from fluorouracil-containing chemotherapy were randomly assigned to receive 0.1 mg of subcutaneous octreotide twice daily for 3 days or to 4 mg of oral loperamide initially and then 2 mg every 6 hours for 3 days. Diarrhea resolved in 19 (91%) of the 21 patients in the octreotide arm compared with three (15%) of the 20 patients in the loperamide arm ($p = 0.005$). No side effects were observed in either treatment arm.[89]

TABLE 18-13 Incidence of Diarrhea for Drugs to Treat Metastatic Colorectal Cancer[55]

Drug	Diarrhea Any Grade	Diarrhea Grade 3 or 4
Irinotecan		
Early-onset diarrhea	50%	10%
Late-onset diarrhea	90%	30%
Topotecan	30%	5%

A double-blind, randomized clinical trial of octreotide involved patients receiving cisplatin. All of the patients enrolled in the study had had diarrhea as a result of a prior course of cisplatin therapy. A total of 43 patients were randomly assigned to receive either octreotide (0.1 mg) or placebo (1 cc of saline solution) by subcutaneous injection 15 minutes before and 6 hours after cisplatin therapy. Diarrhea, defined as more than two loose bowel movements per day, occurred for 75% of patients who received placebo and for 5% of patients who received octreotide ($p = 0.01$). Side effects were minimal. These findings suggest that octreotide is useful for the secondary prevention of cisplatin-induced diarrhea for patients with a history of diarrhea during prior courses of cisplatin.[90]

Treatment of chemotherapy-induced diarrhea can follow an algorithmic approach, as shown in Table 18-12 and Fig. 18-1.[88]

RADIATION-INDUCED DIARRHEA

Etiology and Incidence

Diarrhea is the most common adverse effect of pelvic radiation therapy. Such therapy damages the mucosa of the small or large intestine and thereby produces secretory or other forms of diarrhea. The incidence and severity increases with the addition of fluorouracil. For example, in one study, the combination of fluorouracil and radiation therapy produced a significantly higher rate of acute diarrhea at any time during treatment than radiation therapy alone (79% compared with 41%; $p = 0.001$). The difference between the two groups was particularly large for grades 3 and 4 diarrhea combined (22% compared with 4%; $p = 0.001$).[91]

Treatment

A number of placebo-controlled clinical trials have been unable to identify a drug that can be used to prevent diarrhea induced by pelvic radiation therapy. The findings from one

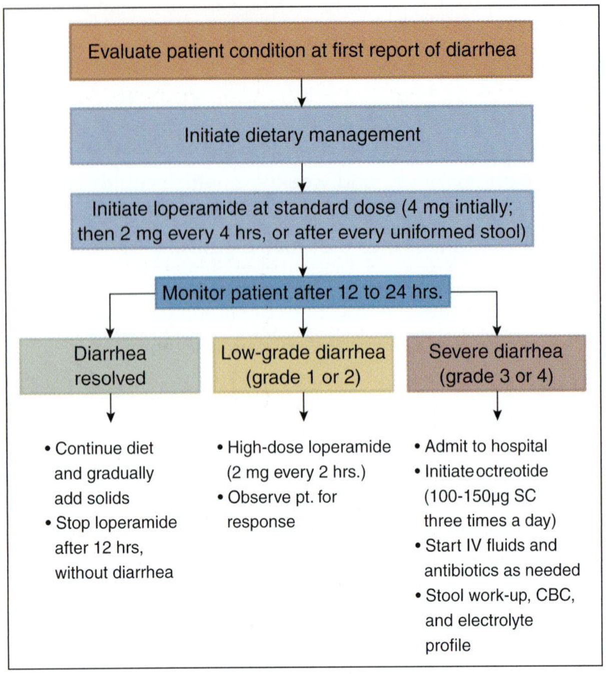

FIG. 18-1 Algorithm for the treatment of chemotherapy-induced diarrhea.[88]

trial of olsalazine actually showed that it increased diarrhea.[92] Another trial demonstrated that cholestyramine decreased diarrhea but at the cost of other toxicities that canceled out the benefit.[93] Trials of sucralfate have provided mixed results that preclude its recommendation for clinical practice use.[92,94] A recently completed, randomized, placebo-controlled, double-blinded clinical trial was unable to demonstrate any benefit for octreotide as an agent to prevent radiation-induced diarrhea.[95]

Preliminary evidence suggests that octreotide, however, may have a role in the treatment of diarrhea induced by pelvic radiation therapy. Thirty-two patients with grade 2 or 3 diarrhea associated with pelvic radiation therapy were randomly assigned to receive either 0.1 mg of subcutaneous octreotide three times daily or 10 mg of oral diphenoxylate (with atropine) daily. Diarrhea resolved within 3 days for 13 of the 16 patients in the octreotide arm and for three of the 16 patients in the diphenoxylate arm (81% compared with 19%; $p = 0.005$).[96]

The most important lesson to be learned from clinical trials designed to evaluate diarrhea prevention in patients receiving pelvic radiation therapy is that the use of pharmacologic agents on an ad hoc basis outside of a clinical trial may be inappropirate. Virtually all of the various categories of agents evaluated in clinical trials consistently failed to show a benefit with an acceptable safety profile. In some cases, agents actually made diarrhea worse (olsalazine) or were associated with unacceptable adverse effects (cholestyramine and sucralfate). As these findings demonstrate, using seemingly benign drugs to prevent diarrhea during pelvic radiation therapy may expose patients to toxicity without any corresponding benefit.

GRAFT-VERSUS-HOST DISEASE-ASSOCIATED DIARRHEA

For patients who have received a bone marrow transplant, diarrhea may result from graft-versus-host disease or from infections related to the use of immunosuppressive therapy. The epithelial damage caused by high-dose chemotherapy can serve as a stimulus for activation of alloreactive cytotoxic T cells, which release a cascade of inflammatory cytokines that contribute to necrosis of epithelial crypt cells.

At the first sign of acute gastrointestinal symptoms that may signify a graft-versus-host reaction, a stool specimen should be evaluated for bacterial, fungal, and viral pathogens and supportive management should be initiated. In addition, the other general measures for managing diarrhea should be used (Table 18-12). Consultation with a gastroenterologist should be considered.

If the findings on stool evaluation are positive for bacteria, a course of appropriate antibiotics should be started. For patients with a diagnosis of graft-versus-host disease (established by biopsy), corticosteroids should be used at a dose of 1 to 2 mg/kg daily (prednisolone or methylprednisolone), and prophylactic immunosuppressive therapy should be continued. Octreotide should be considered at an intravenous dose of 500 mg three times daily. If the patient has a response within 4 days, octreotide should be discontinued in order to avoid ileus. However, if there is no response to octreotide, second-line therapy with antithymocyte globulin or with infliximab should be considered. Alternatively, participation in a clinical trial regarding this problem is quite reasonable as there is no uniform agreement on the ideal treatment of this problem.

CANCER-ASSOCIATED DIARRHEA

Cancer itself, rather than its treatment, may cause diarrhea. For example, in pancreatic cancer, the presence of inadequate digestive enzymes may lead to osmotic diarrhea. For patients who have an increased stool odor, an empiric trial of exogenous pancreatic enzyme should be considered.

Secretory diarrhea may occur in thyroid cancer as a result of the overproduction of calcitonin and prostaglandins, in carcinoid syndrome as a result of the increased secretion of prostaglandins and serotonin, and with pancreatic islet cell cancers. In these situations, octreotide is generally the best option for controlling diarrhea. Cyproheptadine also may be helpful for carcinoid syndrome-related diarrhea.

DYSPNEA

ETIOLOGY AND EVALUATION

Dyspnea is a subjective sensation experienced by patients. It has been defined as the uncomfortable awareness of breathing, shortness of breath, or an inability to get enough air. Patients may describe it as a smothering, suffocating, or drowning feeling.

KEY POINTS

- Dyspnea can be a prominent symptom for many patients with cancer as they near the end of life.
- Patient reports of dyspnea do not always correlate with measures of blood oxygen.
- Oxygen can provide symptomatic relief for patients with dyspnea. Cool air blown across the face also can be a helpful therapy.
- Opioids are the mainstay of pharmacologic management of cancer-associated dyspnea after other causes, such as effusions, pneumania, airway obstructions, or anemia, are treated
- Anxiolytics can be helpful for some patients with breathlessness and anxiety, although they generally are not as helpful as opioids.
- Anticholinergic medications, such as scopolamine, glycopyrrolate, or atrophine, can be helpful for patients with oral secretions that are bothersome.

There is no diagnostic test that reliably confirms the presence of dyspnea. Thus, the patient's self-report is the gold standard for its presence and its relief. Commonly measured parameters such as respiratory rate, partial pressure of oxygen, blood gases, and pulse oximetry do not always correlate with patients' perceptions of their degree of shortness of breath.

Dyspnea is a common symptom of advanced cancer. In various studies, its incidence ranges from 21% to 90%. It is reported by many patients with lung cancer and is particularly prevalent among patients with advanced lung cancer. However, it also is associated with a variety of noncancer illnesses, such as congestive heart failure and chronic obstructive pulmonary disease situations, that may be comorbidities for patients with advanced cancer.

The pathophysiologic basis for a patient's report of breathlessness is incompletely understood. There are at least three components of respiratory drive: central, peripheral, and emotional. Disturbances in any component can result in the report of breathlessness.[97]

The respiratory center in the medulla coordinates the activity of the diaphragm, the intercostal muscles, and the accessory muscles of respiration. It receives information from central and peripheral chemoreceptors, peripheral mechanoreceptors, and the cerebral cortex. However, there is no direct correlation between stimulation of respiratory drive and breathlessness. Although one can demonstrate that metabolic derangements, such as hypercarbia, hypoxemia, and metabolic acidosis, are associated with increased respiratory drive, the converse is not always true. Patients who report having breathlessness may or may not have derangements in these parameters.[98]

Many causes of breathlessness are treatable or, at minimum, have a reversible component. In one study of patients with cancer, potentially correctable elements included hypoxia (40%), anemia (20%), pleural effusions, and bronchospasm.

The patient's history may be useful in determining the etiology of dyspnea. Some patients may not report breathlessness in response to direct questions. However, specific questions about their activities may elicit situations in which breathlessness prevents them from performing their usual activities. The usual descriptors of onset (acute or chronic), severity, aggravating and mitigating factors, associated symptoms, and response to prior treatment may be helpful. Elicitation of other medical problems could demonstrate comorbidities that may be contributing to dyspnea. Information about prior or current cancer treatment is useful for determining whether pulmonary fibrosis, radiation pneumonitis/fibrosis, or allergic reactions could be contributing. Sudden-onset symptoms, accompanying pleuritic pain, or leg edema may suggest the possibility of pulmonary embolus. Occupational and smoking history also may be important etiologic clues.

Severity of symptoms may be reported in a variety of ways. Several authors recommend measuring breathlessness and other symptoms in a manner similar to that recommended for pain, and often the same scale is appropriate for both. One dyspnea scale is the modified Borg scale that has a vertical axis labeled 0 to 10 with corresponding verbal descriptions of intensity (e.g., weak, moderate, and strong).[99] It is reproducible, easy to use, and correlates well with dyspnea during exercise testing. Many, more involved, dyspnea scales exist, but none have been validated for patients with cancer, and their results do not correlate with the specific level of treatment needed.

The level of work-up to determine the cause of breathlessness is dependent on the goals for the patient's care. A decision to treat a reversible cause should be reached only after general goals of care are determined. The burden of diagnostic tests and treatments may outweigh the benefit for an individual patient.[100]

TREATMENT

The major treatment modalities for symptomatic relief of dyspnea include oxygen, opioids, anxiolytics, and nonpharmacologic measures. The cornerstones are treatment of the underlying cause and management of symptoms. It is important for the clinician to direct care at managing symptoms while waiting for specific therapy to be effective. Regardless of the stage of cancer, relief of dyspnea must be of utmost concern. The patient with curable cancer who is dyspneic at presentation or as a complication of treatment needs prompt relief of breathlessness, as does a patient with an incurable cancer who is on hospice.

If the underlying cause can be treated, the prospect for long-term relief of dyspnea improves. If the cancer can be treated effectively, the chances for eventual relief are, of course, higher than if no effective treatment exists. However, even in end-stage lung cancer that cannot be treated directly, relief of symptoms might be able to be provided by using such measures as stents and laser therapy.

Oxygen therapy has been a mainstay for the treatment of dyspnea of all causes. The evidence for beneficial effects of oxygen on dyspnea is based primarily on studies in chronic obstructive pulmonary disease and congestive heart failure. Its effectiveness for patients with cancer who were hypoxemic was demonstrated in a randomized, double-blind crossover study.[101] However, in another controlled study of patients with dyspnea, delivered oxygen and air reduced symptoms to a similar degree, regardless of whether the patient was hypoxemic.[102]

Because breathlessness frequently is perceived to be a lack of air, it would seem to be quite reasonable to suppose that the administration of supplemental oxygen would relieve a patient's sense of breathlessness. Yet, research has shown that most patients who report breathlessness are not hypoxemic and measures of hypoxemia, such as pulse oximetry and determination of arterial blood gas values, may not correlate with the patient's self-report. Some patients who are weak or deconditioned will report dyspnea on exertion yet will have a normal saturation. Thus, these measures are not helpful for assessing relief because the tests do not reliably reflect breathlessness or its relief. In addition, they may be uncomfortable, expensive, and may divert the focus away from the symptom. If the patient feels fine, it does not help symptom management to know that the oxygen saturation is 86%.

When a patient reports breathlessness, a therapeutic trial of supplemental oxygen may be beneficial, regardless of whether hypoxemia is present. Relief of dyspnea may be the result of various effects other than correction of hypoxemia. There is a prominent placebo effect for patients without hypoxemia. Supplemental oxygen frequently is viewed as a potent symbol of contemporary medical care. The continued use of supplemental oxygen is expensive and not reimbursed by all insurance. However, if it is effective, rational treatment includes its continued use.

Cool air moving across a patient's face (e.g., from compressed air or a fan) may, for the symptom of breathlessness, provide as much relief as oxygen.[102] This finding has been explained by the physiologic effect of stimulating the V2 branch of the fifth cranial nerve that has a centrally inhibitory effect on the sensation of breathlessness.

The benefit of opioids for the relief of dyspnea was demonstrated in a number of randomized controlled trials. Findings from an initial study showed the effectiveness of a subcutaneous bolus dose of 5 mg of morphine for 20 patients with cancer-related dyspnea. The results of a study reported in 1993 showed that an increased dose of morphine, 50% higher than the dose the patient was already receiving, was effective for relieving dyspnea.[103]

For patients receiving an opioid on a fixed schedule, an additional oral dose of a short-acting oral opioid (e.g., morphine), equivalent to 10% to 15% of the total daily morphine dose, can be tried every hour and titrated to effect. These agents can be administered intravenously (at 5- to 10-minute intervals) or subcutaneously (at 15-minute intervals) for urgent situations or when the oral route is not available or advisable. For patients who have not previously received opioids, one dosing scheme for intravenous infusion features a bolus of 2 mg repeated every 5 to 10 minutes until efficacy is noted, followed by a continuous infusion at an hourly rate equal to 50% of the loading dose.

Dose-limiting adverse effects of opioids are the same as when these agents are used for pain. In general, pharmacologic tolerance to all of the adverse effects (except constipation) usually develops in a patient within 1 or 2 weeks of initiating opioid therapy.

Research shows that opioids relieve the distress of breathlessness for many patients without having a measurable effect on the respiratory rate or arterial blood gas concentrations. For some patients, relief also may be associated with a measurable increase in exercise tolerance and mobility. The precise mechanism by which opioids exert this influence is unclear because there may be both central and peripheral effects. The patient may have a reduction in respiratory drive, experience an altered perception of dyspnea, and oxygen consumption may be reduced.

Concerns that the use of opioids will hasten death or cause addiction are not relevant. When opioid-dosing guidelines are followed, respiratory depression has not been demonstrated at the doses used to relieve breathlessness.

When opioids are used appropriately to relieve a symptom, as with the management of pain or dyspnea, opioid treatment is consistent with good medical practice. Its use is ethical when the intent is to relieve suffering and when clinicians follow widely accepted dosing guidelines. When used in this setting under such guidelines, opioid use is very unlikely to be associated with abuse. Doses are based on severity of symptoms and opioid tolerance.

Nebulized opioids have been widely reported to be effective in anecdotal reports and phase II studies.[104] However, in placebo-controlled studies, nebulized saline and nebulized morphine were shown to relieve breathlessness equally well.[105,106] Chlorpromazine and promethazine both have been reported to improve breathlessness, particularly when combined with opioids.

Breathlessness, particularly when it is acute or severe, may cause severe anxiety and panic. Opioid and nonpharmaceutical therapies may relieve both breathlessness and resultant anxiety. Anxiolytics are not recommended as first-line pharmacologic therapy for breathlessness.[107] However,

TABLE 18-14 Anxiolytic Drugs for Treatment of Breathlessness

Drug	Dose Range (Route)	Dosing Schedule
Lorazepam	0.5–2 mg (PO; SL, against the buccal mucosa; IV)	Every hour as needed until settled, then every 4–6 hours as needed
Diazepam	5–10 mg (PO, IV)	Every hour until settled, then every 6–8 hours as needed
Clonazepam	0.25–2 mg (PO)	Every 12 hours
Midazolam	0.5 mg (IV)	Every 15 minutes until settled, then continuous infusion (SC or IV)

Abbreviations: PO, orally; SL, sublingually; IV, intravenously.

some patients who are breathless and anxious may need treatment for the anxiety because the opioids themselves, especially with continued dosing, are not particularly anxiolytic.

Benzodiazepines are highly effective anxiolytic medications (Table 18-14). Drugs that have relatively longer half-lives avoid pronounced peak and trough effects that may lead to rebound anxiety. Therapy should start with low doses and be titrated to effect, and the drugs may be combined safely with opioids. An algorithm for the management of breathlessness has been developed by Thomas Smith, MD (Fig. 18-2).[108]

A variety of nonpharmacologic interventions may provide additional relief of breathlessness. These interventions include the following: limiting the number of people in the patient's room; reducing the room temperature (without chilling the patient); opening windows and keeping an unobstructed line of sight between the patient and the outside; minimizing the number of machines and sounds; eliminating environmental irritants, such as smoke or pet dander; maintaining sufficient humidity in the air; repositioning the patient by elevating the head of the bed, or moving him or her to one side or the other; and encouraging relaxation, distraction, massage, or hypnotic therapy. The physician should take time to explain the situation and the various interventions, as well as provide understanding and support to the patient and family. Other members of the interdisciplinary team should be included to increase interaction, minimize loneliness, explore issues of meaning and value, and provide counseling for family because financial, legal, spiritual, or practical issues may be exacerbating the symptom.

As patients approach the last hours of life, family members and caregivers need education about the breathing patterns they may witness. Breathing may become very shallow and frequent. Periods of apnea or Cheyne-Stokes pattern respirations may develop. Accessory respiratory muscle use may become prominent. A few (or many) last reflex breaths may signal death. Families and professional caregivers may perceive that patients will experience these

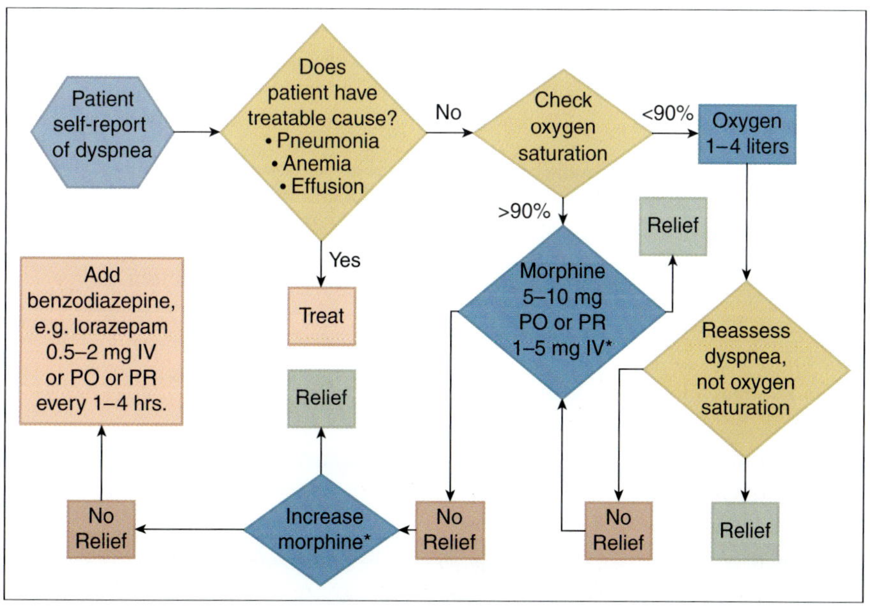

FIG. 18-2 Algorithm for the treatment of breathlessness in patients with cancer.[107]

**To titrate the dose of morphine in patients with severe pulmonary disease, such as chronic obstructive pulmonary disease, the first dose should be at the lower end of the range and be titrated upward every 24 hours, increasing the dose approximately 25% until relief is achieved or adverse effects become limiting. For patients without pulmonary disease, upward increments of 50% to 100% are appropriate for titration.*

expected changes in breathing pattern as a sense of suffocation. Consequently, it is of critical importance that the physician elicit and acknowledge the misperception and provide the information that the comatose patient is not experiencing breathlessness or suffocation and may not benefit from additional therapies. In some cases, low doses of opioids or benzodiazepines are appropriate to manage any perception of breathlessness.

As patients approach death, the gag reflex and reflexive clearing of the oropharynx may decline, and secretions from the tracheobronchial tree may accumulate. Buildup of saliva and oropharyngeal secretions may lead to gurgling, crackling, or rattling sounds with each breath. Some have called this noise the "death rattle," a term frequently disconcerting to families and caregivers. For unprepared families and professional caregivers, it may sound like the patient is choking or suffocating.

Anticholinergic medications may be used to dry secretions in order to prevent and treat these distressing sounds and to minimize coughing and the effort of breathing in those patients with excess secretions. Subcutaneous doses of 0.2 to 0.4 mg of scopolamine every 4 hours (or one to three transdermal patches every 72 hours or 0.1 to 1.0 mg every hour by continuous intravenous or subcutaneous infusion) or of 0.2 mg of subcutaneous glycopyrrolate every 4 to 6 hours (or 0.4 to 1.2 mg daily by continuous intravenous or subcutaneous infusion) will effectively reduce the production of saliva and other secretions. These agents will minimize or eliminate the gurgling and crackling sounds and may be used prophylactically for the dying patient who is unconscious. Anecdotal evidence suggests that the earlier treatment is initiated, the better it works, as larger amounts of secretions in the upper aerodigestive tract are more difficult to eliminate. However, premature use for patients who are still alert may lead to unacceptable drying of oral and pharyngeal mucosa. Atropine may be equally effective and is available as a 1% ophthalmic solution that can be given as one to two drops sublingually every 1 to 4 hours.

If excessive fluid accumulates in the back of the throat and upper airways, it may need to be cleared by repositioning the patient. Turning patients onto one side or placing them into a semiprone position may reduce gurgling. Lowering the head and raising the foot of the bed while the patient is in a semiprone position may cause fluids to move into the oropharynx from which they can be easily removed. Do not maintain this position for more than a few minutes at a time, as stomach contents also may move unexpectedly.

Oropharyngeal suctioning is not recommended. It is frequently ineffective, as fluids are beyond the reach of the catheter. This procedure may only stimulate an otherwise peaceful patient and distress family members who are watching.

CANCER FATIGUE

Fatigue is one of the most bothersome symptoms in patients with cancer.[109–111] It affects patients receiving adjuvant chemotherapy and those with advanced disease. Fatigue has been noted to occur in anywhere from 60% to 90% of patients receiving chemotherapy and in 65% to 100% of patients receiving radiation therapy. The NCCN[111] has defined cancer fatigue as "a persistent subjective sense of tiredness related to cancer or cancer treatment that interferes with usual functioning." This problem is often times not relieved with rest.

Evaluation of this problem should consist of a history, physician examination, and screening blood work that includes a complete blood count and chemistry evaluation of renal function, thyroid function, liver function, calcium, and electrolytes. Adrenal function tests also may be indicated in selected situations, and screening for depression also is appropriate. If any abnormalities are noted from the screening evaluation, then reasonable attempts to correct these abnormalities are, of course, recommended.

Exercise appears to be the best therapy for cancer-related fatigue.[112–119] Psychostimulants such as methylphenidate have been studied but, to date, the bulk of evidence suggests that they are not very helpful. Ongoing research is investigating a longer-acting methylphenidate preparation. Modafinil has been studied but, as of yet, no published manuscripts have reported data from definitive double-blind, placebo-controlled trials to demonstrate that it is beneficial in patients with cancer.[120] Further placebo-controlled trials are ongoing. Ginseng has also been studied based on preliminary clinical information and animal data.[121–125] A randomized, pilot, dose-seeking NCCTG trial, which accrued 282 patients, was presented at the 2007 ASCO meeting.[126] This report provided positive pilot information, supporting that a formal phase III trial should be performed to delineate whether ginseng was helpful for alleviating cancer-related fatigue.

KEY POINTS

- Cancer fatigue is very common and often multifactorial.
- Patients with cancer-associated fatigue should be evaluated for coexisting conditions, such as depression, anemia, thyroid dysfunction, and electrolyte disorders.
- In patients with cancer fatigue, consider instituting an exercise program.
- Promising agents under study for treating cancer fatigue include modafinil and ginseng.

SKIN RASH AND EPIDERMAL GROWTH FACTOR RECEPTOR (EGFR) INHIBITORS

Epidermal growth factor receptor (EGFR) inhibitors, now approved by the U.S. Food and Drug Administration (FDA) for use in a variety of cancers, are commonly used for patients with cancer.[127–130] One of the most common toxicities of many of the EGFR inhibitors is a prominent skin rash, affecting up to 50% of patients treated with these drugs.[130–132] This rash has acne-like characteristics, but is not considered to be acne.

Although there are a number of antidotal therapies that have been reported to be potentially useful for this situation, there is a paucity of clinical trial data to dictate appropriate therapy.

Planned accrual has been completed on at least two randomized, double-blinded, placebo-controlled clinical trials that have looked at tetracycline or a tetracycline derivative as a potential means for preventing this rash in patients starting EGFR inhibitors. Abstract presentation of both of these trials suggested that tetracycline or minocycline might decrease rash severity, moderately.[133] Additional work is ongoing to try to better determine the benefit of this approach. Another NCCTG trial has been initiated regarding a sunscreen preparation as another potential way to decrease this toxicity. Of note, there is an interesting phenomenon whereby, in several different study situations, patients who developed a rash actually appeared to have more antitumor activity with the EGFR inhibitor than did those patients who did not develop a rash. This may be related to pharmacogenetic factors.[129,134]

SEXUAL HEALTH

As evidenced in an article in the "Art of Oncology" section of the *Journal of Clinical Oncology*, "The Sounds of Silence. Sexuality Information for Cancer Patients,"[135] discussion of sexual health is not something that often happens in oncologists' offices. There are at least two reasons why this topic rarely is addressed. Oncologists have limited experience and/or comfort with discussing this issue, and there are limited proven therapies available for patients with cancer who have sexuality concerns — at least regarding those therapies that an oncologist can administer. However, it is recommended that this issue be raised for discussion because recommendations are available.[135]

KEY POINTS

- EGFR inhibitors commonly cause rashes.
- Patients with rashes may be more likely to have EGFR inhibitor-induced tumor regression or stability.
- As of yet, there is no proven therapy to prevent or alleviate this problem.

KEY POINTS

- Sexual health concerns are common in patients with cancer.
- Sexual health is not commonly discussed by oncologists.
- Testosterone, without the addition of estrogen replacement therapy, does not appear to help libido in postmenopausal women with cancer.

A recently completed study looking at sexuality issues in patients with cancer evaluated transdermal testosterone in women with complaints of decreased libido. A number of prior trials had evaluated testosterone in a similar dose and formulation in women who did not have cancer. The results of these trials had been positive, suggesting that testosterone did improve libido, at least to some degree.[136,137] The results of this double-blinded, randomized, placebo-controlled trial in women with cancer was, however, convincingly negative.[138] One potential explanation for the reason why this trial was negative in patients with cancer is that the women involved in this trial were postmenopausal and did not receive supplemental estrogen. In all of the previous trials in other patient groups, women had been premenopausal and/or had been receiving estrogen replacement therapy.

OSTEOPOROSIS

Bone health issues in the general population are receiving more attention with the recognition of fracture problems associated with osteopenia/osteoporosis, the aging population, and the availability of treatment options for prevention and/or treatment of this situation. Additional issues regarding osteoporosis — other than those found in the general population — are prominent in woman with breast cancer and men with prostate cancer.

KEY POINTS

- Bone loss is common with estrogen depletion in women.
- Bone loss is common in men receiving androgen ablation therapy.
- Calcium (1,200 to 1,500 mg daily), vitamin D (800 IU daily), and weight-bearing exercise are recommended in patients at risk for bone loss.
- Bisphosphonates should be reserved for patients with osteoporosis or with marked osteopenia with risk factors for bone fractures.
- Bisphosphonates can cause jaw osteonecrosis.

BREAST CANCER

Women with breast cancer are at increased risk for osteoporotic troubles because of treatment-induced menopause in women who are premenopausal. This treatment-induced menopause can occur as a result of chemotherapy or from oophorectomies done for therapeutic or preventative reasons. In addition, aromatase inhibitors lower estrogen levels in women who are postmenopausal and, by this means, increase the risk of osteoporosis and subsequent fractures.

Given these increased risks, ASCO guidelines recommend interval bone mineral density screening for woman with breast cancer after they have become menopausal.[139]

Current recommendations in women with osteopenia or osteoporosis include weight-bearing physical activity, a calcium intake of 1,200 to 1,500 mg per day (in diet and supplements), and vitamin D 800 IU per day. Smoking cessation and moderate or less alcohol intake also is recommended. Bisphosphonates, available in intravenous or oral formulations, also are recommended for woman diagnosed with osteoporosis.

A number of clinical trials have been developed and/or conducted to examine osteoporosis issues in women with breast cancer. Regarding women receiving chemotherapy who are premenopausal, more than 200 patients have been entered on an NCCTG clinical trial that randomly assigns the participants to receive calcium and vitamin D versus the same plus a bisphosphonate. The aim of this trial is to determine whether a bisphosphonate can attenuate the bone loss in this group of patients and prevent bone fractures. The results of this trial should be available by 2008.

A number of trials also have examined the prevention of bone loss associated with aromatase inhibitor therapy. Large trials of women receiving aromatase inhibitors have been conducted in which patients were randomly assigned to receive a bisphosphonate (either intravenous zolendronic acid or oral residronate) or to no treatment. Early results from a few of these trials have demonstrated that bisphosphonate therapy does attenuate the bone loss seen with use of an aromatase inhibitor.[140] However, a substantial reduction in bone fractures has not been reported from these trials, and, therefore, it is not routinely recommended that such patients receive a bisphosphonate as part of standard therapy. In addition, there are ongoing phase II trials, including an NCCTG trial, investigating the use of an aromatase inhibitor in women who currently have marked osteopenia or osteoporosis and who are deemed appropriate for aromatase inhibitor therapy. Results from these trials are pending.

PROSTATE CANCER

It has been well appreciated that men with prostate cancer receiving androgen ablation therapy have an increased risk of bone loss. Studies have randomly assigned men to receive androgen ablation therapy, a bisphosphonate, or to no treatment. The results from these trials demonstrate an attenuation of bone loss with the use of a bisphosphonate. No clear evidence of decreased bone fractures, however, has been reported.[141] Thus, the current recommendations for patients with prostate cancer include screening for bone density and treatment with a bisphosphonate if they become markedly osteopenic or osteoporotic.

OSTEONECROSIS OF THE JAW

Recently, a new side effect of intravenous bisphosphonate therapy, osteonecrosis of the jaw, was recognized.[142,143] This condition is considered to be relatively rare but can be clinically devastating when it occurs. It is particularly problematic in patients with poor dentition and/or in those patients requiring dental work. There has been increased interest in the duration of the bisphosphonate therapy. Oncologists are less cavalier about the routine use of long-term bisphosphonate therapy for patients with cancer, based on this newly described toxicity. The safest and most effective interval for treatment with bisphosphonates is yet to be defined.

ANEMIA

Anemia is a common problem in patients with cancer. Multiple causes for anemia include bleeding, hemolosis, deficiency of a micronutrient (e.g., iron, folate, or vitamin B12), anemia of chronic disease, and other causes from chemotherapy and radiation therapy.

Anemia can cause many symptoms including fatigue, shortness of breath, and angina. Appropriate evaluation of patients with anemia is important and includes evaluation for sites of blood loss, hemolosis, or deficiencies of iron, folate, and/or vitamin B12.

Erythropoietic agents, such as erythropoietin and darbopoiten, are commonly used in treatment of patients with

KEY POINTS

- Anemia is common in patients with cancer.
- Anemia is caused by multiple factors including anticancer therapy with chemotherapy, radiation therapy, or surgery.
- Transfusions are recommended for patients with symptomatic anemia.
- For less severe anemia, erythropoietic agents do decrease transfusion requirements, increase hemoglobin levels, and potentially improve quality of life.
- Both darbopoetin and erythropoietin are relatively similar regarding efficacy and safety.
- Current recommendations are to cease use of erythropoietin products when the hemoglobin level is greater than or equal to 12 g/dL.

chemotherapy-induced anemia. Although they appear to be helpful for increasing hemoglobin concentrations in patients with cancer-associated but not chemotherapy-associated anemia, there is evidence that these agents may stimulate tumor growth and decrease survival in some patients; therefore, this indication is not approved by the FDA. Currently, there is no convincing evidence that one agent is particularly better than the other agent — both of these agents increase hemoglobin levels as well as decrease transfusion requirements. There is information suggesting that both also can improve quality of life, but this has not been shown in all trials.[144]

Initially erythropoietin was administered three times per week, but currently this is rarely the case. Schedules of every week compared with every 2 and every 3 weeks have been studied to varying degrees with both erythropoietin and darbopoiten. In the United States, the choice of erythropoietin agents in different practices is oftentimes determined based on contract issues with pharmaceutical companies.

There are data to demonstrate that erythropoietic agents increase the risk of thromboembolic complications, and there are data that suggest that this might be a problem with higher hemoglobin levels. For this reason, erythropoietic agents should be stopped when hemoglobin levels reach 12 mg/dL or higher. There are very rare cases of red cell aplasia that have been reported in conjunction with use of some erythropoietic agents.

Some trials have suggested that erythropoietic agents could adversely affect survival.[145,146] Although a meta-analysis of trials investigating erythropoietic products did not suggest that these agents had a detrimental effect on survival,[147] additional trials[148] have shown that erythropoietic products can have a negative effect on survival, especially, it seems, if used without concomitant chemotherapy. NCCN guidelines suggest that, although it is reasonable to consider erythropoietic therapy with hemoglobin levels between 10 and 11 g/dL, it also is reasonable to consider these agents for asymptomatic patients only if the hemoglobin level drops lower than 10 g/dL.

Given the new data on erythropoietic products and the high profile they carry, the FDA has reissued its stance that the use of these drugs in the oncology setting should be restricted to patients receiving chemotherapy. In addition, these agents should not be administered to patients with hemoglobin levels greater than 12.0 g/dL, and doses should be withheld or reduced if hemoglobin levels increase more than 1 g/dL in any 2-week period.

REFERENCES

1. Mortimer JE, Bartlett NL. Assessment of knowledge about cancer pain management by physicians in training. *J Pain Symptom Manage.* 1997; 14(1):21–28.
2. Von Roenn JH, Cleeland CS, Gonin R, et al. Physician attitudes and practice in cancer pain management. A survey from the Eastern Cooperative Oncology Group. *Ann Intern Med.* 1993;119(2):121–126.
3. Cleeland CS, Janjan NA, Scott CB, et al. Cancer pain management by radiotherapists: a survey of radiation therapy oncology group physicians. *Int J Radiat Oncol Biol Phys.* 2000;47(1):203–208.
4. Indelicato RA, Portenoy RK. Opioid rotation in the management of refractory cancer pain. *J Clin Oncol.* 2002; 20(1):348–352.
5. Ryan M, Moynihan TJ, Loprinzi CL. As-needed morphine: yes, but at what dose and at what interval? *J Clin Oncol.* 2005;23(16):3849–3852.
6. Lauretti GR, Oliveira GM, Pereira NL. Comparison of sustained-release morphine with sustained-release oxycodone in advanced cancer patients. *Br J Cancer.* 2003; 89(11):2027–2030.
7. Payne R, Mathias SD, Pasta DJ, et al. Quality of life and cancer pain: satisfaction and side effects with transdermal fentanyl versus oral morphine. *J Clin Oncol.* 1998; 16(4):1588–1593.
8. Smith TJ, Staats PS, Deer T, et al. Randomized clinical trial of an implantable drug delivery system compared with comprehensive medical management for refractory cancer pain: impact on pain, drug-related toxicity, and survival. *J Clin Oncol.* 2002;20(19):4040–4049.
9. Nicholson AB. Methadone for cancer pain. *Cochrane Database Syst Rev.* 2004; (2)CD003971.
10. Cleeland CS, Gonin R, Hatfield AK, et al. Pain and its treatment in outpatients with metastatic cancer. *N Engl J Med.*1994;330(9):592–596.
11. Portenoy RK, Miransky J, Thaler HT, et al. Pain in ambulatory patients with lung or colon cancer. Prevalence, characteristics, and effect. *Cancer.* 1992; 70(6):1616–1624.
12. Grossman S, Benedetti C, Payne R, et al. NCCN practice guidelines for cancer pain. *Oncology.* 1999;13:33–44.
13. Levy MH. Pharmacologic treatment of cancer pain. *N Engl J Med.* 1996;335(15):1124–1132.
14. Gardell LR, King T, Ossipov MH, et al. Opioid receptor-mediated hyperalgesia and antinociceptive tolerance induced by sustained opiate delivery. *Neurosci Lett.* 2006;396(1):44–49.
15. Gralla RJ, Osoba D, Kris MG, et al. Recommendations for the use of antiemetics: evidence-based, clinical practice guidelines. American Society of Clinical Oncology. *J Clin Oncol.*1999;17(9):2971–2994.
16. Hesketh PJ. Comparative review of 5-HT3 receptor antagonists in the treatment of acute chemotherapy-induced nausea and vomiting. *Cancer Invest.* 2000,18(2):163–173.
17. Hesketh PJ, Kris MG, Grunberg SM, et al. Proposal for classifying the acute emetogenicity of cancer chemotherapy. *J Clin Oncol.* 1997;15(1): 103–109.
18. Kris MG, Hesketh PJ, Somerfield MR, et al. American Society of Clinical Oncology guideline for antiemetics in oncology: update 2006. *J Clin Oncol.* 2006;24(18):2932–2947.
19. Eisenberg P, Figueroa-Vadillo J, Zamora R, et al. Improved prevention of moderately emetogenic chemotherapy-induced nausea and vomiting with palonosetron, a pharmacologically novel 5-HT3 receptor antagonist: results of a phase III, single-dose trial versus dolasetron. *Cancer.* 2003;98(11):2473–2482.
20. Aapro MS, Bertoli L, Lyer P. Palonosetron is an effective as ondansetron in preventing chemotherapy-induced nausea and vomiting in patietns receiving highly emetogenic chemotherapy: results of a phase III trial. *Supportice Care in Cancer.* 2003; Berlin, Germany.
21. Vardy J, Chiew KS, Galica J, et al. Side effects associated with the use of dexamethasone for prophylaxis of delayed emesis after moderately emetogenic chemotherapy. *Br J Cancer.* 2006;94(7):1011–1015.
22. Poli-Bigelli S, Rodrigues-Pereira J, Carides AD, et al. Addition of the neurokinin 1 receptor antagonist aprepitant to standard antiemetic therapy improves control of chemotherapy-induced nausea and vomit-

ing. Results from a randomized, double-blind, placebo-controlled trial in Latin America. *Cancer.* 2003;97(12):3090–3098.

23. Loprinzi CL, Alberts SR, Christensen BJ, et al. History of the development of antiemetic guidelines at Mayo Clinic Rochester. *Mayo Clin Proc.* 2000;75(3):303–309.

24. Roila F, Hesketh PJ, Herrstedt J. Prevention of chemotherapy- and radiotherapy-induced emesis: results of the 2004 Perugia International Antiemetic Consensus Conference. *Ann Oncol.* 2006; 17(1): 20–28.

25. Gralla RJ, Roila F, Tonato M. The 2004 Perugia Antiemetic Consensus Guideline process: methods, procedures, and participants. *Support Care Cancer.* 2005;13(2):77–79.

26. Kris MG, Hesketh PJ, Herrstedt J, et al. Consensus proposals for the prevention of acute and delayed vomiting and nausea following high-emetic-risk chemotherapy. *Support Care Cancer.* 2005;13(2):85–96.

27. Ventafridda V, Ripamonti C, Caraceni A, et al. The management of inoperable gastrointestinal obstruction in terminal cancer patients. *Tumori.* 1990; 76(4):389–393.

28. Feuer DJ, Broadley KE, Shepherd JH, Barton DP. Systematic review of surgery in malignant bowel obstruction in advanced gynecological and gastrointestinal cancer. The Systematic Review Steering Committee. *Gynecol Oncol.* 1999;75(3):313–322.

29. Ripamonti C. Bowel obstruction. Philadelphia, PA: Lippincott-Raven: 1998.

30. Riley J, Fallon MT. Octreotide in terminal malignant obstruction of the gastrointestinal tract. *Eur J Palliat Care.* 1994;1:23–25.

31. Mangili G, Franchi M, Mariani A, et al. Octreotide in the management of bowel obstruction in terminal ovarian cancer. *Gynecol Oncol.* 1996; 61(3):345–348.

32. Mercadante S, Maddaloni S. Octreotide in the management of inoperable gastrointestinal obstruction in terminal cancer patients. *J Pain Symptom Manage.* 1992; 7(8):496–498.

33. Couzi RJ, Helzlsouer KJ, Fetting JH. Prevalence of menopausal symptoms among women with a history of breast cancer and attitudes toward estrogen replacement therapy. *J Clin Oncol.* 1995;13(11):2737–2744.

34. Charig CR, Rundle JS. Flushing. Long-term side effect of orchiectomy in treatment of prostatic carcinoma. *Urology.* 1989; 33(3):175–178.

35. Vassilopoulou-Sellin R, Zolinski C. Estrogen replacement therapy in women with breast cancer: a survey of patient attitudes. *Am J Med Sci.* 1992; 304(3):145–149.

36. O'Meara ES, Rossing MA, Daling JR, et al. Hormone replacement therapy after a diagnosis of breast cancer in relation to recurrence and mortality. *J Natl Cancer Inst.* 2001;93(10):754–762.

37. Loprinzi CL, Michalak JC, Quella SK, et al. Megestrol acetate for the prevention of hot flashes. *N Engl J Med.*1994;331(6):347–352.

38. Barton D, Loprinzi C, Quella S, et al. Depomedroxyprogesterone acetate for hot flashes. *J Pain Symptom Manage.* 2002;24(6):603–607.

39. Loprinzi CL, Levitt R, Barton D, et al. Phase III comparison of depomedroxyprogesterone acetate to venlafaxine for managing hot flashes: North Central Cancer Treatment Group Trial N99C7. *J Clin Oncol.* 2006; 24(9):1409–1414.

40. Loprinzi CL, Kugler JW, Sloan JA, et al. Venlafaxine in management of hot flashes in survivors of breast cancer: a randomised controlled trial. *Lancet.* 2000; 356(9247):2059–2063.

41. Stearns V, Beebe KL, Iyengar M, Dube E. Paroxetine controlled release in the treatment of menopausal hot flashes: a randomized controlled trial. *JAMA.* 2003; 289(21):2827–2834.

42. Loprinzi CL, Sloan JA, Perez EA, et al. Phase III evaluation of fluoxetine for treatment of hot flashes. *J Clin Oncol.* 2002;20(6):1578–1583.

43. Kimmick GG, Lovato J, McQuellon R, et al. Randomized, double-blind, placebo-controlled, crossover study of sertraline (Zoloft) for the treatment of hot flashes in women with early stage breast cancer taking tamoxifen. *Breast J.* 2006;12(2):114–122.

44. Borges S, Desta Z, Li L, et al. Quantitative effect of CYP2D6 genotype and inhibitors on tamoxifen metabolism: implication for optimization of breast cancer treatment. *Clin Pharmacol Ther.* 2006; 80(1):61–74.

45. Guttuso TJ Jr. Gabapentin's effects on hot flashes and hypothermia. *Neurology.* 2000; 54(11):2161–2163.

46. Loprinzi CL, Barton DL, Sloan JA, et al. Pilot evaluation of gabapentin for treating hot flashes. *Mayo Clin Proc.* 2002; 77:1159-1163.

47. Guttuso T Jr., Kurlan R, McDermott MP, Kieburtz K. Gabapentin's effects on hot flashes in postmenopausal women: a randomized controlled trial. *Obstet Gynecol.* 2003; 101(2):337–345.

48. Pandya KJ, Morrow GR, Roscoe JA, et al. Gabapentin for hot flashes in 420 women with breast cancer: a randomised double-blind placebo-controlled trial. *Lancet.* 2005; 366(9488):818–824.

49. Reddy SY, Warner H, Guttuso T Jr. et al. Gabapentin, estrogen, and placebo for treating hot flushes: a randomized controlled trial. *Obstet Gynecol.* 2006; 108(1):41–48.

50. Goldberg RM, Loprinzi CL, O'Fallon JR, et al. Transdermal clonidine for ameliorating tamoxifen-induced hot flashes. *J Clin Oncol.* 1994; 12(1):155–158.

51. Quella SK, Loprinzi CL, Barton DL, et al. Evaluation of soy phytoestrogens for the treatment of hot flashes in breast cancer survivors: A North Central Cancer Treatment Group Trial. *J Clin Oncol.* 2000; 18(5):1068–1074.

52. Nelson HD, Vesco KK, Haney E, et al. Nonhormonal therapies for menopausal hot flashes: systematic review and meta-analysis. *JAMA.* 2006; 295(17):2057–2071.

53. Loprinzi CL, Abu-Ghazaleh S, Sloan JA, et al. Phase III randomized double-blind study to evaluate the efficacy of a polycarbophil-based vaginal moisturizer in women with breast cancer. *J Clin Oncol.* 1997; 15(3):969–973.

54. Bygdeman M, Swahn ML. Replens versus dienoestrol cream in the symptomatic treatment of vaginal atrophy in postmenopausal women. *Maturitas.* 1996; 23(3):259–263.

55. Vivino FB, Al-Hashimi I, Khan Z, et al. Pilocarpine tablets for the treatment of dry mouth and dry eye symptoms in patients with Sjogren syndrome: a randomized, placebo-controlled, fixed-dose, multicenter trial. P92-01 Study Group. *Arch Intern Med.* 1999; 159(2):174–181.

56. le Veque G, Hendrix S. Oral pilocarpine to treat vaginal xerosis associated with chemotherapy-induced amenorrhea in pre-menopausal women. *J Clin Oncol.* 2004;22:749.

57. Rubenstein EB, Peterson DE, Schubert M, et al. Clinical practice guidelines for the prevention and treatment of cancer therapy-induced oral and gastrointestinal mucositis. *Cancer.* 2004; 100(9 Suppl): 2026–2046.

58. Mahood DJ, Dose AM, Loprinzi CL, et al. Inhibition of fluorouracil-induced stomatitis by oral cryotherapy. *J Clin Oncol.* 1991; 9(3):449–452.

59. Cascinu S, Fedeli A, Fedeli SL, Catalano G. Oral cooling (cryotherapy), an effective treatment for the prevention of 5-fluorouracil-induced stomatitis. *Eur J Cancer B Oral Oncol.* 1994; 30B(4):234–236.

60. Edelman MJ, Gandara DR, Perez EA, et al. Phase I trial of edatrexate plus carboplatin in advanced solid tumors: amelioration of dose-limiting mucositis by ice chip cryotherapy. *Invest New Drugs.* 1998; 16(1): 69–75.

61. Gandara DR, Edelman MJ, Crowley JJ, et al. Phase II trial of edatrexate plus carboplatin in metastatic non-small-cell lung cancer: a Southwest Oncology Group study. *Cancer Chemother Pharmacol.* 1997; 41(1):75–78.

62. Dreicer R, Propert KJ, Kuzel T, et al. A phase II trial of edatrexate in patients with advanced renal cell carcinoma. An Eastern Cooperative Oncology Group study. *Am J Clin Oncol.* 1997;20(3):251–253.

63. Spielberger R, Stiff P, Bensinger W, et al. Palifermin for oral mucositis after intensive therapy for hematologic cancers. *N Engl J Med.* 2004; 351(25):2590–2598.

64. Loprinzi CL, Martenson JA. Keratinocyte growth factor: not yet ready for prime time. *J Clin Oncol.* 2003; 21(8):1429–1430.

65. Stiff P, Emmanouilides C, Bensinger W, et al. Palifermin (Kepivance) reduces patient reported mouth and throat soreness and improves patient functioning in the hematopoietic stem cell transplantation setting: phase 3 trial results. *J Clin Oncol.* 2006; In Press.

66. Loprinzi C, Barton D, Sloan JA. Whose opinion counts? *J Clin Oncol.* 2006; 24(33):5183–5185.

67. McGinnis WL, Loprinzi CL, Buskirk SJ, et al. Placebo-controlled trial of sucralfate for inhibiting radiation-induced esophagitis. *J Clin Oncol.* 1997;15(3):1239–1243.

68. Komaki R, Lee JS, Kaplan B, et al. Randomized phase III study of chemoradiation with or without amifostine for patients with favorable performance status inoperable stage II-III non-small cell lung cancer: preliminary results. *Semin Radiat Oncol.* 2002;12(1 Suppl 1):46–49.

69. Antonadou D, Coliarakis N, Synodinou M, et al. Randomized phase III trial of radiation treatment ± amifostine in patients with advanced-stage lung cancer. *Int J Radiat Oncol Biol Phys.* 2001; 51(4):915–922.

70. Williams JWJ, Simel DL. Does this patient have ascites? How to divine fluid in the abdomen. JAMA 1992;267: 2645–2658.

71. Murphy M, Rossi M. Managing ascites via the Tenckhoff catheter. *Medsurg Nurs.* 1995; 4(6):468–471.

72. Cairns W, Malone R. Octreotide as an agent for the relief of malignant ascites in palliative care patients. *Palliat Med.* 1999; 13(5):429–430.

73. DeWys WD, Begg C, Lavin PT, et al. Prognostic effect of weight loss prior to chemotherapy in cancer patients. Eastern Cooperative On cology Group. *Am J Med.* 1980; 69(4):491–497.

74. Tisdale MJ. Biology of cachexia. *J Natl Cancer Inst.* 1997; 89(23): 1763–1773.

75. McGeer AJ, Detsky AS, O'Rourke K. Parenteral nutrition in cancer patients undergoing chemotherapy: a meta-analysis. *Nutrition.* 1990; 6(3):233–240.

76. Jatoi A, Kumar S, Sloan JA, Nguyen PL. On appetite and its loss. *J Clin Oncol.* 2000; 18(15):2930–2932.

77. Loprinzi CL, Ellison NM, Schaid DJ, et al. Controlled trial of megestrol acetate for the treatment of cancer anorexia and cachexia. *J Natl Cancer Inst.* 1990;82(13):1127–1132.

78. Rowland KM, Jr., Loprinzi CL, Shaw EG et al. Randomized double-blind placebo-controlled trial of cisplatin and etoposide plus megestrol acetate/placebo in extensive-stage small-cell lung cancer: a North Central Cancer Treatment Group study. J Clin Oncol 1996;14: 135–141.

79. Jatoi A, Loprinzi CL. Loss of appetite and weight. Cambridge, UK: Cambridge University Press 2003.

80. Moertel CG, Schutt AJ, Reitemeier RJ, Hahn RG. Corticosteroid therapy of preterminal gastrointestinal cancer. Cancer 1974;33: 1607–1609.

81. Loprinzi CL, Kugler JW, Sloan JA et al. Randomized comparison of megestrol acetate versus dexamethasone versus fluoxymesterone for the treatment of cancer anorexia/cachexia. *J Clin Oncol.* 1999; 17(10):3299–3306.

82. Kardinal CG, Loprinzi CL, Schaid DJ, et al. A controlled trial of cyproheptadine in cancer patients with anorexia and/or cachexia. *Cancer.* 1990;65(12):2657–2662.

83. Loprinzi CL, Kuross SA, O'Fallon JR, et al. Randomized placebo-controlled evaluation of hydrazine sulfate in patients with advanced colorectal cancer. *J Clin Oncol.* 1994; 12(6):1121–1125.

84. Loprinzi CL, Goldberg RM, Su JQ, et al. Placebo-controlled trial of hydrazine sulfate in patients with newly diagnosed non-small-cell lung cancer. *J Clin Oncol.* 1994;12(6):1126–1129.

85. Goldberg RM, Loprinzi CL, Mailliard JA, et al. Pentoxifylline for treatment of cancer anorexia and cachexia? A randomized, double-blind, placebo-controlled trial. *J Clin Oncol.* 1995; 13(11):2856–2859.

86. Jatoi A, Windschitl HE, Loprinzi CL, et al. Dronabinol versus megestrol acetate versus combination therapy for cancer-associated anorexia: a North Central Cancer Treatment Group study. *J Clin Oncol.* 2002; 20(2):567–573.

87. Jatoi A, Dakhil SR, Kugler JW, et al. A placebo-controlled trial of etanercept, a tumor necrosis factor (TNF) inhibitor, in patients with the cancer anorexia/weight loss syndrome. North Central Cancer Treatment Group (NCCTG) trial N00C1. *J Clin Oncol.* 2006; 24: 476s.

88. Wadler S, Benson AB 3rd, Engelking C, et al. Recommended guidelines for the treatment of chemotherapy-induced diarrhea. *J Clin Oncol.* 1998; 16(9):3169–3178.

89. Cascinu S, Fedeli A, Fedeli SL, Catalano G. Octreotide versus loperamide in the treatment of fluorouracil-induced diarrhea: a randomized trial. *J Clin Oncol.* 1993;11(1):148–151.

90. Gebbia V, Carreca I, Testa A, et al. Subcutaneous octreotide versus oral loperamide in the treatment of diarrhea following chemotherapy. *Anticancer Drugs.* 1993;4(4):443–445.

91. Miller RC, Martenson JA, Sargent DJ, et al. Acute treatment-related diarrhea during postoperative adjuvant therapy for high-risk rectal carcinoma. *Int J Radiat Oncol Biol Phys.* 1998;41(3):593–598.

92. Martenson JA Jr, Hyland G, Moertel CG, et al. Olsalazine is contraindicated during pelvic radiation therapy: results of a double-blind, randomized clinical trial. *Int J Radiat Oncol Biol Phys.* 1996; 35(2):299–303.

93. Heusinkveld RS, Manning MR, Aristizabal SA. Control of radiation-induced diarrhea with cholestyramine. *Int J Radiat Oncol Biol Phys.* 1978;4(7-8):687-690.

94. Kozelsky TF, Meyers GE, Sloan JA et al. Phase III double-blind study of glutamine versus placebo for the prevention of acute diarrhea in patients receiving pelvic radiation therapy. *J Clin Oncol.* 2003, 21(9):1669–1674.

95. Martenson JA, Sloan J, Deming RL et al. Phase III double-blind study of depot octreotide versus placebo in the prevention of acute diarrhea during pelvic radiation therapy: results of North Central Cancer Treatment Group protocol N00CA. *J Clin Oncol.* 2006; 24:469s.

96. Yavuz MN, Yavuz AA, Ilis E, et al. A randomized study of the efficacy of octreotide versus diphenoxylate on radiation-induced diarrhea. *Proc Am Soc Clin Oncol.* 2000; 19:602a.

97. Ripamonti C, Bruera E. Dyspnea: pathophysiology and assessment. *J Pain Symptom Manage.* 1997; 13(4) 220–232.

98. Dudgeon DJ, Lertzman M. Dyspnea in the advanced cancer patient. *J Pain Symptom Manage.* 1998; 16(4):212–219.

99. Borg G. Borg's perceived exertion and pain scales. Champaign, IL:1998.

100. Dudgeon DJ, Rosenthal S. Management of dyspnea and cough in patients with cancer. *Hematol Oncol Clin North Am.* 1996; 10(1): 157–171.

101. Bruera E, de Stoutz N, Velasco-Leiva A, et al. Effects of oxygen on dyspnoea in hypoxaemic terminal-cancer patients. *Lancet.* 1993; 342(9962):13–14.

102. Schwartzstein RM, Lahive K, Pope A, et al. Cold facial stimulation reduces breathlessness induced in normal subjects. *Am Rev Respir Dis.* 1987;136(1):58–61.

103. Allard P, Lamontagne C, Bernard P, Tremblay C. How effective are supplementary doses of opioids for dyspnea in terminally ill cancer patients? A randomized continuous sequential clinical trial. *J Pain Symptom Manage.* 1999;17(4):256–265.

104. Chandler S. Nebulized opioids to treat dyspnea. *Am J Hosp Palliat Care.* 1999;16(1):418–422.

105. Foral PA, Malesker MA, Huerta G, Hilleman DE. Nebulized opioids use in COPD. *Chest.* 2004;125(2):691–694.

106. Joyce M, McSweeney M, Carrieri-Kolhman VL, Hawkins J. The use of nebulized opioids in the management of dyspnea: evidence synthesis. *Oncol Nurs Forum.* 2004;31(3):551–561.

107. Thomas JR, von Gunten CF. Clinical management of dyspnoea. *Lancet Oncol.* 2002;3(4):223–228.

108. Smith TJ, Loprinzi CL, von Gunten CF, et al. ASCO Cirriculum: Optimizing cancer care—the importance of symptom management. Dubuque, IA: Kendall/Hunt Publishing 2001.

109. Mock V. Fatigue management: evidence and guidelines for practice. *Cancer.* 2001; 92(6 Suppl):1699–1707.

110. Fulton C, Knowles G. Cancer fatigue. *Eur J Cancer Care (Engl).* 2000; 9(3):167–171.

111. NCCN cancer related fatigue clinical practice guidelines. Oncology 2003; V.

112. Mock V, Burke MB, Sheehan P, et al. A nursing rehabilitation program for women with breast cancer receiving adjuvant chemotherapy. *Oncol Nurs Forum.* 1994; 21(5):899–907; discussion 908.

113. Schwartz AL, Mori M, Gao R, et al. Exercise reduces daily fatigue in women with breast cancer receiving chemotherapy. *Med Sci Sports Exerc.* 2001; 33(5):718–723.

114. Mock V, Pickett M, Ropka ME, et al. Fatigue and quality of life outcomes of exercise during cancer treatment. *Cancer Pract.* 2001; 9(3):119–127.

115. Stevinson C, Lawlor DA, Fox KR. Exercise interventions for cancer patients: systematic review of controlled trials. *Cancer Causes Control.* 2004; 15(10):1035–1056.

116. Stricker CT, Drake D, Hoyer KA, Mock V. Evidence-based practice for fatigue management in adults with cancer: exercise as an intervention. *Oncol Nurs Forum.* 2004; 31(5):963–976.

117. Galvao DA, Newton RU. Review of exercise intervention studies in cancer patients. *J Clin Oncol.* 2005;23(4):899–909.

118. Knols R, Aaronson NK, Uebelhart D, et al. Physical exercise in cancer patients during and after medical treatment: a systematic review of randomized and controlled clinical trials. *J Clin Oncol.* 2005; 23(16):3830–3842.

119. Schmitz KH, Holtzman J, Courneya KS, et al. Controlled physical activity trials in cancer survivors: a systematic review and meta-analysis. *Cancer Epidemiol Biomarkers Prev.* 2005; 14(7): 1588–1595.

120. Stankoff B, Waubant E, Confavreux C, et al. Modafinil for fatigue in MS: a randomized placebo-controlled double-blind study. *Neurology.* 2005; 64(7):1139–1143.

121. Tadano T, Nakagawasai O, Niijima F et al. The effects of traditional tonics on fatigue in mice differ from those of the antidepressant imipramine: a pharmacological and behavioral study. *Am J Chin Med.* 2000; 28(1):97–104.

122. Banerjee U, Izquierdo JA. Antistress and antifatigue properties of Panax ginseng: comparison with piracetam. *Acta Physiol Lat Am.* 1982; 32(4):277–285.

123. Younus J, Collins A, Wang X, et al. A double-blind, placebo-controlled pilot study to evaluate the effect of singseng on fatigue and quality of life in adult chemo-naive cancer patients. *Proc Am Soc Clin Oncol.* 2003; 22.

124. Engels HJ, Fahlman MM, Wirth JC. Effects of ginseng on secretory IgA, performance, and recovery from interval exercise. *Med Sci Sports Exerc.*2003; 35(4):690–696.

125. Engels HJ, Kolokouri I, Cieslak TJ 2nd, Wirth JC. Effects of ginseng supplementation on supramaximal exercise performance and short-term recovery. *J Strength Cond Res.*2001; 15(3):290–295.

126. Barton DL. A pilot, multi-dose, placebo-controlled evaluation of American ginseng (panax quinquefolius) to improve cancer-related fatigure: NCCTG trial N03CA. 2007 ASCO Annual Meeting. Abstract 9001.

127. Baselga J, Rischin D, Ranson M, et al. Phase I safety, pharmacokinetic, and pharmacodynamic trial of ZD1839, a selective oral epidermal growth factor receptor tyrosine kinase inhibitor, in patients with five selected solid tumor types. *J Clin Oncol.* 2002; 20(21): 4292–4302.

128. Fukuoka M, Yano S, Giaccone G, et al. Multi-institutional randomized phase II trial of gefitinib for previously treated patients with advanced non-small-cell lung cancer (The IDEAL 1 Trial) [corrected]. *J Clin Oncol.* 2003;21(12):2237–2246.

129. Cohen EE, Rosen F, Stadler WM, et al. Phase II trial of ZD1839 in recurrent or metastatic squamous cell carcinoma of the head and neck. *J Clin Oncol.* 2003;21(10):1980–1987.

130. Herbst RS, Maddox AM, Rothenberg ML, et al. Selective oral epidermal growth factor receptor tyrosine kinase inhibitor ZD1839 is generally well-tolerated and has activity in non-small-cell lung cancer and other solid tumors: results of a phase I trial. *J Clin Oncol.* 2002; 20(18): 3815–3825.

131. Kris MG, Natale RB, Herbst RS, et al. Efficacy of gefitinib, an inhibitor of the epidermal growth factor receptor tyrosine kinase, in symptomatic patients with non-small cell lung cancer: a randomized trial. *JAMA.* 2003;290(16):2149–2158.

132. Saltz LB, Meropol NJ, Loehrer PJ Sr, et al. Phase II trial of cetuximab in patients with refractory colorectal cancer that expresses the epidermal growth factor receptor. *J Clin Oncol.* 2004;22(7):1201–1208.

133. Jatoi A, Rowland K, Sloan A, et al. Does tetracycline prevent/palliate epidermal growth factor receptor (EGFR) inhibitor-induced rash? A phase III trial from the North Central Cancer Treatment Group (N03CB). 2007 ASCO Annual Meeting. Abstract LBA 9006.

134. Perez-Soler R. Can rash associated with HER1/EGFR inhibition be used as a marker of treatment outcome? Oncology (Williston Park) 2003;17: 23–28.

135. Katz A. The sounds of silence: sexuality information for cancer patients. *J Clin Oncol.* 2005;23(1):238–241.

136. Shifren JL, Braunstein GD, Simon JA, et al. Transdermal testosterone treatment in women with impaired sexual function after oophorectomy. *New Engl J Med.* 2000;343(10):682–688.

137. Nathorst-Boos J, Floter A, Jarkander-Rolff M, et al. Treatment with percutaneous testosterone gel in postmenopausal women with decreased libido—effects on sexuality and psychological general well-being *Matuiras.* 2006; 53(1):11–18.

138. Barton DL, Loprinzi CL, Winder D et al. Transdermal testosterone in female cancer survivors with decreased libido. J Clin Oncol 2006; 24: 469s.

139. Hillner BE, Ingle JN, Berenson JR, et al. American Society of Clinical Oncology guideline on the role of bisphosphonates in breast cancer. American Society of Clinical Oncology Bisphosphonates Expert Panel. *J Clin Oncol.* 2000;18:1378–1391.

140. Brufsky A. Management of cancer-treatment-induced bone loss in postmenopausal women undergoing adjuvant breast cancer therapy: a Z-FAST update. *Semin Oncol.* 2006; 33(2 Suppl 7):S13–17.

141. Smith MR, Eastham J, Gleason DM, et al. Randomized controlled trial of zoledronic acid to prevent bone loss in men receiving androgen deprivation therapy for nonmetastatic prostate cancer. *J Urol.* 2003; 169(6):2008–2012.

142. Ruggiero SL, Mehrotra B, Rosenberg TJ, Engroff SL. Osteonecrosis of the jaws associated with the use of bisphosphonates: a review of 63 cases. *J Oral Maxillofac Surg.* 2004; 62(5):527–534.

143. Woo SB, Hellstein JW, Kalmar JR. Narrative [corrected] review: bisphosphonates and osteonecrosis of the jaws. *Ann Intern Med.* 2006; 144(10):753–761.

144. Witzig TE, Silberstein PT, Loprinzi CL, et al. A Phase III randomized double-blind study of epoetin alfa versus placebo in anemic patients with cancer undergoing chemotherapy. *J Clin Oncol.* 2005;12(12):2606–2617.

145. Henke M, Laszig R, Rube C, et al. Erythropoietin to treat head and neck cancer patients with anaemia undergoing radiotherapy: randomised, double-blind, placebo-controlled trial. *Lancet.* 2003; 362 (9392):1255–1260.

146. Leyland-Jones B. Breast cancer trial with erythropoietin terminated unexpectedly. *Lancet Oncol.* 2003;4(8):459–460.

147. Bohlius J, Langensiepen S, Schwarzer G, et al. Erythropoietin for patients with malignant disease. *Cochrane Database Syst Rev.* 2004; (3)CD003407.

148. Wright JR, Ung YC, Julian JA, et al. Randomized, double-blind, placebo-controlled trial of erythropoietin in non-small-cell lung cancer with disease-related anemia. *J Clin Oncol.* 2007;25:1027-1032.

19

CANCER IN THE ELDERLY

Joanne Mortimer, MD

LEARNING OBJECTIVES

After reviewing this chapter, the reader should be able to

- Evaluate how the physiologic changes of aging affect the treatment of cancer and palliation of symptoms
- Explain the distinction between physiologic age and chronologic age
- Use the Comprehensive Geriatric Assessment as a way to define physiologic functional reserve and frailty
- Critically evaluate the available "evidence-based" data for treating individual cancers in older patients

More than 60% of all cancers are diagnosed in individuals who are age 65 or older, and cancer is 11 times more likely to develop in people in that age group than in people younger than 65. In addition, patients with cancer who are older than 65 are 16 times more likely to die of the disease.[1, 2] This disproportionately high death rate may be attributed in part to comorbid conditions that may be more life-threatening than the cancer itself; comorbidities may impede the aggressive multidisciplinary treatment of cancer. It has been estimated that by the year 2030, 20% of the U.S. population (70 million people) will be older than 65. By the year 2020, the population will have increased by 12%, but because of the large numbers of older individuals, the incidence of cancer in the overall population is expected to increase by 60%.[3] Such projections highlight the enormity of the incidence of cancer in the older population. Although the median age at which cancer develops is 68, cancer in the elderly has only recently emerged as a subspecialty. For most malignancies, the death rate is disproportionately higher for the elderly population. Possible explanations include an altered natural history of some cancers, competing comorbid medical conditions, decreased physiologic reserve compromising the ability to tolerate therapy, physicians' reluctance to provide aggressive therapy, and barriers in the elderly's access to care. Communication between health care providers and elderly patients may be hampered by deficits in hearing, vision, and cognition. Organ decline and the coexistence of other chronic medical conditions may make it difficult not only to give aggressive cancer treatment but also to give optimal palliative care. These challenges contribute to defining cancer in the elderly as a true subspecialty.

KEY POINTS

- Cancer is a disease of the older population.
- The cancer-related or cause-specific mortality rate for patients who are older than 65 is disproportionally higher than the incidence.

For both the geriatrician and the oncologist, the expectation of high-quality medical care is to maximize the duration of life while maintaining its quality. An understanding of the biology of aging, an appreciation of the effect of comorbidities, and a willingness to spend time with the patient and his or her family are essential to providing care for older patients.

BIOLOGY

The physiologic changes of telomere shortening and defective DNA repair mechanisms are common to both aging and cancer and may partially explain the high incidence of cancer in the older population. This functional decline begins at age 30 and continues at a loss of approximately 1% per year. The aging process occurs at a different rate in each person, and the loss of individual organ reserve occurs at different rates within the same person.[4,5] In most cases, these physiologic changes are clinically imperceptible. However, the delicate balance of functioning can be severely disrupted by an illness and the consequent medical intervention. Once this balance is upset, the patient's physiology may not return to its baseline.

The physiologic changes of aging that lead to decreased functional reserve have an effect on every organ system. The percentage of body fat increases while total body water and muscle mass decrease. Hormone dysfunction can be measured as decreases in renin, aldosterone, dehydroepiandrosterone (DHEA), sex hormones, and triiodothyronine; however, insulin, norepinephrine, parathyroid hormone (PTH), vasopressin, and atrial natriuretic peptide increase. Senescent production of hormones results in a decrease in protein synthesis and contributes to the age-related loss of strength and muscle mass known as sarcopenia.[6] The integument of the skin changes, becoming increasingly dry as sweat glands are lost. The thinning of skin and loss of subcutaneous connective tissue and fat expose blood vessels and contribute to tears and bruising.

Functional decline in the gastrointestinal tract manifests as a decrease in motility and absorption. As blood flow and liver mass decrease, hepatic function declines. Metabolism through the cytochrome P450 microsomal enzyme system also decreases, thus impairing the body's ability to convert some drugs to their active metabolite and compromising the elimination of other drugs. In the kidney, renal blood flow decreases, and both kidney mass and glomeruli are lost and replaced by fat and fibrotic tissue. These changes cause a decrease in the kidney's ability to concentrate urine, excrete water, and eliminate toxins.

KEY POINTS

- Physiologic changes of aging begin at age 30.
- The rate of physiologic change with aging varies by organ system and individual.

The senescent brain undergoes a number of changes. The weight of the brain, blood flow, and the amount of neurotransmitters produced decline with age. This decrease in neurotransmitters may explain the high incidence of Parkinson's disease in the older population; it has been estimated there is clinical evidence of this disease in 30% of individuals older than 70. Both the speed of walking and trunkal stability have been correlated with longevity, and the slowing of gait, coordination, and trunkal stability may reflect the decline in the number of Purkinje cells within the cerebellum. Neuronal loss may lead to decreased levels of neuroreceptors, such as mu and delta. The loss of these receptors provides one potential mechanism for enhanced sensitivity to opioid analgesics in older individuals. The loss of sensory neurons contributes to a decreased ability to perceive pain and also may contribute to compromised wound healing.

The changes in the immune system are more complicated than mere decline in lymphocyte functioning and are most consistent with an immunologic "dysregulation." Declines in both thymic mass and thymic hormones lead to a decrease in the number of so-called naïve lymphocytes and an increase in memory cells. The total lymphocyte count remains normal, but the response to mitogens decreases. The levels of inflammatory cytokines interleukin [IL]-6 and IL-1beta, C-reactive protein (CRP), and transforming growth factor (TGF)-beta increase with age. Elevations of IL-6 and D-dimer have been associated with both a shorter survival and an increased functional dependency. The level of IL-2 decreases with age, contributing to a loss of lymphocyte proliferation. Although the etiology for the increased levels of cytokines is uncertain, it has been proposed that incompletely healed inflammatory reactions throughout a lifetime result in an accumulation of certain cytokines. These cytokines contribute to an overall catabolic state and to sarcopenia. The levels of immunoglobulins increase, but antibody response decreases. This immunologic dysregulation leads to increasing susceptibility to infection and may be responsible for the altered natural history of certain malignant diseases in the older population.

In general, breast and prostate cancers have a more indolent course in older patients. However, hematologic malignancies tend to be more aggressive and less responsive to therapy, possibly because of the increases in the level of IL-6. In the older population, the levels of hemoglobin, the

KEY POINT

- For elderly patients, chemotherapy doses and schedules may need to be modified according to the agent and its route of activation, metabolism, and excretion.

number of white blood cells, and platelet counts are usually within the normal range, despite the fact that marrow mass is lost over time and is then replaced by fat. The marrow reserve is compromised, and with the stress of illness or treatment, blood counts can decline disproportionately compared with those counts in younger individuals.

PHARMACOLOGY

The physiologic changes associated with aging alter pharmacokinetics and contribute to increased toxicity from pharmacologic intervention. Decline in intestinal absorption may compromise the bioavailability of oral agents and may cause a decline in renal excretion of drugs, and as such, their metabolites may increase toxicity. Decreases in the volume of distribution (V_d) may occur as a result of a decrease in total body water, and hypoproteinemia may further lower the V_d for protein-bound drugs. Lower levels of albumin result in higher levels of free drugs and contribute to increased toxicity to normal tissue. Anemia also may decrease the V_d for agents such as the epipodophyllins and anthracyclines that bind to erythrocytes. With these changes in V_d, normal tissues are more likely to be affected by toxicity.

As mentioned previously, the metabolism by cytochrome P450 (CYP) enzymes in the liver is decreased, so agents that require these enzymes for activation or elimination should be used with caution. Some drugs, such as codeine and tramadol, require activation by the CYP enzymes, and thus may have limited utility depending on other factors that affect enzyme activity, including genotype and concomitant medications.

CLINICAL GERIATRIC ASSESSMENT

Typically, older patients minimize their vulnerability and hide it from others (including physicians) in an attempt to avoid being exploited and to protect their families. Feeling like a burden on the family is common and can have many negative consequences, such as lack of medical care, social isolation, and concealment of deteriorating physical health. On one level, an older patient feels guilt and shame about being dependent on his or her children. An older patient also may perceive that overwhelming demands on the family may lead to rejection and abandonment. Clinicians must have an adequate understanding of what "being a burden" means within the social context of each patient. An objective assessment of the patient's function is an essential component of an oncology consultation. Older patients may appear well and function normally until they must deal with the physical and emotional stress of illness and the stress of medical intervention.

The Comprehensive Geriatric Assessment (CGA) is a fundamental tool in the evaluation of an older patient. Its application can help determine the patient's ability to tolerate treatment and can identify potential problems when medical stressors offset the delicate physiologic balance of life. The CGA should include evaluation of function, assessment of comorbidity and frailty, identification of so-called geriatric syndromes, consideration of socioeconomic issues, analysis of polypharmacy (treatment with multiple medications for various illnesses), and nutritional assessment (Table 19-1). Although not considered a component of the CGA, objective measures also may provide prognostic information. A low albumin level and a hemoglobin level of less than 12 g/dL have been associated with shorter survival. Anemia also has been linked to an increased risk for dementia, chronic heart failure, and cardiac deaths.

The treatment plan should be determined only after comparing the comorbidities with the expectations of therapeutic intervention and the potential toxicities related to that intervention. Studies correlating the CGA with outcomes and ability to tolerate aggressive therapies are ongoing.

FUNCTION

Because functional decline is a predictor of early mortality, the patient's functional reserve factors prominently into the determination of treatment options and overall prognosis. The ability to perform activities of daily living, as well as to demonstrate a rapid and steady gait and a strong handgrip, are predictors of greater physical strength during the aging process, and patients with these characteristics live longer than individuals of the same age who have lost these abilities.

COMORBIDITY

Coexistent medical problems in older patients with cancer may be more life-threatening than the cancer itself. Several different indices have been tested to objectively determine

KEY POINTS

- The Comprehensive Geriatric Assessment assists in defining physiologic reserve.
- Comorbid medical conditions increase the physiologic age.
- Depression and delirium are distinct entities, and both are common in the elderly.
- Frailty defines a severe loss of functional reserve and lack of tolerance to intervention.

TABLE 19-1 Components of the Comprehensive Geriatric Assessment

Function	Activities of daily living Eating, dressing, continence, grooming, transferring from the bed to a chair, and going to the bathroom Instrumental activities of daily living Use of transportation, money management, shopping, laundry and household chores, use of the telephone
Comorbidity	Performance status Number of comorbid conditions Seriousness of comorbid conditions
Geriatric Syndromes	Dementia Depression Delirium Falls (one or more per month) Osteoporosis (spontaneous fractures) Neglect and abuse Failure to thrive
Socioeconomic Issues	Living conditions Presence and adequacy of caregiver Income Access to transportation
Polypharmacy	Number of medications Drug–drug interactions
Nutrition	Nutritional risk

the effect of individual comorbidities on overall survival. To identify comorbidities of high and moderate effect, Yancik et al[7] used Surveillance, Epidemiology and End Results (SEER) registry data for patients older than 55 who were diagnosed with colon cancer. They found that, in the presence of this cancer, some comorbid conditions were more life-threatening than others (Table 19-2). For example, liver disease conferred an increased mortality of 3.04 compared with 1.67 for emphysema. A number of comorbidity scales have been developed, but there is no consensus on which is most accurate and useful.

FRAILTY

The term "frailty" has been used to describe a decline in functional reserve that is so severe that the patient cannot tolerate stress. Many factors contribute to the determination of frailty, which is made on clinical assessment (Fig. 19-1). The risks of therapeutic interventions in frail older patients generally outweigh any benefits, and palliation of symptoms is recommended. Although a standard definition of frailty does not exist, most physicians agree that it indicates the presence of at least one of the following: dependence for one or more activities of daily living, three or more comorbid conditions, and one or more geriatric syndromes (Table 19-2).

GERIATRIC SYNDROMES

The prevalence of depression in the older population has been estimated to range from 15% to 40%. In a population with multiple chronic medical problems, symptoms of an underlying mood disorder may not be obvious, especially because many symptoms, such as decreasing activity level, amplification of pain, increasing social isolation, and worsening self-care, are common symptoms of both depression and aging. Medical management is generally successful in relieving depression.

Dementia and delirium should not be confused with each other. Dementia is a chronic degenerative problem evident in almost 10% of patients older than 65 and in 30% to 40% of

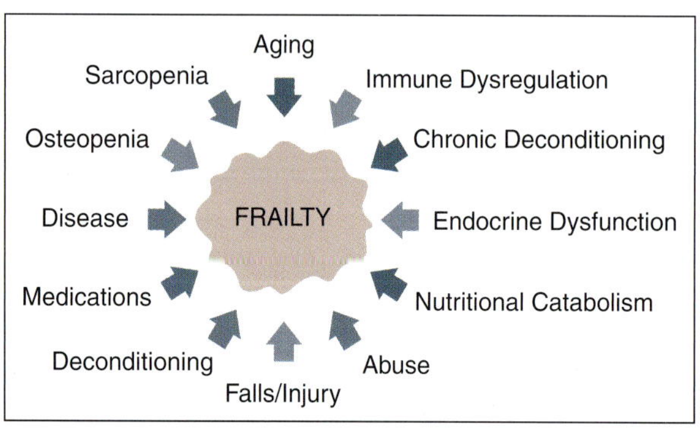

FIG. 19-1 *Many factors contribute to the determination of frailty, which is made on clinical assessment.*

TABLE 19-2 Effect of Comorbidities on Survival[8]

Comorbidities with High Effect

Cardiac History

- Cardiac arrest
- Congestive heart failure
- Chronic obstructive lung disease
- Renal failure

Conditions Requiring Active Therapy

- Angina
- Arrhythmia
- Myocardial infarction
- Valve disease
- Type I diabetes
- Prior malignant disease

Comorbidities with Moderate Effect

Cardiac History

- Angina
- Myocardial infarction
- Valvular disease

Conditions Requiring Active Therapy

- Alcohol abuse
- Anemia
- Asthma
- Deep-vein thrombosis
- Depression
- Hypertension
- Lipid abnormalities
- Liver problems
- Mental illness
- Stroke or transient ischemic attack

Reprinted with permission from Yancik R, Wesley MN, Ries LA, et al. Comorbidity and age as predictors of risk for early mortality of male and female colon carcinoma patients: a population-based study. *Cancer.* 1998;82:2123–2134.

patients older than 80. In addition to the loss of recent memory, patients with dementia have a change in personality and deterioration of motor skills. However, the level of consciousness remains normal with dementia. In contrast, the level of consciousness fluctuates with delirium. The onset of this altered level of consciousness or of disorganized thinking is acute. The prevalence of delirium in hospitalized older patients is as high as 65%. Factors that contribute to delirium include age, heart disease, stroke, multiple medications, infection, nutritional compromise or malnutrition, electrolyte imbalance, sensory deprivation, and change in environment. Delirium is generally reversible, whereas dementia is not.

SOCIOECONOMIC ISSUES

A determination of the patient's living situation is essential because many older people live alone or with a spouse who also has medical needs. It is important to ensure that the family plays an active role in the patient's care and decision making because many patients have a spouse who also is sick or are widowed (25% of men and 50% of women older than age 65 are widowed). Financial concerns and limited health insurance coverage may further compromise the delivery and continuity of care.

TREATMENT APPROACHES

MANAGEMENT OF PAIN

Pain is consistently undertreated for older patients, especially for women and underserved minorities.[9] There are several challenges in managing pain in the older population. First, the loss of sensory neurons with aging may compromise the patient's ability to perceive pain and may raise the threshold for pain recognition. For example, the incidence of pain associated with rectal cancers or peritonitis is substantially lower for older patients than for younger patients.

Second, identifying the source and severity of pain may be complicated by a patient's confusion and dementia, making it difficult to obtain a history and to assess pain. In addition, comorbid conditions, such as prior injury or degenerative joint disease, often complicate the identification of the source of the pain. The clinician should be attentive to nonverbal communication of discomfort, such as a decrease in functional ability, social isolation, increased fatigue, facial grimacing, delirium, and depression. Despite these difficulties, the most accurate pain assessment comes from the patient, and tools that measure the severity of pain, such as thermometers or numeric scales, may be helpful. Clinicians also can ask patients to point to the sites of pain.

A third challenge is the pharmacologic management of pain in the context of aging physiology and the use of multiple medications for comorbidities. Optimal palliation requires an accurate clinical assessment and a knowledge of the physiology and pharmacology associated with aging. Lastly, persistent pain may contribute to the development of depression, and depression, in turn, may amplify the pain. It may be necessary to treat both the pain and the depression.[10,11]

The complications of opioids, which may be used for more severe pain, also are challenging. Older patients are hypersensitive to opioid analgesics, and use of these drugs may worsen already compromised cognitive functioning. In addition, delirium and agitation are side effects of opioids and may be confused with inadequate pain control. Sedative medications, such as benzodiazepines, can often paradoxically increase agitation as a result of worsening delirium. Lowering the dose of opioids or initiating more frequent dosing can minimize these problems. According to the World Health Organization three-step analgesic ladder, which designates the type of analgesic based on the severity of pain, management of cancer-related

KEY POINTS

- Assessment and treatment of pain require an appreciation of aging physiology.
- A higher postoperative mortality rate in the elderly may be attributed to decreased wound healing, a number of comorbidities, and decreased physiologic reserve.
- When chemotherapy and radiation are administered concurrently in the elderly, chemotherapy doses and radiation field size may require modification.

pain is the same for younger and for older patients. (A more detailed discussion of this ladder is available in Chapter 18, Symptom Management.) For older patients, acetominophen is the mainstay of analgesia. Anti-inflammatory agents are beneficial for the management of pain related to bone metastases. The different types of cyclooxygenase (COX) inhibitors, COX-1 and COX-2, are equally effective and equally nephrotoxic; however, COX-2 inhibitors are preferable when gastrointestinal bleeding is a concern.

Oxycodone, hydromorphone, morphine, and methadone are easy to titrate. Morphine is available in a variety of preparations and offers flexibility of administration because it can be administered orally, sublingually, vaginally, or rectally. Its efficacy is predictable. Long-acting preparations provide convenient pain relief with reasonable compliance.

Fentanyl may be administered orally or transdermally. Fentanyl patches provide effective analgesia for 72 hours and are less associated with nausea, pruritus, and constipation than other opioid analgesics. Because of age-related atrophy of the skin, the patch may provide more rapid drug delivery; lower-dose patches may be necessary to help to avoid delirium.

Adjunctive therapies are especially helpful for neuropathic pain. The antiepileptic gabapentin has been shown to be more effective and less toxic than the tricyclic antidepressants. As such, gabapentin is a sound treatment option for older patients because it has no known interactions with other drugs and is not metabolized through the liver.

OPERATIVE INTERVENTION

Generally, the postoperative mortality rate is higher for older patients than for younger patients. An increased number of comorbid medical conditions, decreased wound healing, and lack of physiologic reserve contribute to both prolonged hospital stay and rehabilitation following operative treatment. All phases of healing are compromised by the aging process. Both the inflammatory and proliferative responses are decreased, remodeling occurs to a lesser degree, and the collagen formed is qualitatively different from that in younger individuals. Normally, the repair process initiated by inflammation requires intact sensory nerves that stimulate increased blood flow and growth factor production. The loss of sensory neurons and the coexistence of other medical conditions, such as diabetes and vascular disease, contribute to delayed wound healing. Not surprisingly, complications are more common when surgical intervention is performed on an emergency basis. Often, it is more appropriate to perform an operation as a preventive measure; for example, a hemicolectomy may be performed, even for patients with advanced colorectal cancer, to prevent the need for an emergency operation to treat bowel perforation or obstruction.

CHEMOTHERAPY AND RADIATION THERAPY

Concern about the administration of oral chemotherapy agents appears to be unfounded. Despite decreases in gastric secretions and gastric emptying, oral cytotoxic agents, such as etoposide and cyclophosphamide, are adequately absorbed.

Caution must be exercised when administering cytotoxic drugs that are excreted by the kidney, such as methotrexate, bleomycin, cisplatin, cyclophosphamide, and ifosfamide. Both decreases in the numbers of nephrons and a decline in the glomerular filtration rate may contribute to excess toxicity if these agents are administered in conventional doses. In addition to the renal considerations, the administration of methotrexate is further complicated because the drug accumulates in third-space fluids. As a result, mild edema from heart failure or venous insufficiency can cause the drug and its metabolites to accumulate and to produce mucositis or myelosuppression disproportionate to what would normally be expected.

Although the reason is unclear, acute toxicities such as nausea, vomiting, and alopecia are less likely to occur in older patients than in younger ones; however, the lack of functional reserve in aging may result in increased toxicity to normal tissues. For example, peripheral neuropathy from vincristine, cardiotoxicity from doxorubicin, and mucositis from fluorouracil (5-FU) and leucovorin are all more common and more severe for older patients. Before additional chemotherapy is given, a careful assessment of side effects should be performed, and modifications in dose, schedule, or both, should be made accordingly.[12,13] The use of growth factors also may be helpful in minimizing neutropenic complications without compromising the dose or schedule of chemotherapy.[14]

Few data are available for identifying unique problems associated with radiation therapy in older patients. To minimize toxicity, it is generally recommended to use as small a field as possible when radiating the primary tumor. Newer radiation techniques with intensity-modulated radiation therapy or brachytherapy may provide high doses of radiation while minimizing toxicity to normal tissue.

Combined-modality therapy appears to be more toxic for older patients than for younger patients. In studies involving patients with limited-stage lung cancer treated with concurrent chemotherapy and radiation therapy, mucositis and myelosuppression were found to be more common for patients older than 65 than for younger patients.[15] Such side effects often interrupt the course of radiation therapy and necessitate attenuating the dose of chemotherapy or prolonging the chemotherapy schedule.

SPECIAL CONSIDERATIONS IN COMMON MALIGNANT DISEASES

The randomized controlled trial is the gold standard for investigating new therapies, yet older patients are consistently underrepresented in clinical trials, and much of the treatment data for this population are derived from subset analyses of large studies. Overall survival is a primary endpoint of treatment in most clinical trials; however, for the older population, survival may be compromised more from comorbid medical problems than from cancer. Clinical trials that address cancer treatment in this population should include measures of quality of life and of decrease in cancer-related symptoms. Older patients wish to receive cancer therapy when an intervention can prolong life, but not at the expense of compromising their quality of life. When possible, patients should be encouraged to participate in trials designed to answer how cancers should best be managed.

BREAST CANCER

Almost 50% of all breast cancers develop in women who are age 65 or older, and 13% develop in women older than 80. Recognized prognostic factors, such as estrogen receptor (ER) status, histologic grade, ploidy, *p53* status, epidermal growth factor receptor status, and *HER2* status, suggest that tumors become less aggressive with advancing age.[16,17] Treatment recommendations should be made on an individual basis, taking the patient's comorbid conditions and the expectations of therapy into consideration.

Because of competing comorbid medical problems and less aggressive tumor biology, less invasive approaches to the primary tumor, such as lumpectomy and adjuvant tamoxifen, have been studied. Exclusion of radiation from the treatment plan leads to an increased incidence of recurrence in the ipsilateral breast, and mastectomy is needed for local disease control. Nonetheless, the survival rate for women treated with this less aggressive approach is identical to the rate seen for women treated with conventional surgery and radiation therapy. Resection of the primary tumor and administration of tamoxifen may be appropriate for select women with small, ER-positive breast cancers and a finite life expectancy.[18,19]

Because aromatase inhibitors are associated with greater progression-free survival and less toxicity, they often are used in lieu of tamoxifen in the adjuvant setting. Although only 13% of breast cancers are diagnosed in women older than 80, more than 25% of breast cancer-related deaths occur in this age group. This raises concerns about the undertreatment of

KEY POINTS

- Most of the data for treating cancers in the elderly are derived from subset analyses and may be biased toward healthier, more fit participants.
- The benefits of adjuvant chemotherapy for breast and colon cancer for older patients are similar to those for younger patients.
- Chemotherapy may improve the survival and quality of life for elderly patients with extensive-stage non-small cell lung cancer.

women in this age group. Women age 65 or older are poorly represented in controlled breast cancer trials. In subset analyses of controlled trials of adjuvant therapy, older women appear to derive benefit from both chemotherapy and hormone therapy, although drug delivery may compromise efficacy.[20–23] Therefore, in the absence of severe comorbidities, the guidelines for adjuvant therapy are the same as those that exist for younger women.

Screening

Controlled trials of screening mammography have excluded older women. The efficacy of screening can be assessed only from observational trials, and these data suggest a decrease in breast cancer-related mortality for women aged 70 to 79. The American Geriatrics Society recommends annual screening mammography for women up to age 85 if their life expectancy exceeds 3 years.[24,25]

Chemoprevention

The determination of eligibility for the Breast Cancer Prevention Trial was calculated using the Gail model, and women whose risk for developing breast cancer in 5 years was 1.67% or greater were included for study. Although tamoxifen use reduces the incidence of hormone receptor-positive breast cancer, the potential benefit from chemoprevention for women older than age 55 is outweighed, at least in part, by an increased risk of endometrial cancer and thrombosis for these women. Raloxifene is as effective as tamoxifen for preventing invasive breast cancers and has a lower incidence of thromboembolic events, cataracts, and endometrial cancer.[26]

LUNG CANCER

The median age for patients with newly diagnosed non-small cell lung cancer is 70 years. The prognosis for lung cancer is related to the stage of disease, performance status, sex, and the patient's ability to tolerate adequate treatment.[27]

Controlled trials involving patients age 70 or older confirm a small benefit from chemotherapy for patients with extensive-stage disease. The Elderly Lung Cancer Vinorelbine Italian Study is a comparison of single-agent vinorelbine with best supportive care for patients aged 70 or older.

Vinorelbine led to a statistically significant improvement in median survival (28 weeks compared with 21 weeks; $p = 0.03$) and a reduced relative hazard of death (hazard ratio 0.64; 95% CI 0.45, 0.93). Importantly, the findings of this trial also demonstrated that the quality of life was better for patients who were randomly assigned to vinorelbine.[28,29] Similarly, single-agent gemcitabine and docetaxel also have been shown to produce tumor regression and to prolong survival. Although retrospective studies suggest that the elderly may experience a survival benefit from combination chemotherapy, this has not been demonstrated in prospective studies. Given the side effects of combination chemotherapy, serial monotherapy is reasonable as treatment for advanced non-small cell lung cancer.[30]

One-third of older patients present with locally advanced disease (stages IIIA and IIIB). The available data for the use of concurrent chemotherapy and radiation therapy are derived from subset analyses of older patients enrolled in large controlled trials, rather than from trials designed for that age group. Most of these analyses demonstrate that the "fit older patient" benefits from concurrent chemotherapy and radiation therapy. However, the frequency of grade 4 toxicity — notably hematologic toxicity — is higher for older patients.[15,31,32]

Although age is not an independent prognostic factor, older patients have more side effects from chemotherapy agents used to treat lung cancer, especially when chemotherapy is administered with radiation therapy.

COLORECTAL CANCER

More than two-thirds of all colon cancers develop in patients older than 65. For older patients, lesions are more likely to develop on the right side, and anemia is more likely to occur than pain.[33] Surgical resection of the primary tumor has been the mainstay of treatment. If the primary tumor is not removed, perforation, bleeding, and obstruction may develop, and emergency surgical intervention may be needed. Because the rates of morbidity and mortality associated with emergency operations are higher than expected for patients older than 70, surgery may be advocated for palliation, even for patients with advanced disease.[34]

Adjuvant chemotherapy is offered less frequently to older patients, and as many as 30% who initiate chemotherapy will discontinue treatment prematurely.[35] Non-compliance with adjuvant therapy indications and doses contributes to a higher cancer-related death rate for this population. Subset analyses of controlled trials of adjuvant therapy suggest that chemotherapy yielded the same survival benefit for patients age 70 and older as for younger patients. These trials may be biased because participants met the inclusion criteria and are likely to have included the "fit elderly."

This survival advantage is true for 5-FU and leucovorin regimens, as well as for regimens containing oxaliplatin. An alternative is capecitabine, an oral fluoropyrimidine, which has shown to be at least as effective as bolus 5-FU and leucovorin for adjuvant therapy in stage III colon cancer. Toxicity for all adjuvant regimens is similar to what is observed in younger individuals, with the caveat that all reports represent only the elderly population considered eligible for clinical trials.[36,37]

Similarly, age alone should not affect the recommendation for combined-modality treatment of colorectal cancer. In the Medicare population, the survival and local control advantages of such treatment are similar to the advantages for younger patients.

Patients with advanced colorectal cancer should be offered palliative chemotherapy. The addition of irinotecan to bolus 5-FU and leucovorin has been shown to produce a greater likelihood of tumor regression and possibly a longer survival than 5-FU and leucovorin alone. Among patients age 65 and older, progression-free survival was longer for those treated with bolus 5-FU and leucovorin than for patients treated with standard 5-FU and leucovorin.[38] Because the tolerability of infusional 5-FU is much better than bolus 5-FU, particularly for elderly patients, protracted infusion of 5-FU now forms the backbone of modern combination regimens, such as infusional 5-FU and leucovorin plus oxaliplatin (FOLFOX) and infusional 5-FU and leucovorin plus irinotecan. In a recent meta-analysis, FOLFOX was found to be tolerable and efficacious for patients who were at least 70.[33] Capecitabine or capecitabine plus oxaliplatin combinations can be considered alternatives for 5-FU and leucovorin or FOLFOX. Data specifically addressing the use of cetuximab for the elderly are lacking. The use of bevacizumab for patients older than 65 is associated with an increased risk for arterial thrombotic/thromboembolic events. However, the group of patients at apparent higher risk for thrombotic/thromboembolic events while receiving bevacizumab does not experience the same magnitude of survival benefit as the younger population.

Screening

Colonoscopy has been established as a cost-effective screening tool. Screening should be done every 10 years until age 85. If polyps are identified, the procedure should be repeated every 3 to 5 years.[39]

PANCREATIC CANCER

More than two-thirds of pancreatic cancers develop in individuals age 65 and older. For locally advanced disease, cancer-directed chemotherapy, radiation therapy, or a combination of the two is as effective for older patients as for younger patients.[40,41]

PROSTATE CANCER

Prostate cancer predominantly affects older men, and more than 90% of prostate cancer-related deaths occur in men older than 65. As a result of prostate-specific antigen (PSA) screening, most prostate cancer is diagnosed at an early stage, when it is still confined to the gland. Radiation therapy or radical prostatectomy may provide local control of the cancer. Given the indolent natural history of the disease and competing comorbid conditions, observation only may be appropriate. If "watchful waiting" is assumed to be appropriate for men with lower risk cancers, then as many as 10% of these individuals are currently overtreated by surgery and 45% by radiation therapy.[42] The Scandinavian Prostate Cancer Group conducted a controlled trial of radical prostatectomy compared with watchful waiting for 695 men with localized prostate cancer.[43] For both study arms, the median age was 65. With a median follow-up of 8.2 years, 8.6% of patients undergoing radical prostatectomy died of prostate cancer compared with 14.4% assigned to watchful waiting (relative risk [RR] 0.56; 95% CI 0.36, 0.88; p = 0.01). Distant metastases were more common in the non-surgical arm (RR 0.60; 95% CI 0.42, 0.86; p = 0.004 by Gray's test). Radical prostatectomy is associated with a significant improvement in disease-free and overall survival, as well as a decreased incidence of distant metastasis and local progression.[44] A quality-of-life trial conducted in conjunction with the study determined that radical prostatectomy was associated with an increased frequency of erectile dysfunction and urinary leakage; however, urinary obstruction was more frequent for the observation-only arm.

When the patient's survival is limited by other comorbid conditions, watchful waiting is appropriate, and treatment may be initiated when symptoms develop. Expectant management has been advocated for men older than 70 who had a normal digital rectal exam, who have had no more than two biopsies demonstrating less than 50% cancer, who have a Gleason score of less than 6, and who have clinical T1c disease.[45] Surgery or radiation therapy should be offered to patients with large tumors or to patients with symptoms of urinary obstruction.

Widespread prostate cancer is initially managed with combined hormone therapies. The use of antiandrogens, such as flutamide, in combination with bilateral orchiectomy or a luteinizing hormone-releasing hormone agonist is more likely to control the disease than surgical or hormone castration alone and also may prolong survival. The findings of a meta-analysis that included more than 8,000 men in 27 controlled trials suggest a slight survival advantage to the addition of an antiandrogen.[46] With disease progression, cessation of flutamide may produce a hormone withdrawal response.[47] Once the disease has become resistant to hormone therapy, chemotherapy with docetaxel has been shown to improve survival and may offer palliation. Single-agent mitoxantrone can provide palliation for select patients.

Screening

Among populations of men who receive regular screening, the lifetime risk of prostate cancer is 16%, and the risk of dying as a result of the disease is 3%.[48] Such data suggest that prostate cancer is a chronic disease that may not shorten life expectancy. Autopsies performed on men who have died of other causes have confirmed the presence of occult prostate cancer in 39% of men aged 70 to 79 and in 43% of men older than 80. It has been estimated that PSA screening results in an overdiagnosis rate of 29% for white men and of 44% for black men aged 60 to 84.[49] Although some organizations, such as the American Cancer Society and the American Urologic Society, support annual screening, others recommend that the decision to measure PSA inovid be made on a case-by-case basis, following a discussion about the potential benefits and harms of treatment if a cancer is diagnosed. Until data from the controlled trials become available, the use of PSA as a screening test is likely to be debated.

LYMPHOMA

More than one-half of the aggressive histologic subtypes are diagnosed in individuals older than age 60. An age of 60 or older has been identified as an independent poor prognostic factor by the International Prognostic Factors Project. Regardless of age, the prognosis is favorable for patients with stages I and II disease who are treated with chemotherapy and radiation therapy. A controlled trial compared four cycles of cyclophosphamide, doxorubicin, vincristine, and prednisone (CHOP) with four cycles of CHOP plus involved-field radiation therapy for patients older than 60 with stages I and II aggressive lymphoma and found no benefit to the addition of radiation therapy.[50] More advanced disease (stages III and IV) is treated with chemotherapy with rituximab if CD20+. For more than 2 decades, CHOP has been the standard chemotherapy for aggressive histology lymphoma. Among patients treated with the CHOP regimen, neutropenia and fever are more likely to occur in those older than age 60. However, when doxorubicin has been omitted from the regimen or the dose has been attenuated, the efficacy has been substantially compromised. After the first cycle of chemotherapy, the use of colony-stimulating factors will decrease the incidence of neutropenia, hospitalizations for fever, and will result in higher relative dose intensity. However, neither the complete response rate nor the survival rate are improved by the administration of these costly agents. It is expected that chemotherapy will produce complete remission of disease for most patients, with 30% to 40% of patients remaining free of disease after 5 years. The benefits of chemotherapy are somewhat less profound for patients who are older than 60 or who have one or more comorbid medical conditions. Conventionally administered CHOP with rituximab (if disease is CD20+) remains the chemotherapy of choice for older patients.[51-53] In a population of patients aged 60 to 80 with diffuse large B-cell lymphoma, the addition of rituxumab to CHOP resulted in higher complete remission, 2-year event-free survival, and overall survival rates compared with CHOP alone.[54,55]

ACUTE MYELOID LEUKEMIA (AML)

The incidence of acute leukemia increases with age, and the prognosis is inversely related to the patient's age. For patients older than age 40, the biologic behavior of AML is more aggressive and less amenable to therapy. For older patients, AML frequently develops after a history of myelodysplasia and cytogenetic abnormalities, and deletions of chromosome 5 or chromosome 7 are common. Leukemic cells from older patients also are more likely to express genes that confer drug resistance.[56,57] Such clinical and genetic factors predict resistance to conventional induction regimens. In addition, the treatment-related mortality rate during induction is as high as 25% for older patients. As a result, complete remission is achieved for only 45% of older patients with AML; long-term remissions are rare. Lower doses of chemotherapy produce less toxicity to normal tissues but also are less likely to lead to complete remission.[58] For frail and older patients with substantial comorbidities, it is reasonable to offer only palliative measures.

The approach to treating older patients with cancer requires an ability to assess the patient's physiologic reserve before initiating a treatment plan. Treatment should be tailored according to the patient's functional age and expectations of therapy. The challenges and goals of intervention are to add "life to years" rather than just "years to life."

REFERENCES

1. Ries LAG, Kosary CL, Hankey BF, et al (eds): SEER Cancer Statistics Review 1973–1996. Bethesda, MD, National Cancer Institute NIH Publication No. 99-27789,1999.
2. Yancik R. Cancer burden in the aged: an epidemiologic and demographic overview. *Cancer.* 1997;80(7):1273–1283.
3. Yancik R, Ries LA. Aging and cancer in America: demographic and epidemiologic perspectives. *Hematol Oncol Clin North Am.* 2000; 14(1):17–23.
4. Harman D. The aging process. *Proc Natl Acad Sci U S A.* 1981; 78(11):7124–7128.
5. Gilchrest BA, Bohr VA. Aging processes, DNA damage, and repair. *FASEB J.* 1997;11(5):322–330.
6. Melton LJ 3rd, Khosla S, Crowson CS, et al. Epidemiology of sarcopenia. *J Am Geriatr Soc.* 2000;48(6): 625–630.
7. Yancik R, Wesley MN, Ries LA, et al. Comorbidity and age as predictors of risk for early mortality of male and female colon carcinoma patients: a population-based study. *Cancer.* 1998;82(11):2123–2134.
8. Yancik R, Wesley MN, Ries LA, et al. Comorbidity and age as predictors of risk for early mortality of male and female colon carcinoma patients: a population-based study. *Cancer.* 1998;82(11):2123–2134.
9. Cleeland CS. Undertreatment of cancer pain in elderly patients. *JAMA.* 1998;279(23):1914–1915.
10. Balducci L. Management of cancer pain in geriatric patients. *J Support Oncol.* 2003;1(3):175–191.
11. American Geriatric Society Panel on Persistent Pain in Older Persons. The management of persistent pain in older persons. *J Am Geriatr Soc.* 2002;50(6 Suppl):S205–S224.
12. Von Hoff DD, Layard MW, Basa P, et al. Risk factors for doxorubicin-induced congestive heart failure. *Ann Intern Med.* 1979;91(5):710–717.
13. Petrelli N, Douglass HO, Herrera L, et al. The modulation of fluorouracil with leucovorin in metastatic colorectal carcinoma: a prospective randomized phase III trail. Gastrointestinal Tumor Study Group. *J Clin Oncol.* 1989;7(10):1419–1426.
14. American Society of Clinical Oncology. Recommendations for the use of hematopoietic colony-stimulating factors: evidence-based, clinical practice guidelines. *J Clin Oncol.* 1994;12(11):2471–2508.
15. Sause WT, Scott C, Taylor S, et al. RTOG 88-08 and ECOG 4588: preliminary results of a phase III trial in regionally advanced unresectable non-small cell lung cancer. *J Natl Cancer Inst.* 1995;87(3):198–205.
16. Diab SG, Elledge RM, Clark GM. Tumor characteristics and clinical outcome of elderly women with breast cancer. *J Natl Cancer Inst.* 2000; 92(7):550–556.
17. Basche M, Byers T. Tumor characteristics and clinical outcome of elderly women with breast cancer. *J Natl Cancer Inst.* 2001;93(1):64–65.
18. Fyles A, McCready D, Manchul L, et al. Tamoxifen with or without breast radiation in women 50 years of age or older with early stage breast cancer. *N Engl J Med.* 2004;351(10):963–967.
19. Hughes KS, Schnaper L, Berry D, et al. Lumpectomy plus tamoxifen with and without radiotherapy in women 70 years of age with early breast cancer. *N Engl J Med.* 2004:351(10):971–977.
20. Ragaz J, Coldman A. Survival impact of adjuvant tamoxifen on competing causes of mortality in breast cancer survivors, with analysis of mortality from contralateral breast cancer, cardiovascular events, endometrial cancer, and thromboembolic episodes. *J Clin Oncol.* 1998; 16(6):2018–2024.
21. Extermann M, Balducci L, Lyman GH. What threshold for adjuvant therapy in older breast cancer patients? *J Clin Oncol.* 2000;18(8): 1709–1717.
22. Desch CE, Hillner BE, Smith TJ, et al. Should the elderly receive chemotherapy for node-negative breast cancer? A cost-effectiveness analysis examining total and active life-expectancy outcomes. *J Clin Oncol.* 1993;11(4):777–782.
23. Muss HB, Woolf S, Berry D, et al. Adjuvant chemotherapy in older and younger women with lymph node-positive breast cancer. *JAMA.* 2005;293(9):1073–1081.
24. May DS, Lee NC, Nadel MR, et al. The National Breast and Cervical Cancer Early Detection Program: report on the first 4 years of mammography provided to medically underserved women. *Am J Roentgenol.* 1998;170(1):97–104.
25. Kerlikowske K, Salzmann P, Phillips KA, et al. Continuing screening mammography in women aged 70 to 79 years: impact on life expectancy and cost-effectiveness. *JAMA.* 1999;282(22):2156–2163.
26. Vogel VG, Costantino JP, Wickerham DL, et al. Effects of tamoxifen vs raloxifene on the risk of developing invasive breast cancer and other disease outcomes: the NSABP Study of Tamoxifen and Raloxifene (STAR) P-2 trial. *JAMA.* 2006;295(23):2727–2741.
27. Johnson DH. Treatment of the elderly patient with small-cell lung cancer. *Chest.* 1993;103(1 Suppl):72S–74S.
28. Non-Small Cell Lung Cancer Collaborative Group. Chemotherapy in non-small cell lung cancer: a meta-analaysis using updated data on individual patients from 52 randomised clinical trials. *BMJ.* 1995;311 (7010):899–909.
29. Effects of vinorelbine on quality of life and survival of elderly patient with advanced non-small cell lung cancer. The Elderly Lung Cancer Vinorelbine Italian Study Group. *J Natl Cancer Inst.* 1999;91(1):66–72.
30. Frasci G, Lorusso V, Panza N, et al. Gemcitabine plus vinorelbine versus vinorelbine alone in elderly patients with advanced non small cell lung cancer. *J Clin Oncol.* 2000;18(13):2529–2536.
31. Langer CJ, Hsu C, Curran W, et al. Do elderly patients (pts) with locally advanced non-small cell lung cancer (NSCLC) benefit from combined modality therapy? A secondary analysis of RTOG 94-10. Paper presented at: American Society for Therapeutic Radiology and Oncology 43rd Annual Meeting; November 4–8, 2001; San Francisco, California. *Int J Radiat Oncol Biol Phys.* 2001;51(suppl 1):30. Abstract 31.

32. Langer CJ, Scott C, Byhardt R, et al. Effect of advanced age on outcome in Radiation Therapy Oncology Group studies of locally advanced NSCLC (LA-NSCLC). *Lung Cancer.* 2000;29(suppl 1);104.

33. Mulcahy HE, Patchett SE, Daly L, et al. Prognosis of elderly patients with large bowel cancer. *Br J Surg.* 1994;81(5):736–738.

34. Vivi AA, Lopes A, Cavalcanti Sde F, et al. Surgical treatment of colon and rectum adenocarcinoma in elderly patients. *J Surg Oncol.* 1992;51 (3):203–206.

35. Neugut AI, Matasar M, Wang X, et al. Duration of adjuvant chemotherapy for colon cancer and survival among the elderly. *J Clin Oncol.* 2006;24(15):2368–2375.

36. Sargent DJ, Goldberg RM, Jacobson SD, et al. A pooled analysis of adjuvant chemotherapy for resected colon cancer in elderly patients. *N Engl J Med.* 2001;345(15):1091–1097.

37. Goldberg RM, Tabah-Fisch I, Bleiberg H, et. Al. Pooled analysis of safety and efficacy of oxaliplatin plus fluorouracil leucovorin administered bimonthly in elderly patients with colorectal cancer. *J Clin Oncol.* 2006;24(25):4085–4091.

38. Saltz LB, Cox JV, Blanke C, et al. Irinotecan plus fluorouracil and leucovorin for metastatic colorectal cancer. Irinotecan Study Group. *N Engl J Med.* 2000;343(13):905–914.

39. Frazier AL, Colditz GA, Fuchs CS, et al. Cost-effectiveness of screening for colorectal cancer in the general population. *JAMA.* 2000;284(15): 1954–1961.

40. Poen JC, Ford JM, Niederhuber JE. Chemoradiotherapy in the management of localized tumors of the pancreas. *Ann Surg Oncol.* 1999; 6(1):117–122.

41. Berlin JD, Catalano P, Thomas JP, et al. Phase III study of gemcitabine in combination with fluorouracil versus gemcitabine alone in patients with advanced pancreatic carcinoma: Eastern Cooperative Oncology Group Trial E2297. *J Clin Oncol.* 2002;20(15):3270–3275.

42. Miller DC, Gruber SB, Hollenbeck BK, et al. Incidence of initial local therapy among men with lower-risk prostate cnacer in the United States. *J Natl Cancer Inst.* 2006;98(16):1134–1141.

43. Holmberg L, Bill-Axelson A, Helgesen F, et al. A randomized trial comparing radical prostatectomy with watchful waiting in early prostate cancer. *N Engl J Med.* 2002;347(11):781–789.

44. Bill-Axelson A, Holmberg L, Ruutu M, et al. Radical prostatectomy versus watchful waiting in early prostate cancer. *N Engl J Med.* 2005; 352(19):1977–1984.

45. Klotz L. Active surveillance for prostate cancer: For whom? *J Clin Oncol.* 2005;23(32):8165–8169.

46. Prostate Cancer Trialists' Collaborative Group. Maximum androgen blockade in advanced prostate cancer: an overview of the randomised trials. *Lancet.* 2000;355(9214):1491–1498.

47. Scher HI, Zhang ZF, Nanus D. Hormone and antihormone withdrawal: implications for the management of androgen-independent prostate cancer. *Urology.* 1996;47(1A Suppl):61–69.

48. Etzioni R, Berry KM, Legler JM, et al. Prostate-specific antigen testing in black and white men: an analysis of medicare claims from 1991–1998. *Urology.* 2002;59(2):251–255.

49. Coley CM. Barry MJ. Fleming C, et al. Early detection of prostate cancer. Part II: Estimating the risks, benefits, and costs. American College of Physicians. *Ann Intern Med.* 1997;126(6):468–479.

50. Bonnet C, Fillet G, Mounier N, et al. CHOP alone compared with CHOP plus radiotherapy for localized aggressive lymphoma in elderly patients: A study by the Groupe d'Etude des Lymphomes de I'Adulte. *J Clin Oncol.* 2007;25(7):787–792.

51. Kouroukis CT, Browman GP, Esmail R, et al. Chemotherapy for older patients with newly diagnosed, advanced-stage, aggressive-histology non-Hodgkin Lymp homa: a systematic review. *Ann Intern Med.* 2002; 136(2):144–152.

52. Meyer RM, Browman GP, Samosh ML, et al. Randomized phase II comparison of standard CHOP with weekly CHOP in elderly patients with non-Hodgkin's lymphoma. *J Clin Oncol.* 1995;13(9): 2386–2393.

53. Bastion Y, Blay JY, Divine M, et al. Elderly patients with aggressive non-Hodgkin's lymphoma: disease presentation, response to treatment, and survival—a Groupe d'Etude des Lymphomes de l'Adulte Study on 453 patients older than 69 years. *J Clin Oncol.* 1997;15(8): 2945–2953.

54. Coiffier B, Lepage E, Briere J, et al. CHOP chemotherapy plus rituximab compared with CHOP alone in elderly patients with diffuse large B-cell lymphoma. *N Engl J Med.* 2002;346(4):235–242.

55. Habermann TM, Weller EA, Morrison VA, et al. Rituximab-CHOP versus CHOP alone or with maintenance rituximab in older patients with diffuse large B-cell lymphoma. *J Clin Oncol.* 2006;24(19): 3121–3127.

56. Leith CP, Kopecky KJ, Godwin J, et al. Acute myeloid leukemia in the elderly: assessment of multidrug resistance MDR1) and cytogenetics distinguishes biologic subgroups with remarkably distinct response to standard chemotherapy. A Southwest Oncology Group study. *Blood.* 1997;89(9):3323–3329.

57. Zhu YM, Das-Gupta EP, Russell NH. Microsatellite instability and p53 mutations are associated with abnormal expression of the MSH2 gene in adult leukemia. *Blood.* 1999;94(2):733–740.

58. Tilly H, Castaigne S, Bordessoule D, et al. Low-dose cytarabine versus intensive chemotherapy in the treatment of acute nonlymphocytic leukemia in the elderly. *J Clin Oncol.* 1990;8(2):272–279.

SELF EVALUATION

CHAPTER 1 QUESTIONS:
EPIDEMIOLOGY AND PREVENTION OF CANCER

1-1 Which of the following describes the difference between efficacy and effectiveness in the interpretation of clinical trial results?

A. Efficacy considers the outcomes of a treatment under carefully controlled conditions, whereas effectiveness considers the outcomes when applying a treatment in the routine (real-world) setting
B. Efficacy considers short- and long-term effects, whereas effectiveness considers long-term effects only
C. Efficacy considers only the effect of survival, whereas effectiveness considers all outcomes
D. Efficacy is a clinical measure, whereas effectiveness is statistic measure

1-2 A 60-year-old woman at high risk of breast cancer (because of an extensive family history and a personal history of lobular carcinoma in situ) asks what her options are for decreasing her risk of the disease.

Which of the following measures has been demonstrated in clinical trials to decrease the 5-year risk of breast cancer for this woman?

A. Tamoxifen therapy
B. Selenium supplements
C. Annual mammography
D. Adoption of a low-fat diet

1-3 Which of the following provides the strongest evidence that a cancer screening test is beneficial?

A. Increased 5-year survival of those screened compared with historical controls
B. Earlier stage at time of diagnosis for those screened compared with those not screened
C. Larger numbers of patients diagnosed with cancer among those undergoing screening
D. Decreased cause-specific mortality for those in the screened arm compared with those in the control arm of a randomized clinical trial

1-4 The introduction of a new large-scale screening test has its greatest immediate effect on which of the following?

A. Mortality rate related to the disease
B. Incidence of the disease
C. Survival rate
D. Morbidity

1-5 Which of the following describes the cancer mortality rate of a country?

A. Percentage of patients with cancer in a country who die from cancer each year
B. Absolute number of patients with cancer in a country who die of cancer in a given year
C. Number of patients with cancer who die per 100,000 individuals living in the country in a given year
D. Number of people diagnosed with potentially fatal cancers per 100,000 cases per year

1-6 Which of the following pairs a proven cancer prevention action and the cancer it prevents?

A. Tobacco cessation and bladder cancer
B. Hepatitis C vaccination and hepatoma
C. Increased fiber consumption and colorectal cancer
D. All of the above

1-7 A total of 100 patients are screened for cancer using a newly developed screening test with the following res ults:

- **8 results are truly positive**
- **1 result is falsely positive**
- **1 result is falsely negative**
- **90 results are truly negative**

Which of the following formulas is used to determine the sensitivity of the test?

A. 90 divided by (1 + 90)
B. 8 divided by (90 + 1)
C. 90 divided by (90 + 8)
D. 8 divided by (8 + 1)

1-8 Racial disparities in survival outcomes for a number of malignancies have been of major concern. Which of the following are likely to be possible explanations for these observed differences?

A. Differences in tumor biology

B. Differences in treatment

C. Differences in stage at diagnosis

D. All of the above

1-9 Which cancer screening is supported by positive randomized clinical trials that demonstrate reductions in mortality?

A. Chest x-rays

B. Prostate-specific antigen

C. Fecal occult blood testing

D. Spiral computerized tomography scans of the lungs

CHAPTER 1 EXPLANATORY ANSWERS:
EPIDEMIOLOGY AND PREVENTION OF CANCER

1-1 A

Educational Objective: To understand the concepts of efficacy and effectiveness as they relate to the interpretation of clinical trials results.

Efficacy is the outcome of a clinical trial. The population enrolled in the study will differ from the population at large. Participants in clinical trials generally have less comorbid disease and, in prevention studies, there is often a "healthy volunteer effect." Volunteers are often more interested in health than the average member of the population. How well the intervention works in the group as a whole in routine practice is termed effectiveness.

There are a few trials with effectiveness endpoints. Such studies are generally large and long-term.

Suggested Reading

Kramer BS, Brawley OW. Cancer screening. *Hematol Oncol Clin North Am.* 2000;14:831–848.

1-2 A

Educational Objective: To understand the known methods of reducing the risk of breast cancer.

In randomized, placebo-controlled trials designed to assess tamoxifen as adjuvant treatment for patients with early-stage breast cancer, women taking the drug were found to have one-third fewer new cancers in the contralateral breast than women taking placebo. The Breast Cancer Prevention Trial was a randomized, placebo controlled study of more than 13,000 women at high risk of breast cancer. After a median treatment of 69 months, tamoxifen was found to decrease the period risk of breast cancer by 49%. Tamoxifen also was associated with a reduction in bone fractures and with a small increase in the risk of endometrial cancer, stroke, pulmonary emboli, and deep-vein thrombosis. A trial to compare tamoxifen with another selective estrogen-receptor modulator, raloxifene, found that raloxifene also reduced breast cancer to a similar extent as tamoxifen, but raloxifene had lower risk of endometrial cancer, thromboembolic events, and cataracts. Mammography does not affect the development of breast cancer, and a lower fat intake in certain populations has been shown to correlate with lower risk of breast cancer; however, no trial has demonstrated that a change to a low-fat diet reduces risk.

Suggested Reading

Fisher B, Costantino JP, Wickerham DL, et al. Tamoxifen for prevention of breast cancer: report of the National Surgical Adjuvant Breast and Bowel Project P-1 Study. *J Natl Cancer Inst.* 1998;90:1371-1388.

Greenwald P, Clifford CK, Milner JA. Diet and cancer prevention. *Eur J Cancer.* 2001;37:948–965.

Thomas DB, Gao DL, Ray RM, et al. Randomized trial of breast self-examination in Shanghai: final results. *J Natl Cancer Inst.* 2002;94:1445–1457.

Vogel VG, Constatnino JP, Wickerham DL, et al. Effects of tamoxifen vs raloxifene on the risk of developing invasive breast cancer and other disease outcomes: the NSABP Study of Tam-oxifen and Raloxifene (STAR) P-2 Trial. *J Am Med Assoc.* 2006; 295:2727–2741.

1-3 D

Educational Objective: To recognize the reasons screening can be controversial and even not recommended, and to appreciate the levels of proof of screening utility.

The major reason to screen for cancer is to decrease mortality. A secondary reason is to decrease morbidity associated with treatment. Assessment of survival outside of a randomized controlled trial is subject to lead-time bias. It is possible to have survival rates increase after screening while mortality also increases.

A screening intervention is best assessed in a randomized, controlled screening trial with cause-specific mortality as the endpoint. Studies showing a reduction in the incidence of advanced-stage disease, improved survival, or a shift in disease stage are weaker and offer potentially misleading evidence of benefit. These latter criteria by themselves are not sufficient to establish the value of a screening test.

Because the gold-standard randomized screening trials are large (often involving thousands of people) and last for years, less definitive study designs are frequently used to estimate the efficacy and effectiveness of screening practices. In order of strength of evidence, efficacy can be assessed by the following:

- Findings of internally controlled trials using intervention-allocation methods other than randomization, such as allocation determined by birth date or date of clinic visit;
- findings of cohort or case-control analytic observational studies;
- results of multiple time-series study with or without the intervention; or
- opinions of respected authorities on the basis of clinical experience, descriptive studies, or consensus reports of experts. (Even experts can easily be misled by biases.)

Suggested Reading

Kramer BS, Brawley OW. Cancer screening. *Hematol Oncol Clin North Am.* 2000;14:831–848.

Kramer BS, Brown ML, Prorok PC, et al. Prostate cancer screening: what we know and what we need to know. *Ann Intern Med.* 1993;119:914–923.

Smith RA, Cokkinides V, Eyre HJ. American Cancer Society guidelines for the early detection of cancer, 2003. *CA Cancer J Clin.* 2003;53:27–43.

1-4 B

Educational Objective: To understand the effect of screening on both cancer and population statistics.

Screening, regardless of whether it provides a benefit, will increase the number of specific cancers diagnosed in a population. Any benefit, from improvement in survival beyond the lead-time bias of screening to a decrease in morbidity or mortality, will only be seen much later. Some of the additional cancers may be more indolent and less aggressive and would not have been clinically diagnosed later in life. This is the concept of length bias and, more specifically, the more extreme form of length bias known as overdiagnosis.

Length bias occurs when slow-growing, less aggressive cancers are detected during screening. Cancers diagnosed as a result of the onset of symptoms between scheduled screenings tend to be more aggressive, and treatment outcomes are not as favorable. An extreme form of length bias is referred to as overdiagnosis, or detection of pseudodisease. Some undetected slow-growing tumors fulfill the histologic criteria of cancer but will never be clinically significant or cause death.

Suggested Reading

Harris R, Lohr KN. Screening for prostate cancer: an update of the evidence for the U.S. Preventive Services Task Force. *Ann Intern Med.* 2002;137:917–929.

Kramer BS, Brawley OW. Cancer screening. *Hematol Oncol Clin North Am.* 2000;14:831–848.

Kramer BS, Brown ML, Prorok PC, et al. Prostate cancer screening: what we know and what we need to know. *Ann Intern Med.* 1993;119:914–923.

Mandel JS, Church TR, Bond JH, et al. The effect of fecal occult-blood screening on the incidence of colorectal cancer. *N Engl J Med.* 2000;343:1603–1607.

NIH consensus conference. Ovarian cancer. Screening, treatment, and follow-up. NIH Consensus Development Panel on Ovarian Cancer. *JAMA.* 1995;273:491–497.

1-5 C

Educational Objective: To understand concepts used in descriptive epidemiology, such as cancer incidence rate, mortality rate, survival rates, and age adjustment.

The first point to appreciate is that a rate has a denominator population (i.e., it is not an absolute number). Thus, answer C uses the number of 100,000 people per year as the denominator. This is a key concept in epidemiology, which studies statistics in populations. The percentage of patients with cancer who die each year would reflect the mortality rate of those with the disease, not the population mortality rate. The absolute number of patients with cancer who die in a given country each year is a less useful number because it is not a rate — it does not standardize for the size, age, gender distribution, or other characteristics of the population. Finally, the number of patients diagnosed with a potentially fatal cancer does not reflect how many will actually die — some patients may be cured by treatment.

1-6 A

Educational Objective: To understand some of the more common causes and primary preventive strategies for cancer.

These primary prevention topics are discussed in the chapter. Tobacco is discussed as a cause of bladder cancer, among others. It is the most important cause of cancer, and its prevention is paramount. Its impact is greatest for cancers of the upper aerodigestive tract, but it is important to realize that it is a major player for cancers of the pancreas, kidney, and bladder as well. Although hepatitis C is a major cause of hepatoma, there is no vaccine available. On the other hand, hepatitis B causes hepatoma as well, and there is a vaccine in use that is reducing the incidence of hepatoma. Lastly, although fiber consumption has long been touted as an important preventive agent for colorectal cancer, a number of recent cohort studies and trials have shown that its use does not have an effect on preventing this disease.

Suggested Reading

Schatzkin A, Lanza E, Corle D, et al. Lack of effect of a low-fat, high-fiber diet on the recurrence of colorectal adenomas. Polyp Prevention Trial Study Group. *N Engl J Med.* 2000;342:1149–1155.

Park Y, Hunter DJ, Spiegelman D, et al. Dietary fiber intake and risk of colorectal cancer: a pooled analysis of prospective cohort studies. *J Am Med Assoc.* 2005;294:2849–2857.

O'Brien TR, Kirk G, Zhang M. Hepatocellular carcinoma: paradigm of preventive oncology. *Cancer J.* 2004;10:67–73.

1-7 D

Educational Objective: To calculate and understand the concept of sensitivity, specificity, positive predictive value, and negative predictive value.

When screening for a particular condition, the following outcomes are possible:

	Condition Present	Condition Absent
Positive results	True positive (A)	False-positive (B)
Negative results	False negative (C)	True negative (D)

Sensitivity is the proportion of people with the condition who have a positive test result: A divided by (A plus C).

Specificity is the proportion of people without the condition who have a negative test result: D divided by (B plus D).

Positive predictive value is the proportion of people with a positive test result who have the condition: A divided by (A plus B).

Negative predictive value is the proportion of people with a negative test result who do not have the condition: D divided by (C plus D).

1-8 D

Educational Objective: To appreciate the existence of racial disparities and their multifunctional etiologies.

The most common belief is that the bulk of racial disparities stems from differences in early detection with concomitant differences in stage at diagnosis. These do occur but only account for part of the problem. There also are differences in tumor biology that frequently occur. For example, breast cancers in black women are more likely to be estrogen receptor-negative and to have other features that presage a worse outcome. Differences in treatment for black and white women also are a common finding and may stem from many reasons, including socioeconomic differences, patient-physician communication, differences in attitude toward treatment and the medical profession in general, the way the physician tends to approach patients of different races, etc.

Suggested Reading

Chu KC, Lamar CA, Freeman HP. Racial disparities in breast carcinoma survival rates: separating factors that affect diagnosis from factors that affect treatment. *Cancer.* 2003;97:2853–2860.

Chlebowski RT, Chen Z, Anderson GL, et al. Ethnicity and breast cancer: Factors influencing differences in incidence and outcome. *JNCI.* 2005;97:439–448

Hershman D, McBride R, Jacobson JS, et al. Racial disparities in treatment and survival and outcomes among women with early-stage breast cancer. *J Clin Oncol.* 2005;23:6639–6646.

1-9 C

Educational Objective: To recognize that most of the current screening recommendations are based on less than the optimal type of medical evidence.

Fecal occult blood testing has randomized trials that have shown a consistent benefit in reducing disease-specific mortality. All other recommended screening tests have lesser types of evidence to support their use, although numerous randomized trials are in progress.

Suggested Reading

Mandel JS, Bond JH, Church TR, et al. Reducing mortality from colorectal cancer by screening for fecal occult blood. Minnesota Colon Cancer Control Study. *N Engl J Med.* 1993; 328:1365–1371.

de Koning HJ. Mammographic screening: evidence from randomised controlled trials. *Ann Oncol.* 2003;14:1185–1189.

SELF EVALUATION

CHAPTER 2 QUESTIONS:
MOLECULAR BIOLOGY

2-1 A 35-year-old man presents with colorectal cancer. His mother was diagnosed with endometrial carcinoma in her early 20s and was diagnosed colon cancer when she was 48. His maternal grandfather died of colorectal cancer at age 55. His 38-year-old sister recently underwent a screening colonoscopy, which revealed stage I rectal cancer and no additional polyps.

Which of the following mutations is most likely associated with this patient's colon cancer?

A. Germline deletion of the *hMSH2* gene
B. Loss of heterozygosity of the *ATM* gene
C. Germline mutation of a single allele of the *p53* tumor suppressor gene
D. Mutation of the nucleotide excision repair system

2-2 For a patient with colon cancer, which of the following can be done to demonstrate the DNA repair defect associated with hereditary nonpolyposis colorectal cancer (HNPCC)?

A. Measuring DNA synthesis in fibroblasts after gamma radiation
B. Demonstrating microsatellite instability using polymerase chain reaction (PCR) amplification of short tandem repeats in the tumor cell DNA
C. Examining peripheral blood cells for chromosome breakage in response to diepoxybutane
D. Examing DNA repair in UV-radiated fibroblasts

2-3 Which of the following statements best characterizes the role of this patient's DNA repair defect in sporadic colon cancer?

A. This DNA repair pathway defect results from mutation of the *ATM* tumor suppressor in sporadic colon cancers
B. Approximately 15% of sporadic cancers exhibit the same DNA repair defect
C. Patients with sporadic colon cancer exhibit this DNA repair defect in their peripheral blood lymphocytes as well as in their tumor cells

2-4 A 52-year-old woman has recently been diagnosed with chronic myelogenous leukemia. Which of the following statements about the molecular pathogenesis of chronic myelogenous leukemia (CML) is true?

A. The Philadelphia chromosome causes qualitative alterations in c-ABL expression without structural changes in the *ABL* gene
B. The BCR-ABL fusion creates an inactive, but dominant, negative c-ABL protein
C. The BCR-ABL fusion protein has deregulated tyrosine kinase activity

2-5 A patient with CML undergoes allogeneic stem cell transplantation. Restaging studies demonstrate that he is in complete remission. Which of the following methods could be used to detect minimal residual disease?

A. Southern blot analysis of the *BCR-ABL* gene
B. Real-time (RT) PCR analysis of BCR-ABL mRNA
C. Northern blot analysis of the BCR-ABL mRNA
D. Sequencing of c-ABL to identify point mutations associated with drug resistance

2-6 Which of the following chromosome translocations associated with a hematologic cancer produces a fusion protein?

A. t 8:14 (q24;q32)-Burkitts's lymphoma
B. t15:17 (q21;q21)-Acute promyelocytic leukemia (APL)
C. t11:14 (q13;q32)-Mantle cell lymphoma
D. t14:18 (q32;q21)-Follicular lymphoma

2-7 A 36-year-old man is diagnosed with rhabdomyosarcoma. During the past 10 years, two additional family members have been diagnosed with cancer; his sister with breast cancer at age 38 and his father with osteosarcoma. Which of the following *p53* mutations are commonly inherited in this syndrome?

A. Point mutations that inactivate *p53* function
B. Amplification's that increase *p53* expression
C. Translocations to immunoglobulin loci that deregulate *p53* expression
D. All of the above

2-8 Increased *p53* activity promotes which of the following cellular responses?

A. Increased cell proliferation
B. Reduced binding of growth factors to receptor tyrosine kinases
C. Apoptosis
D. Limitless cellular lifespan

2-9 Checkpoint pathways often are implicated in tumorigenesis. Which of the following statements about checkpoint functions is true?

A. Checkpoints help ensure that cell cycle progression depends upon faithful execution of antecedent cell cycle processes
B. Checkpoint pathways only operate in mitosis
C. Oncogenes that function within checkpoint pathways, rather than tumor suppressor genes, are usually dominant
D. The mitotic checkpoint senses DNA damage

2-10 A 55-year-old man is diagnosed with renal cell carcinoma (RCC). Which of the following patients with hereditary cancer syndromes is likely to have a germline mutation in the same tumor suppressor gene that is mutated in this patient's RCC?

A. A 7-year-old boy with AML and peripheral blood lymphocytes that exhibit sensitivity to DNA cross-linking agents
B. A 23-year-old woman with multiple squamous cell skin carcinomas and photosensitivity
C. A 1-year-old boy with bilateral retinoblastomas
D. A 29-year-old woman with a cerebellar hemangioblastoma and retinal angioma

2-11 Which of the following statements about the *RAS* oncogene is true?

A. *RAS* mutations are found in 80% of advanced breast cancers
B. RAS is a nuclear protein
C. *RAS* mutations are easily detected by oligonucleotide hybridization
D. RAS activity is regulated by nucleotide exchange factors that alter the amount of ADP and ATP bound to *RAS*

2-12 A 68-year-old man is diagnosed with myelodysplastic syndrome and is treated with 5-azacytidine. Which of the following best describes the molecular consequence that directly results from treatment with 5-azacytidine?

A. Histone deacetylase inhibition leading to reactivated expression of a silenced tumor suppressor gene
B. Reduced DNA promoter methylation leading to increased expression of a silenced tumor suppressor gene
C. Activation of the spindle checkpoint
D. Inhibition of RAS farnesylation

2-13 Which of the following statements about the *BCL-2* oncogene is true?

A. It is involved in a translocation with the T-cell receptor gene in follicular lymphoma
B. It stimulates cell death caused by the c-*Myc* oncogene
C. It prevents programmed cell death in part by interacting with pro-apoptotic *BCL-2* family members
D. It is localized to the inner surface of the plasma membrane

2-14 A 36-year-old woman is diagnosed with diffuse large B-cell lymphoma. As part of an investigational study, her lymphoma RNA is analyzed with microarray-based RNA expression analyses. Which of the following statements best describes this technology and its uses in molecular pathology?

A. Microarray studies can be used to predict prognosis for this patient
B. Microarrays utilize RT-PCR to quantitate mRNA abundance in tissue samples
C. Microarrays can only measure the expression of up to 50 genes per chip
D. Microarrays utilize differentially labeled protein probes to compare the amount of mRNA expression between two samples

2-15 Which of the following events are stimulated when epidermal growth factor binds to its receptor?

A. Mitogen-activated protein (MAP) kinase activation
B. Transcription of *MYC* and *JUN* target genes
C. Growth factor receptor dimerization and tyrosine phosphorylation
D. All of the above

2-16 A 53-year-old man is diagnosed with B-cell lymphoma. Pathologic studies are consistent with mantle cell lymphoma, and cytogenetics revealed the t11:14 translocation. Which of the following statements best describes the molecular defect in this patient's lymphoma?

A. The t11:14 translocation disrupts the *cyclin B* gene
B. Increased expression of *E2F* target genes
C. Very high levels of unphosphorylated retinoblastoma protein

2-17 A 70-year-old man with multiple myeloma has recently experienced disease progression after prolonged treatment with thalidomide and dexamethasone, and his oncologist has now suggested a trial of bortezomide, which is a proteasome inhibitor. Which statement about the ubiquitin-proteasome statement is correct?

A. Mdm2 is a ubiquitin ligase that targets the retinoblastoma protein for destruction and is frequently amplified in tumors
B. Degradation of proteins by the proteasome is signaled by ubiquitin conjugation
C. Caspases are the enzymes that attach ubiquitin to target proteins
D. Proteasome inhibitors such as bortezomide prevent the attachment of ubiquitin to proteins targeted for degradation by the ubiquitin-proteasome system

2-18 Which of the following statements best describes microRNAs?

A. MicroRNAs encode short peptides
B. MicroRNAs that are overexpressed in cancers may function as dominant oncogenes
C. MicroRNAs catalyze the destruction of target genes in genomic DNA
D. MicroRNAs catalyze the proteasomal degradation of target proteins

2-19 Which of the following phenotypes are commonly involved in multistep tumorigenesis?

A. Insensitivity to antigrowth signals
B. Increased angiogenesis
C. Resistance to apoptosis
D. All of the above

CHAPTER 2 EXPLANATORY ANSWERS:
MOLECULAR BIOLOGY

2-1 A

Educational Objective: To understand the association between HNPCC and defects in the DNA mismatch repair system.

The patient has three relatives affected with colorectal cancer, one of whom (his mother) is a first degree relative of the other two affected individuals. The pattern of inheritance, the finding of colon cancer at an age younger than 50, and the association with endometrial cancer all suggest HNPCC. His sister's colonoscopy that revealed only a single early-stage cancer without additional polyps argues strongly against familial adenomatous polyposis.

HNPCC is a dominant, autosomal disease that is caused by germline mutations in several genes involved in DNA mismatch repair. The first HNPCC gene to be identified was *hMSH2*, and others include *hMLH1*, *hPMS1*, and *hPMS2*. Affected individuals inherit one mutant and one wild-type allele and subsequently lose the normal allele in the target tissue. Although *p53*-loss occurs commonly in colon cancer, the clinical scenario is not consistent with the Li-Fraumeni syndrome, in which individuals inherit an inactive *p53* allele. Inherited *ATM* mutations are associated with ataxia telangiectasia, whereas mutations within the nucleotide excision repair system cause sun-sensitive diseases such as xeroderma pigmentosum.

Suggested Reading

de la Chapelle A. Genetic predisposition to colorectal cancer. *Nature Reviews: Cancer.* 2004;4(10):769–780.

2-2 B

Educational Objective: See question 1.

Defective DNA mismatch repair results in genetic instability at short tandem repeat sequences, termed microsatellite instability (MIN) (Fig. 2-6). MIN causes a "mutator phenotype" that leads to oncogene mutations. Although PCR amplification of microsatellites is an important diagnostic strategy for HNPCC, diagnoses often are made by directly sequencing mismatch repair genes (most commonly *hMSH2* and *hMLH1*). The other tests described measure repair defects in pathways other than mismatch repair. Radioresistant DNA synthesis is characteristic of ataxia telangiectasia and other diseases with defective double-stranded break repair; sensitivity to cross-linking agents is characteristic of Fanconi anemia; and defective DNA repair of UV treatment is characteristic of xeroderma pigmentosum.

Suggested Reading.

Kaz AM, Brentnall TA. Genetic testing for colon cancer. *Nat Clin Pract Gastroenterol Hepatol.* 2006;3(12):670–679.

2-3 B

Educational Objective: To recognize that microsatellite instability also occurs in sporadic colon cancer.

Approximately 15% of sporadic colon cancers exhibit defective mismatch repair and MIN. However, in these cases, mutations within the mismatch repair genes are rare, and the loss of mismatch repair results from epigenetic changes, such as promoter hypermethylation, which inactivate mismatch repair gene expression. However, because HNPCC accounts for approximately 3% of colon cancers, sporadic cancers account for the majority of cases that exhibit MIN. The *ATM* gene is involved in double-strand break repair and does not play a role in MIN.

Suggested Reading

Kane MF et al. Methylation of the hMLH1 promoter correlates with lack of expression of hMLH1 in sporadic colon tumors and mismatch repair-defective human tumor cell lines. *Cancer Res.* 1997;57: 808–811.

2-4 D

Educational Objective: To understand the molecular basis of CML.

The Philadelphia chromosome defines CML and results in a fusion between the *BCR* and *ABL* genes (Fig. 2-13). The *BCR-ABL* gene produces an mRNA that encodes a fusion protein containing sequences derived from both *BCR* and *ABL*. c-ABL is a tyrosine kinase, and the *BCR* fusion leads to an active and deregulated kinase. Imatinib directly binds to the BCR-ABL protein and prevents ATP from accessing the kinase's active site.

2-5 B.

Educational Objective: To recognize the sensitivity of various molecular methods and their use in detecting residual disease.

The ability of real-time PCR to accurately measure small amounts of the BCR-ABL transcript is a vital tool for CML management. These methods can detect a single CML cell within up to a million normal cells and are the most sensitive means of detecting residual disease. In contrast, Northern and Southern blotting techniques have sensitivities on the order of four to five logs less and are not appropriate methods for detecting rare tumor cells. Finding *ABL* point mutations that prevent imatinib from inhibiting the BCR-ABL protein is an indication for the use of alternate tyrosine kinase inhibitors but is not used to monitor for residual disease.

Suggested Reading.

Oehler VG, Radich JP. Monitoring bcr-abl by polymerase chain reaction in the treatment of chronic myeloid leukemia. *Curr Oncol Rep.* 2003;5(5):426–435.

2-6 B

Educational Objective: To recognize that chromosome translocations activate oncogenes by two distinct mechanisms.

Chromosome translocations found in hematologic cancers activate oncogenes in two ways. The most common way involves creation of fusion genes, as seen in CML (*BCR-ABL,* t9:22). However, in many lymphomas, translocations activate oncogenes by placing them under the transcriptional control of elements contained within the immunoglobulin and T-cell receptor loci. These cases do not result in a fusion protein, but instead cause altered expression of the normal oncoprotein. Three of the examples shown are translocations between proto-oncogenes and immunoglobulin loci (t8:14 involves c-Myc and IgG in Burkett's lymphoma; t11:14 involves cyclin D1 and IgG in mantle cell lymphoma; and t14:18 involves BCL-2 and IgG in follicular lymphoma). In contrast, t15:17 produces a fusion protein derived from the *PML* and *RARalpha* genes, and this fusion protein is the molecular target for all trans-retinoic acid in the treatment of APL (Fig. 2-21).

2-7 A

Educational Objective: To recognize the role of inherited p53 mutations in Li-Fraumeni syndrome (LFS).

The family described displays the characteristics that define LFS, an inherited cancer syndrome characterized by early-onset sarcomas and a wide range of other tumors. The molecular defect in LFS involves inheriting a germline *p53* mutation in one allele and the loss of the remaining *p53* allele in somatic tissues. A large number of *p53* mutations in families with LFS have been described, and these mutations have helped define key functional domains of the p53 protein. These mutations inactivate p53 function and include point mutations, insertions/deletions, and transversions. In contrast, amplifications and translocations would be expected to increase *p53* expression and are not characteristic of LFS.

Suggested Reading

Varley JM. Germline TP53 mutations and Li-Fraumeni syndrome. *Hum Mutat.* 2003;21(3):313–320.

2-8 C

Educational Objective: To understand the cellular functions of the p53 tumor suppressor.

The p53 protein plays a central role in checkpoint pathways that respond to diverse physiologic stresses. p53 serves an effector function in these pathways and instigates complex cellular responses including apoptosis (Figs. 2-25 and 2-26). p53 activation does not promote cell proliferation, but instead inhibits cell division, largely by activating transcription of the p21Cip CDK inhibitor protein. p53 activation also can provoke cellular senescence, and conversely, p53 loss may increase cellular lifespan. In contrast, p53 does not regulate the interactions between growth factors and their receptors.

Suggested Reading

Lane DP. Exploiting the p53 pathway for the diagnosis and therapy of human cancer. *Cold Spring Harb Symp Quant Biol.* 2005;70:489.

Vousden KH, Lu X. Live or let die: the cell's response to p53. *Nat Rev Cancer.* 2002 (8):594–560.

2-9 A

Educational Objective: To understand the functions of checkpoint pathways.

Checkpoints are biochemical pathways that maintain genetic stability by ensuring the cell cycle progresses only when previous cell cycle events have been successfully completed (Fig. 2-25). Loss of checkpoint control is a fundamental feature of cancer and leads to genomic instability. Checkpoints operate in each phase of the cell cycle, and DNA damage can trigger checkpoint responses in both G1 and S-phases. DNA damage in G1 activates p53, and this halts G1 progression through increased transcription of the p21Cip cyclin-dependent kinase inhibitor. Thus, the G1 checkpoint affords cells the opportunity to repair DNA damage before DNA replication begins. In contrast, the mitotic checkpoint senses unattached kinetochores and ensures that mitosis will not proceed until all of the chromosomes are correctly aligned and attached to the spindle.

Suggested Reading

Kastan MB, Bartek J. Cell-cycle checkpoints and cancer. *Nature.* 2004;432(7015):316–323.

2-10 D

Educational Objective: To recognize the role of the Von Hippel-Lindau (VHL) protein in sporadic and hereditary renal cancer.

Most sporadic renal cell cancers contain mutations in the *VHL* gene, which is the tumor suppressor responsible for VHL syndrome, a rare disease characterized by many tumor types, including renal cancers and hemangioblastomas. The VHL protein functions as part of a ubiquitin ligase that catalyzes the addition of ubiquitin to its protein targets, thus causing them to be degraded by the proteasome. One key VHL target is hypoxia-inducible factor alpha (HIF-alpha), a transcription factor that activates a number of genes in hypoxic conditions, including angiogenic growth factors such as vascular endothelial growth factor (VEGF). When VHL is inactivated in renal cancers, HIF-alpha expression increases, leading to increased VEGF production. The patient described in answer D has a clinical history consistent with VHL syndrome. The patients described in answers A, B, and C have Fanconi anemia, xeroderma pigmentosum, and hereditary retinoblastoma, respectively, and none of these syndromes are associated with VHL mutations.

Suggested Reading

Kim, WY, Kaelin, WG. Molecular pathways in renal cell carcinoma –rationale for targeted treatment. *Semin Oncol.* 2006; 33(5):588–595.

2-11 C

Educational Objective: To understand *RAS* functions and mutations in cancers.

RAS genes are mutated in cancers by point mutations that target only a few key amino acids. The highly restricted nature of these mutations allows their detection in cancers by hybridization with oligonucleotide probes that can discriminate between wild-type and mutant alleles. The RAS protein is localized at the plasma membrane by farnesylation, and compounds that inhibit RAS farnesylation are being evaluated as antineoplastic drugs. RAS activity is regulated by being bound to either GDP or GTP, and the amount of GTP and GDP bound to RAS is regulated by proteins that function as GTPase-activating proteins and GTP-exchange factors (Fig. 2-15). *RAS* mutations are found in up to 80% of pancreatic cancers, but they are uncommon in breast cancer.

2-12 B

Educational Objective: To understand the role of DNA methylation in regulating gene expression.

Epigenetic chromatin modifications play important roles in regulating gene expression. DNA methylation in promoter regions reduces gene transcription and is a mechanism leading to silencing of some tumor suppressor genes in cancer cells. 5-azacytidine inhibits DNA methylation and reactivates genes silenced by methylation. Histone acetylation increases gene expression, and drugs that inhibit histone deacetylases are being investigated in clinical trials. However, 5-azacytidine does not alter histone acetylation. Chemotherapeutic drugs that bind to the mitotic spindle, such as the vinca alkaloids and taxanes, trigger the spindle checkpoint, but 5-azacytidine does not. 5-azacytidine does not affect RAS farnesylation.

Suggested Reading

Jones PA. Epigenetic therapy of cancer: past, present and future. *Nat Rev Drug Discov.* 2006;5(1):37–50.

2-13 C

Educational Objective: To understand the role of the *BCL-2* oncogene in suppressing apoptosis.

Many oncogenic stimuli induce programmed cell death, and disabling apoptotic responses is a key event in multistep tumorigenesis (Fig. 2-28). The *BCL-2* oncogene is the founding member of a class of genes that regulate apoptosis, and *BCL-2* expression protects cells from apoptosis induced under many different contexts. For example, deregulated c-Myc activity provokes apoptosis, and this is prevented by *BCL-2* expression. *BCL-2* is involved in the t14:18 characteristic of follicular lymphoma, in which its expression is deregulated by juxtaposition next to immunoglobulin (not T-cell receptor) transcriptional elements. BCL-2 is a mitochondrial protein that interacts with a number of proapoptotic BCL-2 family members, and BCL-2 likely prevents apoptosis by other activities as well, including affects within mitochondria (Fig. 2-19).

Suggested Reading

Chao DT, Korsmeyer SJ. BCL-2 family: regulators of cell death. *Annu Rev Immunol.* 1998;16:395–419.

2-14 A

Educational Objective: To understand the uses of microarrays and global analyses of gene expression.

Microarrays utilize chips that contain spotted arrays of DNA or oligonucleotides and can be used to assess patterns of gene expression in tumor tissues. These arrays are used most commonly to measure mRNA abundance, and modern chips can simultaneously measure the expression of tens of thousands of genes. The chips are hybridized to cDNA probes that are prepared from tumor mRNA and differentially labeled with fluorescent dyes. The amount of relative fluorescent reveals differences in mRNA abundance between samples (Fig. 2-7). Investigators have used these methods to define transcriptional signatures that predict outcome in diseases such as breast cancer and lymphoma (Fig. 2-8). Molecular pathologists are developing microarray analyses that can differentiate diseases that are clinically heterogeneous — yet morphologically similar — such as large cell lymphomas.

Suggested Reading

van't Veer LJ, et al. Expression profiling predicts clinical outcome of breast cancer. *Nature.* 2002;415(6871):530–536.

Rosenwald A, et al. The use of molecular profiling to predict survival after chemotherapy for, diffuse large-B-cell lymphoma. *N Engl J Med.* 2002;346(25):1937–1947.

2-15 D

Educational Objective: To recognize the importance of tyrosine phosphorylation and mitogenic signaling pathways in mediating growth factor activities.

The binding of growth factors to their receptors triggers protein phosphorylation cascades that stimulate cell division (Fig. 2-14). Some growth factors, like epidermal growth factor, bind to receptors termed receptor tyrosine kinases (RTKs). Growth factor binding causes RTKs to dimerize, which results in RTK autophosphorylation on tyrosine residues. These phosphotyrosine motifs function as the recognition motifs that recruit signaling proteins with SH2 domains, and tyrosine phosphorylation is the critical event that sets these signaling pathways in motion. Important downstream events in these signaling chains include MAP kinase activation, and ultimately, activation of transcription factors such as MYC and JUN. Other tyrosine kinases that are not growth factor receptors also are important oncogenes, such as *BCR-ABL*.

2-16 B

Educational Objective: To recognize the role of cyclin D1 in mantle cell lymphoma.

Mantle cell lymphomas are characterized by t11:14, which involves the *cyclin D1* gene, and expresses high levels of cyclin D1 protein. Like other cyclins, cyclin D1 activates cyclin-dependent kinases — in this case, CDK4 and CDK6. The key substrate of cyclin D1 is the retinoblastoma protein (pRb), and phosphorylation of pRb by cyclin-dependent kinases causes it to release E2F transcription factors, which stimulate the onset of S-phase by activating the transcription of E2F target genes. Thus, mantle cell lymphomas exhibit increased pRb phosphorylation. Although Burkitt's lymphomas frequently exhibit translocations involving chromosome 14, the activated oncogene in t8:14 is the *c-myc* gene on chromosome 8 and not *cyclin D1*. The role of the chromosome 14 sequences in both cases is to provide the DNA transcriptional control elements derived from immunoglobulin genes on chromosome 14 that deregulate oncogene expression.

2-17 B

Educational Objective: To understand the principles underlying protein degradation by the ubiquitin-proteasome system.

A large number of cellular proteins are degraded by the ubiquitin-proteasome system. The basic logic of this system involves a series of enzymatic reactions that add chains of ubiquitin, a 76-amino acid protein, to target proteins. Polyubiquitinated proteins are then recognized and rapidly degraded by proteases contained within the 26S proteasome. Protein ubiquitination is a highly regulated process and regulates the activity of many short-lived proteins, such as transcription factors and cell cycle proteins. The Mdm2 ubiquitin ligase ubiquitinates p53, and increased Mdm2 activity disables p53 in tumors. Caspases are proteases that execute the apoptotic program specified by cell death pathways, but they are not found within the proteasome. Proteasome inhibitors, such as bortezomide, do not affect the ubiquitination pathways that target specific proteins for degradation, but instead inhibit the activity of proteases contained within the proteasome itself. These drugs will affect the stability of many proteins, and their specific targets in cancer cells are unknown.

Suggested Reading

Reinstein E, Ciechanover A. Narrative review: protein degradation and human diseases: the ubiquitin connection. *Ann Intern Med.* 2006;145(9):676–684.

Richardson PG, Mitsiades C, Hideshima T, et al. Borte-zomib: proteasome inhibition as an effective anticancer therapy. *Annu Rev Med.* 2006;57:33–47.

2-18 B

Educational Objective: To recognize the functions of microRNAs.

MicroRNAs are a newly discovered class of small RNA molecules that play key roles in regulating gene expression (Fig. 2-9). MicroRNAs do not encode peptides, but instead function by base pairing with their target mRNAs and inhibiting their expression. MicroRNAs inhibit gene expression by both catalyzing mRNA destruction and by inhibiting mRNA translation. In contrast, microRNAs do not cause either DNA or proteins to be degraded. MicroRNA is often overexpressed in cancer, and it has been shown to function as an oncogene in experimental systems.

Suggested Reading

Calin GA, Croce CM. MicroRNA signatures in human cancers. *Nat Rev Cancer.* 2006;6(11):857–866.

2-19 D

Educational Objective: To recognize phenotypes that contribute to multistep tumorigenesis.

Cancer results from the accumulated action of multiple and independent mutations. Although many different mutations contribute to tumorigenesis in different organ sites and individuals, all cancers share many fundamental biologic characteristics. Weinberg and Hanahan articulated 6 "hallmarks of cancer," which include each of the indicated choices (Fig. 2-28).

Suggested Reading

Hanahan D, Weinberg RA. The hallmarks of cancer. *Cell.* 2000; 100(1):57–70.

SELF EVALUATION

CHAPTER 3 QUESTIONS:
CLINICAL PHARMACOLOGY

3-1 A 62-year-old woman will begin capecitabine for metastatic colon cancer. She is taking a beta blocker for hypertension, warfarin for atrial fibrillation, and estrogen for postmenopausal symptoms. You plan on closely monitoring the international normalized ratio (INR).

Which of the following is appropriate?

A. Change the beta blocker to an angiotensin converting enzyme (ACE) inhibitor
B. 50% dose reduction of capecitabine
C. Stop estrogen-replacement therapy
D. Begin full-dose capecitabine

3-2 A 50-year-old man is seen after receiving the first cycle of infusional fluorouracil, leucovorin, and irinotecan for metastatic colon cancer. During this first cycle, which was given 2 weeks ago, he developed febrile neutropenia, with an absolute neutrophil count (ANC) nadir of 100 cells/µL. Results of a complete blood cell count today show a total white blood cell count of 1,200/µL with an ANC of 450 cells/µL, a platelet count of 175,000/µL, and a hematocrit of 36 g/dL. He has had no mucositis, nausea, vomiting, bloody stool, or rash. The results of baseline liver and renal function studies (obtained before the first cycle of treatment) were normal, except for a total bilirubin of 1.5 mg/dL. His only other medication is metoprolol for hypertension

Which of the following would you recommend once the neutrophil count recovers to a normal value?

A. Give no additional fluorouracil
B. Give capecitabine instead of the fluorouracil-based combination
C. Reduce subsequent doses of irinotecan

3-3 In the clinical scenario described in question 2, what is the most likely reason for the severe toxicity observed?

A. A polymorphism in the promoter of the UDP-Glucuronosyltransferase gene (UGT1A1*28)
B. Deficiency in dihydropyrimidine dehydrogenase
C. Metoprolol-induced inhibition of fluorouracil metabolism

3-4 The hospital tumor board asks you to review the findings of a phase III trial that was recently published in a respected peer-reviewed journal. The authors claim that the new treatment is superior to the current standard of care and should become the treatment of choice for patients with this disease. The trial enrolled 300 patients (150 on each study arm) in 60 centers across North America including Canada and Mexico. The two arms were evenly balanced for the important disease characteristics. The trial was designed to detect an improvement in time to disease progression of 50% (median time to disease progression with the standard of care, 6 months; median time to disease progression with the new treatment, 9 months) with 0.80 power at a statistic significance level of 0.05 (two-sided test). Secondary endpoints included overall survival, cost, quality of life, and toxicity. The investigators claim a significant result, with a median time to disease progression for the new treatment of x months compared with a median time to disease progression of y months for the standard of care ($p = 0.02$).

Which of the following conclusions can you draw from the results of this trial?

A. The trial is too small to make any conclusions, regardless of the p value
B. Time to progression is not a valid endpoint; therefore, the results are meaningless
C. The difference in the time to disease progression of 3 months is not a clinically meaningful difference; therefore, the results are invalid
D. Differences in clinical research practices in different countries make this trial impossible to interpret
E. The new treatment is a reasonable option for treatment and may be used as a new standard of care

3-5 Which of the following best describes a pharmacodynamic endpoint?

A. The relationship between an administered dose and the maximum plasma concentration achieved
B. The relationship between an administered dose and an observed toxicity
C. The pharmacokinetic interaction of two drugs administered simultaneously
D. The relationship of an administered dose of a drug and a change in a biologic target
E. The pharmacokinetic impact of a drug on the clearance mechanisms in a patient

3-6 A 60-year-old man with a metastatic sarcoma to the lung and left-sided pleural effusion is being treated with high-dose methotrexate. Following the treatment, he is treated with leucovorin as a rescue agent. The presence of the pleural effusion will have which of the following effects?

A. No effect on the methotrexate clearance or area under the curve
B. Increase the clearance of methotrexate
C. Decrease the clearance of methotrexate
D. No effect on the clearance of methotrexate, but will increase the area under the curve
E. Decrease the clearance of methotrexate and the area under the curve

3-7 A 43-year-old premenopausal female with surgically resected ER-positive, stage II breast cancer is placed on adjuvant tamoxifen. Shortly after beginning tamoxifen, she develops moderate hot flashes and requests pharmacotherapy to reduce their severity and intensity. Which of the following do you recommend?

A. Estrogen replacement for hot flashes for a duration of 1 year
B. Stopping tamoxifen and placing the patient on an aromatase inhibitor
C. Beginning paroxetine, 20 mg/day for hot flashes
D. Beginning venlafaxine XR, 75 mg daily for hot flashes

3-8 A 70-year-old woman presents with recurrent ovarian cancer 2 months after finishing paclitaxel and carboplatin as adjuvant therapy for stage III ovarian cancer. A CT demonstrates extensive peritoneal carcinomatosis, ascites, retroperitoneal adenopathy, and bilateral hydronephrosis. She has an ischemic cardiomyopathy (ejection fraction of 25%). Physical examination demonstrates abdominal distention and a fluid wave. The serum creatinine is 2.5 mg/dL. Which of the following do you recommend?

A Doxorubicin 40 mg/m^2, administered once every 3 weeks
B Carboplatin AUC 5, administered once every 3 weeks
C Topotecan, administered at full dose, daily for 5 days, every 3 weeks
D Topotecan, administered with a 50% dose reduction, daily for 5 days, every 3 weeks

CHAPTER 3 EXPLANATORY ANSWERS:
CLINICAL PHARMACOLOGY

3-1 D

Educational Objective: To understand the drug interactions of capecitabine and warfarin.

This patient is taking warfarin and will begin oral capecitabine. The substantial interactions between these two compounds are difficult to predict. It is not recommended necessarily to reduce the doses of capecitabine, but instead to closely monitor the coagulation status following the initiation of capecitabine. Therefore, the correct answer is to administer the full dose of capecitabine and to closely monitor the coagulation parameters.

Suggested Reading

Copur MS, Ledakis P, Bolton M, et al. An adverse interaction between warfarin and capecitabine: a case report and review of the literature. *Clin Colorectal Cancer.* 2001;1(3):182–184.

Reigner B, Blesch K, Weidekamm E. Clinical pharmacokinetics of capecitabine. *Clin Pharmacokinet.* 2001;40(2):85–104.

3-2 C

Educational Objective: To understand the metabolism of irinotecan and the management of chemotherapy-associated neutropenia.

See 3-3 A for explanatory answer.

3-3 A

Educational Objective: To understand the metabolism of irinotecan.

This 50-year-old patient had marked neutropenia and infection following treatment with fluorouracil, leucovorin, and irinotecan. The results of laboratory studies demonstrate an elevated total bilirubin, consistent with Gilbert syndrome. Patients with these laboratory parameters are frequently found to be homozygous for the UGT1A1*28 allele, a common polymorphism which decreases UGT1A1 enzyme function and, therefore, the efficiency of bilirubin glucuronidation. In the case of irinotecan, patients with this genetic variant have impaired SN38 glucuronidation and a higher risk of severe neutropenia. This patient is unlikely to be dihydropyrimidine dehydrogenase deficient, given the lack of severe diarrhea, the quick recovery phase, and the absence of mucositis.

For question 2, answer D is the best answer, as irinotecan dose reduction will reduce the risk of severe neutropenia for subsequent cycles without compromising the exposure to the active metabolite, SN38.

Suggested Reading

Pizzolato JF, Saltz LB. The camptothecins. *Lancet.* 2003;361 (9376): 2235–2242.

Innocenti F, Undevia SD, Iyer L, et al. Genetic variants in the UDP-glucuronosyltransferase 1A1 gene predict the risk of severe neutropenia of irinotecan. *J Clin Oncol.* 2004;22(8):1382–1388.

3-4 E

Educational Objective: To understand reports of phase III clinical trials.

This question reviews a typical phase III clinical trial performed in oncology. The endpoint of time to disease progression is a new endpoint that is increasing in acceptance. Option A is incorrect because the size of the trial is dictated by the power; therefore, p value is reflective of that. The time to disease progression is a valid endpoint, although the U.S. Food and Drug Administration does not always recognize this when deciding on approval. Option C is incorrect because the difference in time to disease progression of 3 months is typically considered clinically significant. Option D is incorrect because there is good standardization in clinical research across different countries.

Suggested Reading

Ma BB, Britten CD, Siu LL. Clinical trial designs for targeted agents. *Hematol Oncol Clin North Am.* 2002;16(5):1287–1305.

Stadler W. New trial designs to assess antitumor and antiproliferative agents in prostate cancer. *Invest New Drugs.* 2002;20(2):201–208.

3-5 D

Educational Objective: To understand the definition of a pharmacodynamic endpoint.

Pharmacodynamic endpoints are increasingly important in clinical research, and it is important to understand their precise meaning. The relationship between the dose and plasma concentration achieved is a pharmacokinetic endpoint. Toxicity can sometimes be used as a pharmacodynamic endpoint, but the definition is specifically the effect of a drug on a particular biologic target, making D the best option. Options C and E are incorrect, as these are pharmacokinetic interactions.

Suggested Reading

Colburn W, Lee J. Biomarkers, validation and pharmacokinetic-pharmacodynamic modeling. *Clin Pharmacokinet.* 2003;42 (12): 997–1022.

Workman P. How much gets there and what does it do? The need for better pharmacokinetic and pharmacodynamic endpoints in contemporary drug discovery and development. *Curr Pharm Des.* 2003;9(11):891–902.

3-6 D

Educational Objective: To understand the effect of a pleural effusion on the pharmacokinetics of methotrexate.

Third-space fluids must be recognized to influence and alter the clearance of methotrexate, as well as of other drugs. Methotrexate diffuses into the third-space fluid, which then is preserved as a reservoir for prolonged diffusion back into the circulation. Therefore, for this patient, option D is correct. Methotrexate will be cleared at the same rate through the kidney and the liver, but the third-space fluid will increase the area under the curve, in essence, increasing the exposure of the patient to the drug over time and requiring prolonged leucovorin rescue. For this reason, methotrexate is often contraindicated in patients with pleural effusions.

Suggested Reading

Li J, Gwilt P. The effect of malignant effusions on methotrexate disposition. *Cancer Chemother Pharmacol.* 2002;50(5):373–382.

3-7 D

Educational Objective: To understand the metabolism of tamoxifen and the potential for drug interactions.

The patient is taking tamoxifen and develops hot flashes. Recent data have demonstrated that tamoxifen is activated from a weak antiestrogen to a potent antiestrogen, endoxifen. This activation step is dependent upon CYP2D6, a phase I enzyme which is highly variable. Approximately 7% to 10% of white patients lack functional CYP2D6 enzyme (poor metabolizers) and are at higher risk of recurrence. Additionally, a substantial number of medications potently inhibit CYP2D6, and for patients with "normal' levels of the enzyme (extensive metabolizers) the coadministration of potent CYP2D6 inhibitors, such as paroxetine or fluoexetine, will inhibit the metabolic activation of tamoxifen. An analysis of a retrospective phase III tamoxifen adjuvant trial demonstrated that women who were CYP2D6 poor metabolizers or who were administered potent CYP2D6 inhibitors had a 3-fold higher risk of breast cancer relapse than patients with extensive CYP2D6 metabolism who were not administered an inhibitor. The only correct answer is D: begin venlfaxine. Venlafaxine is a weak CYP2D6 inhibitor with preliminary data demonstrating little or no difference in endoxifen plasma levels for patients taking tamoxifen.

Suggested reading

Jin Y, Desta Z, Stearns V, et al. CYP2D6 genotype, antidepressant use, and tamoxifen metabolism during adjuvant breast cancer treatment. *J Natl Cancer Inst.* 2005;97(1):30–39.

Goetz MP, Rae JM, Suman VJ, et al. Pharmacogenetics of tamoxifen biotransformation is associated with clinical outcomes of efficacy and hot flashes. *J Clin Oncol.* 2005;23(36):9312–9318.

Goetz MP, Knox SK, Suman VJ, et al. The impact of cytochrome P450 2D6 metabolism in women receiving adjuvant tamoxifen. *Breast Cancer Res Treat.* 2007;101(1):113–121.

3-8 D

Educational Objective: To understand the excretion of topotecan.

Topotecan is a topoisomerase I inhibitor that is approved for the treatment of metastatic ovarian cancer after failure of first- or second-line therapy. Topotecan is excreted, in part, by the kidney, and a 50% dose reduction is recommended for patients with moderate renal impairment. Therefore, answer C is incorrect, as any patient with moderate renal impairment should not receive full-dose topotecan. Answer A is incorrect, as the patient has pre-existing cardiomyopathy; therefore, doxorubicin is contraindicated. Answer B is incorrect, as the patient experienced disease progression while recieving platinum-containing adjuvant therapy within the last 2 months; therefore, there would be no expected benefit of single-agent carboplatin in this setting.

Suggested Reading

Creemers GJ, Bolis G, Gore M, et al. Topotecan, an active drug in the second-line treatment of epithelial ovarian cancer: results of a large European phase II study. *J Clin Oncol.* 1996;14(12): 3056–3061.

O'Reilly S, Rowinsky EK, Slichenmyer W, et al. Phase I and pharmacologic study of topotecan in patients with impaired renal function. *J Clin Oncol.* 1996;14(12):3062–3073.

SELF EVALUATION

CHAPTER 4 QUESTIONS:
BIOLOGIC THERAPY

4-1 You have observed a sustained, complete clinical response in one of your patients with a solid tumor. Which of the following biologic agents provides the best evidence that antitumor immunity was generated?

A. Aldesleukin
B. Bevacizumab
C. Interferon-alpha 2a
D. Trastuzumab
E. Denileukin diftitox

4-2 A 60-year-old man with metastatic melanoma has been enrolled in a clinical trial investigating the effects of a novel interleukin that has been shown in preclinical studies to enhance the cytotoxic activity of lymphocytes. Which of the following is likely to be true regarding this interleukin's activity?

A. It is produced in a single organ
B. It will induce other cytokines
C. It will act on only one cell type
D. The duration of its immunologic activity will parallel serum levels

4-3 You are designing a combination chemotherapy protocol for refractory lung cancer. Preclinical studies suggest that the greatest antitumor effects are achieved with weekly administration. Thus, you plan to administer the combination on days 1, 8, 15, 22, 29, and 36. Weekly administration is predicted to produce significant neutropenia and thrombocytopenia. Which of the following regimens of hematopoietic factors could you consider incorporating into your protocol to deal with these toxicities?

A. Filgrastim administered days 2 to 50
B. Filgrastim administered days 3 to 5, 10 to 12, 17 to 19, 24 to 26, 31 to 33, and 38 to 40
C. Pegfilgrastim administered days 1, 8, 15, 22, 29, and 36
D. Oprelvekin administered when platelet counts reach less than 50,000/mm^3
E. Sargramostim administered days 1to 36

4-4 You are discussing the benefits and risks of a standard adjuvant interferon-alpha regimen for a patient with stage III melanoma who has undergone wide excision and complete lymphadenectomy. Which of the following side effects is anticipated to abate as therapy proceeds during the 12 months of administration?

A. Fatigue
B. Hepatotoxicity
C. Fever
D. Depression
E. Neutropenia

4-5 A 56-year-old woman has stage IV head and neck cancer that progressed after chemotherapy. She then received palliative radiotherapy to a painful vertebral metastasis. Thereafter, she began cetuximab. She is premedicated with diphenhydramine and has received eight weekly infusions. Except for a rash, she is tolerating it well. Recent scans document stable disease. Which of the following is true?

A. Because of short elimination $t^{1/2}$, daily dosing of monoclonal antibodies is necessary
B. Because they represent immune-mediated effects, the development of rash predicts resistance to cetuximab
C. Because it may dampen immune responses, premedication is contraindicated
D. Radiotherapy is not administered in combination with cetuximab
E. Monoclonal antibodies may be able to improve survival in the absence of tumor regression

4-6 A 71-year-old woman is presented to you for evaluation of supraclavicular and axillary adenopathy. Follicular lymphoma was diagnosed. She was observed with no therapy for 6 months, at which time she became more symptomatic and began rituximab therapy. During her first infusion, she developed dyspnea. The infusion was stopped until dyspnea resolved. Rituximab was restarted at a slower rate, and she was able to complete this and five other weekly infusions. She achieved a complete clinical response. On follow-up 14 months later, new mediastinal adenopathy was found, in addition to recurrence in the axillary and supraclavicular nodes. The findings of repeat biopsy confirmed follicular lymphoma. When considering treatment options, which of the following should influence your decision, regarding retreatment with rituximab?

A. Neutralizing antibodies that will negate therapeutic activity are likely
B. The reaction to the initial infusion is a contraindication for retreatment
C. Response rates associated with retreatment are essentially equivalent to those for initial treatment
D. Administering a non-cross-reactive antibody to CD20, such as alemtuzumab, is preferred
E. Retreating with rituximab is likely to cause neutropenia

4-7 In which of the following disseminated malignant processes has there been approval of a monoclonal antibody that may elicit direct antiproliferative effects?

A. Colorectal cancer
B. Diffuse large B-cell lymphoma
C. Breast cancer
D. Follicular lymphoma
E. All of the above

4-8 There are numerous reports of the benefit of donor lymphocyte infusions (DLI) for patients undergoing homologous stem cell transplantion (HSCT). Which of the following is *true* with regard to the activity of DLI?

A. It will usually occur in the absence of graft-versus-host disease (GVHD)
B. It depends on complete replacement of host immune cells with those of the donor
C. It requires that the malignancy be responsive to the chemotherapy used in the conditioning regimen
D. It is more frequently observed for patients with chronic rather than acute leukemia
E. It is limited to patients with hematologic malignancies undergoing HSCT

4-9 You are the director of a small biotechnology company that has identified a novel glycoprotein that is highly expressed on the surface of breast cancer cells. Subsequent studies have indicated low-level expression on some normal epithelial cells in the upper airway. The DNA sequences of both the factor produced by breast cancers and the normal epithelial cells are identical. Your clinical director is suggesting that this substance be developed as a target for a cancer vaccine. Which of the following statements is a correct assumption?

A. Expression on normal cells will preclude an immune response
B. Membrane expression will promote cytotoxic T-lymphocyte (CTL) recognition
C. Absence of mutations will preclude a vaccine approach
D. Absence of mutations will promote CD4-positive/CD25-positive T-reg cells
E. The carbohydrate component will preclude antibody recognition

CHAPTER 4 EXPLANATORY ANSWERS:
BIOLOGIC THERAPY

4-1 A

Educational Objective: To understand the indirect and direct antitumor mechanisms of biologic agents.

As most solid tumors do not express the interleukin (IL)-2 receptor (CD25), including both renal cell carcinoma and melanoma for which it is approved, aldesleukin does not directly affect the growth of tumors; rather, it functions indirectly. Although the mechanism of aldesleukin has not been established, its primary antitumor function is considered to be activating cytotoxic lymphocytes (e.g., CTL and natural killer cells). The generation of antitumor immunity is not necessary for antitumor effects with bevacizumab, interferon-alpha 2a, trastuzumab, and denileukin diftitox. Bevacizumab can mediate antitumor activity by neutralizing vascular endothelial growth factor and inhibiting tumor angiogenesis. Interferon-alpha 2a can directly modulate the growth of tumor cells and inhibit angiogenesis, as can trastuzumab. Denileukin diftitox uses IL-2 to deliver a toxin to CD25-positive cells.

Suggested Reading

Foss FM. Immunologic mechanisms of anti-tumor activity. *Semin Oncol.* 2002;29(3 Suppl 7):5–11.

Eklund JW, Kuzel TM. Interleukin-2 in the treatment of renal cell carcinoma and malignant melanoma. *Cancer Treat Res.* 2005; 126:263–287.

4-2 B

Educational Objective: To understand the spectrum of cytokine activity.

The administration of a cytokine will initiate a cascade of cytokine production and both stimulatory and inhibitory/antagonistic effects. Although cytokines share many features with hormones; however, in contrast to hormones they are not produced by specific, specialized organs, but rather by cells thoughout the body. Cytokines are characterized by pleiotropy. The serum half-life of cytokines is typically very short, on the order of hours, but the immunologic effects can persist for months.

Suggested Reading

Waller EK, Ernstoff MS. Modulation of antitumor immune responses by hematopoietic cytokines. *Cancer.* 2003;97(7):1797–1809.

Zlotnik A. Chemokines and cancer. *Int J Cancer.* 2006;119(9): 2026–2029.

4-3 B

Educational Objective: To understand the benefit and risks of administering hematopoietic cytokines.

Because of the sensitivity of rapidly dividing myeloid cells, filgrastim and sargramostim should be administered no earlier than 24 hours after the administration of cytotoxic chemotherapy and no later than 24 hours before the administration of chemotherapy. Pegfilgrastim should not be administered in the period between 14 days before and 24 hours after administration of cytotoxic chemotherapy. Oprelvekin must be administered to patients sufficiently in advance of the platelet nadir to allow adequate time for megakaryocyte maturation and platelet formation.

Suggested Reading

Smith TJ, Khatcheressian J, Lyman GH, et al. 2006 update of recommendations for the use of white blood cell growth factors: an evidence-based clinical practice guideline. *J Clin Oncol.* 2006;24(19):2975–2977.

4-4 C

Educational Objective: To understand the side effects of cytokine therapy with interferon.

Although its impact on overall survival is not clear, interferon is routinely applied in the adjuvant setting for patients with stage III melanoma after primary surgery. Flu-like symptoms usually abate as interferon therapy is continued. Fatigue and depression usually develop later and progress with continued therapy. Frequent laboratory assessments are necessary to monitor hepatic function and granulocyte counts.

Suggested Reading

Kirkwood JM, Manola J, Ibrahim J, et al. Eastern Cooperative Oncology Group. A pooled analysis of Eastern Cooperative Oncology Group and intergroup trials of adjuvant high-dose interferon for melanoma. *Clin Cancer Res.* 2004;10(5): 1670–1677.

Hurley KE, Chapman PB. Helping melanoma patients decide whether to choose adjuvant high-dose interferon-alpha2b. *Oncologist.* 2005;10(9):739–742.

4-5 E

Educational Objective: To understand the application of therapeutic monoclonal antibodies.

Through effects on the growth cycle, the antitumor effects of monoclonal antibodies can be cytostatic. Antibodies against growth factor receptors also may modify other important processes in cancer progression, such as invasion and metastasis. Thus, improved survival can be achieved in the absence of tumor regression. Antibodies have elimination half-lives often on the order of days to weeks and usually are not administered daily. Premedication is recommended to reduce infusion reactions prior to the initial infusion for most of the monoclonal antibodies in clinical use. Although active as monotherapy, monoclonal antibodies have been effectively applied with myelosuppressive/immunosuppresive treatment modalities and are usually applied clinically with chemotherapy and radiotherapy. Cetuximab is approved for use with radiotherapy for patients with head and neck cancer. There is evidence that the development of a skin rash for patients receiving cetuximab is predictive of treatment benefit.

Suggested Reading

Adams GP, Weiner LM. Monoclonal antibody therapy of cancer. *Nat Biotechnol.* 2005;23(9):1147–1157.

4-6 C

Educational Objective: To identify the potential immunologic sequelae that can complicate the use of rituximab.

Response rates associated with retreatment have been essentially the same as with initial cycles of treatment (40% to 50%). Although neutralizing antibodies to the chimeric protein are possible, they have rarely been reported. Dyspnea, although common during initial infusion, does not presage more serious sequelae, and treatment can usually continue uninterrupted. Alemtuzumab is a monoclonal antibody directed at CD52, not CD20. It is approved for use to treat chronic lymphocytic leukemia. CD20 is not expressed by neutrophils, and neutropenia would not be predicted with rituximab monotherapy. Rituximab will cause lymphopenia.

Suggested Reading

Davis TA, Grillo-Lopez AJ, White CA, et al. Rituximab anti-CD20 monoclonal antibody therapy in non-Hodgkin's lymphoma: Safety and efficacy of re-treatment. *J Clin Oncol.* 2000;18(17):3135–3143

Hainsworth JD, Litchy S, Shaffer DW, et al. Maximizing therapeutic benefit of rituximab: maintenance therapy versus re-treatment at progression in patients with indolent non-Hodgkin's lymphoma–a randomized phase II trial of the Minnie Pearl Cancer Research Network. *J Clin Oncol.* 2005;23(6):1088–1095

4-7 E

Educational Objective: To understand the mechanism of antitumor activity of clinically applicable monoclonal antibodies.

Monoclonal antibodies can mediate antitumor effects by activating host effector mechanisms such as antibody-dependent cell-mediated cytotoxicity. Also, several have demonstrated the ability to directly inhibit the growth of tumor cells. Trastuzumab has been shown to directly inhibit the growth of breast cancer cells. Similarly, cetuximab has been shown to directly inhibit the growth of colorectal tumor cells. Both function by inhibiting signaling mediated through the epidermal growth factor family of tyrosine kinases, activation of which is implicated in oncogenesis. The mechanism of the direct antiproliferative effects of rituximab compared with malignant B cells has not established but also may involve inhibition of signaling pathways.

Suggested Reading

Adams GP, Weiner LM. Monoclonal antibody therapy of cancer. *Nat Biotechnol.* 2005;23(9):1147–1157.

Maloney DG. Immunotherapy for non-Hodgkin's lymphoma: monoclonal antibodies and vaccines. *J Clin Oncol.* 2005;23(26): 6421–6428.

4-8 D

Educational Objective: To understand the mechanism of activity of an adoptive cellular therapy program in clinical practice.

To date, responses with DLI in the setting of HSCT have been most favorable for patients with chronic myelogenous leukemia. Graft-versus-leukemia (GVL)/graft-versus-tumor (GVT) effects of currently applied DLI programs are usually accompanied by GVHD. Research efforts are focusing on promoting GVL/GVT versus tumor over GVHD. Myeloablation with complete replacement of host immune cells with those of the donor is not necessary. Nonmyeloablative conditioning regimens have been applied to allow for DLI. Antitumor activity is not limited to patients with hematologic malignancies undergoing HSCT. The cancer does not need to be responsive to the chemotherapy used in the conditioning regimen. Tumor regressions, which are usually delayed, have been effected in patients with solid tumors, such as renal cell carcinoma, who are receiving conditioning chemotherapy and whose disease is not shown to be active. Tumor responses are usually observed several months after the chemotherapy is administered.

Suggested Reading

Porter D, Levine JE. Graft-versus-host disease and graft-versus-leukemia after donor leukocyte infusion. *Semin Hematol.* 2006;43(1):53–61.

Childs R, Chernoff A, Contentin N, et al. Regression of metastatic renal-cell carcinoma after nonmyeloablative allogeneic peripheral-blood stem-cell transplantation. *N Engl J Med.* 2000;343(11): 175–183

4-9 D

Educational Objective: To understand potential targets for cancer vaccines.

The expression on normal tissues of the identical species identified in the breast cancer cells would indicate that the glycoprotein is a self-antigen. Although the mechanism is not clear, CD4-positive/CD25-positive T-reg cells have been shown to suppress the activity of self-reactive lymphocytes and have been implicated in the suppression of immune response elicited by vaccines. Strategies are under investigation to address the expansion of T-reg cells in cancer vaccine approaches. T-cell recognition requires presentation of the protein as peptide fragments within the context of major histocompatibility complex molecules. The glycoprotein on the surface of breast cancer cells does not indicate that it is necessarily expressed within the context of MHC molecules. Many substances that are only preferentially expressed on tumors can be targeted by vaccine approaches. Vaccine strategies that can break tolerance to nonmutated, self antigens have been developed and have been shown to be able to stimulate immune responses. Cancer vaccines that stimulate antibody responses have demonstrated promise. Antibodies will recognize polysaccharides as well as protein determinants exposed on cell membranes in their native conformation.

Suggested Reading

Lizee G, Radvanyi LG, Overwijk WW, Hwu P. Improving antitumor immune responses by circumventing immunoregulatory cells and mechanisms. *Clin Cancer Res.* 2006;12(16): 4794–4803

Ribas A, Butterfield LH, Glaspy JA, Economou JS. Current developments in cancer vaccines and cellular immunotherapy. *J Clin Oncol.* 2003;21(12):2415–2432.

Graziano DF, Finn OJ. Tumor antigens and tumor antigen discovery. *Cancer Treat Res.* 2005;123:89–111

Reilly RT, Emens LA, Jaffee EM. Humoral and cellular immune responses: independent forces or collaborators in the fight against cancer? *Curr Opin Investig Drugs.* 2001;2(1): 133–2135.

SELF EVALUATION

CHAPTER 5 QUESTIONS:
BREAST CANCER

5-1 Which of the following statements most accurately describes trends in the incidence of breast cancer?

A. The incidence of breast cancer is higher in developing countries than in the industrialized world
B. The incidence of breast cancer has recently decreased in the United States
C. In Western industrialized countries, breast cancer is the third most common cancer among women
D. Lung cancer has displaced breast cancer as the most common cancer among women in the United States

5-2 The incidence of breast cancer in the United States varies among ethnic groups.

Which of the following statements accurately describes this variation?

A. The highest incidence of breast cancer is found among American Indian women
B. The incidence of breast cancer is lower among black women than white women
C. When Asian people immigrate to the United States, their incidence of breast cancer drops

5-3 Which of the following statements regarding risk factors for breast cancer is true?

A. The incidence of breast cancer is higher for women taking long-term hormone-replacement therapy
B. A history of ovarian cancer on the maternal side of the family — but not on the paternal side — is associated with a 4-fold increase in the risk of breast cancer
C. *BRCA1* mutations are present in 12% of all patients with breast cancer
D. *BRCA2* mutations occur most commonly in Hispanic populations

5-4 Which of the following statements best describes the association of genetic abnormalities with specific familial breast cancer syndromes?

A. *RB* translocation is associated with Cowden syndrome
B. *BRCA2* mutations are associated with Li-Fraumeni syndrome
C. *AKT* mutations are associated with familial estrogen-excess syndrome
D. *TP53* mutations are associated with Li-Fraumeni syndrome
E. The estrogen receptor (ER) gene is hypermethylated and inactive in tumors with *BRCA2* mutations

5-5 Which of the following statements about reproductive risk factors for breast cancer is true?

A. Early onset of menarche, late onset of menopause, and greater number of years with ovulatory cycles are all associated with an increased risk of breast cancer
B. Nulliparity is associated with a reduced risk for breast cancer
C. Lactation, especially for long duration, is associated with a modest increased risk for breast cancer
D. Pregnancy after treatment for breast cancer reduces survival

5-6 Which of the following statements regarding the association of behavior and breast cancer incidence is true?

A. Strenuous physical activity increases the risk of breast cancer
B. Obesity in premenopausal women is associated with a 4-fold increase in the risk of breast cancer
C. Obesity is not a risk factor for postmenopausal women
D. Regular consumption of even one or two alcoholic drinks daily significantly increases the risk of breast cancer

5-7 The risk of breast cancer can be reduced by several medical interventions.

Which of the following statements is true?

A. Prophylactic bilateral ovarian ablation before age 45 is associated with a substantial reduction in risk for women with familial breast cancer
B. For postmenopausal women, hormone-replacement therapy reduces the risk of breast cancer
C. Tamoxifen administered for 5 years is associated with a 30% to 50% reduction in the risk of developing both ER-positive and ER-negative breast cancer
D. Aromatase inhibitors have no effect on the incidence of second primary breast cancers

5-8 Which of the following statements regarding recurrence risk for breast cancer is true?

A. Involvement of the axillary lymph nodes is the most important predictor of both local recurrence and systemic metastasis
B. Expression of the ER or progesterone receptor (PR) is correlated with a lower short-term survival rate than the rate associated with ER-negative and PR-negative tumors
C. Quantitative *cathepsin D*, *Bcl-2*, and *p53* expression provide an excellent reproducible prognostic index

5-9 A 37-year-old premenopausal woman is found to have a 2.5-cm tumor in the upper outer quadrant of her left breast. There is also a 1.5-cm mobile, firm, nontender node in the left axilla that is positive for malignancy on fine needle aspiration. The appropriate staging work up ruled out distant metastasis. The patients prefers breast conservation if it is medically safe.

Which of the following would be the most appropriate regional therapeutic option for this patient?

A. Lumpectomy, axillary dissection, radiation therapy to the breast
B. Lumpectomy, sentinel node biopsy, radiation therapy to the breast
C. Mastectomy and axillary node dissection
D. Lumpectomy followed by breast and axillary radiation

5-10 You are treating a 40-year-old premenopausal woman with stage IIb breast cancer. The tumor is hormone receptor and *HER2* negative.

Which of the following therapeutic options would you recommend?

A. Six cycles of classic cyclophosphamide, methotrexate, and fluorouracil (CMF)
B. Six cycles of fluorouracil, doxorubicin, and cyclophosphamide (FAC) followed by 5 years of anastrozole
C. Four cycles of doxorubicin and cyclophophamide (AC)
D. Four cycles of AC followed by four cycles of paclitaxel administered in a dose-dense schedule
E. Goserelin for 2 years and tamoxifen for 5 years

5-11 A 59-year-old woman who has taken combined hormone-replacement therapy since the onset of menopause 8 years earlier has abnormal findings on screening mammogram. Clusters of suspicious calcifications are identified, covering a 1.2-cm area of the lower, inner quadrant of the right breast. The results of needle-localization biopsy indicate a ductal carcinoma in situ (DCIS) (1.2 cm in largest diameter) that is nuclear grade 2. The medial margin is positive for disease. The ER assay is negative.

Which of the following is the most appropriate treatment plan?

A. Modified radical mastectomy
B. Bilateral subcutaneous mastectomy
C. Lumpectomy with clear surgical margins and radiation therapy to the breast
D. Lumpectomy and axillary dissection, radiation therapy to the breast
E. Lumpectomy alone

5-12 A 53-year-old premenopausal woman is found to have a 1.2-cm mass in the upper, outer quadrant of the left breast. No regional lymph nodes are palpable. Bilateral mammography confirms the presence of a stellate mass in the upper, outer quadrant of the left breast. There are diffuse calcifications throughout the upper, inner quadrant of the left breast. The right breast is unremarkable.

Stereotactic core biopsy of the left breast mass shows an infiltrating ductal cancer that is hormone receptor-positive admixed with DCIS. The findings of biopsy of two areas of calcifications in the left breast demonstrate mixed ductal and lobular carcinoma in situ.

Which of the following is the preferred surgical treatment option for this patient?

A. Left lumpectomy, radiofrequency ablation of the DCIS, with sentinel node biopsy followed by radiation
B. Left lumpectomy with sentinel node biopsy and immediate reconstruction
C. Bilateral mastectomies with left sentinel node biopsy and immediate reconstruction
D. Left mastectomy with immediate axillary node dissection

5-13 During an evaluation for pneumonia, a 42-year-old premenopausal woman is found to have a large mass (7 cm by 9 cm) in the left breast. The mass does not involve the skin or underlying structures. There are multiple enlarged, firm, ipsilateral axillary lymph nodes. The findings of core-needle biopsy demonstrate an infiltrating ductal cancer, nuclear grade 3, that is ER-negative, PR-negative, and *HER2*-negative. Staging work-up does not indicate distant metastasis.

Which of the following is the most appropriate therapeutic plan?

A. Lumpectomy and axillary dissection followed by four cycles of AC, followed by radiation therapy to the breast, with subsequent tamoxifen for 5 years
B. Modified radical mastectomy with sentinel lymph node biopsy followed by four cycles AC and goserelin for 2 years
C. Four cycles of FAC, followed by surgical resection definitive local therapy (breast conservation depending on response), followed by four cycles of a taxane
D. Four cycles of FAC followed by four cycles of a taxane followed by surgical resection, definitive local therapy (breast conservation depending upon response), followed by radiation therapy
E. Subcutaneous mastectomy with placement of a breast implant, followed by radiation therapy, goserelin for 2 years, and trastuzumab for 1 year

5-14 In addition to a history and physical examination, which of the following procedures should be included for the optimal surveillance of patients with primary breast cancer after local, regional, and systemic therapies have been completed?

A. History and physical examination every 4 to 6 months during the first 5 years and yearly thereafter. Annual mammography of the remaining breast tissue
B. History and physical examination, complete blood count, and liver function tests every 4 to 6 months during the first 5 years and yearly thereafter. Annual mammography of the remaining breast tissue
C. History and physical examination, complete blood count, liver function tests, and tumor markers every 4 to 6 months during the first 5 years and yearly thereafter. Annual mammography of the remaining breast tissue
D. History and physical examination, complete blood count, liver function tests, tumor markers, bone scan, and abdominal imaging every 4 to 6 months during the first 5 years and yearly thereafter. Annual mammography of the remaining breast tissue
E. Whole body positron emission tomography (PET) every 4 to 6 months during the first 5 years, then yearly thereafter

5-15 Which of the following statements regarding hormone therapy for metastatic breast cancer is true?

A. Ovarian ablation is only effective for premenopausal patients
B. Aromatase inhibitors are equally effective for pre- and postmenopausal women
C. Women with high endogenous estrogen levels do not respond to tamoxifen
D. Women with hormone-receptor positive breast cancers that overexpress *HER2* do not respond to endocrine therapy.

5-16 A 54-year-old postmenopausal woman is seen in consultation after the diagnosis and surgical removal of a 0.8-cm grade 2 invasive lobular cancer of the right breast that was ER-positive, PR-positive, and HER2-negative. The Recurrence Score on her tumor was 10. She had deep-vein thrombosis 18 months earlier. Lumpectomy was carried out with clear surgical margins, and two sentinel lymph nodes had no disease. Planned treatment will include radiation therapy to the breast.

Which of the following systemic treatment strategies is the best choice?

A. Tamoxifen for 5 years, followed by letrozole for 5 years
B. Tamoxifen for 5 years
C. Six cycles of fluorouracil, epirubicin, and cyclophosphamide, followed by anastrozole for 5 years
D. Anastrozole for 5 years
E. Four cycles of AC

5-17 A 38-year-old premenopausal woman is referred for treatment of metastatic breast cancer. She was diagnosed 18 months earlier with a T1, N0, M0, poorly differentiated invasive ductal cancer that was ER-negative, PR-negative, and *HER2*-positive (3+ staining). The primary tumor was 0.6 cm in the largest diameter. She was treated with a total mastectomy and axillary dissection; of 16 lymph nodes removed, all were negative for disease. No adjuvant systemic therapy was recommended.

She now has bilateral, asymptomatic pulmonary metastases, a small left pleural effusion, several hepatic metastases, and multiple areas of increased uptake on bone scan involving the ribs, spine, and pelvis. X-rays of the bone are remarkably unimpressive, showing one 5-cm lytic lesion in the right ileum. Cytologic analysis of pleural fluid is positive for adenocarcinoma cells, consistent with the earlier diagnosis of breast cancer.

In addition to intravenous bisphosphonate therapy, which of the following would you recommend?

A. Classic CMF
B. Anastrozole with trastuzumab
C. Paclitaxel combined with trastuzumab
D. AC combined with trastuzumab
E. AC alone

CHAPTER 5 EXPLANATORY ANSWERS:
BREAST CANCER

5-1 B

Educational Objective: To recognize the public health importance of breast cancer.

The incidence of breast cancer, which had increased over the past 5 decades throughout industrialized countries, has started to decrease. Approximately half of all new cases worldwide occur in developing countries and the other half in Western industrialized nations. The American Cancer Society (ACS) estimates that 180,000 new cases of breast cancer will be diagnosed in the United States in 2007, and 40,000 women will die. Breast cancer continues to be the most common cancer among women in the United States and represents the second most common cause of cancer death.

Suggested Reading

Jemal A, Siegel R, Ward E, et al. Cancer Statistics. *CA Cancer J Clin.* 2006;56(2):106–130.

ACS: *Cancer Facts and Figures 2006.* Atlanta, American Cancer Society, 2006.

ACS: American Cancer Society: *Breast Cancer Facts & Figures 2005-2006.* Atlanta, American Cancer Society, Inc., 2006.

Ravdin PM, Cronin KA, Howlader N, et al. The dec rease in breast-cancer incidence in 2003 in the United States. *N Engl JMed.* 2007;356(16):1670–1674.

5-2 B

Educational Objective: To identify geographic and ethnic variations in the incidence of breast cancer.

In the United States, the incidence of breast cancer is highest among white women, followed by black, Hispanic, American Indian, and Asian women. Mortality, on the other hand, is highest among black women, followed by white, Hispanic, American Indian, and Asian women. Some of these differences in mortality are thought to be related to differences in socioeconomic level and access to care, whereas others appear to be related to biologic differences. In general, the incidence is greater among higher socioeconomic groups, whereas mortality is higher among lower socioeconomic groups. The rates of breast cancer for Asian populations are traditionally much lower than Western populations; however, the incidence increases for Asian immigrants to the United States, suggesting a correlation with lifestyle and environmental influences.

Suggested Reading

ACS: American Cancer Society: *Breast Cancer Facts & Figures 2005-2006.* Atlanta, American Cancer Society, Inc., 2006.

Smith-Bindman R, Miglioretti DL, Lurie N, et al. Does utilization of screening mammography explain racial and ethnic differences in breast cancer? *Ann Intern Med.* 2006;144(8):541–553.

Kolonel LN, Altshuler D, Henderson BE. The multiethnic cohort study: exploring genes, lifestyle and cancer risk. *Nat Rev Cancer.* 2004;4(7):519–527.

5-3 B

Educational Objective: To identify the most common risk factors for breast cancer and evaluate their relative contribution to overall risk.

Sex is clearly the most significant risk factor; for every man with breast cancer there are approximately 100 women with the disease. The incidence also increases substantially with age; it is rare in women younger than age 40 and common among women in the seventh decade of life. There are multiple hormone associations with breast cancer risk, including early age of menarche, nulli- or late parity, and late menopause. Long-term use of hormone replacement therapy, particularly combined estrogen-progestins, is associated with increased risk of breast cancer. Less than 10% of breast cancers appear to be familial (predisposition is inherited). Familial clustering is a warning sign, but some family histories are more strongly suggestive of inherited breast cancer than others. For instance, a history of unilateral breast cancer detected at age 78 in a second cousin increases the risk of breast cancer only marginally, whereas the history of bilateral breast cancer at a young age (younger than age 40) in two or three first-degree relatives (mother, sister, daughter) increases the lifetime risk to more than 50%. It also increases the risk of bilateral breast cancer and disease occurring at an early age. Familial breast cancer also is associated with increased risk of other cancers. Most cases are explained by mutations in two genes: *BRCA1* and *BRCA2.* Mutations in *BRCA1* are associated with a markedly increased risk of breast and ovarian cancer. *BRCA2* mutations are associated with a marked increase in breast cancer risk but not an increase risk of ovarian cancer. In addition, *BRCA2* mutations are linked to breast cancer in men as well as to an increased incidence of prostate cancer. Familial breast cancers appear to have similar penetrance for the maternal and paternal side, emphasizing the need for a complete family history. Jewish ancestry, especially Ashkenazi ancestry (Eastern European), is associated with a higher likelihood of *BRCA1* and *BRCA2* mutations. There are specific founder mutations detected in various ethnic populations, but there is no known increase in *BRCA1* or *BRCA2* mutations in Hispanic populations.

Suggested Reading

Nathanson KL, Wooster R, Weber BL. Breast cancer genetics: what we know and what we need. *Nat Med.* 2001;7(5):552–556.

Dumitrescu RG, Cotarla I. Understanding breast cancer risk—where do we stand in 2005? *J Cell Mol Med.* 2005;9(1): 208–221.

Grann VR, Whang W, Jacobson JS, et al. Benefits and costs of screening Ashkenazi Jewish women for BRCA1 and BRCA2. *J Clin Oncol.* 1999;17(2):494–500.

Collaborative Group on Hormonal Factors in Brest Cancer. Familial breast cancer: collaborative reanalysis of individual data from 52 epidemiological studies including 58,209 women with breast cancer and 101,986 women without the disease. *Lancet.* 2001;358(9291):1389–1399.

Newman B, Mu H, Butler LM, et al. Frequency of breast cancer attributable to BRCA1 in a population-based series of American women. *JAMA.* 1998;279(12): 915–921.

5-4 D

Educational Objective: To recognize the role of germ-line mutations in breast cancer and their association with familial clustering.

BRCA1 mutations are most often linked to the breast and ovarian cancer syndrome, representing a marked increased in the risk for both cancers. The lifetime risk of breast cancer for carriers of *BRCA1* or *BRCA2* mutations is between 50% and 85%, and both carry an increased risk for ovarian cancer. The breast cancers that develop in *BRCA1* carriers are usually poorly differentiated ER- and *HER2*-negative tumors. *BRCA2* mutations also are associated with an increased risk of breast cancer for both women and men; the breast cancers in *BRCA2* carriers are usually ER-positive and *HER2*-negative. *BRCA1* and *BRCA2* mutations are associated with early-onset breast cancer and an increased frequency of bilateral tumors. For families with *BRCA1* mutations, the frequency of colorectal and prostate cancers also is found to be increased. Mutations in the *BRCA2* gene are linked to increased risk of colorectal, pancreatic, gastric, and prostate cancers. The basic molecular genetic lesion for the Li-Fraumeni syndrome is a germ-line mutation in *TP53*. In addition to breast cancer, a broad spectrum of cancers, including sarcoma, brain tumors, lung and laryngeal cancers, leukemia, lymphoma, and adrenocortical cancers, develop in families with this condition. Mutations in *PTEN* lead to Cowden syndrome, also known as multiple hamartoma syndrome. It is inherited as an autosomal dominant trait and is characterized by distinctive mucocutaneous lesions, as well as by cancers of the breast, thyroid, and the genitourinary tract for women. Abnormalities in the *STK11* gene are associated with the Peutz-Jegher syndrome.

Suggested Reading

Nathanson KL, Wooster R, Weber BL. Breast cancer genetics: what we know and what we need. *Nat Med.* 2001;7(5):552–556.

Frank TS, Deffenbaugh AM, Reid JE, et al. Clinical characteristics of individuals with germline mutations in BRCA1 and BRCA2: analysis of 10,000 individuals. *J Clin Oncol.* 2002;20(6):1480–1490.

Tonin PN. Genes implicated in hereditary breast cancer syndromes. Semin Surg Oncol. 2000;18:281–286; 10,000 individuals. *J Clin Oncol.* 2002;20:1480–1490.

5-5 A

Educational Objective: To identify the influence of reproductive risk factors on breast cancer risk.

Early onset of menarche and late onset of menopause are associated with an increased risk of breast cancer. This finding is thought to be the consequence of a higher number of years with ovulatory cycles. Nulliparity is a risk factor for breast cancer, whereas having a full-term pregnancy before age 20 is protective. It is hypothesized that early pregnancy has a maturing effect on breast glandular tissue, making it more refractory to carcinogenic stimuli. However, having the first full-term pregnancy after age 34 increases the risk of breast cancer. It has been observed that lactation has a protective effect. However, because different studies have provided conflicting results, it is likely that this protective benefit is of modest magnitude. There is evidence that ovarian ablation before natural menopause begins is protective. Ovarian ablation is presumed to shorten the number of ovulatory cycles and lifetime exposure to endogenous estrogens. Conversely, postmenopausal hormone-replacement therapy is associated with a substantial increase in the risk of breast cancer, probably because it prolongs lifetime exposure to estrogens.

Suggested Reading

Col NF, Hirota LK, Orr RK, et al. Hormone replacement therapy after breast cancer: a systematic review and quantitative assessment of risk. *J Clin Oncol.* 2001;19(8): 2357–2363.

Morimoto LM, White E, Chen Z, et al. Obesity, body size, and risk of postmenopausal breast cancer: the Women's Health Initiative (United States). *Cancer Causes Control.* 2002;13(8): 741–751.

Velie EM, Nechuta S, Osuch JR. Lifetime reproductive and anthropometric risk factors for breast cancer in postmenopausal women. *Breast Dis.* 2005;24:17–35.

ACS: American Cancer Society: *Breast Cancer Facts & Figures 2005–2006.* Atlanta, American Cancer Society, Inc., 2006.

5-6 D

Educational Objective: To identify the role of behavioral factors in the modulation of breast cancer risk.

For women who became engaged in regular, strenuous physical activity early in life, the risk of breast cancer is lower. Because strenuous physical activity around and shortly after puberty is associated with delayed puberty, irregular menses, and sometimes amenorrhea, exercise would be equivalent to late menarche and, therefore, a shorter lifetime exposure to estrogens. Obesity in premenopausal women has not been associated with an altered risk of breast cancer; however, there is solid evidence to support the adverse effect of postmenopausal obesity on breast cancer risk. Because obesity is related to eating behavior, it might be one opportunity for behavioral prevention of breast cancer. Epidemiologic studies have suggested a correlation between increased dietary fat intake and breast cancer. However, prospective interventional studies, including low-fat diets, have not confirmed any role for dietary fat intake in modulating breast cancer risk. There have been multiple case-control studies conducted to assess the correlation between postmenopausal hormone-replacement therapy and the risk of postmenopausal breast cancer. The results of several of these studies, as well as a meta-analysis, have suggested an increased risk of breast cancer for women taking long-term (more than 5 years) hormone-replacement therapy. The Women's Health Initiative included a randomized assessment of hormone-replacement therapy compared with placebo for postmenopausal women with an intact uterus. After a mean follow-up of approximately 5 years, a significant 26% increase in the risk of breast cancer was seen among patients receiving hormone-replacement therapy. The consistent intake of alcohol in amounts that exceed one or two drinks a day (12 to 24 grams or 30 to 60 millimeters per day) also has also been associated with a significant increase in the risk of breast cancer. Obesity, hormone-replacement therapy, and alcohol intake are behavioral risk factors that lend themselves to modification, likely resulting in a reduction in the risk of the disease.

Suggested Reading

Rossouw JE, Anderson GL, Prentice RL, et al. Risks and benefits of estrogen plus progestin in healthy postmenopausal women: principal results From the Women's Health Initiative randomized controlled trial. *JAMA.* 2002;288(3):321–333.

Ballard-Barbash R, Forman MR, Kipnis V. Dietary fat, serum estrogen levels, and breast cancer risk: a multifaceted story. *J Natl Cancer Inst.* 1999;91(6):492–494.

Holmes MD, Hunter DJ, Colditz GA, et al. Association of dietary intake of fat and fatty acids with risk of breast cancer. *JAMA.* 1999;281(281):914–920.

Willett WC. Dietary fat and breast cancer. *Toxicol Sci.* 1999; 52(2 Suppl):127–146.

Prentice RL, Caan B, Chlebowski RT, et al. Low-fat dietary pattern and risk of invasive breast cancer: the Women's Health Initiative Randomized Controlled Dietary Modification Trial. *JAMA.* 2006;295(6):629–642.

5-7 A

Educational Objective: To recognize the various options of breast cancer prevention and select the most appropriate option for individual patients.

Removal of all mammary gland tissue (bilateral mastectomy) reduces the risk of breast cancer by up to 90%, even for women with familial or hereditary disease. Prophylactic bilateral ovarian ablation before age 45 also is known to reduce the incidence by at least 50%, even for women with *BRCA1* or *BRCA2* mutations who are at high risk. The results of a number of epidemiologic studies as well as the Women's Health Initiative randomized trial illustrate the association of hormone-replacement therapy with increased breast cancer risk. This increase is especially prominent for women who took a combination of estrogen and progestin. The results of prospective randomized clinical trials of women at high risk have demonstrated that tamoxifen administered daily for 5 years significantly reduces the risk of breast cancer. In the largest randomized trial, this risk reduction approached 50%. In recent randomized investigations in the postoperative adjuvant setting, both anastrozole and letrozole have been associated with a 40% to 50% reduction in incidence of second primary breast cancer.

Suggested Reading

Hartmann LC, Schaid DJ, Woods JE, et al. Efficacy of bilateral prophylactic mastectomy in women with a family history of breast cancer. *N Engl J Med.* 1999; 340(2):77–84.

Rebbeck TR, Lynch HT, Neuhausen SL, et al. Prophylactic oophorectomy in carriers of BRCA1 or BRCA2 mutations. *N Engl J Med.* 2002;346(21):1616–1622.

Fisher B, Costantino JP, Wickerham DL, et al. Tamoxifen for the prevention of breast cancer: current status of the National Surgical Adjuvant Breast and Bowel Project P-1 study. *J Natl Cancer Inst.* 2005;97(22):1652–1662.

Baum M, Budzar AU, Cuzick J, et al. Anastrozole alone or in combination with tamoxifen versus tamoxifen alone for adjuvant treatment of postmenopausal women with early breast cancer: first results of the ATAC randomised trial. *Lancet.* 2002;359 (9324):2131–2139.

5-8 A

Educational Objective: To identify commonly used prognostic factors for primary breast cancer.

Tumor size, involvement of axillary lymph nodes, and high nuclear and histologic grade are all directly related to risk of recurrence. The number of involved axillary lymph nodes provides a semiquantitative assessment of risk of recurrence and death from breast cancer. An increasing number of positive lymph nodes is associated with increased risk of recurrence. The expression of ER or PR by the tumor is a short-term favorable prognostic factor. Recurrent disease tends to develop more slowly during the first 4 to 5 years for patients with ER-positive or PR-positive tumors. Although several genomic-based assays provide independent prognostic information, none of the individual markers listed (*cathepsin D, bcl-2,* and *p53*) are of known value.

Suggested Reading

Olivotto IA, Bajdik CD, Ravdin PM, et al. Population-based validation of the prognostic model ADJUVANT! for early breast cancer. *J Clin Oncol.* 2005;23(12):2716–2725.

Hess KR, Pusztai L, Buzdar AU, et al. Estrogen receptors and distinct patterns of breast cancer relapse. *Breast Cancer Res Treat.* 2003;78(1):105–118.

Fan C, Oh DS, Wessels L, et al. Concordance among gene-expression-based predictors for breast cancer. *N Engl J Med.* 2006;355(6):560–569.

5-9 A

Educational Objective: To determine the choice of local-regional therapy for patients with operable breast cancer.

A breast cancer measuring 2.5-cm is a T2 lesion. The presence of a palpable ipsilateral axillary lymph node represents clinical N1 disease, in this case, confirmed by fine needle aspirate. The absence of evidence of metastases on clinical evaluation would represent an M0 breast cancer. A small T2, N1, M0 breast cancer can be treated with a lumpectomy (wide excision with negative margins) or a total mastectomy. The preferred approach—if the breast-to-tumor ratio permits a good cosmetic result—is a lumpectomy. Axillary staging can be done by an axillary dissection, the standard of care for patients with a palpable axillary node. Sentinel lymphadenectomy is not appropriate for patients with known axillary metastases. The options provided are associated with different risks of local-regional recurrence: a lumpectomy alone without radiotherapy would be associated with higher risk of ipsilateral recurrence than a lumpectomy followed by radiotherapy, although the two procedures would provide equivalent survival. This lesion could be treated with exclusive radiotherapy, without surgical resection, but local recurrence risk would be higher, and the long-term cosmetic results would probably be compromised by the much higher doses of radiotherapy needed for optimal local control. A mastectomy removes the maximum amount of breast tissue and is associated with the lowest risk of local recurrence. However, for patients with a unifocal, small breast cancer and without known *BRCA1* or *BRCA2* mutations, mastectomy is unnecessary and represents excessive therapy.

Suggested Reading

Greene F, Page D, Fleming I, et al. AJCC Cancer Staging Handbook, 6th ed., Philadelphia, Pa: Lippincott Raven Publishers; 2002.

Fisher B, Anderson S, Bryant J, et al. Twenty-year follow-up of a randomized trial comparing total mastectomy, lumpectomy, and lumpectomy plus irradiation for the treatment of invasive breast cancer. *N Engl J Med.* 2002;347(16):1233-1241.

5-10 D

Educational Objective: To identify systemic therapeutic options for primary breast cancer.

In the absence of systemic adjuvant therapy, this patient has a 5-year risk of recurrent disease that exceeds 60%. Because this was a poorly differentiated, ER-, PR-, and *HER2*-negative tumor, the only reasonable treatment options are in the chemotherapy group. Neither endocrine therapy (anastrozole, goserelin, tamoxifen) nor trastuzumab are indicated. Of the three chemotherapy regimens provided as options, the most modern and effective is likely to be four cycles of AC followed by four cycles of paclitaxel, given in a dose-dense fashion (every 2 weeks with hematopoietic growth factor support).

Suggested Reading

Citron ML, Berry DA, Cirrincione C, et al. Randomized trial of dose-dense versus conventionally scheduled and sequential versus concurrent combination chemotherapy as postoperative adjuvant treatment of node-positive primary breast cancer: first report of Intergroup Trial C9741/Cancer and Leukemia Group B Trial 9741. *J Clin Oncol.* 2003;21 (8):1431–1439.

Berry DA, Cirrincione C, Henderson IC, et al. Estrogen-receptor status and outcomes of modern chemotherapy for patients with node-positive breast cancer. *JAMA.* 2006;295 (14):1658–1667.

5-11 C

Educational Objective: To identify therapeutic options for patients with primary operable breast cancer.

This patient had a single, small, mammographically detected noninvasive breast cancer. The standard of care would be a lumpectomy with clear surgical margins followed by radiation therapy to the breast. No axillary staging is needed. Radiation therapy to regional lymph nodes is not indicated. Both a modified-radical mastectomy and bilateral subcutaneous mastectomy are considered overtreatment. Lumpectomy alone, although advocated by some members of the surgical community, is not considered the standard of care.

Suggested Reading

Fisher B, Dignam J, Wolmark N, et al. Lumpectomy and radiation therapy for the treatment of intraductal breast cancer: findings from National Surgical Adjuvant Breast and Bowel Project B-17. *J Clin Oncol.* 1998;16(2): 441–452.

5-12 B

Educational Objective: To identify surgical therapeutic options for patients with primary operable breast cancer.

This patient was found to have a multicentric DCIS, with a separate area of invasive cancer measuring 1.2 cm. Because of the multifocal involvement, resection of all cancer would require multiple lumpectomies with the uncertainty of total resection. Therefore, a total mastectomy is the preferred surgical intervention for this woman. Most would regard bilateral mastectomy as too radical, particularly given the absence of findings on the contralateral side. Radiofrequency ablation is being explored in clinical trials, but its role in routine clinical use is undefined.

Suggested Reading

Rosen PR, Groshen S, Saigo PE, et al. A long-term follow-up study of survival in stage I (T1N0M0) and stage II (T1N1M0) breast carcinoma. *J Clin Oncol.* 1989;7(3): 355–366.

5-13 D

Educational Objective: To determine the optimal therapeutic option for patients with stage III breast cancer.

This stage III breast cancer represents a high-risk lesion. Although it is technically operable, most experts would prefer to start treatment with neoadjuvant chemotherapy. In its current state, this tumor cannot be resected with a lumpectomy. A modified radical mastectomy would be an alternative approach. High-risk tumors with multiple positive axillary lymph nodes necessitate the use of radiation therapy following surgical removal, so even after a mastectomy, delayed reconstruction is preferred to avoid the changes that occur in the reconstructed breast after radiation. A subcutaneous mastectomy would be a completely inadequate intervention for this large, high-risk breast cancer. State-of-the-art chemotherapy would include an anthracycline-based regimen and a taxane, either concurrently or sequentially.

Suggested Reading

Kaufmann M, Hortobagyi GN, Goldhirsch A, et al. Recommendations from an international expert panel on the use of neoadjuvant (primary) systemic treatment of operable breast cancer: an update. *J Clin Oncol.* 2006;24(12): 1940–1949.

Cance WG, Carey LA, Calvo BF, et al. Long-term outcome of neoadjuvant therapy for locally advanced breast carcinoma: effective clinical downstaging allows breast preservation and predicts outstanding local control and survival. *Ann Surg.* 2002;236(3):295–302; discussion 302–303.

Recht A. Locally advanced breast cancer and postmastectomy radiotherapy. *Surg Oncol Clin N Am.* 2000;9(3):603–620, x–xi.

5-14 A

Educational Objective: To identify the recommended practices of surveillance following completion of combined-modality therapy for patients with primary breast cancer.

Randomized clinical trials have not shown a survival benefit associated with the performance of multiple diagnostic tests following completion of optimal combined-modality treatment of primary breast cancer. Most recurrences are detected on the basis of new symptoms or findings on physical examination. Thus, performing blood counts, blood chemistry, tumor markers, chest x-ray, or imaging of the chest, abdomen, pelvis, or bones is not associated with patient benefit. Whereas frequent, extensive testing may disclose asymptomatic metastases earlier for some patients, earlier institution of treatment for metastatic breast cancer did not prolong survival in randomized clinical trials. ASCO recommends a periodic history, physical examination, and yearly mammogram of the remaining breast tissue. There is much interest in assessing the value of whole-body PET scans to stage and monitor the clinical course of breast cancer. However, it has not been shown to be a necessary or useful part of surveillance for patients without evidence of recurrent or metastatic breast cancer.

Suggested Reading

Khatcheressian JL, Wolff AC, Smith TJ, et al. American Society of Clinical Oncology 2006 update of the breast cancer follow-up and management guidelines in the adjuvant setting. *J Clin Oncol.* 2006;24(31):5091–5097.

5-15 A

Educational Objective: To identify the indications for endocrine therapy for breast cancer.

Endocrine therapy has antitumor efficacy by blocking the signaling of the estrogen receptor or the endogenous production of the natural ligand for the estrogen receptor, estrogen. Therefore, in the absence of an estrogen receptor, endocrine therapy has no target and no effect. Ovarian ablation is effective for premenopausal women because it removes or suppresses endogenous estrogen production by the ovary. For postmenopausal women, the ovary does not produce estrogen in sufficient amounts to stimulate breast cancer growth. Most of the estrogen is produced in muscle, peripheral fat, and the adrenal cortex in postmenopausal women. Therefore, suppressing or ablating the ovaries in a postmenopausal woman has no therapeutic effect. Aromatase inhibitors have been tested almost exclusively in postmenopausal women. There is no evidence that they have therapeutic effects for women who are premenopausal. The aromatase inhibitors have not been systematically tested for men with breast cancer either. Levels of endogenous estrogen have no correlation with response to tamoxifen. In fact, tamoxifen results in marked increases in estrogen concentration in premenopausal women, regardless of the antitumor response. Overexpression of HER2 may be associated with relative resistance to antiestrogens in preclinical models; however, clinical data are not definitive.

Suggested Reading

Buzdar A, Howell A. Advances in aromatase inhibition: clinical efficacy and tolerability in the treatment of breast cancer. *Clin Cancer Res.* 2001;7(9):2620–2635.

Osborne CK, Shou J, Massarweh S, et al. Crosstalk between estrogen receptor and growth factor receptor pathways as a cause for endocrine therapy resistance in breast cancer. *Clin Cancer Res.* 2005;11(2 Pt 2):865s–870s.

5-16 D

Educational Objective: To identify the indications for adjuvant systemic therapy.

This patient has a primary breast cancer with a good prognosis and an estimated 5-year risk of recurrence of approximately 15%. Adjuvant chemotherapy is not justified, especially since the tumor was ER-positive and PR-positive, so adjuvant endocrine therapy will provide substantial benefit. Dose-dense therapy would certainly be overtreatment. Most invasive lobular cancers are ER-positive, PR-positive, and *HER2*-negative. Medically reasonable options might include no adjuvant therapy or endocrine therapy alone. Endocrine therapy would reduce the odds of recurrence by approximately 50%. The additional benefit of chemotherapy is very modest in the setting of a low Recurrence Score, which is a genomic-based tool that predicts risk of recurrence despite endocrine therapy in node-negative, hormone receptor-positive breast cancer. Aromatase inhibitors (i.e., anastrozole, letrozole) have a small benefit compared with tamoxifen for postmenopausal women. Tamoxifen is associated with a slight increase in risk of thromboembolic complications and would be relatively contraindicated for this low-risk patient. The aromatase inhibitors (i.e., anastrozole, letrozole, exemestane) are somewhat more effective than tamoxifen for postmenopausal women and are devoid of the increased risk of thromboembolic complications, so they may be a preferred choice for this patient.

Suggested Reading

Olivotto IA, Bajdik CD, Ravdin PM, et al. Population-based validation of the prognostic model ADJUVANT! for early breast cancer. *J Clin Oncol.* 2005;23(12):2716–2725.

Hanrahan EO, Valero V, Gonzalez-Angulo AM, et al. Prognosis and management of patients with node-negative invasive breast carcinoma that is 1 cm or smaller in size (stage 1; T1a,bN0M0): a review of the literature. *J Clin Oncol.* 2006;24(13):2113–2122.

Paik S, Shak S, Tang G, et al. A multigene assay to predict recurrence of tamoxifen-treated, node-negative breast cancer. *N Engl J Med.* 2004;351(27):2817–2826.

Winer EP, Hudis C, Burstein HJ, et al. American Society of Clinical Oncology technology assessment on the use of aromatase inhibitors as adjuvant therapy for postmenopausal women with hormone receptor-positive breast cancer: status report 2004. *J Clin Oncol.* 2005;23(3):619–629.

5-17 C

Educational Objective: To identify the treatment approaches for patients with *HER2*-positive breast cancer.

This premenopausal woman now presents with multiorgan metastatic disease, probably ER-negative, PR-negative, and strongly *HER2*-positive. Data from clinical trials suggest that for optimal therapy, trastuzumab, a monoclonal antibody that targets the extracellular domain of the HER2 oncoprotein, must be a part of the treatment. Single-agent trastuzumab is effective for some patients with *HER2*-positive breast cancer and might be a consideration for this asymptomatic patient; however, her visceral involvement would lead many to incorporate chemotherapy at least for several cycles. Given the ER- and PR-negative nature of her tumor, anastrozole is not indicated. Data from a randomized trial showed a significant prolongation of survival when trastuzumab was combined with chemotherapy. Because of an adverse cardiac interaction between trastuzumab and anthracyclines, it is recommended that these two classes of drugs not be administered simultaneously. Trastuzumab in combination with taxanes has been shown to be safe and effective. In view of the significant survival benefit from the combination of chemotherapy and trastuzumab, it is inappropriate to offer chemotherapy alone to such a patient except in the presence of specific contraindications to trastuzumab. Because of the presence of bone metastases, an intravenous bisphosphonate should be an integral part of the treatment program.

Suggested Reading

Jackisch C. HER-2-positive metastatic breast cancer: optimizing trastuzumab-based therapy. *Oncologist.* 2006;11 Suppl 1:34–41.

Slamon DJ, Leyland-Jones B, Shak S, et al. Use of chemotherapy plus a monoclonal antibody against HER2 for metastatic breast cancer that overexpresses HER2. *N Engl J Med.* 2001;344(11):783–792.

Vogel CL, Cobleigh MA, Tripathy D, et al. Efficacy and safety of trastuzumab as a single agent in first-line treatment of HER2-overexpressing metastatic breast cancer. *J Clin Oncol.* 2002;20(3):719–726.

SELF EVALUATION

CHAPTER 6 QUESTIONS:
LUNG CANCER

6-1 A 62-year-old man with a 60 pack-year-history of smoking presents with a 1-month history of cough and hemoptysis. On physical examination, he has an Eastern Cooperative Oncology Group (ECOG) performance status of 1. No focal physical findings are noted. Computerized tomography (CT) of the chest shows a right-sided lung mass, bulky, right-sided mediastinal adenopathy, and no other pulmonary, adrenal, or liver lesions. The findings on positron emission tomography (PET) scan and on magnetic resonance imaging (MRI) of the head made with gadolinium contrast are negative. The results of percutaneous needle biopsy show small cell cancer.

Which of the following is the best option for treatment?

A. Cisplatin and etoposide followed by 60 Gy of thoracic radiation therapy administered in daily fractions over 6 weeks
B. Cisplatin and etoposide plus concurrent thoracic radiation therapy at 45 Gy administered in daily fractions over 5 weeks
C. Cisplatin and etoposide followed by 45 Gy of thoracic radiation therapy administered twice daily over 3 weeks
D. Cisplatin and etoposide plus concurrent thoracic radiation therapy at 45 Gy administered twice daily over 3 weeks
E. Cisplatin and etoposide, with radiation therapy at 45 Gy administered on relapse of disease

6-2 The patient described in Question 1 has a complete response to your initial treatment. What do you tell him regarding the role of cranial radiation in his treatment?

A. Prophylactic cranial radiation decreases the morbidity associated with brain metastases but at the price of a decrease in cognitive function and with no improvement in survival
B. Prophylactic cranial radiation decreases the morbidity associated with brain metastases without any significant impact on cognitive function and no improvement in survival
C. Prophylactic cranial radiation decreases the morbidity associated with brain metastases and improves survival but with increased long-term cognitive defects
D. Prophylactic cranial radiation decreases the morbidity associated with brain metastases and improves survival, with minimal long-term cognitive defects

6-3 A 72-year-old man with a 40-pack-year history of smoking presents with increasing shortness of breath. He worked in a factory fitting insulation on pipes for more than 30 years before becoming a truck driver 10 years ago. A chest x-ray shows a large right-sided pleural effusion; a thoracentesis is done. On evaluation, the fluid is found to contain cells consistent with mesothelioma. CT scan of the chest shows extensive, diffuse right-sided pleural thickening and hilar and mediastinal adenopathy, but no parenchymal nodules. The results of pulmonary function tests include a forced vital capacity of 1.5 mL. The findings of pleural biopsy are positive for epithelial-type mesothelioma.

Which of the following is the most appropriate treatment for this patient?

A. Cisplatin
B. Cisplatin/doxorubicin/etoposide
C. Cisplatin/gemcitabine
D. Cisplatin/pemetrexed

6-4 A 56-year-old woman with a 30 pack-year smoking history presents with a 3-month history of cough and shortness of breath. During the past 4 weeks, the cough has produced copious amounts of blood-tinged sputum. On physical examination, she has fine, bilateral rales. CT scan of the chest demonstrates small bilateral pulmonary nodules without mediastinal or hilar adenopathy and no signs of metastases in the liver or adrenal glands. Thoracotomy is performed, and one of the nodules shows pure bronchioloalveolar cancer as defined by the World Health Organization.

Which of the following is the most appropriate therapy for this patient?

A. Carboplatin plus paclitaxel
B. Carboplatin, paclitaxel, and bevacizumab
C Carboplatin, paclitaxel, and gemcitabine
D. Erlotinib
E. Carboplatin, paclitaxel, and erlotinib

6-5 Which of the following describes some of the differences between atypical carcinoid and small cell lung cancer?

A. Small cell lung cancer cells have a greater number of neuroendocrine granules as detected by electron microscopy
B. Small cell lung cancer cells have a greater number of mitoses found by light microscopy
C. Atypical carcinoids found in the lung are likely to represent metastases from the gastrointestinal tract, whereas small cell lung cancer is almost always primary to the lung
D. Atypical carcinoids are more likely to be associated with smoking

6-6 You are treating a 55-year-old woman with carboplatin and paclitaxel for squamous cell carcinoma of the lung. The patient had presented with a peripheral, 3-cm mass, mediastinal adenopathy, and bilateral pulmonary nodules. Both the primary tumor and the pulmonary metastases have partially responded to two cycles of therapy, and disease stabilized after an additional four cycles. She is tolerating the chemotherapy well. Her performance status is ECOG 0 to 1; she does not report pain, shortness of breath, or cough.

Which of the following is the most appropriate treatment for this patient?

A. Stop therapy and start chemotherapy at the time of disease progression
B. Continue with maintenance therapy of weekly paclitaxel until disease progression
C. Continue carboplatin and paclitaxel until disease progression
D. Begin maintenance therapy with erlotinib until disease progression
E. Begin radiation of the primary tumor

6-7 A 62-year-old man presents with a 3-month history of chronic cough recently associated with scant hemoptysis. He smokes 2 packs a day. A chest x-ray shows a large right hilar mass with multiple, large (5 cm) mediastinal nodes that is confirmed by CT of the chest. PET demonstrates activity in the primary tumor and the right mediastinum, but nowhere else. Evaluation of a biopsy specimen of the mass indicates squamous cell cancer, and a mediastinoscopy confirms the presence of squamous cell cancer within the lymph nodes on the right only.

Which of the following is most likely to yield an improved survival benefit?

A. Surgery followed by postoperative adjuvant chemotherapy
B. Preoperative chemotherapy and radiation therapy, followed by surgery
C. Chemotherapy followed by 60 Gy of thoracic radiation over 6 weeks
D. Chemotherapy administered concurrently with 60 Gy of thoracic radiation therapy over 6 weeks

6-8 A 50-year-old woman who smoked one pack per day from age 18 to 35 comes to your office asking to be screened for lung cancer. Her father, a heavy smoker, recently died at the age of 70. Your patient has read the recent material in the media regarding screening for lung cancer and is concerned. She is feeling well, has no symptoms, and no other active medical problems.

Which of the following do you tell her regarding screening with low-dose, spiral CT?

A. Screening CTs have not been proven to be helpful in either detecting small, asymptomatic lung cancers, or in decreasing the chance of dying from lung cancer
B. Although screening CTs detect small, asymptomatic lung cancers early, they have not been proven to reduce the chances of dying from lung cancer
C. Screening CTs have been shown to detect small, asymptomatic lung cancers early, as well as to reduce the chances of dying from lung cancer

6-9 A 65-year-old patient who has never smoked presents with a new diagnosis of adenocarcinoma of the lung. A CT/PET scan reveals a 4-cm tumor with bulky mediastinal adenopathy, as well as liver and adrenal metastases. A head MRI is negative for metastases. His ECOG performance status is 1. His health has been good up to this point, he is taking no medication, and his only symptoms are mild, right, upper-quandrant abdominal pains.

The patient is very anxious. His primary goal is to attend the wedding of his granddaughter next year, and he wants the "best" treatment that is most likely to allow him to live longer so that he can achieve his goal. Based upon Level 1, phase III data, which of the following treatments do you recommend?

A. Carboplatin/paclitaxel
B. Carboplatin/paclitaxel/erlotinib
C. Carboplatin/paclitaxel followed by erlotinib
D. Erlotinib
E. Carboplatin/paclitaxel/bevacizumab

6-10 A 60-year-old man presents with a 6-week history of cough, shortness of breath, fatigue, anorexia, and a 15-pound weight loss. In reviewing symptoms, he reports that he also has mild headaches and a vague right-sided abdominal pain. He has smoked two packs of cigarettes daily since the age of 15. On physical examination, he appears cachetic and ill; his performance status is 2. There is no swelling of the right arm or neck, and no venous distension of anterior chest wall veins. A chest x-ray shows a large mass in the right upper lobe. A percutaneous biopsy of the lung mass confirms small cell lung cancer. The results of CT of the chest demonstrate slight compression of the superior vena cava, as well as bulky, right-sided mediastinal adenopathy and liver metastasis.

Which of the following is the appropriate initial treatment for this patient?

A. Emergency radiation therapy to the thorax
B. Chemotherapy
C. Stenting the superior vena cava, followed by chemotherapy
D. Radiation therapy to the thorax, followed by chemotherapy

6-11 Given the above patient's performance status of 2 (Karnofsky performance status of 60%), which of the following is the optimal systemic treatment?

A. Single-agent paclitaxel
B. Single-agent etoposide
C. Single-agent carboplatin
D. Carboplatin and paclitaxel
E. Carboplatin and etoposide

6-12 Which of the following is true regarding the role of such epidermal growth factor (EGF) receptor tyrosine kinase inhibitors as erlotinib for the treatment of non-small cell lung cancer (NSCLC)?

A. Patients should have their tumor analyzed for EGF receptor mutations before initiating erlotinib therapy
B. Erlotinib is ineffective for anyone who has ever smoked cigarettes
C. Erlotinib plus chemotherapy is an appropriate first-line treatment for all newly diagnosed patients with good performance status who have NSCLC
D. Single-agent erlotinib is an option as a first-line treatment for older patients or patients with poor performance status who have NSCLC
E. Single-agent erlotinib improves survival for patients with NSCLC that has progressed following one or more chemotherapy regimens

6-13 Which of the following is true regarding neoadjuvant (preoperative) chemotherapy for stages I, II, and III NSCLC?

A. Neoadjuvant chemotherapy has been shown to improve survival compared with surgery alone in large randomized phase III trials

B. Neoadjuvant chemotherapy has been shown to improve survival compared with postoperative (adjuvant) chemotherapy in large, randomized phase III trials

C. The primary role of neoadjuvant chemotherapy is to render unresectable disease resectable

D. Survival is better for patients whose N2 nodes are pathologically downstaged to N0 following neoadjuvant chemotherapy compared with patients whose nodes did not clear

6-14 A 65-year-old man presents with a 6-cm adenocarcinoma of the lung with ipsilateral hilar lymph node involvement based on CT and PET. You stage his disease as a clinical T2, N1, M0 (stage IIB) NSCLC. He is otherwise in good health and has no contraindications to surgery. A mediastinoscopy is negative for mediastinal lymph node metastases. At surgery, all disease is completely resected, and the clinical stage is confirmed pathologically (IIA, T2N1M0). Which of the following do you recommend?

A. No postoperative treatment

B. Postoperative mediastinal radiation

C. Postoperative cisplatin-based chemotherapy

D. Postoperative cisplatin-based chemotherapy followed by mediastinal radiation

6-15 Carboplatin, paclitaxel, and bevacizumab therapy is indicated for a patient with a new diagnosis of metastatic NSCLC. For which of the following situations would you *not* use bevacizumab?

A. The patient is female

B. The tumor is centrally located

C. The tumor is a squamous cell cancer

D. The patient has controlled essential hypertension

CHAPTER 6 EXPLANATORY ANSWERS:
LUNG CANCER

6-1 D

Educational Objective: To recognize the appropriate therapy for a patient with limited-stage small cell lung cancer.

Combined chemoradiotherapy improves survival for patients with limited-stage small cell lung cancer by approximately 5% at 3 years. The chemotherapy of choice is cisplatin and etoposide because these agents are much better tolerated with radiation therapy than doxorubicin-based regimens, and the combination of cisplatin and irinotecan has not yet been tested in this setting.

Until recently, there have been no randomized studies designed to evaluate the dose and schedule of radiation therapy to the thorax. Traditionally, the schedule of radiation has been concurrent chemotherapy plus radiation therapy at 45 Gy administered in daily fractions over 5 weeks; 45 Gy has been empirically chosen because of the marked in vitro sensitivity of small cell lung cancer cell lines to even small doses of radiation. This sensitivity is theoretically caused by the lack of a shoulder on radiation dose-response curves for small cell lung cancer, meaning that at even relatively low doses per fraction, small cells are killed exponentially; large doses of radiation are needed for more radiation-resistant cells to overcome the shoulder on the dose-response curve. Thus, multiple small fractions of radiation therapy can kill small cell lung cancer cells while simultaneiously reducing permanent damage to normal tissues.

In 1999, Turrisi, et al reported that twice-daily radiation (45 Gy over 3 weeks) beginning with the first cycle of chemotherapy significantly improved survival compared with concurrent once-daily radiation therapy (45 Gy over 5 weeks). The 2-year survival rate was 47% for twice-daily radiation and 41% for once-daily radiation. Five-year survival was 26% and 16%, respectively. Esophagitis occurred more frequently for patients receiving twice-daily treatment (grade 3 esophagitis occurring in 27% and 11% of patients in the once-daily and twice-daily groups, respectively; $p < 0.001$), although there was no difference in pulmonary complications or myelosuppression.

It is not known whether higher doses of radiation (e.g., 60 Gy) administered on a daily schedule for 6 weeks concurrently with chemotherapy is as effective as twice-daily doses of 45 Gy over 3 weeks.

Suggested Reading

Pignon J, Arriagada R, Ihde D, et al. A meta-analysis of thoracic radiotherapy for small-cell lung cancer. *N Engl J Med.* 1992; 327(23):1618–1624.

Turrisi AT, Kim K, Blum R, et al. Twice-daily compared with once-daily thoracic radiotherapy in limited small-cell lung cancer treated concurrently with cisplatin and etoposide. *N Engl J Med.* 1999;340(4):265–271.

6-2 D

Educational Objective: To recognize the role of prophylactic cranial irradiation for patients with limited-stage small cell lung cancer.

Findings from numerous trials have demonstrated that prophylactic cranial irradiation decreases the risk of brain metastases for patients with small cell lung cancer who have had a favorable response to primary chemotherapy. Although reports originally described a decrease in mental function, this side effect was primarily observed for patients who had been originally treated with doxorubicin; the incidence of substantial long-term neurologic defects is much lower for patients treated with the combination of cisplatin and etoposide. A recent meta-analysis of seven randomized trials demonstrated that prophylactic cranial irradiation was associated with a significant increase in 3-year survival, with a net gain of 5.4%. The optimal dose and duration of prophylactic cranial irradiation is under investigation in randomized trials.

Suggested Reading

Auperin A, Arriagada R, Pignon J, et al. Prophylactic cranial irradiation for patients with small cell lung cancer in complete remission. *N Engl J Med.* 1999;341(7):476–484.

6-3 D

Educational Objective: To recognize the optimal treatment of inoperable mesothelioma

Mesothelioma is a rare disease, occurring in approximately 5,000 patients each year. Most patients present within advanced disease, advanced age, or poor pulmonary function, which means that they are not candidates for surgery. Thus, no randomized studies have been carried out for patients with good performance status who have more limited disease. However, long-term survival has been reported with a surgical-based approach; for younger patients with a good performance status and the pulmonary reserve to tolerate surgery, an extrapleural pneumonectomy should be attempted. Patients with negative mediastinal nodes and an epithelial histology are most likely to benefit from surgery.

The chemotherapy used for mesothelioma has typically involved cisplatin, although it results in a response rate of only 10% to 20%. Gemcitabine also has single-agent activity in this range. However, the only randomized clinical trial in mesothelioma was for patients with advanced disease who were not candidates for surgery, and patients were randomly assigned to cisplatin alone or cisplatin plus pemetrexed. Pemetrexed targets several key enzymes in the purine-synthesis pathway, such as thymidylate synthase, dihydrofolate reductase, and glycinamideribonucleotide formyltransferase. The combination of pemetrexed plus cisplatin resulted in a 12-month median survival compared with 9-month median survival for cisplatin alone.

Suggested Reading

Vogelzang NJ. Emerging insights into the biology and therapy of malignant mesothelioma. *Semin Oncol.* 2002;29(6 Suppl 18): 35–42.

Vogelzang NJ, Rusthoven JJ, Symanowski J, et al. Phase III study of pemetrexed in combination with cisplatin versus cisplatin alone in patients with malignant pleural mesothelioma. *J Clin Oncol.* 2003;21(14):2636–2644.

6-4 A

Educational Objective: To recognize the standard first-line therapy for NSCLC.

Single-agent therapy has been compared with platinum-based doublets for the treatment of metastatic NSCLC, and combination therapy has been found to be more effective. Bevacizumab is contraindicated for patients with hemoptysis, thus, eliminating option B. Most clinical trials have shown triplets to be more toxic and less effective than platinum-based doublets and as such, option C is generally considered incorrect. Although patients with bronchioalveolar cancer may respond better to single-agent erlotinib than other histologic subtypes, this has not been proven to result in improved survival compared with chemotherapy in randomized phase III clinical trials. Furthermore, erlotinib is approved only in the recurrent-disease setting and thus, would not be appropriate for this patient. In addition, in randomized trials, erlotinib did not add any benefit to platinum-based doublets as first-line therapy, particularly for smokers. There does not appear to be a clinically significant difference between platinum-based doublets in terms of survival; therefore, option A is the appropriate answer.

Suggested Reading

Baggstrom M, Socinski M, Hensing T, et al. Addressing the optimal number of cytotoxic agents in stage IIIB/IV non-small cell lung cancer: A meta-analysis of the published literature. *Proc Am Soc Clin Oncol.* 2003;22(abstract 2510).

Herbst RS, Giaccone G, Schiller JH, et al. Gefitinib in combination with paclitaxel and carboplatin in advanced non-small-cell lung cancer: a phase III trial–INTACT 2. *J Clin Oncol.* 2004;22(5):785–794.

Delbaldo C, Michiels S, Syz N, et al. Benefits of adding a drug to a single-agent or a 2-agent chemotherapy regimen in advanced non-small-cell lung cancer: a meta-analysis. *JAMA.* 2004;292 (4): 470–484.

Herbst RS, Prager D, Hermann R, et al. TRIBUTE: a phase III trial of erlotinib hydrochloride (OSI-774) combined with carboplatin and paclitaxel chemotherapy in advanced non-small-cell lung cancer. *J Clin Oncol.* 2005;23(25):5892–5899.

Lilenbaum RC, Herndon JE, 2nd, List MA, et al. Single-agent versus combination chemotherapy in advanced non-small-cell lung cancer: the cancer and leukemia group B (study 9730). *J Clin Oncol.* 2005;23(1):190–196.

6-5 B

Educational Objective: To recognize some of the clinical and pathologic differences between atypical carcinoid and small cell lung cancer.

Neuroendocrine lung tumors represent a spectrum of pathologic entities characterized by the presence of neurosecretory granules seen on electron microscopy. They range in aggressiveness from low-grade typical carcinoid, atypical carcinoid (intermediate grade), large cell neuroendocrine cancer (high grade), and small cell lung cancer (high grade). High-grade, more aggressive tumors are characterized by the number of mitoses seen by light microscopy; there is no correlation between the number of neuroendocrine granules and grade. Approximately 20% to 40% of patients with both typical and atypical carcinoid are nonsmokers, whereas virtually all patients with small cell lung cancer and large cell neuroendocrine cancer are cigarette smokers.

Suggested Reading

Travis W. High-grade neuroendocrine tumors: what we know and important unanswered questions. *Lung Cancer.* 2003;41:S101.

6-6 A

Educational Objective: To recognize the optimal duration of treatment for patients with NSCLC.

Three randomized trials have evaluated the issue of the appropriate duration of chemotherapy. In one study, four cycles of paclitaxel and carboplatin were compared with continuous therapy; in a second trial, three cycles of mitomycin, vinblastine, and cisplatin were compared with six cycles; and in a third study, vinorelbine and four cycles of induction chemotherapy were compared with the combination of mitomycin, ifosfamide, and cisplatin followed by observation. None of the three trials showed any survival benefit with the prolonged regimen. Investigators are exploring the role of maintenance erlotinib in ongoing randomized trials, but no data are available yet to support this approach. Radiating a primary tumor for cure of a patient with metastatic NSCLC does not prolong survival.

Suggested Reading

Depierre A, Quoix E, Mercier M. Maintenance chemotherapy in advanced non-small cell lung cancer (NSCLC): a randomized study of vinorelbine (v) versus observation (ob) in patients (pts) responding to induction therapy (French Cooperative Oncology Group). *Proc Am Soc Clin Oncol.* 2001;20:309a.

Smith IE, O'Brien MER, Talbot DC, et al. Duration of chemotherapy in advanced non-small-cell lung cancer: a randomized trial of three versus six courses of mitomycin, vinblastine, and cisplatin. *J Clin Oncol.* 2001;19(5):1336–1343.

Socinski MA, Schell MJ, Peterman A, et al. Phase III trial comparing a defined duration of therapy versus continuous therapy followed by second-line therapy in advanced-stage IIIB/IV non-small-cell lung cancer. *J Clin Oncol.* 2002;20(5): 1335–1343.

6-7 D

Educational Objective: To recognize the optimal treatment for patients with bulky stage IIIA non-small cell lung cancer who have good performance status.

This patient has bulky, multilevel mediastinal disease, making her stage IIIA (N2) and inoperable. Adjuvant therapy has been explored for the treatment of patients with stages II and microscopic IIIA disease, but not for patients with bulky stage IIIA or stage IIIB. A subset analysis of a randomized study suggests that patients who have clearing of their ipsilateral mediastinal N2 nodes with chemoradiation may do well with surgery, but this is a subset analysis; therefore, surgery cannot be routinely recommended for patients with bulky N2 disease.

Findings from two randomized studies have shown a survival advantage for concurrent chemoradiation therapy compared with a sequential approach. In a Japanese trial, two cycles of mitomycin-C, vindesine, and cisplatin (MVP) were given concurrently or sequentially with radiation therapy at 56 Gy. Patients in either arm who had a response received another two cycles of MVP after radiation therapy was completed. In a confirmatory randomized trial conducted by the Radiation Therapy Oncology Group, the combination of cisplatin, vinblastine, and radiation therapy was compared with sequential chemoradiation therapy. Both studies demonstrated a survival advantage for concurrent chemoradiation therapy compared with a sequential approach, albeit at the expense of increased toxicity.

Chemotherapy can be given in full systemic doses with radiation therapy or in weekly radiosensitizing doses. However, if given in weekly low doses, standard chemotherapy also should be administered either before or after the thoracic radiation therapy, as there are no data from phase III trials to suggest that weekly, low-dose chemotherapy is adequate. Randomized trials are ongoing to determine whether pre-chemoradiation ("induction") or post-chemoradiation ("consolidative") chemotherapy is optimal.

Suggested Reading

Albain K, Swann R, Rusch VR, et al. Phase III study of concurrent chemotherapy and radiotherapy (CT/RT) vs CT/RT followed by surgical resection for stage IIIA(pN2) non-small cell lung cancer (NSCLC): Outcomes update of North American Intergroup 0139 (RTOG 9309). *J Clin Oncol.*, 2005 ASCO Annual Meeting Proceedings. 2005;23:7014.

Curran WJ, Scott C, Langer C, et al. Phase III comparison of sequential vs. concurrent chemoradiation for patients with unresected stage III non-small cell lung cancer (NSCLC): initial report of Radiation Therapy Oncology Group (RTOG) 9410. *Proc Am Soc Clin Oncol.* 2000;19:484a.

Furuse K, Fukuoka M, Kawahara M, et al. Phase III study of concurrent versus sequential thoracic radiotherapy in combination with mitomycin, vindesine, and cisplatin in unresectable stage III non-small-cell lung cancer. *J Clin Oncol.* 1999;17(9): 2692–2699.

6-8 B

Educational Objective: To recognize that screening has not been proven to decrease the mortality from lung cancer.

Five randomized screening studies in the 1980s of chest x-rays with or without cytologic analysis of sputum failed to detect an effect on mortality by screening patients at high risk, although earlier stage cancers were detected in the screened group. Presumably, this discrepancy was related to lead-time bias, length-time bias, and overdiagnosis. Similarly, low-dose, thin-slice, spiral CT, without the use of contrast medium, is more sensitive than chest x-rays in detecting lung nodules and lung cancer at early stages but has not yet been shown to have an effect on mortality related to lung cancer in randomized studies. Furthermore, spiral CT is unable to distinguish small tumors from benign inflammatory or granulomatous nodules, making it necessary for many patients to follow up with serial scans, which, in turn, makes the cost of this screening modality extremely high. In nonrandomized studies, patients whose lung cancer is diagnosed by spiral CT screening appear to have a long survival, but that may be because of lead-time bias, length-time bias, or overdiagnosis. To determine whether CT screening decreases the number of deaths because of lung cancer, the results of the randomized studies must be awaited. Until then, no screening method for lung cancer can be routinely recommended, and the advantages and disadvantages of screening should be discussed with patients. Chest x-ray screenings are being compared with spiral CT in an ongoing large, national, randomized study.

Suggested Reading

Bach PB, Kelley M, Tate RC, et al. Screening for lung cancer: a review of the current literature. *Chest.* 2003;123(1 Suppl): 72S–82S.

Bach PB, Jett JR, Pastorino U, et al. Computed tomography screening and lung cancer outcomes. *JAMA.* 2007;297(9):953–961.

Henschke CI, Yankelevitz DF, Libby DM, et al. Survival of patients with stage I lung cancer detected on CT screening. *N Engl J Med.* 2006;355(17):1763–1771.

6-9 E

Educational Objective: To recognize that the state-of-the-art, first-line treatment for NSCLC is carboplatin, paclitaxel, and bevacizumab for appropriately selected patients.

Numerous phase III studies have been conducted during the past several decades to identify the optimal therapy for first-line treatment of metastatic NSCLC. In general, these studies have shown that doublet chemotherapy is more effective than single-agent chemotherapy; that treatment with three drugs is not more effective than two drugs and is associated with more toxicity and expense; that the addition of erlotinib to front-line chemotherapy does not prolong survival; and that the addition of the antiangiogenic agent bevacizumab to carboplatin and paclitaxel for appropriate patients significantly increases the response rate, progression-free survival, and overall survival compared with carboplatin and paclitaxel alone, despite the increase in grades IV to grade V bleeding episodes and neutrapenic fevers. Given that the patient does not have brain metastases, squamous cell carcinoma, hemoptysis, and is not receiving anticoagulants, Option E has the best level 1 evidence for improved survival. Although single-agent erlotinib has been shown to have high response rates in first-line single arm phase II studies of patients with *EGFR*-mutated disease, it has not been studied as a single agent in first-line phase III unselected patients with NSCLC.

Suggested Reading

Sandler A, Gray R, Perry MC, et al. Paclitaxel-carboplatin alone or with bevacizumab for non-small-cell lung cancer. *N Engl J Med.* 2006;355(24):2542–2550.

6-10 B

Educational Objective: To recognize the optimal treatment for superior vena cava syndrome for patients with small cell lung cancer.

Although superior vena cava syndrome was previously considered an oncologic emergency, an appreciation of the chemosensitivity of small cell lung cancer has resulted in the initial use of chemotherapy as first-line treatment when superior vena cava syndrome is caused by the disease. Occasionally, a short course of radiation therapy to the thorax in severe cases may be indicated while awaiting the results of biopsy, as the differential diagnosis includes thymomas, lymphomas, and NSCLC, and the treatment would change for each of these diagnoses. However, once the biopsy results are available, systemic chemotherapy for small cell lung cancer is likely to be as effective as thoracic radiation therapy unless the patient was in extreme distress, in which case both thoracic radiation therapy and chemotherapy would likely be indicated. If the subsequent staging work-up failed to show any signs of distant metastases, radiation therapy to the thorax could be added at that time.

Placement of a stent is generally reserved for patients with small cell lung cancer for whom radiation therapy to the thorax failed or for patients with NSCLC who present with such bulky disease that thoracic radiation therapy is deemed unlikely to be helpful immediately.

Suggested Reading

Kvale PA, Simoff M, Prakash UB. Lung cancer. Palliative care. *Chest.* 2003; 123(1 Suppl):284S–311S.

6-11 E

Educational Objective: To recognize the optimal chemotherapy regimen for extensive-stage small cell lung cancer.

Small cell lung cancer is a rapidly progressive disease and, in many cases, the symptoms and poor performance status of the patient can be attributed to the cancer itself. Although the response rate is 30% for single-agent etoposide, in two randomized studies, this treatment was inferior to two-drug therapy, even for older patients or patients with poor performance status. Both of the studies were closed early because of ethical considerations, in that overall survival, improvement in side effects, and tolerability were unfavorable for patients in the experimental group. Although paclitaxel has single-agent activity in small cell lung cancer, it has not been extensively studied in phase III trials, and thus, cannot be routinely recommended. Indeed, it has not been shown to add any benefit to the standard combination of cisplatin and etoposide for previously untreated patients. In North America, the standard therapy for extensive-stage disease is a plat inum agent plus etoposide. Although findings from a recent randomized phase III Japanese study showed a survival benefit for irinotecan plus cisplatin when compared with etoposide plus cisplatin, these results have not been confirmed in a randomized trial in the United States. Thus, Option E is the best choice.

Suggested Reading

Ettinger D, Finkelstein D, Sarma R, Johnson D. Phase II study of paclitaxel in patients with extensive-disease small-cell lung cancer: an Eastern Cooperative Oncology Group study. *J Clin Oncol.* 1995;13(6):1430–1435.

Girling DJ, for the Medical Research Council Lung Cancer Working Party. Comparison of oral etoposide and standard intravenous multidrug chemotherapy for small-cell cancer: a stopped multicentre randomized trial. *Lancet.* 1996;348:(9027) 563–566.

Grant S, Gralla R, Kris M, et al. Single-agent chemotherapy trials in small-cell lung cancer, 1970 to 1990: the case for studies in previously treated patients. *J Clin Oncol.* 1992;10(3): 484–498.

Harper P, Underhill C, Ruiz de Elvira MC, et al. A randomised study of oral etoposide versus combination chemotherapy in poor prognosis small cell lung cancer. *Proc Am Soc Clin Oncol.* 1996;15:abst 2019.

Niell H, Herndon J, Miller A, et al. Randomized phase III Intergroup trial (CALGB 9732) of etoposide (vp-16) and cisplatin (DDP) with or without paclitaxel (tax) and G-CSF in patients with extensive stage small cell lung cancer (ed-SCLC). *Proc Am Soc Clin Oncol.* 2002;21:293a.

Noda K, Nishiwaki Y, Kawahara M, et al. Irinotecan plus cisplatin compared with etoposide plus cisplatin for extensive small-cell lung cancer. *N Engl J Med.* 2002;346(2):85–91.

Hanna N, Bunn PA, Jr., Langer C, et al. Randomized phase III trial comparing irinotecan/cisplatin with etoposide/cisplatin in patients with previously untreated extensive-stage disease small-cell lung cancer. *J Clin Oncol.* 2006;24(13):2038–2043.

6-12 E

Educational Objective: To understand the role of erlotinib for the treatment of NSCLC.

In two randomized phase II trials for patients with recurrent NSCLC, erlotinib significantly improved symptoms for approximately one-third of patients. A phase III trial of erlotinib in previously treated, unselected NSCLC showed a survival advantage compare with best supportive care. Although patients with EGFR mutations often have dramatic responses to EGFR inhibitors, overexpression of either the EGFR protein, as detected by immunohistochemistry, or amplification of the *EGFR* gene, as detected by fluorescent in-situ hybridization (FISH), also correlates with survival. Thus, mutation status should not be used as the sole criterion for treatment with these agents. Improved survival was observed with erlotinib in all clinical subsets studied, including men, squamous cell carcinoma, and smokers (although the magnitude of benefit was lower for smokers).

The role of erlotinib as a first-line therapy for NSCLC is under evolution. Single-arm phase II studies have demonstrated promising survival results with single-agent erlotinib for patients with *EGFR* mutations, although this has not yet been confirmed in randomized trials, either as a single agent or when combined with chemotherapy. Erlotinib has not been assessed as a single agent in first-line therapy in a phase III randomized trial, and thus, cannot be routinely recommended as a first-line therapy, even for older patients or patients with a poor performance status. In fact, in a randomized phase II study of erlotinib compared with chemotherapy for treatment-naïve patients with poor performance status, patients with a performance status of 2 appeared to do better with standard carboplatin/paclitaxel than with erlotinib. Erlotinib has been evaluated in combination with chemotherapy compared with chemotherapy alone in the first-line setting for unselected patients in phase III trials, with no observed improvement in survival, response rate, or symptom control and as such, cannot be recommended for concurrent use with chemotherapy, although its role as a maintenance agent is being explored.

Suggested Reading

Fukuoka M, Yano S, Giaccone G, et al. Multi-institutional randomized phase II trial of gefitinib for previously treated patients with advanced non-small-cell lung cancer. *J Clin Oncol.* 2003; 21:2237–2246.

Shepherd FA, Rodrigues Pereira J, Ciuleanu T, et al. Erlotinib in previously treated non-small-cell lung cancer. *N Engl J Med.* 2005;353:123–132.

Lilenbaum R, Axerold R, Thomas S, et al. Randomized phase II trial of single agent erlotinib vs. standard chemotherapy in patients with advanced non-small cell lung cancer (NSCLC) and performance status (PS) of 2. *Journal of Clinical Oncology,* 2006 ASCO Annual Meeting Proceedings Part I. 2006;24: abstract number 7022.

Cappuzzo F, Hirsch FR, Rossi E, et al. Epidermal growth factor receptor gene and protein and gefitinib sensitivity in non-small-cell lung cancer. *J Natl Cancer Inst.* 2005;97:643–655.

6-13 D

Educational Objective: To understand the role of neoadjuvant chemotherapy for patients with operable NSCLC.

The role of neoadjuvant chemotherapy reached clinical interest when findings from two small (60 patients each) randomized studies published in 1994 showed improved survival compared with surgery alone. Since then, however, three much larger randomized trials have failed to report a survival benefit, caused in part by increased postoperative mortality, particularly for patients undergoing right-sided pneumonectomy. The most recent study from the Medical Research Council and the European Organisation for Research and Treatment of Cancer randomly assigned more than 500 patients with stages I to III disease to surgery or three cycles of chemotherapy. Survival was nearly identical between the two arms, with a hazard ratio of 1.02 (95% CI 0.80,1.31; $p = 0.86$). The estimated median and 5-year survival rates were 55 months and 45%, respectively, for patients in the surgery arm, and 54 months and 44%, respectively, for the neoadjuvant arm.

Retrospective analyses that have suggested that downstaging to N0 to N1 at surgery is prognostic and significantly correlates with event-free survival and overall survival. Hence, resection is recommended only for patients with mediastinal downstaging after chemotherapy.

Suggested Reading

Albain K, Scott C, Rusch V, et al. Phase III comparison of concurrent chemotherapy plus radiotherapy (ct/RT) and ct/RT followed by surgical resection for stage IIIA (pn2) non-small cell lung cancer (NSCLC): initial results from Intergroup trial 0139 (RTOG 93-09). *Proc Am Soc Clin Oncol.* 2003; 22:621.

Betticher D, Schmitz SH, Totsch M, et al. Mediastinal lymph node clearance after docetaxel-cisplatin neo-adjuvant chemotherapy is prognostic of survival in patients with stage IIIA pN2 non-small-cell lung cancer: a multi center phase II trial. *J Clin Oncol.* 2003;21: 1752–1759.

Depierre A, Milleron B, Moro-Sibilot D, et al, for the French Thoracic Cooperative Group. Preoperative chemotherapy followed by surgery compared with primary surgery in resectable stage I (except T1N0), II, and IIIA non-small cell lung cancer. *J Clin Oncol.* 2002;20(1):247–253.

Gilligan D, Nicolson M, Smith I, et al: Preoperative chemotherapy in patients with resectable non-small cell lung cancer: results of the MRC LU22/NVALT 2/EORTC 08012 multicentre randomised trial and update of systematic review. *Lancet.* 2007;369(9577):1929–1937.

Rosell R, Gomez-Codina J, Camps C, et al. A randomized trial comparing preoperative chemotherapy plus surgery with surgery alone in patients with non-small-cell lung cancer. *N Engl J Med.* 1994;330:153–158.

Roth J, Fossella F, Komaki R, et al. A randomized trial comparing perioperative chemotherapy and surgery with surgery alone in resectable stage IIIA non-small-cell lung cancer. *J Natl Cancer Inst.* 1994;86(9):673–680.

6-14 C

Educational Objective: To recognize the role of adjuvant treatment in resectable NSCLC.

Positive results from three randomized trials comparing adjuvant chemotherapy with surgery alone have resulted in adjuvant chemotherapy emerging as the standard of care for patients with stage II and minimal IIIA NSCLC. Although earlier studies were negative, an updated meta-analysis confirmed the benefit of adjuvant cisplatin-based adjuvant chemotherapy. The role of adjuvant therapy for stage IB is more controversial; the one study which looked specifically at patients with IB was statistically negative, with a p value of 0.10. However, there was a trend for improved survival (hazard ratio of 0.8), the study was relatively small and, therefore, probably underpowered, and it was the only study that utilized carboplatin instead of cisplatin. The role of postoperative radiation therapy is not indicated for patients with node-negative disease; a meta-analysis showed that postoperative radiation therapy could prove detrimental.

Suggested Reading

Douillard JY, Rosell R, De Lena, M, et al. Adjuvant vinorelbine plus cisplatin versus observation in patients with completely resected stage IB-IIIA non-small-cell lung cancer (Adjuvant Navelbine International Trialist Association [ANITA]): a randomised controlled trial. *Lancet Oncol.* 2006;7(9):719–727.

Strauss G, Herndon J, Maddaus, MA, et al. Adjuvant chemotherapy in stage IB non-small cell lung cancer (NSCLC): Update of Cancer and Leukemia Group B (CALGB) protocol 9633. *Journal of Clinical Oncology, 2006 ASCO Annual Meeting Proceedings Part I.* 2006;24.

Winton T, Livingston R, Johnson D, et al. Vinorelbine plus cisplatin vs. observation in resected non-small-cell lung cancer. *N Engl J Med.* 2005;352(25):2589–2597.

Arriagada R, Bergman, B Dunant, A, et al. Cisplatin-based adjuvant chemotherapy in patients with completely resected non-small-cell lung cancer. *N Engl J Med.* 2004;350(4):351–360.

Hotta K, Matsuo K, Ueoka H, et al. Role of adjuvant chemotherapy in patients with resected non-small-cell lung cancer: reappraisal with a meta-analysis of randomized controlled trials. *J Clin Oncol.* 2004;22(19):3860–3867.

6-15 C

Educational Objective: To recognize the contraindications for bevacizumab.

E4599 was the ECOG study that demonstrated that the addition of bevacizumab to paclitaxel and carboplatin prolonged survival, progression-free survival, and improved the response rate compared with paclitaxel and carboplatin alone. Because of the preceding phase II study, which showed that approximately one-third of all patients with squamous cell histology developed severe or fatal hemoptysis, patients with a history of hemoptysis, squamous cell carcinoma, thromboembolic events, brain metastases, or those requiring therapeutic anticoagulants were excluded. Patients with central tumors were allowed on study; therefore, central tumors are not part of the exclusion criteria. With those exclusion criteria, the incidence of severe or fatal hemoptysis was 1.4% for the bevacizumab group, compared with 0% for the control group. Patients with brain metastases were empirically excluded, but clinical studies are ongoing to determine if patients with radiated brain metastases can be safely treated. In a retrospective subset analysis, women assigned to the bevacizumab arm were found to have improved response rates and progression-free survival — but not improved overall survival compared with women assigned to the chemotherapy alone arm. Given that this was an unplanned, retrospective analysis, and that women with colon cancer were found to have an improved survival when treated with chemotherapy and bevacizumab, female sex is not a contraindication to bevacizumab unless these findings are observed in other ongoing prospective studies.

Suggested Reading

Sandler A, Gray,R, Perry MC, et al. Paclitaxel-carboplatin alone or with bevacizumab for non-small-cell lung cancer. *N Engl J Med.* 2006;355(4):2542–2550.

SELF EVALUATION

CHAPTER 7 QUESTIONS:
HEAD AND NECK CANCER

7-1 **A 58-year-old Asian man presents with a 3-month history of an enlarging mass on the left side of the neck. He reports that he has had no anorexia or weight loss, but he has had a mild headache intermittently during the past month.**

On assessment of the neck, there is a 2- to 3-cm, mobile, upper cervical lymph node on the left. Examination of the tympanic membranes reveals serous otitis media on the left side. Fiberoptic examination shows a left-sided nasopharyngeal mass obstructing the left eustachian tube.

Computerized tomography (CT) of the neck confirms a left-sided nasopharyngeal mass and two enlarged lymph nodes in the left side of the neck; erosion of the skull base adjacent to the mass is noted. Fine-needle aspiration reveals a poorly differentiated tumor. The findings of biopsy of the nasopharynx are interpreted as lymphoepithelioma. Testing reveals no evidence of distant metastatic disease.

Which of the following is the most appropriate therapy for this patient?

A. Nasopharyngectomy with a left modified-radical neck dissection, followed by adjuvant radiotherapy to the primary site and ipsilateral neck
B. Induction cisplatin and fluorouracil for three cycles, followed by hyperfractionated radiotherapy in a curative dose to the primary site and to both sides of the neck
C. Concurrent cisplatin with curative-dose radiotherapy to the primary site and both sides of the neck, followed by adjuvant cisplatin and fluorouracil for three cycles
D. Curative-dose radiotherapy alone to the primary site and the ipsilateral neck
E. High-dose carboplatin-based chemotherapy with stem cell rescue followed by curative-dose radiotherapy to the primary site and both sides of the neck

7-2 **A 69-year-old man presents with a new cough. Three years previously, he was treated with concurrent platinum-based chemoradiotherapy for T3, N2b, M0 squamous cell cancer of the base of the tongue on the right side. He was free of disease after treatment. At the time of this follow-up visit, a chest x-ray shows a new 2-cm nodule in the left upper lobe of the lung.**

The physical examination is normal. CT of the chest shows no additional nodules, no abnormal hilar, and no mediastinal adenopathy. Positron emission tomography reveals abnormal uptake with a standard uptake value of 9.8 corresponding to the left upper lobe mass. Bronchoscopy with transbronchial fine-needle aspiration of the lung mass reveals poorly differentiated squamous cell cancer cells on cytologic examination.

Which of the following is the most appropriate next step in management?

A. Palliative radiotherapy to the lung nodule
B. Referral to a thoracic surgeon
C. Platinum-based concurrent chemotherapy with curative-dose radiotherapy to the lung nodule and hilar and mediastinal lymph nodes
D. Palliative chemotherapy with paclitaxel
E. Platinum-based combination chemotherapy followed by curative-dose radiotherapy to the lung nodule and hilar and mediastinal lymph nodes

7-3 **A 59-year-old man presents with a 3-month history of hoarseness. He has a 20 pack-year history of smoking. Mirror examination reveals a nodule in the middle of the left vocal cord, but normal mobility is preserved. The remainder of the physical examination and the routine lab tests are normal.**

The chest x-ray shows no cardiopulmonary disease. CT scan of the neck reveals a mass on the left vocal cord with no evidence of supraglottic or extralaryngeal extension; no pathologic adenopathy is noted in the neck. Examination under anesthesia documents the vocal cord lesion. The findings on examination of a biopsy specimen indicate a moderately to poorly differentiated squamous cell cancer.

Which of the following is the most appropriate therapy for this patient?

A. Curative-dose radiotherapy to the larynx alone
B. Curative-dose radiotherapy to the larynx and ipsilateral neck
C. Combination chemotherapy with cisplatin and fluorouracil followed by curative-dose radiotherapy to the larynx and both sides of the neck
D. Concurrent cisplatin with curative-dose radiotherapy to the larynx and both sides of the neck
E. Hemilaryngectomy and left modified-radical neck dissection

7-4 **A 62-year-old man presents for routine follow-up 8 months after completing treatment with chemoradiotherapy for T3, N2b, M0 squamous cell cancer of the right tonsil. He was rendered free of disease. He has had mild dysphagia and odynophagia for approximately 3 weeks. He continues to work full-time.**

On physical examination, an ulcerated mass is seen in the area of the right tonsil, with extension into the soft palate; it is clinically T3 in extent. Evaluation of the neck shows no adenopathy. The remainder of the physical examination is unremarkable.

CT of the neck confirms the recurrent tonsillar mass and regional nodes are not enlarged or necrotic. Biopsy of the tonsillar mass demonstrates a poorly differentiated squamous cell cancer. Consultation with a radiation oncologist indicates that the recurrence is squarely within the prior radiation field.

Which of the following is the most appropriate therapy for this patient?

A. Single-agent chemotherapy
B. Combination chemotherapy
C. Salvage-combined chemoradiotherapy with intensity-modulated radiotherapy
D. Referral to a head and neck surgeon

7-5 **A 64-year-old woman presented with a 3-cm mass on the hard palate that was found to be adenoid cystic cancer on examination of a biopsy specimen. No cranial nerve palsies or focal neurologic findings were present. Extent of disease evaluation demonstrates no other disease sites. After primary surgical treatment, adjuvant radiotherapy was administered. The radiation field included nerve pathways to the base of skull.**

Four years later, she returns to your office with a chest x-ray from her primary care physician that shows a possible left lung nodule. She is entirely asymptomatic, and she continues to work full-time. Physical examination, including evaluation of the original primary site, is normal. CT of the chest confirms a 1-cm nodule in the left lower lobe, and approximately 10 subcentimeter bilateral pulmonary nodules. A thoracoscopic biopsy was performed. Two nodules were removed, both showing metastatic adenoid cystic cancer.

Which of the following is the most appropriate next step in management?

A. Imatinib
B. Chemotherapy with cyclophosphamide, doxorubicin, and cisplatin
C. Immunotherapy with interferon-alpha
D. Watchful waiting with serial imaging of the chest
E. Referral to thoracic surgeon for staged bilateral thoracotomy and metastectomy

7-6 **A 70-year-old man presents with a 3-month history of an enlarging mass on the anterior part of the neck, and the new development of hoarseness. He reports a 15-pound weight loss during that time.**

On physical examination, he appears to have mild respiratory discomfort. There is an obvious mass in the anterior part of the neck, measuring 7 cm. Mirror examination reveals a paralyzed left vocal cord. No stridor is audible. A CT scan demonstrates a large mass arising from the thyroid, with destruction of thyroid cartilage and early invasion into the larynx. There are multiple bilateral pulmonary nodules. Core-needle biopsy shows a pure anaplastic thyroid cancer.

Which of the following is the most appropriate next intervention for this patient?

A. Surgical debulking followed by adjuvant radioactive iodine
B. Radioactive iodine
C. Concurrent chemoradiotherapy
D. Doxorubicin-based chemotherapy
E. Prophylactic tracheostomy

7-7 **A 30-year-old woman is referred by her primary care physician for evaluation of bilateral lung nodules. Five years ago, she had total thyroidectomy for a 2.5-cm papillary thyroid cancer and subsequent ablation of residual thyroid tissue with radioactive iodine. She has had no subsequent treatment and was lost to follow-up. Two weeks ago, she presented to her primary care physician with nasal congestion and a cough. A chest x-ray showed small bilateral pulmonary nodules, which were confirmed by CT of the chest with intravenous contrast. The serum thyroglobulin level was elevated (227 ng/mL). The results of thoracoscopic biopsy of two nodules demonstrated papillary histology. A diagnostic whole-body scan with injection of radioactive iodine, after recombinant thyrotropin stimulation, revealed no evidence of iodine-avid disease.**

Which of the following is the most appropriate management?

A. Chemotherapy with a doxorubicin-based regimen
B. Repeat whole-body scan with injection of radioactive iodine in 6 to 8 weeks
C. Surgical resection of the dominant pulmonary nodule
D. External beam radiation therapy to the dominant pulmonary nodule
E. Octreotide scan and treatment with somatostatin if the scan is positive for disease

CHAPTER 7 EXPLANATORY ANSWERS:

HEAD AND NECK CANCER

7-1 C

Educational Objective: To recognize the appropriate management of advanced local-regional nasopharyngeal cancer.

This patient has advanced, local-regional nasopharynx cancer (T3, N1, M0, stage III). The report of lymphoepithelioma is consistent with World Health Organization type II or III histology and is a carcinoma, not a lymphoma. This subtype is particularly common in endemic areas of southern China and the Mediterranean basin; unlike for other upper aerodigestive tract cancers, tobacco use does not appear to be a major risk factor. Nasopharyngeal cancer commonly presents with unilateral serous otitis media, and such a symptom, particularly for an adult, warrants examination of the nasopharynx. Therapy with curative intent should be recommended if there is no evidence of disease below the clavicles. Complete resection of even small disease is technically difficult, so primary surgery is not pursued for previously untreated patients, except to obtain a biopsy. Integrated chemoradiotherapy has become the standard of care for these patients, largely based on the results of the Intergroup study 0099, in which patients with stage III and stage IV diseases were randomly assigned to receive radiotherapy alone (70 Gy in 35 fractions over 7 weeks) or the same radiotherapy schedule with three planned cycles of concurrent cisplatin (100 mg/m2) administered every 21 days, followed by three planned cycles of adjuvant cisplatin and fluorouracil. Despite the fact that only 63% of patients received the full three cycles of concurrent cisplatin with radiotherapy and only 55% of patients received the full three cycles of adjuvant chemotherapy, the 3 year overall survival rate was significantly better for patients who received chemoradiotherapy (78% vs. 47%). Available data suggest that inclusion of concurrent chemoradiotherapy is particularly important.

The remaining choices are incorrect for the following reasons: Induction chemotherapy approaches followed by hyperfractionated radiotherapy alone have not received scrutiny in a randomized trial; curative-dose radiotherapy alone is appropriate for patients with early-stage disease (e.g., T1, N0, M0), but not for a patient with involvement of the lymph nodes in the neck. Of note, given that the nasopharynx is rich in lymphatic vessels, nodes in both sides of the neck are at risk for microscopic disease, even when clinically negative, so bilateral treatment is required, which is another reason why choices A and D are incorrect. There are no data to support improved outcomes with high-dose chemotherapy followed by stem cell rescue with radiation.

Suggested Reading

Al-Sarraf M, Leblanc M, Giri PG, et al. Chemoradiotherapy versus radiotherapy in patients with advanced nasopharyngeal cancer: phase III randomized Intergroup study 0099. *J Clin Oncol.* 1998;16(4):1310–1317.

Lin JC, Jan JS, Hsu CY, et al. Phase III study of concurrent chemoradiotherapy versus radiotherapy alone for advanced nasopharyngeal cancer: positive effect on overall and progression-free survival. *J Clin Oncol.* 2003;21(4):631–637.

7-2 B

Educational Objective: To recognize the high probability of second primary cancers for patients with a history of squamous cell cancer of the head and neck.

The patient could have metastatic cancer of the base of the tongue, particularly because the neck nodes were involved at the time of presentation. However, the long disease-free interval and tobacco history, as well as the presence of a solitary new lesion are all also consistent with new, early-stage lung cancer. This disease is associated with a much better prognosis than a metastatic head and neck cancer. The risk for second primary cancers is high for patients with a history of squamous cell cancer of the upper aerodigestive tract, particularly of related body sites also exposed to tobacco and alcohol, such as the lung and esophagus. This well-documented field cancerization effect leads to an incidence rate of second primary cancers of 3% to 7% per year. The fact that this patient resumed smoking increased his already elevated baseline risk for a second malignancy. There is no clear consensus on what routine screening program should be instituted for these patients. Isotretinoin has received considerable attention as a potential chemopreventive agent, but the results of randomized trials do not show a benefit in overall survival.

It is crucial to have this patient evaluated for what could be a potentially curative resection of the solitary lung mass. Assuming that he has incurable disease is the most important mistake to avoid. As such, choices A and D are incorrect. Choices C and E would be appropriate considerations for a newly diagnosed stage III non-small cell lung cancer.

Suggested Reading

Yamamoto E, Shibuya H, Yoshimura R, Miura M. Site specific dependency of second primary cancer in early stage head and neck squamous cell carcinoma. *Cancer.* 2002;94(7): 2007–2014.

7-3 A

Educational Objective: To understand the appropriate therapy of early-stage squamous cell cancer of the larynx.

This patient has early-stage squamous cell cancer of the true vocal cord. He has T1a, N0, M0 stage I disease on the basis of a solitary vocal cord-limited tumor, with preservation of vocal cord mobility and lack of disease in the neck lymph nodes. For T1 lesions, the 5-year overall survival rates associated with primary surgery (cordectomy, hemilaryngectomy) and with primary radiotherapy with salvage surgery as necessary have been comparable (approximately 90%). The better approach is a frequently debated issue, although many clinicians assert that functional outcomes are better with radiotherapy than with surgical management, particularly if a primary hemilaryngectomy is performed or a repeat cordectomy is required. An important anatomic consideration in the larynx is that the paucity of lymphatic drainage of the true vocal cords makes nodal metastases from early glottic lesions extremely infrequent. Elective, comprehensive neck management for this early-stage lesion is not required, making choices B and E incorrect. Also, if surgery to the primary site is pursued, a less-extensive procedure than hemilaryngectomy with follow-up would be preferred for a T1a lesion.

In the Department of Veterans Affairs Larynx Study Group trial, induction chemotherapy followed by radiotherapy offered potential larynx preservation for patients with stage III or IV disease without compromising overall survival, but this approach is not appropriate for a stage I lesion. More recent data suggest that concurrent chemoradiotherapy is preferable to the sequential approach for patients with advanced local-regional disease, but again, it would not be appropriate for this patient with early-stage disease.

Suggested Reading

Forastiere AA, Goepfert H, Maor M, et al. Concurrent chemotherapy and radiotherapy for organ preservation in advanced laryngeal cancer. *N Engl J Med.* 2003;349(22):2091–2098.

Hinerman RW, Mendenhall WM, Amdur RJ, et al. Early laryngeal cancer. *Curr Treat Options Oncol.* 2002;3(1):3–9.

Induction chemotherapy plus radiation compared with surgery plus radiation in patients with advanced laryngeal cancer. The Department of Veterans Affairs Laryngeal Cancer Study Group. *N Engl J Med.* 1991;324(24):1685–1690.

7-4 D

Educational Objective: To recognize the appropriate management of locally recurrent, squamous cell cancer of the head and neck.

This patient has locally recurrent, squamous cell cancer of the oropharynx. The recurrent tumor is advanced but not T4 in extent, and the absence of neck disease increases the likelihood of successful surgical salvage. It cannot be assumed this patient has incurable disease. Evaluation by a head and neck surgeon for possible salvage surgery is clearly indicated and is the correct choice.

The remaining choices are incorrect for the following reasons: intensity-modulated radiotherapy may facilitate repeat radiation therapy, and the disease-free interval will be longer for a small group of selected patients receiving concurrent chemotherapy with repeat radiation therapy compared with chemotherapy alone. Even if feasible, however, this approach would represent a second-tier choice for this patient. Chemotherapy alone, either as a single agent or in combination, is palliative and should not be pursued as primary therapy if a potentially curative option exists. Combination chemotherapy maximizes response rate in the recurrent setting compared with single-agent chemotherapy. Toxicity is greater, however, and the effect on survival is disappointing. Gene therapy to address mutations in the *p53* gene has been shown to induce tumor regression for patients with refractory local disease but would not be appropriate outside a research protocol.

Suggested Reading

Clavel M, Vermorken JB, Cognetti F, et al. Randomized comparison of cisplatin, methotrexate, bleomycin and vincristine (CABO) versus cisplatin and 5-fluorouracil (CF) versus cisplatin (c) in recurrent or metastatic squamous cell carcinoma of the head and neck. A phase III study of the EORTC Head and Neck Cancer Cooperative Group. *Ann Oncol.* 1994;5(6): 521–526.

De Crevoisier R, Bourhis J, Domenge C, et al. Full dose reirradiation for unresectable head and neck carcinoma. Experience at the Gustave Roussy Institute in a series of 169 patients. *J Clin Oncol.* 1998;16(11):3556–3562.

Khuri FR, Nemunaitis J, Ganly I, et al. A controlled trial of intratumoral ONYX-015, a selectively-replicating adenovirus, in combination with cisplatin and 5-fluorouracil in patients with recurrent head and neck cancer. *Nat Med.* 2000;6(8): 879–885.

7-5 D

Educational Objective: To understand the role of observation for the management of metastatic adenoid cystic cancer of the head and neck.

This patient has recurrent, metastatic adenoid cystic cancer to the lung. Adenoid cystic cancer is the most common malignant histologic subtype of tumors of the minor salivary glands. Neoplasms of this histologic subtype have a characteristic propensity for perineural spread, and skip lesions can represent pitfalls during primary treatment. Whenever possible, wide surgical excision is the treatment of choice. Well-established criteria for postoperative radiotherapy have not been defined, but an inadequate surgical margin would certainly justify adjuvant radiotherapy. Again, given the propensity for perineural spread, radiation portals should incorporate relevant nerve pathways, so inclusion of the base of the skull for this patient was appropriate.

Recurrent, metastatic adenoid cystic cancer is generally considered incurable. However, an indolent natural history is not uncommon especially in the case of isolated lung disease following a long disease-free interval. Data regarding the activity of chemotherapy is limited for adenoid cystic cancer, and available series commonly include mixed histologic subtypes of salivary gland tumors. The combination of doxorubicin, cisplatin, and cyclophosphamide has been reported to have activity. Other active agents include fluorouracil, mitoxantrone, and vinorelbine. Overall, chemotherapy is not curative, and only a few patients will have a complete or partial response even with combination chemotherapy.

Although a potential role for immune factors is commonly postulated for this disease, interferon is not an established standard agent. The c-kit target has been reported to be expressed in most adenoid cystic cancers, so there is interest in imatinib as a therapeutic option. However, there is insufficient evidence to support its role as a standard treatment option. Given that the multiple lung nodules represent hematogenous spread of disease, the likelihood that surgery could render this patient free of disease in the long term is very unlikely.

Taken together, especially in the context of this entirely asymptomatic patient, close watchful waiting with serial imaging would be the preferred approach. The other choices would likely result in an unfavorable toxicity-benefit ratio for the patient at this juncture.

Suggested Reading

Gedlicka C, Schüll B, Formanek M, et al. Mitoxantrone and cisplatin in recurrent and/or metastatic salivary gland malignancies. *Anticancer Drugs.* 2002;13(5):491–495.

Licitra L, Cavina R, Grandi C, et al. Cisplatin, doxorubicin and cyclophosphamide in advanced salivary gland carcinoma. A phase II trial of 22 patients. *Ann Oncol.* 1996;7(6):640–642.

Penner CR, Folpe AL, Budnick SD. C-kit expression distinguishes salivary gland adenoid cystic carcinoma from polymorphous low-grade adenocarcinoma. *Mod Pathol.* 2002;15(7):687–91.

Spiro RH. Management of malignant tumors of the salivary glands. *Oncology.* 1998;12(5):671–680.

7-6 C

Educational Objective: To identify the appropriate management of anaplastic thyroid cancer.

This patient has metastatic, anaplastic thyroid cancer to the lung. In contrast to the excellent long-term survival for patients with well-differentiated thyroid cancer, the median survival for patients with this disease in most series is less than 1 year from the time of diagnosis. Long-term survivors are rare. Because of the poor prognosis, pathology review is crucial to ensure that more curable and treatable diagnoses, such as large cell lymphoma, are not missed. Fortunately, the incidence of anaplastic thyroid cancer is low, estimated as representing 1% to 3% of all thyroid cancers. Also, in contrast to the situation with well-differentiated thyroid cancers, the median age of the patient at the time of presentation is 20 to 30 years older, and the female-to-male ratio is significantly more balanced. An association with prior well-differentiated thyroid cancer or benign thyroid nodule disease is not uncommon.

Anaplastic thyroid cancer is characterized by rapidly growing primary lesions with locally invasive characteristics. Despite the fact that 20% to 50% of patients have distant metastases at the time of presentation, patients commonly die as the result of upper airway consequences of aggressive local-regional disease. As such, aggressive treatment of local disease is appropriate even if there are distant metastases, if the local disease at presentation appears most immediately worrisome for disease-related morbidity. Although the results of clinical series show that the best outcomes occur in patients who have successful resection combined with adjuvant therapy, these patients commonly have unresectable disease when first seen.

Unlike with differentiated thyroid cancers, radioactive iodine is not useful in pure anaplastic thyroid cancer. Radiotherapy has had some success as a single modality, and the use of concurrent chemotherapy may improve control of local disease. However, long-term survival remains poor. Given the presumed distant metastases in this case, chemotherapy as a single modality is a reasonable consideration, but response rate in the neck will likely be higher with combined-modality therapy, and this is the site of greatest initial clinical concern in this patient.

Tracheostomy is sometimes necessary for these patients, but is not routinely pursued prophylactically because tumors may fungate through the stoma. Also, the potential adverse quality-of-life consequences of tracheostomy placement must be carefully reviewed with the patient in light of the overall poor prognosis.

Suggested Reading

Tan RK, Finley RK, Driscoll D, et al. Anaplastic carcinoma of the thyroid: a 24-year experience. *Head Neck.* 1995;17(1):41–47.

Tennvall J, Lundell G, Hallquist A, et al. Combined doxorubicin, hyperfractionated radiotherapy, and surgery in anaplastic thyroid carcinoma. Report on two protocols. The Swedish Anaplastic Thyroid Cancer Group. *Cancer.* 1994;74(4):1348–1354.

7-7 **B**

Educational Objective: To recognize that radioactive iodine is the treatment of choice for metastatic, differentiated thyroid cancer and that recent use of iodinated contrast can interfere with the interpretation of a diagnostic whole-body scan using radioactive iodine.

This patient has recurrent thyroid cancer with metastases to the lung. Although the diagnostic radioactive iodine scan was interpreted as showing no evidence of iodine-avid disease, the scan was performed shortly after the administration of iodinated contrast. Iodinated contrast increases the circulating iodine pool and interferes with uptake on the radioactive iodine scan, rendering it nondiagnostic. The whole-body scan should be repeated after 6 to 8 weeks.

Radioactive iodine is the treatment of choice for metastases that take up iodine. Complete responses to treatment have been observed for 45% of patients with distant metastases. A higher frequency of complete responses has been noted for younger patients and for those with small pulmonary metastases.

The other choices are incorrect for the following reasons: although doxorubicin-based chemotherapy regimens have been most extensively studied for metastatic thyroid cancer, responses are generally transient and incomplete. As a result, cytotoxic chemotherapy should generally be reserved for patients with demonstrated radioactive iodine-resistant progressive disease. Whereas there is a role for surgical resection or radiation therapy for the management of locally recurrent disease and for symptomatic metastatic lesions, there is no indication for such treatment in this case. Somatostatin is a consideration for tumors revealing uptake on octreotide scintigraphy. However, such an approach is reserved for patients with clearly documented radioactive iodine-resistant disease.

Suggested Reading

England RJ, Atkin SL. Somatostatins and their role in thyroid cancer. *Clin Otolaryngol.* 2002;27:120–123.

Haugen BR. Management of the patient with progressive radioiodine non-responsive disease. *Semin Surg Oncol.* 1999;16(1): 34–41.

Mazzaferri EL, Kloos RT. Current approaches to primary therapy for papillary and follicular thyroid cancer. *J Clin Endocrinol Metab.* 2001;86(4):1447–1463.

Schlumberger M, Challeton C, De Vathaire F, et al. Radioactive iodine treatment and external radiotherapy for lung and bone metastases from thyroid carcinoma. *J Nucl Med.* 1996;37(4): 598–605.

SELF EVALUATION

CHAPTER 8 QUESTIONS:
GASTROINTESTINAL CANCERS

8-1 A 55-year-old man presents because of an elevated carcinoembryonic antigen (CEA) level (15 ng/mL) at his last routine visit. The patient has a history of a T3, N1, M0 adenocarcinoma of the colon, which was diagnosed 24 months previously. The tumor was resected, and the patient received postoperative treatment with fluorouracil leucovorin plus oxaliplatin (FOLFOX) for 6 months. He has returned for regular follow-up visits every 6 months. Previous CEA levels had all been less than 2 ng/mL.

At the present time, the findings on physical examination are normal. There are no abnormalities noted on chest x-ray. Findings on computerized tomography (CT) show a 3-cm lesion in the right lobe of the liver. Positron emission tomography (PET) demonstrates a positive signal correlating precisely with the lesion seen on the CT scan and no other uptake.

Which of the following would you recommend?

A. Chemotherapy with fluorouracil, leucovorin, and irinotecan (FOLFIRI) plus bevacizumab
B. Biopsy of the liver lesion
C. Referral to a surgeon for resection of the liver lesion
D. No treatment because of the lack of symptoms

8-2 A 68-year-old woman is referred to you for additional treatment 4 weeks after surgical resection for a tumor in the ascending colon that was determined on pathologic evaluation to be a moderately differentiated adenocarcinoma of the colon arising from a villous adenoma. The tumor had penetrated through the serosa, and three of 12 lymph nodes were positive for metastatic cancer. No other disease was seen at the time of surgery.

Preoperatively, the CEA level was 1.2 ng/mL, and CT of the chest, abdomen, and pelvis demonstrated no metastasis.

She has recovered from surgery well except for a slow recovery of normal bowel function, with two to three stools a day, compared with one stool per day preoperatively. Her history includes diabetes controlled with oral agents, hypertension poorly controlled with a beta blocker and a diuretic, and a hysterectomy for fibroids. She lives with her husband, is physically active, and is able to drive and maintain her own household.

Which of the following would you recommend?

A. 6 months of treatment with fluorouracil/leucovorin (Roswell Park of Mayo Clinic regimen)
B. 6 months of treatment with capecitabine
C. 6 months of treatment with fluorouracil/leucovorin and irinotecan (FOLFIRI)
D. 6 months of treatment with fluorouracil/leucovorin and oxaliplatin (FOLFOX or FLOX)
E. No treatment

8-3 A 35-year-old woman presents after colonoscopy examination revealed a solitary lesion in the ascending colon, with no other polyps or signs of inflammatory bowel disease noted. Evaluation of a biopsy sample obtained during colonoscopy showed adenocarcinoma, poorly differentiated histology, and no evidence of a pre-existing polyp.

The patient is married and has two children, ages 10 and 6. Her mother died at age 48 of uterine cancer. Her father is alive and healthy. Her 40-year-old sister was diagnosed with an early-stage colon cancer 2 years ago and has been followed up with no recurrence of new cancers. The patient has no other siblings and no further family history was elicited.

A right hemicolectomy is done. At surgery, the lesion is determined to be a T3, N1, M0 adenocarcinoma. She recovered well and presents to you for further recommendations regarding treatment options. She is also concerned that her children are at increased risk for colon cancer.

You recommend genetic testing. Which of the following is the most likely familial cancer syndrome affecting this family?

A. *BRCA* 2 mutation
B. Hereditary nonpolyposis colorectal cancer (HNPCC)
C. Familial adenomatous polyposis (FAP)
D. Li-Fraumeni syndrome

8-4 A 55-year-old man presents because of multiple lung and liver metastases found on routine follow-up CT 2 years after treatment for stage III cancer of the sigmoid colon. At that time, he was treated with resection of the primary tumor and postoperative adjuvant chemotherapy with fluorouracil and leucovorin. Examination of a biopsy sample of the liver lesion now demonstrates adenocarcinoma consistent with a primary cancer of the colon. The results of laboratory tests are as follows: total bilirubin, 2.1 mg/dL; direct bilirubin 0.2 mg/dL; creatinine, 0.8 mg/dL; alkaline phosphatase, 108 U/L; aspartate aminotransferase, 22 U/L; alanine aminotransferase, 12 U/L; and albumin, 4.0 g/dL. The patient has a very good performance status, is eager to begin treatment, and understands that no treatment offers curative potential.

Which of the following would you recommend?

A. FOLFOX plus bevacizumab
B. FOLFIRI plus bevacizumab
C. Capecitabine and oxaliplatin (XELOX)
D. FOLFOX plus cetuximab
E. No therapy because the patient is asymptomatic and chemotherapy offers no survival benefit

8-5 **A 45-year-old man presents to his primary care physician because of darkening urine, mild pruritis, and his wife's concerns about his "color." A review of systems was positive for low-level back pain, mild early satiety, and a 15-pound weight loss in the past 2 months. The physical examination revealed scleral icterus, hepatomegaly, and bilateral edema (1+) in the lower extremities. CT demonstrated biliary constriction, a 5-cm mass in the pancreatic head, and multiple lesions (2 to 4 cm) on the liver. Endoscopic retrograde cholangiopancreatography (ERCP) allowed for the placement of a biliary stent, resulting in the normalization of the jaundice and pruritis. Oxycodone, 5 mg every 6 hours, was started for the back pain. Brushings obtained during the ERCP were positive for a cluster of poorly differentiated adenocarcinoma. The patient and his wife now ask you for treatment advice. He has a performance status of 90%, his pain is controlled, and he continues to work but has reduced his hours to part-time.**

Which of the following would you recommend?

A. Gemcitabine as single-agent chemotherapy
B. Initial radiation therapy to the primary pancreatic tumor, given concurrently with chemotherapy, followed by gemcitabine as single-agent therapy
C. Gemcitabine and fluorouracil combination chemotherapy
D. Gemcitabine and oxaliplatin combination chemotherapy
E. No therapy and referral to hospice

8-6 **A 70-year-old woman is referred to you after a diagnosis of a pancreatic mass and two lesions on the left lobe of the liver. The lesions were found on CT that was done as part of a general health screening because the patient was concerned that there was "something wrong," even though she had no specific symptoms. She has no significant medical history and takes no medications. Findings of other testing included no evidence of cancer on ERCP, increased PET signal from the pancreatic mass and the hepatic lesions consistent with cancer, and negative findings on evaluation of a sample obtained by percutaneous ultrasound-guided biopsy of the liver lesions. Serologic testing for selected tumor markers revealed elevated levels of carbohydrate antigen 19-9 (85 U/mL; normal, 0 to 37 U/mL) and CEA (12 ng/mL; normal, 0 to 3 ng/mL). She is referred to you for consideration of treatment options.**

Which of the following would you recommend?

A. Chemotherapy with gemcitabine
B. Exploratory laparotomy, with resection of the pancreatic mass and the hepatic lesions
C. Radiation therapy to the pancreatic mass, given concurrently with gemcitabine
D. Repeat biopsy

8-7 **A 42-year-old man presents 4 weeks after successful partial gastrectomy for adenocarcinoma of the stomach because his surgeon has suggested the need for chemotherapy. Preoperative staging after diagnostic upper endoscopy was negative for metastatic disease. He recovered well after the surgery, with his weight stabilizing. (He had had a 15-pound weight loss at initial presentation.) Pathologic evaluation of the surgical specimen demonstrates a transmurally penetrating, moderately differentiated adenocarcinoma, and one of 15 lymph nodes is positive for metastatic disease. The proximal margin is read as "close" but negative (1 cm). The findings of physical examination are normal, including a well-healed mid-line scar.**

Which of the following would you recommend?

A. No further treatment
B. Radiation therapy to the upper abdomen with fluorouracil as a radiation sensitizer
C. Adjuvant chemotherapy with fluorouracil and cisplatin for 4 to 6 months
D. Chemotherapy with fluorouracil plus leucovorin for one cycle, followed by combined radiation therapy and fluorouracil, followed by three more cycles of fluorouracil plus leucovorin
E. Adjuvant chemotherapy with fluorouracil for 6 months

8-8 **A 65-year-old man with locally-advanced adenocarcinoma of the esophagus has recently completed treatment consisting of radiation, fluorouracil, and cisplatin. Pretreatment CT demonstrated an esophageal mass and a 3-cm celiac lymph node. Endoscopic ultrasound confirms a T3, N1 tumor. A specimen from the celiac node, obtained by transgastric biopsy, was positive for adenocarcinoma (M1). The patient tolerated the chemotherapy regimen and recovered well. His weight is stable, and he is swallowing adequately. A CT scan made after the completion of treatment showed considerable regression of the tumor and the lymph node. Repeat upper endoscopy showed complete regression of the esophageal lesion, and the findings on random biopsy specimens were negative. The patient seeks your advice regarding further treatment.**

Which of the following do you recommend?

A. Distal esophagectomy
B. Continuation of chemotherapy
C. Close follow-up without further treatment

8-9 **A 42-year-old man presents because of rectal bleeding and tenesmus. He reports having substantial abdominal distention, narrowed stools, and difficulty with bowel movements. On colonoscopy, a large friable lesion is found 4 cm from the anal verge; it was difficult to pass the colonoscope because of the lesion. The findings on biopsy were positive for adenocarcinoma. Staging CT demonstrated more than 10 hepatic lesions with substantial hepatic replacement. The levels of aspartate aminotransferase and alkaline phosphatase were 3 times the upper limit of normal. A surgeon recommended a diverting colostomy, but the patient is reluctant. He presents to you for chemotherapy instead.**

Which of the following would you recommend?

A. Radiation and fluorouracil for local control of the rectal lesion, followed by irinotecan, fluorouracil, leucovorin, and bevacizumab
B. Abdominoperineal resection of the primary lesion followed by systemic chemotherapy
C. Initial chemotherapy with oxaliplatin, fluorouracil, leucovorin, and bevacizumab
D. Diverting colostomy followed by chemotherapy

8-10 **A 54-year-old woman complains about a 10-year history of intermittent diarrhea, which was initially classified as irritable bowel syndrome. The frequency and severity of diarrhea has gradually increased in recent years. Now, the patient has noticed intermittent flushing and increased abdominal cramping. Upon physical exam, the liver is palpable 4 cm below the right costal margin. A CT scan demonstrates multiple intrahepatic lesions in all segments replacing about 40% of the total liver parenchyma. Laboratory values show only slightly elevated liver function tests; a 24-hour urine reveals significantly elevated levels of 5-HIAA. The patient is referred to you for further management of her disease.**

Which of the following should be done?

A. Systemic chemotherapy
B. Hepatic arterial infusional chemotherapy
C. Somatostatin
D. PET/CT scan

CHAPTER 8 EXPLANATORY ANSWERS:
GASTROINTESTINAL CANCERS

8-1 C

Educational Objective: To understand the resectability of metastatic colon cancer.

The appearance of a PET-positive solitary liver lesion concomitant with a rise in the tumor marker carcinoembryonic antigen in a patient with stage III colon cancer diagnosed 2 years ago strongly suggests liver metastasis from his colon cancer. To understand whether the patient has a potentially curative option, a surgeon should review the patient's history and the results of CT. Decisions about chemotherapy before or after surgery and the need for biopsy should await surgical opinion. Given that this patient has a potentially curative option, it is inappropriate to postpone treatment. Although a liver biopsy is not the best answer, it is true that confirmation of diagnosis is important; however, for this patient, who appears to have a clearly resectable lesion with substantial suggestion of recurrent disease before the biopsy, a surgical resection should be considered. The role of systemic chemotherapy in this scenario as neoadjuvant treatment is not yet well defined and is the subject of ongoing clinical trials

Suggested Reading

Fong Y, Kemeny N, Paty P, et al. Treatment of colorectal cancer: hepatic metastasis. *Semin Surg Oncol.* 1996;12(4):219–252.

Charnsangavej C, Clary B, Fong Y, et al. Selection of patients for resection of hepatic colorectal metastases: Expert Consensus Statement. *Ann Surg Oncol.* 2006;13(10):1261–1268.

Poston, GJ, Adam, R, Alberts S, et al. OncoSurge: a strategy for improving resectability with curative intent in metastatic colorectal cancer. *J Clin Oncol.* 2005;23(28):7125–7134

8-2 D

Educational Objective: To define the role of adjuvant chemotherapy for stage III colon cancer.

It is recognized that patients with stage T3, N1-2, M0 adenocarcinoma of the colon should receive adjuvant chemotherapy because the patient is at substantial risk for relapse. Recent studies confirmed that 6 months of either FOLFOX or FLOX is superior to fluorouracil/leucovorin alone in terms of disease-free survival. Thus, adjuvant therapy with FOLFOX or FLOX can be considered standard of care for a stage III patient without obvious contraindications against chemotherapy in general and oxaliplatin in particular. Capecitabine has been shown to be a reasonable alternative to fluorouracil/leucovorin, but should be reserved for patients who are not considered candidates for an oxaliplatin-based regimen. Irinotecan-containing treatment approaches have failed to significantly affect disease-free survival in clinical trials and play no role in the adjuvant treatment of colon cancer.

Suggested Reading

Andre T, Boni C, Mounedji-Boudiaf L, et al. Oxaliplatin, fluorouracil, and leucovorin as adjuvant treatment for colon cancer. *N Engl J Med.* 2004;350(23):2343–2351.

Kuebler JP, Wieand HS, O'Connell M et al. Oxaliplatin combined with weekly bolus fluorouracil and leucovorin as surgical adjuvant chemotherapy for stage II and III colon cancer: results from NSABP C-07. *J Clin Oncol.* 2007;25(16):2198–2204.

Sargent DJ, Wieand HS, Haller DG, et al. Disease-free survival versus overall survival as a primary end point for adjuvant colon cancer studies: individual patient data from 20,898 patients on 18 randomized trials. *J Clin Oncol.* 2005;23(34):8664–8670.

Twelves C, Wong A, Nowacki MP, et al. Capecitabine as adjuvant treatment for stage III colon cancer. *N Engl J Med.* 2005;352 (26):2696–2704.

8-3 B

Educational Objective: To understand the genetic syndromes associated with colon cancer and explain their implications to patients.

This patient is likely a member of a family with type II HNPCC (Lynch syndrome II), given that gastric cancer was diagnosed in her mother at a young age, that early-stage colon cancer was diagnosed in a sister at age 40, and that the patient presents with stage III disease with a tumor location in the ascending colon. Genetic testing is now available for this type of hereditary cancer. The uterine cancer and the colon cancer track together in this genetic syndrome. The absence of a pre-existing polyp is typical for familial cancers of this type, and further screening is not likely to detect additional polyps because this type of tumor rarely—if ever—arises from a polyp. Further surgery may be warranted as hemicolectomy is often believed to be inadequate, and a subtotal or near-total colectomy should be done. In addition, hysterectomy and oophorectomy should be considered because the incidence of uterine and ovarian cancers is higher for patients with this genetic syndrome. The woman's children are at increased risk for colon cancer, and they should be monitored closely.

Suggested Reading

Hendriks YM, de Jong AE, Morreau H, et al. Diagnostic approach and management of Lynch syndrome (hereditary nonpolyposis colorectal carcinoma): a guide for clinicians. *CA Cancer J Clin.* 2006;56(4):213–225.

Grady WM. Genetic testing for high-risk colon cancer patients. *Gastroenterology.* 2003;124(6):1574–1594.

Lindor NM, Petersen GM, Hadley DW, et al. Recommendations for the care of individuals with an inherited predisposition to Lynch syndrome: a systematic review. *JAMA.* 2006;296(12): 1507–1517.

Lynch HT, Lynch JF, Lynch PM. Toward a consensus in molecular diagnosis of hereditary nonpolyposis colorectal cancer (Lynch syndrome). *J Natl Cancer Inst.* 2007;99(4):261–263.

8-4 A

Educational Objective: To recognize appropriate choices for chemotherapy for patients with metastatic colon cancer.

Systemic chemotherapy in advanced colorectal cancer has shown significant improvements in overall survival and quality of life compared with best supportive care. All listed chemotherapy options could represent reasonable choices as first-line therapy. Because the addition of bevacizumab to fluorouracil-based first-line chemotherapy has been associated with improved outcome (particularly in terms of prolonged overall survival), a bevacizumab-containing approach would be preferable. For this patient with elevated bilirubin, further aspects must be considered. Patients with abnormal end-organ function (abnormal renal or hepatic function) may have different adverse reactions to either irinotecan, capecitabine, or oxaliplatin. The elevated bilirubin could be a result of the presence of metastatic disease or Gilbert syndrome. Irinotecan should not be given to patients with Gilbert syndrome and/or elevated bilirubin without significant dose reductions. Cetuximab has documented efficacy as a salvage therapy option either as single agent or in combination with irinotecan. Its role as component of upfront chemotherapy is studied in ongoing clinical trials. Thus, FOLFOX plus bevacizumab appears to be the best alternative in this scenario.

Suggested Reading

Innocenti F, Ratain MJ. Irinotecan treatment in cancer patients with UGT1A1 polymorphisms. *Oncology.* 2003(5 Suppl 5);17:52–55.

Cunningham D, Humblet Y, Siena S, et al: Cetuximab monotherapy and cetuximab plus irinotecan in irinotecan-refractory metastatic colorectal cancer. *N Engl J Med.* 2004;351(4): 337–345.

Giantonio BJ, Catalano PJ, Meropol NJ et al. Bevacizumab in combination with oxaliplatin, fluorouracil, and leucovorin (FOLFOX4) for previously treated metastatic colorectal cancer: results from the Eastern Cooperative Oncology Group Study E3200. *J Clin Oncol.* 2007; 25(12):1539–1544.

Goldberg RM, Sargent DJ, Morton RF, et al. A randomized controlled trial of fluorouracil plus leucovorin, irinotecan, and oxaliplatin combinations in patients with previously untreated metastatic colorectal cancer. *J Clin Oncol.* 2004;22(1):23–30.

Hurwitz H, Fehrenbacher L, Novotny W, et al. Bevacizumab plus irinotecan, fluorouracil, and leucovorin for metastatic colorectal cancer. *N Engl J Med.* 2004;350(23):2335–2342.

8-5 A

Educational Objective: To understand the appropriate therapy for patients with metastatic pancreatic cancer.

The stent and pain medication has provided effective palliation for this patient. Gemcitabine as single-agent chemotherapy for patients with metastatic pancreatic cancer is the appropriate choice on the basis of the findings from a randomized trial in which relief of symptoms and survival were better for gemcitabine than for fluorouracil. Studies to evaluate gemcitabine-based combination therapy have so far produced only disappointing results, including combinations with fluorouracil and oxaliplatin. Concurrent radiation and chemotherapy followed by gemcitabine is not appropriate for this patient with distant metastases and should be reserved for patients with intractable pain, and possibly, for locally advanced pancreatic cancer. Referral to hospice with no further treatment can be appropriate for patients who are not considered candidates for chemotherapy at all because of poor performance status or comorbidities. Since gemcitabine offers a survival advantage and is generally well tolerated, it should be considered for most patients with metastatic pancreatic cancer.

Suggested Reading

Hochster HS, Haller DG, de Gramont A, et al. Consensus report of the international society of gastrointestinal oncology on therapeutic progress in advanced pancreatic cancer. *Cancer.* 2006;107(4):676–685.

Cardenes HR, Chiorean EG, Dewitt J, et al. Locally advanced pancreatic cancer: current therapeutic approach. *Oncologist.* 2006;11(6):612–623.

8-6 D

Educational Objective: To identify the appropriate tests for confirming a diagnosis of cancer.

Despite findings suggestive of metastatic pancreatic cancer on several tests, no evaluation of a biopsy specimen has confirmed the diagnosis to this point in the evaluation of the patient. No imagine scan including PET/CT fusion scans can identify the histo-origin of metastatic disease. Thus, a repeat biopsy should be done, as it is possible that the patient has another type of cancer, such as neuroendocrine tumor, which is associated with a more favorable prognosis and different treatment options. Before a diagnosis of an "incurable" cancer can be given, a confirmatory biopsy is required. Exploratory laparotomy with resection of the lesions is not appropriate, as resection of liver metastasis is inappropriate for patients with metastatic pancreatic cancer. Chemotherapy and radiation should not be given prior to establishing a definitive diagnosis.

Suggested Reading

Chamlou R, Matos C, Nagy N, et al. Pitfalls on frozen section of a hepatic lesion in the management of a pancreatic tumor. *Surgery.* 2003;133(5):599–600.

Jhala NC, Jhala DN, Chhieng DC, et al. Endoscopic ultrasound-guided fine-needle aspiration. A cytopathologist's perspective. *Am J Clin Pathol.* 2003;120(3):351–367.

Maemura K, Takao S, Shinchi H, et al. Role of positron emission tomography in decisions on treatment strategies for pancreatic cancer. *J Hepatobiliary Pancreat Surg.* 2006;13(5):435–441.

8-7 D

Educational Objective: To fully understand the data supporting adjuvant therapy for gastric cancer.

This individual represents a classic example of successful resection of stage III gastric cancer. In 2001, the results of a study were published and showed a survival advantage to fluorouracil/leucovorin, followed by combined fluorouracil-based chemoradiation, followed by fluorouracil/leucovorin compared with surgery alone. Radiation therapy without additional chemotherapy is not indicated, nor is fluorouracil and cisplatin or fluorouracil and leucovorin alone, as none of these has shown a benefit. Therefore, for this young patient, adjuvant chemotherapy would,be the appropriate recommendation. If he had been seen by a medical oncologist before surgery, perioperative chemotherapy using epirubicin, fluorouracil, and cisplatin (ECF) could have been considered based on convincing phase III data that demonstrate a survival advantage of this approach compared with surgery alone. Clinical trials investigating ECF in the adjuvant setting as a substitute for fluorouracil/leucovorin are underway.

Suggested Reading

Van Laethem JL, Demols A. Adjuvant therapy in gastric and cardia cancer: should we irradiate? *Curr Opin Oncol.* 2006;18(4): 381–385.

Macdonald JS, Smalley SR, Benedetti J, et al. Chemoradiotherapy after surgery compared with surgery alone for adenocarcinoma of the stomach or gastroesophageal junction. *N Engl J Med.* 2001;345(10):725 730.

Cunningham D, Allum WH, Stenning SP, et al. Perioperative chemotherapy versus surgery alone for resectable gastroesophageal cancer. *N Engl J Med.* 2006;355(1):11–20.

8-8 C

Educational Objective: To understand the staging and management of esophageal cancer.

Metastatic disease must be immediately recognized in this patient because a celiac lymph node with this disease is categorized as M1. Therefore, in this palliative situation, surgery will not play a role in the overall survival and relapse rate and is not indicated. Close follow-up (with surgery considered if local relapse occurs) is a possible option, but surgery would be done only if no other palliative means such as stent placement were available to control local esophageal recurrence. If the celiac node had not been present, surgical resection of the esophagus would have been an acceptable—although controversial—choice.

Suggested Reading

Bedenne L, Michel P, Bouche O, et al. Chemoradiation followed by surgery compared with chemoradiation alone in squamous cancer of the esophagus: FFCD 9102. *J Clin Oncol.* 2007;25(10): 1160–1168.

Lightdale CJ, Kulkami KG. Role of endoscopic ultrasonography in the staging and follow-up of esophageal cancer. *J Clin Oncol.* 2005;23:4483–4489.

Leonard GD, McCaffrey JA, Maher M. Optimal therapy for oesophageal cancer. *Cancer Treat Rev.* 2003;29:275–282.

Makary MA, Kiernan PD, Sheridan MJ, et al. Multimodality tre-atment for esophageal cancer: the role of surgery and neoadjuvant therapy. *Am Surg.* 2003; 69:693–700; discussion 700–702.

8-9 D

Educational Objective: To summarize the management of a newly diagnosed rectal cancer.

The substantial primary tumor of the rectum is a problem, but more pressing is the substantial liver lesions and the hepatic replacement. Because of this, effective systemic chemotherapy should be initiated as soon as possible. Trying to avoid a diverting colostomy by beginning with radiation and fluorouracil is inappropriate because this does not include—and thus delays—optimum systemic chemotherapy. The response rate associated with chemotherapy alone with regard to the advanced primary tumor is similarly inadequate, given the bleeding, tenesmus, and likelihood of abdominal obstruction caused by the progressing cancer. An abdominoperineal resection will not help in the long-term and will only delay chemotherapy. Therefore, an initial diverting colostomy and initiating definitive chemotherapy is the most appropriate choice. A rectal stent could be another alternative for this patient, but the technology for this procedure is not available at all cancer centers.

Suggested Reading

Chawla AK, Kachnic LA, Clark JW, et al. Combined modality therapy for rectal and colon cancer. *Semin Oncol.* 2003;30: 101–112.

Sauer R, Becker H, Hohenberger W, et al. Preoperative versus postoperative chemoradiotherapy for rectal cancer. *N Engl J Med.* 2004;351:1731–1740.

Terstriep S, Grothey A. First- and second-line therapy of metastatic colorectal cancer.

Expert Rev Anticancer Ther. 2006;6:921–930.

8-10 C

Educational Objective: To understand the most management of advanced carcinoid tumors.

The patient suffers from a metastatic neuroendocrine tumor with carcinoid syndrome (long-standing diarrhea, flushing). Somatostatin is used to suppress circulating serotonin levels and provide symptomatic relief of the carcinoid syndrome, which can be associated with significant impairment of the patient's quality of life. In select cases, tumor debulking procedures, either in the form of surgical debulking or hepatic chemoemboliztion, can likewise reduce the overall serotonin production of the tumor and improve symptom control. However, the pattern of metastatic spread would preclude any surgical approach with curative intent (i.e., with the goal to remove all metastatic lesions). Differentiated neuroendocrine tumors such as metastatic carcinoids are relatively chemorefractory so that systemic chemotherapy is not indicated here. The most sensitive imaging options are MRI to evaluate the extent of liver metastasis and octreotide scan to detect distant metastases. If CT imagining is utilized, it should be performed as a triple-phase CT to evaluate the liver in an optimal way.

Suggested Reading

Lal A, Chen H. Treatment of advanced carcinoid tumors. *Curr Opin Oncol.* 2006;18:9–15.

de Herder WW, Kwekkeboom DJ, Valkema R, et al. Neuroendocrine tumors and somatostatin: imaging techniques. *J Endocrinol Invest.* 2005;28(11 Suppl):132–136.

SELF EVALUATION

CHAPTER 9 QUESTIONS:
GENITOURINARY CANCERS

9-1 A 52-year-old man presents for the first time for a routine physical examination and is found to have a prostate-specific antigen (PSA) level of 4.1 ng/mL. He has no urinary symptoms or erectile dysfunction. No abnormalities are found on physical examination. On digital rectal examination, the prostate appears to be of normal size with no abnormalities. There are no associated medical comorbidities.

Which of the following would you advise for the patient at this point?

A. Repeat PSA test
B. Transrectal ultrasound-guided biopsy of the prostate
C. Free PSA test
D. Computerized tomography (CT) scan of the abdomen and pelvis, and a bone scan
E. Follow-up evaluation in 1 year

9-2 A 58-year-old man is found to have a PSA level of 4.8 ng/mL on routine examination, which is increased from the level a year previously (3.4 ng/mL). He has no urinary symptoms or erectile dysfunction. On digital rectal examination, the prostate appears to be of normal size with no abnormalities. He was referred for a urologic evaluation; the findings of a transrectal ultrasound-guided biopsy of the prostate indicated adenocarcinoma, Gleason grade 6 in two of six cores from the right, and none of six cores from the left. It is estimated that 10% of each of the two cores is involved by cancer. There are no associated medical comorbidities.

Which of the following would you advise for the patient at this point?

A. CT of the abdomen and pelvis only
B. Bone scan only
C. CT scan of the abdomen and pelvis and bone scan
D. Capromab pendetide imaging
E. None of the above

9-3 A 72-year-old man presents with symptomatic bone metastases secondary to prostate cancer. The baseline hemoglobin was 11 g/dL, and the PSA level at the start of hormone treatment was 250 ng/mL. Androgen ablation was initiated with a 3-month depot of goserelin, a gonadotropin-releasing hormone analogue, and the antiandrogen, bicalutamide. After 6 months of therapy, the symptoms improved, and the PSA level was undetectable. He continued to be monitored every 3 months. At month 18, the PSA level was 10 ng/mL, with no change in other parameters. A repeat PSA level was 15 ng/mL. A testosterone level is at castrate level. Bisphosphonate therapy was initiated recently.

Which of the following should be the next intervention?

A. Change to a different antiandrogen
B. Ketoconazole and hydrocortisone
C. Change to a different bisphosphonate
D. Discontinue bicalutamide, but continue therapy with goserelin
E. Strontium-89 or samarium-153

9-4 A 46-year-old male smoker presents with hematuria. The findings of cytologic analysis of a urine sample indicate the presence of malignant cells, and CT demonstrates no masses in the kidney, bladder, or lymph nodes. An examination under anesthesia and a bimanual assessment reveal no palpable masses, whereas the endoscopic evaluation reveals a 2-cm lesion obscuring the right ureteral orifice. Evaluation of a biopsy specimen demonstrates grade 2, infiltrating urothelial carcinoma of the bladder. Muscle is not present in the submitted surgical specimen. Results of repeat urine cytology show no malignant cells.

Which of the following would you recommend?

A. Observation
B. Evaluation of the ureters and renal pelvis
C. Administration of intravesical mitomycin-C
D. Administration of intravesical bacille Calmette-Guérin (BCG)
E. Repeat cystoscopy and biopsy

9-5 A 46-year-old man has urinary frequency and is found to have a mass in the bladder on examination under anesthesia and cystoscopy. A clinical T3 lesion is diagnosed, and invasive urothelial carcinoma is confirmed on biopsy.

Which of the following statements concerning the use of chemotherapy for invasive bladder cancer is correct?

A. Neoadjuvant chemotherapy with a cisplatin-based combination regimen has been shown to improve survival when given to patients with invasive bladder cancer
B. Chemotherapy with gemcitabine and cisplatin should be administered to all patients with invasive disease after radical cystectomy
C. Randomized comparisons of a regimen of methotrexate, vinblastine, doxorubicin, and cisplatin (M-VAC) followed by cystectomy compared with cystectomy alone; and a regimen of cisplatin, methotrexate, and vinblastine (CMV) followed by radiation or surgery compared with radiation or surgery alone have shown no benefit for early chemotherapy
D. For patients with impaired renal function, non-cisplatin–containing regimens have demonstrated a survival benefit in the perioperative setting

9-6 A 52-year-old man had a radical cystectomy with creation of an internal urinary reservoir for a T4, node-positive urothelial carcinoma of the bladder. Two of 12 lymph nodes were positive for metastatic disease. One year after the surgery, a pulmonary lesion was identified in the upper lobe of the right lung, which was biopsy-confirmed metastatic urothelial carcinoma. The patient received three cycles of systemic chemotherapy with gemcitabine and cisplatin, which produced a 60% reduction in the size of the pulmonary lesion. Three additional cycles of therapy were then administered with no further change in the size of the lesion and no new lesions present.

Which of the following would you recommend?

A. Add single-agent paclitaxel
B. Continue the same chemotherapy regimen
C. Surgically resect the metastatic lesions
D. Change to the M-VAC regimen
E. Change to a combination of paclitaxel and carboplatin

9-7 A 24-year-old man presented with a left testicular mass and underwent a radical inguinal orchiectomy. The preoperative level of human chorionic gonadotropin (HCG) was 224 IU/mL. Pathologic evaluation of the resected specimen revealed choriocarcinoma and embryonal carcinoma with evidence of vascular invasion. The HCG level 10 days and 20 days after surgery were 224 IU/mL and 110 IU/mL, respectively. The alpha-fetoprotein level is within normal limits. The findings on CT of the chest, abdomen, and pelvis prior to orchiectomy were normal.

Which of the following would you advise?

A. Three cycles of bleomycin, etoposide, and cisplatin
B. A nerve-sparing retroperitoneal lymph node dissection
C. Three cycles of etoposide and cisplatin
D. Radiation therapy to the abdomen
E. Observation

9-8 A 32-year-old man presents with a 4-week history of a cough and an enlarging testicular mass. The evaluation shows five pulmonary nodules in the left lung; the largest is 1.5 cm. A CT scan of the abdomen shows multiple enlarged nodes in the retroperitoneum (maximum size, 10 cm). Laboratory values include a lactate dehydrogenase level of 800 U/L, an alpha-fetoprotein level of 3,500 units, and an HCG level of 4 mIU/mL. The testicular mass is removed and the pathologic diagnosis is embryonal carcinoma with elements of choriocarcinoma and teratoma. He receives three cycles of cisplatin, etoposide, and bleomycin, with resolution of symptoms and normalization of markers. Imaging studies after the three cycles of chemotherapy show no evidence of disease in the chest, but the abdominal CT reveals a 3-cm residual mass in the retroperitoneum.

Which of the following would you recommend?

A. 18-fluorodeoxyglucose (FDG)-positron emission tomography (PET) and observation to ensure there is no residual disease
B. Change in therapy to vinblastine, ifosfamide, and cisplatin
C. Two additional cycles of cisplatin, etoposide, and bleomycin
D. Surgical exploration of the abdomen with retroperitoneal lymph node dissection with resection of the abdominal mass
E. Radiation therapy to the abdomen

9-9 A 27-year-old man presents with a left testicular mass. A radical orchiectomy is done, and pathologic evaluation reveals embryonal carcinoma with yolk sac elements and mature and immature teratoma. Postoperatively, the physical examination is normal. The alpha-fetoprotein level is 400 ng/dL, and the HCG level is 25 mIU/mL. CT scans of the abdomen and pelvis demonstrate an 8-cm para-aortic mass with minimal hydronephrosis. Standard cisplatin-based chemotherapy is started. On day 22, the alpha-fetoprotein level is 248 ng/dL, and the level of HCG is undetectable. At that time, a mass is palpated in the left upper quadrant. Repeat CT scans of the abdomen and pelvis show a 17-cm para-aortic mass deviating the aorta medially, with moderate hydronephrosis extending inferiorly to the bifurcation of the aorta.

Which of the following is the most appropriate treatment?

A. Change in chemotherapy regimen to ifosfamide plus cisplatin
B. Retroperitoneal lymph node dissection
C. High-dose chemotherapy with peripheral stem cell support
D. Continuation of standard treatment
E. Radiation therapy for palliation

9-10 A 47-year-old woman presents with right flank pain. She has no associated fever, chills, or weight loss. The findings on physical examination are remarkable for a palpable mass in the right upper quadrant. No costovertebral angle tenderness is noted. The results of laboratory tests include hemoglobin, 11 g/dL; alkaline phosphatase, normal; aspartate aminotransferase, 180 U/L; lactate dehydrogenase, 300 U/L; and partial thromboplastin time, 1.5 times normal.

Diagnostic studies show a right-sided mass originating in the kidney, with a question of extension into the perirenal fat. There is no adenopathy and no evidence of invasion into the inferior vena cava. No focal abnormalities were observed in the liver.

Which of the following should be included in the management of disease?

A. Bone scan
B. Intravenous pyelography
C. Resection of the right renal mass
D. Interferon-alpha
E. Interleukin-2 (aldesleukin)

9-11 A 60-year-old man was diagnosed with a renal tumor in 2001 and underwent a resection of a 9-cm clear cell renal cell carcinoma. In 2006, he presented to his doctor complaining of a 2-month history of a non-productive cough, a 15-pound weight loss, and right-side posterior rib discomfort. A metastatic work-up showed multiple pulmonary nodules from 5 to 20 mm in diameter in both lungs and metastases to multiple ribs and the distal left humerus. Biopsy of a pulmonary nodule confirmed recurrent clear cell renal cell carcinoma. The patient was treated with two cycles of high-dose interkeukin-2. Follow-up CT scan showed multiple new pulmonary nodules. Which of the following is the most appropriate treatment recommendation at this time?

A. Interferon-alpha
B. Surgical resection of all pulmonary nodules
C. Retreatment with two additional cycles of high-dose aldesleukin
D. Chemotherapy
E. Sunitinib malate or sorafenib tosylate

CHAPTER 9 EXPLANATORY ANSWERS:
GENITOURINARY CANCERS

9-1 A

Educational Objective: To understand how PSA testing is used to diagnose localized prostate cancer and to recognize the need for repeat testing.

Although a 52-year-old man with no associated comorbidities is likely to benefit from early diagnosis and treatment of prostate cancer, a single determination of the serum PSA level is not sufficient to justify additional diagnostic testing unless the level has been confirmed. In a study of 772 men followed for a 4-year period, 68 of 154 (44%) participants with a PSA level higher than 4 ng/mL had a normal level on a subsequent test. Isolated abnormalities in PSA levels should be confirmed before additional testing is advised. Measuring free PSA levels may help determine who is at a higher risk for the development of cancer, because the level of the free enzyme is reduced when cancer is present.

Suggested Reading

Catalona WJ, Partin AW, Slawin KM, et al. Use of the percentage of free prostate-specific antigen to enhance differentiation of prostate cancer from benign prostatic disease: a prospective multicenter clinical trial. *JAMA.* 1998;279:1542–1547.

Eastham JA, Riedel E, Scardino PT, et al. Variation of serum prostate-specific antigen levels: an evaluation of year-to-year fluctuations. *JAMA.* 2003;289:2695–2700.

Magklara A, Scorilas A, Catalona WJ, et al. The combination of human glandular kallikrein and free prostate-specific antigen (PSA) enhances discrimination between prostate cancer and benign prostatic hyperplasia in patients with moderately increased total PSA. *Clin Chem.* 1999;45:1960–1966.

9-2 E

Educational Objective: To identify the best method to determine the pathologic stage of prostate cancer.

The yield of the staging procedures outlined is limited in the setting of a tumor with a Gleason grade 6 histology and a low PSA level. CT scans of the abdomen and pelvis do not have the resolution to accurately predict whether there has been spread to or through the capsule, to the seminal vesicles, or to lymph nodes. CT is used for radiation treatment planning; however, the results will not affect the choice of primary treatment. Magnetic resonance imaging with an endorectal probe provides better resolution and a better estimate of the size and local spread of the tumor around the prostate. Similarly, capromab pendetide imaging does not permit an accurate determination of nodal spread. On the basis of this presentation, the probability of spread to bone is 0.3%. As such, a bone imaging modality is not required to make a therapeutic decision. Some physicians order a bone scan to provide a baseline measurement because of the high frequency of noncancerous changes, but this is not required. The probability that a prostate tumor has spread to the capsule, seminal vesicles, lymph nodes, and bone can be estimated by combining the findings of the digital rectal examination, PSA level, and Gleason score.

Suggested Reading

Partin A, Yoo J, Carter HB, et al. The use of prostate specific antigen, clinical stage and Gleason score to predict pathologic stage in men with localized prostate cancer. *J Urol.* 1993; 150:110–114.

Ross PL, Scardino PT, Kattan MW. A catalog of prostate cancer nomograms. *J Urol.* 2001;165:1562–1568.

9-3 D

Educational Objective: To recognize the appropriate evaluation of a patient in whom prostate cancer progresses during treatment with hormones, and to recognize the importance of documenting castrate status.

The first therapeutic intervention for this patient is to discontinue the antiandrogen, bicalutamide, which has been associated with a decline in the PSA level, improvement in symptoms (if present), and regression of measurable lesions for a proportion of patients. This response is part of the steroid hormone-withdrawal syndrome, the mechanisms for which are under investigation.

The other interventions can be considered after a period of observation for response to discontinuation of the antiandrogen. Similarly, in randomized comparisons, bisphosphonate therapy has been shown to delay skeletal events and to reduce bone loss associated with androgen ablation, and this addition is appropriate. Stontium-89 and samarium-153 are approved for the palliation of pain but have minimal effects on the growth of established tumors.

Suggested Reading

Saad F, Gleason DM, Murray R, et al. A randomized, placebo-controlled trial of zoledronic acid in patients with hormone-refractory metastatic prostate carcinoma. *J Natl Cancer Inst.* 2002;94:1458–1468.

Schellhammer P, Kolvenbag GJ. Serum PSA decline after casodex withdrawal. *Urology.* 1994;44:790–791.

Scher HI, Kolvenbag GJ. The antiandrogen withdrawal syndrome in relapsed prostate cancer. *Eur Urol.* 1997;31:3–7.

Small EJ, Carroll PR. Prostate-specific antigen decline after casodex withdrawal: evidence for an antiandrogen withdrawal syndrome. *Urology.* 1994;43:408–410.

9-4 E

Educational Objective: To recognize the importance of adequate sampling of the bladder wall with inclusion of muscle for proper staging and clarification of T1 disease.

The patient appears to have T1 disease that was resected on the basis of the pathologic description, absence of a palpable mass, and negative findings on postoperative urinary cytologic analysis. If T1 disease were confirmed, BCG would be an appropriate therapeutic choice. However, the degree of infiltration by the tumor cannot be assessed unless muscle is present in the transurethral resection. Thus, repeat cystoscopy and biopsy are required before a therapeutic recommendation can be made. If muscle invasion is documented, standard therapy is neoadjuvant chemotherapy followed by a radical cystectomy. The staging errors associated with attempts to assess the depth of invasion by endoscopic means are highest in the T3a to T3b range. Evaluation of the ureters and renal pelvis is not indicated on the basis of the data presented. Observation is not appropriate because the depth of invasion has not been fully assessed.

Suggested Reading

Herr HW. The value of a second transurethral resection in evaluating patients with bladder tumors. *J Urol.* 1999;162:74–76.

Stein JP, Skinner DG. Results with radical cystectomy for treating bladder cancer: a 'reference standard' for high-grade, invasive bladder cancer. *BJU Int.* 2003;92:12–17.

9-5 A

Educational Objective: To recognize the role for neoadjuvant cisplatin combination chemotherapy in patients with invasive bladder cancer.

Chemotherapy has been integrated into the management of invasive bladder cancer in both the preoperative (neoadjuvant) and postoperative (adjuvant) settings. Initial studies evaluating neoadjuvant chemotherapy for invasive bladder cancer showed downstaging in the primary tumor with complete pathologic responses in 20% of cases. Early randomized comparisons involved small numbers of patients and overestimated the potential effect of the approach and, as such, were largely inconclusive. Many did not include cisplatin-based combination regimens. Recently, two large-scale trials were reported. In the first, patients were randomly assigned to either three cycles of M-VAC chemotherapy followed by cystectomy or cystectomy alone. The results showed a significant survival benefit in favor of neoadjuvant therapy. In the second study, patients were randomly assigned to either three cycles of CMV chemotherapy followed by surgery or radiation therapy, or surgery or radiation therapy alone. No significant difference was reported initially; however, longer follow-up showed that the chemotherapy led to a significant survival benefit. In the metastatic setting, compared with M-VAC, the combination of gemcitabine and cisplatin has been shown to produce similar anticancer effects with no difference in survival, but this regimen has not been tested definitively in the perioperative setting. Despite these promising results for neoadjuvant therapy, it is not clear whether they can be translated uniformly to the adjuvant setting, where the effect of chemotherapy on survival is less clear. Prospective randomized trials have not evaluated non-cisplatin–containing regimens in the perioperative setting.

Many physicians recommend adjuvant chemotherapy for patients with disease of P3 or greater or for node-positive disease.

Suggested Reading

Advanced Bladder Cancer Meta-Analysis Collaboration. Neoadjuvant chemotherapy in invasive bladder cancer: a systematic review and meta-analysis. *Lancet.* 2003;361:1927–1934.

Grossman HB, Natale RB, Tangen CM, et al. Neo adjuvant chemotherapy plus cystectomy compared with cystectomy alone for locally advanced bladder cancer. *N Engl J Med.* 2003;349:859–866.

Hall RR. Updated results of a randomised controlled trial of neoadjuvant cisplatin (C), methotrexate (M) and vinblastine (V) chemotherapy for muscle-invasive bladder cancer. *Proc Am Soc Clin Oncol.* 2002;21:178a.

von der Maase H, Hansen SW, Roberts JT, et al. Gemcitabine and cisplatin versus methotrexate, vinblastine, doxorubicin, and cisplatin in advanced or metastatic bladder cancer: results of a large, randomized, multinational, multicenter phase III study. *J Clin Oncol.* 2000;18:3068–3077.

9-6 C

Educational Objective: To recognize that resection of responding metastatic bladder cancer after chemotherapy may result in a cure.

The paradigm of a combined-modality approach for germ cell cancers, in which combination chemotherapy is followed by resection of residual disease, may be applied to the management of urothelial tumors. Data from several groups show that a select subset of patients with metastatic disease will have long-term survival after systemic chemotherapy followed by resection of residual disease. The patient described is an appropriate candidate (given the limited metastatic disease), and combined-modality therapy would be the treatment of choice. Although paclitaxel is an active agent as second-line therapy, the probability of a complete remission — a prerequisite for cure — is low whether it is used alone or in combination with cisplatin.

Suggested Reading

Einhorn LH, Roth BJ, Ansari R, et al. Phase II trial of gallium nitrate, vinblastine and ifosfamide in metastatic urothelial cancer. *J Clin Oncol.* 1994;12:2271–2276.

McCaffrey JA, Bajorin DF, Scher HI, et al. Combined-modality therapy for bladder cancer. *Oncology.* 1997;11:18–26.

Sternberg CN, Yagoda A, Scher HI, et al. Preliminary results of methotrexate, vinblastine, adriamycin and cisplatin (M-VAC) in advanced urothelial tumors. *J Urol.* 1985;133:403–407.

Herr HW, Donat SM, Bajorin DF. Post-chemotherapy surgery in patients with unresectable or regionally metastatic bladder cancer. *J Urol.* 2001;165(3):811–814.

Siefker-Radtke AO, Walsh GL, Pisters LL, et al. Is there a role for surgery in the management of metastatic urothelial cancer? The M. D. Anderson experience. *J Urol.* 2004;171(1):145–148.

Rasco DW, Assikis V, Marshall F. Integrating metastatectomy in the management of advanced urological malignancies-where we are in 2005? *J Urol.* 2006;176(5):1921–1926.

9-7 A

Educational Objective: To identify residual disease based on persistent marker elevation for a patient who has had primary therapy for a germ cell tumor.

The patient presents with persistent disease after radical orchiectomy, as shown by the prolonged decline in the levels of HCG. If no residual diseases were present, the levels should have declined by more than five half-lives to less than 2.5 IU/mL. Although the CT scan of the chest and abdomen are negative before orchiectomy, patients with persistently elevated alpha-fetoprotein and/or HCG after orchiectomy will often have disease outside of the retroperitoneum and should undergo primary chemotherapy rather than initial retroperitoneal lymph node dissection. The patient could be treated with three cycles of bleomycin, etoposide, and cisplatin or four cycles of etoposide and cisplatin. These regimens have produced similar long-term outcomes when given in adequate doses to patients with favorable-risk germ cell tumors. Three cycles of etoposide and cisplatin are inadequate therapy, and observation has no role in the setting of residual disease. Additionally, external beam radiation therapy serves no role in the management of nonseminomatous germ cell tumors.

Suggested Reading

Davis BE, Herr HW, Fair WR, Bosl GJ. The management of patients with nonseminomatous germ cell tumors of the testis with serologic disease only after orchiectomy. *J Urol.* 1994; 152:111–114.

Saxman SB, Nichols CR, Foster RS, et al. The management of patients with clinical stage I nonseminomatous testicular tumors and persistently elevated serologic markers. *J Urol.* 1996;155:587–589.

Williams SD, Birch R, Einhorn LH, et al. Treatment of disseminated germ-cell tumors with cisplatin, bleomycin, and either vinblastine or etoposide. *N Engl J Med.* 1987;316(23): 1435–1440.

Loehrer PJ Sr, Johnson D, Elson P, et al. Importance of bleomycin in favorable-prognosis disseminated germ cell tumors: an Eastern Cooperative Oncology Group trial. *J Clin Oncol.* 1995;13(2):470–476.

de Wit R, Stoter G, Kaye SB, et al. Importance of bleomycin in combination chemotherapy for good-prognosis testicular nonseminoma: a randomized study of the European Organization for Research and Treatment of Cancer Genitourinary Tract Cancer Cooperative Group. *J Clin Oncol.* 1997;15(5): 1837–1843.

Kondagunta GV, Bacik J, Bajorin D, et al. Etoposide and cisplatin chemotherapy for metastatic good-risk germ cell tumors. *J Clin Oncol.* 2005;23(36):9290–9294.

9-8 D

Educational Objective: To describe the importance of resection of residual disease for patients with germ cell tumors.

The patient should have a retroperitoneal lymph node dissection and resection of the residual mass because there are no definitive predictors that allow clinicians to predict the presence of residual viable germ cell tumor or teratoma. Approximately 45% of residual masses will consist of necrotic debris or fibrosis, 40% will consist of mature teratoma, and 15% will harbor viable germ cell tumor. Neither normalization of previously elevated tumor markers nor a percentage of reduction in the size of the mass is predictive. Although histologically benign, teratoma arises from malignant germ cells and may grow over time. Additionally, teratoma may undergo malignant transformation to incurable cell types, such as rhabdomyosarcoma or adenocarcinoma. An additional concern includes the poor outcome associated with late relapses and the finding that an inadequately controlled retroperitoneum is a major predisposing factor. Radiation therapy has no role in the management of this disease. FDG-PET scans may not detect residual teratoma.

Suggested Reading

Oldenburg J, Alfsen GC, Lien HH, et al. Postchemotherapy retroperitoneal surgery remains necessary in patients with nonseminomatous testicular cancer and minimal residual tumor masses. *J Clin Oncol.* 2003;21(17):3310–3317.

Oldenburg J, Alfsen GC, Waehre H, Fossa SD. Late recurrences of germ cell malignancies: a population-based experience over three decades. *Br J Cancer.* 2006;94(6):820–827.

Carver BS, Motzer RJ, Kondagunta GV, et al. Late relapses of testicular germ cell tumors. *Urol Oncol.* 2005;23(6):441–445.

Carver BS, Shayegan B, Serio A, et al. Long-term clinical outcome after postchemotherapy retroperitoneal lymph node dissection in men with residual teratoma. *J Clin Oncol.* 2007;25(9): 1024–1025.

9-9 B

Educational Objective: To recognize the growing teratoma syndrome.

The patient presents with signs and symptoms of a growing teratoma syndrome. Although the markers appear to be declining slowly, there is typically an initial increase in markers such that a level measured 1 week after the initiation of chemotherapy is often higher than the baseline value (before therapy). Thus, there is no indication that the patient is refractory to primary therapy, which will ultimately need to be continued. More emergent at this point are the symptoms related to the growing mass, which most likely represents a teratoma. This neoplasm must be removed surgically because it does not respond to chemotherapy or to radiation treatment.

Suggested Reading

Oldenburg J, Alfsen GC, Lien HH, et al. Post chemotherapy retroperitoneal surgery remains necessary in patients with nonseminomatous testicular cancer and minimal residual tumor masses. *J Clin Oncol.* 2003;21:3310–3317.

Vuky J, Bains M, Bacik J, et al. Role of postchemotherapy adjunctive surgery in the management of patients with nonseminoma arising from the mediastinum. *J Clin Oncol.* 2001;19: 682–688.

Speiss PE, Kassouf W, Brown GA, et al. Surgical management of growing teratoma syndrome: the M.D. Anderson cancer experience. *J Urol.* 2007;177(4):1330–1334.

9-10 C

Educational Objective: To recognize that a paraneoplastic syndrome associated with renal cell tumors does not preclude definitive therapy.

The patient presents with Stauffer syndrome, which is a hepatopathy associated with renal cell cancer. This paraneoplastic syndrome occurs in 3% to 6% of cases and is reversible on resection of the primary tumor. The findings on the CT scan with respect to the hepatic lesion are nonspecific. Similarly, the findings according to CT scan are not definitive with respect to extension into the renal capsule and are not accurate enough to preclude definitive surgery, which is the only hope for a long-term response or cure in this patient. In addition, cytoreductive nephrectomy should be considered as initial treatment for suitable patients with metastatic disease; two prospective randomized studies demonstrated improved survival for patients subsequently treated with interferon, with a combined analysis showing a median survival of 13.6 months for patients undergoing nephrectomy plus treatment with interferon compared with 7.8 months for patients receiving interferon alone, despite similar low response rates to interferon.

Suggested Reading

Flanigan RC, Salmon SE, Blumenstein BA, et al. Nephrectomy followed by interferon alpha-2b compared with interferon alpha-2b alone for metastic renal-cell cancer *N Engl J Med.* 2001;345(23):1655–1659.

Kim HL, Belldegrun AS, Freitas DG, et al. Paraneoplastic signs and symptoms of renal cell carcinoma: implications for prognosis. *J Urol.* 2003;170:1742–1746.

Ritchie AWS, Chisholm GD. The natural history of renal carcinoma. *Semin Oncol.* 1983;10:390–400.

Stauffer MH. Nephrogenic hepatosplenomegaly. *Gas troenterology.* 1961;40:694.

Flanigan RC, Mickisch G, Sylvester R, et al. Cytoreductive nephrectomy in patients with metastatic renal cancer: a combined analysis. *J Urol.* 2004;171:1071–1076.

Stauffer MH. Nephrogenic hepatosplenomegaly. *Gas troenterology.* 1961;40:694.

9-11 E

Educational Objective: To describe the management of metastatic renal cell cancer refractory to cytokine therapy.

The patient has metastatic clear cell renal cell carcinoma that progressed on first-line therapy with high-dose aldesleukin. Patients who progress on aldesleukin rarely experience a response to interferon-alpha, and no improvement in survival has been demonstrated. Similarly, additional cycles of aldesleukin for a patient who rapidly progressed following two cycles are not indicated. Two trials have demonstrated improvement in progression-free survival for patients with cytokine refractory renal cancer treated with either sorafenib tosylate or with sunitinib malate. Both agents are approved by the U.S. Food and Drug Administration for this indication. The agents have not been directly compared with each other in a clinical trial, and each would be appropriate. Therapy with this class of agents is generally well tolerated with manageable toxicity.

Suggested Reading

Escudier B, Chevreau C, Lasset C, et al. Cytokines in metastatic renal cell carcinoma: is it useful to switch to interleukin-2 or interferon after failure of a first treatment? Groupe Francais d'Immunotherape. *J Clin Oncol.* 1999;17:2039–2043.

Motzer RJ, Rini BI, Bukowski RM, et al. Sunitinib in patients with metastatic renal cell carcinoma. *JAMA.* 2006;295: 2516–2524.

Escudier B, Eisen T, Stadler WM, et al; TARGET Study Group. Sorafenib in advanced clear-cell renal-cell carcinoma. *N Engl J Med.* 2007;356:125–134.

SELF EVALUATION

CHAPTER 10 QUESTIONS:
GYNECOLOGIC CANCERS

10-1 A 68-year-old woman presents with a 3-week history of abdominal pain and nausea. A computerized tomography (CT) scan of the abdomen and pelvis shows ascites, a large omental mass, and an enlarged right ovary. During an exploratory laparotomy, the patient is found to have a poorly differentiated adenocarcinoma of the ovary. At completion of surgery, the largest residual tumor is more than 3 cm in maximum diameter.

Which of the following would you recommend as the next course of action?

A. Six cycles of carboplatin (area under the curve [AUC] 6) plus 3-hour infusional paclitaxel plus gemcitabine
B. Six cycles of cisplatin plus 3-hour infusional paclitaxel
C. Six cycles of single-agent carboplatin (AUC, 12)
D. Six cycles of carboplatin (AUC, 6) plus 3-hour infusional paclitaxel
E. Six cycles of carboplatin (AUC, 6) plus cyclophosphamide

10-2 A 62-year-old woman who has had pelvic discomfort for several months is found to have an enlarged left ovary. The CA-125 antigen level is 97 U/mL. The patient is referred to a gynecologic oncologist who performs a laparotomy with a definitive resection of the mass. Pathologic review indicates a stage I (grade 3) epithelial ovarian cancer.

Which of the following is the most appropriate next step for the treatment of this patient?

A. Computerized tomography (CT) of the abdomen and pelvis every 6 months for 5 years
B. Six courses of carboplatin plus paclitaxel
C. Physical examination and measurement of the CA-125 antigen level every 3 months for 5 years
D. Repeat exploration by laparotomy in 1 year
E. Whole abdomen radiotherapy

10-3 A 35-year-old woman presents with abnormal vaginal bleeding. Pelvic examination and the findings on analysis of a biopsy specimen indicate a squamous cell malignant lesion, which, on further evaluation, is found to be a stage IIB cervical cancer.

Which of the following is the most appropriate next step for the treatment of this patient?

A. External beam radiation therapy
B. Six cycles of cisplatin and paclitaxel
C. Three cycles of cisplatin and fluorouracil followed by radiation therapy to the pelvis
D. External beam radiation therapy followed by five cycles of cisplatin and ifosfamide
E. External beam radiation therapy with concurrent weekly cisplatin

10-4 Abnormal uterine bleeding develops in a 72-year-old woman who is taking tamoxifen as adjuvant treatment for a stage II estrogen receptor (ER)-positive breast cancer. On examination, an adenocarcinoma (grade 1) of the endometrium is found. Other than mild hypertension, the patient has no substantial comorbid medical conditions.

Which of the following is the most appropriate next step for the treatment of this patient?

A. Hysterectomy, omentectomy, bilateral oophorectomy, retroperitoneal lymph node dissection, followed by six cycles of adjuvant chemotherapy with cisplatin and paclitaxel
B. Total abdominal hysterectomy and bilateral salpingo-oophorectomy followed by six cycles of adjuvant chemotherapy with cisplatin and doxorubicin
C. Total abdominal hysterectomy, bilateral salpingo-oophorectomy and paraaortic lymph node dissection
D. Initiation of medroxyprogesterone therapy
E. Discontinuation of tamoxifen and re-evaluation in 6 months.

10-5 A 58-year-old woman is diagnosed with stage III epithelial ovarian cancer. Following surgical cytoreduction, the diameter of the largest residual tumor nodule is less than 1 cm.

Based on currently available data, which of the following chemotherapy regimens might be considered for intraperitoneal (IP) treatment in clinical setting?

A. IP cisplatin plus IP topotecan
B. IP cisplatin plus IP doxorubicin
C. IP cisplatin plus IP paclitaxel
D. IP carboplatin plus IP docetaxel
E. IP cisplatin plus IP mitoxantrone

10-6 A 49-year-old woman is seen by her family physician because of lower abdominal discomfort lasting for 3 months. Physical examination and CT of the abdomen and pelvis demonstrate a large (8 cm by 12 cm) pelvic mass. The lymph nodes are not enlarged, and there is no evidence of ascites. The CA-125 antigen level is 47 U/mL. During exploratory laparotomy, a stage I granulosa cell tumor is found and is completely resected.

Which of the following is the most appropriate next step for the treatment of this patient?

A. No further treatment
B. Six cycles of carboplatin plus paclitaxel
C. Four cycles of cisplatin plus etoposide
D. Radiation therapy to the whole abdominal cavity

10-7 A 20-year-old woman with a 1-week history of fairly intense pelvic pressure is seen by a physician at the student health center at her college. On palpation, the physician feels a mass, and a CT scan of the abdomen and pelvis demonstrates a large cyst on the right ovary. During exploratory surgery, a benign cyst is found, but a small portion (less than 10%) of the mass is found to be an endodermal sinus tumor. There is no evidence of disease outside of the ovary. Postoperatively, the beta-human chorionic gonadotropin (HCG) and alpha-fetoprotein levels are within normal limits.

Which of the following is the most appropriate next step for the treatment of this patient?

A. Observation with monthly monitoring of beta-HCG and alphafetoprotein.
B. Chemotherapy with bleomycin, etoposide, and cisplatin (BEP)
C. Chemotherapy with carboplatin and paclitaxel
D. Chemotherapy with carboplatin and paclitaxel, followed by high-dose chemotherapy with autologous peripheral stem cell rescue

10-8 A 45-year-old woman is found to have stage IIB cervical cancer that is treated with external beam radiation therapy along with weekly cisplatin (40 mg/m^2). At the completion of radiation therapy, the patient's condition appears to be improved, but she has persistent disease, which is confirmed by CT. Two months after the completion of chemoradiotherapy, the patient reports back pain that prevents her from sleeping. She also notes a major decrease in appetite and a loss of 15 pounds during the past month. A repeat CT scan demonstrates a number of newly enlarged retroperitoneal lymph nodes (3 cm to 4 cm in diameter), a growing pelvic mass (4 cm by 5 cm), and several pulmonary nodules (1 cm to 3 cm), which were not present on the previous CT scan.

Which of the following would you recommend?

A. Surgery to remove the pelvic mass and enlarged nodes, followed by chemotherapy with cisplatin and paclitaxel
B. Chemotherapy with cisplatin and ifosfamide
C. Pelvic exenteration followed by surgical removal of the pulmonary nodules
D. Palliative measures to treat symptoms only
E. Whole abdomen radiation therapy followed by cisplatin-based chemotherapy

10-9 An 87-year-old woman is seen because of shortness of breath, abdominal pain, and bloating. The patient lives with her granddaughter and had been fairly independent in her daily activities. However, for the last few weeks she has spent most of the day in bed. The patient has well-controlled hypertension and adult-onset diabetes. She had a minor stroke 4 years ago, from which she recovered completely.

On physical examination, breath sounds are decreased at both lung bases, and there is marked ascites. The findings of CT of the abdomen and pelvis confirm the presence of ascites and show diffuse carcinomatosis. There also is evidence of a large pelvic mass that is consistent with an ovarian neoplasm. The CA-125 antigen level is 5,700 U/mL. A paracentesis is performed, with removal of 5 L of fluid. The findings of cytologic analysis of the peritoneal fluid indicate adenocarcinoma.

Which of the following is the most appropriate next step for the treatment of this patient?

A. A combination regimen consisting of a platinum agent and a taxane delivered without dose modification
B. Single-agent carboplatin followed by paclitaxel if the response is inadequate
C. Single-agent paclitaxel
D. Hospice referral

10-10 A 65-year-old woman with stage III ovarian cancer has a clinically defined complete response following surgery and treatment with carboplatin and paclitaxel. Other than moderate fatigue, the patient tolerated the chemotherapy regimen without major side effects, such as emesis, neuropathy, or arthralgias/myalgias. Three years after the completion of primary chemotherapy, the patient has intermittent diffuse abdominal discomfort. Repeat CT demonstrates moderate ascites and possible small peritoneal implants. The CA-125 antigen level is 575 U/mL. The gynecologic oncologist does not believe that repeat surgery will be of any clinical value.

Which of the following treatment strategies would you recommend for this patient?

A. Single-agent cisplatin
B. Single-agent carboplatin
C. Carboplatin and paclitaxel
D. Whole abdomen radiation therapy
E. Single-agent paclitaxel

CHAPTER 10 EXPLANATORY ANSWERS:
GYNECOLOGIC CANCERS

10-1 D

Educational Objective: To recognize standard management of suboptimal residual advanced ovarian cancer following primary surgery.

The findings of two well-designed randomized trials involving patients with advanced ovarian cancer have shown that cisplatin and paclitaxel is better than cisplatin and cyclophosphamide in terms of response rate, time to disease progression, and overall survival. Recent randomized trials have confirmed that cisplatin with paclitaxel and carboplatin plus paclitaxel are equivalent, but the carboplatin-based regimen is associated with a more favorable toxicity profile.

The delivery of cisplatin (75 mg/m^2) and 3-hour infusional paclitaxel (175 mg/m^2) is associated with a substantial risk of grade 3 peripheral neuropathy (20% to 30%) and should not be used in this clinical setting. If a regimen of cisplatin and paclitaxel is used, the paclitaxel should be delivered as a 24-hour infusion.

Because there is no evidence to suggest that so-called high-dose, platinum-based chemotherapy results in a superior outcome compared with more conventional dosing, there is no reason, to administer carboplatin at an area under the curve (AUC) of 12.

There also is no evidence that adding a third drug to a platinum/taxane primary chemotherapy regimen improves outcome in advanced ovarian cancer.

Suggested Reading

Covens A, Carey M, Bryson P, et al. Systematic review of first-line chemotherapy for newly diagnosed postoperative patients with stage II, III, or IV epithelial ovarian cancer. *Gynecol Oncol.* 2002;85(1):71–80.

du Bois A, Luck HJ, Meier W, et al. A randomized clinical trial of cisplatin/paclitaxel versus carboplatin/paclitaxel as first-line treatment of ovarian cancer. *J Natl Cancer Inst.* 2003;95(17): 1320–1330.

McGuire WP, Hoskins WJ, Brady MF, et al. Cyclophosphamide and cisplatin compared with paclitaxel and cisplatin in patients with stage III and stage IV ovarian cancer. *N Engl J Med.* 1996;334(1):1–6.

Ozols RF, Bundy BN, Greer BE, et al. Phase III trial of carboplatin and paclitaxel compared with cisplatin and paclitaxel in patients with optimally resected stage III ovarian cancer: a Gynecologic Oncology Group study. *J Clin Oncol.* 2003;21(17):3194–3200.

Piccart MJ, Bertelsen K, James K, et al. Randomized intergroup trial of cisplatin-paclitaxel versus cisplatin-cyclophosphamide in women with advanced epithelial ovarian cancer: three-year results. *J Natl Cancer Inst.* 2000;92(9):699–708.

10-2 B

Educational Objective: To recognize the role of adjuvant platinum-based chemotherapy in the management of high-risk, early-stage ovarian cancer.

Data from randomized phase III clinical trials have demonstrated the favorable effect on overall survival (8% improvement at 5 years) associated with the adjuvant delivery of platinum-based chemotherapy for high-risk, early-stage ovarian cancer compared with observation until documented recurrence. Chemotherapy should be given to patients with stage II disease or stage I, grade 3 cancer. Chemotherapy is not necessary for patients with appropriately staged disease who have stage I, grade 1 ovarian cancers. It is uncertain whether adjuvant treatment should be given to patients with stage I, grade 2 cancers.

Although no randomized trial has involved a direct comparison between whole abdomen radiation therapy and currently used chemotherapy regimens of a platinum agent and a taxane, the documented survival benefits (noted previously) associated with cytotoxic drug delivery suggest it is appropriate to use chemotherapy in this specific clinical setting.

Suggested Reading

International Collaborative Ovarian Neoplasm 1 (ICON1) and European Organization for Research and Treatment of Cancer Collaborators-Adjuvant ChemoTherapy in Ovarian Neoplasm (EORTC-ACTION). International Collaborative Ovarian Neoplasm Trial 1 and Adjuvant ChemoTherapy in Ovarian Neoplasm trial: two parallel randomized phase III trials of adjuvant chemotherapy in patients with early-stage ovarian carcinoma. *J Natl Cancer Inst.* 2003;95(2):105–112.

International Collaborative Ovarian Neoplasm (ICON1) Collaborators. International Collaborative Ovarian Neoplasm Trial 1: a randomized trial of adjuvant chemotherapy in women with early-stage ovarian cancer. *J Natl Cancer Inst.* 2003;95(2): 125–132.

Trimbos JB, Vergote I, Bolis G, et al. Impact of adjuvant chemotherapy and surgical staging in early-stage ovarian carcinoma: European Organization for Research and Treatment of Cancer-Adjuvant Chemotherapy. In Ovarian Neoplasm Trial. *J Natl Cancer Inst.* 2003;95(2):113–125.

10-3 E

Educational Objective: To define the role of concurrent chemoradiotherapy in the management of locally-advanced cervical cancer.

Several phase III randomized trials have demonstrated better progression-free and overall survival associated with the concurrent administration of cisplatin-based chemotherapy and external beam radiotherapy for advanced, localized cervical cancer.

Neither the adjuvant (following definitive local treatment) nor the neoadjuvant (prior to definitive local treatment) delivery of cisplatin-based chemotherapy has been shown in randomized trials to have a favorable influence on survival in this clinical setting.

Suggested Reading

Green JA, Kirwan JM, Tierney JF, et al. Survival and recurrence after concomitant chemotherapy and radiotherapy for cancer of the uterine cervix: a systematic review and meta-analysis. *Lancet.* 2001;358(9284):781–786.

Keys HM, Bundy BN, Stehman FB, et al. Cisplatin, radiation, and adjuvant hysterectomy compared with radiation and adjuvant hysterectomy for bulky stage IB cervical carcinoma. *N Engl J Med.* 1999;340(15):1154–1161.

Morris M, Eifel PJ, Lu J, et al. Pelvic radiation with concurrent chemotherapy compared with pelvic and para-aortic radiation for high-risk cervical cancer. *N Engl J Med.* 1999;340(15): 1137–1143.

Peters WA III, Liu PY, Barrett RJ II, et al. Concurrent chemotherapy and pelvic radiation therapy compared with pelvic radiation therapy alone as adjuvant therapy after radical surgery in high-risk early-stage cancer of the cervix. *J Clin Oncol.* 2000; 18(8):1606–1613.

Rose PG, Bundy BN, Watkins EB, et al. Concurrent cisplatin-based radiotherapy and chemotherapy for locally advanced cervical cancer. *N Engl J Med.* 1999;340(15):1144–1153.

10-4 C

Educational Objective: To recognize the management of tamoxifen-associated endometrial cancer.

Most of the available data suggest that the natural history of and prognosis for tamoxifen-associated endometrial cancers are similar to those of endometrial cancers that develop in women who have not previously received this hormonal antineoplastic agent. As a result, patients with tamoxifen-associated endometrial cancer should be treated as if the cancer developed in the absence of this risk factor. Aggressive surgery, avoidance of surgery, or use of adjuvant chemotherapy to treat such patients is inappropriate.

Suggested Reading

Bergman L, Beelen MLR, Gallee MPW, et al. Risk and prognosis of endometrial cancer after tamoxifen for breast cancer. Comprehensive Cancer Centre ALERT Group. Assessment of Liver and Endometrial Cancer following Tamoxifen. *Lancet.* 2000;356(9233):881–887.

Fisher B, Costantino JP, Redmond CK, et al. Endometrial cancer in tamoxifen-treated breast cancer patients: findings from the National Surgical Adjuvant Breast and Bowel Project (NSABP)B-14. *J Natl Cancer Inst.* 1994;86(7):527–537.

Jordan VC, Assikis VJ. Endometrial carcinoma and tamoxifen: clearing up a controversy. *Clin Cancer Res.* 1995;1(5):467–472.

Suh-Burgmann EJ, Goodman A. Surveillance for endometrial cancer in women receiving tamoxifen. *Ann Intern Med.* 1999; 131(2):127–135.

10-5 C

Educational Objective: To identify the cytotoxic agents delivered by the intraperitoneal route for which existing evidence-based data support their use as appropriate components of standard management of small-volume residual advanced ovarian cancer.

Three randomized phase III trials have revealed the administration of cisplatin-based intraperitoneal chemotherapy as primary treatment of small-volume advanced ovarian cancer can improve both progression-free and overall survival. The most recent phase III trial employed intraperitoneal paclitaxel in addition to intraperitoneal cisplatin.

There is no evidence to support the use of intraperitoneal cisplatin (or intraperitoneal carboplatin) with topotecan, doxorubicin, or mitoxantrone.

Suggested Reading

Alberts DS, Liu PY, Hannigan EV, et al. Intraperitonenal cisplatin plus intravenous cyclophosphamide versus intravenous cisplatin plus intravenous cyclophosphamide for stage III ovarian cancer. *N Engl J Med.* 1996;335(26):1950–1955.

Markman M, Bundy BN, Alberts DS, et al. Phase III trial of standard-dose intravenous cisplatin plus paclitaxel versus moderately high-dose carboplatin followed by intravenous paclitaxel and intraperitoneal cisplatin in small-volume stage III ovarian carcinoma: an intergroup study of the Gynecologic Oncology Group, Southwestern Oncology Group, and Eastern Cooperative Oncology Group. *J Clin Oncol.* 2001; 19(4):1001–1007.

Armstrong DK, Bundy B, Wenzel L, et al. Phase III randomized trial of intravenous cisplatin and paclitaxel versus an intensive regimen of intravenous paclitaxel, intraperitoneal cisplatin and intraperitoneal paclitaxel in stage III ovarian cancer: A Gynecologic Oncology Group study. *N Engl J Med.* 2006; 354(1):34–43.

10-6 A

Educational Objective: To identify the management and natural history of early-stage granulosa cell tumors of the ovary.

For most women with this uncommon ovarian neoplasm, the disease is confined to the ovary at the time of diagnosis. The risk of recurrence in this setting is relatively low, and there is no evidence that adjuvant chemotherapy or radiation to the whole abdominal cavity will prolong survival. In addition, there is no rationale for aggressive monitoring for recurrent disease with follow-up CT if there are no new symptoms. If abdominal symptoms develop, a CT scan is an appropriate diagnostic test.

Suggested Reading

Fox H. Pathologic prognostic factors in early stage adult-type granulosa cell tumors of the ovary. *Int J Gynecol Cancer.* 2003; 13:1–4.

Homesley HD, Bundy BN, Hurteau JA, et al. Bleomycin, etoposide, and cisplatin combination therapy of ovarian granulosa cell tumors and other stromal malignancies: a Gynecologic Oncology Group study. *Gynecol Oncol.* 1999;72(2):131–137.

Schumer ST, Cannistra SA. Granulosa cell tumor of the ovary. *J Clin Oncol.* 2003;21(6):1180–1189.

10-7 B

Educational Objective: To recognize the appropriate management of endodermal sinus tumors and other nondysgerminomatous germ cell tumors of the ovary.

Endodermal sinus tumors are uncommon but extremely aggressive ovarian neoplasms. Even if apparently localized at the time of surgical exploration, most of these cancers will have micrometastatic spread beyond the confines of the ovary at the time of initial diagnosis.

Before the introduction of cisplatin-based combination chemotherapy, most young women with this disease died of complications related to progressive cancer. Following the administration of adjuvant standard-dose BEP chemotherapy, cure is the expected outcome for more than 90% of patients with endodermal sinus and other nondysgerminomatous germ cell tumors who have no gross macroscopic disease present when cytotoxic therapy is initiated.

Suggested Reading

Lokey JL, Baker JJ, Price NA, et al. Cisplatin, vinblastine, and bleomycin for endodermal sinus tumor of the ovary. *Ann Intern Med.* 1981;94(1):56–57.

Williams S, Blessing JA, Liao S-Y, et al. Adjuvant therapy of ovarian germ cell tumors with cisplatin, etoposide, and bleomycin: a trial of the Gynecologic Oncology Group. *J Clin Oncol.* 1994;12(4):701–706.

10-8 D

Educational Objective: To recognize the rational management of cervical cancer that is resistant to radiation and cisplatin.

Treatment in this setting must focus on comfort measures, particularly pain management. For a patient with cervical cancer in whom disease has progressed shortly after radiation and cisplatin-based chemotherapy, there is a less than 5% to 10% chance that second-line chemotherapy will relieve symptoms. In addition, any objective or subjective benefits of therapy are likely to be brief (less than 2 to 3 months). Patients may understandably wish to receive additional cytotoxic therapy, but it is important to inform them about the limited opportunity for clinical benefit and the substantial risk of toxicity. Patients with a good performance status should be considered for referral to a center where phase I and II trials are conducted.

Surgical resection and radiation therapy to the whole abdominal cavity have no role in the treatment of widespread metastatic cervical cancer. For carefully selected patients, both radiation therapy (to painful areas on bones) and surgery (colostomy in the presence of large bowel obstruction) may be useful in providing short-term — but clinically meaningful — palliation of severe symptoms.

Suggested Reading

Friedlander M, Grogan M.U.S. Preventative Services Task Force. Guidelines for the treatment of recurrent and metastatic cervical cancer. *The Oncologist.* 2002;7(4):342–347.

Vermorken JB. The role of chemotherapy in squamous cell carcinoma of the uterine cervix: a review. Int *J Gynecol Cancer.* 1993;3(3):129–142.

Waggoner SE. Cervical cancer. *Lancet.* 2003;361(9376):2217–2225.

10-9 B

Educational Objective: To recognize the treatment options for older women or women with a poor performance status who have malignant disease consistent with advanced ovarian cancer.

Data support the conclusion that single-agent carboplatin is a reasonable initial treatment option for patients with advanced ovarian cancer who are not considered candidates for combination chemotherapy because of a marginal performance status, substantial comorbid medical conditions, or advanced age. If disease does not respond to the platinum agent, a subsequent decision can be made about whether to use a second-line cytotoxic agent or to provide symptomatic/comfort measures only.

There is no justification for concluding that a woman with malignant disease consistent with ovarian cancer should be denied the opportunity to have clinically meaningful symptomatic benefit (anticipated response rate of 50% to 80%) from treatment based solely on her age. Also, most cases of ovarian cancer develop in women who are older than age 65, and there is considerable data to suggest that many of these women are severely undertreated.

Suggested Reading

Muggia FM, Braly PS, Brady MF, et al. Phase III randomized study of cisplatin versus paclitaxel versus cisplatin and paclitaxel in patients with suboptimal stage III or IV ovarian cancer: a Gynecologic Oncology Group study. *J Clin Oncol.* 2000;18(1):106–115.

The International Collaborative Ovarian Neoplasm (ICON) Group. Paclitaxel plus carboplatin versus standard chemotherapy with either single-agent carboplatin or cyclophosphamide, doxorubicin, and cisplatin in women with ovarian cancer: the ICON3 randomised trial. *Lancet.* 2002;360(9332):505–515.

10-10 C

Educational Objective: To recognize the demonstrated survival benefit associated with the combination of a platinum agent and paclitaxel for recurrent ovarian cancer.

The treatment goals for recurrent ovarian cancer are to improve symptoms related to the disease, prolong the time to progression, and prolong overall survival. There is no evidence for the curative potential of any second-line treatment strategy for ovarian cancer. However, the reported results of a randomized phase III trial involving women with recurrent ovarian cancer indicate that the combination of carboplatin and paclitaxel leads to improved progression-free and overall 2-year survival (57% and 50%, respectively; $p = 0.02$) compared with carboplatin alone. Of note, the incidence of grade 2 or 3 neuropathy was higher for the combination regimen (20% compared with 1%). For this patient, neuropathy had not occurred during the prior chemotherapy; thus, it would be reasonable to conclude that she has limited potential risk for neuropathy from a similar regimen administered 3 years subsequently. The issue of neuropathy should not interfere with a recommendation that she be given a regimen associated with a demonstrated survival benefit.

No data are available to support the use of nonplatinum-based chemotherapy or whole abdomen radiation therapy for this patient. Whole abdomen radiation therapy may be associated with major morbidity, such as bowel obstruction, for an individual who has previously had one or more laparotomies.

Suggested Reading

Markman M, Bookman MA. Second-line treatment of ovarian cancer. *Oncologist.* 2000;5(1):26–35.

Parmar MK, Ledermann JA, Colombo N, et al. Paclitaxel plus platinum-based chemotherapy versus conventional platinum-based chemotherapy in women with relapsed ovarian cancer: the ICON4/AGO-OVAR-2.2 trial. *Lancet.* 2003;361(9375):2099–2106.

SELF EVALUATION

CHAPTER 11 QUESTIONS: MALIGNANT MELANOMA

11-1 A 26-year-old woman presents for a second opinion regarding the management of melanoma. Five years ago, she was treated for a malignant melanoma on the lower part of the abdomen. The melanoma was 0.9 mm thick, there was no ulceration, and the Clark level was III. She was treated with wide excision that showed no residual melanoma and was then monitored. She now has an enlarged right inguinal lymph node that measures 2.5 cm by 2.0 cm. The lymph node is removed and is positive for melanoma. A staging work-up, including computerized tomography (CT) of the chest, abdomen, and pelvis, is negative for metastatic disease.

Which of following treatment options would you now recommend to this patient?

A. Isolated limb perfusion
B. Complete inguinal lymph node dissection
C. High-dose interferon therapy
D. No further therapy
E. Radiation therapy to the inguinal lymph node basin

11-2 A mutation in which of the following genes is most commonly associated with malignant melanoma?

A. Tumor suppressor gene *TP53*
B. *HER2/neu*
C. *EGFR* receptor
D. *BRAF* gene
E. *RET* proto-oncogene

11-3 A 52-year-old woman with stage III melanoma is receiving high-dose interferon therapy. She has completed the 4 weeks of daily intravenous therapy and is now in the fifth month of maintenance subcutaneous therapy with interferon. Laboratory analyses performed on the previous day demonstrated a normal complete blood count and differential count, but the serum bilirubin was 1.9 mg/dL, the asparate aminotransferase was 420 U/L, and the alanine aminotransferase was 380 U/L. The patient feels well at this time except for fatigue. A physical examination performed last week was normal.

Which of the following treatment options would you recommend?

A. Continue with the current treatment plan
B. Discontinue interferon therapy permanently
C. Continue interferon, but reduce the dose by 50%
D. Discontinue interferon and start treatment with aldesleukin (interleukin-2)
E. Discontinue interferon until the liver function tests normalize, then restart interferon at a 50% dose reduction

11-4 A 34-year-old woman was recently diagnosed with a 0.83-mm thick melanoma. There was no ulceration, and the Clark level was III. The melanoma arose from the posterior part of the right calf. Complete blood counts and chemistry blood tests, which were done preoperatively, were within normal limits.

Which of the following radiologic procedures is appropriate for this patient?

A. Chest-x-ray
B. Magnetic resonance imaging (MRI) of the brain; CT scan of the chest, abdomen, and pelvis
C. Positron emission tomography (PET) scan and MRI of the brain
D. Bone scan and CT of the chest, abdomen, and pelvis

11-5 A 28-year-old woman recently had a mole removed from the back (Fig. 11-1). She described it as light brown in color and as having increased in size during the past year. On physical examination, there are numerous flat light brown to dark moles over the trunk, which range in size from 7 to 15 mm. Biopsy results indicate a dysplastic nevus with mild atypia; the lesion did not extend to the margins. Her family history is remarkable for a paternal uncle with a history of melanoma and a father with numerous moles.

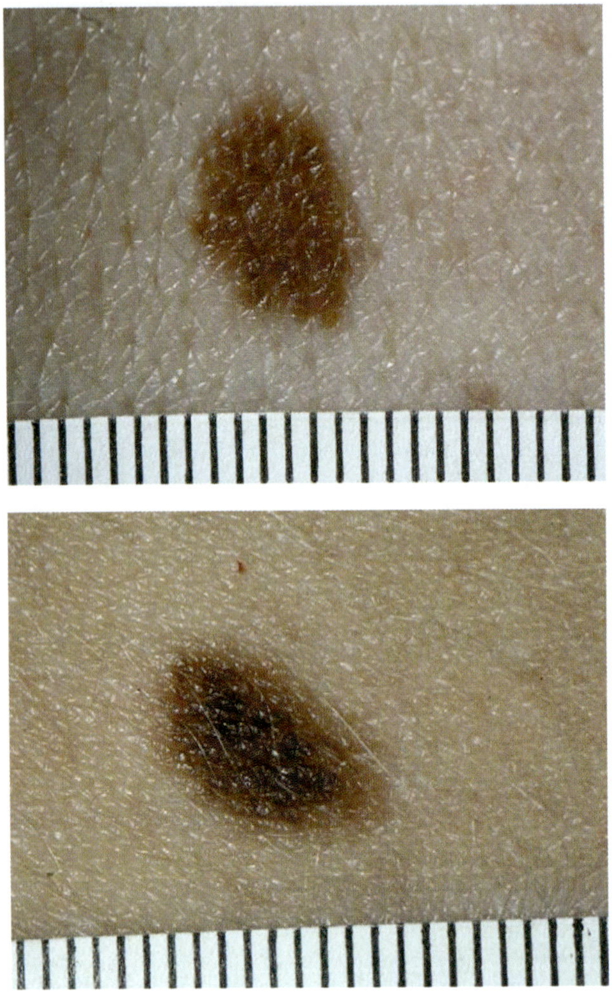

FIG. 11.1 Mole on the back of the patient before (top) and after (bottom) progression. Each line indicates 1 mm.

What would you recommend for this patient?

A. Wide excision of the biopsy site, with 1-cm to 2-cm margins
B. No further surgery
C. Wide excision of the original lesion with 1-cm to 2-cm margins and excision of all the remaining moles on her trunk
D. Local radiation therapy to the biopsy site
E. Liquid nitrogen freezing at the biopsy site

11-6 A 45-year-old man was recently diagnosed with malignant melanoma. He had first presented with a changing mole on the left anterior chest. The findings on biopsy indicated a superficial spreading melanoma, with a depth of 1.6 mm; ulceration was present. A sentinel lymph node biopsy of the left axilla was positive for melanoma involving two lymph nodes. Completion lymph node dissection showed no additional lymph nodes involved with melanoma. A staging work-up with CT of the chest, abdomen, and pelvis was negative.

Which of the following options would you now advise?

A. Begin treatment with dacarbazine
B. Consider treatment with high-dose interferon-alfa
C. Begin radiation therapy to the left axilla
D. Begin treatment with aldesleukin

11-7 A 58-year-old woman presents for a routine check-up, and the physical examination reveals an enlarged 2-cm left axillary lymph node. She was diagnosed 2 years previously with a superficial spreading malignant melanoma with a depth of 1.6 mm on her left scapula. Sentinel lymph node biopsy from the left axilla at that time was negative for melanoma, and the wide excision showed no residual melanoma.

Which of the following options would you now advise?

A. Continue with close follow-up
B. Arrange for lymph node biopsy or fine-needle aspiration of the lymph node
C. Begin treatment with high-dose interferon
D. Begin radiation therapy to the left axilla

11-8 You are treating a 55-year-old woman with melanoma, and you recommend high-dose interferon.

Which of the following side effects of interferon treatment will you discuss with her?

A. Fever, hair loss, congestive heart failure, and diarrhea
B. Myalgia, numbness and tingling, and chills
C. Fever, chills, depression, neutropenia, and abnormal liver function tests
D. Neutropenia, peripheral edema, and pleural effusion
E. Constipation and myelosuppression

11-9 Which of the following statements is true regarding the use of interferon in the adjuvant setting for patients with high-risk melanoma?

A. High-dose interferon improves relapse-free survival by approximately 10% and possibly improves overall survival
B. Low-dose interferon improves both relapse-free survival and overall survival by approximately 10%
C. There is no difference in the side-effect profile between low- dose and high-dose interferon regimens
D. Clinical trials with peptide-based melanoma vaccines show improved relapse-free survival compared with high-dose interferon
E. Four weeks of intravenous interferon have been shown to be equivalent to 1 year of interferon therapy

CHAPTER 11 EXPLANATORY ANSWERS:
MALIGNANT MELANOMA

11-1 B

Educational Objective: To recognize that surgery is potentially curative for patients with regional lymph node recurrence.

Surgery is the appropriate treatment for this patient, and the only potentially curative approach. If the staging work-up is negative for metastatic disease, then the patient should have a therapeutic dissection of the lymph nodes (in this case, dissection of the right inguinal nodes). Radiation therapy could be considered after a therapeutic lymph node dissection, but it should not replace surgery. Some clinicians consider postoperative radiation therapy if many nodes are involved and/or if there is evidence of extracapsular extension, although there is no evidence that radiation therapy improves overall survival. Regional radiation increases the risk of lymphedema. Isolated limb perfusion is a surgical procedure for regional intravascular delivery of chemotherapeutic agents to an extremity with in-transit cutaneous melanoma metastases. This patient has no evidence of in-transit metastases, so there is no role for this treatment. Following surgery, interferon or participation in a clinical trial can be considered, but surgery should be completed before adjuvant therapy is initiated.

Suggested Reading

McMasters KM, Sondak VK, Lotze MT, et al. Recent advances in melanoma staging and therapy. *Ann Surg Oncol.* 1999;6(5):467–475.

Pawlik TM, Sondak VK. Malignant melanoma: current state of primary and adjuvant treatment. *Crit Rev Oncol Hematol.* 2003;45(3):245–264.

11-2 D

Educational Objective: To identify important genetic abnormalities in melanoma.

Mutation in *TP53* is found in approximately half of all non-small cell lung cancers and does not play a role in melanoma. Overexpression of *HER2/neu* occurs in breast cancer, not melanoma. An activating mutation in *BRAF* has been identified in 60% of primary melanomas, particularly in those that are associated with intermittent sun exposure. *BRAF* is an important therapeutic target as well, with ongoing trials involving *BRAF* inhibitors (i.e., sorafenib) for patients with metastatic melanoma. The *RET* proto-oncogene is associated with medullary thyroid cancer and multiple endocrine neoplasias (MEN) type 2, and mutations in *EGFR* receptor are associated with lung cancer.

Suggested Reading

Curtin JA, Fridlyand J, Kageshita T, et al. Distinct sets of genetic alterations in melanoma. *N Engl J Med.* 2005;353(20):2135–2147.

11-3 E

Educational Objective: To recognize the toxicities associated with high-dose interferon and the importance of dose modification.

High-dose interferon therapy is associated with significant toxicity. Patients have flu-like symptoms, such as fatigue, fever, chills, myalgias, anorexia, nausea, vomiting, and headache. Laboratory abnormalities include elevated levels of hepatic transaminases, elevated levels of triglycerides, neutropenia, thyroid dysfunction, and anemia. It is critical that patients treated with interferon are closely monitored and that the dose of interferon be modified appropriately for toxicity. Therefore, it is recommended that liver function is monitored weekly during the induction phase of treatment and monthly during the maintenance phase. If the level of hepatic transaminases increases to more than 5 times the upper limit of normal, then interferon treatment should be temporarily discontinued until these values normalize; interferon should then be restarted at 50% of the previous dose. Similarly, if granulocytes decrease to less than 500/mm^3, treatment should be held until normalization, and the interferon dose should be reduced by 50%.

Suggested Reading

Kirkwood JM, Bender C, Agarwala S, et al. Mechanisms and management of toxicities associated with high-dose interferon alfa-2b therapy. *J Clin Oncol.* 2002;20(17):3703–3718.

Pawlik TM, Sondak VK. Malignant melanoma: current state of primary and adjuvant treatment. *Crit Rev Oncol Hematol.* 2003;45(3):245–264.

11-4 A

Educational Objective: To identify the appropriate staging evaluation for a patient with low-risk melanoma.

The staging evaluation of a patient with a low-risk melanoma should include a physical examination that incorporates a skin examination, chest x-ray, and blood work. Most patients do not have distant metastases at the time of presentation with melanoma; therefore, extensive evaluations with CT, PET scans, MRI or bone scans to search for distant metastases have an extremely low yield are not indicated in asymptomatic patients. More extensive staging evaluation with CT of the chest, abdomen, and pelvis can be considered for patients with high-risk disease (primary melanoma that is more than 4 mm thick or node-positive disease), for whom the risk of distant metastatic disease is increased.

Suggested Reading

National Institutes of Health Consensus Development Conference Statement on Diagnosis and Treatment of Early Melanoma, January 27–29, 1992. *Am J Dermatopathol.* 1993;15(1): 34–43,46–51.

Wang T, Johnson TM, Cascade PN, et al. Evaluation of staging chest radiographs and serum lactate dehydrogenase for localized melanoma. *J Am Acad Dermol.* 2004;51(3):399–405.

NCCN Practice Guidelines for Melanoma. V.2.2006. www.nccn.org/professionals/physian-gls/Pdf melanoma.pdf Accessed December 2006.

11-5 B

Educational Objective: To understand that dysplastic nevi and/or family history of melanoma are important risk factors for melanoma and that such patients require more intensive surveillance and follow-up.

The patient described has dysplastic nevi or atypical moles. Because the pathology report describes only mild atypia and the surgical margins are clear, no additional surgery is needed. Atypical moles or dysplastic nevi are important precursor lesions of melanoma and also serve as markers for increasing melanoma risk. The presence of dysplastic nevi is associated with a 6% lifetime chance of developing melanoma. This risk increases to as much as 80% for individuals who have dysplastic nevi and a family history of melanoma. This patient should have regular skin examinations every 6 to 12 months; overview and close-up photography may aid in the follow-up. Biopsy should be performed on new or changing dysplastic nevi. There is no role for local radiation therapy, and liquid nitrogen should never be used in this setting.

Suggested Reading

Hayward NK. Genetics of melanoma predisposition. *Oncogene.* 2003;22(20):3053–3062.

Tucker MA, Halpern A, Holly EA, et al. Clinically recognized dysplastic nevi. A central risk factor for cutaneous melanoma. *JAMA.* 1997;277(18):1439–1444.

11-6 B

Educational Objective: To understand that high-dose interferon has been approved by the U.S. Food and Drug Administration (FDA) for the treatment of high-risk melanoma.

The FDA recommended approval for interferon-alpha-2b in 1995 based on a study (E1684) conducted by the Eastern Cooperative Oncology Group (ECOG). In that study, 280 patients were randomly assigned to treatment with either an intravenous induction phase of 20 million U/m^2, 5 days a week, for 1 month, followed by an 11-month course of 10 million U/m^2, given subcutaneously 3 days a week, or to observation only. For patients treated with interferon, the median survival was significantly longer than for patients in the observation only arm (3 years vs. 4 years; $p = 0.02$), and the relapse-free survival was better (1 year vs. 2 years; $p = 0.002$). Treatment with interferon was associated with an increase in the 5-year survival rate from 36% to 47%. Subsequent trials confirm the relapse-free survival results, but there are conflicting results regarding the effect of high-dose interferon on overall survival. High-dose interferon is the only adjuvant therapy approved in the United States for the treatment of patients with high-risk melanoma (primary melanoma that is more than 4 mm thick or node-positive disease). Dacarbazine is approved for patients with stage IV disease, but there are no data to support the use of dacarbazine in the adjuvant setting. Similarly, there is no evidence that adjuvant IL-2 has an effect on disease-free survival or on overall survival. There is no indication for radiation therapy to the axilla for this patient with only two lymph nodes involved and with no evidence of extracapsular extension.

Suggested Reading

Kefford RF. Adjuvant therapy of cutaneous melanoma: the interferon debate. *Ann Oncol.* 2003;14(3):358–365.

Kirkwood JM, Ibrahim J, Sondak V, et al. High and low-dose interferon alfa-2b in high-risk melanoma: first analysis of Intergroup trial E1690/S9111/C9190. *J Clin Oncol.* 2000;18(12):2444–2458.

Kirkwood JM, Ibrahim JG, Sosman JA, et al. High-dose interferon alfa-2b significantly prolongs relapse-free and overall survival compared with the GM2-KLH/QS21 vaccine in patients with resected stage IIB/III melanoma: results of Intergroup Trial E1694/S9512/C509801. *J Clin Oncol.* 2001;19: 2370–2380.

Kirkwood JM, Strawderman MH, Ernstoff MS, et al. Interferon alfa-2b adjuvant therapy of high-risk resected cutaneous melanoma: the Eastern Cooperative Oncology Group Trial EST 1684. *J Clin Oncol.* 1996;14(1):7–17.

11-7 B

Educational Objective. To recognize that there can be false-negative findings of sentinel lymph node mapping and that careful monitoring of regional lymph nodes is necessary.

Sentinel lymph node mapping is considered an appropriate surgical staging procedure for patients with melanoma. This technique can identify the draining lymph node most likely to be involved with melanoma. Sentinel lymph node mapping may be considered for melanomas that are more than 1 mm thick or for thinner lesions with worrisome histologic features, such as ulcerations or lesions that are Clark level IV or V. The false-negative rate for sentinel lymph node mapping is approximately 4%. For this patient who has palpable adenopathy, a biopsy should be done to confirm the clinical suspicion of recurrent melanoma. If the results of fine-needle aspiration or biopsy are positive for melanoma, a therapeutic lymph node dissection should be performed, which is potentially curative. Interferon therapy, participation in a clinical trial, or observation could be considered after the surgery has been completed.

Suggested Reading

Allen PJ, Coit DG. The surgical management of metastatic melanoma. *Ann Surg Oncol.* 2002;9(8):762–770.

Morton DL, Cochran AJ, Thompson JF, et al. Lymphatic mapping and sentinel lymphadenectomy for early-stage melanoma: accuracy and morbidity in MSLT-1, an international multicenter trial. *Ann Surg.* 2005;242:302–311.

11-8 C

Educational Objective: To recognize the side effects of high-dose interferon.

High-dose interferon therapy is associated with a number of side effects. Patients have profound flu-like symptoms such as fatigue, fever, chills, myalgias, anorexia, nausea, vomiting, and headache. Interferon may cause or exacerbate depression. Suicidal ideation and suicide have been associated with interferon therapy. Significant laboratory abnormalities include elevated levels of hepatic transaminases, neutropenia, elevated triglyceride levels, and anemia. It is critical that patients being treated with interferon are monitored closely and that the dose of interferon is modified appropriately for toxicity.

Suggested Reading

Kirkwood JM, Bender C, Agarwala S, et al. Mechanisms and management of toxicities associated with high-dose interferon alfa-2b therapy. *J Clin Oncol.* 2002;20(17):3703–3718.

Pawlik TM, Sondak VK. Malignant melanoma: current state of primary and adjuvant treatment. *Crit Rev Oncol Hematol.* 2003;45(3):245–264.

11-9 A

Educational Objective: To understand the benefits of high-dose interferon for patients with melanoma.

The FDA recommended approval for interferon-alpha-2b in 1995 based on the results of study E1684 conducted by the Eastern Cooperative Oncology Group (ECOG). In that study, 280 patients were randomly assigned to treatment with an intravenous induction phase of 20 million U/m^2, 5 days a week, for 1 month, followed by an 11-month course of 10 million U/m^2, given subcutaneously 3 days a week, or to observation only. The median survival was significantly longer for patients who received interferon (3 years compared with 4 years; $p = 0.02$), and relapse-free survival was also better (1 year compared with 2 years; $p = 0.002$). Treatment with interferon was associated with an increase in the 5-year survival rate from 36% to 47%. Subsequent trials have confirmed the relapse-free survival results, but there are conflicting results regarding the impact of high-dose interferon on overall survival. High-dose interferon is the only adjuvant therapy approved in the United States for the treatment of patients with high-risk melanoma (primary melanoma that is more than 4 mm thick or node-positive disease). Randomized clinical trials have shown no survival benefit associated with low-dose interferon for patients with high-risk melanoma. The side effect profile of high-dose interferon is less favorable than low-dose interferon because the toxicities are dose related. At this time, there is no evidence that vaccines are superior to interferon, but ongoing clinical trials are investigating the use of vaccines in the adjuvant setting.

Suggested Reading

Hancock BW, Wheatley K, Harris S, et al. Adjuvant interferon in high-risk melanoma: the AIM HIGH study—United Kingdom Coordinating Committee on Cancer Research randomized study of adjuvant low-dose extended-duration interferon alfa-2a in high-risk resected malignant melanoma. *J Clin Oncol.* 2004;22(1):53–61.

Pawlik TM, Sondak VK. Malignant melanoma: current state of primary and adjuvant treatment. *Crit Rev Oncol Hematol.* 2003;45(3):245–264.

Lens MB, Dawes M. Interferon alpha therapy for malignant melanoma: A systematic review of randomized clinical trials. *J Clin Oncol.* 2002;27(7):1818–1825.

Kirkwood JM, Manola J, Ibrahim J, et al. A pooled analysis of eastern cooperative oncology group and intergroup trials of adjuvant high-dose interferon for melanoma. *Clin Cancer Res.* 2004;10(5):1670–1677.

SELF EVALUATION

CHAPTER 12 QUESTIONS:
SARCOMA

12-1 A radiograph of the right humerus of an 18-year-old woman with pain just distal to the shoulder shows a sclerotic humeral lesion with evidence of destruction of the cortex and a surrounding soft tissue component. A computerized tomography (CT) scan of the chest showed no evidence of metastatic disease. A core needle biopsy of the mass demonstrated a high-grade osteogenic sarcoma.

Which of the following would be appropriate treatment for this patient?

A. Surgery only
B. Surgery and radiation therapy
C. Surgery and chemotherapy
D. Surgery, radiation therapy, and chemotherapy

12-2 A 53-year-old male with a gastrointestinal stromal tumor (GIST) of the stomach resected 5 years ago is found to have an isolated metastatic GIST lesion in the left lobe of the liver. The patient has a successful left hepatectomy with negative margins. A postoperative CT scan with intravenous contrast shows no evidence of disease.

Which of the following the best next option for care?

A. Imatinib, 400 mg daily for 1 year
B. Imatinib, 400 mg daily indefinitely
C. Radiation to the surgical margin
D. Close follow-up only

12-3 A 62-year-old woman presents with a 6-cm mass in the upper portion of the left trapezius muscle. The mass is found to be a low-grade fibrosarcoma, deep to investing fascia. The mass is removed with a minimum 8-mm margin in all directions.

Which of the following is the most appropriate postoperative treatment for this patient?

A. Chemotherapy
B. Radiation therapy
C. Chemotherapy followed by radiation
D. Close follow-up with no further intervention at the present time

CHAPTER 12 EXPLANATORY ANSWERS: SARCOMA

12-1 C

Educational Objective: To identify the optimal treatment of osteogenic sarcoma (osteosarcoma), the most common primary bone tumor.

Osteogenic sarcoma is a rare cancer in the adult population but one of the more common sarcomas in the adolescent and pediatric populations. The differential diagnosis for a primary bone tumor typically includes Ewing's sarcoma, chondrosarcoma, malignant fibrous histiocytoma of bone, primary bone lymphoma, and metastatic disease to bone. Ewing's sarcoma tends to occur in the diaphysis of bone and is characterized by an infiltrative pattern known as "onion-skinning." Chondrosarcoma is more common in the older population. It typically appears as a radiolucent area with a moderate number of discrete calcified areas and often involves the medullary cavity of the bone. Osteogenic sarcomas involve the metaphysis of long bones, in general, and display a cortical/soft tissue reaction (sunburst pattern) if they extend into soft tissue.

Adjuvant therapy for osteogenic sarcoma typically includes neoadjuvant chemotherapy and surgery, followed by additional adjuvant chemotherapy; radiation is almost never used because it has not been shown to improve local control for patients with osteogenic sarcoma. The standard drugs used for adjuvant chemotherapy in osteogenic sarcoma include the combination of doxorubicin and cisplatin, with or without high-dose methotrexate. The role of ifosfamide is not yet clearly defined in treating osteogenic sarcoma. In contrast, chemotherapy, surgery, and radiation are all used for the adjuvant therapy of Ewing's sarcoma. The standard chemotherapy used for Ewing's sarcoma involves five drugs (alternating cycles of vincristine/doxorubicin/cyclophosphamide with ifosfamide/etoposide).

Suggested Reading

Souhami RL, Craft AW, Van der Eijken JW, et al. Randomised trial of two regimens of chemotherapy in operable osteosarcoma: a study of the European Osteosarcoma Intergroup. *Lancet.* 1997;350(9082):911–917.

12-2 D

Educational Objective: To determine the best course of action for a patient with GIST rendered without evidence of disease by surgery after a long disease-free interval.

Imatinib has been approved in various countries, including the United States, as a standard of care for metastatic GIST based on two large international phase III studies. The standard starting dose is 400 mg oral daily, with an increase in the dose to 800 mg daily before switching to sunitinib for disease progression. Surgery can be considered for limited disease progression (continuing with imatinib therapy thereafter), because it appears such patients have a significant time to progression compared with patients who have multiple sites of progressing disease and who undergo surgery. Radiation plays a minor role in the treatment of GIST because a tumoricidal dose of radiation cannot usually be delivered to the liver or to the abdominal cavity.

In this case, the patient has had evidence of disease progression after many years without evidence of disease. Although imatinib could be employed in this setting (stage IV, without evidence of disease), there appears to be no clear urgency in starting such therapy and no evidence that a course of imatinib in this setting would change the patient's outcome. In addition, the long-term side effects, such as the description of a small number of cases of heart failure for patients receiving imatinib, remain unknown. Although imatinib is approved for this indication, given this clinical scenario, the best course of action is observation alone.

Suggested Reading

Bonvalot S, Eldweny H, Pechoux CL, et al. Impact of surgery on advanced gastrointestinal stromal tumors (GIST) in the imatinib era. *Ann Surg Oncol.* 2006;13(12):1596–1603.

Berman E, Nicolaides M, Maki RG, et al. Altered bone and mineral metabolism in patients receiving imatinib mesylate. *N Engl J Med.* 2006; 354(19):2006–2013.

Kerkela R, Grazette L, Yacobi R, et al. Cardiotoxicity of the cancer therapeutic agent imatinib mesylate. *Nat Med.* 2006; 12(8):908–916.

12-3 B

Educational Objective: To understand how to manage a completely resected low-grade, soft-tissue sarcoma.

The only curative therapy for the vast majority of adult patients with sarcomas is surgical resection. Adjuvant radiation therapy has been shown to be helpful in decreasing the local rate of recurrence by one-third to one-half. Adjuvant radiation can be in the form of brachytherapy for high-grade sarcomas or external beam radiation for high- and low-grade sarcomas. In the case presented, the tumor is larger than 5 cm, a situation in which radiation therapy has been shown to be helpful. If the tumor is smaller than 5 cm, one reasonable standard of care is observation alone for a favorable tumor site (e.g., lower extremity) because the risk of local recurrence is only 10% to 15%. Thus, 85% to 90% of patients would be spared radiation and could have another resection and subsequent radiation if there were a local recurrence. Given that the tumor is low-grade, the potential benefit of chemotherapy is limited and, as such, this treatment should be avoided.

Suggested Reading

Pisters PW, Harrison LB, Leung DH, et al. Long-term results of a prospective randomized trial of adjuvant brachytherapy in soft tissue sarcoma. *J Clin Oncol.* 1996;14(3):859–868.

Yang JC, Chang AE, Baker AR, et al. Randomized prospective study of the benefit of adjuvant radiation therapy in the treatment of soft tissue sarcomas of the extremity. *J Clin Oncol.* 1998;16(1):197–203.

SELF EVALUATION

CHAPTER 13 QUESTIONS:

AIDS-RELATED MALIGNANCIES: NON-HODGKIN'S LYMPHOMA AND KAPOSI'S SARCOMA

13-1 A 42-year-old patient with a history of intravenous drug use presents with a 3-week history of an enlarging mediastinal mass. Infection with human immunodeficiency virus (HIV) was diagnosed 3 years earlier and treated with highly active antiretroviral therapy (HAART) consisting of zidovudine (AZT), epivir (3TC), and atazanavir (aprotease inhibitor). The patient's initial CD4-positive count was 50 cells/L, but during the course of 4 years, his CD4-positive count improved to 150 cells/L. Since initiation of HAART, his HIV viral load has remained consistently nondetectable.

Physical examination is unremarkable. A computerized tomography (CT) scan demonstrates a 6-cm by 8-cm anterior mediastinal mass and mild splenomegaly. A bone marrow biopsy is normal. A core-needle biopsy of the anterior mediastinal mass is done.

What is the most likely histologic diagnosis?

A. Thymoma
B. Large B-cell lymphoma
C. Non-T cell, non-B-cell lymphoma
D. Metastatic seminoma

13-2 A 35-year-old homosexual man with a history of HIV infection, a CD4-positive count of 450 cells/L, and an HIV viral load of 30,000 copies/mm^3 presents to medical attention with 20 scattered pigmented skin lesions on his arms. He has not previously received antiretroviral therapy. A skin biopsy confirms the presence of Kaposi's sarcoma, and a physical exam does not identify other sites of disease. What treatment do you recommend?

A. Velban and bleomycin
B. HAART
C. Liposomal doxorubicin
D. Radiation therapy to the largest lesions

13-3 A 50-year-old man with HIV with a CD4-positive count of 180 cells/L and an HIV viral load of 145,000 copies/mL began HAART, consisting of zidovudine, epivir, and efavirenz (a non-nucleoside reverse transcriptase inhibitor) 2 years ago. He seeks medical attention because of the emergence of pigmented skin lesions on his legs and arms. The lesions are not painful. On physical exam, more than 60 cutaneous lesions are appreciated. Laboratory studies are unremarkable; his CD4-positive count is 315 cells/L, and his HIV viral load is less than 75 copies/mL. A skin biopsy confirms a clinical suspicion of Kaposi's sarcoma.

Which of the following is the best treatment option for this patient with Kaposi's sarcoma?

A. A combination of doxorubicin, bleomycin, and velban
B. Prednisone
C. Single-agent liposomal anthracycline
D. A change in HAART

13-4 A 46-year-old man receving HAART for the past 5 years experiences fevers and night sweats for 1 month before seeking medical attention. A CT scan reveals extensive lymphadenopathy. A bone marrow biopsy reveals diffuse large B-cell lymphoma. His CD4-positive count is 380 cells/L, and his HIV viral load is less than 75 copies/mL.

Which of the following statements regarding this patient is true?

A. His expected prognosis is similar to patients diagnosed with AIDS-related lymphoma in the pre-HAART era
B. The likelihood that this patient will respond to anti-lymphoma chemotherapy is dramatically different than if he was HIV-seronegative
C. Patients with AIDS generally do not tolerate standard antilymphoma chemotherapy regimens
D. Rituximab is an important component of the treatment of AIDS-related non-Hodgkin's lymphoma

CHAPTER 13 EXPLANATORY ANSWERS:

AIDS-RELATED MALIGNANCIES: NON-HODGKIN'S LYMPHOMA AND KAPOSI'S SARCOMA

13-1 D

Educational Objective: To understand that most cases of AIDS-related non-Hodgkin's lymphoma are the B-cell type.

The most common form of lymphoma among patients with HIV is the B-cell form. Both flow cytometry and immunostaining are likely to show cell-surface staining for CD19 or CD20, but not for CD3, CD4, or CD8. Similarly, studies of immunoglobulin gene rearrangement will show clonal expansion of the B cell. T-cell lymphoma has been reported in 10% or less of AIDS-lymphoma cases. Primary effusion lymphoma, also known as body cavity lymphoma, is a lymphoma subtype which is seen very rarely for patients with HIV. Primary effusion lymphoma typically lacks CD19 and CD20, but it expresses CD45 and carries immunoglobulin rearrangement. Cells of this variant contain the human herpes virus type-8 and, on occasion, Epstein-Barr virus.

Suggested Reading

Knowles DM. Etiology and pathogenesis of AIDS-related non-Hodgkin's lymphoma. *Hematol Oncol Clin North Am.* 2003; 17:785–820.

Carbone A, Cloghini A. AIDS-related lymphoma: from pathogenesis to pathology. *B J Haematol.* 2005;130:662–670.

Mbulaiteye SM, Biggar RJ, Goedert JJ, et al. Pleural and peritoneal lymphoma among people with AIDS in the United States. *J Acquir Immune Defic Syndr.* 2002;29:418–421.

13-2 B

Educational Objective: To understand that HAART is a first-line treatment for HIV-associated Kaposi's sarcoma.

The patient described should receive HAART. Such therapy leads to Kaposi's sarcoma regression in more than 60% of cases. In the setting of aggressive and rapidly progressive disease, HAART may not be sufficient. The decision to provide local or systemic therapy should be based on several factors, including assessment of disease abundance, site of the disease, disease progression, patient concern regarding the effect Kaposi's sarcoma has on their appearance, and presence of organ dysfunction. Although HAART is the mainstay of treatment for Kaposi's sarcoma, individuals infrequently experience Kaposi's sarcoma flare during the first 2 months after initiation of an effective HAART regimen, representing another protein manifestation of immune reconstitution inflammatory syndrome. Close clinical supervision is warranted for the patient with Kaposi's sarcoma who is initiating, changing, or resuming HAART. Fatalities in this setting are associated with progressive pulmonary Kaposi's sarcoma, the diagnosis of which has proven problematic and, on occasion, may require open-lung biopsy. Systemic chemotherapy appears to be effective in suppressing immune reconstitution inflammatory syndrome-associated Kaposi's sarcoma. For some patients, chemotherapy may be later withdrawn. As immune reconstitution continues to improve with antiretroviral therapy, the patient's Kaposi's sarcoma lesions often will continue to regress independently of chemotherapy. Randomized clinical trials have shown that single-agent liposomal doxorubicin or daunorubicin has comparable response rates with combination chemotherapy regimens, but pegylated anthracyclines are associated with less toxicity.

Suggested Reading

Aversa SM, Cattelan AM, Salvagno L, et al. Treatments of AIDS-related Kaposi's sarcoma's. *Cnt Rev Oncol Hematol.* 2005;53: 253–265.

Aboulafia DM. Kaposi's sarcoma. *Clinics in Dermatology.* 2001;19: 269–283.

Leidner R, Aboulafia DM. Recrudescent Kaposi 's sarcoma after initiation of HAART: a manifestation of immune reconstitution syndrome. *AIDS Patient Care and STDs.* 2005;19: 635–644.

Gill PS, Wernz J, Scadden DT, et al. Randomized phase III trial of liposomal daunorubicin versus doxorubicin, bleomycin, and vincristine in AIDS-related Kaposi's sarcoma. *J Clin Oncol.* 1996;14:2353–2364.

Northfelt DW, Dezube BJ, Thommes JA, et al. Pegylated-liposomal doxorubicin versus doxorubicin, bleomycin, and vincristine in the treatment of AIDS-related Kaposi's sarcoma: results of a randomized phase III clinical trial. *J Clin Oncol.* 1998;16:2445–2451.

13-3 C

Educational Objective: To understand the optimal treatment for AIDS-associated Kaposi's sarcoma in the setting of tumor progression and despite optimal HAART.

Liposomal daunorubicin and doxorubicin are well-tolerated options for patients with AIDS-associated Kaposi's sarcoma who require chemotherapy. Patients with disease that does not respond to these agents experience a favorable response to paclitaxel at a dose of 135 mg/m^2 every 3 weeks or 100 mg/m^2 every 2 weeks. The lower-dose regimen appears to be very well tolerated and has a favorable toxicity profile. A report suggested that gemcitabine may have significant antitumor effects, although further investigations will be required to know where it will sit on the hierarchy of appropriate chemotherapy options for the disease. Factors that may contribute to intercurrent illness, such as pneumonia, or the use of corticosteroids may exacerbate Kaposi's sarcoma growth. A change in antiretroviral therapy is not likely to be useful given that the patient's current antiviral regimen has resulted in immune reconstitution and a nondetectable HIV viral load. None of the recent and novel pathogenesis-based therapies that have been studied for the treatment of Kaposi's sarcoma have received U.S. Food and Drug Administration approval for this clinical indication (e.g., thalidomide, Col-3, imatinib mesylate), but this is an area of active investigation.

Suggested Reading

Cheung MC, Pantanowitz L, Dezube BJ. AIDS-related malignancies: emerging challenges in the era of highly active antiretroviral therapy. *The Oncologist.* 2005;10:412–426.

Gill PS, Tulpule A, Espina BM, et al. Paclitaxel is safe and effective in the treatment of advanced AIDS-related Kaposi's sarcoma. *J Clin Oncol.* 1999;17:1876–1883.

Dezube BJ, Pantanowitz L, Aboulafia DM. Management of AIDS-related Kaposi's sarcoma: Advances in target discovery and treatment. *AIDS Reader.* 2004;14:236–253.

13-4 D

Educational Objective: To define emerging paradigms in the treatment of AIDS-related non-Hodgkin's lymphoma.

Recent retrospective epidemiologic studies and phase II clinical trials have highlighted the improved response associated with standard chemotherapy when administered to patients with AIDS-related non-Hodgkin lymphoma. In particular, patients with diffuse large B-cell non-Hodgkin's lymphoma are achieving response rates that are similar to patients without HIV. Popular regimens include rituximab, cyclophosphamide, doxorubicin, vincristine, and prednisone as an outpatient regimen, every 3 weeks, or rituximab given in conjunction with dose-adjusted cyclophosphamide, coupled with continuous infusion etoposide, vincristine, and doxorubicin. In addition, several recent studies have highlighted the utility of incorporating rituximab monoclonal antibody therapy with conventional chemotherapy options.

Suggested Reading

Cheung MC, Pantanowitz L, Dezube BJ. AIDS-related malignancies: emerging challenges in the era of highly active antiretroviral therapy. *The Oncologist.* 2005;10:412–426.

Little RF, Pittaluga S, Grant N, et al. Highly effective treatment of acquired immunodeficiency syndrome-related lymphoma with dose-adjusted EPOCH: impact of antiretroviral therapy suspension and tumor biology. *Blood.* 2003;101:4653–4659.

Kaplan LD, Lee JY, Ambinder RF, et al. Rituximab does not improve clinical outcome in a randomized phase 3 trial of CHOP with or without rituximab in patients with HIV-associated non Hodgkins lymphoma: AIDS-Malignancy Consortium Trial 010. *Blood.* 2005;106:1538–1543.

Bove F, Gabarre J, Gisselbrecht C, et al. Phase II trial of CHOP plus rituximab in patients with HIV-associated non-Hodgkins lymphoma. *J Clin Oncol.* 2006;24:4123–4128.

Dunleavy K, Wilson WH, Kaplan LD. The case for rituximab in AIDS-related lymphoma. *Blood.* 2006;107:3014–3015.

Bower M, Gazzard B, Mandalia S, et al. A prognostic index for systemic AIDS-related non-Hodgkin lymphoma treated in the era of highly active antiretroviral therapy. *Ann Intern Med.* 2005;143:265–273.

SELF EVALUATION

CHAPTER 14 QUESTIONS:
CENTRAL NERVOUS SYSTEM TUMORS

14-1 A 35-year-old previously healthy man was seen in the emergency room after a sudden onset grand mal seizure that occurred while he was at work. The findings on physical examination in the ER, including neurologic evaluation, are normal.

Anticonvulsant medications are prescribed. The patient has magnetic resonance imaging (MRI) of the head (Fig. 14-1, 14-2). The patient has a subtotal resection of the tumor. Pathology reveals an anaplastic oligodendroglioma. Cytogenetic analysis of tissue from the lesion obtained by biopsy demonstrates loss of the short arm of chromosome 1 and loss of the long arm of chromosome 19.

Which of the following are true?

A. The clinical presentation is typical for oligodendroglioma
B. Deletions of chromosomes 1p and 19q are common in oligodendroglioma
C. Patients whose tumors demonstate 1p and 19q deletions have a better prognosis than those that do not
D. The patient is likely to benefit from chemotherapy
E. All of the above

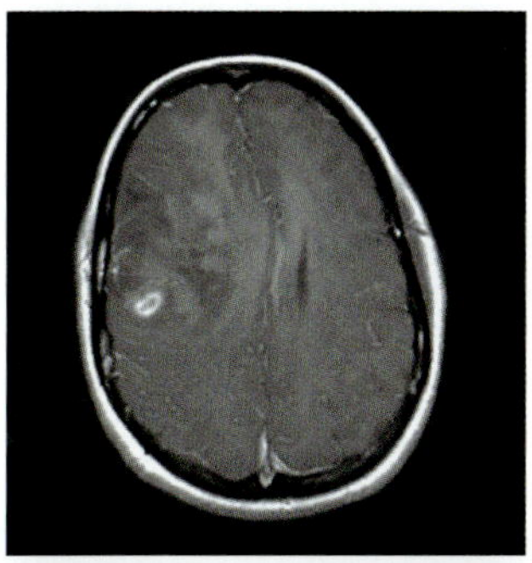

FIG. 14.1

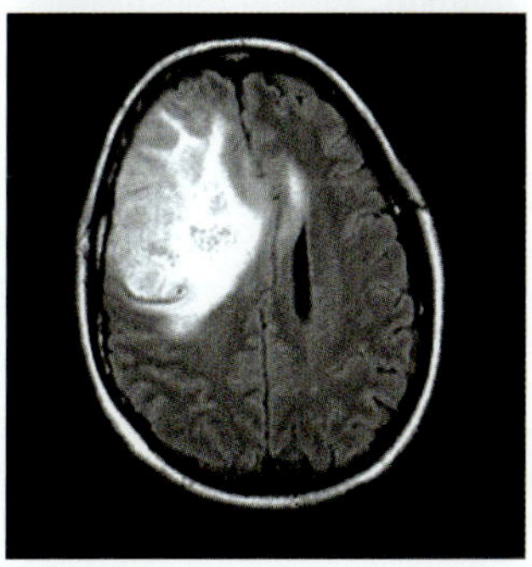

FIG. 14.2

14-2 A 68-year-old woman slips on ice and hits the back of her head on the sidewalk. She is unconscious for less than a minute. In the emergency room, she has pain and swelling on the occiput. She was treated for stage I breast cancer 7 years ago. Routine follow-ups with her oncologist have been normal.

On physical examination, a subgaleal hematoma is found on the occipital region of the scalp, and there are no abnormalities on neurologic evaluation. The remainder of her examination and all routine admission labs are normal.

A Computed Tomography (CT) scan of the head demonstrates a dural-based mass with calcification. A MRI scan shows a contrast-enhanced dural-based mass (Fig. 14-3).

Which of the following is the most appropriate intervention?

A. Repeat MRI of the head in 2 to 3 months
B. Whole-brain radiation therapy
C. Surgical excision of the mass lesion
D. 18-fluorodeoxyglucose (FDG)-positron emission tomography

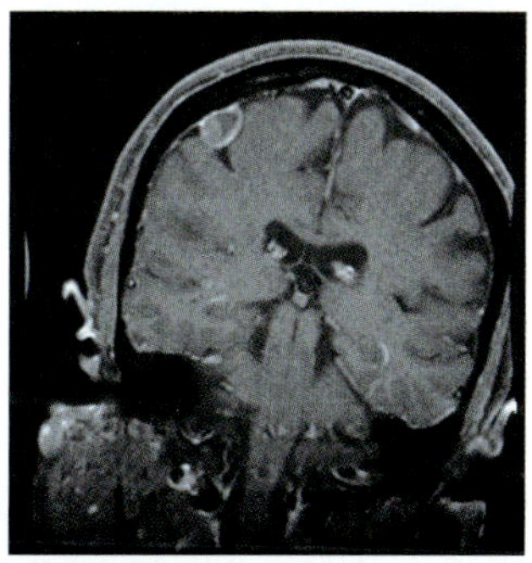

FIG. 14.3 Reprinted with permission from Cheson, BD, ed. Oncology MKSAP, 3rd ed. Philadelphia, PA: American College of Physicians; 2004: 357.

14-3 **A 70-year-old man presents with a 3-week history of increasing weakness of the left arm and leg. The medical history indicates no evidence of prior malignant disease, recent infection, or use of immunosuppressive medications. On physical examination, he has reduced strength in the left arm and leg, but there are no other abnormal findings.**

MRI shows a solitary, uniformly contrast-enhanced mass lesion in the right posterior frontal lobe (Fig. 14-4). Tumor specimen obtained by biopsy indicates large B-cell lymphoma. The complete blood count, serum chemistries levels — including liver enzymes, lactate dehydrogenase, and human immunodeficiency virus (HIV) serology — are normal, as well as the findings on slit lamp eye examination. The results of CT of the chest, abdomen, and pelvis are normal. The results of MRI of the spine are unremarkable, and no malignant cells are found on cytologic analysis of cerebrospinal fluid.

Which of the following is the best treatment option?

A. Whole-brain radiation therapy
B. Excision of the mass lesion
C. Chemotherapy with cyclophosphamide, doxorubicin, vincristine, and prednisone (CHOP)
D. High-dose methotrexate-based chemotherapy
E. Concurrent methotrexate-based chemotherapy and whole-brain radiation therapy

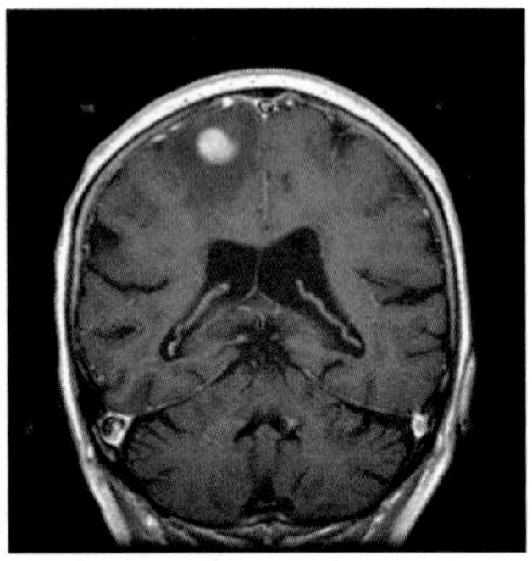

FIG. 14.4 Reprinted with permission from Cheson, BD, ed. Oncology MKSAP, 3rd ed. Philadelphia, PA: American College of Physicians; 2004: 357.

14-4 **A 53-year-old man presents with a 4-day history of a new onset of slurred speech and tingling on the right side of the face and the right upper extremity. Physical examination is notable for dysarthria and mild left facial weakness, but no other abnormalities. T1-weighted MRI scans of the head, made with use of gadolinium, show a ring-enhanced mass lesion with substantial surrounding low attenuation (Fig. 14-5). The presumptive diagnosis is glioblastoma multiforme.**

What is the appropriate action at this time?

A. Biopsy followed by radiation therapy
B. Biopsy followed by radiation therapy and corticosteroids
C. Surgical debulking followed by chemotherapy
D. Surgical debulking followed by radiation therapy and chemotherapy

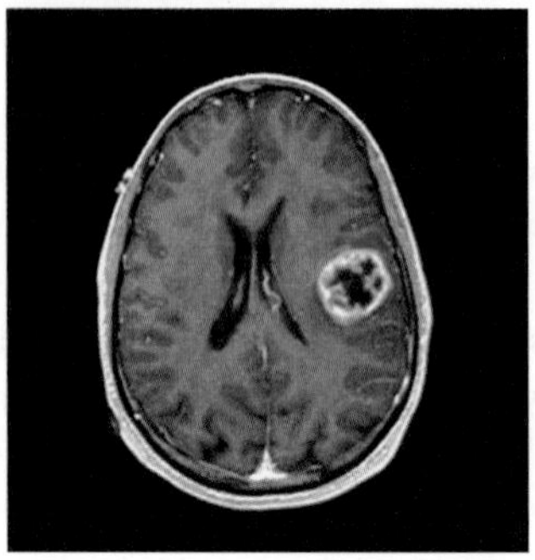

FIG. 14.5 Reprinted with permission from Cheson, BD, ed. Oncology MKSAP, 3rd ed. Philadelphia, PA: American College of Physicians; 2004: 358.

14-5 **A 60-year-old woman had a right upper lobectomy for a T2, N1, M0 adenocarcinoma of the right lung 1 year ago. She had no other treatment for the lung cancer. She presents now with gradual onset of increasing headache and slight weakness of the left upper extremity over the past 3 to 4 weeks. On physical examination, there is minimal left upper extremity neglect and paresis. She has stable diminished breath sounds, no adenopathy, and no other physical findings indicative of metastases. MRI of the head demonstrates a solitary, uniformly contrast-enhanced mass lesion at the junction of gray and white matter in the right frontal lobe. CT scans of the chest and upper abdomen show no evidence of metastatic lung cancer.**

Which of the following therapeutic approaches is most likely to extend her life and to reduce the risk of long-term neurologic deterioration?

A. Corticosteroids and observation
B. Whole-brain radiation therapy
C. Surgical excision and observation
D. Surgical excision and whole-brain radiation therapy
E. Surgical excision and adjuvant chemotherapy

CHAPTER 14 EXPLANATORY ANSWERS:
CENTRAL NERVOUS SYSTEM TUMORS

14-1 E

Educational Objective: To recognize the clinical presentation of oligodendroglioma, diagnostic and prognostic implications of 1p and 19q deletions, and chemosensitivity.

New onset of seizures in a young adult suggests a diagnosis of primary brain tumor. MRI scan reveals an infiltrating, contrast-enhancing, mass lesion and is characteristic of oligodendroglioma. Loss of chromosomes 1p and 19q has been found to be associated with oligodendroglioma but this loss is uncommon with astrocytoma. Loss of 1p and 19q also is associated with longer survival and, possibly, an increased likelihood of response to chemotherapy. Recently, a translocation of 19q to 1p t(1p;19q) was confirmed to mediate loss of 1p and 19q and is associated with improved prognosis. Retrospective studies and the intergroup prospective trial of adjuvant chemotherapy suggest that patients with 1p and 19q deletions/translocations may predict for greater chemosensitivity.

Suggested Reading

van den Bent MJ, Taphoorn MJ, Brandes AA, et al. Phase II study of first-line chemotherapy with temozolomide in recurrent oligodendroglial tumors: the European Organization for Research and Treatment of Cancer Brain Tumor Group Study 26971. *J Clin Oncol.* 2003;21(13):2525–2528.

Cairncross G, Berkey B, Shaw E, et al. A randomized clinical trial of chemotherapy plus radiotherapy (RT) versus RT alone for pure and mixed anaplastic oligodendroglioma: an Intergroup trial by the RTOG, NCCTG, SWOG, NCIC CTG and ECOG. *J Clin Oncol.* 2006;24(18):2707–2714.

Jenkins RB, Blair H, Ballman KV, et al. A t(1;19)(q10;p10) mediates the combined deletions of 1p and 19q and predicts a better prognosis of patients with oligodendroglioma. *Cancer Res.* 2006; 66(20):9852–9861.

Smith JS, Alderete B, Minn Y, et al. Localization of common deletion regions on 1p and 19q in human gliomas and their association with histologic subtype. *Oncogene.* 1999;18(28):4144–4152.

14-2 A

Educational Objective: To identify the clinical presentation and management of meningioma.

Meningiomas are relatively common, asymptomatic lesions found incidentally on neuroimaging for other indications. This patient had no neurologic symptoms either before or after the fall. The MRI scan shows the characteristic dural-based contrast-enhanced solitary lesion with contrast enhancement extending from the mass along the dura, known as the "dural tail." For this patient who was treated for breast cancer 7 years ago, the risk of metastatic breast cancer is low. A dural-based lesion in the absence of any other evidence of metastatic disease and the absence of parenchymal disease is evidence against the diagnosis of metastatic breast cancer. Moreover, if she had asymptomatic breast cancer, the follow-up MRI scan would likely show growth and prompt more invasive, diagnostic, and therapeutic interventions. Therefore, immediate radiation therapy or surgical intervention is not warranted based on the clinical presentation. Although FDG PET may be useful for detecting metastases, it may be positive for nonmalignant conditions and does not provide histologic diagnosis. Because both meningioma and breast cancer are relatively common, it is important to understand the different clinical presentations of each.

Suggested Reading

Go RS, Taylor BV, Kimmel DW. The natural history of asymptomatic meningiomas in Olmsted County, Minnesota. *Neurology.* 1998;51(6):1718–1720.

14-3 D

Educational Objective: To recognize appropriate treatment options for patients with primary central nervous system (CNS) lymphoma.

Recent studies of primary CNS lymphoma have shown that patients treated with regimens containing high-dose methotrexate live longer compared with patients who receive radiation alone or chemotherapy with CHOP plus radiation therapy. Historically, the median survival associated with radiation alone or radiation plus CHOP is about 1 year. More recent series in which high-dose methotrexate-based regimens have been used demonstrate a median survival of more than 30 months. Although phase III trials in which various options are compared have not been completed, the consistency of both single- and multi-institution studies suggests that high-dose methotrexate either alone or with other drugs, given intravenously or intra-arterially, produces similar outcomes. Surgical excision does not improve the outcome. Whole-brain radiation therapy has been reported to result in a substantial risk of delayed cognitive decline. Concurrent methotrexate and radiation therapy are known to increase the risk of leukoencephalopathy, so this combination would not be appropriate in this setting.

Suggested Reading

Abrey LE, Yahalom J, DeAngelis LM. Treatment for primary CNS lymphoma: the next step. *J Clin Oncol.* 2000;18(17): 3144–3150.

DeAngelis LM, Seiferheld W, Schold SC, et al. Combination chemotherapy and radiotherapy for primary central nervous system lymphoma: Radiation Therapy Oncology Group Study 93–10. *J Clin Oncol.* 2002;20(24):4643–4648.

Nelson DF, Martz KL, Bonner H, et al. Non-Hodgkin's lymphoma of the brain: can high dose, large volume radiation therapy improve survival? Report on a prospective trial by the Radiation Therapy Oncology Group (RTOG): RTOG 8315. *Int J Radiat Oncol Biol Phys.* 1992;23(1):9–17.

O'Neill BP, Wang CH, O'Fallon JR, et al. Primary central nervous system non-Hodgkin's lymphoma (PCNSL): survival advantages with combined initial therapy? A final report of the North Central Cancer Treatment Group (NCCTG) Study 86–72–52. *Int J Radiat Oncol Biol Phys.* 1999;43(3):559–563.

Schultz C, Scott C, Sherman W, et al. Preirradiation chemotherapy with cyclophosphamide, doxorubicin, vincristine, and dexamethasone for primary CNS lymphomas: initial report of Radiation Therapy Oncology Group protocol 88–06. *J Clin Oncol.* 1996;14(2):556–564.

14-4 D

Educational Objective: To explain the clinical presentation, diagnostic findings, and management of glioblastoma multiforme.

From the history, physical examination, and findings on MRI, the most likely diagnosis is glioblastoma multiforme or another high-grade glioma. The patient has no substantial comorbid illness, the neurologic status is largely intact, and the tumor is technically resectable, especially with the advent of stereotactic and cortical mapping techniques. Therefore, debulking surgery will allow for sufficient tissue to be obtained for diagnosis and to relieve mass effect. There also is ample evidence that survival is longer when more complete surgery is done, although there is uncertainty regarding what the better survival is truly associated with—the surgery itself or the clinical presentation that permits the more aggressive surgery. Randomized trials have established that radiation therapy prolongs survival compared with surgery alone, but the addition of corticosteroids alone does not. Surgery followed by chemotherapy alone produces inferior outcomes compared with surgery plus radiation therapy. There is evidence that the addition of chemotherapy to surgery and radiation therapy is associated with slightly greater survival at 1 and 2 years. It is entirely reasonable to add chemotherapy, such as placement of carmustine-impregnated wafers at the time of surgery or the addition of temozolomide.

Suggested Reading

Westphal M, Hilt DC, Bortey E, et al. A Phase 3 trial of local chemotherapy with biodegradable carmustine (BCNU) wafers (Gliadel wafers) in patients with primary malignant glioma. *Neuro Oncol.* 2003;5(2):79–88.

Stupp R, Mason WP, van den Bent MJ. Raiotherapy plus concomitant and adjuvant temozolomide for glioblastoma. *N Engl J Med* 2005;35(10):987–996.

14-5 D

Educational Objective: To identify the clinical presentation and management of solitary brain metastases.

Randomized trials have demonstrated that the resection of solitary metastases prolongs survival for a patient with a solid tumor who has both a good performance status and controlled or absent primary tumor. A randomized trial also has demonstrated that whole-brain radiation therapy following surgical resection results in fewer brain metastases and a lower frequency of neurologic deterioration compared with surgery alone; however, whole-brain radiation did not increase the length of survival. Because of concerns that radiation may result in an unacceptable incidence of dementia, some advocate avoiding radiation. This practice is reasonable, as radiation does not prolong survival. However, the patient should be informed that the risk of future neurologic problems from recurrent brain metastases is greater without cranial radiation. There is no evidence that adjuvant chemotherapy improves survival for this group of patients.

Suggested Reading

Patchell RA, Tibbs PA, Regine WF, et al. Postoperative radiotherapy in the treatment of single metastases to the brain: a randomized trial. *JAMA.* 1998;280(17):1485–1489.

Patchell RA, Tibbs PA, Walsh JW, et al. A randomized trial of surgery in the treatment of single metastases to the brain. *N Engl J Med.* 1990;322(8):494–500.

SELF EVALUATION

CHAPTER 15 QUESTIONS:

LEUKEMIAS

15-1 A 59-year-old man is referred for evaluation of persistent lymphocytosis. On physical examination, he is found to have cervical, axillary, and inguinal lymphadenopathy. The white blood cell count is 19,000/mm^3, with 65% mature-appearing lymphocytes but occasional large atypical lymphocytes as well.

Which of the following should be done next to establish a diagnosis?

A. Lymph node biopsy
B. Bone marrow biopsy
C. Cytogenetic examination of peripheral blood
D. Immunophenotyping of peripheral blood lymphocytes
E. Polymerase chain reaction (PCR) examination of peripheral blood for BCL-2 translocation

15-2 A 28-year-old man presents with fever and bleeding gums. The results of laboratory studies include a white blood cell count of 60,000 mm^3, of which most are blasts. Immunophenotyping shows the blasts to express myeloid antigens CD33 and CD13 and to coexpress the B-cell antigen CD19. Cytogenetic analysis shows inv(16) in 20 of 20 metaphases.

Which of the following is most important for estimating the likelihood of achieving a sustained complete response with chemotherapy?

A. Age of the patient
B. Cytogenetic features of the blasts
C. White blood cell count at the time of presentation
D. Presence of a lymphoid marker on the myeloblasts

15-3 A 59-year-old man is diagnosed with chronic lymphocytic leukemia (CLL). Because of disease-related symptoms and a rapidly increasing lymphocyte count, therapy is initiated with fludarabine and rituximab. After six cycles of therapy, the blood counts normalize and his symptoms disappear. In 10 months, however, the white blood cell count is 27,000 mm^3, and he reports having drenching night sweats. He has cervical and inguinal lymphadenopathy. Results of a node biopsy show CLL, with no evidence of transformation to large cell lymphoma.

Which of the following is the best treatment option?

A. Repeat treatment with fludarabine and rituximab
B. Chlorambucil
C. Lenalidomide
D. Alemtuzumab
E. Interferon-alpha

15-4 A 41-year-old man has been diagnosed with acute myeloid leukemia (AML). The white blood cell count is 30,000 mm^3 and cytogenetic analysis shows t(8;21). A complete remission is achieved with treatment with daunomycin and standard-dose cytarabine. He has no human leukocyte antigen (HLA) matched siblings.

According to the results of randomized trials, which of the following would prolong the duration of complete remission for this patient?

A. Central nervous system (CNS) prophylaxis with intrathecal methotrexate and cranial radiation
B. Maintenance therapy with low-dose interleukin (IL)-2
C. Consolidation therapy with multiple cycles of high-dose cytarabine
D. Maintenance therapy with all-trans retinoic acid
E. Autologous marrow transplantation while in first remission

15-5 A 43-year-old man with AML, who initially presented with a white blood cell count of 42,000 mm^3 and blasts characterized as having trisomy 8, is treated with daunomycin and standard-dose cytarabine. A complete remission is achieved with a single cycle of therapy. He then is treated with three cycles of high-dose cytarabine. Shortly after completing the third cycle (5 months after diagnosis), a repeat bone marrow examination is performed because of a declining platelet count. Although no blasts are seen in the peripheral smear, the marrow shows 20% myeloblasts, again with trisomy 8. Repeat induction therapy with daunomycin and cytarabine is proposed.

Which of the following is most important in assessing the likelihood of achieving a second remission?

A. Duration of the first remission
B. Achievement of the first remission with a single cycle of induction therapy
C. Age of the patient
D. Cytogenetic characteristics of the leukemia
E. Detection of relapse before there were circulating blasts

15-6 A 47-year-old woman presents 2 years after completing therapy for stage II breast cancer. Treatment included lumpectomy, radiation therapy, and chemotherapy with cyclophosphamide and doxorubicin. She now has anemia and thrombocytopenia and is found to have AML with inv(16).

Which of the following statements is true?

A. Because of the timing of the leukemia, it is unlikely that it is associated with the previous therapy
B. Because of the cytogenetic characteristics of the leukemia, it is unlikely that it is associated with the previous therapy
C. Although inv(16) is usually associated with a high rate of complete response, that is not the case for this previously treated patient
D. The leukemia may be associated with the previous therapy, but given the inv(16), a high rate of complete response can be expected

15-7 Which of the following is the most favorable cytogenetic finding in patients with CLL?

A. Normal cytogenetics
B. Trisomy 12
C. del(11q)
D. del(13q)

15-8 A 34-year-old woman with chronic myeloid leukemia (CML) in chronic phase has received an allogeneic bone marrow transplant without depletion of the T cells. The transplant donor is a HLA-identical brother. The preparative regimen included busulfan and cyclophosphamide. One year after the transplant, disease is in morphologic and cytogenetic complete remission, but a PCR assay performed for the first time is positive for BCR-ABL.

Which of the following statements best describes the significance of the positive assay?

A. It has no significance
B. It increases the risk of relapse to 40%
C. It increases the risk of relapse to 80%
D. It represents a 100% risk of relapse

15-9 A 56-year-old man presents with a persistent cough, dyspnea, and an elevated eosinophil count. Six months earlier, an elevated eosinophil count was noted on routine screening but no work-up was performed. The current white blood cell count is 25,000 mm^3 with 40% eosinophils and no peripheral blasts. Examination of the bone marrow shows hypercellular marrow with eosinophils or their precursors constituting 50% of the marrow elements. The patient takes no medications, and multiple stool samples are negative for evidence of parasitic infection.

Which of the following therapies is most appropriate?

A. Gemtuzumab
B. Imatinib mesylate
C. All-trans retinoic acid
D. Interferon-alpha
E. Cyclosporine

15-10 **A 59-year-old man presents with a history of several weeks of progressive fatigue and easy bruising. A complete blood count demonstrates pancytopenia, with a platelet count of 52,000/mm^3, a neutrophil count of 900/mm^3, and a hemoglobin of 8.1 g/dL. Evaluation of bone marrow aspirate indicates hypercellularity with occasional ringed sideroblasts on an iron stain. The differential count on the bone marrow shows 6% blasts. Cytogenetic analysis identifies an abnormality of chromosome 7.**

According to the International Prognostic Scoring System, which of the following categories describes the likelihood of his disease progressing to AML and his median survival?

A. Low-risk disease
B. Intermediate-1 disease
C. Intermediate-2 disease
D. High-risk disease

15-11 **A 21-year-old man presents with a white blood cell count of 38,000/mm^3, of which 90% are lymphoblasts, a platelet count of 110,000, and a hematocrit of 38%. Cytogenetics demonstrate the Ph chromosome in 19 of 20 metaphases. He is treated with induction chemotherapy including imatinib, cyclophosphamide, vincristine, prednisone, and daunomycin. He achieves a complete remission based on morphology, cytogenetics, and PCR assays of peripheral blood and marrow. He does not have a matched sibling.**

What should be recommended now?

A. Imatinib alone
B. Imatinib plus consolidation and maintenance chemotherapy
C. Autologous hematopoietic cell transplantation
D. Reduced-intensity unrelated donor hematopoietic cell transplantation
E. Standard-intensity unrelated donor hematopoietic cell transplantation

15-12 **A 60-year-old male presents with fatigue and easy bruising and is found to have a white blood cell count of 110,000/mm^3, a hematocrit of 26%, and platelets of 40,000/mm^3. Bone marrow examination shows 85% blasts with normal cytogenetics, and an immunophenotype that is positive for the myeloid marker CD13, CD33, and CD34 and for the lymphoid marker CD19. The patient is treated with idarubicin and cytarabine.**

What approach should be taken toward CNS prophylaxis?

A. Intrathecal methotrexate
B. Intrathecal methortrexate plus cranial radiation
C. Craniospinal radiation
D. High-dose systemic methotrexate
E. No therapy is required

15-13 **A 39-year-old woman presents with a white blood cell count of 24,000/mm^3, a platelet count of 22,000/mm^3, and is found to have acute promyelocytic leukemia. She begins all-trans retinoic acid, daunomycin, and cytarabine thearpy. On day 10 of therapy, her white blood cell count is 6,000/mm^3, the majority of which are myeloid forms of varying maturity. During the next 24 hours, despite being on broad spectrum antibiotics, she develops fever, respiratory distress, and pulmonary infiltrates. Bronchoalveolar lavage is performed without an immediate diagnosis, but cultures are pending.**

Which of the following would be the next appropriate step?

A. Discontinue the all-trans retinoic acid
B. Dexamethasone
C. Voriconazole
D. Bactrim

15-14 A 49-year-old man with newly diagnosed chronic phase CML is begun on imatinib at 400 mg once daily. After 6 months of therapy, his white blood cell count has normalized, but a bone marrow shows that 20% of metaphases continue to be Ph positive.

Which of the following would represent appropriate management at this time?

A. Continue imatinib at 400 mg once daily
B. Increase imatinib to 800 mg once daily
C. Add alfa interferon
D. Switch to dasatinib

15-15 A 62-year-old man is found to be anemic on a routine blood test with a hematocrit of 34%, a platelet count of 110,000/mm^3, and a white blood cell count of 2,800/mm^3 with 40% neutrophils. A bone marrow shows trilineage dysplasia with 3% blasts, and cytogenetics show del(20q) in 17 of 20 metaphases. He has three healthy siblings.

Which of the following would represent appropriate treatment for this patient?

A. Observation
B. Lenalidomide
C. 5-azacytadine
D. Decitabine
E. Reduced-intensity allogeneic hematopoietic cell transplantation

15-16 A 56-year-old woman presents with fatigue and easy bruising for 2 weeks duration. Her white blood cell count is 12,500/mm^3 with 40% myeloblasts. A bone marrow is hypercellular with 60% myeloblasts. Cytogenetics are 46XX in all 20 metaphases. Additional molecular studies show a mutation in the *NPM1* gene but no mutation in *FLT3*.

Which of the following do the additional molecular studies suggest?

A. Her prognosis is somewhat better than average for those with normal cytogenetics
B. Her leukemia will be specifically sensitive to anthracyclines
C. Her leukemia will be specifically sensitive to high-dose cytarabine
D. There is a high likelihood that she will develop extramedullary disease

15-17 A 52-year-old man with chronic phase CML is treated with imatinib at 400 mg once daily. His peripheral blood counts normalize, and after 1 year of therapy, he has a partial cytogenetic remission with 80% Ph-negative metaphases in his marrow. After 2 years of therapy, his counts remain normal, and a bone marrow reveals no metaphases with a Ph chromosome, but 3 out of 20 metaphases now show trisomy 8.

What is the appropriate treatment for this patient?

A. Continue imatinib at 400 mg once daily
B. Increase imatinib to 800 mg once daily
C. Switch to dasatinib
D. Switch to interferon-alfa
E. Allogeneic hematopoietic cell transplantion

15-18 A 44-year-old man presents with a white blood cell count of 28,000/mm^3 most of which are lymphoblasts, a platelet count of 45,000/mm^3, and hematocrit of 30%. Bone marrow examination shows 90% lymphoblasts and cytogenetics show 20 of 20 meta-phases with t(4;11).

Which of the following do the cytogenetic findings imply?

A. A worse prognosis than average for adult ALL
B. A high likelihood for sensitivity to imatinib
C. A T-cell phenotype with mediastinal involvement
D. They no significance

CHAPTER 15 EXPLANATORY ANSWERS:
LEUKEMIAS

15-1 D

Educational Objective: To identify the appropriate studies required for the diagnosis of CLL.

The diagnosis of CLL requires a lymphocytosis of at least 5,000/mm^3. The morphology of the peripheral blood lymphocytes should demonstrate primarily mature-appearing cells. However, a number of entities can be confused with CLL, including hairy cell leukemia, prolymphocytic leukemia, and non-Hodgkin's lymphoma in a leukemic phase. Histologic assessment of lymph node or bone marrow biopsy samples will not provide sufficient information to distinguish among these entities. Immunophenotyping provides the best information to successfully distinguish them. CLL cells characteristically express CD19, CD20, CD23, CD5, and surface immunoglobulins, although these tend to be relatively low in intensity. The expression of CD5 differentiates CLL from other B-cell malignant diseases with the exception of mantle cell lymphoma, which also is CD5+. However, in contrast to CLL cells, MCL cells are negative for CD23 and stain for cyclin D1.

Suggested Reading

Argatoff LH, Connors JM, Klasa RJ, et al. Mantle cell lymphoma: a clinicopathologic study of 80 cases. *Blood.* 1997;89(6): 2067–2078.

Cheson BD, Bennett JM, Grever M, et al. National Cancer Institute-Sponsored Working Group guidelines for chronic lymphocytic leukemia: Revised guidelines for diagnosis and treatment. *Blood.* 1996;87(12):4990–4997.

15-2 B

Educational Objective: To identify the important prognostic factors associated with initial therapy for AML.

The results of initial treatment of AML are best predicted by the cytogenetic features of the leukemia blasts. For patients with AML characterized by inv(16) or t(8;21) that is treated with conventional therapy, the likelihood of complete remission is 85%, and the probability of 5-year survival is 60%. In contrast, for patients with leukemias characterized by abnormalities in chromosomes 5 or 7 or with complex abnormalities, the likelihood of complete remission is 50%, and the probability of survival at 5 years is 12%. Increased age, a history of myelodysplasia, and a high white blood cell count at diagnosis are all predictors for a worse outcome but none so powerfully as cytogenetic findings. The presence of lymphoid markers on myeloid blasts is of no prognostic significance.

Suggested Reading

Grimwade D, Walker H, Oliver F, et al. The importance of diagnostic cytogenetics on outcome in AML: analysis of 1,612 patients entered into the MRC AML 10 trial. The Medical Research Council Adult and Children's Leukaemia Working Parties. *Blood.* 1998;92(7):2322–2333.

Slovak ML, Kopecky KJ, Cassileth PA, et al. Karyotypic analysis predicts outcome of preremission and postremission therapy in adult acute myeloid leukemia: a Southwest Oncology Group/Eastern Cooperative Oncology Group study. *Blood.* 2000;96(13): 4075–4083.

15-3 D

Educational Objective: To recognize the role of alemtuzumab in the treatment of CLL.

Fludarabine or fludarabine-containing combinations have become the initial treatment of choice for most patients with CLL. However, relapse is inevitable, and subsequent treatment options are needed. Repeat treatment with the same regimen, used initially is a reasonable option for patients with a response that has lasted longer than 1 year. Approximately two-thirds of such patients will have a second response. However, the response in the described patient was less than 1 year. Chlorambucil has limited activity in disease that has relapsed after fludarabine therapy. In a multicenter randomized trial, only 7% of patients had a partial response to chlorambucil after treatment with fludarabine had failed. Lenalidomide is being studied in CLL, but only limited data are available about its utility. Interferon-alpha has limited activity in CLL. In the pivotal trial of alemtuzumab for patients with disease refractory to fludarabine and who also had received chlorambucil, the response rate was 33%, including a 2% rate of complete response. Response rates varied with a number of clinical factors, notably the size of the lymph nodes. Because this man did not have massive lymphadenopathy, response to alemtuzumab would be expected.

Suggested Reading

Keating MJ, Flinn I, Jain V, et al. Therapeutic role of alemtuzumab (CAMPATH-1H) in patients who have failed fludarabine: Results of a large international study. *Blood.* 2002;99(10):3554–3561.

Rai KR, Peterson BL, Kolitz J, et al. Fludarabine compared with chlorambucil as primary therapy for chronic lymphocytic leukemia. *New Engl J Med.* 2000;343(24):1750–1757.

Byrd JC, Rai K, Peterson BL, et al. Addition of rituximab to fludarabine may prolong progression-free survival and overall survival in patients with previously untreated chronic lymphocytic leukemia: an updated retrospective comparative analysis of CALBG 9712 and CALBG 9011. *Blood.* 2005; 105(1):49–53

15-4 C

Educational Objective: To select appropriate therapy for patients with AML.

Prospective randomized trials have explored a variety of therapies administered after remission for younger patients with AML. When such patients are not candidates for transplant, the best results have been achieved when multiple cycles of consolidation therapy, including high-dose cytarabine, are administered. This seems to be particularly true for patients with favorable-risk disease, including patients with t(8;21) and inv(16). There is no role for CNS prophylaxis in AML. Although IL-2 and all-trans retinoic acid have been explored as maintenance therapy, neither has yet been shown to affect disease-free or overall survival. Results from prospective randomized trials have generally not identified a clear advantage for autologous transplantation for patients with favorable-risk disease in first remission.

Suggested Reading

Marcucci G, Mrózek K, Ruppert AS, et al. Prognostic factors and outcome of core binding factor acute myeloid leukemia patients with t(8;21) differ from those of patients with inv(16): a Cancer and Leukemia Group B study. *J Clin Oncol.* 2005;23(36):5705–5717.

Schlenk RF, Benner A, Krauter J, et al. Individual patient data-based meta-analysis of patients aged 16 to 60 years with core binding factor acute myeloid leukemia: a survey of the German Acute Myeloid Leukemia Intergroup. *J Clin Oncol.* 2004;22(18):3741–3750.

15-5 A

Educational Objective: To recognize the prognostic factors for achieving a second remission in relapsed AML.

Overall, repeat treatment with an anthracycline and cytarabine leads to a second remission for approximately 30% to 50% of patients with AML in first relapse. The duration of first remission is the strongest single predictor of the likelihood of a second complete response. If the initial remission was longer than 18 months, the complete response with repeat induction therapy may be as high as 65%, whereas if the first remission was shorter than 18 months the probability of successful repeat induction is less, averaging only 25%. Once the duration of the first complete response is accounted for, other factors, such as age, cytogenetic features, and the white blood cell count at relapse, have much less prognostic importance.

Suggested Reading

Estey EH. Prognostic factors in acute myelogenous leukemia. *Leukemia.* 2001;15(4):670–672.

Estey EH. Treatment of relapsed and refractory acute myelogenous leukemia. *Leukemia.* 2000;14(3):476–479.

15-6 D

Educational Objective: To recognize the various syndromes of treatment-related AML.

Patients treated with aggressive anthracycline therapy are at risk of leukemia typical of previous exposure to topoisomerase II inhibitors. Such leukemias have a shorter latency period than seen after exposure to alkylating agents and often have cytogenetic abnormalities involving the long arm of chromosome 11 (band q23), although other abnormalities can be seen, including inv(16). In general, the overall response rate of therapy-related AML to initial chemotherapy is lower than seen in de novo disease, averaging 35% to 40% in several large series. Furthermore, the duration of complete remission tends to be short. Important exceptions are patients with secondary leukemias that have favorable cytogenetic abnormalities. The complete response rate for such patients is indistinguishable from that for patients with de novo leukemia with similar karyotypes, and, although data are limited, survival also appears to be similar.

Suggested Reading

Andersen MK, Larson RA, Mauritzson N, et al. Balanced chromosome abnormalities inv(16) and t(15;17) in therapy-related myelodysplastic syndromes and acute leukemia: report from an international workshop. *Genes Chromosomes Cancer.* 2002; 33(4):395–400.

Shepherd L, Ottaway J, Myles J, et al. Therapy-related leukemia associated with high-dose 4-epi-doxorubicin and cyclophosphamide used as adjuvant chemotherapy for breast cancer. *J Clin Oncol.* 1994;12(11):2514–2515.

15-7 D

Educational Objective: To recognize the prognostic importance of cytogenetics in CLL.

Before the availability of fluorescent in situ hybridization (FISH), trisomy 12 was considered the most common cytogenetic abnormality in CLL. However, with this newer technology has come a recognition that other abnormalities occur with greater frequency. Notably, del(13q) occurs, either alone or in combination with other abnormalities, in more than half of patients and is associated with a more favorable outcome. This finding is in striking contrast to the situation of multiple myeloma, in which abnormalities of chromosome 13 are one of the most adverse prognostic features. Normal cytogenetic characteristics and del(11q) occur in approximately 18%, with trisomy 12 in 16% of patients. Patients with an del(11q) abnormality often have disproportionately large lymphadenopathy related to the lymphocyte count. Although cytogenetic characteristics are one of the strongest predictors of outcome, testing is expensive, and the results do not yet have an effect on treatment decisions. Therefore, testing with FISH is not routinely recommended.

With the recognition of the importance of immunoglobulin heavy-chain gene mutations, the more favorable cytogenetic abnormalities tend to occur in the mutated group, and the most unfavorable occur in the unmutated group. However, these unfavorable cytogenetic abnormalities are independent prognostic features, and their absence indicates a modestly improved outcome for those patients with unmutated heavy chain genes.

Suggested Reading

Döhner H, Stilgenbauer S, Benner A, et al. Genomic aberrations and survival in chronic lymphocytic leukemia. *New Engl J Med.* 2000;343(26):1910–1916.

Kröber A, Seiler T, Benner A, et al. Vh mutation status, CD38 expression level, genomic aberrations, and survival in chronic lymphocytic leukemia. *Blood.* 2002;100(4):1410–1416.

15-8 B

Educational Objective: To identify the risk associated with a positive PCR assay for BCR ABL after transplantation for CML.

PCR assay, if performed at 6 or 12 months after transplantation, is a powerful predictor of outcome, with a risk of relapse of 42% for patients with a positive assay compared with 3% for patients with a negative assay. If the assay is performed earlier — for example, at 3 months — it has no predictive power. These results suggest that a considerable amount of time is required for the preparative regimen and the allogeneic graft-versus-leukemia effect to completely eradicate the malignant clone.

Suggested Reading

Radich JP, Gehly G, Gooley T, et al. Polymerase chain reaction detection of the BCR-ABL fusion transcript after allogeneic marrow transplantation for chronic myeloid leukemia: results and implications in 346 patients. *Blood.* 1995;85(9): 2632–2638.

Radich JP, Gooley T, Bryant E, et al. The significance of bcr-abl molecular detection in chronic myeloid leukemia patients "late," 18 months or more after transplantation. *Blood.* 2001; 98(6):1701–1707.

15-9 B

Educational Objective: To select the appropriate therapy for hypereosinophilic syndrome.

Given the duration of disease, the peripheral blood and marrow findings, and the lack of other causes, this patient meets the criteria for idiopathic hypereosinophilic syndrome. Recently, this syndrome has been shown to be associated with a novel fusion tyrosine kinase, FIP1L1-PDGFR-alpha, which is a consequence of an interstitial chromosome deletion. The fusion results in a constitutively activated tyrosine kinase. Imatinib mesylate, a specific tyrosine kinase inhibitor, leads to a complete response for more than 50% of patients. It is yet unclear how enduring these responses will be, and disease recurrence associated with further mutations in PDGFR-alpha has been documented.

Suggested Reading

Cools J, DeAngelo DJ, Gotlib J, et al. A tyrosine kinase created by fusion of the PDGFRA and FIP1L1 genes as a therapeutic target of imatinib in idiopathic hypereosinophil syndrome. *N Engl J Med.* 2003;348(13):1201–1214.

15-10 C

Educational Objective: To understand the use of the International Prognostic Index for determining the prognosis of patients with myelodysplastic syndromes.

An international group of investigators in myelodysplastic syndromes developed a prognostic scoring system designed to improve the other systems in use around the world at the time. They combined cytogenetic, morphologic, and clinical data for 816 patients. The factors that best predicted outcome in a multivariate analysis included percent of blasts, number of peripheral blood cytopenias, and cytogenetic findings. Age also was an important predictor. Different numeric weights were assigned to the various levels of abnormality. Low-risk disease is associated with a median survival of 12 years and with more than 9 years for a 25% likelihood of transformation to acute leukemia. Intermediate-1 myelodysplastic syndrome is associated with a 5-year median survival and 7 years for a 25% likelihood of transformation. Intermediate-2 disease has a 1.8-year median survival, with 1.3 years for a 25% likelihood of transformation. High-risk disease is associated with a 0.3-year median survival and 0.2 years for a 25% likelihood of transformation. The patient described is younger than 60 years old, had 6% blasts (0.5 point), pancytopenia (0.5 point), and a chromosome 7 abnormality (1.0 points). The total score of 2.0 points represents the high end of the Intermediate-2 risk group.

Suggested Reading

Greenberg P, Cox C, LeBeau M, et al. International scoring system for evaluating prognosis in myelodysplastic syndromes. *Blood.* 1997;89(6):2079–2088.

15-11 E

Educational Objective: To select the appropriate therapy for Ph+ ALL.

Ph+ ALL has a very poor prognosis when treated with conventional chemotherapy. In two large prospective studies, both disease-free and overall survival were improved with allogeneic hematopoietic cell transplantation performed in first remission. The addition of imatinib appears to improve the initial complete remission rate of Ph+ ALL but there is, as yet, inadequate data about the long-term outcome of patients with Ph+ ALL treated with imatinib-containing combination chemotherapy. The role of autologous hematopoietic cell transplantation in Ph+ ALL is not established.

Suggested Reading

Dombret H, Gabert J, Boiron JM, et al. Outcome of treatment in adults with Philadelphia chromosome-positive acute lymphoblastic leukemia--results of the prospective multicenter LALA-94 trial. *Blood.* 2002;100(7):2357–2366.

Lee S, Kim YJ, Min CK, et al. The effect of first-line imatinib interim therapy on the outcome of allogeneic stem cell transplantation in adults with newly diagnosed Philadelphia chromosome-positive acute lymphoblastic leukemia. *Blood.* 2005; 105(9):3449–3457.

15-12 E

Educational Objective: To understand the indications for CNS prophylaxis in adults with AML.

Prospective randomized trials have not found any evidence that CNS prophylaxis improves either disease-free or overall survival for adults with AML. The finding of a single lymphoid marker on otherwise classic AML does not alter the behavior of the disease or the risk for CNS involvement.

Suggested Reading

Morrison FS, Kopecky KJ, Head DR, et al. Late intensification with POMP chemotherapy prolongs survival in acute myelogenous leukemia - Results of a Southwest oncology group study of rubidazone vs. adriamycin for remission induction, prophylactic intrathecal therapy, late intensification, and levamisole maintenance. *Leukemia.* 1992;6(7):708–714.

15-13 B

Educational Objective: To recognize symptoms of the retinoic acid syndrome and its appropriate treatment.

During induction therapy of APL with either all-trans retinoic acid or arsenic, some patients will have a syndrome of fever, weight gain, respiratory distress, pulmonary infiltrates, episodic hypotension, and renal failure. The syndrome is thought to be related to the sudden maturation of promyelocytes. If untreated, the syndrome can be fatal. However, if treated with dexamethasone most disease will rapidly respond within 1 to 3 days. Development of the retinoic acid syndrome is not a contraindication to further therapy with all-trans retinoic acid.

Suggested Reading

Tallman MS, Andersen JW, Schiffer CA, et al. Clinical description of 44 patients with acute promyelocytic leukemia who developed the retinoic acid syndrome. *Blood.* 2000;95(1):90–95.

15-14 A

Educational Objective: To understand appropriate management of chronic phase chronic myelogenous leukemia.

Imatinib has become the initial treatment of choice for most patients with chronic phase CML. Complete hematologic responses are seen in almost all patients using a dose of 400 mg once daily, and complete cytogenetic remissions occur for more than 75% of patients. However, complete cytogenetic responses frequently take 12 or more months to achieve, and the presence of 20% Ph-positive metaphases after 6 months of therapy is no reason to alter therapy. If, however, a complete cytogenetic response is not achieved in 18 months, the dose of imatinib should be increased or consideration be given to alternative therapies including dasatinib, nilotinib, and allogeneic hematopoietic cell transplantation.

Suggested Reading

Baccarani M, Saglio G, Goldman J, et al. Evolving concepts in the management of chronic myeloid leukemia recommendations from an expert panel on behalf of the European leukemianet. *Blood.*2006;108(1):1809–1820.

15-15 A

Educational Objective: To select appropriate therapy for patients with low-risk myelodysplasia.

According to the International Prognostic Scoring System, this patient has low-risk disease, and a median survival without specific therapy of more than 5 years. Lenalidomide is appropriate therapy for patients with 5q- myelodysplasia, but there is no established role in other forms of MDS. 5-azacytadine and decitabine are reserved for patients with intermediate-risk 2 disease. Allogeneic transplantation is potentially curative for MDS, but is generally withheld until patients progress to intermediate stage 1 disease with life-threatening cytopenias or intermediate-risk 2 disease.

Suggested Reading

Greenberg P, Cox C, LeBeau M, et al. International scoring system for evaluating prognosis in myelodysplastic syndromes. *Blood.* 1997;89(6):2079–2088.

15-16 A

Educational Objective: To understand the implications of the mutational status of *NPM1* and *FLT3* in adult AML.

FLT3 is a receptor tyrosine kinase that is mutated either as an internal tantem repeat or a point mutation in 20% to 40% of AML cases. Mutations in *FLT3* are somewhat more common for older patients, and they are associated with a higher white blood cell count at diagnosis and with a poorer response to therapy, particularly if there is a high ratio of abnormal-to-normal alleles among leukemic blasts. Mutations in the nucleophosmin gene (*NPM1*) can be found in 20% to 40% of adult AML cases, usually those with a normal karyotype, and cases with *NPM1* mutations appear to do somewhat better than average. In several studies, patients who have normal cytogenetics, are *FLT3* negative, and are *NPM1* positive have a more favorable outcome than other patients with a normal karyotype.

Suggested Reading

Falini B, Mecucci C, Tiacci E, et al. Cytoplasmic nucleophosmin in acute myelogenous leukemia with a normal karyotype. *N Engl J Med.* 2005;352(3):254–66.

Thiede C, Koch S, Creutzig E, et al. Prevalence and prognostic impact of NPM1 mutations in 1485 adult patients with acute myeloid leukemia (AML). *Blood.* 2006;107(10):4011–4020.

15-17 A

Educational Objective: To understand the significance of cytogenetic changes in non Ph-positive cells in patients with CML being treated with imatinib.

In approximately 5% of cases, patients with chronicphase CML being treated with imatinib will develop other chromosome abnormalities (OCA) in Ph-negative cells. Approximately 50% of these changes are trisomy 8 alone, another 10% will be trisomy 8 with other abnormalities, and 15% will involve chromosome 7. In some cases, particularly those involving chromosome 7, patients with OCA will go on to develop myelodysplasia. But in other cases, patients remain clinically stable and the OCA clone will disappear. Thus, there is no evidence that the development of OCA, particularly OCA without involvement of chromosome 7, should signal a change in the treatment of the patient.

Suggested Reading

Baccarani M, Saglio G, Goldman J, et al. Evolving concepts in the management of chronic myeloid leukemia recommendations from an expert panel on behalf of the European leukemianet. *Blood.* 2006;108(1):1809–1820.

15-18 A

Educational Objective: To recognize the prognostic significance of 11q23 abnormalities in adult ALL.

Between 60% and 70% of adult ALL cases will have a recurrent cytogenetic abnormality. The most common abnormality seen is t(9;22) (the Philadelphia chromosome). Abnormalities involving the mixed lineage leukemia gene MLL at 11q23 are seen in 5% to 10% of adult ALL cases, and the most common translocation is t(4;11). Adults with this translocation tend to be older, have a higher white blood cell count, an organomegaly, and have a higher likelihood of CNS involvement. The immunophenotype is typically a pro-B cell negative for CD10. ALL with t(4;11) carries a poor prognosis, and so, if the patient achieves a complete remission and is healthy enough to undergo transplantation, an allogeneic hematopoietic cell transplant should be considered.

Suggested Reading

Pui CH, Relling MV, Downing JR. Acute Lymphoblastic Leukemia. *N Engl J Med.* 2004;350(15):1535–1548.

Mancini M, Scappaticci D, Cimino G, et al. A comprehensive genetic classification of adult acute lymphoblastic leukemia (ALL): analysis of the GIMEMA 0496 protocol. *Blood.* 2005;105(9):3434–-3441.

SELF EVALUATION

CHAPTER 16 QUESTIONS:
LYMPHOMAS AND MYELOMA

16-1 A 52-year-old woman notices several new, enlarged inguinal lymph nodes but otherwise has no symptoms. On physical examination, she is found to have bilateral enlarged cervical axillary and inguinal lymph nodes. There is no hepatoplenomegaly. The results of excisional biopsy of a lymph node are consistent with the diagnosis of follicular non-Hodgkin's lymphoma, grade II. She is evaluated again in 3 months. The nodes have increased in size, and she reports that she has begun to have night sweats. Treatment with cyclophosphamide/vincristine/prednisone (CVP) and rituximab is administered with a complete response.

Which of the following statements is true about maintenance rituximab in this setting?

A. Rituximab maintenance has not been shown to prolong survival following an initial rituximab-based chemotherapy regimen
B. Rituximab therapy is associated with an increased risk of transformation to large cell lymphoma
C. Rituximab therapy will not prolong disease-free survival
D. Rituximab maintenance is associated with late cardiac toxicity

16-2 A 27-year-old woman presents with shortness of breath and cough. A chest radiograph reveals a mediastinal mass. Physical examination identifies several enlarged cervical lymph nodes and splenomegraly. Biopsy demonstrates nodular sclerosing Hodgkin's lymphoma. Her bone marrow biopsy is negative, and she is staged IIIA. She is given six cycles of doxorubicin/bleomycin/vinblastine/dacarbazine chemotherapy with resolution of her lymphadenopathy, splenomegaly on physical examination, and disappearance of her symptoms. Two months after completion of chemotherapy, a computerized tomography (CT)/positron emission tomography (PET) scan shows an ^{18}F-fluorodeoxyglucose(FDG)-avid mass in her mediastinal region.

Which of the following should be done?

A. Change to nitrogen mustard/vincristine/prednisone/procarbazine (MOPP) chemotherapy
B. Radiation therapy to the mediastinum
C. High-dose chemotherapy with autologous stem cell transplantation
D. No intervention; repeat the scan in 3 months

16-3 A 59-year-old woman with excellent performance status is found to have an elevated serum protein concentration at the time of a routine examination. Immunoelectrophoresis reveals a monoclonal IgG with a concentration of 2,764 mg/dL. Although her renal function is normal, her hemoglobin concentration is 11.6 g/dL. Bone survey shows a few lytic lesions in the calvarium. A bone marrow is notable for 50% plasma cells in sheets and clusters. The diagnosis of multiple myeloma is made.

Which of the following should you recommend?

A. Vincristine/adriamycin/dexamethasone (VAD)
B. Thalidomide plus dexamethasone
C. Single-agent dexamethasone
D. Single-agent bortezomib
E. Melphalan and prednisone

16-4 Which of the following histologic subtypes of Hodgkin's lymphoma is most likely to respond to treatment with rituximab?

A. Nodular sclerosing
B. Nodular lymphocyte-predominant
C. Mixed cellularity
D. Lymphocyte-depleted

16-5 **A 63-year-old man presents with pain in the lower back that is responsive to nonsteroidal anti-inflammatory agents. Compression fractures of the vertebrae are seen on x-rays. Neurologic examination is normal and magnetic resonance imaging shows no evidence of cord compression. Additional findings include a hemoglobin of level 10.0 g/dL, an IgG level of 3,500 mg/dL, a serum calcium level of 10.9 mg/dL, and a uric acid level of 2.7 mg/dL. Renal function is normal. Evaluation of bone marrow aspirate indicates sheets of plasma cells. The results of a bone survey are remarkable for numerous lytic bone lesions. The diagnosis of multiple myeloma is made.**

Additional management at this time should include all of the following except:

A. Monthly zoledronic acid
B. Thalidomide and dexamethasone
C. Daily aspirin
D. Radiation therapy to the area of back pain

16-6 **For which of the following diseases in relapse is bortezomib most active?**

A. Mantle cell lymphoma
B. Diffuse large B-cell lymphoma
C. Hodgkin lymphoma
D. Chronic lymphocytic leukemia

16-7 **Which of the following is a side effect of Yttrium-90-labeled (^{90}Y)-ibritumomab tiuxetan radioimmunotherapy used for follicular and low-grade non-Hodgkin lymphoma?**

A. Congestive heart failure
B. Hypothyroidism
C. Hemorhhagic cystitis
D. Secondary acute leukemia

16-8 **Which cytogenetic abnormality and resulting protein are associated with the lymphoma most likely to be cured with therapy?**

A. t(11;14) and cyclin D1
B. t(14;18) and BCL-2
C. t(2;5) and ALK
D. t(9;14) and PAX-5
E. t(1;14) and CARD

16-9 **A 46-year-old woman undergoes kidney transplantation and is subsequently treated with immunosuppressive agents in an attempt to prevent graft rejection. After 3 years, she begins to note fevers, night sweats, and abdominal bloating. A CT scan of the abdomen demonstrates a gastric mass. The results of biopsy indicate an aggressive lymphoma.**

Which of the following would be a characteristic of this lymphoma?

A. Findings on polymerase chain reaction (PCR) are positive for Epstein-Barr virus (EBV)
B. Withdrawal of immunosuppression results in resolution of the lymphoma
C. It exhibits a polymorphic histologic appearance
D. Immunophenotyping identifies a T-cell origin

16-10 **A 70-year-old woman describes symptoms of fevers and night sweats, a diffuse rash, and some arthralgias. On physical examination, in addition to the macular rash, there is diffuse lymphadenopathy and mild hepatosplenomegaly. The findings of laboratory testing include a hemoglobin level of 9.8 g/dL, a hematocrit of 31%, and normal white blood cell and platelet counts. Further assessment reveals hypergammaglobulinemia, an LDH level of 460 U/L, and an erythrocyte sedimentation rate of 78 mm/hour. She also has positive results on Coombs testing.**

The results of fine-needle biopsy of one of the lymph nodes are nondiagnostic. The findings on excisional biopsy are notable for partial effacement with decreased B-cell follicles. There is vascular proliferation with perivascular, atypical, medium-sized lymphoid cells, as well as eosinophils and plasma cells, with Reed-Sternberg-like cells. Immunohistochemistry results are CD3+, CD4+, CD8+, and CD10+, with proliferation of follicular dendritic cells (CD21+). The bone marrow is also involved.

Which of the following is the most likely diagnosis?

A. Angioimmunoblastic T-cell lymphoma
B. Anaplastic large T-cell lymphoma
C. Hodgkin's lymphoma
D. Mycosis fungoides
E. Reactive hyperplasia

CHAPTER 16 EXPLANATORY ANSWERS:
LYMPHOMAS AND MYELOMAS

16-1 A

Educational Objective: To discuss the role of maintenance rituximab therapy for patients with previously untreated, follicular non-Hodgkin's lymphoma.

Rituximab is now a standard component of the initial treatment of patients with follicular and low-grade non-Hodgkin's lymphoma. In addition, the use of continued rituximab following attainment of at least stable disease with initial CVP chemotherapy is a U.S. Food and Drug Administration (FDA)-approved indication. These data were based, in large part, on a trial conducted by the Eastern Cooperative Oncology Group and Cancer and Leukemia Group B in which patients with follicular and low-grade non-Hodgkin's lymphoma were treated with CVP, and those who did not progress were randomly assigned to rituximab maintenance or to observation. Benefit was seen for progression-free survival; however, a survival advantage is not apparent at this time. Nevertheless, there are a number of issues that remain. First, there are multiple maintenance strategies that have been employed, including four weekly doses every 6 months for 2 years, one dose every 2 months for 8 months, one dose every 3 months for 2 years, one dose every 3 months until disease progression, four weekly doses months 3 and 9, and dosing by blood levels. There is no information as to which is clearly preferable. In addition, there are, as of yet, no data on the benefit of maintenance therapy for patients who have received chemotherapy plus rituximab for induction as part of the initial therapy for the disease, although the results of such a trial are pending. A study from the European Organization for Research and Treatment of Cancer has demonstrated a survival advantage to rituximab therapy for previously treated patients who upon relapse received either rituximab, cyclophosphamide, doxorubicin, vincristine, and prednisire (R-CHOP) or CHOP followed by maintenance rituximab or observation. Nevertheless, in several studies exploring the role of maintenance therapy, there has been neutropenia and an increased number of infections, even in the absence of neutropenia, including progressive multifocal leukoencephalopathy. Thus, recommendations of this therapy include a discussion of the potential benefits, many of which are as of yet unknown, with the risks that are being increasingly recognized.

Suggested Reading

Hochster HS, Weller E, Gascoyne RD, et al. Maintenance rituximab after CVP results in superior clinical outcome in advanced follicular lymphoma (FL): results of the E1496 phase III trial from the Eastern Cooperative Oncology Group amd the Cancer and Leukemia Group B. *Blood.* 2005;106 (11 pt 1): 106a (abstr 349).

Hainsworth JD, Litchy S, Barton JH, et al. Single-agent rituximab as first-line and maintenance treatment for patients with chronic lymphocytic leukemia or small lymphocytic lymphoma: a phase II trial of the Minnie Pearl Cancer Research Network. *J Clin Oncol.* 2003;21(9):1746-1751.

Hainsworth JD, Litchy S, Shaffer DW, et al. Maximizing therapeutic benefit of rituximab: maintenance therapy versus retreatment at progression in patients with indolent non-Hodgkin's lymphoma: a randomized phase II trial of the Minnie Pearl Cancer Research Network. *J Clin Oncol.* 2005;23(6):1088-1095.

Ghielmini M, Schmitz SF, Cogliatti SB, et al. Prolonged treatment with rituximab in patients with follicular lymphoma significantly increases event-free survival and response duration compared with weekly × 4 schedule. *Blood.* 2004;103(12):4416-4423.

Gordan LN, Grow WB, Pusateri A, et al: Phase II trial of individualized rituximab dosing for patients with CD20-positive lymphoproliferative disorders. *J Clin Oncol.* 2005;23(6):1096-1102.

16-2 D

Educational Objective: To define the role of FDG-PET scanning in response assessment of patients with Hodgkin's lymphoma.

PET and PET/CT scans have proven to be a valuable adjunct for select patients with Hodgkin's lymphoma and non-Hodgkin's lymphoma. Although this test is very sensitive, it is not as specific, and a number of false positive findings can result in clinical confusion. For example, patients with Hodgkin's lymphoma who present with a mediastinal mass may experience a complete remission with standardchemotherapy.

However, after several months following treatment, a CT may reveal a mediastinal mass that is FDG-avid on a PET scan. This finding is generally the result of thymic hyperplasia. As a result, no diagnostic or therapeutic intervention is generally warranted. A scan repeated in 2 to 3 months will generally show resolution of the FDG-avidity and, perhaps, even the mass.

Suggested Reading

Juweid M, Cheson BD. Positron emission tomography and assessment of cancer therapy. *N Engl J Med.* 2006;354(5): 496-507.

Juweid ME, Stroobants S, Hoekstra OS, et al. Use of positron emission tomography for response assessment of lymphoma: consensus recommendations of the Imaging Subcommittee of the International Harmonization Project in Lymphoma. *J Clin Oncol.* 2007;25(5):571-578.

16-3 B

The traditional initial therapy for patients with multiple myeloma had included melphalan and prednisone. Single-agent dexamethasone has been reported to induce responses in more than half of patients who are older or who have significant comorbidities. Although the VAD regimen was initially considered promising, its activity was shown to primarily reflect the activity of the dexamethasone. Recent randomized trials have clearly demonstrated a survival advantage for patients who received the combination of thalidomide and dexamethasone compared with dexamethasone alone. Thus, this combination has emerged as a current standard for such patients as the one in this example. However, there are a number of risks, such as thromboembolic events, that are markedly increased with the combination and that require prophylactic anticoagulation. The combination of lenalidomide and dexamethasone is promising but must be directly compared with a thalidomide-based regimen. Bortezomib, although quite active in the relapsed setting, has not been adequately evaluated as a single agent in the initial therapy of this disease.

Rajkumar SV, Blood E, Vesole D, et al. Phase III clinical trial of thalidomide plus dexamethasone compared with dexaametha-sone alone in newly diagnosed multiple myeloma: A clinical trial coordinated by the Eastern Cooperative Oncology Group. *J Clin Oncol.* 2006;24(3):431-436.

16-4 B

Educational Objective: To recognize the immunophenotypic differences between classical Hodgkin's lymphoma and nodular lymphocyte-predominant Hodgkin's lymphoma.

Hodgkin's lymphoma is subclassified into two sets of diseases: nodular lymphocyte-predominant Hodgkin's lymphoma and classic Hodgkin's lymphoma. Nodular lymphocyte-predominant Hodgkin's lymphoma represents approximately 5% of Hodgkin's lymphoma and occurs most often in men ages 30 to 50 years. Mediastinal, spleen, and bone marrow involvement are much less common than for classic Hodgkin's lymphoma. Most patients present with localized, early-stage disease. Indeed, the propensity for this type of Hodgkin's to exhibit an indolent course with late relapses suggest a similarity with follicular center cell B-cell lymphomas. There are number of important differences between nodular lymphocyte-predominant Hodgkin's lymphoma and classical Hodgkin's lymphoma. For example, classic Hodgkin's lymphoma cells are positive for the antigens CD15 and CD30 and negative for CD20; in contrast, nodular lymphocyte-predominant Hodgkin's lymphoma is positive for CD20 and negative for CD15 and CD30. In addition, nodular lymphocyte-predominant Hodgkin's lymphoma is associated with a higher response rate than that for classic Hodgkin's lymphoma, with a greater propensity for relapse (particularly late relapse), and occasionally, with a large B-cell non-Hodgkin's lymphoma. Because nodular lymphocyte-predominant Hodgkin's lymphoma is CD20-positive, several recent studies have evaluated rituximab in this disorder, and significant activity has been found. Although this agent is currently used for patients at the time of relapse, attempts are being made to incorporate the antibody as part of initial treatment.

Suggested Reading

Diehl V, Sextro M, Franklin J, et al. Clinical presentation, course, and prognostic factors in lymphocyte-predominant Hodgkin's disease and lymphocyte-rich classical Hodgkin's disease: report from the European Task Force on Lymphoma project on lymphocyte-predominant Hodgkin's disease. *J Clin Oncol.* 1999;17(3):776-783.

Ekstrand BC, Lucas JB, Horwitz SM, et al. Rituximab in lymphocyte-predominant Hodgkin disease: results of a phase II trial. *Blood.* 2003;101(11):4285-4289.

16-5 D

Educational Objective: To recognize the importance of supportive therapy for the treatment of patients with multiple myeloma.

The combination of thalidomide and dexamethasone has emerged, based on results from both nonrandomized and randomized studies, as a treatment of choice for patients with previously untreated multiple myeloma. Bisphosphonates — either pamidronate or zoledronate — have been demonstrated to delay the time to a major skeletal event for patients with multiple myeloma. Therefore, treatment with one of these agents should be routinely initiated for all patients with myeloma. Zoledronate is more convenient because of its shorter time of administration, but it is much more expensive. At present, there is no clear evidence of clinical superiority between the two agents. The combination of thalidomide and dexamethasone, although more effective than either as single agent, is associated with an increased risk of thrombosis (as high as 20% to 50%) compared with that observed for either agent. As a result, prophylaxis against thrombosis is recommended. There is no uniformly accepted agent; low molecular weight heparin, coumadin, or a single 81-mg aspirin tablet daily can reduce the likelihood of a thrombotic event by more than half.

Patients with multiple myeloma are at increased risk for recurrent bacterial infections. Available data fail to demonstrate that prophylactic antibiotics reduce the incidence of these infections or infectious mortality. Similarly, intravenous immunoglobulins are not recommended for routine use but are reserved for patients with documented, recurrent bacterial infection. Radiation therapy does not have an impact on compression fractures. Unless there is an impending fracture of a weight-bearing bone, radiation should be delayed for patients during initial therapy, as radiation may reduce bone marrow tolerance of systemic chemotherapy.

Suggested Reading

Berenson JR, Hillner BE, Kyle RA, et al. American Society of Clinical Oncology Clinical Practice Guidelines: the role of bisphosphonates in multiple myeloma. *J Clin Oncol.* 2002;20(17):3719-3736.

Rajkumar SV, Blood E, Vesole D, et al. Phase III clinical trial of thalidomide plus dexamethasone compared with dexaamethasone alone in newly diagnosed multiple myeloma: A clinical trial coordinated by the Eastern Cooperative Oncology Group. *J Clin Oncol.* 2006;24(3):431-436.

16-6 A

Educational Objective: To recognize the diseases for which bortezomib is an active agent and its prominent adverse events.

Bortezomib (PS341) is the first proteasome inhibitor in clinical trials. Proposed mechanisms of action include inhibition of nuclear factor-kappa B, which leads to apoptosis, increased sensitivity to a variety of chemotherapy drugs, and impairment of elaboration of a number of cytokines and factors that favor the growth and proliferation of the malignant cells. Based on a study in which 202 patients with relapsed and refractory myeloma were treated with bortezomib, the overall response rate was 35%, including a 3% rate of complete response. In addition, myeloma protein was detectable only by immunofixation in 6% of patients. The median overall survival was 16 months, with a median duration of response of 12 months. Thrombocytopenia and neuropathy were the most frequent serious adverse events.

More recently, several phase I and II trials of bortezomib have demonstrated response rates of 25% to 50% for patients with relapsed and refractory mantle cell lymphoma, with activity against follicular and marginal zone lymphomas as well. In contrast, activity is minimal in diffuse large B-cell non-Hodgkin's lymphoma, small lymphocytic lymphoma/chronic lymphocytic leukemia, and is virtually absent in Hodgkin's lymphoma.

The most problematic side effects of bortezomib include thrombocytopenia and peripheral neuropathy.

Suggested Reading

Mileshkin L, Biagi JJ, Mitchell P, et al. Multicenter phase 2 trial of thalidomide in relapsed/refractory multiple myeloma: adverse prognostic impact of advanced age. *Blood.* 2003;102(1):69-77.

Richardson PG, Barlogie B, Berenson J, et al. A phase 2 study of bortezomib in relapsed, refractory myeloma. *N Engl J Med.* 2003;348(26):2609-2617.

Weber D, Rankin K, Gavino M, et al. Thalidomide alone or with dexamethasone for previously untreated multiple myeloma. *J Clin Oncol.* 2003;21(1):16-19.

O'Connor OA, Wright J, Moskowitz C, et al. Phase II clinical experience with the novel proteasome inhibitor bortezomib in patients with indolent non-Hodgkin's lymphoma and mantle cell lymphoma. *J Clin Oncol.* 2005;23(4):676-684.

Goy A, Younes A, McLaughlin P, et al. Phase II study of proteasome inhibitor bortezomib in relapsed or refractory B-cell non-Hodgkin's lymphoma. *J Clin Oncol.* 2005;23(4): 667-675.

Fisher RI, Bernstein SH, Kahl BS, et al. Multicenter phase II study of bortezomib in patients with relapsed or refractory mantle cell lymphoma. *J Clin Oncol.* 2006;24(30):4867-4874.

16-7 D

Educational Objective: To understand the role of radioimmunotherapy in follicular, low-grade non-Hodgkin's lymphoma.

Radioimmunotherapy, with ^{90}Y-ibritumomab tiuxetan and iodine-131-labeled (^{131}I) tositumomab, have been approved for the treatment of follicular and low-grade non-Hodgkin's lymphoma. ^{90}Y-ibritumomab localizes to bone; therefore, the major adverse effect is myelosuppression. ^{131}I-tositumomab localizes primarily to the thyroid leading to hypothyroidism, and it also results in myelosuppression. Both agents have been associated with an increased risk of secondary acute myelogenous leukemia and myelodysplastic syndrome. These drugs induce responses for more than 60% of patients with relapsed or refractory disease following rituximab, although the complete response rate is only in the range of 25%. Because of the associated myelosuppression, these drugs should be restricted to patients who have less than 25% bone marrow involvement. In general, the nadir following administration of these agents occurs at around 6 to 9 weeks, yet growth factor support is necessary for fewer than 15% of patients, with fewer than 10% of patients requiring hospitalization for infections. In a randomized study, rituximab-naive patients were randomly assigned to treatment with either rituximab or ^{90}Y-ibritumomab tiuxetan therapy. In a phase III randomized trial in which ^{90}Y-ibritumomab tiuxetan was compared with rituximab, the radioimmunoconjugate was associated with better rates of complete response (34% and 20%) and overall response (80% and 56%); however, no advantage in time-to-progression was detected as the study was not sufficiently powered for that endpoint.

Suggested Reading

Cheson BD. Radioimmunotherapy of non-Hodgkin lymphomas. *Blood.* 2003;101(3):391-398.

Witzig TE, Flinn IW, Gordon LI, et al. Treatment with ibritumomab tiuxetan radioimmunotherapy in patients with rituximab-refractory follicular non-Hodgkin's lymphoma. *J Clin Oncol.* 2002;20(15):3262-3269.

Witzig TE, Gordon LI, Cabanillas F, et al. Randomized controlled trial of yttrium-90-labeled ibritumomab tiuxetan radioimmunotherapy versus rituximab immunotherapy for patients with relapsed or refractory low-grade, follicular, or transformed B-cell non-Hodgkin's lymphoma. *J Clin Oncol.* 2002; 20(10):2453-2463.

Witzig TE, White CA, Gordon LI, et al. Safety of yttrium-90 ibritumomab tiuxetan radioimmunotherapy for relapsed low-grade, follicular, or transformed non-Hodgkin's lymphoma. *J Clin Oncol.* 2003;21(7):1263-1270.

Cheson BD. Radioimmunotherapy of non-Hodgkin's lymphomas. *Curr Drug Targets.* 2006;7(10):1293-1300.

Witzig TE, Gordon LI, Cabanillas F, et al. Randomized controlled trial of yttrium-90-labeled ibritumomab tiuxetan radioimmunotherapy versus rituximab immunotherapy for patients with relapsed or refractory low-grade, follicular, or transformed B-cell non-Hodgkin's lymphoma. *J Clin Oncol.* 2002; 20(10):2453-2463.

16-8 C

Educational Objective: To recognize the prognostic importance of molecular findings in non-Hodgkin's lymphoma.

The t(2;5) is a feature of anaplastic large cell non-Hodgkin's lymphoma, the most favorable of the peripheral T-cell non-Hodgkin's lymphomas. At the time of presentation, a large proportion of patients are in a favorable risk group, according to the International Prognostic Index. With chemotherapy regimens such as CHOP, approximately 70% of patients have long-term disease-free survival. Of patients with a score of 0 to 1 on the International Prognostic Index, more than 90% may be cured. The outcome is not as favorable for patients who are treated with an alkylating agent.

The t(11;14) is the site of the BCL-1 oncogene. It is associated with mantle cell lymphoma, with the diagnostic feature being positive staining for cyclin D1. Mantle cell lymphoma is considered one of the most unfavorable lymphomas. It is incurable with current therapies and exhibits an aggressive course, with a median survival of 3.5 to 4.0 years.

The t(14;18) is the site of the BCL-2 gene, which is overexpressed in 80% to 90% of follicular lymphomas, almost all patients with chronic lymphocytic leukemia (CLL), and one-fourth of patients with large cell non-Hodgkin's lymphoma. In general, overproduction of the protein is associated with an unfavorable outcome.

The t(9;14) is associated with production of PAX-5 which is a feature of immunocytoma. These indolent non-Hodgkin's lymphomas are incurable. The t(1;14) is a feature of marginal zone non-Hodgkin's lymphoma, with the BCL-10 gene resulting in Caspase recruitment domaine. Marginal zone lymphomas are indolent lymphomas that are generally incurable.

Suggested Reading

Falini B, Mason DY. Proteins encoded by genes involved in chromosomal alterations in lymphoma and leukemia: Clinical value of their detection by immunocytochemistry. *Blood.* 2002;99(2): 409-426.

Gascoyne RD, Aoun P, Wu D, et al. Prognostic significance of anaplastic lymphoma kinase (ALK) protein expression in adults with anaplastic large cell lymphoma. *Blood.* 1999;93(11):3913-3921.

Hill ME, MacLennan KA, Cunningham DC, et al. Prognostic significance of bcl-2 expression and bcl-2 major breakpoint region rearrangement in diffuse large cell non-Hodgkin's lymphoma: a British National Lymphoma Investigation study. *Blood.* 1996;88(3):1046-1051.

Kauh J, Baidas SM, Ozdemirli M, et al. Mantle cell lymphoma: clinicopathologic features and treatments. *Oncology (Williston Park).* 2003;17(6): 879-896.

Stein H, Foss H D, Dùrkop H, et al. CD30+ anaplastic large cell lymphoma: a review of its histopathologic, genetic, and clinical features. *Blood.* 2000;96(12):3681-3695.

16-9 D

Educational Objective: To understand the characteristics of lymphoproliferative disorder after transplantation.

Lymphoproliferative disorder after transplantation is an entity similar to lymphomas that are associated with human immunodeficiency virus infection. These lymphomas develop in the setting of immunosuppression and often occur in extranodal sites. They have a heterogeneous morphology, ranging from a polyclonal lymphocytosis to a monoclonal lymphoid tumor. These lymphomas can be divided into two groups: the more common are lymphomas that occur early (1 year or less after transplantation) or lymphomas that occur later (more than 1 year). The tumors that occur early are generally of B cell origin and uniformly positive for EBV, and the tumors that occur late may be negative for EBV and of T-cell origin. The early-occurring tumors often regress following withdrawal of immunosuppression. In contrast, withdrawal of immunosuppression for the monoclonal tumors may result in resolution of the tumor, but that is generally short-term. In general, tumors that develop late require treatment with aggressive chemotherapy. Additional treatment strategies currently being studied include the use of rituximab alone or in combination with chemotherapy, and EBV-specific cytotoxic T-lymphocytes.

Suggested Reading

Ambinder R. Posttransplant lymphoproliferative disease: pathogenesis, monitoring, and therapy. *Curr Onc Rep.* 2003;5(9): 359-363.

Leblond V, Davi F, Charlotte F, et al. Posttransplant lym phoproliferative disorders not associated with Ebstein-Barr virus: a distinct entity? *J Clin Oncol.* 1998;16(3):2052-2059.

Leblond V, Dhedin N, Mamzer Bruneel MF, et al. Identification of prognostic factors in 61 patients with posttransplantation lymphoproliferative disorders. *J Clin Oncol.* 2001;19(3):772-778.

Soler MJ, Puig JM, Mir M, et al. Posttransplant lymphoproliferative disease: treatment and outcome in renal transplant patients. *Transpl Proc.* 2003;35(5):1709-1713.

Porcu P. New approaches to posttransplant lymphoproliferative disorder (PTLD). *Clin Adv Hematol Oncol.* 2005;3(1):24-26.

16-10 A

Educational Objective: To recognize the unique features of angioimmunoblastic T-cell lymphoma.

Angioimmunoblastic T-cell lymphoma was formerly known as angioimmunoblastic lymphadenopathy with disproteinemia. It tends to occur in older patients and has no known etiology. It accounts for 15% to 20% of T-cell malignant diseases in adults. At the time of presentation, patients most often have generalized lymphadenopathy, hepatosplenomegaly, and skin rash. The clinical course tends to be aggressive, and median survival is less than 3 years. A variety of therapies have been used, including CHOP, fludarabine, and interferon, but infectious complications are common and interfere with therapy.

Anaplastic large T-cell lymphoma also may have R–S-like cells but is characteristically CD30-positive, and it is positive for the ALK protein in most cases. The malignant cells tend to be large with horseshoe-shaped nuclei. Patients with this disease also tend to have disease-related symptoms and advanced-stage disease at the time of presentation. There is no vascular proliferation as with the angioimmunoblastic T-cell lymphoma. In 75% of cases, CD3 and CD8 are negative. Anaplastic large T-cell lymphoma may be morphologically confused with Hodgkin's lymphoma; however, the latter, is a B-cell disease.

The phenotype rules out mycosis fungoides, which is CD2-positive, CD3-positive, CD4-positive, but usually CD8-negative. The cells tend to be cerebriform in appearance. The clonality of the T-cells is evidence that this process is not merely a reactive one.

Suggested Reading

Dogan A, Attygalle AD, Kyriakou C. Angioimmunoblastic lymphadenopathy. *Br J Haematol.* 2003;121(5):681-691.

SELF EVALUATION

CHAPTER 17 QUESTIONS:
HEMATOPOIETIC CELL TRANSPLANTATION

17-1 A 48-year-old man was initially treated for stage III diffuse large cell lymphoma 6 years earlier and complete remission was achieved with six cycles of combination chemotherapy with cyclophosphamide, vicristine, prednisone, and doxorubicin.

Eighteen months after diagnosis, the patient had relapse, with disease in previously involved nodes, and received treatment with two cycles of ifosfamide, etoposide, and carboplatin followed by peripheral stem cell collection and autologous transplantation. The preparative regimen included cyclophosphamide and total body radiation. The patient had a complete remission and remained well until now. He now presents with new-onset anemia and thrombocytopenia. His physical examination is normal. His complete blood count shows a hematocrit of 29%, a mean corpusular value of 102 fL, a reticulocyte count of 0.1%, a leukocyte count of 3.9 × $10^3/\mu L$ with a normal differential, and a platelet count of 62 × $10^3/\mu L$.

Which of the following is the most likely reason for the anemia and thrombocytopenia?

A. Myelodysplasia
B. Graft failure
C. Recurrent lymphoma
D. Epstein-Barr virus (EBV)-related lymphoproliferative syndrome

17-2 A 45-year-old man presents with oral sicca and elevated serum levels of liver function tests 90 days after receiving a transplant from a matched sibling for chronic myeloid leukemia in chronic phase. The preparative regimen involved busulfan and cyclophosphamide. A pathologically confirmed diagnosis of chronic graft-versus-host disease limited to skin and liver is made, and prednisone (1 mg/kg per day) is added to a stable dose of cyclosporine. Ten days later, cytomegalovirus (CMV) antigens are detected in the peripheral blood for the first time following transplantation, and treatment with intravenous ganciclovir (5 mg/kg twice daily) is begun. Ten days later, the granulocyte count has decreased from a normal value to 0.7 × $10^3/\mu L$.

Which of the following is the most likely cause of the granulocytopenia?

A. Chronic graft-versus-host disease
B. CMV infection of the marrow
C. Ganciclovir toxicity
D. Recurrence of leukemia
E. Graft rejection

17-3 A 56-year-old woman with multiple myeloma underwent an autologous peripheral blood transplant after a preparative regimen of melphalan 200 mg/m^2. The patient had an uneventful early post-transplant course, but on day 28 developed new onset anorexia and vomiting. An upper endoscopy showed gross and microscopic changes consistent with graft-versus-host disease.

Which of the following is the most appropriate next step?

A. Human leukocyte antigen (HLA) type the patient's peripheral blood to rule out transfusion-induced graft-versus-host disease
B. Treat with fluids and gut rest
C. Begin cyclosporine
D. Begin a short course of prednisone

17-4 A 49-year-old woman presents with newly diagnosed acute myeloid leukemia (AML). Bone marrow cytogenetics show complex chromosome abnormalities. The patient is married with three children and has two full siblings. Both parents are deceased.

Concerning HLA typing, which of the following is the best course to take?

A. Delay drawing blood for typing from the patient until achievement of first remission
B. Type patient and her siblings now
C. Type patient, her siblings, and her children now
D. Type patient, her siblings, and her husband now

17-5 Fourteen days ago, a 40-year-old man with acute lymphocytic leukemia in second relapse received an infusion of granulocyte-colony stimulating factor (G-CSF)-mobilized peripheral blood stem cells from a matched unrelated donor following a conditioning regimen of cyclophosphamide and total body radiation. Prophylaxis against graft-versus-host disease is with methotrexate and cyclosporine. He is now being evaluated for the recent onset of jaundice.

On physical examination, scleral icterus is noted. A mild erythematous rash is also observed on the upper part of the back, and the patient reports that it has been present for 2 days. The liver is palpable two fingerbreadths below the right costal margin and is tender to palpation. There is a suggestion of ascites. He is febrile (38.2°C), and he had a weight gain of approximately 9 pounds during the past week. After a nadir peripheral white blood cell count following transplantation, the count has recovered to 0.7 × 10^3/μL, and the platelet count is 40 × 10^3/μL. The results of liver function tests have become increasingly abnormal, with a serum bilirubin of 6 mg/dL, a serum aspartate aminotransferase of 160 L, and a serum alanine aminotransferase of 420 L.

Which of the following is the most likely cause of the patient's clinical condition?

A. Allogeneic engraftment syndrome
B. Graft-versus-host disease
C. Biliary sludge associated with hyperalimentation
D. Veno-occlusive disease of the liver
E. Cyclosporine toxicity

CHAPTER 17 EXPLANATORY ANSWERS:
HEMATOPOIETIC CELL TRANSPLANTATION

17-1 A

Educational Objective: To recognize the potential complications of autologous hematopoietic cell transplantation.

A high incidence of myelodysplasia (nearly 10%), has been reported following autologous transplantation for lymphoma. Whether myelodysplasia is a consequence of the transplant or the long-term effects of chemotherapy received before the transplantation is uncertain, and retrospective analyses have reported that the risk of myelodysplasia is related to the total amount of therapy received by the patient. Graft failure as a result of stem cell exhaustion, if it occurs at all, is extremely rare. Large cell lymphoma recurring solely in the marrow would also be uncommon. EBV-related lymphoproliferative syndrome is not generally a complication seen after autologous transplantation.

Suggested Reading

Metayer C, Curtis RE, Vose J, et al. Myelodysplastic syndrome and acute myeloid leukemia after autotransplantation for lymphoma: a multicenter case-control study. *Blood.* 2003;101(5):2015–2023.

Pedersen-Bjergaard J, Andersen MK, Christiansen DH. Therapy-related acute myeloid leukemia and myelodysplasia after high-dose chemotherapy and autologous stem cell transplantation. *Blood.* 2000;95(11):3273–3279.

17-2 C

Educational Objective: To recognize the myelosuppressive effects of ganciclovir.

Ganciclovir frequently results in myelosuppression when used following transplantation. Most experts recommend continuing the drug and treating the neutropenia with G-CSF, if possible. Chronic graft-versus-host disease can be associated with marrow suppression, but that disease usually affects platelets more than neutrophils. CMV can occasionally affect the marrow, but is far less common than ganciclovir-related toxicity. Recurrence of chronic myeloid leukemia is uncommon after transplantation and should not cause neutropenia. Graft failure following non-T cell-depleted transplants after a full conditioning regimen is uncommon.

Suggested Reading

Goodrich JM, Bowden RA, Fisher L, et al. Ganciclovir prophylaxis to prevent cytomegalovirus disease after allogeneic marrow transplant. *Ann Intern Med.* 1993;118(3):173–178.

17-3 D

Educational Objective: To recognize the syndrome of autologous graft-versus-host disease and its appropriate treatment.

A syndrome of autologous graft-versus-host disease occurs in 10% to 15% of patients undergoing high-dose therapy followed by autologous stem cell transplantation. The most common presentation is persistent or new-onset anorexia and can be confirmed by intestinal biopsy. The syndrome is more common in women, virtually always responds to a short course of prednisone, and does not affect overall survival.

Suggested Reading

Holmberg L, Kikuchi K, Gooley TA, et al. Gastrointestinal graft-versus-host disease in recipients of autologous hematopoietic stem cells: incidence, risk factors, and outcome. *Biol Blood Marrow Transplant.* 2006;12(2):226–234.

17-4 B

Educational Objective: To recognize appropriate steps to take to identify potential hematopoietic cell donors.

Patients with AML who are potential transplant candidates are best typed at diagnosis so that if their disease fails to achieve a complete remission, they can still proceed to transplantation without unnecessary delay. The presence of leukemic blasts usually does not interfere with typing results. The patient's siblings also should be typed. Typing the children (or the husband as a surrogate) is much less likely to yield an appropriate donor and is generally recommended only if the patient has a very common HLA allele.

Suggested Reading

Biggs JC, Horowitz MM, Gale RP, et al. Bone marrow transplants may cure patients with acute leukemia never achieving remission with chemotherapy. *Blood.* 1992;80(4):1090–1093.

Fung HC, Stein A, Slovak M, et al. A long-term follow-up report on allogeneic stem cell transplantation for patients with primary refractory acute myelogenous leukemia: impact of cytogenetic characteristics on transplantation outcome. *Biol Blood Marrow Transplant.* 2003;9(12):766–771.

17-5 D

Educational Objective: To distinguish clinical features of veno-occlusive disease of the liver.

Veno-occlusive disease of the liver can be seen within 1 to 4 weeks after a transplant conditioning regimen. Signs include weight gain, ascites, tender hepatomegaly, and jaundice. The overall incidence of veno-occlusive disease is approximately 10% but varies according to the preparative regimen. The incidence is higher for patients with abnormal results of liver function tests before transplant. No therapy has been demonstrated to be effective, although results with defibrotide have been encouraging. Acute graft-versus-host disease (and the so-called engraftment syndrome) can cause elevated levels of liver enzymes but is not associated with tender hepatomegaly or weight gain. The same is true for the elevated levels of liver enzymes associated with hyperalimentation or cyclosporine-related toxicity.

Suggested Reading

Bearman SI. The syndrome of hepatic veno-occlusive disease after marrow transplantation. *Blood.* 1995;85(20):3005–3020.

Richardson PG, Elias AD, Krishnan A, et al. Treatment of severe veno-occlusive disease with defibrotide—compassionate use results in response without significant toxicity in a high-risk population. *Blood.* 1998;92(3):737–744.

SELF EVALUATION

CHAPTER 18 QUESTIONS:
SYMPTOM MANAGEMENT

18-1 A 62-year-old woman presents with a 6-year history of ovarian cancer. At the time of the initial diagnosis, she had an exploratory laparotomy with debulking, followed by platinum-based chemotherapy. Two years later, disease recurred, and she had a recurrent laparotomy with a debulking. She then received chemotherapy with topotecan. Over the past 1.5 years, she has had intermittently progressing ovarian cancer signaled by rising CA-125 levels, despite treatment with hexamethylmelamine and tamoxifen. She now has symptoms suggestive of small bowel obstruction. She has never taken opioids.

The findings on physical examination are remarkable for mild cachexia and a distended abdomen with quiet bowel sounds. There is no evidence of rebound or tenderness. A radiograph of the abdomen shows small bowel obstruction. A nasogastric tube is inserted. Surgeons have been consulted and have recommended against any surgical procedure. Clamping of the nasogastric tube after 5 days results in recurrent symptoms of nausea and vomiting. The patient has had no flatus.

Which of the following medications has been shown to provide symptomatic improvement in this setting?

A. Amoxicillin
B. Senna laxative
C. Octreotide
D. Nalaxone

18-2 A 57-year-old man with prostate cancer that is metastatic to the bone is receiving hospice care.

Immediate-release morphine sulphate has been prescribed at a dose of 30 mg every 4 to 6 hours as needed for pain. He has been taking an average of 120 mg daily for the past several days. He is tolerating it well but still having substantial pain, with an average score of 7 on a pain scale of 0 to 10.

A decision is made to prescribe sustained-release morphine at a dose of 90 mg orally twice a day. An appropriate bowel regimen is prescribed. In addition to the sustained-release morphine, his physician decides to provide an as-needed, 30-mg dose of immediate-release morphine.

At which of the following intervals should this as needed, oral immediate-release morphine be available for the patient to take for unrelieved pain?

A. 15 minutes
B. 1 hour
C. 3 hours
D. 4 hours

18-3 A 55-year-old woman with breast cancer that is metastatic to the bone presents because of substantial pain that is not well controlled with a nonsteroidal anti-inflammatory drug. Her physician decides to begin treatment with an opioid. The patient is educated with regard to the side effects of opioid medications and is told that many of the side effects are temporary. However, you tell her that she should expect one side effect to be chronic and require treatment with other medications.

Which of the following side effects is this chronic toxicity that oftentimes needs ongoing management?

A. Nausea
B. Sedation
C. Constipation
D. Cognitive impairment

18-4 **A 52-year-old woman presents with severe hot flashes that affect her quality of life. She has a history of stage II, estrogen receptorpositive breast cancer that was diagnosed 2 years previously. At that time, she was treated with a lumpectomy, radiation therapy, and adjuvant chemotherapy. She became menopausal shortly after the chemotherapy was started. She now takes tamoxifen. She has had no evidence of recurrent breast cancer since the diagnosis, and the current history and findings on physical examination are normal.**

The patient reports having five or six hot flashes during the day in addition to awaking two or three times each night with drenching night sweats. She has tried vitamin E without relief.

Which of the following is the best choice for treating her hot flashes?

A. Venlafaxine
B. Amitriptyline
C. Lorazepam
D. Soy protein

18-5 **A 53-year-old woman has testing of bone mineral density as part of a general health evaluation. She has a history of stage I breast cancer 5 years ago and has been without recurrence. The results of bone mineral density testing demonstrate a T score of–1.6, which is an indication of mild osteopenia but not osteoporosis. The patient has no family history of osteoporosis. Her diet does not include many dairy products.**

Which of the following should you recommend for this patient?

A. Calcium and vitamin D
B. Calcitonin
C. A bisphosphonate
D. Vitamin E

18-6 **A 60-year-old woman receiving adjuvant tamoxifen has substantial hot flashes for which she desires therapy. Which of the following choices is the best choice to palliate her hot flashes?**

A. Paroxetine (Paxil)
B. Fluoxetine (Prozac)
C. Gabapentin (Neurtontin)
D. Sertraline (Zoloft)

18-7 **A 60-year-old woman is scheduled to receive cisplatin-based chemotherapy. As such, her physician plans to give her a serotonin-3 receptor antagonist and a corticosteroid. Her physician discusses the pros and cons of adding aprepitant. The patient asks her oncologist what additional percent of patients will not vomit in the 5 days after chemotherapy if they use aprepitant. The answer is:**

A. 3%
B. 10%
C. 50%
D. 80%

18-8 **A 50-year-old man is being treated with gemcitabine for metastatic pancreatic cancer. He tolerates the chemotherapy reasonably well but has anorexia and weight loss. The patient asks for something to help him gain weight. Because of a history of thromboembolic complications, he and his physician decide not to use megestrol acetate.**

Which of the following drugs has been shown, in multiple placebo-controlled trials, to stimulate appetite in this setting?

A. A corticosteroid
B. Dronabinol (a cannabinoid)
C. Fluoxymesterone (an androgen)
D. Eicosopentenoic acid

18-9 **Severe diarrhea developed in a 72-year-old patient with rectal cancer, 2 weeks after treatment with an initial course of continuous infusion of fluorouracil and pelvic radiation, given postoperatively. Treatment for the diarrhea is begun with loperamide 2 mg for every loose stool, to a total dose of 20 mg daily.**

Despite this treatment, diarrhea continues to be a substantial problem, with 10 watery stools daily. The patient is otherwise in good condition and is ingesting adequate liquids to maintain normal hydration.

Which of the following medications would you recommend to alleviate this treatment-induced diarrhea?

A. Octreotide
B. Sucralfate
C. Ozalazine
D. Glutamine

18-10 A patient with advanced incurable cancer has been placed on hospice and is being treated at home with substantial support from extended family. The patient had been comfortable but, during the preceding week, has become weaker. As a result of hepatic insufficiency, the patient became comatose 2 days ago. He does not appear to be in any pain and is breathing comfortably. However, during the past 12 hours, a gurgling sound developed in the back of his throat with respirations. He does not appear to be coughing or to be otherwise uncomfortable, but the family is distressed about whether the patient is "drowning in his own secretions." They ask if something can be done.

Which of the following would you recommend to dry the secretions to treat this so-called death rattle?

A. Lorazepam
B. Propranolol
C. Dexamethasone
D. Atropine

CHAPTER 18 EXPLANATORY ANSWERS:
SYMPTOM MANAGEMENT

18-1 C

Educational Objective: To understand the use of octreotide for the treatment of small bowel obstruction.

Somatostatin is the naturally occurring precursor hormone of octreotide. It functions as a neurotransmitter and a neurohormone with regulatory effects in the gastrointestinal tract and has both endocrine and exocrine effects on the pancreas. The net effect of somatostatin is generally inhibitory. It inhibits the glandular secretion of growth hormone, thyrotropin, corticotropin, and prolactin and decreases the release of gastrin, cholecystokinin, insulin, glucagon, gastric acid, and pancreatic enzymes. It also prevents neurotransmission in the peripheral nerves of the gastrointestinal tract leading to decreased peristalsis and a decrease in splanchnic blood flow. There is some indication that somatostatin inhibits the function of activated immune cells and may have a central opioid-like function.

The dosing regimen of octreotide for gastrointestinal obstruction for patients with cancer is not well established. Therapy can be initiated at 10 mg per hour either intravenously or subcutaneously and titrated every 24 hours to control the symptoms of nausea and vomiting. Alternatively, octreotide can be instituted as an intermittent subcutaneous injection at 50 mg every 8 hours and titrated every 24 hours.

Octreotide is generally well tolerated. Most patients describe no side effects. The most common side effect is dry mouth, which is amenable to ice chips and moist troches. Although octreotide has been reported to cause nausea, abdominal pain, and diarrhea (4% to 7%), the results of published studies that have examined the treatment of bowel obstruction show improvement in these symptoms. Long-term therapy has been shown to lead to biliary sludging with actual stone formation (15% to 20%); however, patients in this setting are unlikely to live long enough for these side effects to be a concern. Because of its effects on insulin and glucagon secretion, octreotide has been reported to cause mild hyperglycemia. These possible side effects have not been reported to be of clinical importance in the management of gastrointestinal obstruction even with the use of high doses (up to 150 mg per hour or 3,600 mg daily). There are some patients with obstruction for whom the use of octreotide has been associated with cessation of nausea and vomiting, removal of nasogastric tubes, and, in some cases, the ability to resume modest oral intake. Thus, octreotide appears to be a reasonable therapy to try, pending data from a placebo-controlled evaluation in this setting.

Other treatment strategies in this setting include use of percutaneous endoscopic gastrostomy tube as decompression with connection to intermittent suction on an as-needed basis. This allows patients to take in small amounts of oral intake for the pleasure of taste and eating; gastric contents can then be removed when symptoms redevelop.

Suggested Reading

Mangili G, Franchi M, Mariani A, et al. Octreotide in the management of bowel obstruction in terminal ovarian cancer. *Gynecol Oncol.* 1996;61(3):345–348.

Mercadante S, Maddaloni S. Octreotide in the management of inoperable gastrointestinal obstruction in terminal cancer patients. *J Pain Symptom Manage.* 1992;7(8):496–498.

Riley J, Fallon MT. Octreotide in terminal malignant obstruction of the gastrointestinal tract. *Eur J Palliat Care.* 1994;1(1): 23–25.

18-2 B

Educational Objective: To understand that the use of as-needed, immediate-release morphine should be prescribed based on time to maximal response, not on the half-life of the drug.

A common mistake is prescribing as-needed medications at 3- to 4-hour intervals based on the half-life of morphine. Rather, in a situation where morphine is being titrated for pain relief, the more appropriate time to dose this medication is based on the time-to-peak effect from the last dose, which occurs by 30 to 60 minutes. Thus, an interval of 1 hour is a reasonable time frame for giving the next dose of as-needed immediate-release oral morphine. If subcutaneous morphine is used, the interval should be every 15 minutes; if intravenous morphine is used, the interval should be every 5 minutes.

Suggested Reading

Davis T, Miser AW, Loprinzi CL, et al. Comparative morphine pharmacokinetics following sublingual, intramuscular and oral administration in patients with cancer. *Hosp J.* 1993;9(1): 85–90.

18-3 C

Educational Objective: To understand that constipation is a chronic toxicity to which the patient does not develop tolerance.

Many of the toxicities of narcotics are relatively temporary. Generally, the patient will become accustomed to mild nausea, sedation, and cognitive impairment. However, constipation is a long-term toxicity that must be managed appropriately.

Suggested Reading

Cleeland C, Gonin R, Hatfield A, et al. Pain and its treatment in outpatients with metastatic cancer. *N Engl J Med.* 1994;330(9): 592–596.

Grossman S, Benedetti C, Payne R, et al. NCCN practice guidelines for cancer pain. *Oncology.* 1999;13:33–44.

Levy MH. Pharmacologic treatment of cancer pain. *N Engl J Med.* 1996;335(15):1124–1132.

Portenoy R, Miransky J, Thaler H, et al. Pain in ambulatory patients with lung or colon cancer: prevalence, characteristics, and effect. *Cancer.* 1992;70(6):1616–1624.

18-4 A

Educational Objective: To understand that the newer antidepressants are effective nonhormonal agents for treating hot flashes for many women.

Multiple double-blind, placebo-controlled clinical trials have demonstrated that newer antidepressants decrease hot flashes substantially more often than placebo. This outcome is true for patients with a history of breast cancer or for women in general. It also is true for patients receiving tamoxifen compared with patients not receiving tamoxifen.

There is no good indication that the older tricyclic antidepressants are effective in this regard. Some older clinicians might be tempted to choose bellergal or a soy product. Nonetheless, there is little information to suggest that bellergal is helpful. Most of the data regarding soy products find them to be ineffective for alleviating hot flashes for women.

The choice of antidepressant is important, especially for women receiving tamoxifen because some antidepressants influence the activity of CYP 2D6 required for the activation of tamoxifen into the active form of the drug. Venlafaxine does not appear to substantially affect CYP 2D6 activity and therefore, is the drug of choice in this category. Paroxetine is a potent inhibitor of CYP 2D6; sertraline and fluoxetine are moderate inhibitors of this enzyme. Therefore, these latter drugs should not be used for women taking tamoxifen.

Suggested Reading

Barton DL, Loprinzi CL, Sloan JA, et al. Pilot evaluations of newer antidepressants for hot flashes. *Proc Am Soc Clin Oncol.* 2002;21:366a (suppl abstr 1463).

Loprinzi CL, Kugler JW, Sloan JA, et al. Venlafaxine in management of hot flashes in survivors of breast cancer: a randomised controlled trial. *Lancet.* 2000;356(9247):2059–2063.

Loprinzi CL, Pisansky TM, Fonseca R, et al. Pilot evaluation of venlafaxine hydrochloride for the therapy of hot flashes in cancer survivors. *J Clin Oncol.* 1998;16(7):2377–2381.

Loprinzi CL, Sloan JA, Perez EA, et al. Phase III evaluation of fluoxetine for treatment of hot flashes. *J Clin Oncol.* 2002;20(6): 1578–1583.

Stearns V, Beebe KL, Iyengar M, et al. Paroxetine controlled release in the treatment of menopausal hot flashes: a randomized controlled trial. *JAMA.* 2003;289(21):2827–2834.

Stearns V, Isaacs C, Rowland J, et al. A pilot trial assessing the efficacy of paroxetine hydrochloride (Paxil) in controlling hot flashes in breast cancer survivors. *Ann Oncol.* 2000;11(1): 17–22.

Borges S, Desta Z, Li L, et al. Quantitative effect of CYP2D6 genotype and inhibitors on tamoxifen metabolism: Implication for optimization of breast cancer treatment. *Clin Pharmacol Ther.* 2006;80(1):61–74.

18-5 A

Educational Objective: To understand that calcium and vitamin D should be the mainstay for maintaining appropriate bone health for women.

This patient clearly must maintain optimal calcium and vitamin D intake, which can be a combination of both dietary and supplemental sources. This patient should take 1,200 to 1,500 mg daily of elemental calcium along with 400 to 800 IU of daily vitamin D. Vitamin E has no role for bone health in this setting. Calcitonin and bisphosphonates might be used for some patients with osteoporosis (T score of –2.5 or worse); however, they are not generally indicated for osteopenia.

Suggested Reading

Bruning PF, Pit MJ, de Jong-Bakker M, et al. Bone mineral density after adjuvant chemotherapy for premenopausal breast cancer. *Br J Cancer.* 1990;61(2):308–310.

Delmas PD, Fontana A. Bone loss induced by cancer treatment and its management. *Eur J Cancer.* 1998;34(2):260–262.

Kanis JA, McCloskey EV, Powles T, et al. A high incidence of vertebral fracture in women with breast cancer. *Br J Cancer.* 1999;79(7-8):1179–1181.

NIH Consensus Development Panel on Osteoporosis Prevention, Diagnosis, and Therapy. Osteoporosis prevention, diagnosis, and therapy. *JAMA.* 2001;285(6):785–795.

18-6 C

Educational Objective: To understand that CYP2D6 inhibitors should not be given with tamoxifen.

Tamoxifen itself is relatively inactive against breast cancer. However, its active metabolite, endoxifen, appears to be the most important component to show activity against breast cancer. The tamoxifen is converted to endoxifen by an enzyme labeled CYP2D6. There are several drugs which can inhibit CYP2D6 activity. Paroxetine is a potent inhibitor of CYP2D6. Fluoxetine and sertraline are moderate inhibitors of CYP2D6. To date there is no suggestion that gabapentin affects CYP2D6 activity. Of note, venlafaxine also does not appear to substantially inhibit CYP2D6 activity, so this would be another potential option for this patient.

Suggested Reading

Borges S, Desta Z, Li L, et al. Quantitative effect of CYP2D6 genotype and inhibitors on tamoxifen metabolism: implication for optimization of breast cancer treatment. *Clin Pharmacol Ther.* 2006;80(1):61–74.

Jin Y, Desta Z, Stearns V, et al. CYP2D6 genotype, antidepressant use, and tamoxifen metabolism during adjuvant breast cancer treatment. *J Natl Cancer Inst.* 2005;97(1):30–39.

Goetz MP, Loprinzi CL. A hot flash on tamoxifen metabolism. *J Natl Cancer Inst.* 2003;95(23):1734–1735.

18-7 B

Educational Objective: To understand that the degree of benefit for aprepitant.

Aprepitant does increase the percentage of patients who will not vomit for 5 days after chemotherapy. This increases by about 10% to 15%.

Suggested Reading

Kris MG, Hesketh PJ, Somerfield MR, et al. American Society of Clinical Oncology guideline for antiemetics in oncology: update 2006. *J Clin Oncol.* 2006;24(18):2932–2947.

Hesketh PJ, Grunberg SM, Herrstedt J, et al. Combined data from two phase III trials of the NK1 antagonist aprepitant plus a 5HT 3 antagonist and a corticosteroid for prevention of chemotherapy-induced nausea and vomiting effect of gender treatment response. *Support Care Cancer.* 2006;14(4):354–360.

18-8 A

Educational Objective: To recognize that the findings from several placebo-controlled trials demonstrate that both corticosteroids and progestational agents improve appetite for patients with cancer-related anorexia and cachexia.

The results from more than 10 placebo-controlled clinical trials show that megestrol acetate stimulates the appetites of patients with advanced cancer-induced anorexia and cachexia. It also leads to weight gain. Findings from a smaller number of trials have shown the same results with a cousin medication, medroxyprogesterone acetate. In addition, evidence from five placebo-controlled trials indicates that corticosteroids stimulate the appetites of patients with advanced cancer-induced anorexia and cachexia.

Megestrol acetate is better tolerated than dexamethasone because it does not generally have steroid toxicities. Nonetheless, it causes adrenocortical suppression that may require stress doses of corticosteroids if patients undergo a trauma, infection, or a surgical procedure while receiving this drug, or if they recently stopped taking this agent.

A corticosteroid such as dexamethasone is a reasonable alternative for treating patients if a patient has a history of thromboembolic complications; it is only likely to be given for a short period of time (before steroid toxicities are likely to become problematic); or if expense is a major factor in the decision-making process.

Although findings from pilot studies suggested that cannabinoids (i.e., dronabinol), androgenic agents (i.e., fluoxymesterone), and eicosopentenoic acid might be helpful for treating cancer-induced anorexia and cachexia, controlled trials have failed to substantiate these claims.

Suggested Reading

Jatoi A, Kumar S, Sloan J, et al. On appetite and its loss. *J Clin Oncol.* 2000;18(15):2930–2932.

Jatoi A, Windschitl HE, Loprinzi CL, et al. Dronabinol versus megestrol acetate versus combination therapy for cancer-associated anorexia: a North Central Cancer Treatment Group study. *J Clin Oncol.* 2002;20(2):567–573.

Loprinzi CL, Bernath AM, Schaid DJ, et al. Phase III evaluation of megestrol acetate as therapy for patients with cancer anorexia and/or cachexia. *Oncology.* 1994;51 Suppl 1:2–7.

Loprinzi CL, Ellison NM, Schaid DJ, et al. Controlled trial of megestrol acetate for the treatment of cancer anorexia and cachexia. *J Natl Cancer Inst.* 1990;82(13):1127–1132.

Loprinzi CL, Kugler JW, Sloan JA, et al. Randomized comparison of megestrol acetate versus dexamethasone versus fluoxymesterone for the treatment of cancer anorexia/cachexia. *J Clin Oncol.* 1999;17(10):3299–3306.

18-9 A

Educational Objective: To understand that octreotide is an effective means to treat cytotoxic therapy-induced diarrhea.

The results of a randomized trial indicated that subcutaneous octreotide (0.1 mg three times a day) was more effective than 10 mg of daily diphenoxylate for the treatment of radiation-induced diarrhea. Diarrhea resolved within 3 days for 81% of the octreotide group compared with 19% of patients in the diphenoxylate group.

There are some agents that have been shown, in placebo-controlled trials, to actually increase diarrhea (e.g., ozalazine) or to have unacceptable side effects (e.g., sucralfate) for patients with radiation-induced diarrhea. Therefore, these agents should be avoided. A placebo-controlled trial demonstrated that glutamine was not helpful in this situation, even though it did not cause toxicity.

In addition, findings from other studies have indicated that octreotide was beneficial for patients with chemotherapy-induced diarrhea.

Suggested Reading

Cascinu S, Fedeli A, Fedeli SL, et al. Control of chemotherapy-induced diarrhea with octreotide: a randomized trial with placebo in patients receiving cisplatin. *Oncology.* 1994;51(1):70–73.

Gebbia V, Carreca I, Testa A, et al. Subcutaneous octreotide versus oral loperamide in the treatment of diarrhea following chemotherapy. *Anticancer Drugs.* 1993;4(4):443–445.

Wasserman E, Hidalgo M, Hornedo J, et al. Octreotide (SMS 201-995) for hematopoietic support-dependent high-dose chemotherapy (HSD-HDC)-related diarrhoea: dose finding study and evaluation of efficacy. *Bone Marrow Transplant.* 1997;20(9):711–714.

18-10 D

Educational Objective: To understand that either scopolamine or atropine can be used to appropriately treat the "death rattle."

As patients approach death, the gag reflex and reflexive clearing of the oropharynx decline, and secretions from the tracheobronchial tree accumulate. Buildup of saliva and oropharyngeal secretions may lead to gurgling, crackling, or rattling sounds with each breath. Some have called this noise the "death rattle," a term frequently disconcerting to families and caregivers. For unprepared families and professional caregivers, it may sound like the patient is choking or suffocating.

Anticholinergic medications may be used to dry secretions in order to prevent or treat the distressing sounds. Sublingual atropine (1% ophthalmic solution; one to two drops every 1 to 4 hours) can effectively dry up oral moisture. Subcutaneous scopolamine 0.2 to 0.4 mg every 4 hours (or one to three transdermal patches every 72 hours or 0.1 to 1.0 mg each hour by continuous intravenous or subcutaneous infusion) or subcutaneous doses of glycopyrrolate 0.2 mg every 4 to 6 hours or 0.4 to 1.2 mg daily by continuous intravenous or subcutaneous infusion will effectively reduce the production of saliva and other secretions. They will minimize or eliminate the gurgling and crackling sounds and may be used prophylactically for the dying patient who is unconscious. Anecdotal evidence suggests that the earlier treatment is initiated, the better it works, as larger amounts of secretions in the upper aerodigestive tract are more difficult to eliminate. However, premature use for patients who are still alert may lead to unacceptable drying of oral and pharyngeal mucosa.

Suggested Reading

Davis CL. Palliation of breathlessness. In: von Gunten CF, ed. *Palliative Care and Rehabilitation of Cancer Patients.* Boston, Ma: Kluwer Academic Publishers; 1999:59–74.

Thomas JR, von Gunten CF. Clinical management of dyspnea. *Lancet Oncol.* 2002;3(4):223–228.

Thomas JR, von Gunten CF. Treatment of dyspnea in cancer patients. *Oncology.* 2002;16(6):745–750.

SELF EVALUATION

CHAPTER 19 QUESTIONS:

CANCER IN THE ELDERLY

19-1 A 73-year-old woman with a 40 pack-year history of smoking presents with pain in her back. Plain films show a lytic lesion consistent with metastatic disease. A chest radiograph demonstrates a right upper lobe mass. Bronchoscopy and biopsy confirm non-small cell lung cancer (NSCLC). The remainder of her metastatic workup is negative, including an x-ray of her spine. Her labwork is remarkable for a serum creatinine of 1.6 mg/dL.

The patient lives alone, still drives, and cares for herself. Her back pain is controlled with oral Tylenol. She is interested in chemotherapy if it will improve her quality of life.

Which of the following should be recommended?

A. Cisplatin/vinorelbine
B. Single-agent vinorelbine
C. Vinorelbine/gemcitabine
D. Gemcitabine/carboplatin
E. No therapy has been shown to sustain her quality of life

19-2 On routine blood screening, a 74-year-old man is found to have an elevated prostate-specific antigen. He reports no nocturia or urinary frequency. On clinical examination, the prostate is soft. Four quadrant biopsies are performed, and two cores identify cancer in 20% and 40% of the specimen. The Gleason score is 6. The patient is being treated for congestive heart failure secondary to long-standing hypertension. He has mild dementia, and because he has fallen once or twice a month, he and his wife moved into an assisted-living facility.

Which of the following would you recommend?

A. Watchful waiting
B. Radical prostatectomy
C. Cryosurgery
D. Radiation therapy
E. Brachytherapy

19-3 A 75-year-old man presents with cervical adenopathy, mediastinal adenopathy, and fevers for 3 months duration. He denies significant weight loss. A cervical lymph node biopsy confirms a diffuse large B-cell lymphoma that is CD20-positive. Marrow biopsy is negative for lymphomatous involvement, lactate dehydrogenase is 300μL, and hemoglobin is 14.7 g/dL. The patient is fully ambulatory. He is presently on an ACE inhibitor for hypertension. His white blood cell (WBC) is 7.3K/μL, his hemoglobin is 14.0 g/dL, and his platelet count is 167,000K/μL.

Which of the following do you recommend?

A. Cyclophosphamide, vincristine, and prednisone for six cycles
B. Cyclophosphamide, adriamycin, vincristine, and prednisone for six cycles
C. Cyclophosphamide, adriamycin, vincristine, and prednisone for six cycles with rituximab
D. Rituximab as a single agent
E. Hospice referral

19-4 An 81-year-old woman presents after having a lumpectomy in the upper outer quadrant of the left breast with sentinel node mapping. The findings of bilateral diagnostic mammography confirmed a spiculated lesion in the area of concern. No other abnormalities were identified in either breast. The results of an excisional biopsy demonstrated that the tumor was a grade 1 infiltrating ductal cancer, measuring 1.6 centimeters in maximum dimension. The margins of resection exceeded 4 millimeters. The primary tumor was estrogen receptor (ER) positive, progesterone receptor (PR) positive, and *HER2* negative. The sentinel node was negative.

The woman had an osteoporotic fracture of a lumbar vertebra 2 years ago and has lived with her daughter and son-in-law since then. Her medical history includes a hysterectomy for uterine fibroids and a bladder suspension procedure. Her active medical problems include mild renal failure, hypertension, and diabetes.

Which of the following would you recommend?

A. Radiation therapy to the breast
B. Mastectomy with lymph node dissection
C. Chemotherapy
D. Hormone therapy
E. Repeat excision of the biopsy cavity to achieve wider clear margins followed by no further treatment

19-5. A 78-year-old woman had a lumpectomy and axillary dissection for breast cancer. The primary tumor measures 3.5 centimeters in maximum dimension, is ER negative, PR negative, and *HER2* negative. The margins of resection are free of cancer. Two of 10 lymph nodes were involved with cancer. The patient is in excellent health, with the exception of mild hypertension for which she takes hydrochlorthiazide. She is widowed and lives in the home she shared with her husband for 35 years.

Radiation therapy to the breast is planned. What other, if any, therapy is appropriate?

A. Anastrozole
B. Tamoxifen
C. Chemotherapy
D. No additional therapy

CHAPTER 19 EXPLANATORY ANSWERS:
CANCER IN THE ELDERLY

19-1 B

Educational Objective: To identify chemotherapy with proven efficacy for elderly patients with extensive NSCLC.

This patient is an appropriate candidate for chemotherapy as her performance status is 1, and she is motivated to receive therapy. Because of renal insufficiency, cisplatin should not be considered. The Elderly Lung Cancer Vinorelbine Italian Study (ELVIS) demonstrated that single-agent vinorelbine produced an improvement in progression-free survival, overall survival, and quality of life compared with supportive care. Gemcitabine also has been shown to be well tolerated and to improve disease-free and overall survival for elderly patients with extensive NSCLC. Two separate trials have addressed the value of adding gemcitabine to vinorelbine therapy. The Multicenter Italian Lung Cancer in the Elderly Study (MILES) study randomly assigned 698 patients older than age 70 to vinorelbine or vinorelbine plus gemcitabine and found no benefit to the combination. In contrast, the Southern Italian Cooperative Oncology Group (SICOG) conducted a smaller trial in 120 patients with stage IIIB or IV NSCLC age 70 years and older and reported both improved symptom management and 1-year survival for the combination. This was a smaller study, and patients in the single-agent vinorelbine arm did more poorly than expected from other trials such as ELVIS. A Southwest Oncology Group (SWOG) trial utilized sequential vinorelbine and docetaxel with a reported response rate of 21% and median survival of 9 months. In the Cancer and Leukemia Group B study 9730, patients with IIIB and IV disease were randomly assigned to single-agent paclitaxel or paclitaxel combined with carboplatin. A preplanned subset analysis for age found that for both younger and older patients, the combination of paclitaxel and carboplatin improved response rate and failure-free survival. The most robust data support single-agent therapy for the elderly. However, data using the combination of a taxane and a platinum salt suggest that the combination is superior to a taxane alone. Given this patient's underlying renal insufficiency, single-agent vinorelbine may be prudent.

Suggested Reading

The Elderly Lung Cancer Vinorelbine Italian Study Group. Effects of vinorelbine on quality of life and survival of elderly patients with advanced non-small cell lung cancer. *J Natl Cancer Inst.* 1999;91(1):66–72.

Kanard A, Jotoi A, Castillo R, et al. Oral vinorelbine for the treatment of metastatic non-small cell lund cancer in elderly patients: a phase II trial of efficacy and toxicity. *Lung Cancer.* 2004;43(3):345–353.

Frasci G, Lorusso V, Panza N, et al. Gemcitabine plus vinorelbine versus vinorelbine alone in elderly patients with advanced non-small-cell lung cancer. *J Clin Oncol.* 2000;18(13):2529–2536.

Hesketh PJ, Chanksky L, Lau DH, et al. Sequential vinorelbine and docetaxel in advanced non-small cell lung cancer patients > 70, or with performance status 2: A SWOG phase II trial. *Proc Amer Soc Clin Oncol.* 2004;23 (Suppl abst 7056):627.

Lilenbaum RC, Herndon JE, 2nd, List MA, et al. Single-agent versus combination chemotherapy in advanced non-small-cell lung cancer: the Cancer and Leukemia Group B (study 9730). *J Clin Oncol.* 2005;23(1):190–196.

19-2 A

Educational Objective: To recognize that frail older patients should be treated with palliative measures only.

Although this patient is relatively young, he has two geriatric syndromes (frequent falls and dementia). Thus, he meets the criteria for frailty, which is defined as a functional reserve that is substantially compromised; therefore, palliative measures alone are indicated.

The Scandinavian Prostate Cancer Group conducted a trial to address the question of whether any treatment is necessary for early-stage prostate cancer. Radical prostatectomy was compared with so-called watchful waiting (observation only) in a controlled trial involving 695 men with localized prostate cancer. After 6 years of follow-up, the overall survival for the observation-only arm was equivalent to that for the radical prostatectomy arm. However, the patients who had surgery were less likely to die of prostate cancer. A quality-of-life trial conducted in conjunction with that study demonstrated that radical prostatectomy was associated with a greater frequency of erectile dysfunction and urinary leakage but with a lower frequency of urinary obstruction. After 2 additional years of follow-up, this trial demonstrated that patients randomly assigned to radical prostatectomy had a significant improvement in cancer-specific and overall survival, fewer distant metastases, and superior local disease control. When the patient's survival is limited by other comorbid conditions, watchful waiting is appropriate; treatment may be initiated when symptoms develop. Watchful waiting has been advocated for men older than age 70, with a normal digital rectal exam, who have had two biopsies or less that demonstrate cancer and that contain less than 50% cancer, a Gleason score of less than 6, and clinical T1c disease. Surgery or radiation therapy should be offered to patients with large tumors or with symptoms of urinary obstruction. Treatment decisions should be made with the patient and his family after informing them of the expectations and limitations of each modality.

Suggested Reading

Holmberg L, Bill-Axelson A, Helgesen F, et al. A randomized trial comparing radical prostatectomy with watchful waiting in early prostate cancer. *N Engl J Med.* 2002;347(11):781–789.

Bill-Axelson A, Holmberg L, Ruutu M, et al. Radical prostatectomy versus watchful waiting in early prostate cancer. *N Engl J Med.* 2005;352(19):1977–1984.

Klotz L. Active surveillance for prostate cancer: For whom? *J Clin Oncol.* 2005;23(32):8165–8169.

19-3 C

Educational Objective: To identify appropriate therapy for elderly patients with diffuse B-cell lymphoma.

A phase III trial of cyclophosphamide, doxorubicin, vincristine, and prednisone (CHOP) compared with CHOP plus rituximab was conducted for the treatment of patients age 60 to 80 with diffuse B-cell lymphoma. The complete response rate (76% vs. 63%), 2-year event-free survival, and overall survival favored the group receiving the antibody.

Suggested Reading

Coiffier B, Lepage E, Briere J, et al. CHOP chemotherapy plus rituximab compared with CHOP alone in elderly patients with diffuse large B-cell lymphoma. *N Engl J Med.* 2002;346(4):235–242.

19-4 D

Educational Objective: To recognize that less aggressive therapies may be appropriate in frail women with breast cancer without compromising survival.

Adjuvant treatment with tamoxifen alone is reasonable. Breast cancers in older women tend to have a unique and seemingly less aggressive behavior. When prognostic factors such as ER status, histologic grade, ploidy, TP53 status, epidermal growth factor receptor status, and HER2 status are assessed, it appears that tumors become less aggressive with advancing age. Although the biologic behavior of breast cancer is less aggressive, 60% of the deaths from breast cancer occur in women older than age 65.

More conservative approaches to the treatment of the primary tumor have been addressed in controlled clinical trials. The data from these studies suggest that following surgical removal of the primary tumor, tamoxifen without radiation therapy may be adequate for select patients. However, by eliminating radiation therapy, recurrence in the ipsilateral breast is more common and is generally treated by mastectomy for local control of the primary cancer. Despite the higher rate of so-called in-breast recurrences, the survival rate associated with this less aggressive approach is identical to that associated with conventional surgery and radiation therapy. Resection of the primary tumor and administration of tamoxifen may be appropriate for selected women with small, ER-positive breast cancers and a finite life expectancy. Older women with a favorable long-term outlook should be treated as aggressively as younger women. However, this patient has three comorbid conditions and one geriatric syndrome (osteoporosis) and should be considered frail. Tamoxifen is a reasonable adjuvant therapy and has the potential for increasing bone density as well.

Suggested Reading

Basche M, Byers T. Tumor characteristics and clinical outcome of elderly women with breast cancer. *J Natl Cancer Inst.* 2000;93(1): 64–65.

Fyles A, McCready D, Manchul L, et al. Tamoxifen with or without breast radiation in women 50 years of age or older with early stage breast cancer. *N Engl J Med.* 2004;351(10): 963–967.

Hughes KS, Schnaper L, Berry D, et al. Lumpectomy plus tamoxifen with and without radiotherapy in women 70 years of age with early breast cancer. *N Engl J Med.* 2004:351(10): 971–977.

19-5 C

Educational Objective: To understand that the benefits from chemotherapy for older women with a favorable long-term outcome are comparable with those for younger women.

This older woman is healthy; she has one comorbid condition (hypertension) and no geriatric syndromes. Therefore, treatment should be the same as that recommended for any other postmenopausal woman with ER-negative disease. When chemotherapy is indicated, the reduction in recurrence and the survival advantage are similar to that found for younger women. Although the comorbid conditions must be factored into the treatment decision, appropriately administered adjuvant therapy has been shown to be cost-effective. In the absence of severe comorbidities, the guidelines for adjuvant therapy are identical to those used to treat younger women.

Suggested Reading

Desch C, Hillner BE, Smith TJ, et al. Should the elderly receive chemotherapy for node-negative breast cancer? A cost-effectiveness analysis examining total and active life-expectancy outcomes. *J Clin Oncol.* 1993;11(4):777–782.

Extermann M, Balducci L, Lyman GH. What threshold for adjuvant therapy in older breast patients. *J Clin Oncol.* 2000;18(8): 1709–1717.

Muss HB, Woolf S, Berry D, et al. Adjuvant chemotherapy in older and younger women with lymph node-positive breast cancer. *JAMA.* 2005;293(9):1073–1081.

Warren JL, Brown ML, Fay MP, et al. Costs of treatment for elderly women with early-stage breast cancer in fee-for-service settings. *J Clin Oncol.* 2001;20(1):307–316.

NORMAL LABORATORY VALUES

Lab Test	Reference Range, Conventional Units	Reference Range, SI Units
Hematologic Values		
D-dimer	< 0.5 μg/mL	< 500 mg/L
Erythrocyte count		
Men	4.7–6.1 × 10^6/μL	4.7–6.1 × 10^6/μL
Women	4.2–5.4 × 10^6/μL	4.2–5.4 × 10^6/μL
Erythrocyte sedimentation rate		
Men	0–15 mm/hr	0–15 mm/hr
Women	0–20 mm/hr	0–20 mm/hr
Erythropoietin	5–36 mU/mL	5–36 IU/L
Ferritin		
Men	12–300 ng/mL	12–300 μ/L
Women	10–150 ng/mL	10–150 μg/L
Hematocrit		
Men	41%–50%	0.41–0.50
Women	35%–45%	0.35–0.45
Hemoglobin		
Men	14.0–17.5 g/dL	140–175 g/L
Women	12–15 g/dl	120–150 g/L
Leukocyte count	4,500–11,000/μL (4,500–11,000/mm^3)	4.5–11.0 x 10^9/L
Lymphocytes		
$CD4^+$ cell count	640–1175/mm^3	0.64–1.18 × 10^9/L
$CD8^+$ cell count	335–875/mm^3	0.34–0.88 × 10^9/L
CD4:CD8 ratio	1.0–4.0	1.0–4.0
Partial thromboplastin time	25–40 seconds	25–40 seconds
Platelet count	130–400 × 10^3/μL (130,000–400,000/mm^3)	130–400 × 10^9/L
Prothrombin time	10–13 seconds	10–13 seconds
Whole Blood, Serum, and Plasma Values		
Acid phosphatase	0.0–0.6 U/L	0.0–0.6 U/L
Albumin	3.5–5.5 g/dL	35–50 g/L
Aminotransferase, serum alanine (ALT, SGPT)	10–40 U/L	10–40 U/L

Aminotransferase, serum aspirate (AST, SGOT)	20–48 U/L	20–48 U/L
Aldosterone		
Supine	2–5 ng/dL	55–138 pmol/L
Standing	7–30 ng/dL	0.19–0.83 nmol/L
Alkaline phosphatase	50–120 U/L	50–120 U/L
Alpha-fetoprotein	0–20 ng/mL	0–20 μg/L
Amylase	25–85 U/L	25–85 U/L
Bilirubin		
Total	0.3–1.2 mg/dL	5–21 μmol/L
Direct	< 0.2 mg/dL	< 3.4 μmol/L
C-reactive protein	< 0.8 mg/dL	< 8 mg/L
CA 19-9	< 37 U/mL	< 37 kU/L
CA 125	0–35 U/mL	< 35 kU/L
Calcitonin	< 19 pg/mL	< 19 ng/L
Calcium	8.2–10.2 mg/dL	2.05–2.55 mmol/L
Carcinoembryonic antigen	< 3 ng/mL	< 3 μg/L
Catecholamines (norepinephrine)	50–440 ng/L	296–2600 pmol/L
Chloride	96–106 mEq/L	96–106 mmol/L
Creatinine	0.6–1.2 mg/dL	53–106 μmol/L
Creatinine clearance	75–125 mL/min	1.24–2.08 mL/s
Dehydroepiandrosterone sulfate		
Men	50–450 μg/dL	1.6–12.2 μmol/L
Women	0.6–3.3 mg/mL	1.6–8.9 μmol/L
Folate, serum	5–25 ng/mL	11–57 nmol/L
Human chorionic gonadotropin (adult female, not pregnant)	< 3 mIU/mL	< 3 IU/L
Immunoglobulins, serum		
IgA	113–563 mg/dL	1.1–5.6 g/L
IgD	0.5–3.0 mg/dL	5–30 mg/L
IgE	0.01–0.04 mg/dL	0.1–0.4 mg/L
IgG	800–1800 mg/dL	8–18 g/L
IgG_1	280–1020 mg/dL	2.8–10.2 g/L
IgG_2	60–790 mg/dL	0.6–7.9 g/L
IgG_3	14–240 mg/dL	0.14–2.4 g/L
IgG_4	11–330 mg/dL	0.11–3.3 g/L
IgM	54–222 mg/dL	0.5–2.2 g/L
Insulin, plasma	11–240 μU/mL	35–139 pmol/L
Lactate dehydrogenase, serum	50–200 U/L	50–200 U/L
Lipase, serum	0–160 U/L	0–160 U/L
Parathyroid hormone (intact), serum	10–50 pg/mL	1.1–5.3 pmol/L

Phosphorus	3–45 mg/dL	0.97–1.45 mmol/L
Potassium, plasma	3.5–5.0 mEq/L	3.5–5.0 mmol/L
Prostate-specific antigen (PSA)	0–4 ng/mL	0–4 μg/mL
Protein, serum		
Total	6–8 g/dL	60–80 g/L
Globulins	2.5–3.5 g/dL	25–35 g/L
Alpha1	0.2–0.4 g/dL	2–4 g/L
Alpha2	0.5–0.9 g/dL	5–9 g/L
Beta	0.6–1.1 g/dL	6–11 g/L
Gamma	0.7–1.7 g/dL	7–17 g/L
Renin, plasma	1–6 ng/mL/hr	0.77–4.6 nmol $\times$ $L^{-1} \times h^{-1}$
Sodium, plasma	136–142 mEq/L	136–142 mmol/L
Testosterone, serum		
Men	300–1200 ng/dL	10.4–41.6 nmol/L
Women	20–75 ng/dL	0.7–2.6 nmol/L
Thyroglobulin, serum	3–42 ng/mL	3–42 μg/L
Thyroid function tests		
Thyroid-stimulating hormone (TSH)	0.5–5.0 μU/mL	0.5–5.0 mU/mL
Thyroxine (T4), serum		
Total	5.5–12.5 μg/dL	71–160 nmol/L
Free	0.9–2.3 ng/dL	12–30 pmol/L
Free T4 index	4–11	4–11
Triiodothyronine, resin uptake	25%–35%	0.25–0.35 Proportion of 1
Triiodothyronine, serum (total T3)	70–200 ng/dL	1.08–3.14 nmol/L
Triglycerides, plasma, serum	10–190 mg/dL	0.11–2.15 mmol/L
Urea nitrogen, serum	8–23 mg/dL	2.9–8.2 mmol/L
Uric acid, serum	4.0–8.5 mg/dL	0.24–0.51 mmol/L
Vasopressin	1–5 pg/mL	0–1.5 ng/L
Urine/Miscellaneous		
Catecholamines, total	< 100 μg/m^2 per 24 hr	< 591 nmol/m^2 per 24 hr
Metanephrines (total), urine	< 1 mg/24 hr	< 5 μmol/24 hr
Beta$_2$-microglobulin	0–2 μg/mL	0–170 nmol/L
Forced vital capacity (FVC)	> 80% predicted	> 0.80 (Proportion of 100) predicted

DRUG REFERENCE LIST

Generic Name	Trade Name	Chapter(s)
5-azacytidine		2, 15
13-*cis*-retinoic acid (isotretinoin)	Acutane	7, 9
4-hydroperoxycyclophosphamide (4-HC)		15
^{131}I tositumomab	BEXXAR	4, 16
6-mercaptopurine	6-MP, Purinethol	3, 15
^{90}Y-labeled ibritubomab tiuxetan	Zevalin	4, 16
acetaminophen	Tylenol, Panadol, and others	4, 15, 18
acyclovir	Zovirax	15, 17
aldesleukin (interleukin [IL]-2)	Proleukin	3, 4, 9, 11, 13, 15, 18
alemtuzumab	Campath	4, 15, 16
alitretinoin gel	Panretin	13
allopurinol	Zyloprim	15, 18
all-*trans* retinoic acid		15
amifostine	Ethyol	7, 15, 18
amiloride	Midamor	18
amoxicillin	Amoxil	16
amphotericin	Amphocin	17
anastrozole	Arimidex	5
antithymocyte globulin	Atgam	15, 17, 18
aprepitant	Emend	18
arsenic trioxide	Trisenox	15
asparaginase	Elspar, L-Asparaginase	15
aspirin (acetylsalicylic acid)	Bayer, Bufferin, various other	1, 18
atropine	Atropine	18
azathioprine	Imuran	1, 3, 17
axitinib		7
bacille Calmette-Guérin	BCG, TheraCys	9
bendamustine	Treanda	16
beta-carotene	Lumitene, Max-Caro	1, 5, 6
bevacizumab	Avastin	3, 4, 5, 6, 7, 8, 9
bexarotene	Targretin	16
bicalutamide	Casodex	9
bimolane (AT-1727)		15

bisacodyl	Dulcolax, Fleet enema	18
bleomycin	Blenoxane	6, 7, 9, 10, 13, 16, 19
bortezomib (PS-341)	Velcade	16
bromocriptine	Parlodel	14
busulfan	Myleran (PO), Busulfex (IV)	15, 17
calcitonin	Miacalcin	18
calicheamicin		15
capecitabine	Xeloda	3, 4, 5, 8, 19
carbamazepine	Tegretol	14
carboplatin	Paraplatin	3–7, 9, 10, 11, 14
carmustine, impregnated wafer	BCNU, Glidel wafer	11, 14
casanthranol		18
celecoxib	Celebrex	1
cetuximab (C225)	Erbitux	2, 3, 4, 7, 8
chlorambucil	Leukeran	15
chlorhexidine	Perio-Chip	18
chlorpromazine	Thorazine	18
cholestyramine	Questran	18
cisapride	Propulsid	18
cisplatin	Platinol, CDDP	3–12, 14, 18, 19
cladribine (2-chlorodeoxyadenosine [2-CdA])	Leustatin	4, 15
clarithromycin	Biaxin	16
clodronate	Bonefos	5
clonidine	Catapres	18
codeine		18, 19
COL-3		13
colchicine	Colchicine	16
cyclophosphamide	Cytoxan, Neosar	4–6, 9, 10, 12–19
cyclosporine	Neoral	1, 15, 17
cyproheptadine	Periactin	18
cytarabine (cytosine arabinoside)	Cytosar-U, Depocyt (liposomal)	4, 13, 14, 15
dacarbazine	DTIC	7, 11, 12, 16
dactinomycin-D	Actinomycin-D, Cosmegen	12
dapsone	Sprycel	17
darbopoiten		18
dasatinib	Sprycel	15
daunorubicin (daunomycin)	Cerubidine, Daunomycin	13, 15
daunorubicin, liposomal	DaunoXome	13
decitabine	Dacogen	15
defibrotide		17
dehydroepiandrosterone		5

demeclocycline	Declomycin	6
denileukin diftitox	Ontak	4, 16
depsipeptide		15
dexamethasone	Decadron	15, 16, 18
didanosine	Videx	13
diethylstilbestrol		1
diphenhydramine	Benadryl	4, 15
diphenoxylate	Lofene	7, 18
docetaxel	Taxotere	5–9, 12, 19
docusate	various	18
dolasetron	Anzemet	18
domperidone	Motilium	18
doxorubicin	Adriamycin, DOX, Doxil (liposomal)	4–10, 12–16, 18, 19
doxycycline	Vibramycin, various other	6
dronabinol	Marinol	18
droperidol	Inapsine	18
epirubicin	Ellence, EPI	5, 7, 8, 9, 10, 12
epratuzumab		16
erlotinib (OSI-774)	Tarceva	2, 6, 7, 8
erythropoietin	EPO, Epogen, Procrit, Exprex, Neorecormon, Aranesp	13, 15, 16, 18
etoposide	VePesid	6, 8–10, 12–17, 19
etretinate	Tegison	7
exemestane	Aromasin	5
famciclovir	Famvir	4
fenretinide		5
fentanyl	Actiq	18, 19
filgrastim	Neupogen	4, 6
finasteride	Proscar	1, 9
flavopiridol		15
floxuridine	FUDR	9
fluconazole	Diflucan	13, 17
fludarabine	Fludara	4, 15–17
fluorouracil (5-fluorouracil)	Efudex	3, 5, 7–9, 18, 19
fluoxetine	Prozac, Sarafem	18
fluoxymesterone	Halotestin	5
flutamide	Eulexin	9, 18, 19
foscarnet	Foscavir	17
fotemustine		11
fulvestrant	Faslodex	5
furosemide	Lasix	18

gabapentin	Neurontin	18, 19
galiximab		16
ganciclovir	Cytovene, Cymevene	15, 17
ganglioside GM2 vaccine		11
gefitinib	Iressa	2, 6, 7
gemcitabine	Gemzar	4–10, 12, 13, 16, 18, 19
gemtuzumab (ozogamicin)	Mylotarg	4, 15
genistein		5
gimeracil		8
glutamine		18
glycopyrrolate	Robinul	18
goserelin	Zoladex	5
granisetron	Kytril	18
haloperidol	Haldol	18
heparin	Calceparine, Liquaemin	14
hexamethylmelamine	Hexalen	18
hydrazine sulfate		18
hydrocortisone	Cortef, Hydrocortone, Cortisol	4, 9, 15
hydromorphone	Dilaudid	18, 19
hydroxyurea	Hydrea	7, 15
idarubicin	Idamycin	15
ifosfamide	Ifex	3, 6, 7, 9, 10, 12, 19
imatinib mesylate	Gleevec	2, 4, 7, 12, 13, 15, 17
Infliximab	Remicade	18
interferon-alpha (interferon, IFN-α)	Roferon (2a), Intron A (2b)	3, 4, 7, 8, 9, 11, 15, 16, 18
irinotecan (CPT-11)	Camptosar	3–6, 7, 8, 14, 18, 19
ketoconazole	Nizoral	9
lactulose	various	18
lapatinib	Tykerb	5, 7
lenalidomide	Revlimid	15, 16
letrozole	Femara	5
leucovorin	Folinic Acid, Leucovorin	8, 18, 19
leuprolide	Lupron	5
levamisole	Ergamisol	8
levetiracetam	Keppra	14
Levo-hyoscyamine		18
lomustine	CCNU	11, 14
loperamide	Imodium	18
lorazepam	Ativan	18
magnesium citrate		18
magnesium hydroxide	Milk of Magnesia	18

mAMSA		15
mannitol	Osmitrol	14
mechlorethamine (nitrogen mustard)	Mustargen,	16
medroxyprogesterone acetate	Provera, Cycrin, Amen	5, 9, 18
megestrol acetate	Megace	5, 6, 18
melphalan (also referred to as phenylalanine mustard)	Alkeran, L-PAM	5, 11, 15, 16, 17
meperidine	Demerol	18
methadone	Dolophine	18, 19
methotrexate	Amethopterin, MTX	3, 5, 7–9, 12–15, 17–19
methoxypsoralen (methoxsalen, topical)	Oxsoralen	16
metoclopramide	Octamide	18
metronidazole	MetroGel	16
mitomycin-C	Mitomycin, Mutamycin	5, 6, 8, 9
mitoxantrone	Novantrone	5, 7, 9, 15, 16, 19
modafinil	Provigil	18
morphine	MS-Contin	18, 19
mycophenolate mofetil	CellCept	15, 17
n-acetylcysteine		7
nelarabine	Arranon	16
Nilotinib	Tasigna	15
nilutamide	Nilandron	9
Oblimersen	Genasense	11
Octreotide	Sandostatin	7, 8, 18
olsalazine	Dipentum	18
oltipraz		5
olsalazine	Dipentum	18
omeprazole	Prilosec	16
ondansetron	Zofran	18
oprelvekin	Neumega	4
oteracil		8
oxaliplatin	Eloxatin	7, 8, 9, 19
oxandrolone	Oxandrin	18
oxycodone	OxyContin	18, 19
paclitaxel	Taxol	3–10, 13, 14
palifermin	Kepivance	7, 17, 18
palonosetron	Aloxi	18
pamidronate (disodium)	Aredia	5, 6, 16
panitumumab	Vectibix	4, 8
paroxetine	Paxil	18
pegfilgrastim	Neulasta	4

Pemetrexed	Alimta	6, 7, 8, 9
penicillin	Various	17
pentostatin (2′-deoxycoformycin [DCF])	Nipent	4, 15
pentoxifylline	Trental	18
phenacetin		1
phenobarbital	Solfotou	14
phenothiazine	Thorazine	18
phenytoin	Dilantin	14
pilocarpine	Salagen	7, 18
piroxicam	Feldene	1
polyethylene glycol	Miralax	18
pralatrexate		16
prednisolone	Medrol, Prelone, Prednisolone Tablets	4, 18
prednisone	Deltasone, Liquid Pred	4, 9, 13–17, 19
procarbazine	Matulane	14, 16
prochlorperazine		18
promethazine	Phenergan	18
propoxyphene	Darvon	18
raloxifene (keoxifene)	Evista	1, 5, 19
risedronate	Actonel	18
rituximab	Rituxan	4, 13, 14, 15, 16, 19
samarium-153	Quadramet	5, 9
sargramostim	Leukine	4
scopolamine	Transderm Scop	18
selenium sulfide	various	1, 9
senna	various	18
somatostatin		7, 18
sorafenib tosylate	Nexavar	3, 7, 8, 9, 11
spironolactone	Aldactone	18
streptozocin, streptozotocin	Zanosar	3,7, 8
strontium-89	Metastron	5, 9
sucralfate	Carafate	18
sulindac	Clinoril	1
sunitinib, sunitinib malate	Sutent	3, 4, 9, 12
tacrolimus	Prograf	15, 17
talc	Schlerosol	6
tamoxifen	Nolvadex	1, 2, 3, 5, 10, 11, 18, 19
temozolomide	Temodar	11, 14, 16
temsirolimus	Torisel	9, 16
thalidomide	Thalomid	11, 13, 15–16

thioguanine	6-TG	15
thiotepa (triethylenethiophosphoramide)	Thioplex, TSPA	9, 14
thrombopoietin		4
thyroxine		7
tipifarnib	Zarnestra	2
tirapazamine	Tirazone	6
topotecan	Hycamtin	6, 7, 10, 14, 15, 18
toremifene	Fareston	5
tositumomab	Bexxar	4
tramadol	Ultram	19
trastuzumab	Herceptin	2–6
trimethoprim sulfamethoxazole	Proloprim	4, 13, 15, 17
uracil/tegafur (S1)	Uftoral	8
valrubicin	Valstar	9
venlafaxine	Effexor	18
vinblastine	Velban	6, 9, 11, 13, 16
vincristine	Oncovin	4, 5, 6, 12–16, 19
vindesine	Eldisine	6
vinorelbine	Navelbine	4–7, 10, 12, 19
vitamin A (retinyl palmitate, retinol)	various	1, 5, 6, 7
vitamin D	various	1, 18
vitamin E (alpha tocophorol)	various	1, 5, 7, 18
voriconazole	VFEND	17
Vorinostat	Zolinza	16
warfarin	Coumadin	14
zoledronate, zoledronic acid	Zometa	5, 6, 9, 18

INDEX

In this index "*f*" and "*t*" refer to figures and tables, respectively.

PARTICIPANT EVALUATION OF *ASCO-SEP*™

Please complete and return the following pages of the evaluation. For credit, complete *both* the Evaluation and Request for Credit Forms. Please fax, mail, e-mail, or return online to: ASCO/CME, 1900 Duke St., Ste. 200, Alexandria, VA 22314; Fax: 703-686-5482; E-mail: CME@asco.org; URL: www.asco.org/ascosep.

Demographic Information

Please indicate your primary professional role (*select only one*)

- Physician
- Pharmacist
- Nurse
- Physician Assistant
- Researcher
- Student
- Fellow, Resident or Beginning Practitioner
- Other________________________

Where does your professional activity primarily occur? (*select only one*)

- Private Practice
- Hospital or Clinical Facility
- Academic Facility/Medical School
- Research Institute (nonprofit or corporate)
- Government Agency
- Training Program (resident, fellow, student)
- Biotechnology or Pharmaceutical Company
- Other________________________

Physicians, please indicate your Board Certification or International Equivalent? (*select only one*)

- Dermatology
- Gynecologic Oncology
- Hematology (only)
- Medical Oncology (only)
- Medical Oncology & Hematology
- Nuclear Medicine
- Pathology
- Pediatrics (including Pediatric Oncology, Pediatric Hematology, Pediatric Oncology/Hematology)
- Radiation Oncology
- Surgery (including Surgical Oncology and Surgical Specialties)
- Gastroenterology
- Radiology (Diagnostic and Interventional)
- Urology/Urological Oncology

Overall Evaluation

Please identify your level of agreement for each area listed below.

⑤ = Strongly Agree ④ = Agree ③ = Neutral ② = Disagree ① = Strongly Disagree

1. I would recommend that others participate in this educational activity. ⑤ ④ ③ ② ①
2. *ASCO-SEP*™ helped me to assess my current level of knowledge and identify areas of educational need. ⑤ ④ ③ ② ①
3. The content was relevant to my professional role and educational need. ⑤ ④ ③ ② ①
4. The content was scientifically rigorous and based on the best available evidence. ⑤ ④ ③ ② ①
5. Information was presented in an objective and educationally balanced manner. ⑤ ④ ③ ② ①
6. I gained new insight and knowledge that will be of benefit to me in my professional role. ⑤ ④ ③ ② ①
7. The content was free from commercial influence or bias. ⑤ ④ ③ ② ①
8. The self-assessment examination added to the educational value of this activity. ⑤ ④ ③ ② ①
9. I preferred the comprehensive self-assessment examination as opposed to test items contained within each chapter. ⑤ ④ ③ ② ①
10. The print/web-based content delivery format met my educational needs. ⑤ ④ ③ ② ①
11. I updated and/or validated my knowledge and understanding of current cancer research and best practices in care for cancer patients or survivors. ⑤ ④ ③ ② ①
12. I plan to implement revisions to my current practice or institute new practices based on the knowledge acquired from my participation in this activity. ⑤ ④ ③ ② ①
13. Overall, this resource provided a high-quality overview of the current state of oncology. ⑤ ④ ③ ② ①

Chapter 1: Epidemiology and Prevention *(2.0 CME credits)*

- The content presented in the chapter was well organized. ⑤ ④ ③ ② ①
- The information presented graphically (tables, figures, charts, etc.) added value to the content ⑤ ④ ③ ② ①
- Overall, the quality of the chapter was of a high standard. ⑤ ④ ③ ② ①
- Describe one area of new knowledge or validated existing knowledge you acquired upon reading this chapter.

  ____

  ____

  ____

- Briefly explain how this chapter's content applies to your work and practice. Please indicate if there are additional content areas you would like to see included in future editions.

  ____

  ____

  ____

Chapter 2: Molecular Biology *(3.5 CME credits)*

- The content presented in the chapter was well organized. ⑤ ④ ③ ② ①
- The information presented graphically (tables, figures, charts, etc.) added value to the content ⑤ ④ ③ ② ①
- Overall, the quality of the chapter was of a high standard. ⑤ ④ ③ ② ①
- Describe one area of new knowledge or validated existing knowledge you acquired upon reading this chapter.

  ____

  ____

  ____

- Briefly explain how this chapter's content applies to your work and practice. Please indicate if there are additional content areas you would like to see included in future editions.

  ____

  ____

  ____

Chapter 3: Clinical Pharmacology *(1.0 CME credits)*

- The content presented in the chapter was well organized. ⑤ ④ ③ ② ①
- The information presented graphically (tables, figures, charts, etc.) added value to the content ⑤ ④ ③ ② ①
- Overall, the quality of the chapter was of a high standard. ⑤ ④ ③ ② ①
- Describe one area of new knowledge or validated existing knowledge you acquired upon reading this chapter.

  ____

  ____

  ____

- Briefly explain how this chapter's content applies to your work and practice. Please indicate if there are additional content areas you would like to see included in future editions.

  ____

  ____

  ____

Chapter 4: Biologic Therapy

(2.5 CME credits)

- The content presented in the chapter was well organized. ⑤ ④ ③ ② ①
- The information presented graphically (tables, figures, charts, etc.) added value to the content ⑤ ④ ③ ② ①
- Overall, the quality of the chapter was of a high standard. ⑤ ④ ③ ② ①
- Describe one area of new knowledge or validated existing knowledge you acquired upon reading this chapter.

___

___

___

- Briefly explain how this chapter's content applies to your work and practice. Please indicate if there are additional content areas you would like to see included in future editions.

___

___

___

Chapter 5: Breast Cancer

(3.5 CME credits)

- The content presented in the chapter was well organized. ⑤ ④ ③ ② ①
- The information presented graphically (tables, figures, charts, etc.) added value to the content ⑤ ④ ③ ② ①
- Overall, the quality of the chapter was of a high standard. ⑤ ④ ③ ② ①
- Describe one area of new knowledge or validated existing knowledge you acquired upon reading this chapter.

___

___

___

- Briefly explain how this chapter's content applies to your work and practice. Please indicate if there are additional content areas you would like to see included in future editions.

___

___

___

Chapter 6: Lung Cancer

(3.0 CME credits)

- The content presented in the chapter was well organized. ⑤ ④ ③ ② ①
- The information presented graphically (tables, figures, charts, etc.) added value to the content ⑤ ④ ③ ② ①
- Overall, the quality of the chapter was of a high standard. ⑤ ④ ③ ② ①
- Describe one area of new knowledge or validated existing knowledge you acquired upon reading this chapter.

___

___

___

- Briefly explain how this chapter's content applies to your work and practice. Please indicate if there are additional content areas you would like to see included in future editions.

___

___

___

Chapter 7: Head and Neck Cancers *(3.0 CME credits)*

- The content presented in the chapter was well organized. ⑤ ④ ③ ② ①
- The information presented graphically (tables, figures, charts, etc.) added value to the content ⑤ ④ ③ ② ①
- Overall, the quality of the chapter was of a high standard. ⑤ ④ ③ ② ①
- Describe one area of new knowledge or validated existing knowledge you acquired upon reading this chapter.

___

___

___

- Briefly explain how this chapter's content applies to your work and practice. Please indicate if there are additional content areas you would like to see included in future editions.

___

___

___

Chapter 8: Gastrointestinal Cancers *(2.0 CME credits)*

- The content presented in the chapter was well organized. ⑤ ④ ③ ② ①
- The information presented graphically (tables, figures, charts, etc.) added value to the content ⑤ ④ ③ ② ①
- Overall, the quality of the chapter was of a high standard. ⑤ ④ ③ ② ①
- Describe one area of new knowledge or validated existing knowledge you acquired upon reading this chapter.

___

___

___

- Briefly explain how this chapter's content applies to your work and practice. Please indicate if there are additional content areas you would like to see included in future editions.

___

___

___

Chapter 9: Genitourinary Cancers *(3.0 CME credits)*

- The content presented in the chapter was well organized. ⑤ ④ ③ ② ①
- The information presented graphically (tables, figures, charts, etc.) added value to the content ⑤ ④ ③ ② ①
- Overall, the quality of the chapter was of a high standard. ⑤ ④ ③ ② ①
- Describe one area of new knowledge or validated existing knowledge you acquired upon reading this chapter.

___

___

___

- Briefly explain how this chapter's content applies to your work and practice. Please indicate if there are additional content areas you would like to see included in future editions.

___

___

___

Chapter 10: Gynecologic Cancers *(1.0 CME credits)*

- The content presented in the chapter was well organized. ⑤ ④ ③ ② ①
- The information presented graphically (tables, figures, charts, etc.) added value to the content ⑤ ④ ③ ② ①
- Overall, the quality of the chapter was of a high standard. ⑤ ④ ③ ② ①
- Describe one area of new knowledge or validated existing knowledge you acquired upon reading this chapter.

___

___

___

- Briefly explain how this chapter's content applies to your work and practice. Please indicate if there are additional content areas you would like to see included in future editions.

___

___

___

Chapter 11: Malignant Melanoma *(1.0 CME credits)*

- The content presented in the chapter was well organized. ⑤ ④ ③ ② ①
- The information presented graphically (tables, figures, charts, etc.) added value to the content ⑤ ④ ③ ② ①
- Overall, the quality of the chapter was of a high standard. ⑤ ④ ③ ② ①
- Describe one area of new knowledge or validated existing knowledge you acquired upon reading this chapter.

___

___

___

- Briefly explain how this chapter's content applies to your work and practice. Please indicate if there are additional content areas you would like to see included in future editions.

___

___

___

Chapter 12: Sarcoma *(1.0 CME credits)*

- The content presented in the chapter was well organized. ⑤ ④ ③ ② ①
- The information presented graphically (tables, figures, charts, etc.) added value to the content ⑤ ④ ③ ② ①
- Overall, the quality of the chapter was of a high standard. ⑤ ④ ③ ② ①
- Describe one area of new knowledge or validated existing knowledge you acquired upon reading this chapter.

___

___

___

- Briefly explain how this chapter's content applies to your work and practice. Please indicate if there are additional content areas you would like to see included in future editions.

___

___

___

Chapter 13: AIDS-Related Cancer

(1.5 CME credits)

- The content presented in the chapter was well organized. ⑤ ④ ③ ② ①
- The information presented graphically (tables, figures, charts, etc.) added value to the content ⑤ ④ ③ ② ①
- Overall, the quality of the chapter was of a high standard. ⑤ ④ ③ ② ①
- Describe one area of new knowledge or validated existing knowledge you acquired upon reading this chapter.

____

____

____

- Briefly explain how this chapter's content applies to your work and practice. Please indicate if there are additional content areas you would like to see included in future editions.

____

____

____

Chapter 14: Central Nervous System Tumors

(2.0 CME credits)

- The content presented in the chapter was well organized. ⑤ ④ ③ ② ①
- The information presented graphically (tables, figures, charts, etc.) added value to the content ⑤ ④ ③ ② ①
- Overall, the quality of the chapter was of a high standard. ⑤ ④ ③ ② ①
- Describe one area of new knowledge or validated existing knowledge you acquired upon reading this chapter.

____

____

____

- Briefly explain how this chapter's content applies to your work and practice. Please indicate if there are additional content areas you would like to see included in future editions.

____

____

____

Chapter 15: Leukemias

(3.0 CME credits)

- The content presented in the chapter was well organized. ⑤ ④ ③ ② ①
- The information presented graphically (tables, figures, charts, etc.) added value to the content ⑤ ④ ③ ② ①
- Overall, the quality of the chapter was of a high standard. ⑤ ④ ③ ② ①
- Describe one area of new knowledge or validated existing knowledge you acquired upon reading this chapter.

____

____

____

- Briefly explain how this chapter's content applies to your work and practice. Please indicate if there are additional content areas you would like to see included in future editions.

____

____

____

Chapter 16: Lymphomas and Myelomas

(2.0 CME credits)

- The content presented in the chapter was well organized. ⑤ ④ ③ ② ①
- The information presented graphically (tables, figures, charts, etc.) added value to the content ⑤ ④ ③ ② ①
- Overall, the quality of the chapter was of a high standard. ⑤ ④ ③ ② ①
- Describe one area of new knowledge or validated existing knowledge you acquired upon reading this chapter.

___

___

___

- Briefly explain how this chapter's content applies to your work and practice. Please indicate if there are additional content areas you would like to see included in future editions.

___

___

___

Chapter 17: Hematopoietic Cell Transplantation

(1.0 CME credits)

- The content presented in the chapter was well organized. ⑤ ④ ③ ② ①
- The information presented graphically (tables, figures, charts, etc.) added value to the content ⑤ ④ ③ ② ①
- Overall, the quality of the chapter was of a high standard. ⑤ ④ ③ ② ①
- Describe one area of new knowledge or validated existing knowledge you acquired upon reading this chapter.

___

___

___

- Briefly explain how this chapter's content applies to your work and practice. Please indicate if there are additional content areas you would like to see included in future editions.

___

___

___

Chapter 18: Symptom Management

(3.5 CME credits)

- The content presented in the chapter was well organized. ⑤ ④ ③ ② ①
- The information presented graphically (tables, figures, charts, etc.) added value to the content ⑤ ④ ③ ② ①
- Overall, the quality of the chapter was of a high standard. ⑤ ④ ③ ② ①
- Describe one area of new knowledge or validated existing knowledge you acquired upon reading this chapter.

___

___

___

- Briefly explain how this chapter's content applies to your work and practice. Please indicate if there are additional content areas you would like to see included in future editions.

___

___

___

Chapter 19: Cancer in the Elderly

(1.0 CME credits)

- The content presented in the chapter was well organized. ⑤ ④ ③ ② ①
- The information presented graphically (tables, figures, charts, etc.) added value to the content ⑤ ④ ③ ② ①
- Overall, the quality of the chapter was of a high standard. ⑤ ④ ③ ② ①
- Describe one area of new knowledge or validated existing knowledge you acquired upon reading this chapter.

___

___

___

- Briefly explain how this chapter's content applies to your work and practice. Please indicate if there are additional content areas you would like to see included in future editions.

___

___

___

Comprehensive Self-Assessment Examination

(3.0 CME credits)

- Exam items were clearly stated. ⑤ ④ ③ ② ①
- Item rationales provided sufficient explanation of correct answers. ⑤ ④ ③ ② ①
- The exam was a useful tool for self-assessment and/or Board and MOC preparation. ⑤ ④ ③ ② ①
- The exam was representative of the entire *ASCO-SEP*™ chapter content.

Comments:

___

___

Comments

What was your primary reason for purchasing *ASCO-SEP*™? (i.e. self-learning, board preparation, teaching/training tool, etc.)

Additional Comments:

Thank You!

REQUEST FOR CONTINUING MEDICAL EDUCATION (CME) CREDIT

Instructions

To receive credit, please complete both the Request for CME Credit and Evaluation for the *ASCO-SEP*™: *Medical Oncology Self Evaluation Program* based on your participation. Upon completion of the form, please fax, mail, or submit online to:

ASCO / CME
1900 Duke Street; Suite 200
Alexandria, VA 22314
Fax: 703-684-5482
Email: cme@asco.org
URL: www.asco.org/ascosep

Approximate times required for completion of individual chapters noted in parentheses.

Chapter	Title	CME Credits Claimed
1	Epidemiology and Prevention (2.0)	
2	Molecular Biology (3.5)	
3	Clinical Pharmacology (1.0)	
4	Biologic Therapy (2.5)	
5	Breast Cancer (3.5)	
6	Lung Cancer (3.0)	
7	Head and Neck Cancers (3.0)	
8	Gastrointestinal Cancers (2.0)	
9	Genitourinary Cancers (3.0)	
10	Gynecologic Cancers (1.0)	
11	Malignant Melanoma (1.0)	
12	Sarcoma (1.0)	
13	AIDS-Related Cancers (1.5)	
14	Central Nervous System Tumors (2.0)	
15	Leukemias (3.0)	
16	Lymphomas and Myelomas (2.0)	
17	Hematopoietic Cell Transplantation (1.0)	
18	Symptom Management (3.5)	
19	Cancer in the Elderly (1.0)	
	Comprehensive Self-Assessment (3.0)	
	Total:	

I claim ________ *AMA PRA Category 1 credit(s)*™ for my participation as a learner in this activity (1 credit per hour, not to exceed 43.5 credits)

Signature:

Name (please print): ASCO Member ID:

Address:

City: State/Country: Zip:

Email: Date:

For ASCO members, a certificate for CME credit will be available to print within two weeks on ASCO's CME bank. Nonmember certificates will be emailed within two to three weeks.